MEDICAL INFORMATICS EUROPE '99

Studies in Health Technology and Informatics

Editors

Volume 68

Earlier published in this series

Vol. 34. J. Brender, J.P. Christensen, J.-R. Scherrer and P. McNair (Eds.), Medical Informatics Europe '96
Vol. 35. M. Di Rienzo, G. Mancia, G. Parati, A. Pedotti and A. Zanchetti (Eds.), Frontiers of Blood Pressure and Heart Rate Analysis
Vol. 36. M. Sosa-ludicissa, N. Oliveri, C.A. Gamboa and J. Roberts (Eds.), Internet, Telematics and Health
Vol. 37. J.A. Sevastik and K.M. Diab (Eds.), Research into Spinal Deformities 1
Vol. 38. R.A. Mortensen (Ed.), ICNP in Europe: TELENURSE
Vol. 39. K.S. Morgan, H.M. Hoffman, D. Stredney and S.J. Weghorst (Eds.), Medicine Meets Virtual Reality
Vol. 40. G. Lowet, P. Rüegsegger, H. Weinans and A. Meunier (Eds.), Bone Research in Biomechanics
Vol. 41. J. Mantas (Ed.), Health Telematics Education
Vol. 42. J. Brender, Methodology for Assessment of Medical IT-Based Systems
Vol. 43. C. Pappas, N. Maglaveras and J.-R. Scherrer (Eds.), Medical Informatics Europe '97
Vol. 44. G. Riva (Ed.), Virtual Reality in Neuro-Psycho-Physiology
Vol. 45. J. Dudeck, B. Blobel, W. Lordieck and T. Bürkle (Eds.), New Technologies in Hospital Information Systems
Vol. 46. U. Gerdin, M. Tallberg and P. Wainwright (Eds.), Nursing Informatics
Vol. 47. W. Ceusters, P. Spyns, G. De Moor and W. Martin (Eds.), Syntactic-Semantic Tagging of Medical Texts: The Multi-TALE Project
Vol. 48. J. Graafmans, V. Taipale and N. Charness (Eds.), Gerontechnology
Vol. 49. L. van den Broek and A.J. Sikkel (Eds.), Health Cards '97
Vol. 50. J.D. Westwood, H.M. Hoffman, D. Stredney and S.J. Weghorst (Eds.), Medicine Meets Virtual Reality
Vol. 51. J. Mantas (Ed.), Advances in Health Telematics Education
Vol. 52. B. Cesnik, A.T. McCray and J.-R. Scherrer (Eds.), MedInfo '98
Vol. 53. M.C. Sievert, D.E. Moxley, N.J. Ogg and T.B. Patrick, Thesaurus of Health Informatics
Vol. 54. O. Ferrer-Roca and M. Sosa-Iudicissa (Eds.), Handbook of Telemedicine
Vol. 55. H.M.J. Goldschmidt, M.J.T. Cox, R.J.E. Grouls, W.A.J.H. van de Laar and G.G. van Merode, Reference Information Model for Clinical Laboratories
Vol. 56. I. Iakovidis, S. Maglavera and A. Trakatellis (Eds.), User Acceptance of Health Telematics Applications
Vol. 57. In production
Vol. 58. G. Riva, B.K. Wiederhold and E. Molinari (Eds.), Virtual Environments in Clinical Psychology and Neuroscience
Vol. 59. I.A.F. Stokes (Ed.), Research into Spinal Deformities 2
Vol. 60. M. Di Rienzo, G. Mancia, G. Parati, A. Pedotti and A. Zanchetti (Eds.), Methodology and Clinical Applications of Blood Pressure and Heart Rate Analysis
Vol. 61. R.A. Mortensen (Ed.), ICNP® and Telematic Applications for Nurses in Europe
Vol. 62. J.D. Westwood, H.M. Hoffman, R.A. Robb and D. Stredney (Eds.), Medicine Meets Virtual Reality
Vol. 63. R. Rogers and J. Reardon, Recommendations for International Action
Vol. 64. M. Nerlich and R. Kretschmer (Eds.), The Impact of Telemedicine on Health Care Management
Vol. 65. In production
Vol. 66. In production
Vol. 67. In production

ISSN: 0926-9630

Medical Informatics Europe '99

Edited by

Peter Kokol

University of Maribor, Slovenia

Blaž Zupan

University of Ljubljana, Slovenia

Janez Stare

University of Ljubljana, Slovenia

Marjan Premik

University of Ljubljana, Slovenia

Rolf Engelbrecht

European Federation for Medical Informatics

IOS Press

Ohmsha

Amsterdam • Berlin • Oxford • Tokyo • Washington, DC

ISBN 0 9673355 1 5 (IOS Press)
ISBN 4 274 90313 3 C3047 (Ohmsha)
Library of Congress Catalog Card Number: 99-65239

Publisher
IOS Press
Van Diemenstraat 94
1013 CN Amsterdam
Netherlands
fax: +31 20 620 3419
e-mail: order@iospress.nl

Distributor in the UK and Ireland
IOS Press/Lavis Marketing
73 Lime Walk
Headington
Oxford OX3 7AD
England
fax: +44 1865 75 0079

Distributor in the USA and Canada
IOS Press, Inc.
5795-G Burke Centre Parkway
Burke, VA 22015
USA
fax: +1 703 323 3668
e-mail: iosbooks@iospress.com

Distributor in Germany
IOS Press
Spandauer Strasse 2
D-10178 Berlin
Germany
fax: +49 30 242 3113

Distributor in Japan
Ohmsha, Ltd.
3-1 Kanda Nishiki-cho
Chiyoda-ku, Tokyo 101
Japan
fax: +81 3 3233 2426

PRINTED IN THE NETHERLANDS

Preface

The MIE'99 (Medical Informatics Europe) conference is the 15th in the series of conferences organised by European Federation of Medical Informatics and is organised in alternation with the MEDINFO (World Congress on Medical Informatics) organised by IMIA (International Medical Informatics Association). For the last conference in this millennium Ljubljana, the capital of Slovenia has been selected by the EFMI board. The motto of this year's conference "Bridges of Knowledge" reflects this historical event – bridges between millenniums, and bridges between various countries and various disciplines.
The response to the call for papers was overwhelming, 263 contributions from 28 different countries were received and 208 high quality papers were accepted for oral or poster presentations. Each paper has been reviewed by at least two reviewers coming from 35 countries. The quality, clarity and originality were the main criteria for accepting or rejecting a paper.
All accepted presentations presented in this proceedings are divided into following topics:

- Information systems in health care and medicine
- Telemedicine and telematics
- Security
- Biomedical processing, data analysis and image processing
- Data warehousing, data mining and knowledge discovery
- Training and education
- Internet/Intranet
- Resources management
- Intelligent medical systems
- Health guidelines and protocols
- Electronic patient encounter, card technology, electronic data interchange
- Terminology
- Nursing informatics.

The presented papers not only reflect the "state of the art", but present many new exciting ideas that will guide the progress of medical informatics in the new millenium.
The editors of the proceedings would like to thank all that in some or another way contributed in the production of the proceedings. Specially acknowledge goes to:

- All authors for presenting their valuable ideas
- Reviewers and programming committee for selecting the papers and improving their quality
- The staff of Laboratory of System Design (University of Maribor, Slovenia) for managing the contributions from early draft to final camera ready copy
- Organising committee for their support in all stages of the proceeding's production process and
- IOS Press for being so kind to publish it.

Peter Kokol
Blaž Zupan
Janez Stare
Marjan Premik
Rolf Engelbrecht

Contents

Security

Biomedical Processing, Data Analysis and Image Processing

Data Warehousing, Data Mining and Knowledge Discovery

Training and Education

Internet/Intranet

Knowledge Sharing

WWW

Other

Resource Management

Intelligent Medical Systems

Applications

Decision Support Systems

Methods

Electronic Patient Encounter, Card Technology, Electronic Data Interchange

Terminology

Nursing Informatics

Posters

Information Systems in Health Care and Medicine

Medical Informatics Europe '99
P. Kokol et al. (Eds.)
IOS Press, 1999

A matrix-approach proposal for the treatment of contents to be integrated into multimedia health resources for citizens

A Alonso, C Díaz & F Sanz
IMIM – Research Group on Medical Informatics
Carrer Dr Aiguader, 80. E-08003 Barcelona. Spain
e-mail: aalonso@imim.es

It is generally accepted that the improvement on health conditions largely depends on the adoption of healthier life styles and disease prevention attitudes by citizens. This has always been a major concern for authorities, health professionals and other health-related organisations and it has been dealt with by the development of different information delivery strategies. Three factors have generally provided the clue for such strategies: the target audience, the communication channel and the pedagogic model.

Telematics Applications are newcomers to this arena and may mean a total new approach since they are increasingly being used in the fields of health promotion, disease prevention and medical treatment. They are attractive because of their potential for providing information in a tailored way that includes factors such as users' needs and literacy, social conditions or access to technology.

The benefits that can be derived from a wide spread use of such technologies may deeply affect the health status of the population by allowing citizens to take better decisions regarding their health. This could eventually reduce health costs.

There are also drawbacks for their use. Misleading information can imply a serious risk for people accessing it. Also telematic information resources have to be made available to everybody if benefits are sought in large scale.

In the framework of the MELIC Project (funded by the EU Ten-Telecom program, project#45560), our institution has developed a matrix approach methodology to tackle this issue. By doing so, it contributes to the MELIC project's objective of establishing a tested methodology for the development of the most efficient telematic delivery solution to meet citizens' needs on health information.

Methodology

A health information delivery problem or need reported by a client is the starting point. From this point, the successive phases of the methodology take place.

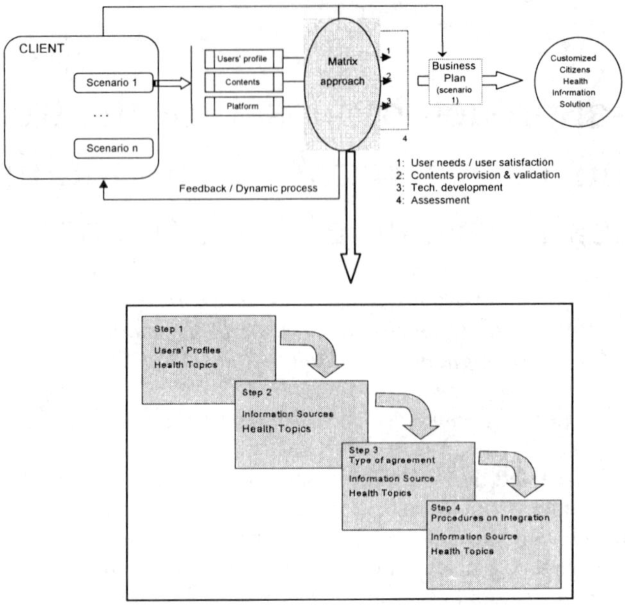

Phase A: Requirement analysis. Every information solution has its own context of use. This implies a particular users' profile defined as a specific combination of users' conditions (age, literacy, interests, disabilities...), selection of contents and technological platform by which these contents are provided to those users.

Phase B: Process of contents. Technical development & assessment . For each user profile a particular set of contents and a technological platform can be established. Collection, elaboration and validation of contents are performed through a matrix approach methodology. The aim is to ensure an adequate combination of Content Units (pieces of information). This implies that: 1) The proper information is gathered, 2) it is addressed to the proper user profile, as specified at the entry point (previous phase), 3) it is guaranteed that the right sources are accessed and 4) it conforms standards on quality of the information.

The process yields a highly customised information package suitable for its implementation on a particular platform. This is a primary component for a successful information-knowledge interaction.

Phase C: Business plan. In this final phase, the information solution to be delivered to the client is further developed in a business plan. At this stage, details for the marketing of the product, the investment needed, the financial plan are established to conform a feasible solution.

Focussing in the process of treatment of contents we have developed a 4-step matrix approach. Users' profiles (equivalent to context of use, a combination of main health goals, scenario and socio-demographic data that are common to a significant group of users), resulting from previous survey investigation are the entry level for this methodology. From this point, 4 subsequent steps follow in a cascade-like fashion:

Step 1 - Matrix 1: Users' Profile – Health Topics. This matrix will define which the general groups of Users' Profiles are and which health topics must be considered inside each group. New categories can be defined at any time, so the growth of the system is assured. An example of such a matrix would be the following:

		Health Topics					
Users' Profile		Health care Services	Chronic Diseases	Drug abuse	Diet	Contraception	---
	---	---	---	---	---	---	---
	Hospital patients and relatives	X	X		X		--
	Adults 40 – 65	X	X		X		---
	Teenagers			X	X	X	---
	---	---	---	---	---	---	---

Note that the same Health Topic can be found associated to different Users' Profile. This conveys the idea of a matrix.

Step 2 – Matrix 2: Information Source – Health Topic. This matrix defines where the information required for all categories must be found. This will make possible to know which is a solid information provider and, if this is the case, to choose among different options. New providers can be incorporated at any time, assuring system's growth. An example of such a matrix would be the following:

		Health Topics					
Information Source		Health care Services	Chronic Diseases	Drug Abuse	Diet	Contraception	---
	---	---	---	---	---	---	---
	WHO recommendations	X	X		X	---	---
	University of Barcelona School of Medicine		X	X	X	---	---
	Merck Igoda Co.	X			X		
	---	---	---	--	---	---	---

Step 3 - Matrix 3: Information Source – Health topic (Types of Agreement). This matrix is intended to clarify the different types of agreements to be established between different information providers and the organisation managing the health information resource. The type of agreement may depend on both the Information Source and the Health Topic. An example of such a matrix would be the following:

Information Source		Health Topics					
		---	---	Chronic diseases	---	---	---
	---	---	---	---	---	---	---
	WHO Recommendations						
	University of Barcelona School of Medicine	---	---	Information will be provided in electronic format (Word 7.0) according to the document xxx on a quarterly basis. The information provision will be free of charge. As a compensation, editorial will allow access of students to the items and a kiosk will be maintained at the Central Hospital.	---	---	---
	Merck Igoda Co.						
	---	---	---	--	---	---	---

Step 4 - Matrix 4: Information Source – Health topic (Procedures on Integration of Contents). Information to be integrated will arrive in different types of formats. This matrix aims at defining a structured list of procedures to cope with such a diversity. As a result, a clear standardised link will join contents, platforms and providers. This will make possible accurate analysis of users' satisfaction with the product and as a result, corrections could be made. An example of such a matrix would be the following:

Information Source		Health Topics					
		---	---	Chronic diseases	---	---	---
	---	---	---	---	---	---	---
	University of Barcelona School of Medicine	---	---	Information provided in electronic format (Word 7.0) will be incorporated to the Internet facilities after completing the following checks: validation of contents by two external reviewers, publishing board advice, inclusion on a web page, final approval. The following presentations are to be considered: "Ask the doctor", BBS, list of servers / newsletter, encyclopaedia-like presentation, disease-file search.	---	---	---
	---	---	---	--	---	---	---

It is our opinion that this is a consistent methodology for content compilation, elaboration and validation. This methodology heavily depends on users' profile identification. This fact guarantees that during the whole process, users' requirements are kept on target. By making use of this methodology, we think that the process of treatment of contents to be integrated in a multimedia health information resource can be significantly improved.

Medical Informatics Europe '99
P. Kokol et al. (Eds.)
IOS Press, 1999

Expanding DIOGENE with a Clinical Information System Based on a New Hospital-Wide Clinical Finding Dictionary

Claudine Bréant, François Borst, Daniel Campi, Vincent Griesser, and Huy Son Le
Division d'Informatique Médicale
University Hospital of Geneva, 1211 Geneva 14, Switzerland

Abstract. The aim of this project is to expand DIOGENE with a centralized and integrated patient clinical database system providing a standardized framework for the building of future clinical databases and for the integration of existing heterogeneous ones. The combined 'across time view' and 'across departments view' generated from the integrated clinical data will enable an evolutionary view of the patient state both across time and across medical specialties. For this purpose and to permit the communication and exchange of data, a new controlled vocabulary for representing clinical data has been created. The construction of this vocabulary is based on the international ICD classification, already being used in DIOGENE for encoding patient diagnosis and procedures. A new extension of the ICD is proposed for medical information that goes beyond diagnosis and procedures encoding. The building of a common clinical finding dictionary recording the definition of findings is based on this newly developed clinical vocabulary. This process is incremental, manual, and significant.

1. Introduction

At the University Hospital of Geneva (HUG), a recent inventory of about 50 clinical databases embedding many different medical fields has been performed. The inability of the DIOGENE [1] hospital information system to provide any framework for the management of clinical data coupled with the advent in the early 80's of personal computers prompted the uncontrolled development of many medical database systems. Indeed, these systems were independently designed and implemented by several medical groups precluding effective data communication and exchange. While fulfilling the immediate needs of each department, many long-term problems linked to the maintenance of such a large and growing heterogeneous environment have become increasingly important.

A four years project has begun in 1997 to expand DIOGENE with a repository of detailed, structured, and standardized clinical data and medical protocols. Detailed clinical data is needed for a complete understanding of quality of care and consumption of resources. Such data describes the precise state of the patient and its evolution beyond diagnosis and therapeutic codes. For instance, it includes items such as the measure of blood pressure, the description of a diabetic retinopathy, and the pulse rate.

The new clinical information system provides a generic and standardized framework to help for the building of future clinical databases and for the integration of existing heterogeneous databases with DIOGENE. This has required the development of a controlled vocabulary representing clinical data. The present work fits into the more general effort for building an integrated electronic patient record system at the HUG.

Motivations to build a centralized clinical information system integrated with DIOGENE can be expressed in two different ways:

a) In terms of electronic patient record functions:

- Reuse and share of the clinical data collected by many different departments mainly to avoid a redundant data capture.
- Automatic link with the DIOGENE hospital information system patient data (admission/discharge data, laboratory, medical records, patient administrative information, image database, etc.).
- Automatic production of textual documents from input data such as letters to referring physicians and patient summary reports.

b) In terms of prospective data processing:

- retrieval of patient data from various points of view:
  - The *'across departments view'*: The state of the patient is described by clinical parameters coming from different medical specialties such as for instance obstetrics, intensive care unit, surgery, etc.
  - The *'across time view'*: This will allow for a evolutionary view of selected patient clinical data through time.

  Both approaches can be combined in order to show for instance the evolution of neonates going from the obstetrics to the pediatrics department.
- Production of federal statistics, clinical studies and medical research queries: the system will enable the mass screening of a large amount of patient data matching certain user-defined criterions.
- Quality of care and consumption of resources: most existing grouping systems, such as Diagnosis-Related Groups (DRG) are based on a few sets of data. An accurate understanding of either the quality of care or the consumption of resources requires more detailed data about the patient. This data goes beyond the 'administrative' medical summary and relies on detailed clinical databases.
- Case-based reasoning or the process of retrieving similar cases [2].

2. Design of the integrated clinical information system

The general functional architecture of the proposed clinical information system is illustrated in figure 1 and characterized by the following features:

- A new common database repository for hospital-wide patient clinical data integrated into DIOGENE.
- A controlled clinical vocabulary built using a bottom-up approach driven by the development of new clinical applications.
- A common hospital-wide clinical finding dictionary defined from the controlled clinical vocabulary.
- A general framework and PC-based graphical tools to design medical questionnaires. The clinical finding dictionary drives the design of a medical questionnaire.

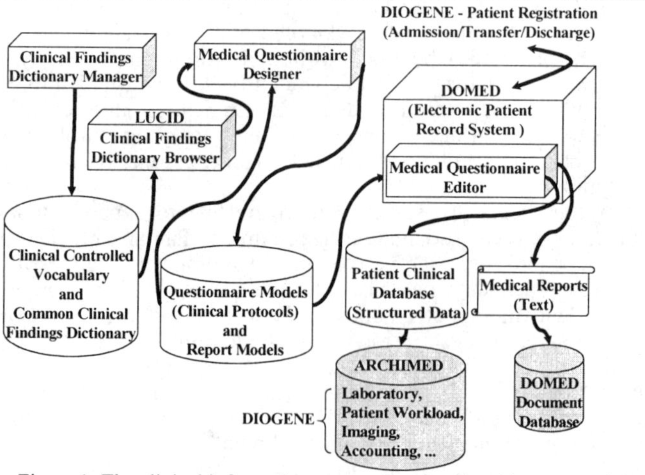

Figure 1: The clinical information system functional architecture and the integration with DIOGENE.

- A centralized and sharable database repository for medical questionnaire models representing medical knowledge about on-going hospital-wide medical protocols and clinical studies. This database includes report models for the automatic generation of textual medical reports, follow-up letters, etc.
- An integration of the questionnaire data entry interface within the framework of the DOMED [3] electronic patient record system currently being implemented at the University Hospital of Geneva.
- Storage and indexation into the DOMED database of automatically generated documents from the clinical database.

The Clinical Findings Dictionary Manager is a tool to facilitate the tasks of adding and/or maintaining the controlled clinical vocabulary as well as of defining new clinical findings.

The Medical Questionnaire Designer is a graphical tool to build questionnaire models detailing a clinical study and/or a medical protocol. The process of establishing a new model is driven by the Common Clinical Findings Dictionary and by the Questionnaire Models database. The Common Clinical Findings Dictionary is accessed through the browser LUCID [4]. The Questionnaire Models database allows previous models of questionnaires to be reused by new applications. Report Models for generating textual documents are built along with a questionnaire model. These allow an automatic production of textual medical documents from data retrieved from the Patient Clinical Database. When a questionnaire model and its report models are published, they can be accessed through DOMED and then through the Medical Questionnaire Editor. An instantiation of a questionnaire is given in figure 2. Signing out a questionnaire triggers the storage of input data into the Patient Clinical Database. Clinical data is subsequently archived into ARCHIMED, the patient information archive gathering data sent or retrieved from DIOGENE remote applications. At the same time, automatically generated medical reports from clinical data are indexed and stored into the DOMED database.

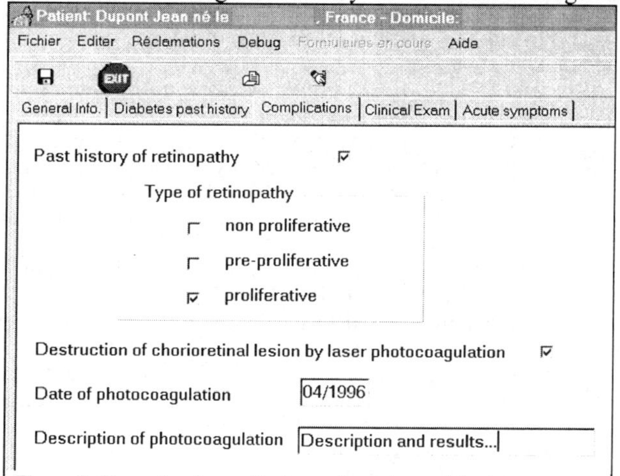

Figure 2: Example of a medical questionnaire and the input of patient data

3. The Hospital-Wide Dictionary for Clinical Findings

Increased interest in decision support, clinical guidelines and protocols requires more detailed, understandable, and sharable clinical vocabulary terms. Much work has been done in order to look for a common and comprehensive clinical controlled vocabulary set. However, the current systems are unable to meet the requirements for clinical data representation [5][6][7]. A general-purpose controlled vocabulary such as the Systematized Nomenclature of Human and Veterinary Medicine (SNOMED International) is multi-axial and cannot be easily used. As for the version 3 of the READ [8] codes classification, it is today limited to a utilization in the UK only. Therefore, it has been necessary to create a centralized controlled vocabulary to support any type of clinical applications developed at the HUG.

The construction of the new clinical controlled vocabulary relies on the ICD classification already being used in DIOGENE to encode patient diagnosis and procedures. More specifically, ICD10 [9] applies for the diagnosis and ICD9CM [10] for the procedures and they both constitute the Swiss standard. ICD has been completed with two extensions that are local to the HUG: the Diagnosis and Procedures Extension (ICD-DPE) and the Clinical Extension (ICD-CE). The process of inserting a new element in the clinical controlled vocabulary is incremental and is performed each time the current version of the vocabulary fails to fulfill the needs of a medical department.

The ICD-DPE was started in 1979 when the hospital diagnosis and procedures encoding process begun [11]. It is concerned with local extensions for diagnosis and procedures only. These are still periodically added to the classification in order to meet specific needs of the medical staff for a more accurate coding. The codes of these extensions end by the character '-' followed by a three digit number. It represents an additional level in the nomenclature. For instance, the ICD10 diagnostic: *H36.0 diabetic retinopathy* has been extended by three local extensions in order to define the more specific following diagnosis:

H36.0X-001 non proliferative diabetic retinopathy
H36.0X-002 pre-proliferative diabetic retinopathy
H36.0X-003 proliferative diabetic retinopathy

The same process is applied to extend a procedure code. For instance, the ICD9CM item: 68.3 *subtotal abdominal hysterectomy,* has been extended by the two following local extensions:

68.3X-001 open subtotal abdominal hysterectomy
68.3X-002 laparoscopic subtotal hysterectomy

The ICD-CE has newly been created to expand the controlled vocabulary beyond diagnosis and procedures proposed by the existing ICD and ICD-DPE classifications. Therefore, the existing approach already in place for the ICD-DPE is generalized and permits the organization of the vocabulary for clinical items like:

type of diabetes
date of destruction of chorioretinal lesion by laser photocoagulation
measure of the body weight

The codes are created in the ICD-CE with a similar syntax to the codes in the ICD-DPE. They end by the character '=' followed by a three digit number. Codes are included in the corresponding chapter of the ICD structure as a matter of priority. When this is not possible, codes are inserted in the "U" (user-defined) chapter. For instance, the following codes have been created in the ICD-CE structure:

E14.9X=004 type of diabetes
14.24=001 date of destruction of chorioretinal lesion by laser photocoagulation
U50.0X=005 measure of the body weight (Kg)

The existing programs for managing the ICD-DPE have been extended for the purpose of managing the ICD-CE and are part of the Clinical Findings Dictionary Manager toolbox. These tools primarily help for checking the non-redundancy and non-ambiguity when some vocabulary is added to the classification.

The Clinical Findings Dictionary records the definition for all the clinical findings. A clinical finding is composed of several attributes including a link to the controlled vocabulary. Clinical findings in the proposed clinical information system are defined from the vocabulary set including the standard ICD and its two local extensions (the ICD-DPE and the ICD-CE). A clinical finding is fully defined by the following attributes:

- The name of the finding, that needs to be self-explanatory and non-ambiguous.
- The context of the finding such as past history, family history, and complaint. It helps to further qualify a finding to avoid tremendous increasing of the list of codes.
- The type of the value: integer, float, text, date/time, enumeration, or boolean.

An enumeration is a set of codes selected among the ICD, ICD-DPE, or the ICD-CE classifications. For instance, the following set of codes defines the type for the clinical finding *type of retinopathy*:

H36.0X-001 non proliferative diabetic retinopathy
H36.0X-002 pre-proliferative diabetic retinopathy
H36.0X-003 proliferative diabetic retinopathy

- The unit, if the type attribute is numeric.
- The link with the corresponding item in ICD, ICD-DPE, or ICD-CE.

Table 1 describes the clinical findings *weight, past history of retinopathy*, and *type of retinopathy.* Once defined, these items become available to the medical staff through the Medical Questionnaire Designer tool as shown in figure 2.

Table 1: Clinical findings *weight, past history of retinopathy*, and *type of retinopathy* as registered in the common clinical finding dictionary

Clinical finding	*weight*	*Past history of retinopathy*	*type of retinopathy*
Type	*float*	*Boolean (y/n)*	enumeration: *H36.0X-001 non proliferative diabetic retinopathy* *H36.0X-002 pre-proliferative diabetic retinopathy* *H36.0X-003 proliferative diabetic retinopathy*
Unit	*Kg*	*n/a*	*n/a*
Context	*n/a*	*Past history*	*n/a*
ICD link	*U50.0X=005 measure of the body weight*	*H36.0 retinopathy*	*H36.0X=002 type of retinopathy*

4. Results and perspectives

Clinical questionnaires in the field of diabetes have been designed at the HUG using this common clinical finding dictionary. Integrating existing heterogeneous clinic data implies a system integration (at the level of patient admission/transfer/discharge data), a data structure integration (with the medical archive system ARCHIMED), and a vocabulary integration (description of items in a common clinical dictionary). A hospital-wide clinical finding dictionary based on extensions of ICD10 and ICD9CM has been developed. This is essential for sharing information between departmental clinical systems. However, in the absence of internationally recognized clinical vocabulary, the work necessary to create such a clinical dictionary is significant. The main tasks have included the setting of manual procedures and algorithms as well as computerized tools such as the Clinical Findings Dictionary Manager and LUCID. Sophisticated vocabulary maintenance tools have yet to be designed and implemented to automate some of the work in adding new terms in the ICD two extensions. This would help to add vocabulary more rapidly with a higher quality than it would be possible manually. Finally, the development of an internationally recognized vocabulary has yet to be done. ICD was not designed for organizing clinical vocabulary. However, its structure makes it possible to simply determine clinical extension codes for element related to the ICD10 and the ICD9CM chapter structures.

References

[1] Borst F., Lovis C., Thurler G., Maricot P., Rossier P., Revillard C., Scherrer J.R. Happy birthday DIOGENE: a Hospital Information System born 20 years ago. *Medinfo 98*. B. Cesnik et al. (editors).

[2] Jaulent M.C., Le Bozec C., Zapletal E., and degoulet P. Case Based Diagnosis in Histopathology of Breast Tumours. *Medinfo 98*. B. Cesnik et al. (editors).

[3] Baud R., Lovis C., Scherrer J.R., Nouvelles perspectives en matière de dossiers patients en réseau. *Journées Francophones d'Informatique Médicale à Lièges, Belgique*, Avril 98.

[4] Michel PA, Lovis C, Baud R. LUCID : a semi-automated ICD-9 encoding system. *Medinfo* 1995.

[5] Hammond WE. Call for a Standard Clinical Vocabulary. *J Am Med Inform Assoc.* 1997 ;4 :254-255.

[6] Campbell JR, Carpenter P, Sneidman C et al. Phase II Evaluation of Clinical coding schemes : completeness, taxonomy, mapping, definitions, and clarity. *J Am Med Inform Assoc.* 1997 ;4 :238-251.

[7] Cimino J.J., Johnson S.B., Hripcsak G., Hill C.L., and Clayton P.D. Managing Vocabulary for a Centralized Clinical System. *Medinfo 95 Proceedings*. R.A. Greenes et al. (editors).

[8] Buckland R. The Language of Health. *British Medical Journal* (1993) 306:287-8.

[9] International Statistical Classification of Diseases and Related Health Problems. *World Health organization*, Geneva, 1992; volume 1 and 3.

[10] International Classification of Diseases Nine[th] Revision. *MedIndex Publications*, Salt Lake City, USA, 1994.

[11] Borst F., Griesser V., RossierP., Bourdillou R., and Scherrer JR. Fifteen Years of Medical Encoding in the Diogene HIS. *Medinfo (Canada),* 1995.

Medical Informatics Europe '99
P. Kokol et al. (Eds.)
IOS Press, 1999

Metabolic Drug Pointing and Information Processing

Ralf Hofestädt, Ulrike Mischke, Manuela Prüß, Uwe Scholz
Institute of Technical and Business Information Systems
Otto-von-Guericke-Universität Magdeburg
P.O. Box 4120, D-39016 Magdeburg
E-mail: {hofestaedt|mischke|pruess|uscholz}@iti.cs.uni-magdeburg.de
Tel.: ++49-391-67-18659 Fax: ++49-391-67-12020

Abstract. Computer supported drug design is based on the biochemical information for the prediction of alternative bio-chemical pathways. Molecular information on genes, proteins, biochemical reactions, mutations, inborn errors and metabolic diseases are available via internet. Based on this information we developed an information retrieval and processing concept combining knowledge about metabolic diseases and biochemical effects.

1. Introduction

Up to now about 450 genetic metabolic defects are known. The most frequent conditions are diseases in the degradation pathway of amino acids or the just recently described fatty acid oxidation disorders. It is estimated that every 4000th newborn is affected with such a disease. For most of these defects dietary and/or medical treatment is available.
Thus by applying modern methods, for many of these metabolic diseases biochemical diagnosis is available, so a rapidly increasing number of diagnosed children and infants is to expect. The most challenging problem is the fact that inborn errors of metabolism are very heterogeneous. Prediction of the phenotype by knowing the genotype has become more and more important since the decision for initiating a certain treatment may be difficult using only biochemical data. The possibility for a genotype-phenotype correlation in a certain disease is dependent from several parameters. However, the number of patients is relatively small and they are widespread, so for making any correlation, an international metabolic diseases database for rare metabolic disorders is very useful.
A lot of different electronical information systems are available which represent the medical level of knowledge. Moreover, different databases concerning data on diseases, genes, enzymes, biochemical reactions, and biochemical effects of drugs are available. The idea of our project was and is to integrate the microscopic and macroscopic knowledge of metabolic diseases pointing out the biochemical effects of drugs.

2. Metabolic Diseases, Diagnosis, and Therapy

Inherited metabolic diseases are a group of disorders characterised by pathological abnormalities of metabolic pathways. Most of them are caused by a block regarding the corresponding metabolic pathway, others by a defect in a transport protein or a defect in the storage of products of the metabolism. The underlying defect leading to this type of disease is mostly an inborn enzyme deficiency, caused by a single gene mutation.
The knowledge of the pathogenesis of these diseases is very important, because it can explain the manifestations of a specific disorder, is necessary in order to reach a decision about rational treatment, and may even suggest that treatment is not feasible. Today, information on metabolic, molecular and genetic details for many metabolic diseases is

available, which brings with it new perspectives concerning the complex biological processes and resulting methods of diagnosis and therapy. At the same time, efforts to understand the biochemical and especially the molecular basis underlying human genetic variation are more vigorous then ever [1].
One of the most common inborn metabolic diseases is the Ornithine Transcarbamylase Deficiency, or OTC Deficiency. The deficient enzyme, Ornithine Transcarbamylase, or OTC, is involved in the urea cycle, and there are more than 60 known mutations of the OTC gene [2]. The OTC gene of the DNA, part of the whole genotype of a person, encodes the enzyme OTC. This enzyme's special task lies in the metabolic pathway, the urea cycle, where it catalyses the reaction from Ornithine to Citrulline. In case of a gene defect, the enzyme will not be produced and the urea cycle is interrupted. As a result, typical pathological effects occur concerning the phenotype of the involved person.
The diagnosis of metabolic diseases generally is based on the detection of metabolites. The reason is that specific metabolites can not be produced, basing on a genetic defect. Beyond these biochemical reactions new methods of biotechnology allow the molecular detection of this metabolites [3]. Therefore, the diagnosis of metabolic processes can be realised on different metabolic levels.
In general, however, efforts are made to intervene therapeutically into the involved pathway, although substitution of the lacking gene product mostly is difficult. In most of the cases a special dietetic treatment is used to prevent the accumulation of undegradable metabolites. If the enzyme activity is reduced, it sometimes can be activated by high-dosed intake of essential cofactors, e.g. of biotin. Another method of degradation of metabolites is the activation of alternative metabolic pathways. Such an activation can occur pharmacologically by supplementation of substances which bind and help to excrete toxic metabolites, or possibly gene therapeutically by the introduction of a new gene respectively a new enzyme which "nudges" a new pathway, resulting in a normal phenotype. Research is undertaken intensively, especially, in the field of metabolic diseases [4].

3. Metabolic Drug Pointing

A drug can be defined as a chemical compound, natural or synthetic, that is used in the prevention, diagnosis, treatment, or cure of disease, for the relief of pain, or to control or improve any physiological or pathological disorder in humans or animals. The effect of a drug depends on its concentration, its reaction with specific receptors and its interaction with different substances. The computer supported drug design is becoming more and more relevant [5].
In case of metabolic diseases, information on drug effects and on specific drug destinations is rare. Here different levels can be important: on the one hand the biochemical level, at which the conversion of the substances takes place. On the other hand, also the DNA level is of great interest, because here methods of gene therapy could be used to replace a defect or deficient gene. Looking at a specific metabolic disorder, e.g. the OTC deficiency, for its understanding and especially for the understanding of its therapy, it is important to know where and how a given drug intervenes in the individual's organism. This is what we call "drug pointing". In the case of OTC deficiency, the urea cycle is blocked at the conversion of ornithine to citrulline and nitrogen can not be excreted as urea. Normally, glutamine is degraded via the urea cycle. An alternative degradation of glutamine is possible: when sodium phenylacetate is given as a drug, it converts glutamine to phenylacetate glutamate, which can be excreted.
It is the aim of our Metabolic Diseases Database (MDDB), to point out not only the regular pathways related to different metabolic diseases, but also alternative pathways and biochemical drug effects, as far as there is information available.

4. Information Systems and Metabolic Diseases

For the detection of inborn errors the database system METAGENE is available [6]. This database system provides medical knowledge of inborn errors (macroscopic knowledge). Our group has extended the METAGENE database system by collecting the molecular knowledge of metabolic diseases (microscopic knowledge). This new database system is called Metabolic Diseases Database (MDDB). Moreover, access to the OMIM database system provides medical knowledge of metabolic diseases, and access to the molecular knowledge (genes, proteins, and pathways) is realised by using the powerful information system KEGG [7] which allows access to every known metabolic pathway including the related genes and proteins. Besides the development of the MDDB, the design and implementation of an integrative molecular knowledge server, called BIOBENCH, for the detection of inborn errors is one of our research goals. The architecture of our system allows automatic access to different database systems.

4.1 Related Works

Today, a new update of P.O.S.S.U.M (Pictures Of Standard Syndromes and diagnoses Malformations) is available. The biochemical genetics unit of the Montreal Children's Hospital is in the process of implementing a database system, that will provide knowledge of Phenylalanine-Hydroxylase (PKU). The University of Nürnberg-Erlangen has started a new project called Computer-Mediated-Communication, which will implement a professional electronic mailing list for the discussion of topics related to inborn errors of the metabolism. Moreover, specific database systems exist which provide medical knowledge, a lot of them are available via the Internet. At a microscopic level, methods of metabolic engineering will allow the analysis and synthesis of metabolic pathways. Different database systems for genes, proteins, and pathways are already available.
Nowadays, specific integrative information systems are implemented which allow specific access to molecular data. For the detection of metabolic diseases typical gene sequences, proteins, and metabolic pathways must be identified and analysed. An electronical representation of the complete metabolic pathway data set does not exist. Boehringer collects all biochemical reactions and presents this data graphically on the so called Boehringer Biochemical Pathway Chart [8]. The electronical representation of this data is the main goal of the KEGG project.

4.2 MDDB - A Molecular Information System for the Prediction of Alternative Pathways

We developed and implemented a database system called Metabolic Diseases Database (MDDB) which provides microscopic and macroscopic knowledge for the detection of a specific group of inborn errors, the so called hyperammonemias. We want to present not only the medical data, like general information on the disease, symptoms, laboratory findings and therapy, but also the molecular data. This includes information on genes, gene variants and their description, and gene regulation elements, as far as there are data available. The data on enzymes include also general information like EC number, synonyms and structure of the enzyme and information on the catalysed biochemical reaction, with structural formulas of the substances. Additionally, we collect data about drugs which are of therapeutic use in different cases, and we try to show their effects on the metabolic pathways, as described in section 3. The related pathways are shown, and possible alternative pathways will be predicted.
Thus using different information systems and literature, we are extending medical knowledge (macroscopic knowledge) as presented in the METAGENE database systematically by adding information about molecular processes. The MDDB has been developed to simplify data collection and to support the persistent storage of information about metabolic diseases. Moreover the user of the MDDB can obtain access to the various data in a uniform and integrated form.

5. BIOBENCH - a Knowledge Server for the Detection of Inborn Errors

The MDDB is integrated into the BIOBENCH system; a prototype of it is available via Internet. Its key idea is to develop and implement an information tool for the detection of inborn errors which is based on new technology, using methods of *information fusion* [9]. Therefore, we will combine the basic knowledge of medicine and molecular biology using a multi-database system. The basic module of our molecular knowledge server is the MDDB database system. Moreover, automatic access to the KEGG information system and the TRANSFAC database system is implemented. KEGG represents the molecular knowledge of metabolic pathways and TRANSFAC the molecular knowledge of gene regulation processes. Using our knowledge server, the information stored in these systems can easily be used. Communication between the user and our knowledge based server is founded on an uniform user interface. Regarding the current version, the user can ask for diseases, enzymes, and pathways. Asked for example for the OTC deficiency, the system will automatically create agents which will contact all the linked databases and information systems. The created agents will automatically identify every relevant entry, which will be sent to the server of our system, followed by the server's realisation of the information fusion between the data collected by the agents. At the end of that process an information window, which represents the selected information, will be presented to the user.

6. Discussion

Today, methods of biotechnology enable the systematic investigation of metabolic diseases, and gene therapy is becoming popular. This does not only influence the molecular diagnostics in a positive way, but also the therapy of this diseases. As a result of this research a huge amount of data arose and is still growing. There are different information systems available, which manage and offer this data via Internet.

The idea of our work is to expand the macroscopic knowledge about metabolic diseases by collecting molecular information, too. This process is what we call information fusion. Therefore, we have developed and implemented the Metabolic Disease Database (MDDB). Regarding a metabolic disease, our information system presents information about the corresponding metabolic pathways, genes, enzymes, and medicine (drugs). Moreover, relevant references and therapy plans are offered. The special feature of the MDDB we are working at will be the realisation of the so called drug pointing. This data will be of great relevance for the computation of alternative pathways and for the tuning of gene therapy.

We embedded our MDDB system in an integrative molecular information system, the BIOBENCH, which provides a connection to the KEGG information system and the TRRD database system. It enables an easy access to relevant biochemical and genetic data concerning metabolic diseases.

Acknowledgement

This work is supported by the Kurt-Eberhard-Bode-Stiftung in the Stifterverband für die Deutsche Wissenschaft.

References

[1] A. L. Beaudet *et al.*, Genetics, biochemistry, and Molecular Basis of Variant Human Phenotypes. In: C. R. Scriver *et al.* (eds.), The Metabolic and Molecular Bases of Inherited Disease (7. ed.). McGraw-Hill, New York, 1995, pp. 53-118.

[2] M. Tuchmann and R. J. Plante, Mutations and Polymorphisms in the Human Ornithine Transcarbamylase Gene: Mutation Update Addendum. *Hum. Mut.* **5** (1995) 293-295.

[3] C. Perez-Carda *et al.*, An Unusual Late-Onset Case of Propionic Acidaemia: Biochemical Investigations, Neuroradiological Findings and Mutation Analysis. *Eur. J. Pediatr.* **157** (1998) 50-52.

[4] K. Overturf *et al.*, Ex Vivo Hepatic Gene Therapy of a Mouse Model of Hereditary Tyrosinemia Type I. *Hum. Gene Ther.* **9** (1998) 295-304.

[5] H.-J. Böhm *et al.*, Wirkstoffdesign. Spektrum Akademischer Verlag, Heidelberg, Berlin, Oxford, 1996.

[6] U. Mischke *et al.*, KBS-DIAMET: Database and Expert System for Diagnosis and Treatment of Patients with Inborn Errors of Metabolism. *J. Inherit. Metab. Dis.* **18** (1995) 224-226.

[7] S. Goto *et al.*, Organizing and Computing Metabolic Pathway Data. In: R. Altman et al. (eds.), Proceedings of the Pacific Symposium on Biocomputing. (World Scientific), 1997, pp. 175-186.

[8] G. Michal (ed.), Biochemical Pathways. Böhringer Mannheim, Penzberg, 1993.

[9] R. Hofestädt and U. Scholz, Information Processing for the Analysis of Metabolic Pathways and Inborn Errors. *Biosystems* **47** (1998) 91-102.

Medical Informatics Europe '99
P. Kokol et al. (Eds.)
IOS Press, 1999

MedicDAT
- Making Information Available -

C.-M. Reng, A. Tsakpinis, J. Schoelmerich
Dpt. of Internal Medicine 1 and DV-Med, University of Regensburg, Germany

1. Introduction

Today most hospitals use computer-based systems for administrative purposes. Electronic patient-records exist in highly specialised versions mostly limited to the needs of single departments. In contrast integrative systems that allow a hospital-wide documentation of medical data are rare. Also electronic systems are used in practices, hospitals and medical schools to gain non-patientspecific medical information. Drug-index-systems, handbooks or scientific publications on CD are available. Access to the Internet to search online-databases is at more and more physicians disposal.

2. The problem

However the acceptance of these electronic media is poor. There are several reasons that keep healthcare-professionals away from using the majority of the offered electronic tools regularly and frequently. Whereas the global performance of database-research used to be a major problem in former times the technical aspect of performance becomes less and less important today. The different user-interfaces, the often complex navigation within the various systems and the increasing amount of redundant or worthless information that is presented especially by the internet limits the use of electronic media in everyday use. The efficiency of using electronic information systems is often too low compared to traditional media therefore the use of these systems costs the most expensive good that is at the user's disposal - his time.

3. The MedicDAT-project

The aim of the MedicDAT(Interface for Medical Documents, Scientific Abstracts and Text Books)-project is to increase the acceptance of electronic media in clinical medicine. MedicDAT shall reach this aim by simplifying the acquisition of qualified information in the electronical media environment. The University of Regensburg is initiator and leader of the MedicDAT-project. The scientific publishing houses Urban & Fischer (München) and Springer (Heidelberg), the online content-provider HOS-Multimedica, the SAP related software-developer GSD (Berlin) and the medical informatics section of the University of Lübeck are partners in the project. The project is granted as "Leitprojekt" of the German federal ministery of education, science, research and technology (bmb+f).

4. Communication of electronical media in medicine today

Although electronic media in medicine are used in diagnosis, therapy and education, there is hardly any communication between the different programmes and machines. Only structured data like monitor values or laboratory results can be transported from application to application using standard exchange-protocols like HL7. Nevertheless most of the applications are typical "island"-solutions that deal with their own data but - besides a minimal data-set like patient's name and address - cannot share or exchange data or functionality with any other application. When looking at electronic media holding non-patientspecific medical data, no common interface to link similar, extended or supplemental information exists. In the majority of cases each data-source provides it's own method and user-interface to navigate within this application and to present the requested information. So it costs an increasing lot of time to look for information at more than one data-source. The users' acceptance to ask for a comprehensive "second electronic opinion" therefore is little. Even the world wide web with it's millions of references usually only links one homepage to the other instead of a closer content-oriented linking. The need of redundant navigation is the unfavourable result.

5. What can be the benefit of electronically available information

The use of books and newspapers instead of electronic media is easier, as no costly and unwieldy machine is necessary to present the contents. Therefore there must be a an additional benefit to change to the new media. Such benefit can be the availability of all latest information at all computers at the same time in a network. Another benefit can be the possibility of electronically collecting and linking information from different sources. This can easily be illustrated with two examples:

It is of no special interest to the student to find virtual lectures on the net, if this information can be brought to him by the "real professor". So the use of such services is limited to special circumstances like long-distance-education. A benefit of virtual lectures - besides these special circumstances and the effect of revision - could be the possibility to look for further information. The lecture's topic may be found in scientific papers, text-books or other additional sources of information. A consolidation or expansion of the obtained information according to the actual needs of the student with an increase of the quality of education could result from this.

In everyday's work the clinician already sits at his computer for diagnosis, therapy-planing or documentation. He or she would greatly appreciate to navigate right from this application to look up additional information that might be needed right at that moment. If high-quality information could be obtained quick and preselected from various data-sources, according exactly to the actual needs of the user, a lot of time could be saved compared to the traditional way of gathering information.

6. Why another interface for medical data

A lot of highly developed interfaces for medical data exist. But all these interfaces refer to structured information. It is easy to exchange patient's names, birthdays, insurances etc. and there is no problem to communicate laboratory data from one system to the other, but there is no interface for medical contents. No existing interface or technology provides a link between similar or extended medical information. There is no technology in use that keeps in mind, what the specific requirements of the user are. Of course a student needs other information than an attending physician while doing the same job. There is no technology in use that is able to check what is done at a computer at the moment and use this context to judge what specific information therefore may be relevant to the user. MedicDAT wants to provide a technology and an interface that helps to find medical information that is text-related, user-specific and context-orientated. This is what we call a content-based linking.

7. What is the MedicDAT functionality

MedicDAT wants to improve the search within electronic media. Not all possible results shall be displayed. MedicDAT shall help to preselect reliable information that is fitting in the context of the actual workflow. To make a complete search possible besides the search's headwords also its synonyms have to be processed. This leads straight to the technical and logical possibility of translating the headwords to other languages, forming the language-independent concept of the MedicDAT-research. To find the required information, not only conventional database-indexes can be used. Also new indexes - that can be compared to the tables of contents in the first pages of most scientific books - must be used by the MedicDAT "intelligent meta-search-engine" to make sure that more than just the headword can be found in the potential data-source. The presentation of information has to be homogeneous. The user does not want to navigate through different graphically decorated applications when quickly searching for information. He needs a standardised form of presentation. MedicDAT therefore will display the gathered information in a standard user-environment independent from the data-source. MedicDAT has to "keep in mind", what information the user needed when finishing his query. Based on this information MedcDAT can be able to lead him quicker to the required information when he starts his next MedicDAT-query. MedicDAT also has to provide billing functionality, as parts of the displayed information - especially when searching across the web - will not be for free. So the user will have to decide whether he wants to see what is offered and whether he accepts to pay for the information, if it is not for free. Including the billing functionality multiple login-procedures can be avoided. Finally MedicDAT integrates a tool for the efficiency control of its functions. During the phase of development and further on the project wants to make sure to produce a useful tool for everyday-practice, not just an academic toy.

8. Technical realisation

Applications that call MedicDAT to fetch information are called MedicDAT-Clients, applications that serve information are called MedicDAT-Servers in the project-terminology. The technical realisation is possible since intra- and internet-technology are available. An independent technical platform can be defined to allow access to most existing data-sources. Also the technology for the knowledge-based functions already exists and only has to be adapted to the MedicDAT-requirements. More complex is the context-based indexing and structuring of information to make the MedicDAT search-functions possible. This is the reason for the primary partnership including three providers of medical contents. The content-providers take part in the project with adapting their potential sources of information - the MedicDAT-Servers - with the necessary additional content-based structures. The manufacturers of potential MedicDAT-Clients integrate the link to MedicDAT into their products. This includes the integration of functionality to submit information about the user's workflow. The University of Regensburg will provide the MedicDAT core-technology and is responsible for project co-ordination and final definition of the data-structures. Six project-phases are planned. The prephase with the project-definition is already finished. The first MedicDAT-release will connect the clinic communication system IS-H*med to certain intranet-informations provided on MedicDAT-adapted customary CDs. The second project-phase will allow other communication-systems to use MedicDAT, then also gaining information from the web. The third project-phase will add the knowledge based functions. In the following phase the automatic or semi-automatic adaption of any data-source to MedicDAT shall be established. At the same time MedicDAT shall be tested at various hard- and software-platforms. On from the beginning MedicDAT will be available to a selected number of pilot-users. Finally after the fifth project-phase MedicDAT will be commercially available.

9. Economic realisation

The yearly releases of MedicDAT force the project to focus on fixed product-cycles that always result in an application ready to use. This shall prevent an escalation of useless high-tech development without final benefit to the user. The distribution of MedicDAT - once commercially available - will be provided by the manufacturers of MedicDAT-compatible products. MedicDAT simply will be shipped with their products either MedicDAT-Servers or -Clients. The MedicDAT-license itself will be for free to the end-user. MedicDAT will be financed by the manufacturers of MedicDAT-compatible products and by taking money for billing-services. Primary financing of the project is guaranteed by the grant of the bmb+f. An amount of 4.2 million Euro can be spent during the next five years. After that time the organisation of the MedicDAT-project will consist of three administrative structures. The MedicDAT-company as the commercial copyright-holder, being responsible for development and product-support. The MedicDAT-consortium representing the producers of MedicDAT-compatible products. The MedicDAT-association as the scientific board to keep the project under an independent control.

10. What is the aim and perspective of MedicDAT

According to the Announcement of the bmb+f's competition about "world-wide knowledge" that was won by MedicDAT, it shall be a structured information- and knowledge-system based upon modern information- and communication-technology. MedicDAT shall be an independent and strategic product that can be used in medical science and hospitals just as in the practice of a general practitioner. It shall revaluate compatible products so that their acceptance by the professional user increases. The aim of MedicDAT is that someone buying a MedicDAT compatible CD knows that on from the moment when he puts this CD in his computer or his net, the contained knowledge is available together with and linked to all other previously installed MedicDAT-compatible data-sources.

As a perspective the project-partners hope that in the future the MedicDAT-integration will be a standard-feature of all high-quality software in medicine.

MedicDAT on a portable computer is technically also already possible today. If MedicDAT can provide real quick highly specialised medical information to nearly every place in the world this could open a new dimension especially to emergency- and out-patient treatment. The capability of MedicDAT to link between languages makes it a primarily international product. The acceptance of MedicDAT throughout the “medical world” will be directly depending on the benefit of MedicDAT to the user. Only if MedicDAT will help to save time and increase the quality of work, it will be a successful bridge of knowledge.

Medical Informatics Europe '99
P. Kokol et al. (Eds.)
IOS Press, 1999

How to structure clinical information: A practical example

Schweiger R[1], Bürkle T[1], Köhn F[2], Dudeck J[1]
[1]*Department of Medical Informatics, University of Gießen, Heinrich-Buff-Ring 44, D-35392 Gießen, Germany*
[2]*Department for Dermatology and Andrology, University of Gießen*

Abstract. In the frame of an European telemedicine project, we have designed and implemented an Andrology server that provides the user (e.g. physicians, students) with a set of anonymized andrology cases. Within this context we faced the problem of re-structuring existing clinical information sources and gained some experience on how much of the problem might be solved by the software engineer. This paper presents a method that partially automates the maintenance of the andrology case collection. Moreover, the potential benefit of XML for information representation will be discussed.

1. Pushing the border to structured information

Clinical information can be split into two large partitions. The first is patient related data which may be contained e.g. in an electronic patient record [1]. The second partition comprises clinical information sources such as electronic textbooks, electronic dictionaries or electronic guidelines [2,3,4]. Both types of information are relevant for clinical staff and must be available at the clinical workstation. Many authors have emphasized the necessity to capture and to store clinical patient data in a structured fashion and to avoid free text entries [5,6,7,8]. Cimino for example depicts a transition from unstructured patient data to more structured and coded data and emphasizes the significance of universal codes (see fig. 1) [9].

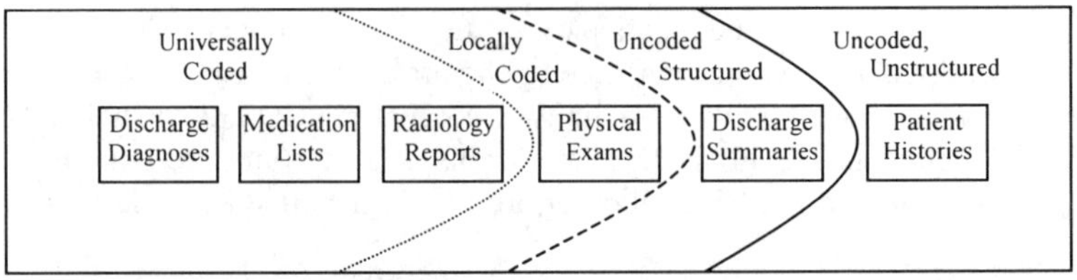

Fig. 1: Pushing the border to more structured data. Taken from [9].

However, far less has been published about the structuring of clinical information sources. Many commercial information sources have been made available only inside application programs. Others have tried to achieve structure by implementing information sources on top of databases [2,3,4]. But to achieve this database structure is often a difficult process. If information sources cannot be transformed easily into a good structure, electronic support for information management (retrieval, reuse in knowledge based functions) will be limited.

2. An example to better structured clinical information sources

Inside a European research project the task was to implement an electronic information source for a medical subspeciality. We have implemented successfully what we call an Andrology case atlas. It contains a set of case descriptions derived from different andrology patients (andrology deals with problems of male fertility) and is available on the Internet [10]. To implement and fill this case atlas we received the clinical information in shape of narrative unstructured text documents together with a set of slides from each of the participating andrology specialists. For each case the responsible physician usually provides a wordprocessor file and several slides. In this situation our basic idea was to automate the implementation and maintenance of the case collection as far as possible.

Some manual preparation proved unavoidable. First of all, the slides have to be scanned to convert them into an electronic format (we choose JPEG). To enable automated processing the wordprocessor file must be converted to plain text, preserving however the basic structure of the document. The automating processor must know where to include non-text elements such as tables and images. This is currently done manually, marking the proper location with predefined white space characters such as tabs and new lines. Reference to pictures is included using Uniform Resource Locators.

The remaining tasks are performed automatically by a compiler. This compiler performs several tasks. Parsing the text, it automatically inserts appropriate HTML (Hyper Text Markup Language) tags. It recognizes automatically headers and paragraphs and takes care that they appear accordingly in the resulting document. The structure of the case description in terms of chapters can differ from author to author. Besides, the compiler creates and updates several indices. For each case description it constructs an index of chapters, tables and images. Moreover, common indices (images, keywords and diagnoses) are updated automatically each time a new case is delivered.

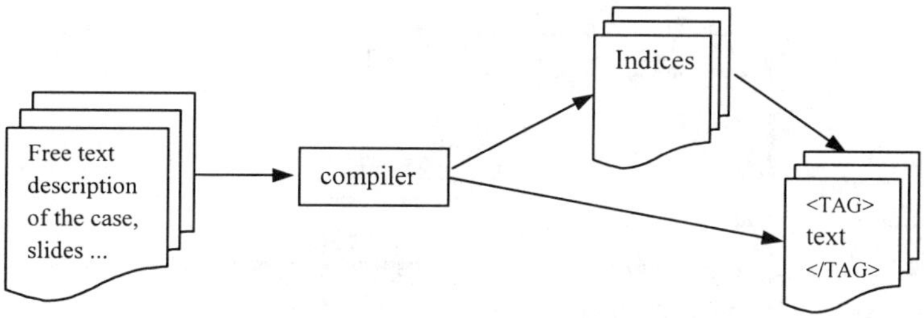

Fig. 2: A compiler supports the re-structuring of legacy data (markup) and the maintenance of indices (access of case descriptions by diagnosis, therapy, image, keyword).

3. The result: A well structured Andrology case atlas

The task of the Andrology server is to make specialist knowledge of a small medical field known to a larger community. Internet technology has been used to allow a wide variety of interested persons to access the information. Cases have been anonymized for privacy reasons. The available case descriptions cover a wide spectrum of reproductive diseases ranging from malignant tumors to infections.

Based on well structured information, several access paths to the cases have been established to enable an appropriate access to the knowledge for different types of users. A student for example might want to train his diagnostic capabilities and conclude from clinical information such as the patient's history and findings (textual description, ultrasound image) to the correct andrologic diagnosis. An urologist however could try to match one of his patients with one of the cases and afterwards might want to contact the respective specialist by email.

Figure 3 shows a screenshot of the Andrology case atlas. The top part of the screen contains potential navigation pathways across all cases of the case atlas. As mentioned above, those pathways are updated automatically once a new case is inserted. The *Case* link allows the search in a list of available cases (a case is usually identified by the diagnosis). The *Search* link allows to enter a plain text search phrase. A search engine will look up this phrase in all case descriptions and return a list of cases containing the phrase. The *Image* link leads to a list of all available images of all cases. Since those images are crosslinked, a click on an image will link to the respective case. The *About* link provides some introduction to the Andrology atlas. The case itself consists of chapters, tables and images. A table of contents for the selected case is therefore displayed in the lower left window. It permits access to any part of a specific case at any time. The case description itself appears in the lower right frame. It contains inline images which can be enlarged on double click. The user can scroll through this window in order to read the complete case description. A link has been established, so that the author of the case can be contacted by email.

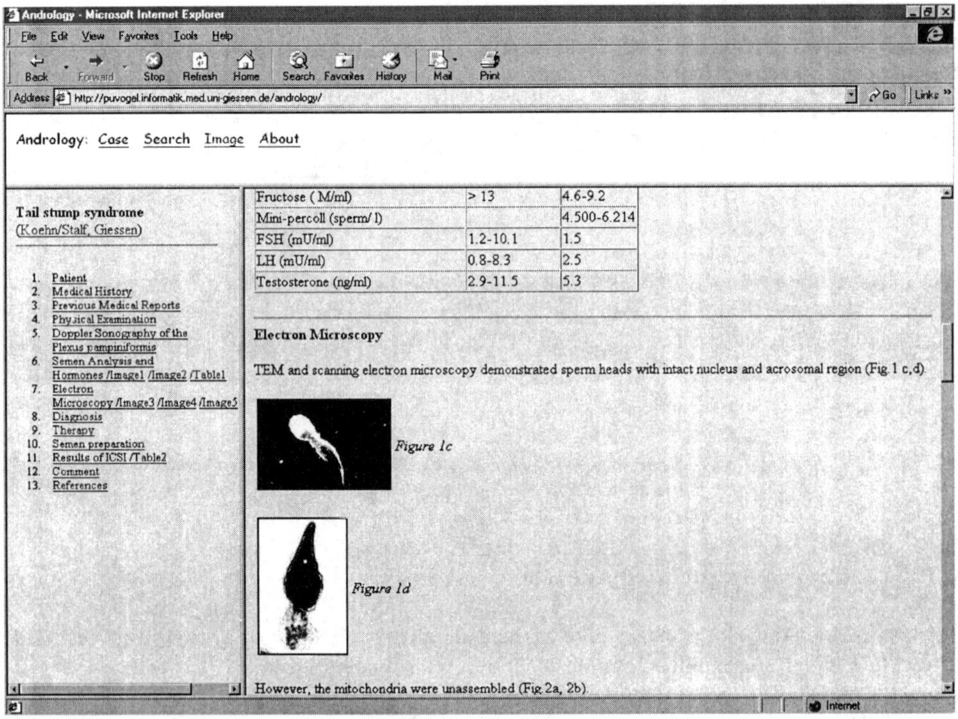

Fig 3.: Screenshot of the Andrology case atlas.

Our Web server registered about 2523 external accesses to the Andrology case atlas within a period of 17 months. A more sophisticated statistic that distinguishes the different user groups and their access pathways is desirable.

4. Discussion

There are many successful examples for Internet based information engineering [2,3,4]. We don't want to add just another example of an Internet based information source Instead, our goal was to automate the re-structuring process of existing documents in order to produce well structured case descriptions with a large variety of access paths to the stored medical knowledge. For our Andrology server we used the Hypertext Markup Language (HTML), mainly because the presentation of the information was supported by existing Web browsers (HTTP, multimedia, links, ...). Our compiler supported us not only in the markup process, but also in the maintenance of several access pathways (indices) each time a new case description was delivered.

One limitation of the HTML approach is that we cannot capture much meaning from the documents yet. Let's assume we want to find the cases of all patients with an age between 40 and 50. For this task we would need something like an <age> element. Limitations of the document based approach can be overcome when tags can be freely defined and are not restricted to presentation. For this reason, we also considered the eXtensible Markup Language (XML) [11] as an alternative to HTML, because it allows to define more meaningful elements such as diagnosis and therapy and, as a consequence, enables a more meaningful information retrieval. However, the software support for XML at this time was rather low.

The problem remains to get the HTML/XML markup into the case descriptions. Most of our case descriptions were derived from scientific publications and presentations and were delivered as wordprocessor files. In the case of the Andrology case collection, the tagging respectively re-structuring of the text was rendered by the software engineer, mainly to reduce the burden of contribution. We asked for example our physicians to mark up important catchwords inside the document with ampersands: @phrase@. Such markup would enable the compiler to construct a better keyword index. But the medical specialists had not even considered this option. On the other hand, the possibilities of the software engineer are rather limited due to his medical knowledge. Input forms e.g. could make the structuring process more transparent so that the medical expert would do it. An input form for a contribution to the Andrology atlas could be generated automatically from a so-called XML schema, i.e. a XML document that describes a document structure such as the structure of an andrology case description. Such a schema could be very flexible in terms of structure (options, repeating groups), extensibility (invent new elements if necessary) and software support (browser, search engine, parser).

In any case, manual effort has to be invested in order to re-structure legacy data. The basic structuring of the text remained manual work, although the compiler made some of it easier (white space structure versus markup structure). The role of our compiler was mainly to create and update several access pathways. Thus we can accommodate the requirements of experienced urologists as well as those of less experienced medical students.

5. Conclusion

We would like to conclude this paper with the statement that more structure should be introduced not only in patient data but also in information sources. Only then the large body of clinical knowledge will become easier to handle and automated functions can make use of such knowledge. It turned out that the re-structuring of legacy data will always require manual effort. Some of the manual effort, however, can be automated as our compiler has proven. Beside of that, markup languages will play an important role in the structuring process. XML e.g. not only allows to capture meaningful structures such as exams, findings, diagnoses and therapies, but also offers a considerable software support.

References

[1] Borst F: Computer-based patient records, Synopsis. Yearbook of Medical Informatics 95, 191-194.
[2] Bittorf A, Krejci-Papa NC, Diepgen TL: Development of a dermatological image atlas with worldwide access for the continuing education of physicians. Journal of Telemedicine and Telecare 1995, 45-53.
[3] Quade G, Püschel N, Far F: CancerNetTM Redistribution via WWW. Journal of the American Medical Informatics Association, 1996, 403-407.
[4] Bürkle T, Prokosch H-U, Dudeck J. Knowledge and Information Based Functions in the Gießen Hospital Information System - Present and Future. Toward An Electronic Health Record Europe '96 Proceedings London, 100-107.
[5] Moorman PW, van Ginneken AM, van der Lei J, van Bemmel JH: A Model for Structured Data Entry Based on Explicit Descriptional Knowledge. Yearbook of Medical Informatics 95, 195-204.
[6] McDonald CJ, Blevins L, Tierney WM, Martin DK: The Regenstrief Medical Records. MD Computing 5, 1988, 34-47.
[7] Stead WW, Hammond WE: Computer-based medical records: the centerpiece of TMR. MD Computing 5, 1988, 48-62.
[8] McDonald CJ, Tierney WM, Overhage JM, Martin DK, Wilson GA: The Regenstrief medical record system: 20 years of experience in hospitals, clinics and neighborhood health centers. MD Computing: 9, 1992, 206-215.
[9] Cimino JJ: Data storage and knowledge representation for clinical workstations. Yearbook of Medical Informatics, 1995, 289-298.
[10] www.med.uni-giessen.de/imi/neu/forschung/index.html
[11] www.w3.org

Medical Informatics Europe '99
P. Kokol et al. (Eds.)
IOS Press, 1999

Hospital Information Systems: Chances and Obstacles on the Way to Integration

Richard Lenz, Rainer Blaser, Klaus A. Kuhn
Philipps-University, Marburg, Germany

Abstract. Today, most large hospital information systems (HIS) comprise many heterogeneous application systems, loosely coupled via interfaces. Integration could offer many advantages, like the support of interdepartmental workflows or a consistent patient record. This cannot be achieved, however, by simply interfacing originally unrelated component systems. In this paper, we present relevant concepts of integration, the autonomy/consistency tradeoff, and technical alternatives in some detail. Based on our recent experiences in analyzing an existing HIS and selecting adequate vendors for the needs of our 1250-bed hospital, we then discuss strategies and tradeoffs on the way to a HIS that utilizes state-of-the-art technology to fill the users' needs.

1. What does integration mean?

The term "integrated system" is used in various different meanings. Actually, numerous different aspects should be expected from an integrated system. Some of them are:

- *Ubiquity*: Data stored at one place should be available elsewhere [1, 5, 7]
- *Consistency and Integrity*: Different data items stored within the system should not be contradictory and integrity constraints should be maintained [6]. In particular, concurrent data access should not result in inconsistent data (Synchronization)
- *Single system image*: The user should be able to interact with the system via a singe standard user interface [5]. Moreover, the user should not be aware of heterogeneous system components (transparency) [6, 7]

The main purpose of a hospital information system, however, is to capture and store data consistently in order to rearrange and display the data as needed [1]. Increasingly, organizational aspects and the support of workflows have to be covered. It is important to remember, that a common – not necessarily physically centralized – database shared by the entire hospital information system is the main characteristic and most important requirement for a truly integrated system [1]. A proper schema design should ensure that the part of the real world to be mapped into the database is not redundantly described (one fact in one place) [6]. The purpose of the common database is to ensure consistent access to commonly used data items by concurrently running applications.

So far we emphasized the data integration aspect. Leguit [7] defines data integration as "Data stored in one subsystem is available for other subsystems", which corresponds to the ubiquity aspect of distributed data management. True data integration, however, also implies data consistency. Other "classes of integration" mentioned by Leguit are presentation integration (uniform interaction with the system) and functional integration (combining different functions still guarantees a coherent result). Both aspects correspond to the requirement of a single system image. We would like to add an additional class of integration, namely organizational and workflow integration. This aspect emphasizes the adaptation of the system to the organizational structure and business processes of the hospital, including data protection and security.

2. Heterogeneity in hospital information systems

HISs are characterised by various degrees of heterogeneity on different levels. We will not focus on heterogeneity of networks, hardware and operating systems, which impose integration problems that are not domain specific. The core problem are application systems from different vendors. Usually each software product stores its "own" data and comes with a database of its own. As a result, the data stored within the HIS is redundantly distributed over different databases with different data models, independently developed database schemas, and managed by different database management systems with different query languages and synchronization mechanisms. One of the most serious problems in this context is the *semantic heterogeneity* of overlapping database schemas. As defined in [11] semantic heterogeneity occurs when there is a disagreement in the meaning, interpretation, or intended use of the same or related data.

As we recapitulate the reasons for heterogeneity, it becomes clear that it is difficult to avoid:

- *Organizational structure of the hospital*: Decisions in hospital departments are often driven by departmental needs in the first place rather than by hospital needs.
- *Medical devices*: Cardiac catheter, ECG, or EEG devices etc. often come with "in-built" database systems as well as specific documentation software. Measurement data are directly written into this database and the documentation software accesses these data in order to generate reports.
- *System vendors:* Two kinds of vendors can be distinguished: generalists (total system vendors) and specialists (niche vendors) [1]. Niche vendors have specialized products for some dedicated purpose (e.g. laboratory systems). Generalists, offer a full range of functionality for a HIS but often lack in specialized functionality.
- *"Best of breed" philosophy*: It is often believed that buying the best software for each purpose or each department will result in the best overall HIS. The additional functionality provided by an integrated system (consistency, cross departmental workflow support, single system image, etc.) is lost if this is the dominant philosophy to build a HIS.
- *Legacy applications*: Legacy systems often are very old, written in some proprietary programming language and use hierarchical databases or no database at all. Substituting these systems can be very difficult, especially when valuable information is hidden within the application code.

These aspects of "grown" HISs are serious obstacles on the way to a more or less integrated system. In some cases the organizational structure of a hospital requires a certain degree of autonomy for some departmental systems. However, autonomy and global consistency are contradictory goals.

3. Autonomy and consistency tradeoff

Building an integrated system by combining independently developed autonomous component systems is an illusion, because there is a tradeoff between *autonomy* on the one hand and *consistency* and *transparency* on the other hand. Different types of autonomy, like *design, communication, execution* and *association autonomy* [11] can be distinguished. At this point we only pick out the *execution autonomy*, which refers to the ability of a component database system to execute a local operation independently from external operations. In particular, each component system can decide independently in which order the local operations are executed.

If global consistency has to be preserved for some data item replicated in two systems, an update can only be successful if it is executed in both systems (*synchronous update*). This requires a (global) distributed transaction with subtransactions in each system. The typical correctness criterion for concurrent execution of transactions is *serializability*. Serialization of such distributed global transactions, however, can only be achieved if the corresponding subtransactions are executed in the same order at each participating site. Therefore consistency in the sense of traditional transaction correctness can only be achieved if execution autonomy is violated. Even if it were possible to compromise execution autonomy in order to synchronize replicated objects, this would cause new problems. Replication is useful to increase availability of read operations but reduces availability of update operations, thus replication is only helpful with data objects that are rarely updated. In autonomous systems, however, replication is not introduced where it is needed, but is simply given due to overlapping database schemas. Therefore, enforcing synchronous updates on replicated objects in autonomous systems might result in reduced availability. Asynchronous updates, on the other hand, might result in global inconsistencies, as explained before. If updates on the same object are allowed in more than one system even diverging instances of the object might occur.

The computer science and medical informatics research community have worked for a long time on integration concepts that either allow for combining preexisting subsystems or that help avoiding integration problems as described above for newly developed system components. Some of these concepts currently being discussed are described within the next section.

4. Technical alternatives in the context of integration

Speaking about integration of HISs, the most frequently mentioned concept is the so called *communication server*. With a growing number of subsystems interfaced among each other, managing the interfaces becomes difficult. A communication server is a tool that helps with the management of interfaced systems. The number of interfaces can be reduced, because each system only needs an interface to the communication server and not to all the other systems it communicates with. However, interfaced systems remain interfaced systems with all inherent shortcomings and are not integrated just because some sophisticated tool is used to manage and monitor the interfaces.

WWW together with *HTML* and *Java* are also often mentioned in the context of integration. This technology is most useful for realizing platform independent solutions (e.g. [8]). However, different systems from different vendors will necessarily lead to inconsistent data as a consequence of their autonomy and are not integrated just because they provide a web interface and can be accessed by the same web browser at the same terminal.

Multi-Database Systems (MDBS) are intended to provide global access to several component database systems while preserving the autonomy of the component systems. Different classifications of MDBS can be found in the literature [3, 11]. In the context of HISs *federated database systems* are probably the most prominent variant of MDBSs. A *federation* provides a global schema based on the export schemas of the participating component systems. The *schema integration* process, which is needed to resolve semantic heterogeneity of the export schemas, cannot be automated and has to be repeated whenever one of the participating component databases changes its local database schema. Moreover, the integrity of the global schema cannot be guaranteed when the component systems remain autonomous. Due to these circumstances FDBS do not play a major role in the context of HIS so far.

Data warehousing is a concept intended for decision support [4]. The *operational systems* within a HIS are targeted to support OLTP applications which require detailed and up-to-date data and which perform reads and updates on these data. The data warehouse, in contrast, collects data from the operational databases in order to provide summarized and consolidated read only data for online analytical processing (OLAP). The operational systems which are sources for the data warehouse remain autonomous and are neither integrated nor substituted by the data warehouse.

One key problem of different independently developed operational systems within a hospital information system is the *overlapping functionality,* which results in overlapping database schemas and diverging instances of common objects. This can be avoided if updates on these common data objects are always performed on a *primary copy* stored in a *reference system.* To realize such a functional separation of systems requires either a high programming effort and cooperating system vendors or must be enforced by simply disabling certain functions in the subsystems. In [9] Ohly points out the "*extreme practical difficulties in achieving the functional integration of applications that were never designed for this purpose*" concerning the BERMED project.

Heterogeneous HISs have a lot of disadvantages compared to a truly integrated system. Each of the concepts discussed so far contributes to minimizing some of these disadvantages. However, none of the concepts comes close to a truly integrated system. The reason for this is, that the operational systems in a hospital are originally designed and built as stand alone systems and are not intended as one component that performs a dedicated task within a distributed information system.

Novel middleware technologies provide means for building more cooperative systems (*open systems).* The most prominent of these middleware technologies is *CORBA* (Common Object Request Broker Architecture) [2, 10], a standardized framework for distributed object computing. The specification of a CORBA Object is separated from its implementation. A client can refer to any object without any knowledge about the objects location or implementation. This feature eases replacement of object implementations and helps to avoid future legacy applications. The functionality provided by existing legacy applications can be used within a CORBA environment, if the legacy system is embedded in an object oriented front-end (*wrapper* or *adapter*) [2]. Yet, as long as legacy component systems are characterized by design and execution autonomy, the essential tradeoffs and resulting consistency problems will necessarily occur.

Building an integrated HIS using independently developed object components would require semantically standardized objects. CORBAmed is a current standardization effort in which health care semantics are brought to a CORBA-based distributed object environment. Unfortunately, most healthcare system vendors have not adopted this distributed object technology yet and the standardization process is far from what would be needed.

5. Conclusion and strategies

We have pointed out that integrating heterogeneous system components within a HIS is an extremely challenging task. There are numerous concepts and well established standards like HL7 or DICOM that help to manage or even hide aspects of heterogeneity to the user. We conclude, however, that today there is no concept that turns a number of originally unrelated systems into an integrated system. The remaining question is, which strategy should a hospital use to build up a HIS that comes close to the ideal of a truly integrated system. Such strategic approaches can be characterized by two extremes, which we would like to call best of breed vs. homogeneity

Best of breed approach: As a consequence of the resulting heterogeneity, interconnection standards have to be introduced as a minimum means for communication and information processing across the system borders. This approach seems to offer flexibility and functionality advantages. There are, however, several severe disadvantages. Costly interfaces have to be supported, while surprisingly often the connectivity offered by specialized (niche) vendors is low, and to a considerable degree even widely accepted standards like HL7 or DICOM are only rudimentarily supported.

In a distributed HIS with autonomous components, inconsistencies on various levels cannot be avoided. The same or similar functionality is often bought in different systems, and considerable efforts are necessary to build at least roughly consistent databases. Minimum need is a central administrative patient database. A communication server is useful to manage the interfaces. Altogether, costs for the resulting low level of integration are high. In addition, error handling among different vendors is extremely complicated and costly.

To some degree, strategic considerations of this kind are unavoidable, especially when the necessary functionality is only offered by some specific specialist vendor, or when a system comes connected to a medical device. As a primary strategy, however, it shows critical weaknesses.

Homogeneity approach: A modular system is built on top of a central database. The typical start would be to buy a system with full functionality or at least a patient database system from some generalist vendor. The potential for connecting future applications directly to this database should be extremely carefully considered; technical criteria like inspection of concepts, tools, and modularity, as well as application criteria like check of functionality, flexibility, and genericity have to be applied. Then, many evident advantages will result: We have the chance to achieve the highest level of integration at even lower costs. Widely different, demanding and innovative technologies are needed in order to make such a holistic approach flexible enough: generic modular implementation (generic functions), adaptive user interfaces and openess (CORBA / OLE etc.) are key requirements.

This need for new technologies may be considered as one disadvantage, the other one is certainly the lack of existing products covering the necessary range of functionality. Our market analysis showed that vendors increasingly try to follow this integration approach, although not always modern and available technologies are utilized yet. For various reasons (as described above) still some heterogeneous subsystems might remain which have to be interfaced to the central database. However, as soon as a subsystem is to be replaced the strategy is not to buy the best available stand alone system but rather to prefer a module that directly operates on the central database.

References

[1] H. L. Bleich and W. V. Slack, Designing a hospital information system: a comparison of interfaced and integrated systems *MD Comput.* vol. 9, pp. 293-296, 1992.

[2] A. Bouguettaya, et.al. *Interconnecting Heterogeneous Information Systems*, Boston: Kluwer, 1998.

[3] M. W. Bright, A. R. Hurson, S. H. Pakzad, A Taxonomy and Current Issues in Multidatabase Systems *IEEE Computer*, vol. 25, pp. 50-60, 1992.

[4] S. Chaudhuri, U. Dayal, An Overview of Data Warehousing and OLAP Technology *SIGMOD Record*, vol. 26, pp. 65-74, 1997.

[5] P. D. Clayton, R. V. Sideli, and S. Sengupta, Open architecture and integrated information at Columbia-Presbyterian Medical Center *MD Comput.* vol. 9, pp. 297-303, 1992.
[6] C. J. Date. *An Introduction to Database Systems*, Reading: Addison-Wesley Publishing Company, 1995.
[7] F. A. Leguit. Interfacing Integration. In: *Hospital Information Systems: Scope-Design-Architecture*, eds. A. R. Bakker, C. T. Ehlers, J. R. Bryant, and W. E. Hammond. Amsterdam: North-Holland, 1992. pp. 141-148.
[8] P. R. Norris, B. M. Dawant, and A. Geissbuhler, Web-based data integration and annotation in the intensive care unit *Proc. AMIA. Annu. Fall. Symp.* vol. :794-8, pp. 794-798, 1997.
[9] M. J. Ohly. Information Management in Patient Care. In: *Open Systems in Medicine*, ed. E. Fleck. Amsterdam: IOS Press, 1995. pp. 55-62.
[10] R. Orfali, D. Harkey, and J. Edwards. *Instant CORBA*, John Wiley & Sons, Inc. 1997.
[11] A. Sheth and J. Larson, Federated Database Systems for Managing Distributed, Heterogeneous, and Autonomous Databases *ACM Computing Surveys*, vol. 22, pp. 183-235, 1990.

Medical Informatics Europe '99
P. Kokol et al. (Eds.)
IOS Press, 1999

A Simulation of Dynamic Tasks Routing to Improve Cooperation in Intensive Care Units

J-M. Renard*, N. Bricon-Souf*, J-M. Geib**, R. Beuscart*
**CERIM, Faculté de médecine - Université de Lille 2 - 59045 Lille - FRANCE*
***LIFL, Université de Lille 1, 59655 Villeneuve d'ascq - France*
E-mail : renard@univ-lille2.fr

Abstract. Cooperation between Health Care Professionals is essential for the quality of care. Workflow systems could improve the transfer of informations and responsibilities within Health Care Actors. We have proposed a conversation-based Workflow in order to modelize the therapeutics plan in the ICU. In such a complex field, the flexibility of the workflow system is essential for the system to be usable. We have introduced some dynamicity by adding roles in the model. With the use of roles, the dynamicity of the workflow is assumed by the routing process. We need to use simulation to be able to study the impact of routing algorythms on the efficiency of the coordination.

1. Introduction

The evolution of medical activities improve the need of cooperation between specialists. But the need of cooperation concerns the whole medical team. In intensive care units, breakdowns could occur in the communication between all the actors involved in the care delivery. These breakdowns are the result of a lack of transmission of the information or the result of breaks in the coordination between the care-providers[1]. The CSCW (Computer Supported Cooperative Work) searches to solve such problems with the use of computer based tools[7]. In intensive care units, we need tools that will be able to assume the support of the coordination and the access to the right information. The paradigm of cooperation in ICU is to coordinate the access to the information in a way that enables the right actor to use the right information at the right time and the right place[7].The goal of the project Placo is to improve the coordination between the actors in Intensive care units. After the analysis of breakdowns we have proposed an asynchronous model based on conversation-oriented workflow. The need of flexibility is a very important feature of this model and we used a dynamic approach to link the task to the actors. But the choice of a routing algorythm to link the tasks with the actors is not obvious. As testing the effects of coordination tools like placo in real medical units could not be safe for patients, we built a simulator to study the impact of different routing algorythms on the coordination.

2. Conceptual framework

The health care is a field where close collaboration between all the members of the medical team is a rule. But collaboration is not obvious : The analysis of the breakdowns observed in ICU was performed by a team of psychologists during the first part of the project[1]. They come either from synchronisation failures between people or from the absence of useful informations (excess, lack or distorsion of informations). Groupware should be efficient to solve such problems. The Team of the Intensive Care Unit is composed of physicians and nurses. But at one moment the basic element of coordination is the transfer of informations and the transfer of responsibilities between two actors. Let's take the example of a physician diagnosing an arterial pressure excess. He decides to start an infusion with calcic inhibitors and makes the prescription. This prescription is adressed to a nurse. The nurse adjusts the time delivery of the infusion. The same nurse or another one starts the infusion. A few hours later the physician evaluates the effect of the drog and changes the prescription if needed. Each drug administration in the ICU can be split in scenarii like this one. We used the workflow analysis based on the language/action perspective developed by Winograd and Flores to build our model[5]. The structure of our workflow cycle is made up of four steps or phases and four transitions[2]. It is initialised by a prescription. Prescriptions are usually made by physicians, but sometimes nurses do acts that could be assimilated to prescriptions. In our model a prescription is a request to start a therapeutic action. This is the first phase. In the second phase, the request (for example: starting an infusion) is confronted to practical constraints. In our example some constraints could be : is there an infusion pump available in the unit? or is there a veinous access on the patient? or is there another infusion which could be incompatible with the request? In the third phase the request is carried out. This is the operational phase. The fourth phase is the assessment. The result of the actions are analysed and they are compared with the expected ones. The transitions (four) represent the agrement between the actors involved in the coordination. This is a control component.

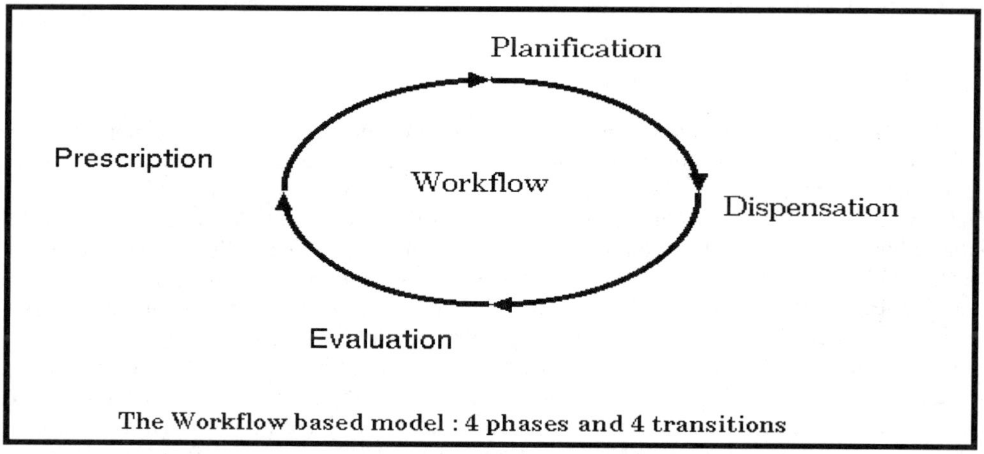

figure 1.

In the ICU, the coordination software cannot control all the human activities. One reason is that sometimes emergencies occur. Another one is that the time needed for an actor to execute his tasks is not forseeable with a strong presision. Even if the Placo system proposes a task to an actor, this actor can chose another one. The human choices depends on the knoweldge of the activity process and the information domain. In such a context, it is very difficult to anticipate about the real disponibility of the actors, and affecting a task in advance to an actor will be inefficient especially when crisis occur. The solution we have implemented is to introduce some roles[6]. The coordination module does not allocate in advance a task to an actor but allocates the task to a role. Primary roles are for prescription, planification, dispensation, evaluation but each role can be specialized.Thanks to roles, the visibility of the data is reduced to the competent and authorized persons. And human control over the workflow is still allowed. The workflow improves the coordination between actors without preventing them from making decisions. With this model the dynamicity and the flexibility resides in the routing process. Our current focus is to determine how the tasks must be routed to the actors. We need to simulate the intensive care unit to study the impact of algorythms on the coordination of the actors.

3. The role of routing in Placo efficiency

The goal of the workflow kernel is to control the execution of the tasks. This control focuses on sychronisation and time constraints. Time constraints depend on the nature of the tasks and the state of the patient. The time properties of the task are variable. Some needs a very strict respect of the planification with tolerances under the minute (ie adrenaline infusion). Others are very low binded with the planification and accept gaps in hours or days (ie some nutrition elements). Another factor involved in time constraints is the state of the patient: unstable or stable. This one in not easy to predict. If the patient is unstable, tasks cannot be planified a long time before they occur. Morever changes will appear and will need modifications of the planification or will need modification of the actor who will do the task. The workflow have to control the level of the emergency of the tasks. If a task is not done at the right time, the workflow kernel increases her priority. This introduces the synchronisation action of the workflow. Synchonisation applies at two levels : the first one is at the patient one and the second one is at the unit one. At this two levels the most urgent tasks must be done before the less ones, and the ordered tasks must be done in order.All modifications of the priority of a task could change the affectation and the order of all the tasks. The same reorganisation is attended when tasks are canceled or added.

With the use of roles, the dynamicity of the workflow is assumed by the routing process. The main difficulty in Placo is to provide a system which involves the coordination without reducing the human control over the tasks. A specificity of the ICU is that the system has to be used either in normal activity when health care actors only have to know about the task they have to perform, or in unusual situations where actors have to make urgent decisions and need to access to all the informations about the authorized system. The system does not prevent actors from making decisions. It does not have any medical knoweldge. So it will be able to let actors make decisions which are inducted by external (human) knoweldge. This means, for each actor, that he can either follow the system propositions and do the next proposed tasks or chose another task on another patient on the base of human knoweldge.

The dynamic routing acts as follow: Placo proposes a list of tasks to each actor. These tasks are ordered by priority or by actors. When the level of the activity is low, each actor does his tasks one after the other. When the level of the activity is high, placo links tasks to roles and the routing algorythm allocates the role to the available actors in real time . When a task is not done at the planified time the routing kernel is able to link the tasks to other actors.

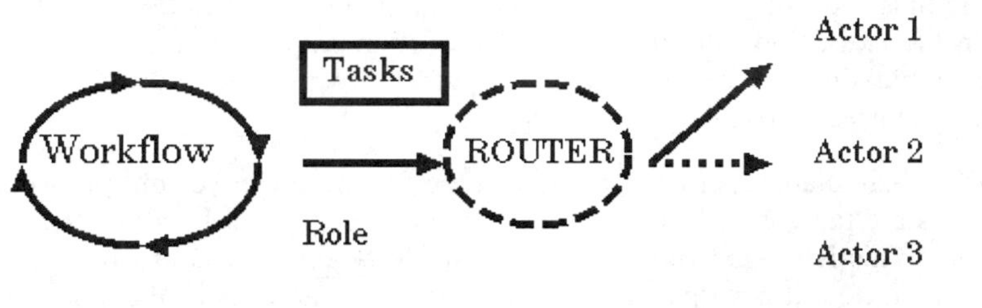

The router links tasks to actors according to their availability and their role

figure 2.

A challenge for the routing mecanism is to sufficiently inform the actors for the tasks to be done whithout overloading them. For this reason, we have to choose very carefully the way the routing process will run. To solve the paradox of informing without overloading, we must focus on the strategies of the routing process. The goal of the routing system is to link the tasks to the actors in the most efficient way. Solutions to dynamically link actors and tasks are numerous. Testing this solutions in actual ICU could be not safe for patients cares. So we decided to use simulation to test routing algorythms.

4. PlacoSim : the simulation to improve coordination

We built a simulator which is written in Java. The simulation describes the tasks flow in the ICU. Each cycle of simulation performs the actions observed in a unit of time. The architecture of the simulator is modular so that it will be easy to plug in the strategies we will test. We use the strategy design pattern to implement the algorythms[4]. We define four families of strategy classes : extraction, presentation, action and aging. Each family encapsulates the algorythms and makes them interchangeable. With this design the algorythms varies independently from the part of the simulator that uses it. In order to test a strategy, we specialize a classe with the algorythm we will test and we plug this strategy in the simulator.

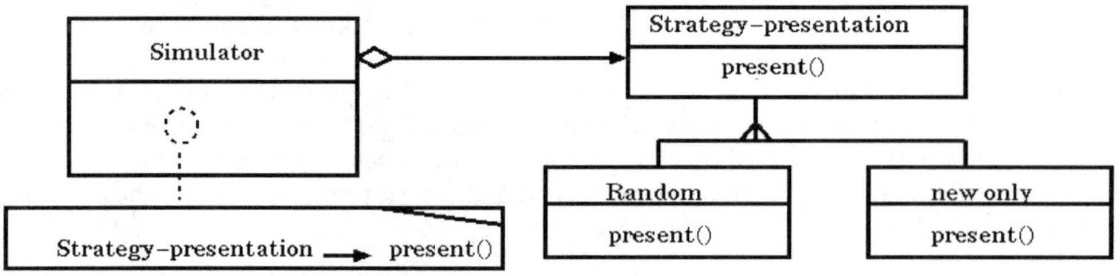

The modular architecture of the simulator use the "strategy design pattern"
The specialisation of the main class allow us to plug in new strategies in the simulator

figure 3.

The output of the simulator consists in statistical data. It displays the initial state of the simulator: how many patients, how many actors, which roles the actors have, what are the initials tasks and the initials workflow cycles on patients. In running mode, the outputs are some informations on the extraction, the presentation, the action and the aging. At the end of the simulation the output displays a summary of the actions performed : distribution of tasks, Statistics on the time needed to execute the tasks.

One cycle of simulation performs a unit of time. In one cycle we split the work in three phases. this phases are the core of the routing principle. The first phase is to determine which task will be routed.This is the extraction phase (of active tasks). If it is obvious that the tasks done will not be extracted, it isn't that obvious to chose the parameters of the other tasks which will be routed. The second phase is to determine which actors will be linked to the previous tasks according to their roles.This is the presentation phase (of extracted tasks). The main issue in this phase is, among other things, the question of the presentation of the tasks in a very emergency level. The third one is to determine which task(s) the actors will carry out. This is the action phase. Between two cycles the tasks are processed with an aging strategy. The aging strategy implements the workflow model and assumes that the tasks follow the workflow cycle. The aging strategy performs the increasement of the priority of the tasks not done. This function depends on the type of task.

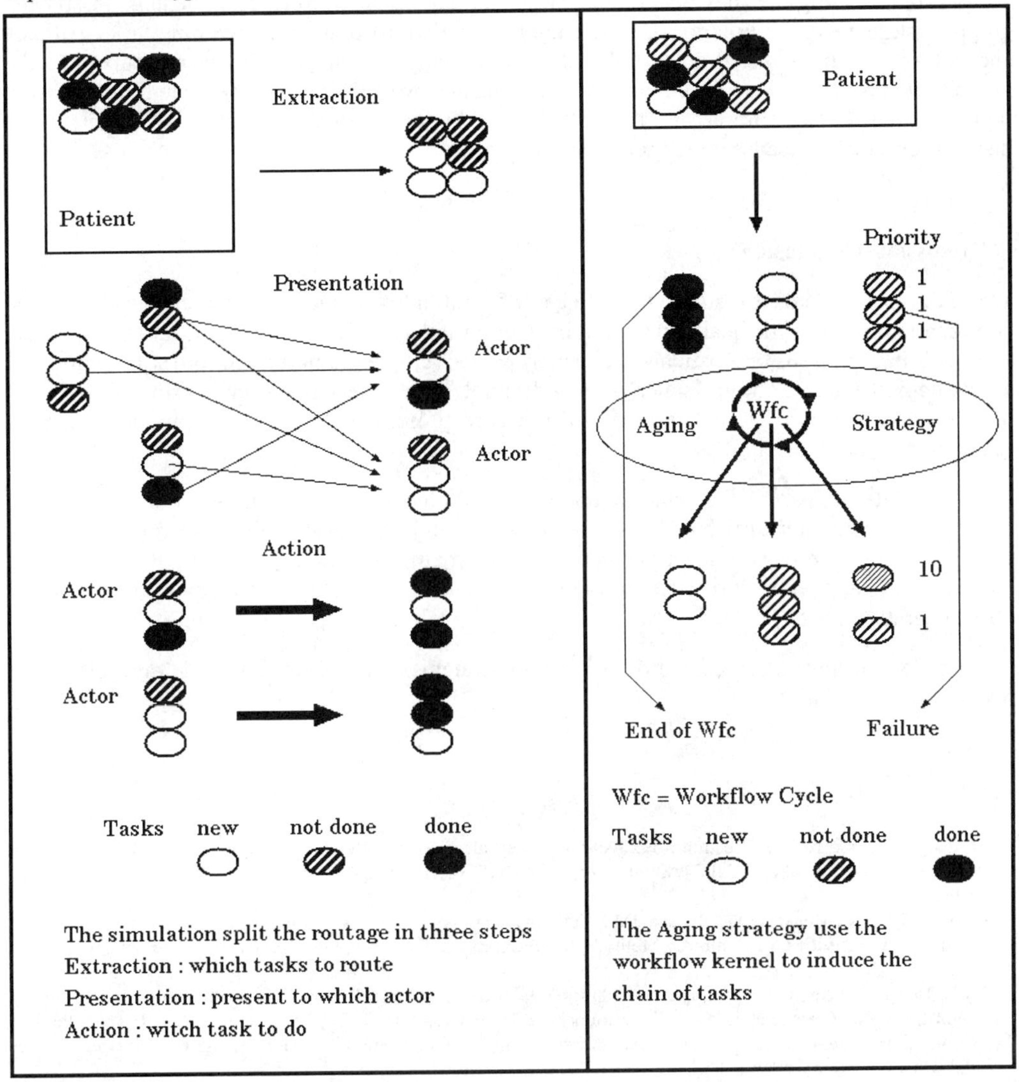

figure 4.

We will analyze strategies to determine which ones are the more efficient. Here are examples of basic strategies we will analyze:

- For the extraction phase : The first strategy is to extract all the tasks to be done. The second one is to extract only the new ones.
- For the presentation phase : The first strategy is to randomize the link to the actor. The second one is to link the task to the first free actor.

- For the action phase : The first strategy is to randomize the task chosen by the actor. The second one is to chose the most urgent one.

Before analysing the statistical output of the simulation we need to describe and classify the group of strategies. The criteria for efficiency is statistical parameters concerning tasks, patients and actors. We trust the ability of the chosen strategies to support the increasement of the number of tasks to be done. The main criteria is the ability of the tasks to be done in the allowed time interval. Other criteria are the distribution on actors and patients. We calculate the distribution of tasks according to their level of delay.

5. Discussion-Conclusion

We built a simulator to study the effects of routing strategies on the efficiency of the coordination because medical constraints in ICU do not allow us to compare the effects of the strategies in a rigorous and patient-safe maner. Moreover using a prototype to test the effects of the strategies will add the influence of non desirable parameters like user interface design and user friendly usage of computer (some health care professionals are very computer friendly, other are not at all).

It will be very interesting to compare our algorythms with those used for process allocation in computer distributed systems. This is mainly the case of the dynammic allocation algorythms. In the process allocation algorythms the main parameters are usually those mesuring the charge of each processor[3]. In our model we focus on the tasks more than on the ditribution of the charge.

We will now focus on the design of our strategies and on the statistical analysis of the result of our simulations.

References

[1] Beuscart R., Carre V., Westrelin F., Dalmas S. et al. "Interim Report on Co-operative Work in CCE (Methodology)". AIM - TANIT (A2036) Project, COOP Workpackage. Deliverable #D2, Public Report, July 1992.

[2] Bricon-Souf N., Beuscart R., Renard JM., Geib JM., An asynchronous co-operative model for co-ordinating medical unit activities. In Computer Methods and Programs in Biomedicine. Elsevier Science Publishers, pp77-83, 1997.

[3] Jean-Luc Dekeyser, Cyril Fonlupt, and Philippe Marquet. Analysis of synchronous dynamic load balancing algorithms. In E. H. D'Hollander, F. J. Joubert, F. J. Peters, and D. Trystram, editors, PARCO'95 Parallel Computing: State-of-the Art Perspective, Advances in Parallel Computing, Gent, Belgium, Elsevier Science Publishers, September 1995.

[4] Erich Gamma, Richard Helm, Ralph Johnson, John Vlissides, Design Patterns: Elements of Reusable Object-oriented Software, Addison-Wesley Publishing 1995.

[5] Medina-mora R. , Winograd T.,. Flores R., Flores F. The Action Workflow Approach to workflow management technology. In proceedings CSCW '92 : shering perspective, J Turner & R. Kraut, Eds., association for computing machinery, pp.281-288, 1992.

[6] Nathalie Bricon-Souf, Jean-Marie Renard, Régis Beuscart, Dynamic Workflow model for complex activity in Intensive Care Unit.in proceedings of Medinfo'98. August 18-22, 1998 SEOUL

[7] Schmidt K., Cooperative Work : A Conceptual Framework. In Distributed Decision Making : Cognitive Models for Cooperative Work. Rasmussen Leplat eds, pp. 76-110, 1991.

Medical Informatics Europe '99
P. Kokol et al. (Eds.)
IOS Press, 1999

A prototype of an information system for assessing the health status of prison inmates

A. Duhamel[1], E. Archer[2], P. Devos[1], M.C. Nuttens[1], R. Beuscart[1]
[1] *Department of Medical Informatics, CHRU LILLE (France)*
[2] *Prison psychiatric unit of Loos-Lez-Lille (France)*

Abstract. A research-action program was established in 1996 between the Loos-Lez-Lille prison psychiatric unit and the Department of Medical Informatics of the University Hospital of Lille (France) : - (1) to investigate the health status and the general characteristics of the prison population - (2) to develop an Information System for improving the prison health care and to facilitate social rehabilitation of convicts. Starting off 1988, all new prisoners are interviewed on their arrival using a standard questionnaire. The transfer of all the information recorded in this questionnaire into a computer base was initiated in 1996, when the research action program began. A statistical analysis was performed on 15200 records (1989-1995) to identify the most informative parameters : 50% of inmates were less than 24 years old; 57% were unemployed; 60% had no professional qualification. 31% of inmates had a psychiatric history and 16% had made a previous suicide attempt. The rate of drug abuse has increased from 24% in 89 to 53% in 95. To analyze the time trends of these parameters, a prototype of Information System was then developed. The system uses the database to product standard reports in real time.

1. Problem

Prison inmates are exposed to major risk factors : suicide attempts, illicit drug use, excessive drinking, psychiatric disorders ... The rise in juvenile delinquency, the modification of the nature of crimes committed as well as the expansion of the prison population all make it increasingly important to produce epidemiological data in this field. In spite of this need however, very few studies concerning the French inmate population have so far been published. Excepted the demographic data provided by the Department of Justice, existing studies were either restricted to small samples or to particular problems such as sexually transmitted diseases. The other published results concern essentially the North American or British prison population and they have focused on the prevalence of mental illness or substance misuse.

In North American studies, between 50% to 80% of prisoners (on remand or sentenced) were diagnosed as having a history of lifetime abuse or of dependence on alcohol and between 30% to 60% abused or were dependent of illicit drugs. Prevalence of mental illness was estimated between 5% to 42% [1]. In a recent study among the inmates in England, 71% of males were considered to require medical help directly for their drug or alcohol abuse and the rate of psychiatric disorders was estimated at 26% [2]. These results show that there is a great variability in the rates of findings reported according the studies and the countries. However it's quite obvious that these disorders far exceed those found in the general population.

2. Objectives

A research-action program was established in 1996 between the prison psychiatric unit of Loos-Lez-Lille and the Department of Medical Informatics of the University Hospital of Lille (France). The Loos-Lez-Lille jail is a French prison for remand and short sentenced prisoners. It houses 1200 inmates and has an average number of 2200 arrivals a year.

The aims of this project were :

(1) to assess the health status and the general characteristics of the prison population
(2) to analyse the time trends of these characteristics
(3) to build an information system intended to contribute to the improvement of prison health care and to facilitate the prevention of the jail recidivism.

3. Method

Starting from the 1st January 1988, all new prisoners are interviewed at their arrival into the prison by the psychiatric doctor or one of two trained clinical psychologists. A pilot study was initially undertaken from January to June 1988 to build a standard questionnaire. The questionnaire gathered information regarding demographic data, education and socio-economic level, arrest charge, social and family history, lifestyle, medical and psychiatric history, suicidal ideation, and drug, alcohol or smoking abuse. During the pilot study, interrater reliability was monitored. This was achieved by a procedure whereby one of the three aforementioned persons (doctor, psychologists) conducted an interview with the new prisoner while the others listened. The three of them subsequently recorded the questionnaire independently. A total of 130 prisoners were interviewed in this manner. For the questions relating to psychiatric disorders, substance abuse as well as for their appreciation of the prisoner's behavior during the interview, the agreement between raters was measured by means of Kappa coefficients. Questions with mean inter-rater reliability less than 90% were either modified or discarded.

Since the 1st July 1988, the "interviewers" (psychiatric doctor or psychologist) have used the questionnaire which requires 30 minutes to administer. Prisoners are informed that the interview is confidential, that any information disclosed will not be passed on to prison staff and that the collected data are included in their medical record.

The prototype was developed between 1996 and 1997. All the questionnaires collected from 1 January 1989 through 30 June 1996 were first anonymously recorded. Data acquisition was performed within the prison by an informatic service company. Statistical analysis was then performed using the SAS software. This analysis allowed to determine the characteristics of the prison population and to identify the most informative variables. The third step involved the transfer of data into a database developed with the ACCESS/WINDOWS DBMS. This database was designed using the questionnaire and the results of the statistical analysis.

Finally, a system for the production of standard reports was designed using EXCEL/WINDOWS and connected to the database. This system gives the possibility of having an comprehensive summary of the jail population (curves, charts ...) in real time and allows for the analysis of the time trends of various variables (Figures 1a, 1b). From the 1st July 1997, the questionnaires of new prisoners are recorded after interview using the database interface (questionnaires from 1 July 96 through 30 June 97 are yet to be recorded).

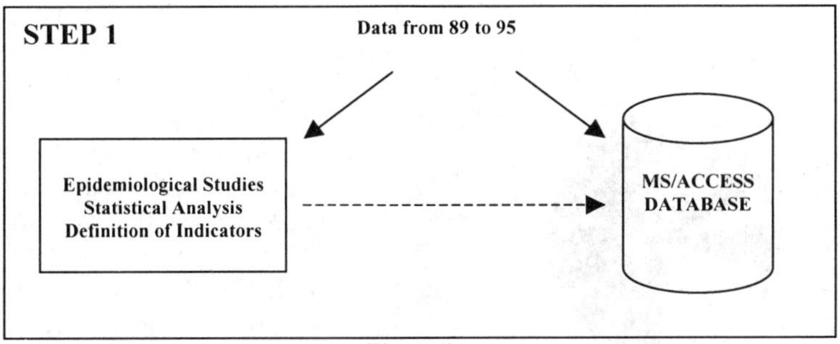

Figure 1a

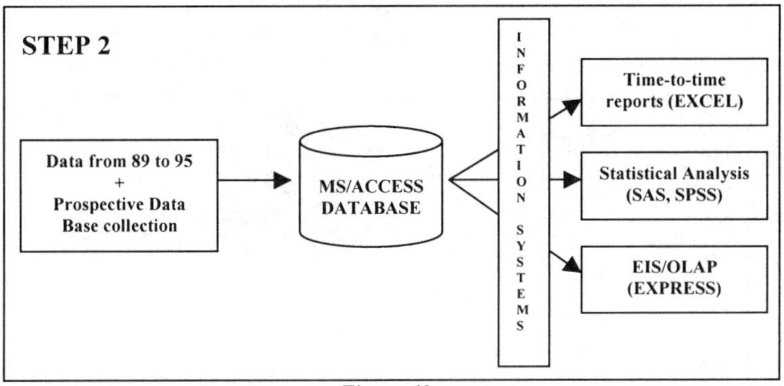

Figure 1b

4. Results

We present the preliminary results of data collected from 1989 to 1995 (15200 records, figures 2a,2b,2c).

Demographic data and arrest charges : The prisoners are young people : 17% were less than 19 years old and 85% were below 35. (mean /median age = 27 /24). More than 97% were male. A lot of them were unmarried (61%). Unemployment rate was extremely high (56.7%). This rate was 65% for the inmates between 25-50 years old in 1995.

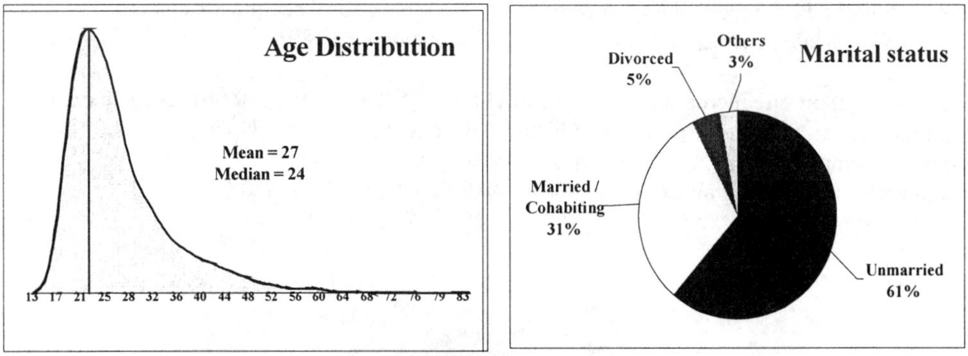

Figure 2a

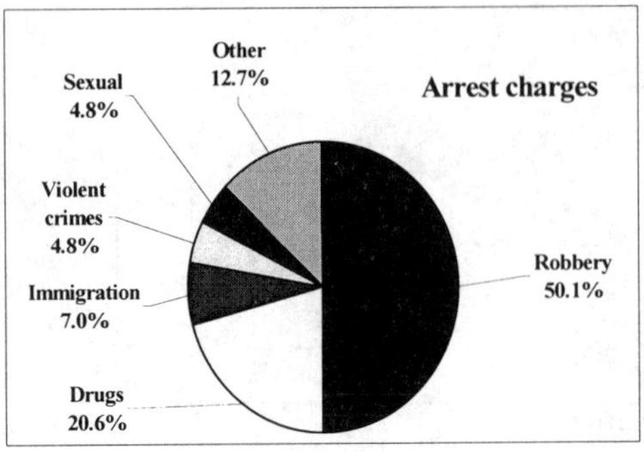

Figure 2b

The rate of robberies was higher than the national figure (50% versus 40%) while the rate of sexual offences was lower (5% versus 13%). The rates of others offences were sufficiently close to the national rates. For all the offences studied, the evolution between 1989 to 1995 as identical to that identified by the Department of Justice : increase in drug related and sexual offences and decrease in robberies.

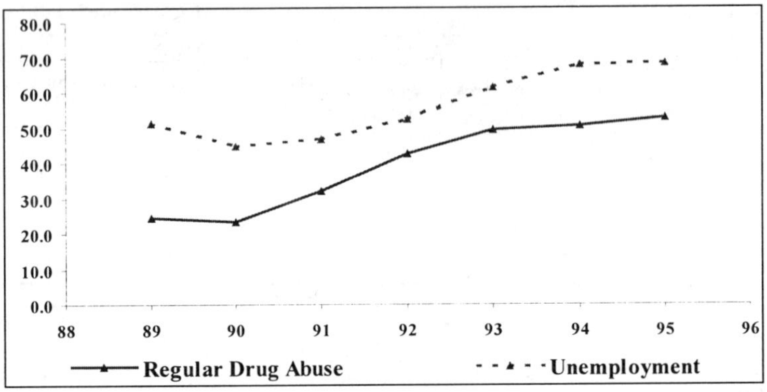

Figure 2c

Education level : 60% of inmates had no professional qualification. 51% had left the education system before 16 years old.

Substance abuse : The rate of substance abuse disorders was extremely high. 21% had a regular alcohol consumption and 40% were regular drug abusers. Amongst them, 77% used heroin.

Medical data : 31% had a psychiatric history. 8% had previous suicidal ideation and 16% a previous suicide attempt. Among the prisoners with psychiatric disorders and/or drug abuse, 69% had not received any form of care from the existing health care system.

Evolutionary Data : the analysis of evolutions between 89 to 95 showed (Figure 2c):

- unemployment rate increased from 45% in 1989 to 68% in 1995 (p<0.001, chi-square test)
- an increase in the rate of psychiatric history (from 27% in 89 to 37% in 95, p<0,001) and suicide attempt (from 15% in 89 to 18% in 95, p<0,001)
- a meteoric rise in drug abuse from 24% in 1989 to 53% in 1995 (p<0,001).

5. Discussion and conclusion

A typical inmate is a young man, with no job and a poor level of education, arrested for robbery or drug misuse. He has often a psychiatric history and/or substance use disorders, is likely to have a multidrug habit and needs multidisciplinary assistance. Some of these findings are not surprising but they had never been quantified before in France. The rate of psychiatric disorders found in our study (31%) is close that observed by Mason [2] in England (26%) and in the range of those reported by Powell [1] in USA. The rate of drug abuse (40%) is in the range of those reported in the USA (30% - 60%) [1]. Our study shows a pronounced increase of this rate from 89 to 95. Most prisoners are released after a short period and without any adequate detoxification program the problem of drug use in prisons will inevitably spill over into the community.

The results of this study demonstrate the relevance of an information system for improving the monitoring of the jail population. It provides information in real time thus enabling the concerned prison personnel to adapt jail management, to improve the health care of prisoners as well as that of released inmates. It can be used to define an efficient policy for the reduction of the recidivism of prison sentences.

References

[1] T.A. Powell, J.C. Holt, K.M. Fondacaro, *The prevalence of mental illness among inmates in rural state*, ***Law and Human Behavior***, Vol. 21, N°4, 427-438, 1997.

[2] D. Mason, L. Birmingham, D. Grubin, *Substance use in remand prisoners : a consecutive case study*, ***BMJ***, Vol. 315, 18-21, 1997.

This work was supported by the Region and the justice department of Nord Pas de Calais.

Medical Informatics Europe '99
P. Kokol et al. (Eds.)
IOS Press, 1999

ArchAIDS connects a clinical department and a virological laboratory to automatize the follow up of AIDS patients

M. Giacomini[1,2,3], C. Ruggiero[1,2], I. Martini[3], J.L. McDermott[3], O.E. Varnier[3,4]
[1]*DIST - Dept. of Communication Computer and System Sciences, University of Genova, Via Opera Pia 13, 16145 Genova – Italy. E-mail: giacomin@dist.unige.it*
[2]*DIST laboratory, Advanced Biotechnology Centre, Genova - Italy*
[3]*Molecular Virology Unit, Advanced Biotechnology Center, Genova - Italy*
[4]*Dept. of Clinical and Experimental Oncology, School of Medicine, Univ. of Genova - Italy*

Abstract. A communication system for the automation of the follow up of AIDS patients set up by DIST at the Molecular Virology Unit in the Advanced Biotechnology Centre of Genova and at the Department of Internal Medicine of the Medical School of Genova is presented. This system includes a distributed database to store both clinical and virological data and a set of procedures to transfer patient data with a complete respect of requirements about completeness and privacy.

1. Introduction

The laboratory management of infections caused by human retroviruses (which produce very important diseases like the AIDS, TSP and ATL) can be divided into two phases: diagnosis and follow-up.

The diagnosis can be further divided into two procedures: a preliminary one based on an enzymatic immuno assay (EIA) to detect the presence of antibodies against retroviral antigens [1] and a confirmatory one based on Western blot [2]. When a person is identified as sero-positive, a follow-up phase begins, during which the specific antigens [3] and nucleic acids [4] levels are measured to monitor disease progression. Some of these tests use the EIA method for analyte detection and at the Advanced Biotechnology Centre a program was set up to automatically quantify analyte amount with a wide dynamic range [5]. The quality of these kits has been continuously improved with close to 100% sensitivity (absence of false negative) and specificity (absence of false positive). Nevertheless the processing itinerary of retroviral diagnosis and follow-up is not error free, specially in crowded working conditions or where technical personnel has limited experience. The use of computer science offers several advantages, although it requires specific training. Sample information and test results can be easily stored, work lists and test summaries can be printed and data can be rapidly analysed. Moreover, automatic quality controls on performed tests can assure the correctness, completeness and safety of the whole information set.

A communication system is presented for the automation of the follow up of AIDS patients set up by DIST at the Molecular Virology Unit in the Advanced Biotechnology Centre of Genova (ABC) and at Department of Internal Medicine (DIMI) of the Medical School of Genova. This system (ArchAIDS) includes a distributed database to store both clinical and virological data and a set of procedures to transfer patient data with a complete respect of requirements about completeness and privacy.

2. Materials and Methods

In both centres patient and sample data were stored in hierarchical databases with known data duplication and possible input error problems. Moreover, the organisation of the two data bases was significatively different. Starting from these previous systems and from user and communication requirements, a new communication system has been developed which contains a relational distributed database (whose structure has been developed in order to make the information management more reliable), and a set of procedures to transfer patient data with a complete respect of requirements about completeness and privacy. Moreover, the new database has the possibility to interface with other software for laboratory automation to acquire test results without human intervention.
The data structure has been designed with the mixed approach, but the presentation follows the top-down approach. Figure 1 presents the overall structure of the data base and the physical location of the tables.

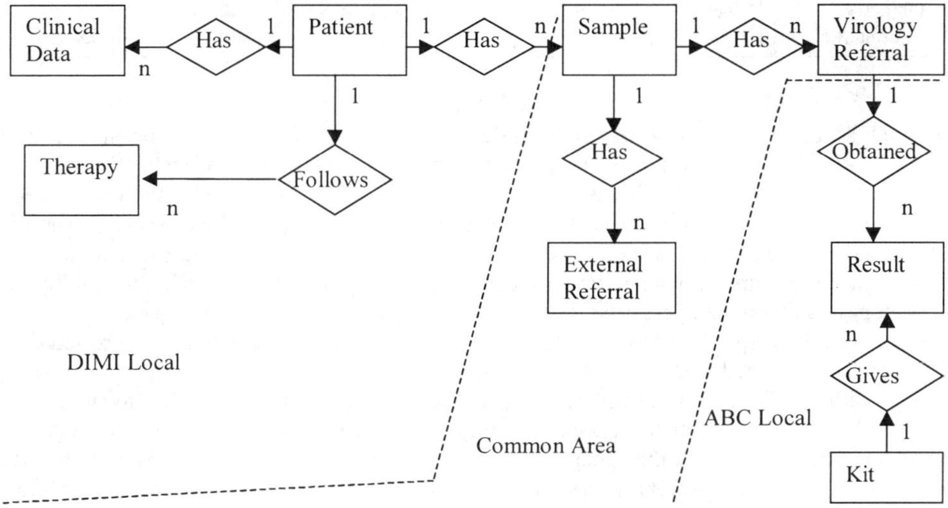

Fig. 1 Entity Relation – Level 0

A deeper insight of the data structure from the point of view of clinical data is presented in figure 2.
At this level of detail more specific information is shown. In the DIMI part tables to record clinical information (CDC category to assess the stage of disease progression, opportunistic infection, number of CD4+) and therapeutical information (therapy protocol, drug, dosage, starting date, previous therapies) are present, directly linked to the patient. Sample information is stored in the common area, as samples are the material treated in both centres. Referrals are divided into virology referrals produced in the virology laboratory, and external referrals, produced in the general laboratory (these data are inserted in the system by a manual procedure).
Result and Kit are then main entities of the ABC part of the database. Many results contribute to produce a complete virology referral for a sample, this referral is produced by an automatic procedure, but it has to be formally approved by the head of the virology unit to be stored in the common area. Kit entity has been divided into two more specific entities to retain the difference in the detection method (EIA – Western Blot). This difference, from a computer science point of view, involves a different amount of information that must be stored for each result: EIA results consist mainly in a number (the O.D. measured for that

sample), western blot results are a series of numbers (the colour level reached for the reaction to each antigen on the strip). Obviously their interpretation is also quite different.

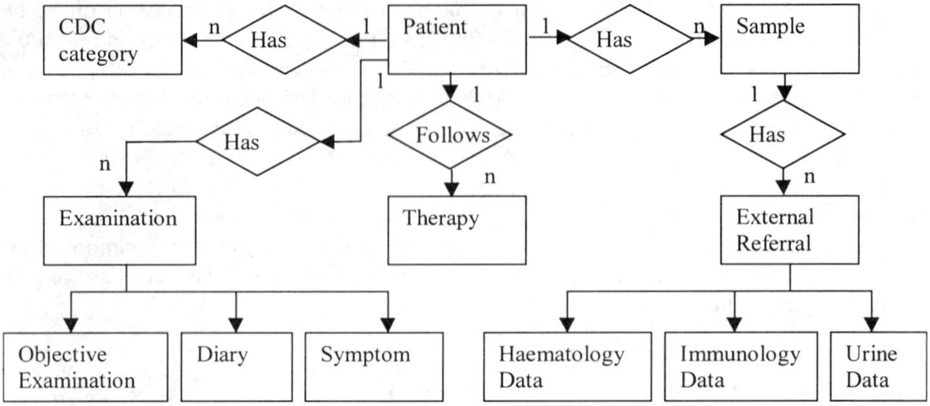

Fig. 2 Entity Relation - Level 1 DIMI part

For each kit all storage problems are considered and for EIA kits, it is also possible to use the same kit with different protocols in order to obtain different kind of tests (for example qualitative or quantitative). The assay tables contain quality control information for each assay performed within the laboratory. The results table are linked both with the sample table and with the assay tables to enable both a patient driven result evaluation (to individual follow-up) and an assay driven result evaluation (to a check the quality of laboratory and technician performance for the specific test).

The database is integrated with a series of automatic procedures to perform controlled data insertion and assisted data consultation. These procedures are shown in the following figures with the Data Flow Diagram method. Figure 3 shows the procedure to produce a new work list. First of all the checks if samples are present with examination requests. Afterwards he/she chooses the specific test to be performed on these samples and chooses the particular lot in the warehouse (mainly according to date criterion). This choice allows the technician to know how many single examinations are possible, with the resources present in the laboratory. This number influences the criteria for sample selection to be applied in the sample choice procedure. In normal situations the oldest samples are chosen, but particular research circumstances can suggest other selection criteria which can be applied via a simple selection mask, based both on patient data (clinical and therapeutical situation) and on sample data (previous results with other tests).

A login procedure (with multiple password system) assigns each user an authorisation level which can limit the access to specific data. For example, students who come to the laboratory can only access the database to insert results of tests they performed or to consult summary forms, not to see patient personal data.

3. Results and conclusion

The presented database has been tested in the virology laboratory of the Molecular Virology Unit of the Advanced Biotechnology Center in Genova and is being validated at the Department of Internal Medicine of the Medical School of Genova.

The first test was a retrospective one in which all old data, stored in the previously described hierarchical database, were inserted in the new one to control the correctness of the selected relations among tables. These data were: 300 patient data, 1000 sample data, 9 ELISA kits, 2 Western Blot kits, 2310 results from screening (antibodies – antigens) test and molecular biology (nucleic acids) test (with ELISA detection method), 107 results from confirmation test (with Western Blot method).

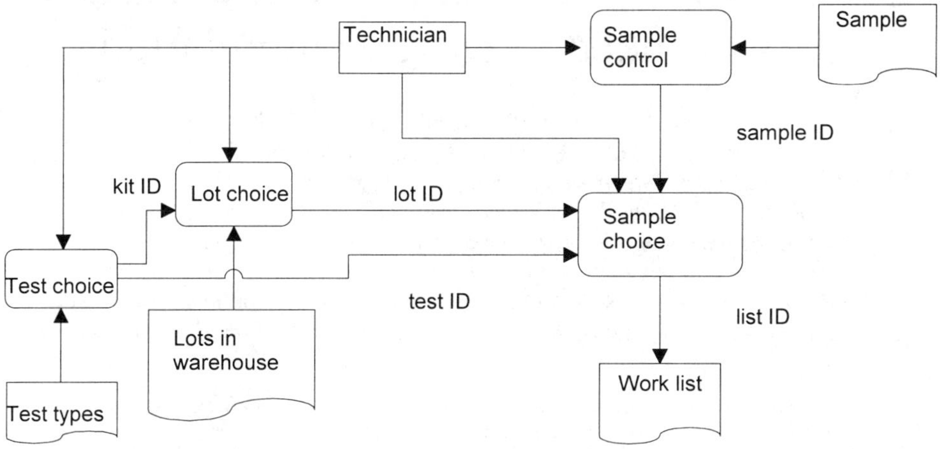

Fig. 3: Work list creation DFD

The second validation phase, which is still in progression, started one year ago, and consists in the routine use of this database in the same laboratory. First impressions both from the medical and the technical personnel are quite good. They mainly appreciate the user-friendly features of the interface and above all the control filters on the patient data which avoid many identification problems which were particularly frequent with the previous database. In this period many new data have been inserted, without any particular problems by the laboratory personnel and only a four hour practical training course by the database designer.

We are now planning the physical installation of data base in the clinical department. We had only local simulation for this part of the system.

Possible future developments are foreseeable in the field of information sharing between the presented system and the general information system of the hospital to automatically obtain anagraphic patient data and general laboratory results.

Acknowledgement

This study was partially supported by a grant of the ''Istituto Superiore di Sanità' National AIDS Program N. 30A/0/71. Mauro Giacomini is supported by a study grant of the 'Istituto Superiore di Sanità' program entitled 'Lotta all'AIDS'.

References

[1] O.E. Varnier, A. Narvanen, M. Korkolainen, F.B. Lillo, S. Kontio, J. Elm, J. Suni, A. Vaheri, M.L. Huhtala: "Synthetic peptides in HIV antibody screening and typing". Ann. of the New York Acadey of Sci., in "Frontiers in Human Reproduction", (M. Seppala and L. Hamberger eds.), 1991, pp. 502-518.

[2] O.E. Varnier, F.B. Lillo, G.C. Schito, A. Lazzarin, ,P.J. Kanki: "Parallel Western blot analysis for HIV-1 and HIV-2 infection in Italian subjects at risk for AIDS". AIDS, 1988, vol. 2, pp. 215-217.

[3] O.E. Varnier, M. Giacomini, F.B. Lillo: "High quantifiable levels of p24 antigenemia are detectable in HIV-1 infected patients". AIDS Res.Hum. Retrov., 1996, vol. 12, pp. 565-566.

[4] J.L: McDermott, A.A. Giri, I. Martini, M. Bono, M. Giacomini, A. Campelli, L. Tagliaferro, A. Cara, O.E. Varnier: "Level of Human Immunodeficiency virus DNA in peripheral blood mononuclear cells correlates with efficacy of antiretroviral therapy". J. of Clin. Microbiology, 1999, vol. 37, n. 7, in press.

[5] M. Giacomini, C. Ruggiero, F.B. Lillo, J.L. McDerrmott, O.E. Varnier: "A software tool to extend the quantitation power of a virological analysis". Med. & Biol. Engineering & Computing, 1996, vol. 34, pp. 71-72.

Medical Informatics Europe '99
P. Kokol et al. (Eds.)
IOS Press, 1999

An Information System on Toxicological Risks Linked to Drug Manipulation

Elaheh POURABBAS*, Nicoletta MUCCI+,
Riccardo MACERATINI^, Maurizio RAFANELLI*
* *Istituto di Analisi dei Sistemi ed Informatica - C.N.R. viale Manzoni 30, 00185 Roma, Italy. E-mail: {pourabbas, rafanelli}@iasi.rm.cnr.it*
\+ *I.S.P.E.S.L.- Dipartimento di Medicina del Lavoro, via di Fontana Candida 1, 00040 Monte Porzio Catone, Italy*
^ *Dipartimento di Scienze Chirurgiche e Tecnologie Mediche, Applicate, Universita' di Roma La Sapienza, viale del Policlinico, 00161 Roma, Italy. E-mail: ricmac@iol.it*

Abstract. Aim of the project is to define and to implement an information system able to help people, who produce chemotherapic antineoplastic drugs, and health care operators, who manipulate such drugs, to prevent short and long term adverse effects connected to the above mentioned activities. The system is able to give a detailed and updated information about these problems, and to give an up-to date, from a professional point of view, to the users of the system. Also an information system prototype was implemented, which consists of an object-oriented database, a decision support system, able to manage and to plan a periodic control of workers, to verify the adverse effects of the antineoplastic chemotherapic drugs, a management system for the network communications.

1. Background

The important progresses during the last few years of the antineoplastic therapies are bringing, as a consequence, a rapid, widespread and progressive increase in the use of chemiotherapics, generally administered for long periods and at high doses. Such drugs, if from a given point of view obtain a high effectiveness in health care, often determine a high toxicity, with immediate and long-term risks for patients, and possibly also for health care operators.

In Italy, the programs for the health care education and for brushing up one's professional knowledge are insufficiently widespread and suitable, so that often chemotherapic drugs are stored, prepared, administered and eliminated by inappropriate procedures.

On the Internet, in the last several years, many drug databases and data banks have been available (e.g. ABDA in Germany, Theriaque in France, Martindale in Grain Britain, First Data Bank in USA, etc.). Other information systems (e.g.RTECS, CCRIS, IRIS) focus on long-term effects of chemical substances, including active ingredients of antineoplastic drugs. These programs, however, need a preliminary subscription and, over all, their consultation is often inadequately oriented in emergency: their multimedial component is minimal and human-computer interface is not "friendly" enough for sanitary personnel (nurses, physicians).

2. Goal of the project

Aim of the project was to define and implement an information system able 1) to help people, who produce chemotherapic drugs and health care operators who use such drugs, to prevent accidents or intoxications using the protocols suggested by the system; 2) to give a detailed and updated information about these problems; 3) give an up-to date, from a professional point of view, to the users of the system.

The implemented system is available (in Italian) through the network for the above mentioned workers.

The problem, which the project faced and solved, at least in its fundamental parts, consists of getting suitable information to the worker in such activities "at risk" whenever he wishes to have an update or in case of an accident.

The most important aims of the project are:

1) to give a contribution to professional updating. To obtain this it was necessary to define the activity model, and in particular, to define the actors (for example, first aid health operator), and methods.

2) to evaluate the micro and macro-emergencies, supporting the prevention and the management of worker accidents.

3) to implement an interactive and multimedial user interface with regard to informative tools.

On these bases, this research projected and implemented an information system, defining a model and implementing a prototype for the management of a database. This database contains information regarding the toxicological characteristics of the mostly used and new antineoplastic chemotherapic drugs and the possible adverse effects on workers.

The system plans also a temporal calendar for the periodic control of the above mentioned workers, in order to verify the above mentioned adverse effects.

The system is, obviously, updatable, and it was projected to be available for other work areas.

3. System description

In order to implement the previously described project, an information system prototype was implemented.

It consists of the following parts:

- an object-oriented database, in which to store information about people who produce and manipulate chemotherapic antineoplastic drugs (people "at risk");
- a decision support system (DSS), able to plan the periodic control of the workers in order to verify the adverse effects of the antineoplastic chemotherapic drugs on them, and to manage casual accidents by its interactive use. In fact, a Listening Center for Emergency (ELC) is continuously active to carry out in real time a teleconsultation between a user and an expert who is in the ELC. As it is known, the management of accidents due to the adverse effects of the antineoplastic chemotherapic drugs requires the availability of appropriate information, such as data on medical management of victims and guidelines for treatment and adequate antidotal drugs, standard treatments, and special treatments. This DSS is connected, through the Internet, to different users, who are in different places of the territory. The DSS has a knowledge base in which information on drugs, protocols for planning the worker's activity and for managing emergencies and follow-ups are stored.
- a management system for the network communications;
- a visual user-friendly interface, with multimedial capabilities, for unexperst end users.

Through it the users ask queries to the system, and, in general, they exchange information. The system is conceptually represented in Figure 1.

Each place connected to the object-oriented database has its own database (for privacy reason), in which each worker at risk stores data which the system requires following a periodic planning purposely defined for them. This means that, for example, every six months the worker has to do some laboratory analyses, when results are stored in database. The DSS controls which stored values are within the regular ranges of these examinations, and, if they are out of these ranges, the relative "alarm protocol" starts. At the end of the planned period of the protocol, the same laboratory analyses are repeated, and so on.

Different is the situation in which an accident occurs. In this case the user (the victim or his colleague) interfaces with the system, that is, the DSS, which is able to help him.

With regard to the information service, the system is connected with the Italian National Inventory of Chemical Substances in which the base set information required to classify a new chemical substance is stored, according to the 7th amendment of directive 67/548/EEC [5].

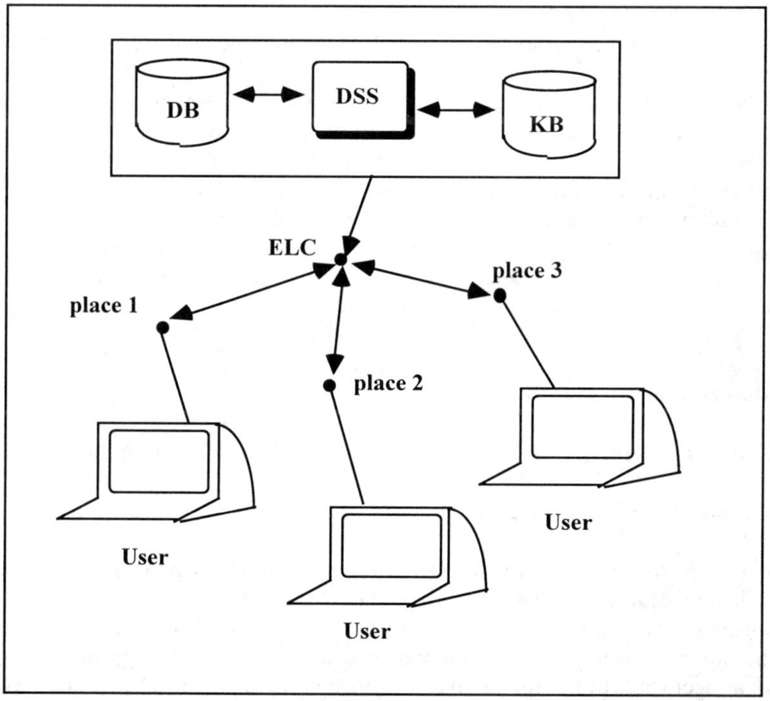

Figure 1

In it, toxicological and ecotoxicological properties are classified. As it is well known, the number of chemicals used in general (and in the medical area in particular) is very high and it is continuously increasing. This situation creates a growing need for assessing the risk posed by the already existing (as well as new) chemicals with the aim of eliminating or reducing their adverse effects on human health. This assessment implies the knowledge of the intrinsic properties, of the risk factors, and exposure of human beings to their effects. This means that it is necessary to know at least the intrinsic properties of chemicals. Recently, the Commission of the European Union (EU) issued a directive on risk assessment [6], which procedure comprises four steps: 1) hazard identification; 2) concentration/effect assessment; 3) exposure assessment; 4) risk characterization. For example, hazard identification is "the identification of the adverse effects which a substance has an inherent capacity to cause toward human health and environment" [5]. At the Italian national level, there is an increasing need of information concerning chemical hazards and chemical risks according to the specific necessities of public and private institutions which have to deal with the management of human health risks.

4. Conclusion

The system, shortly described, was started at the beginning of this year and it is functioning only in a restricted subset of centers (test phase). At present it is not possible to have any evaluation regarding the improvements which this system should bring, but the first comments in its use are in encouraging.

References

[1] Birgham E., Hazards to health workers from antineoplastic drugs. New Eng. J. Med., 7, (1985).1220-1221.
[2] Carere E., Mohn G.R., Parry J.M., et al., Methods and testing strategies for evaluating the genotoxic properties of chemicals. Eureopean Commission, EUR15945, 1995.
[3] Henderson D., McCall J., Boyle J., Decision support system for designing chemotherapeutic regimens. Proceed. MIE'97, C.Pappas et al. (Eds), 1997, pp. 353-357.
[4] Ohman B., Lyrvall H. et al., Clinical pharmacology and the provision of drug information. European Journal of Clinical Pharmacology, pp. 563-568, 1992.
[5] European Communities 1992. Council directive 92/32/EEC of 30 April 1992 amending for the 7th time Council directive 67/548/EEC of the approximation of laws, regulations and administrative provisions relating to the classification, packing and labelling of dangerous substances ("7th amendment"). Off. J. Eur. Communities (L 154 of 5/6/92).
[6] European Communities 1993. Commission directive 93/67/EEC of 20 July 1993 laying down the principles for assessment of risks to man and the environment of substances notified in accordance with Council directive 67/548/EEC. Off. J. Eur. Communities (L 227/9 of 8/9/93).

Medical Informatics Europe '99
P. Kokol et al. (Eds.)
IOS Press, 1999

Outpatient Health Care Statistics Data Warehouse - Implementation

Dejan Zilli
Vizija d.o.o., Ljubljanska 42, Celje, Slovenia

Abstract. Data warehouse implementation is assumed to be a very knowledge-demanding, expensive and long-lasting process. As such it requires senior management sponsorship, involvement of experts, a big budget and probably years of development time. Presented Outpatient Health Care Statistics Data Warehouse implementation research provides ample evidence against the infallibility of the above statements. New, inexpensive, but powerful technology, which provides outstanding platform for On-Line Analytical Processing (OLAP), has emerged recently. Presumably, it will be the basis for the estimated future growth of data warehouse market, both in the medical and in other business fields. Methods and tools for building, maintaining and exploiting data warehouses are also briefly discussed in the paper.

Keywords:
Data warehouse, outpatient health care statistics, On-Line Analytical Processing (OLAP), Decision Support Services (DSS).

1. Introduction

In our country there are several outpatient health care information systems that are used to store medical data in health care centers, private practices and other health care institutions. The Institute of Public Health of the Republic of Slovenia has defined several requirements for collecting outpatient health care statistics data on the state level. Application for statistical data distribution, made according to these requirements, served as a basis for the presented data warehouse solution.

The outpatient health care statistics collects the data about diseases and conditions as well as those about attendance and referrals. The research was limited to diseases and conditions, but can be easily used for the whole outpatient health care statistics eventually. The logical design of Outpatient Health Care Statistics Data Warehouse is discussed in the paper by Natek S. [1]. This paper introduces some methods and tools for building, maintaining and exploiting the data warehouse. It also presents some practical experience gathered during the implementation of Outpatient Health Care Statistics Data Warehouse.

The technology and techniques for building a data warehouse are not new to the world of database experts. They are thoroughly discussed by Inmon [2], Kimball [3] and by lots of others [6, 7]. It is not the intention of this paper to discover any new method or technique for building the data warehouse. The purpose of this research is to show how to effectively employ new inexpensive technology to do the work that took a lot of money and time in the past, with a very small budget and in a short period of time.

To achieve this goal the following hypotheses were proposed:

1) The *PC environment* is mature enough to serve as the basis for our data warehouse solution,
2) *Microsoft SQL Server 7.0* [4] with its *Decision Support Services* [5] can provide a powerful and reliable platform for implementation of almost any OLAP system.

One of the most difficult decisions in designing Outpatient Health Care Statistics Data Warehouse was related to the data granularity [2]. The decision to omit the lowest level of detail from the data warehouse [1] had a major influence upon all further implementation activities. The decision about data sources, data extraction and transformation, the design and population of data cubes, and the exploitation of Outpatient Health Care Statistics Data Warehouse are all the subject of this article.

2. Data Sources

The decision about a higher detail data level was largely influenced by the state level standard for distribution of outpatient health care statistics data. By not having adopted this standard, the data source for Outpatient Health Care Statistics Data Warehouse would be the transaction data from various medical information systems. Such a decision would make the data warehouse implementation much more complex and time-consuming. However, benefit of a lower detail data level would be time dimension (as opposed to half a year period dimension in summarized statistical data). The amount of used disk space would increase considerably, and data sparsity [3] would be much higher.

The state level standard regulates all obligatory statistical data transfer. The statistical data has to be submitted in a fixed format textual file. The data in those transfer files could serve as the data source for the statistical data warehouse. The problem of that solution is the fact that data in transfer files could be of low integrity, therefore complex data cleansing procedures should be developed to check the data integrity. Another deficiency is the lack of dimensional data (diagnoses, reporting units, specialties...) in transfer files. For these reasons the data from statistical data distribution application was used as the data source instead.

The data from statistical data distribution application are in Paradox tables and therefore ODBC readable [8]. Another benefit of this decision is that data from those tables are already checked for consistency by the statistical data distribution application. Every record has a flag stating whether it is consistent. The consistency check verifies the existence of any of the twenty possible kinds of mistakes. The statistical data distribution application also stores dimensional data needed for the data warehouse. For all stated reasons the selected data source is the most suitable for our data warehouse solution.

3. Data Extraction and Transformation

The data from On-Line Transaction Processing (OLTP) systems are almost never in the form suitable for the data warehouse. The same goes for the outpatient health care statistics data. The data transfer data model has several differences from the data warehouse model [1]. Therefore the data extraction and transformation is not trivial. This process usually requires complex programming and the use of data import/export and transformation tools. In our case most of the data cleansing and integration was already performed by the distribution application. Data Transformation Services (DTS), a new facility in Microsoft SQL Server 7.0 [9], was used for the data transformation.

DTS provides a graphical environment for describing data transformation process packages. DTS package stores data source description, data flow description, execution sequence, and transformation description. The transformation is performed by SQL sentences, which are supplemented by VB scripting language and the usage of external transformation tools. DTS package execution scheduling enables total data transformation automation. Four DTS packages were made to extract and transform the fact tables data. The usage of SQL sentences was sufficient for the realization of outpatient health care statistics data transformation.

Several problems were brought to attention during extraction of dimensional data:

1. Overlapping periods in reporting period dimension; there are two standard overlapping reporting periods (first half of the year, whole year). One way of solving this problem would be by calculating the fact data for the second half of the year (the difference between the whole year and the first half of the year). Fortunately, the statistics distribution application also supports the user-defined period, which was set to the second half of the year for the purpose of the data warehouse implementation.
2. Various special values representing the 'NULL' value; all those values had to be translated to 'NULL' value.
3. Dimensions inherent in the data transfer data structure (sex, age group, insurance category, and duration of pregnancy). The data for those dimensions had to be entered into dimensional tables. Modification of those dimensional data would be necessary only in the case of data structure changes.
4. Data integration problem; as the result of the data transfer data model, some of the dimensions could not be integrated in the same data cube. Several data cubes were proposed during logical design [1]. The integration of data cubes in the virtual data cube removes all dimensions, which are not present in all data cubes.

Visual database diagram [9] simplifies the task of changing the data structure. It provides a simple graphical environment for definition of tables, attributes, primary keys, and foreign keys in the SQL Server database.

4. Design and Population of Data Cubes

There are several important decisions that have to be made while designing data cubes [5]:

1. *Storage choice*: DSS offers the possibility to choose between three different storage models: Relational OLAP (ROLAP), Multidimensional OLAP (MOLAP), and Hybrid OLAP (HOLAP). MOLAP model is the most suitable for Outpatient Health Care Statistics Data Warehouse. The data are stored in multidimensional database, which ensures fast response times.
2. *Dimension hierarchy*: some dimensions are hierarchical by their nature. The decision, how to store the data of hierarchical dimensions, was already made during the logical design phase. In the *star schema* the data of all dimension levels are stored in a single table. This solution ensures fast response times for the price of redundancy. *Partial snowflake schema* was adopted in the case of Outpatient Health Care Statistics Data Warehouse, which means that the data of hierarchical dimensions are stored in multiple tables.
3. *Level of preaggregation*: DSS provides the possibility to set the extent of aggregation stored by OLAP server. This can be set with performance gain percent or with maximum storage space. DSS uses heuristics to select and store the most useful aggregations. Full performance gain was set for the sake of this research to achieve the best possible response times.

4. *Virtual data cube design:* the disintegration problem caused by the data source decision can be solved by the means of a virtual data cube. The virtual data cube provides a view over several data cubes, which have shared dimensions. Dimensions that are not common to all data cubes are left out. Measures are summarized over omitted dimensions. In the case of Outpatient Health Care Statistics Data Warehouse virtual data cube can also serve for the verification of the data transformation process (the number of instances of all age groups and sexes must correspond to the number of instances of all insurance categories).

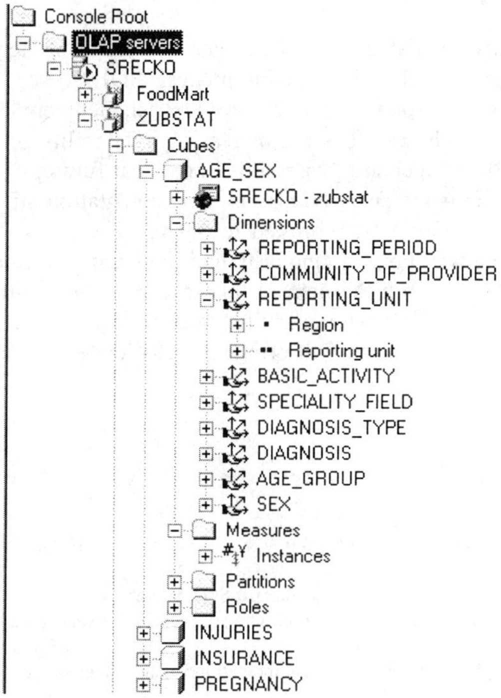

Picture1: Structure of outpatient health care statistics data cubes, dimensions and measures

After data cubes have been designed it is time to populate them. In DSS this is called processing of data cube. The process is fully automated. It can also be scheduled for the off hours period.

5. Exploitation of Outpatient Health Care Statistics Data Warehouse

Every data warehouse solution, simple or complex, is built to support a number of decision support functions that can not be implemented in the OLTP system. Most frequently used function of OLAP systems is *drill-down analysis* [2]. It gives the possibility to overview summarized data and then drill-down in the direction of interest. The summarized medical data of Outpatient Health Care Statistics Data Warehouse could be used for reporting, analysis of known facts, and discovery of unknown facts (Data Mining). However, it is not the scope of this article to examine all possibilities of Outpatient Health Care Statistics Data Warehouse exploitation.

There are already some client tools available on the market that support Microsoft DSS Server. They use interface called Pivot Table Services (PTS), which provides easy access to the whole DSS functionality. Such open client architecture ensures that many other software providers will follow. Arguably the most important OLAP client tool will become Office 2000 with its spreadsheet application Excel. Relative high availability of those tools should bring data warehousing and OLAP systems closer to the average user.

6. Conclusion

The research shows that broadly available PC based data warehousing technology is becoming mature enough to support the decision-making process. SQL Server 7.0 database functionality and included Decision Support Services provide excellent environment for building and maintaining a data warehouse. It is the increasing availability of client tools that will make the expansion of OLAP technology possible in the near future.

The Outpatient Health Care Statistics Data Warehouse implementation study provides several tips for building a data warehouse with limited resources. The decision about the data source and consequential data warehouse granularity had the greatest influence on the choice of implementation techniques. With the help of this research, the experts from the Ministry of Health have finally been given the possibility to analyze the outpatient health care statistics data. The transition to utilization will bring new challenges and could be the subject of another research.

References

[1] Natek S., Data Warehouse for Outpatient Health Care Statistics - Logical Design, MIE 99, 1999.
[2] Inmon W.H., Building the Data Warehouse, 2.ed., John Wiley & Sons, Inc., USA, 1996.
[3] Kimbal R., The Data Warehouse Toolkit, John Wiley & Sons, Inc., USA, 1996.
[4] Microsoft Corporation, http://www.microsoft.com/sql : Microsoft SQL Server 7.0
[5] Microsoft Corporation, Microsoft SQL Server 7.0 Decision Support Services: Lowering the Cost of Business Intelligence, USA, 1998.
[6] Singh H., Data Warehousing Concepts, Technologies, Implementations, and Management, Prentice Hall, USA, 1998.
[7] Anahory S., Murray D., Data Warehousing in the Real World, Addison Wesley, USA, 1997.
[8] Lazar D., Microsoft Strategy for Universal Data Access, USA, 1997.
[9] Microsoft Corporation, The Microsoft Data Warehousing Strategy: A platform for improved decision-making through easier data access and analysis, USA, 1998.

Medical Informatics Europe '99
P. Kokol et al. (Eds.)
IOS Press, 1999

Implementing HISA Standard in the Middleware Layer of Our Applications

Nataša Planinc, Boštjan Berčič, Marjana Pikec
Infonet, Informacijski inženiring, Planina 3, 4000 Kranj, Slovenija
E-mail: info@infonet.si
URL: http://www.infonet.si

Abstract. This article describes our experiences in implementation of the European standard for the architecture of healthcare information systems. The standard was a great help, but this article focuses more on some problems we have encountered.

1. What is HISA?

HISA stands for **Healthcare Information System Architecture**. It is the European prestandard defined by the CEN/TC251 prENV 12967-1, and establishes general principles for the architecture of healthcare information systems.

The architecture of any generic healthcare information system is described through three co-operative layers:

- **Healthcare application layer** models the data, operation on data and interaction with user required to support the processes in the specific healthcare organization.
- **Healthcare middleware layer** models services, which are shared by whole organization and required to support the application layer.
- **Healthcare bitways layer** models technological infrastructure, which provides services to the middleware layer. It hides diverse locations and diverse platforms by providing common facilities for middleware layer.

The scope of HISA is to describe the **middleware** layer. HISA consists of a group of shared services system - **Healthcare Common Services (HCS)**. They provide the rest of the system with services common throughout the whole healthcare information.

Middleware layers conforming to HISA enable integration and communication between individual healthcare units and their applications on local, regional or even national level. This is achieved not only by message exchange but also by a consistent and common information fund. Middleware layers enable interworking of different and heterogeneous applications, letting them behave together as an integrated system towards the environment.

2. The Need for a Standard

Healthcare organisations today face a tendency to change from huge, vertically organized organizations toward a group of mutually complementary, specialized autonomous units, even on different locations. Each of these units has different needs and mode of work, and its own unique requirements. All of them must work effectively, must satisfy health and social needs of the area, must know how to communicate with others, and must be able to provide data important for clinical, management, statistical, and epidemiological activities to actors responsible for them.

One way to achieve this is by creating a big uniform system, which dictates data structures and available operations on them. This approach has been used in the past but has failed to fulfil all the needs of individual users, as well as to ensure optimal procedures.

Another way is to model the hospital information system as a group of independent applications, which are optimised for the needs of each unit, but are also able to intercommunicate. HISA proposes a way of doing that, which also encourages modularity and extensibility of applications.

3. Healthcare Common Services (HCS)

Specification of middleware in HISA consists mainly of description of healthcare common services. There are six groups of services:

- **Subject of care HCS** group the services for identification of subject of care and storing and retrieval of its personal, administrative and epidemiological data. Main entities of information managed are **Subject of care,** his **contacts** and his **cases.**
- **Activity HCS** describe the services for structuring healthcare organization into a set of service points, for classification and description of activities and support of their life-cycle, for clustering activities into groups (protocols and request), and for classification and specification of results of activities (non-health characteristic).
- **Health characteristics HCS** include the description and classification of the various types of health characteristics as well as the actual data relating to the values of such characteristics for the individual subject of care. They may also represent result of the execution of an individual activity or combined group of activities.
- **Resource HCS** groups the services for classification and management of resources, in terms of availability (planning) and actual utilization of them.
- **Authorization HCS** groups services describing individual user's access to various data elements and the execution of different services provided by the system.
- **Concept HCS** groups the services managing vocabulary items and rules for instantiation of particular attributes of objects.

For each entity in the group of services the standard defines essential attributes and relations with other entities. It also defines a set of services for:

- **Retrieval of a list of instances** satisfying some selection criteria based on value of entity's attributes or its' relation with other entities.
- **Maintenance of one instance of the entity**: entering new instance, retrieval of the full set of information of one instance, modification and deletion of one instance.
- **Retrieval and maintenance of relationships** between one entity and another entity connected to it.

4. The Specific Adoption of HISA Standard in Middleware Layer of Our Applications

In developing the applications' middleware layer based on HISA, we have met some general and at the same time some very specific problems.

We had to take into account that there is a gap between the general functionality described in the standard, which is at the conceptual level only, and the particular functionality required by the end-users. The standard is very general and describes only the fundamental set of services and attributes. It does not specify the characteristic of any application or subsystem. Neither it specifies all possible classes of information or services, which are necessary and useful in possible healthcare information systems. Therefore we were faced to the need of allocating and dividing the data into different entities. Sometimes we had to invent new entities and functionality not covered by the standard in order to satisfy the users' needs.

The fact that the standard does not describe the items in consideration sufficiently detailed for direct implementation leaves a lot of space for different interpretations of entities and relations, and as a consequence possible different implementations. Such discrepancies in implementations might jeopardize the benefits of seamless communication between different units in the healthcare information system.

One way to avoid incompatible implementations is common development and joint efforts of all software providers (that work on healthcare information systems). That kind of agreement would unify various interpretations of the standard. We have started such an initiative in our country.

Choosing object-oriented implementation of healthcare middleware layer, as we had, and at the same time being compliant with the HISA standard, we had to implement the mapping between the entities described in the standard and the business objects, which form the corresponding middleware layer. The standard gives only a skeleton of entities, their attributes, and relationships between entities. We have added functionality such as different kind of statistics, various specific views on patient's data (insight into patient's treatment, tracking of some of his or hers health characteristic, view of patient's contacts, cases...), views of group of patients selected by different criteria, accounting of healthcare services etc. Therefore we had to add new attributes and even new entities (classes) to those described in the HISA standard.

Subject of care or patient is probably an object that we supplemented most. We added address as a separate object; we added attributes describing patient's employment, his selected doctor for certain period of time, contracts with payers of the healthcare service patient has received, etc. We developed a new group of classes, which describes the way healthcare service is charged to the payer. This is a part of business objects' layer that is subject to constant change due to the changes in legislation and insurance companies' politics. We have tried to make it as independent and as separate as possible.

We had some problems defining the right relation between contact and case. The standard describes contact as the time period during which subject of care is under active consideration of the healthcare organization and case as an aggregation of several contacts. The dilemma we faced was what happens when the patient is moved between different units in the hospital. Does that mean that his first contact is closed and a new one is created or is this still the same contact? What happens when the patient is transferred, from one department in the hospital to another? HISA standard wisely delegates this decision to designers and programmers of particular application.

We have added quite a few attributes to the health characteristics, as well. We have created sub-entities (in our terminology subclasses) of health characteristic and its type. They describe classification and management of the health characteristics collected in laboratories.

A dynamic part of the system, which is covered in the standard by activity health care common services, lacked some useful details, too. Some requests are addressed to the actors in other healthcare information systems. We had to consider how the execution of such activity and how the results will be reported back. We wanted that such an activity is handled the same way as activity ordered and executed within the system.

5. Conclusion

The static part of health information system described in HISA standard, e.g. entities and their attributes, was relatively easy to extend – we only added data elements when needed. With dynamic part of the system, the workflow of a typical healthcare information system, it was different. Here we were on our own and had to develop our particular solutions.

HISA standard is a good guidance and a great help in developing healthcare applications. It provides a solid basis for integration of information systems in healthcare. As a software solution provider involved in integration of legacy healthcare information systems and the development of new ones we are proud to be a part of the process of quality improvement, modernization, and standardization in this area.

References

[1] CEN/TC 251 Final Draft 2 prENV 12967-1:1997 Healthcare Information System Architecture Part 1 (HISA), 1997. http://www.ehto.be/ikb/standards/centc251/hisa/

[2] F. Ferrara, Healthcare Information System Architecture. In J. Dudeck, B. Blobel, W. Lordieck, T. Bürkle (ed.), New Technologies in Hospital Information Systems. ISBN 90 5199 363 3 45. IOS Press, Amsterdam, 1997, pp. 1-9.

[3] G. Booch, Object Oriented Analysis and Design with Applications. ISBN 0-8053-5340-2 The Benjamin/Cummings Publishing Company Inc., 1994.

Medical Informatics Europe '99
P. Kokol et al. (Eds.)
IOS Press, 1999

European and Latin-American Countries Associated in a Networked Database of Outstanding Guidelines in Unusual Clinical Cases (ELCANO)

C. Ohmann[1,7], H.P. Eich[1], J.J. Sancho[2], C. Diaz[2], G. Faba[3], N. Oliveri[4], S. Clamp[5,7], J.M. Cavanillas[6], E. Coello[6]

[1]*Theoretical Surgery Unit, Dept. of General and Trauma Surgery, Heinrich-Heine University Düsseldorf, Germany*
[2]*Dept. of Medical Informatics, Institut Municipal d'Investigació Mèdica, Barcelona, Spain (project co-ordination)*
[3]*Dirección general de Estadistica e Informática, Centro Nacional de Información y documentación sobre Salud, Mexico-City, Mexico*
[4]*Dept. of Medical Informatics, Fundación de Informática Médica, Buenos Aires, Argentina*
[5]*Clinical Information Science Unit, University of Leeds, United Kingdom*
[6]*División de Ingenieria del Software, SEMA Group sae. SEMA, Madrid, Spain*
[7]*Research and Telemedicine Committee of the World Organisation of Gastroenterology*

Abstract. The aim of ELCANO, an EU - funded project, is to build a virtual multilingual multimedia library of unusual clinical cases related to gastroenterology. Based on a standardisation of the format to report and the representation of clinical information on WWW, the multilingual multimedia case has been developed and till now 350 cases have been included. User satisfaction and user acceptance of ELCANO are under evaluation.

1. Introduction

It has been widely recognised that the morbidity and mortality of unusual clinical cases ranges from five to six times those of usual clinical cases. There is an acute lack of structured information sources on the best managing practices (diagnosis, treatment, patient information, prevention and prognosis) of these unusual cases. In many cases the high mortality and morbidity is due to the lack of knowledge on previous experiences with similar cases.

The aim of ELCANO is to cover this lack of information and communication. ELCANO is an European project funded under the INCO-DC program by the DG XII of the European Commission. The main objective of ELCANO is to build-up and maintain a multilingual virtual library of clinical reports of unusual clinical cases. This virtual library is being distributed across the World Wide Web. The initial area of the clinical practice addressed is gastroenterology. The project consortium consists of different partners from Europe and Latin-America. The project has a funding for 30 months (1st January 1997 – 30th June 1999).

2. Methods

The project plan covers 11 work packages (WP) (table 1) [1]. In WP 1 types of valid clinical cases integrated in the virtual library have been defined. The major obstacle which occurs here is what physicians may characterise as "unusual" [2]. The task is to define a gold-standard when assessing the unusuality of a clinical case. The three main sources of documented prevalence of diseases are scientific clinical journals, textbooks and computer applications for diagnostic support based on a Bayesian approach.

Table 1: Work packages of the project

No	work package
1	definition of unusual cases
2	definition of styles
3	format of graphic part
4	coding standards
5	database and query systems (description and implementation of the database structure)
6	the web server (design, implementation and maintenance of the web server, dissemination of the contents)
7	acquire new cases strategy (analysis and exploration of potential strategies, implementation of strategy for acquisition)
8	mirroring strategy (definition of mirroring scheme and implementation)
9	validation of new cases (definition of criteria, formation of an editorial board, performance and documentation of validation)
10	methodology of translation
11	methodology to monitor the virtual library use

The WPs 2 and 3 deal with the textual and graphical format of the electronic case report. In this part, style and conventions have been defined for a generic case report in order to offer a set of guidelines to build a consistent structure of the clinical report. Some sections have been defined as fixed and mandatory and some other sections are optional. The laboratory values have a unique form and the description of symptoms, diseases, examinations and treatments are set to be reported in non structured form (as opposed to form-based data entry) to allow a rich clinical description. For the graphical part of the case report existing standards for image representation and compression have been thoroughly evaluated. A minimum ground for including images and a recommended range of resolution for each category has to been set-up. Furthermore, guidelines to preserve the privacy of the patient have been adopted.

Objective of WP 4 was the choice of the most appropriate set of coding standards to code the reports of clinical cases. The standard to be adapted to represent clinical data in detail must agree with the CEN published documentation regarding the representation of clinical data.

A database structure and query system (WP 5) has been designed to allocate the clinical cases descriptions and codes. This structure is capable to process the queries obtained from HTML query forms. Its reports are automatically formatted accordingly to HTML format conventions, ready to be sent over the WWW as a report page. A further objective is the design of a secondary database to handle the validation and monitoring of the Web Server, with special emphasis on automatic reporting of the use, hit rate, queries processed and feed-back from Web Clients. The web server design (WP 6) handles queries to search for clinical cases in the database, in-page inclusions of images and templates for each page (multilingual versions). For the different installations of the servers a mirroring strategy has been developed (WP 8). The task of acquiring new cases (WP 7) spanned through the second part of the project life time. The participating partners directly input cases in the virtual library, recruiting clinicians at their respective sites to build clinical reports. The validation of new cases (WP 9) is processed in a similar manner as for peer-reviewed clinical reports submitted for publication in printed form to a scientific journal. An editorial board of reviewers has been set-up to whom the newly submitted cases are forwarded. Furthermore a technical board of reviewers is set-up in order to check the adherence to the guidelines for authors in terms of distribution of material, images format and privacy preservation. Once a case is validated it is translated to English or Spanish (WP 10) depending on the original manuscript's language. To monitor and evaluate the virtual library in use a methodology has to be developed to measure the hit rates, fields of interest and user acceptance (WP 11).

3. Results

Table 2 shows the categories of valid unusual cases integrated in the virtual library. Indicators of how unusual a disease is, are that there are no publications of this case, only some publications of isolated clinical cases but no systematic review, reviews published but obsolete due to advances of medicine or known prevalence lower than 1%. The decision for integrating a case is made by the Editorial board, since also issues like completeness and instructiveness of a case are evaluated.

Table 2: Types of unusual clinical cases to be integrated into the virtual library

No	Types of unusual clinical cases
1	Universal low prevalence
2	Dissimilar incidence among European and Latin-American regions
3	Unusual cluster of symptoms
4	Unusual constraints for its treatment
5	Unusual combinations of different diseases
6	Documented management errors from which to learn

The generic case report covers six sections: identification, brief description, clinical report, discussion, references, images and comments. The identification section consists of the case number, entry date, ELCANO site, category, authors name, address and a brief description of the case. The case report (section 2) covers the history, physical examination, laboratory tests, imaging techniques, endoscopy, additional studies, diagnosis, treatment, evolution and outcome.

To decide which standard for pictures is best for the virtual library of ELCANO, different web sites with medical images were examined. For example, a web site with a large image database can be found at the North-western University Radiology Department[1] with further links to large image databases[2]. Browsing these sites the different formats that were used are: GIF (graphics interchange format) and JPEG (joint photographic expert group). The GIF-format provides a lossless compression of images. JPEG provides a loose compression but with a higher compression rate. For pictures in the virtual library of ELCANO it was decided to use the JPEG format. Images are stored with a compression rate not higher than 1:20 or 1:40, if important medical features are not lost by this loose compression. If diagnostic accuracy is an imperative requisite a loose compression will be avoided. The obvious advantage of a loose compression is the increase of transmission speed over the internet.

The reasons of choosing coding systems for ELCANO are related to the need for a standardisation of the vocabulary used in the unusual medical cases, as well as, codes that allow a codification from more general aspects to smaller details and to reduce the

[1] http://pubweb.acns.nwu.edu/~dbk675/nwu_radiology.html
[2] http://pubweb.acns.nwu.edu/~dbk675/netsites.html

redundancy of the diseases reported for a single patient [3]. Neither of the existing systems in medicine can be identified as a ideal resource for the codification of unusual clinical cases, therefore three coding systems are used in the ELCANO project. In a first step the Spanish version of the Medical Subject Headings (MeSH) (Spanish version: DeSC) is used build-up a lexicon for unusual cases. Then ICD-9/10 (International Classification of Diseases) are assigned and finally an exhaustive and detailed codification of the cases is done using the Systemised Nomenclature of Medicine (SNOMED). This methodology warranties a complete codification of unusual cases and will allow web users a logical and easy search and retrieval of the cases with a wide variety of alternatives. Starting point for codification is the diagnosis noted by the author. These terms are used as descriptor search and standardised with MeSH. The MeSH terms are then used for further codification with ICD-9 and SNOMED.

Three different database structures have been developed for the ELCANO project (cases database, administrative database and web contents database). Microsoft Access version 7.0 is used for all of them. In the cases database all fields are in HTML ready format, and therefore are directly put into the web pages as a user requires to browse a particular case. This structure allows rapid changes in the display format of the database. Each case is uploaded from the database directly to the MS Word template described in the generic case report. Images are kept in different directories and a pointer to their filename and directory is all that is stored in the cases database. The WEB contents database is filled with the non clinical contents of ELCANO. These are documents as the description of the project, the deliverables made public and the profiles of the partners are stored in twin tables for English and Spanish. The administrative database is central to the ELCANO activities regarding collection, revision, translation and publication of the newly acquired cases. It shares a number of fields with the cases database, and it is dynamically linked to the tables of the cases database. It contains the status of the case (reviewed or not, published in Spanish / English), comments of the chief editor, warnings, etc. The search strategy is based upon the Microsoft SQL Server and the Microsoft Internet Server. Search is available from the main page and the cases pages. Two levels of search are available: search in all categories and search in specific categories. When the user chooses to search in all categories, the search engine carries out a search through all ELCANO database case fields, indexed, and non indexed. It shows the result in a screen similar to those used to present the cases when listed for browsing. When the user chooses to search for individual characteristics, the screen is divided in different fields. The user can then introduce full or partial search terms (and use SQL syntax if wanted) in the fields required. The search engine processes the query among fields as a logic AND.

The task of acquiring new cases was solved with different approaches: new submissions, published cases in medical journals, cases books, scientific meetings, existing databases, from the web and via a contest. Until December 1998 350 case reports were introduced in to the virtual library (150 English, 200 Spanish). From this cases 246 belong to diseases with low prevalence, 65 have differential diagnoses, 34 unusual cluster of symptoms, 16 with management errors, 16 different incidences between Europe and Latin-America and 2 with unusual limitations in treatment. The ELCANO web site will be accessible via 5 different severs at the end of the project (Madrid[3], Barcelona[4], Leeds[5], Buenos Aires[6] and Mexico-City[7]).

---

[3] elcano.sema.es
[4] www.imim.es/elcano
[5] www.hci.leeds.ac.uk/elcano
[6] www.pccp.com.ar/elcano
[7] www3.ssa.gob.mx/elcano

4. Discussion

ELCANO encourages collaborative activities over different hemispheres, in synergy with EU policies on development and economic collaboration by taking advantage of the summation of medical knowledge and research capabilities form all partners. The immediate effects can be regarded in two fronts: technical front and medical front. The implementation of existing global network technologies linking separate world regions is a working demonstration of the feasibility of such technology to share clinical information. As an important part of the project ELCANO deals with the standardisation on the format to report and represent clinical information on the WWW, it might represent an important point of reference for future work in transmitting clinical information over the Internet.

An evaluation of the use and acceptance of a web site is an difficult task. An experimental evaluation of ELCANO in a controlled clinical trial would be preferable, is however not feasible. Assess to the World Wide Web and Internet cannot be controlled and there are no restrictions in the use of the ELCANO database. It would be extremely difficult to set up a quasi-experimental trial such as a before/after trial measuring the effects of using ELCANO on clinical care. Instead of looking at the process and outcome of clinical care in a controlled clinical trial, the ongoing evaluation concentrates on whether the system is really used, whether users are satisfied with the systems interface and content and whether they perceive the system as useful. The sharing of medical guidelines to manage clinical cases among partners with different degrees of expertise benefits for the partners participating, as well as for any third party user willing to make a consultation to the virtual library of clinical cases and/or contributing with new cases to the library.

Acknowledgement

The ELCANO project is supported by the INCO-DC program (DG XII) of the European Commission in the 4th Framework Telematics Application Programme (1996-1999) and by the Research and Telemedicine Committee of the World Organisation of Gastroenterology (OMGE).

References

[1] J.J. Sancho, S. Clamp, N. Oliveri, G. Faba, C. Ohmann, J.M. Cavanillas, M. Sosa, E. Coello, F. Sanz, Proyecto Elcano: biblioteca electronica de casos clinicos inusuales en patologia digestiva. *International Telemedicine* **4** (1997) 22-28.

[2] A. Kong, O. Barnett, F. Mosteller, C. Youtz, How medical professionals evaluate expressions of probability. *New England Journal of Medicine* **315** (1986) 740-744.

[3] J.J. Berman, G.W. Moore, W.H. Donnelly, J.K. Massey, B. Craig, A SNOMED analysis of three years' accessioned cases (40.124) of a surgical pathology department: implications for pathology-based demographic studies. *Proceedings of the Annual Symposium of Computer Applications in Medical Care* (1994) 188-192.

Medical Informatics Europe '99
P. Kokol et al. (Eds.)
IOS Press, 1999

A uniform database of rehabilitation as a basis for evaluating the outcome quality

Flierl, S.[1], Alt, B.[1], Hornig, K.[2], Jacobi, E.[1]
[1]*Rehabilitation Research Centre at the University of Ulm, Germany*
[2]*Bliestal Clinic, Department of Orthopaedics, Blieskastel, Germany*

Keywords. Electronic patient register, ORACLE® database, outcome quality, quality assurance.

1. Summary

To make it possible to benefit from patient data recorded in rehabilitation clinics, with regard to outcome quality and scientific investigation, the Rehabilitation Research Centre at the University of Ulm has created a rehabilitation register, a database based on ORACLE®, into which the relevant patient data is transferred, having been made anonymous via an SQL archiving program. The archived data includes the clinical parameters, the running text of the discharge report, and the doctor's and patient's assessment of the rehabilitation outcome. It can be automatically searched for structured data, according to every conceivable criterion and in every conceivable combination, also in combination with a text search in the running text of the admission and discharge reports and the rehabilitation outcome.

With the aid of the rehabilitation register and thanks to the possibilities of EDP (Electronic Data Processing), in future it will be possible to make much more differentiated comments on the rehabilitation outcome than would be the case if the search were restricted to structured data alone. This is essential in order to be able constantly to improve outcome quality and to verify the economic benefit of rehabilitation medicine.

2. Introduction

Outcome quality in rehabilitation medicine is influenced by a variety of factors. In this context, it is important for patient data to be available for scientific consideration (personal data, data on findings on admission and discharge, rehabilitation outcome, therapy, etc.). If deficits are identified, possible improvements can be designed and the outcome quality can thus be improved. Our aim is to provide a convenient, easy-to-use user interface, so that this data can be easily input and optimally evaluated.

3. Methods

Under the global approach of rehabilitation, free formulation of a rehabilitation objective geared to the individual is essential. The approach can be described as global because, unlike acute medicine, rehabilitation medicine is multidimensional. Rehabilitation medicine is defined by the terms “impairment“, “disability“ and, consequently, “handicap“. Thus doctor and patient agree a rehabilitation objective, as an important component of quality assurance, and on completion of the rehabilitation measures, achievement of the objective is documented in writing. At the beginning and end of rehabilitation, the patient answers questions important in assessing the outcome by ticking the appropriate answer from among those provided. The questions relate to assessing his health and capabilities and to his expectations of rehabilitation.

In our research association, around 20 000 data sets a year are available, in the form of structured medical and socio-demographic data, supplemented by the running text from the record of achievement of the rehabilitation objective and from discharge reports.

Text processing via EDP is not sufficient to enable a rational evaluation to be achieved. Instead, it was necessary to switch the entire reporting system over to a database system and to give text processing only the role of an input mask.

The Rehabilitation Research Centre at the University of Ulm has developed a completely new secretariat program. Components consisting of electronic patient register, structured discharge report for pension insurance, variable statistical evaluation and remote data transmission were incorporated into a client-server architecture based on an ORACLE® database.

To make it possible to benefit from this data, with regard to outcome quality and scientific observations, a rehabilitation register was created, a database also based on ORACLE®, into which the relevant patient data is transferred, having been made anonymous via an SQL archiving program.

The archived data includes the clinical parameters, the running text of the discharge report, achievement of the rehabilitation objective, and the patient’s assessment of the rehabilitation outcome. As a result of control mechanisms supported by EDP, the information obtained from the medical routine of rehabilitation is of high quality and facilitates a completely new dimension of statistical evaluation, such as the calling up of data in a few seconds in accordance with the influencing variables of choice (discharge status, fitness for work, cause of disease, periods of unfitness for work, performance capacity, etc.) and the inclusion of linguistic variables.

Since the letter, the agreed objective and achievement of the objective are freely formulated and stored in the database, there are a vast range of options for differentiated evaluations.

4. Results

The program development has not yet been completed, so the applications currently possible will now be presented.

The patient account currently comprises approx. 10 000 entries from various clinics involved in the research association. Research can be carried out either on a clinic-by-clinic basis, or on the basis of all the clinics combined.

The first thing that appears when the rehabilitation register is opened is a greeting mask, on the basis of which one clicks on either pure evaluation of structured data, evaluation of structured data in combination with free texts (this is currently still restricted to evaluation of the free text of achievement of the rehabilitation objective), or diagnostic statistics.

The structured data can be searched according to every conceivable criterion and in every conceivable combination. Diagnostic groups (in accordance with the International Statistical Classification of Diseases and Related Health Problems (ICD-9)) and problem groups can be created. Patient data can be sifted out and directly subjected to statistical processing.

All criteria for selection from among the structured data can be linked to a text search. Two keywords linked with "OR" can each be linked with a blocking word. There are "INSTRING" functions, i.e. the sequence of letters may also occur within a longer word. The program then forms a sentence string with 5 words on the left of the word searched for and 5 words on its right. The blocking words can be checked in the sentence string, with "no" or "not" as the blocking word meaning the opposite. The blocking words can be linked with "AND" or "AND NOT".

As already mentioned, the text search is currently still restricted to the free text describing the achievement of the objective.

If information from several clinics is investigated jointly, the findings in a comparison of the clinics are sorted by differences in the patient questionnaires, in other words assessment of the state of health at the beginning minus assessment of the state of health at the end of rehabilitation. Thus it can immediately be seen, for example, which clinic produces the best outcome from the patient's point of view with a particular diagnosis or in accordance with other selection criteria. Quality assurance can be evaluated for all criteria individually or combined, for individual clinics or for all of them combined. All the outcomes can be schematically displayed and printed out.

The cost unit itself can also evaluate the outcome quality obtained by the affiliated clinics centrally and set them in relation to all the socio-medical variables from the PATIENT ACCOUNT. The evaluation is based on data that have not been made anonymous, in order to identify patients. Using this method, problem groups or problem clinics can be selected.

5. Discussion

The data input into the computer when the doctor's letter is written is stored centrally in the patient account with no further effort required. Following the automated transfer of the data, in anonymous form, to the rehabilitation register, it becomes accessible to scientific investigation. As the data is available in electronic form and owing to the easy-to-use, multilayered enquiry masks, the time taken to survey the data is only a fraction of that required in traditional processes involving study of files and manual evaluation. The questions can be dealt with virtually automatically.

Loss of information is reduced to a minimum, since the loss of files does not involve loss of data, and the input data is largely complete because of the EDP control. The archives are space saving and economical, and save on resources, because almost no consumer materials are involved. The remote data transmission takes only a matter of seconds, thus opening up completely new prospects in the context of co-operation among colleagues and continuity of treatment.

The rehabilitation register permits, on a routine basis and without major and time-consuming effort, monitoring of one's own performance on the basis of a wide range of parameters such as diagnosis, admission of patient fit for work or unfit for work for inpatient treatment, patient motivation, etc.

Thus profiles of the performance of participating clinics can be produced for internal use, but these can also be made available for statistical comparison of the clinics. It becomes possible to compare the outcome of various clinics within the association participating in the rehabilitation register. This objectification of outcome quality may reveal deficits and facilitates continuous and specific influencing of the relevant parameters.

Quality assurance can function only by objectifying quality and by means of appropriate quality control. People who can be monitored are concerned to improve their performance, and this applies just as much to clinics as institutions as to individual employees.

In future, it will be possible to search all free texts not only for individual words, but also for sequences of words of any length. Doctors' comments, directly or stored in encoded form as synonyms, can be sifted out with the aid of thesauri. For example, in an unadorned direct comment, the term "wants pension" appears. In coded form, this would read "The patient is of the opinion that he can no longer perform his previous work". In SQL, all synonyms can be linked with an "OR" command.

It will also be possible to include the therapy and to relate it to the outcome achieved. Thus it will be possible, for example, to compare different therapies for one clinical picture retrospectively, without major effort.

It will be possible to combine any number of diagnoses (ICD). In other words, patients can be selected not only under the main diagnosis, but also under the main diagnosis in combination with various secondary diagnoses. In addition, in view of the imprecision of the ICD (something that also applies to the ICD-10), it will be possible to input all diagnoses in explicit terms.

Checking of the data input for internal consistency can be done automatically whenever anything is input. "Internal consistency" means, for example, that the sense of the rehabilitation outcome formulated should tally with that of the findings on discharge.

With the aid of the rehabilitation register and thanks to the possibilities of EDP, in future it will be possible to make much more differentiated comments on the rehabilitation outcome than would be the case if the search were restricted to structured data alone. This is essential in order to be able constantly to improve outcome quality and to verify the economic benefit of rehabilitation medicine.

References

[1] J. Aigner, Untersuchungen zum Qualitätssicherungsprogramm der LVA Württemberg. Prüfung zweier Dokumentationsinstrumente der Qualitätssicherung auf ihre Reliablilität. Dissertation Medizinische Fakultät Universität Ulm, 1996

[2] N. Domhan, Erprobung eines teilstrukturierten Arztfragebogens als Basisdokumentation in der medizinischen Rehabilitation bei Erkrankungen des Bewegungsapparates. Dissertation Medizinische Fakultät Universität Ulm, 1996

[3] D. Evans, Pragmatically - structured lexical - semantic knowledge based for unified medical language systems. 12th Annual Symposium on Computer Applications in Medical Care, Washington DC (1988) 169-173.

[4] H. Feldweg, Stochastische Wortartendisambiguierung des Deutschen. In H. Feldweg und E. W. Hinrichs (Hrsg.): Lexikon und Text, Niemeyer Tübingen (1996) 217-230

[5] W. Gaus, Dokumentation und Ordnungslehre. Theorie und Praxis des Information Retrival. Springer, Heidelberg, 1995

[6] E. Jacobi, EDV-gestützter ärztlicher Abschlußbericht und Datenfernübertragung mit der LVA Württemberg. Z. Prävention und Rehabilitation (1995) 102-104.

[7] E. Jacobi, J. Schneider, Der ärztliche Entlassungsbericht - erstellt mit Hilfe der Datenverarbeitung. Sonderdruck aus Mitteilungen der LVA Württemberg, 1990.

[8] W. H. Jäckel, R. Cziske, N. Gerdes, E. Jacobi, Überprüfung der Wirksamkeit stationärer Rehabilitations-maßnahmen bei Patienten mit chronischen Kreuzschmerzen: eine prospektive, randomisierte, kontrollierte Studie. Die Rehabilitation 2 (1990) 67-160.

[9] D. von Stetten, Datenerfassung, Datenverarbeitung, Texterstellung und Informationsaustausch in der klinischen Rehabilitation. Z. Prävention und Rehabilitation (1995) 95-101.

[10] G. Vossen, Datenmodelle, Datenbanksprachen und Datenbank-Management-Systeme. Addison-Wesley, Bonn, 1994.

Medical Informatics Europe '99
P. Kokol et al. (Eds.)
IOS Press, 1999

A Unified Framework for Data Modeling on Medical Information Systems

José Neves Paulo Cortez Miguel Rocha António Abelha José Machado
Vitor Alves Sousa Basto Henrique Botelho João Neves
Universidade do Minho, Largo do Paço, Braga, Portugal

Abstract. *Medical Information Systems (MIS)* are seen as a way of optimizing the use of existing health-care infrastructure, without resorting to new and costly hospital (re)construction. The qualitative (re)design of such an environment requires a basic understanding of patient and doctors related characteristics and capabilities. Patient care, patient education, medical education, and clinical research need to be considered to meet the basic requirements on the level of services desirable, determined on the basis of the patient's length of stay; i.e., used for modeling the significant entities of such a world. The aim is to extract conclusions for the level of services provided to the users. One's concept will capture, as well as will integrate, the basic design principles under which *MIS* may be set.

1 Introduction

Medicine has been for some years a very attractive domain for *Computer Science (CS)* researchers, in general. There is a great potential for information automation, and a lot remains to be done. *Medical Informatics (MI)* is indeed becoming an issue of study in which *Medicine* and Computing overlap. Another reason for this increasing interest is costs. Today's strained health-care economics makes it necessary for expensive resources to be efficiently used, and requires a balanced management.

CS researchers have long used *Medicine* to elaborate on their own work. The field is probably one of the most knowledge intensive ones, loaded with human reasoning, with most of the procedure relying exclusively on the clinical experts. This makes health-care a perfect target for *CS*, since conventional systems are naturally bounded by their lack of rich knowledge representation and proof schemes. *Medicine* allows for the testing and exposing of new ideas and techniques by *CS* scientists, which creates a certain complicity between the two communities. Early knowledge-based systems like MYCIN, a medical consultation system for diagnosis of blood infectations (e.g., meningitis) and the recommendation of drug (e.g., antibiotic) treatment, or CADUCEUS, an expert system for medical diagnosis developed by Jack Mayers and Harry Pople at the University of Pittsburgh, 1985, which is an enhancement of INTERNIST, in that it incorporates causal relationships in its diagnosis process, shows the benefits of using *CS* in complex tasks. The proliferation of such systems during the eighties helped, in a certain way, to bridge the gap between theoretical, academia *CS*, and real world applications.

What is the best approach to help doctors and patients? It is believed *Artificial Intelligence (AI)* enters at this point. A system intended to be a support tool for clinicians must have its focus on knowledge representation and reasoning. Such system should be able to explain and justify its conclusions. On the other hand it has to be flexible enough to allow for simulation, training of novices and maintenance.

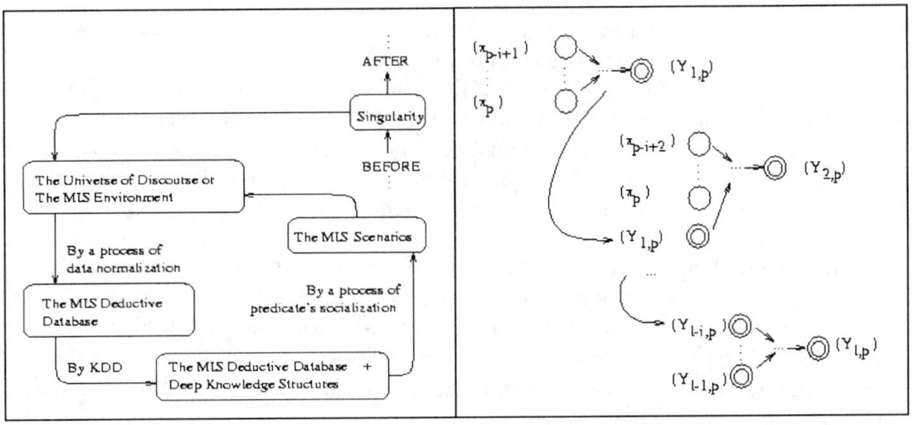

Figure 1: A Cosmic View of the Design Process of *MIS* and Getting *Y*

2 The Methodology

Any complex software system can be viewed as a collection of independent cooperating units or entities, each of which implements a subset of an application's total functionality.In some sense a cooperating unit will be called an agent, where relationships create bridges and methods among them [5].The underlined cognitive architecture will be defined as the portion of the system that provides and manages the primitive resources of such an entity; i.e., the substrate upon which a physical symbol system will be realized. Such a system, part symbolic, part sub-symbolic, will make use of *Neural Networks (NNs),* understood as autonomous agents in their own right. Indeed the concept of intelligence is keen to many different interpretations. In a this setting it may amalgamate the best of two worlds:

- the *symbolic AI* or *deliberate thinking* paradigms, where an agent is assumed to be driven by logic [7], and
- the *nouvelle AI*, *behavior-based AI*, or *situated agents* paradigms, where intelligence comes into being a property exhibited by the system's agents [4][3].

For instance, if one is working in areas such as detection of pathological occurrences in images of cervical smears or breasts images for automatic screening, soon realize that his/her experience and knowledge cannot be easily expressed using exclusively conventional symbolic systems [2].

In the design phase of a *MIS*, strategies need to be developed in order to apply some mitigation measures in the most cost effective manner. The strategy for each situation has to be based on the results of the cost effectiveness of the improvement options, the level of potential state investment required to achieve positive returns, and the potential long term benefits for both the state and the user. The improvements to be implemented may range from simple device enhancements to major reconstruction of facilities. The objective is to improve the quality of health-care, and, consequently, to reduce the loss of lives.

To quantify not only this parameter, and claim cost savings, but also to characterize the improvements to be implemented, and the fact that the data involved in the process has far out paced one's ability to interpret and digest it, it is felt a need for a new generation of tools and techniques for automated and intelligent construction and analysis of *MIS*. These tools and techniques make a new field of *Knowledge Discovery in Databases (KDD)*, and also make the core of one's approach (Figure 1).

KDD is concerned with the identification and description of data patterns [6], which, in this work, are interpreted as classes or concepts. In order to obtain such patterns it was followed the work by Agrawal [1] on association rules, expressions of the form $X \Rightarrow Y$, where X and Y are sets of items (the relations' attributes). The intuitive meaning of such a rule is that database transactions which contain X tend to contain Y.

Definition: Let $I=\{i_1,i_2,...,i_n\}$ be a set of terms, a set of the database's relations attributes. Let D be a set of transactions, where each transaction Tr is an attribute set such that $Tr \subseteq I$; i.e., such that I is a set of attributes over the binary domain $\{0,1\}$. Let a tuple Tu of the database D be represented by identifying its attributes with the binary value 1. Let TID be a unique identifier associated with transaction Tr. Let a set of attributes $X \subset I$ be called an attribute set. It may be claimed that:

- A transaction Tr contains an attribute set X, if $X \subseteq Tr$.
- An *association rule* is an implication of the form $X \Rightarrow I$, where $X \subset I$, $Y \subset I$, and $X \cap Y = \varnothing$ (the empty set).
- The rule $X \Rightarrow Y$ holds in the transaction set D with confidence C, if C% of transactions in D that contain X also contain Y.
- The rule $X \Rightarrow Y$ has support S in the transaction set D, if S% of transactions in D contain $X \cap Y$.

The set D stands for the extension of the relations (or predicates):

- *binary-identify-characteristics()*;

...

- *binary-healthy-and-happy-community()*.

where *binary-*()* stands for a relation whose attributes are defined over the binary domain $\{0,1\}$, and * stands for itself. To get X (from the rule $X \Rightarrow Y$), are used the procedures presented at [1]. To get Y (from the rule $X \Rightarrow Y$), it is followed the *Artificial Neural Network (ANN)* approach to *Time Series Forecasting* presented at [8]. The *ANN* will take the form L_i-L_h-1, for a network with L_i input nodes (or X), L_h hidden nodes, and *one* output node. The training cases, given by X, will take the form:

$$\begin{array}{ccc} x_1, x_2, \ldots, x_i & \rightarrow & x_{i+1} \\ \ldots & \rightarrow & \ldots \\ x_{p-i}, \ldots, x_{p-1} & \rightarrow & x_p \end{array}$$

for a set Y of cardinality p. After training, one-step ahead forecast (i.e., getting $Y_{1,p}$), is produced be feeding the *ANN* with the last known values for set X, namely:

$$Y_{1,p}=ANN(x_{p-i+1},\ldots,x_p)$$

where *ANN()* stands for the function modeled by the *ANN* and $Y_{r,s}$ for the forecast in the s period to r periods ahead of s. Multi-step ahead forecasts (looking at different *Ys*) are done by feedback of the previous ones (Figure 1).

3 Conclusions

For several decades, *CS* scientists and physicians have been building computer programs to diagnose medical illness and to recommend therapy. The resulting work helped to define and seed the development of expert and decision support systems in the area. On the other hand medical diagnosis and patient management procedures assisted to ensure that domain specific assertions and extensive knowledge about a problem domain are more crucial to problem solving, that are domain specific principles of reasoning. Thus, early generation of hypotheses seems to provide leverage for the diagnostician. Building on these results, an approach to data modeling on a *MIS* environment was set. It explores new techniques for the discovered of rules and data, driven by both deliberate thinking and behaviour based *AI*. It makes possible to dig in knowledge without generalization or background knowledge, a step forward in attribute oriented induction in data mining. Besides further advances on *KDD* on the attribute-oriented induction area, we are also investigation other data mining methods potentially applied to *MIS* design, with a particular emphasis on non-destructive worlds with incomplete information.

References

[1] Agrawal, R.; Manila, H.; Srikant, R.; Toivonen, H; and Verkamo, A. I. 1996. Fast Discovery of Association Rules. In *Advances in Knowledge Discovery and Data Mining*, Fayyed, U.M.; Shapiro, G. P.; Smyth, P.; and Uthurusamy, R. eds. The MIT Press, Menlo Park, California, USA.

[2] Anthony, D. *The Use of Artificial Intelligence in Medicine*, Warwick University, September 11, 1994.

[3] Bond A. A Computational Model for Organizations of Cooperating Agents, *SIGOIS Bulletin II*, 1990.

[4] Carbonell, J. *Machine Learning Paradigms and Methods*, The MIT Press, England, 1990.

[5] Cavedon, L. and Tidhar G. A Logical Framework for Multi-Agent Systems and Joint Attitudes, In *Proceedings of the First Australian Workshop on Distributed Artificial Intelligence*, University of New South Wales, Australian Defense Force Academy, Australia, 1995.

[6] Frawley, W.; Piatetsky-Shapiro, G. ; and Mathews, C. Discovery in Databases: An Overview. In *Knowledge Discovery in Databases*, G. Piatetsky-Shapiro and W. Frawley, Eds. The AAAI Press, Menlo Park, California, USA, 1991.

[7] Maes, P. Situated Agents Can Have Goals, In P.Maes ed. *Designing Autonomous Agents: Theory and Practice from Biology to Engineering and Back*, The MIT Press, London, England, 1990.

[8] Neves, J.; and Cortez, P. 1998. Combining Genetic Algorithms, Neural Networks and Data Filtering for Times Series Forecasting. In *Recent Advances in Circuits and Systems*, Mastorakis, N. E. ed. The World Scientific Press, London, UK.

Medical Informatics Europe '99
P. Kokol et al. (Eds.)
IOS Press, 1999

Preliminary study on relevant data for health management in hospitals

Brusaferro S., Scarbolo M.
Hospital Health Direction, Chair of Hygiene, Policlinico Universitario a Gestione Diretta, University of Udine - Italy

Abstract. Data and information are nowadays keys of success. We experienced the building of an hospital *Information System* (IS) selecting data from those already routinely produced and sharing them with health care units and general management. IS should be shaped to accomplish mission, vision and strategic direction of the hospital and in this direction our efforts are oriented.

1. Introduction

In 1992 the Health Reform has set the foundation for the reorganisation of the Italian National Health System[1]. The core of the reform set out to transform the hospitals and local health units into non-profit public enterprises. Hospital resources are now linked to the number Diagnosis Related Groups (DRG) produced and ambulatory patients assisted. This new approach has triggered off a complex process adapting hospital organisation and clinical work. Today, the keys to success in public health as in other fields are related to quality (technical, perceived and management quality[2]) and management. With this in mind, there are some major points that may play a role in the changing process: the IS and the interfaces between health-care units and hospital management. An efficient management of these points can guarantee an effective and continuous monitoring of the activity both in quantitative and qualitative terms and a continuous adaptation process of the strategies, targets and projects.

In our system the *hospital health direction* (HHD) has "the responsibility of running the hospital and the health-care units" [1] and the director is one of the managers of the hospital administration team; HHD has historically been the crossroads between health information and the strategic organisation of a hospital.

It is well known that producing data has a cost [3]. Producing too much data may lead to low quality data, waste of resources which are not used [4,5].

Our experience has taken the first step in attempting to identify, in a hospital, all existing operational data relevant for health management, and to select those capable of summarising the remarkable aspects of the activity.

The aim of our IS is to support strategic management. At the moment we try to give health-care-unit directors, hospital health directors and other hospital managers the possibility to evaluate periodically the work done and to correct possible deviations from the defined targets [6,7].

Developing an efficient IS is a prerequisite towards the realisation of a computerised system for management of health data.

2. Methods

The study has been conducted in a high specialisation teaching hospital with 300 beds in northern Italy between October 1997 and October 1998.

We adopted a structured interview in order to gather all the existing data produced, the technology of data organisation, their storage, retrieval and manipulation. We looked only for data relevant for health management. The items of the interview included: type of information, significance of information, origin of information, people responsible for that flow, destination, frequency of production, dead lines, existence of computerised data-base. What is meant by significance of information is the correlation of the data to relevant hospital operational processes both in health care and logistic/support areas.

We interviewed personnel operating in producing and managing data (n° 15 people). The interviews were repeated 15 days later in order to validate the results.

We analysed the flows to divide them into few categories corresponding to different health management aspects [7,8]. This allowed us to draw a new functional diagram of HHD. At the moment the role of the IS in our organisation is to collect, select and share data with hospital administration, direction, health-care-unit directors, and hospital managers. We developed a reporting system and some feed-back mechanisms were tested.

3. Results

We found 103 informative flows. Many of them managed different databases that can not be interfaced with each other. These flows were classified in eight categories illustrated in table 1.

Each flow was analysed with respect to the relevance it had to health care processes, management functions and/or national/regional laws. We suppressed 29 flows (table 1) as for example, bed rotation index or data on routine environmental microbiological contamination in operating rooms. For each flow we identified a flowchart including check points for quality control (figure 1); flows were classified to fit responsibility areas in the HHD that were ad hoc restructured (figure 2).

For instance the DRGs data flow (output production category) is identified as very important and it reflects all passages in data handling; there are three different categories of quality checks: quality of the clinical data (signature of the health unit responsible, up coding final random control); quality of patient discharging form fill in (control before data entry, software check algorithm), completeness of the data flow (check of all DRGs produced at the end of each month, validation from health care units quarterly) (fig.2).

Table 1: Classification and numbers of informative flows identified before and after revision

CATEGORY	BEFORE REVISION	AFTER REVISION
1. Flows deriving from law obligations (infectious disease surveillance, mortality data, etc.);	31	28
2. Flows related to environmental hygiene (waste disposal, cleaning services, environmental risks, etc.);	9	11
3. Flows related to worker's preventive medicine (vaccination compliance, worker's accidents, etc.);	12	8
4. Flows related to personnel management (personnel turn-over, personnel on duty, etc.);	17	11
5. Flows related to the structure (physical environment, equipment, instruments etc.);	4	4
6. Flows related to resource used (drugs, personnel, diagnostic tests, etc.)	3	1
7. Flows related to output production (DRGs, ambulatory services);	15	4
8. Quality indicators (hospital infections incidence, waiting time for outpatients and inpatients, etc.);	16	11

Table 2: Example of scheme for the DRG informative flow

INFORMATIVE FLOW	FREQUENCY	TRANSMISSION DEADLINE	DOCUMENT PATH		
			SOURCE	OFFICE/ OFFICERS RESPOSIBLE	DESTINATION
DRGs produced per health unit	Monthly	20th following month	Clinical Database	Statistic Office	Health-Care Units

We developed a scheme describing all the steps of the flows with respect to frequency, transmission deadlines, sources, destinations and stating responsibilities for them (table 2). This scheme is official for all personnel operating in the hospital.

A significant part of the information that has been collected is required by law or for administrative use and which is not particularly relevant for health care units, for HHD or for strategic direction (i.e. statistics requested for national/regional purposes).

At the end we developed a reporting system with a minimal set of data [4,9]: output quantity, resources consumes and quality assurance. Due to the nature of the collecting data system and the absence of a linked database reports are published quarterly for the moment.

Data included in the report are: percentage of admission following appropriateness-hospital-use-evaluation protocols [10]; day-hospital activity; ambulatory (outpatient and inpatient) activity; DRGs; health-care-units expense note; n.° of ambulance transports; n° of inpatient's accidents; number of patient's compliance; absenteeism index; number of transfer requests by personnel per health care unit; average waiting time for clinical or laboratory performances; services checks (cleaning, disposables, kitchen, etc.); hospital infections surveys; number of professional accidents.

For some of the still existing flows we tested feedback mechanisms. The use of a quarterly report to health care units on DRGs led to filling in discharge forms more accurately and to a demand for data to analyse (at the moment we send an excel file with all discharging form data and DRGs). A costs report of the single unit strengthened the budget approach in health care workers (HCW) and allowed the hospital administration to correct possible mistakes and to refine the system of attributing costs. The appropriateness-hospital-use-evaluation protocols (regional project) led to a significant reduction of non-acute hospital admissions and to a definition of written clinical protocols (42% 1995 versus 19% 1998 $p < 0.05$).

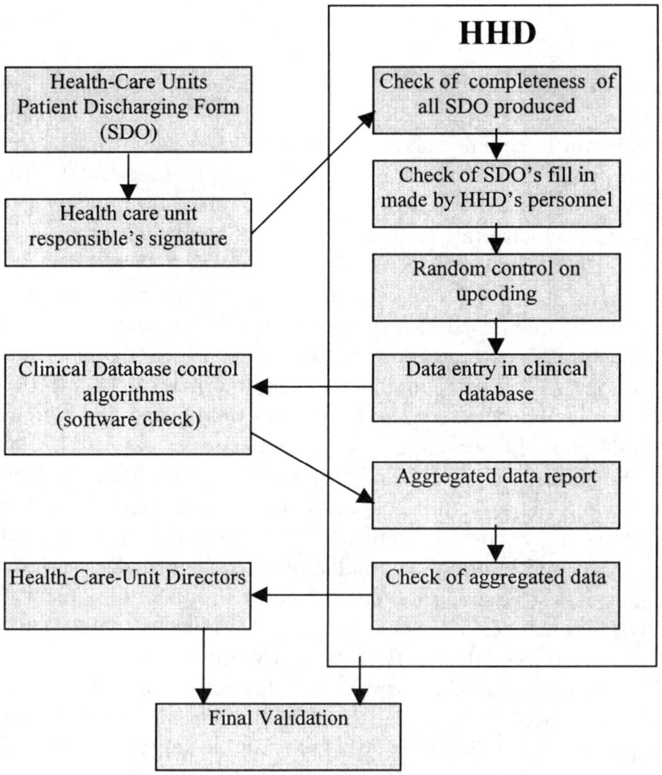

Figure 1: Flow chart for DRG attribution system

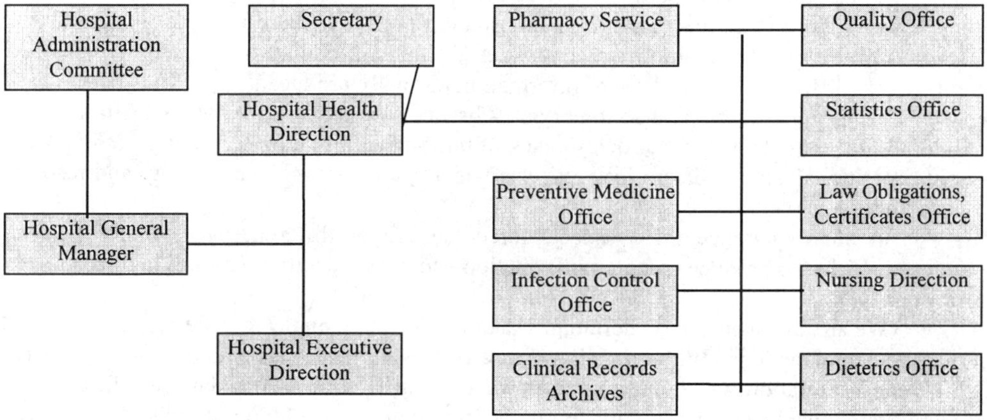

Figure 2: Hospital Health Direction Organisation

4. Discussion

The need for information in modern hospitals is constantly growing, but seldom do we focus our attention on the utility of data already produced and on converting data in information [11]. Our experience shows that most of the existing data are required by-law or for administrative use, not required for management or strategic information. So, if theoretically there is a remarkable amount of data, only a little part are useful to hospital management [4,5,7] and overall few of them are strategic information. Accurate data as well as essential data are major priorities of a management system but there ought to be a common aim among mission, strategies, projects and information collected [12]. In Italy, the IS has historically been used in response to outside necessities (law obligations) rather than to hospital strategies. Another important aspect in managing informative flows are times of production. It is well known that data and information have a cost [3], so it is very important to outline which flow require continuous monitoring and which may be satisfied by periodic evaluation. In our experience data regarding single patients or health care workers must be processed as quickly as possible (i.e. single accident, a surgical site infection, etc..) while data on the hospital output and/or organisation can be evaluated periodically because they must be aggregated to become information. Each hospital has to define the set of data and information and the recurrence needed: it varies in function to the environment, hospital structure, national/regional law obligations, management strategies, etc.... In our system great deal of resources are spent in the attempt to define the operational data flows existing and to model the HHD responsibility areas.

Quality in data is another aspect of information production. It is obvious that information without quality is useless, but also high quality represents an additional expense. It is important to define levels of quality and detail which is needed to reach goals; any additional quality and details represent only additional expenses.

The evolution of the institutional context with laws changing frequently and internal rules require both organisational flexibility and increased collaboration among different functions. This is particularly true for IS. This aspect is particularly relevant if in the hospital there is a lack of uniform informative policy, if there is a prevalence of the "top-down" logic in the informative flow establishment; if data is requested which is completely different from the type of information normally produced.

Technical aspects are also important. Absence of a network for data transmission, in order to prevent data losses and delays, lack of uniform information technology and lack of cost/benefit analysis are determinant aspects which can guarantee data quality and respect dead lines.

In our experience these aspects force the use of different data sources (paper, magnetic disks) to produce complex information and consequently the IS has high costs and low quality [5,13].

We are still working on defining what and how many indicators are really useful for management functions. We are testing the responses of health-care units with respect to different information. Our preliminary tests show that feed-back to a data set often is not enough and must be supported with continuous attention on fixed targets and with tools that leave the user a wide range of possibilities of self analysis.

A last step would be the attempt to transform data produced via a routine process into strategic information.

5. Conclusions

This experience, although specific to an italian context, shows a methodology in defining the amount of existing data flows, the roles and functions of HHD, the existing interfaces inside the hospitals and the role of IS.

This process may lead to different results: suppression of useless data with reduction of costs, improvement in the quality of data, increased capacity to define responsibilities inside the hospital, increased participation of HCW in budget processes, increase in sharing knowledge of operational and management data, a preliminary step for hospital accreditation and/or certification [8].

References

[1] Decreto Legislativo 30/12/1992, n° 502. Supplemento ordinario alla Gazzetta Ufficiale del 30/12/1992, n° 305.
[2] Øvretveit J. : Health Service Quality. Blackwell Scientific Publications. 4.
[3] Archibald R.D. Managing High-Technology Programs and Projects. Second edition Wiley, N.Y. 1992.
[4] Gordon D.; Carter M.; Kunov H.; Dolan A.; Chapman F. A strategic information system to facilitate the use of performance indicators in hospitals. Health Serv Manage Res, 1998 May, 11:2, 80-91.
[5] Minard B.; Fink M.; Brooke G. Deploying a new model for clinical information delivery. Top Health Inf Manage, 1998 Aug, 19:1, 31-8.
[6] Shelton D.; Shen J. A longitudinal analysis of hospital performance using data envelopment analysis. Abstr Book Assoc Health Serv Res, 1997, 14:, 341.
[7] Zanetti M.; Montaguti U. Il medico e il management Accademia Nazionale di Medicina Editore. Modena 1994.
[8] Loiudice M. La gestione del cambiamento in sanità, manuale teorico pratico di project management in sanità. Centro Scientifico Editore. Torino 1998.
[9] Lathrop C.B. Using graphs to consolidate reports to the board. J Healthc Qual, 1997 Jan, 19:1, 26-33
[10] Gertman P.M., Restuccia J. D. The appropriateness Evaluation Protocol: A Technique for Assessing Unnecessary Days of Hospital Care. Medical Care, 1981, 19 855-871.
[11] Peter F. Drucker, "The coming of the New Organisation", Harward Business Review 66, n° 1 (January/February 1988), 45.
[12] Charles J. Austin Information System for Health Services Administration, 4th sd. (Ann Arbor, Michigan: AUPHA Press, 1992), 299.
[13] Zviran M.; Armoni A.; Glezer C. HIS/BUI: a conceptual model for bottom-up integration of hospital information systems. J Med Syst, 1998 Jun, 22:3, 147-59.

Medical Informatics Europe '99
P. Kokol et al. (Eds.)
IOS Press, 1999

An Approach for Access Differentiation Design in Medical Distributed Applications Built on Databases

S. K. Shoukourian, A. M. Vasilyan, A. A. Avagyan, *A. K. Shukurian
Yerevan State University
**Yerevan State Medical University*

Abstract. A formalized "top to bottom" design approach was described in [1] for distributed applications built on databases, which were considered as a medium between virtual and real user environments for a specific medical application.
Merging different components within a unified distributed application posits new essential problems for software. Particularly protection tools, which are sufficient separately, become deficient during the integration due to specific additional links and relationships not considered formerly. E.g., it is impossible to protect a shared object in the virtual operating room using only DBMS protection tools, if the object is stored as a record in DB tables. The solution of the problem should be found only within the more general application framework. Appropriate tools are absent or unavailable.
The present paper suggests a detailed outline of a design and testing toolset for access differentiation systems (ADS) in distributed medical applications which use databases. The appropriate formal model as well as tools for its mapping to a DMBS are suggested. Remote users connected via global networks are considered too.

1. A unified approach for ADS design and testing

An approach (**Figure 1**), suggested in the paper, is to be applied after first steps of the formalized design, including design of an object-oriented model of the system and a preliminary rough distribution of the system functions between a client and a server [1].
The approach allows apply the unified design technique of ADS to various classes of objects within the system. The matter of the technique is a combination of miscellaneous mechanisms and tools for access differentiation, which are usually used separately, within the framework of a unified shell.
It is supposed that as a result of previous steps a specification of ADS, including a tabular description of objects and appropriate limitations for these objects, is already obtained (formulated). The first design stage of the ADS is to define basic data structures and basic algorithms for access differentiation, defined on these structures. Simultaneously a design of corresponding structures and algorithms for the ADS testing has to be carried out. This allows test, reveal and remove mismatches for a given set of limitations at each design stage.
At first design and testing of ADS for users within a local network will be considered. This part of the ADS will be named Internal Security System (ISS).
The limitations considered in [1], lead to an outcome of the target ADS synthesis consisting of two parts: a component of protection control (CPC) and a component of protection generation (CPG). The tools of functional testing of the ADS are also included.
A similar technique will be applied for design and testing of ADS for external users.

2. Key objects of protection

The objects of protection are divided into three classes: functional resources (FR), resources of the information field (IF), time resources and workstations (TR).
Design and synthesis of a ADS for time resources and workstations can be reduced to the creation of interfaces to appropriate services of an operating system and, therefore, to the usage of standard or sufficiently known procedures [2], and these classes are not considered further.

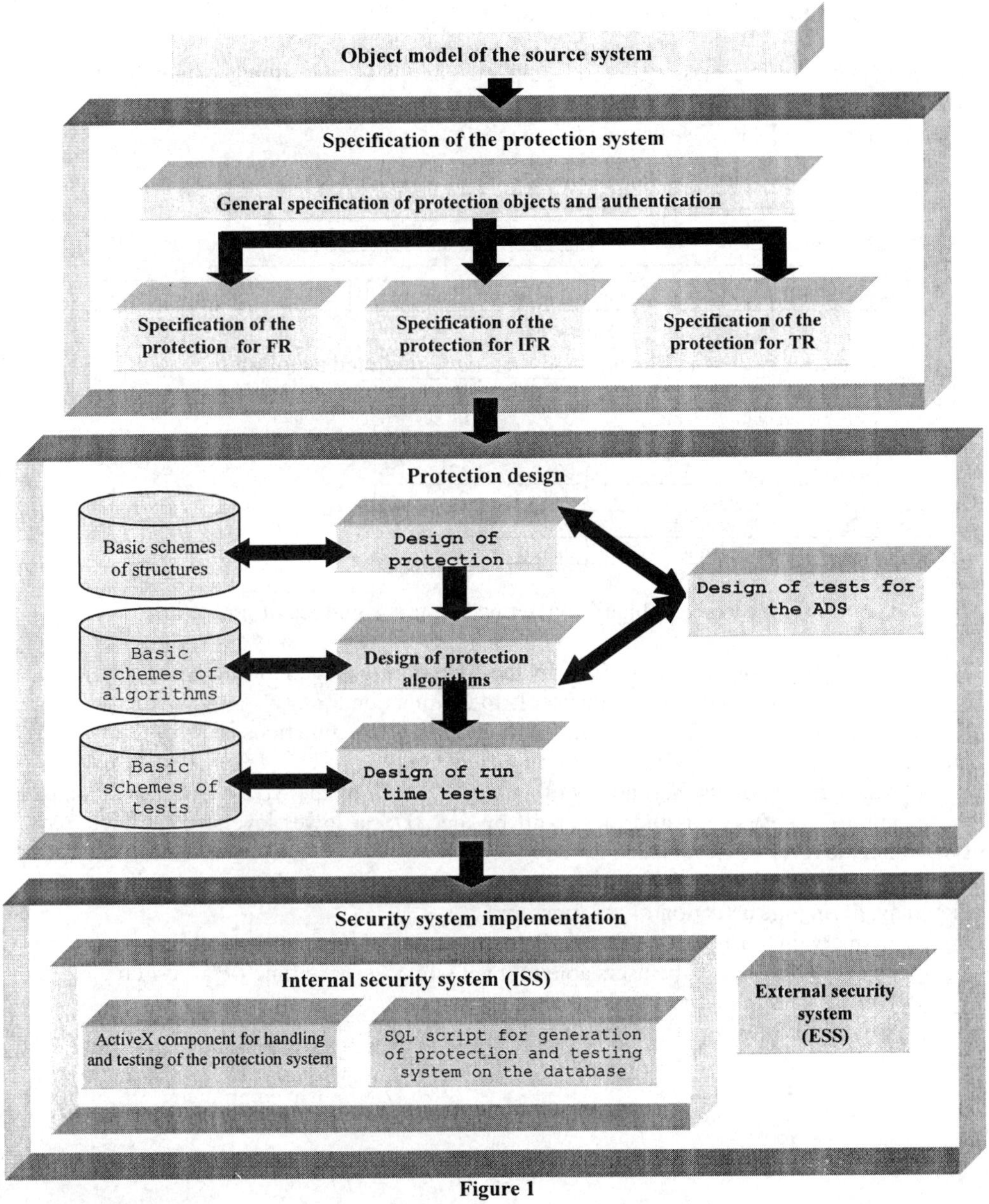

Figure 1

2.1. Design and testing of ADS for the class of functional resources

2.1.1. Specification of the class protection

A specification of the class protection for FR consists of:
- A hierarchical description of FR as a list of units;
- Maximums for embedded levels in a hierarchy of FR, for a total number of functions and users, for a total capacity of required disk memory.

These variable fields and parameters obtain specific values during the design.

2.1.2. Schemes for basic structures of protection

The protection for the class of FR is built on a structure describing a hierarchy of FR (FTREE) and a structure of a protection description for FR (FDESC).
The scheme of the FTREE structure is shown below.

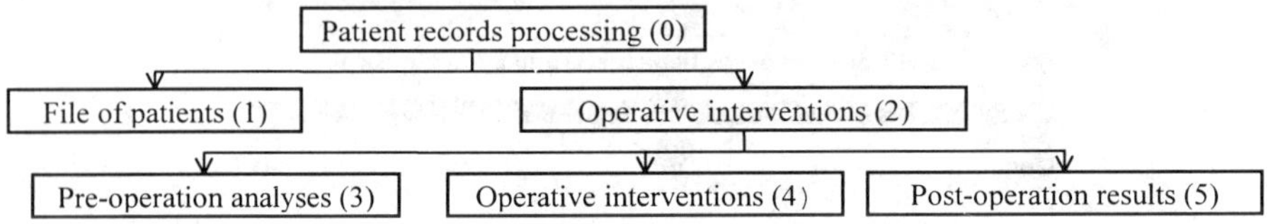

Figure 2

The structure circumscribing this hierarchy can be represented as follows:

F_id	**F_name**	**F_idX**	**F_level**
0	Interaction with patients	0	0
1	File of patients	01	1
2	Operative interventions	02	1
3	Pre-operation analyses	023	2
4	Operative interventions	024	2
5	Post-operation results	025	2

2.1.3. Schemes for basic algorithms (SA) defined on the structures of protection

SA #1. Checking up on authorities built by the ADS during actuation of the function.
SA #2. Changing access rights for the user U to the function F.
SA #3. Optimizing a chain of descriptors for appropriate functions at lower levels of hierarchy, during actuation of the function F for the user U.
SA #4. Checking up on the heritability of authorities, built by the ADS during actuation of the function F, as well as authorities, built by the ADS at lower levels of the hierarchy lower than the level of the actuated function F.
SA #5. Changing access rights for the user U to appropriate functions at lower level hierarchy, during the actuation of the function F.
SA #6. A query on a list of functions available /(not available) for the user U.
SA #7. A query on a list of the users able/(not able) to access the functional resource F.
SA #8. Addition of the user U to the system.
SA #9. Removal of the user U from the system.

2.1.4. Testing of specified limitations

The testing of limitations is reduced to the checking of maximums for total capacity of disk memory, the size of the FTREE, the size of the FDESC.

2.1.5. Basic schemes of testing for protection structures

The scheme of tests #1. Integrity test for structures of the hierarchy description.
The scheme of tests #2. Integrity test for structures of the protection description.

2.1.6. Synthesis of the resulting ADS

The resulting system consists of the ADS and tests on the database server and the ActiveX component, handling protection and testing.
The ActiveX element handles protection and testing and provides a graphic user interface for the dynamic access control, based on calls of algorithms #1 - #9, and for the start of tests #1 and #2. It also allows an administrator to perform an edition of users authorities.
The process of protection design and testing for the class of information filed resources is similar to design and testing of ADS for the class of functional resources.

3. Extension of ISS for external users

A direct addition of the external users to the ISS described above, by increasing parameters of protection, does not seem expedient due to the following basic restriction.
The external connections are performed through existing global computer networks and, in particular, through the highly prevalent Internet network. Difficulties of effective protection methods construction for these networks lead to a significant deterioration of the ISS characteristics and numerous opportunities of the ISS break by the Internet users [3].
Therefore a limited way of access to resources for external users was chosen:
- an external user has access rights only to information, which is exposed in a form of a request for the manipulation from the outside;
- any application to the system is considered only, if it is a response to the previously sent request;
- the exposed information is isolated from the database of local users;
- responses of external users are registered in the appropriate request forms and are brought into the database only as additions, after preliminary testing and checking.

This way of access is realised as a separate External Security System (ESS) of the ADS. It is based on main structural units of request and response schemes or templates.
Design and testing of ADS for the mentioned hierarchy of templates should be done providing heritability of accesses rights from top to bottom on the hierarchy applied.

4. Mathematical model

The constructed model of protection is implemented using an object-oriented technology.
A complete set of equivalent transformations for chains of descriptors is built and problems of their optimisation on criteria of a chain length and time of interpretation are solved. The problem of optimal representation for a given protection process is also solved.

Specific objects corresponding to molds are introduced for protection processes of ESS. Problems of verification and built-in (online) testing for these processes are considered. The mathematical justification is carried out within the model considered in [4].
The detailed description of the mentioned results will be considered in our further publications.

5. Conclusion

The approach proposed here can serve as the foundation of an integrated design and testing tool set supporting access differentiation design for distributed applications built on databases. The approach besides specific medical applications like otosurgery could be used also for more general hospital management systems.

References

[1] S.K.Shoukourian, A.K.Shukurian, A.A.Avagyan, A.M. Vasilyan, Designing a virtual operating room for prediction of operative interventions under some pathologies of middle ear. A case of the database, Proceedings of 9th World Congress on Medical Informatics, Medinfo '98, Seoul, Korea, August 1998.
[2] P.Dusserre, F.-A.Allaert, L.Dusserre, Basic rules for the security of frosen section diagnosis through image transmission between anatomo-pathologists, Proceedings of Medical Informatics Europe' 97 MIE'97, "Studies in Health technology and Informatics", vol.43, pp.171-175, IOS Press, 1997.
[3] M.Norifusa, Internet security: difficulties and solutions, International Journal of Medical Informatics, vol . 49, March 1998, pp.69-74.
[4] S.K.Shoukourian, A Unified Design Methodology for Off-line and On-line testing, IEEE Design and Test of Computers, April-June 1998, pp. 73-79.

Medical Informatics Europe '99
P. Kokol et al. (Eds.)
IOS Press, 1999

Integrated Databases – The Foundation for the Information Linking of the Actors in the National Health Care and Health Insurance Systems

Tomaž Marčun, dipl.ing., Franc Košir, dipl.iur.
Health Insurance Institute of Slovenia

Abstract. Among the characteristics of the present time, we meet the ranking of information among the key resources of effective management of business systems. Up to date, integral and accurate information have gained precedence over conventional economic resources. This applies particularly in the case of large and complex business systems, including the national health care and health insurance systems. High quality and unified databases form the foundation for rational and quality procedures ranging from the operative level to the national strategy level.

The goal of this paper is to demonstrate, on the example of Slovene experience, the importance of keeping quality databases for the purposes of health care and health insurance system management. The paper reviews the achieved level and the plans of further development of unified databases in this sector in Slovenia. The key emphasis in the development of an integrated system has been laid upon establishing uniform primary databases and providing appropriate integration in the area of data interchange among the actors of the health care and health insurance systems and other national systems.

1. Health Insurance and its Role in Penetration of Information Technology into the Health Care Sector in Slovenia

As a Central European country, Slovenia enjoys a tradition of health insurance exceeding one hundred years. After our gaining of political independence in 1991, the general turns in society and development orientation towards a modern European state laid the bases and established prerequisite conditions for a vital modernisation of the existing health care and health insurance system. In February 1992, new legislation was passed. It defined the compulsory health insurance as the primary model of providing social security to the population for the situations of diseases, injuries, and some other further incidences. It further defined the voluntary health insurance as the insurance towards the copayment of the balance between the actual service cost and the amount covered by voluntary health insurance and towards the payment of extra standards services and extra risks. The legislation also instated the Health Insurance Institute of Slovenia as the national provider of compulsory health insurance and appointed it to introduce voluntary health insurance, which can further be provided by other commercial insurance companies. Two major factors of the development of health insurance have been the assertion of private health care practice and implementation of a partnerial approach in the formulation of the scope and the contents of the programme and of the prices of health care services.

Since its foundation, the Health Insurance Institute, in its role of statutory compulsory health insurance provider, has been devoting great attention to the development of the information technology system for its own purposes, as well as actively participating in the formulation of elements of a unified information technology support to all the health care actors in Slovenia. In its strategic development programme, adopted in 1997, the Health Insurance Institute defined databases as the key resource for the carrying out its mission and for a prosperous cooperation with the actors in the health care and other national systems.

From the outset on, the Health Insurance Institute undertook to set up the house information technology system on entirely new foundations, conformant with the new health insurance model and with the Institute's role in this sector. The plan of this radical renovation has been successfully implemented applying the methodologies of project management and methodological support to development. The first objective under this renovation was the establishment of unified and centralised compulsory health insurance and voluntary health insurance databases. This was then followed by the introduction of the health care service provider database, established in the combined effort by the Health Insurance Institute of Slovenia and by the Institute of Health Preservation. All these databases represent the basic groundwork for the information technology solutions in other Health Insurance Institute business functions and for the overall information linking to the health care system and broader environment.

In parallel with the establishment of the house databases, the Health Insurance Institute has been active in the promotion and support of the information technology development in the health care sector and in other sectors. In 1992, an extensive action of equipping of health care service providers with personal computers was carried out, which boosted the equippedness of the Slovene health care sector with information technology to the peak rank among the European countries. This equipment with technology was then followed by the coordination of provision with unified solutions for the keeping of records and accounting of health care services, which represented, to many Slovene health care service providers, the first step towards the building of information technology systems serving to support their business activity. These initial unified information technology solutions were upgraded by a series of solutions providing higher quality operation of the health care service providers and higher quality data gathering for the purposes of health care statistics at the regional and national levels. In 1994, progressive introduction of electronic data interchange was undertaken, for the accounting of health care services, between the service providers and the Health Insurance Institute of Slovenia. This electronic data interchange resulted in a reduction of costs and shortening of procedure times. The year 1996 saw the introduction of a new national health insurance identifier. The health insurance number, being an autonomous unique identifier of an insured person or contribution obligor, provides autonomy of the health care and health insurance systems from other national identifiers of natural and legal persons, which are, from time to time, exposed to political initiatives towards their abolishment.

The latest momentous step in rising the quality and extent of information support of the health care sector is the introduction of the health insurance card. The health insurance card, a smart microprocessor based card, is a personal identifier the insured person, which, in addition to accurate personal details, brings the data on the card holder's status of health insurances to the health care service providers. After the successful introduction in the pilot region last year, the national scope introduction was undertaken early this year.

2. Integrated Health Insurance Databases and the Interchange of Data with External Partners Within and Outside the Health care System

In designing integral health insurance databases, the main goal of was the establishment of unified and integral databases. It was recognised that extensive national scope databases can only be a quality business asset only provided they are set up in an appropriately unified manner. Unification and integration of databases translates to the formulation of common primary data collections, kept in a technologically centralised manner, subsequently enhanced by data collections for individual business sectors. The common primary data records, such as the records of natural and legal persons, serve as the uniform basis for all the other sectoral records. The unification of databases not only ensures an effective source of data, but also contributes towards the reduction of the costs of their management. This reduction of costs arises above all from the fact that with the central records, the need of keeping of the primary data records in every business sector is eliminated and the keeping is reduced to one instance only. Here follows the description of the structure of the integrated databases - starting with the primary data collections and ranging to the separate data collections in particular business sectors.

2.1. Health Insurance Primary data Collections

The primary core of the health care / health insurance databases consists of the persons (physical persons) and organisations (legal entities) data collections. Both collections are complete with address details (address of residence or business seat).

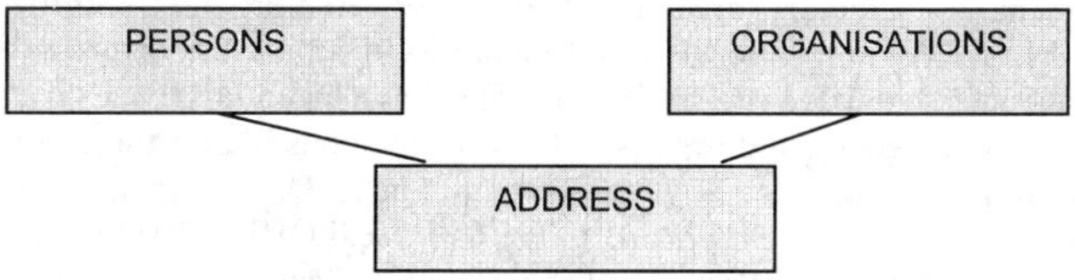

Figure 1. Health insurance primary data collections

The persons data collection serves as the basis to all other data collections denoting physical persons (insured persons, physicians, ...). On the other hand, the organisations data collection serves as the basis to all data collections denoting legal entities in their various roles (contribution obligors, health care service providers, ...).

The above two data collections are maintained in the process of registering of persons into compulsory health insurance and are regularly updated with modifications of data in the population, territorial unit and business enterprise national registers kept by the Ministry of Internal Affairs and by the Statistical Office. These sources provide, on a monthly basis, data on all key changes, and are entered in a corresponding controlled procedure. In this manner, the quality currency of data is ensured, as well as their accordance with official data on persons and enterprises. Upon our integration into the European structures, the link of the persons data collection to the national registers will provide the accordance of data with the unified European Union databases.

2.2. The Basic Health Insurance Sectoral Data Collections

Upon the primary database collections, the basic health insurance sectoral data collections are derived: the data collections of insured persons and of contribution obligors, and the data collection of health care service providers. The *insured persons database* is the register of all persons covered by compulsory health insurance. The comparison of the insured person data collection with the primary data collection of all physical persons offers the means of monitoring of the status of incorporation of the population of Slovenia in compulsory health insurance. The *contribution obligors* are those legal entities or physical persons who are, by statute, bound to register their employees into compulsory health insurance and to settle their health insurance contributions. By means of linking this data collection with the primary registers of persons and organisations, the Health Insurance Institute is enabled to monitor their status and to undertake appropriate measures in the cases of declaration of bankruptcy, death, etc. The *health care service providers* register hosts the details of all institutions providing health care services, of all physicians and of all other health care personnel and their employment details. The health care service providers register is managed by the Institute of Health Preservation, while in terms of technology, the database is set up in the Health Insurance Institute central computer and is used by both organisations.

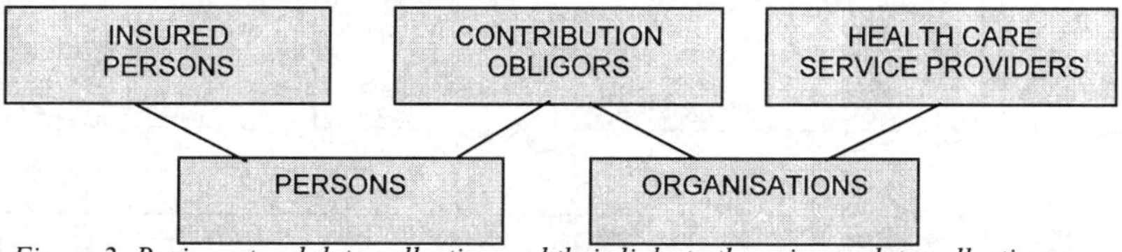

Figure 2: Basic sectoral data collection and their links to the primary data collections

2.3. Integral Business Data Collections

Upon the basic sectoral data collections, the integral business data collections have been set up, hosting the data necessary for efficient information technology support to particular procedures and business areas.

In the segment of collection of income, of a key significance is an integral *compulsory health insurance data collection*, which keeps the details of all compulsory health insurance policies taken by insured persons, together with the details of the corresponding insurance contribution obligors. The compulsory health insurance data collection facilitates the reporting of data on new insurances, modifications and registering out of insurance to the pension and invalidity insurance system and to the employment system, since the effective agreement in Slovenia provides a unified procedure for the registering into health insurance, pension and invalidity insurance, and for the purposes of the Institute of Employment. The unified registering into the above listed insurances is carried out at the Health Insurance Institute counters, and the Institute is also responsible for the entry of data into the information system and the corresponding reporting of data. The compulsory health insurance register also serves as the basis for the reporting to the Statistical Office for the purposes of national statistical processing and to the tax offices for the purposes of accounting supervision, settlement and recovery of compulsory health insurance contributions.

The *register of selected personal physicians* is a unified register of all patients' declarations of general physicians, dentists and gynaecologists opted for by the insured persons pursuant to the regulations. The law provides the personal physician to be an overall custodian of the state of health of the persons declared, and assigns him the task and responsibility of referring the patient to specialists or hospitals, and of prescribing drugs on account of the health insurance funds, of gathering and keeping the medical records and of determining the patient's inability to work. The register of selected personal physicians is linked to the basic sectoral data collections of insured persons and of service providers (including the data collection of physicians). The data on the selections of personal physicians is collected by the Health Insurance Institute from the health care service providers where the selections have been declared.

An extensive data collection serving for the support of the *checking and settling of invoices of the service providers* facilitates a high quality performance of complex procedures of checking and settling of invoices. The invoice checking procedures are tied to the checking of insured persons' insurance statuses, hence this data collection is closely linked to the insured persons data collection. This data collection is of vital importance in the provision of analytical data for the purposes of drafting of health care service expenditure plans and for the purposes of the monitoring of their implementation.

The *signing and monitoring of the contracts with service providers* are supported by the registers kept in this business sector. The registers support the entire cycle of the annual agreement and signing of contracts between the health care service providers and the health insurance provider.

The health insurance information system encompasses, as an integral part, also the segment of *medical boards*. The data collections of this segment are built upon the insured persons and health care service providers data collections.

In the process of introduction of the health insurance cards, the Health Insurance Institute, being their issuer, requires integral records for the purposes of the monitoring of the data cycle of each card. To this end, health insurance card administration registers have been developed. These registers are linked to the insured persons and contribution obligors data collections.

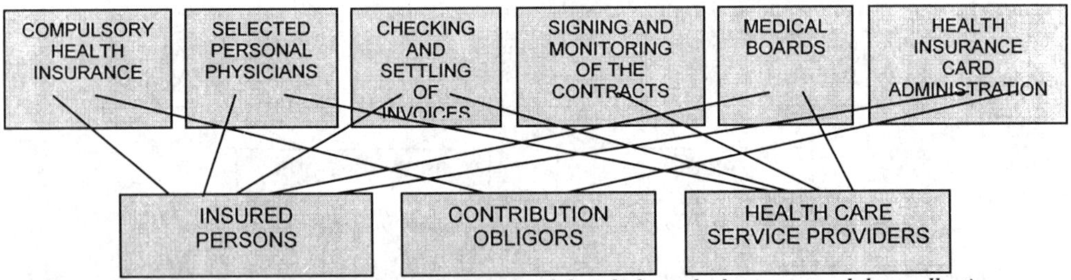

Figure 3: Integral business sector data collections and their links to the basic sectoral data collections

2.4. Planning and analyses, decision making support, support to national statistics

In addition to operative records, the effectiveness of the management of the health insurance system closely depends on the registers serving for the purposes of planning and analyses, and of decision

making processes. The development of extensive databases is in progress, to facilitate the process of interactive data analyses, reporting, statistical processing and data mining on large volumes of data. The results of the said procedures and techniques will facilitate the preparation of high quality data input to the decision making processes.
At the same time, the data methodically gathered from operations registers and databases serve for the purposes of statistical reporting at the national level to the Ministry of Health care and to research organisations.

3. Modern Data Stream Channels

The numerous forms of data interchange between the health insurance and other national systems referred to in this contribution demand high quality approaches in the segment of data transfer as well. Back in 1994, the Health Insurance Institute undertook the introduction of electronic data interchange in the segment of invoices, between the health care service providers and the Institute. This data interchange is based on the international EDIFACT standard and incorporates high quality solutions regarding data security. This particular data interchange has been enhanced, in the recent period, by the data on drug dispensing in pharmacies, and data on the selection of personal physicians. By the end of the year, all the health care service providers under contract are to transfer to this mode of data interchange. Up to now, due to a high initial investment in technology, this mode of data transmission has won recognition most of all with large service providers, but lately, non-expensive solutions are available, which will render the method accessible to small service providers as well.

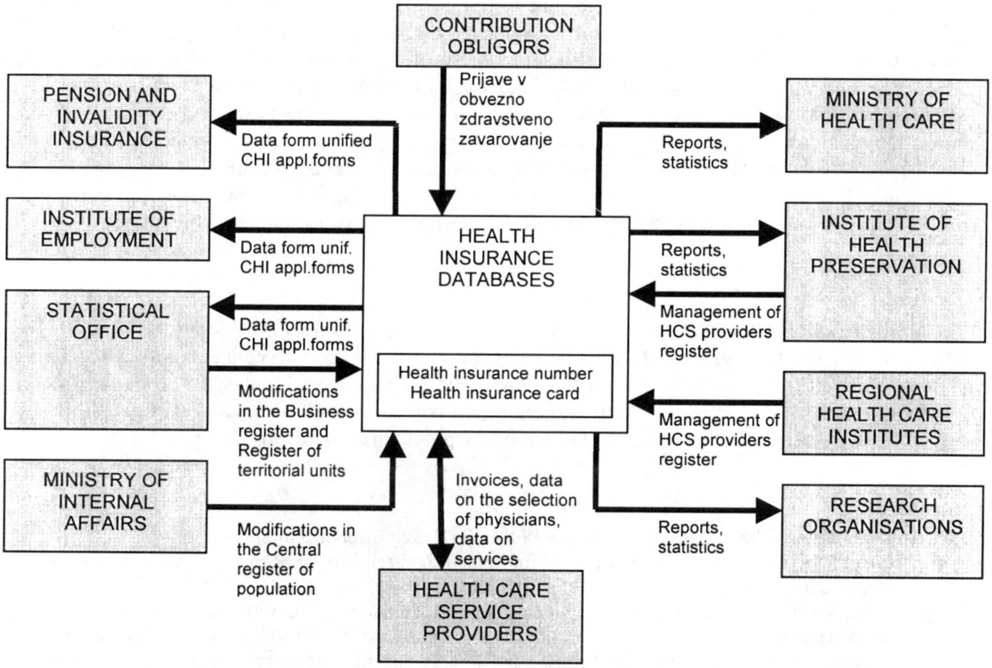

Figure 4: Data interchange between the health insurance databases and the actors within and outside the health care system

Interchange of data with partners outside health care, too, relies, in most cases on the electronic data interchange technology. Particular solutions depend on the technology options of partners.

A further important factor of quality of the interchange of data, particularly in the direction between the health insurance and the health care service providers, is the health insurance card. The card facilitates the transfer of up to date and accurate personal and insurance details of insured persons to the service providers. In this way, a higher quality level of health care service providers' databases is ensured. Applying the health insurance number as the insured persons' identifier, the service providers' databases are turning into a component of the integrated databases of the health care sector in its broadest sense. The transmission of accurate card holders' details provides the health care service providers with the ability of high quality accounting and invoicing of services and facilitates the settling of invoices.

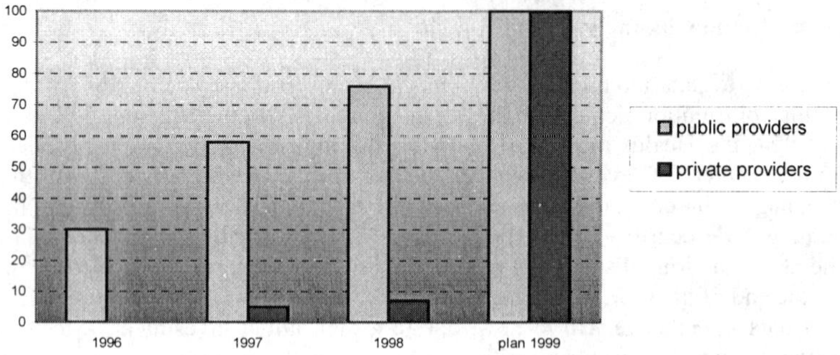

Figure 5: The percentage of service providers practising electronic data interchange

4. Plans for the Future

Even with the predominant part of the health insurance business functions adequately provided in terms of information technology by unified databases, there is no lack of major or minor tasks ahead. In the case of basic operations registers, we aim to participate, in an active manner, in the final setting up of an unified national drug database, to provide the performance of more detailed expenditure analyses, to provide information support to the tasks of supervision of the implementation of contracts with the health care service providers regarding the accounting of health care services and the insured persons' implementation of rights. We are planning, intensively, to expand the contents of the databases and to facilitate the development of new ones - in particular, for the inter-sectoral analyses and reporting for the purposes of decision making processes.

5. Conclusion

The unified national level databases in the sector of health insurance in Slovenia serve as the foundation for the health care databases and facilitate high quality interconnection of information systems. The orderly maintenance of the national data collections facilitates the promotion of the quality of health care services due to the superior quality of data, and the reduction of overall health care costs, due to the efficiency of carrying out of the procedures involved.

References

[1] Franc Košir, Zdravstveno zavarovanje v Sloveniji (Health Insurance in Slovenia), 3/95

[2] doc.dr.Marjan Premik, Javnozdravstveni informacijski sistemi (Information Systems in the Public Health care System), contribution to the DMI congress, 9/96

[3] Franc Košir, Uvajanje elektronskega poslovanja med Zavodom za zdravstveno zavarovanje Slovenije in izvajalci zdravstvenega varstva (Introduction of Electronic Business Conduit between the Health Insurance Institute of Slovenia and the Health Care Service Providers), paper in the "Organizacija" periodical, 3/98

[4] ZZZS, Strateški razvojni program (Strategic Development Programme), 5/97

[5] ZZZS, Zasnova sistema kartice zdravstvenega zavarovanja (Design of the Health Insurance Card), 12/96

[6] ZZZS, Projektna dokumentacija projekta RIP (The EDI Project Design Documents), 01/99

[7] Tone Košir, Meta Mencej, Zdravstveni zakoni – zakoni s pojasnili in komentarjem (The Health Care Laws with Comments), 1992

Medical Informatics Europe '99
P. Kokol et al. (Eds.)
IOS Press, 1999

Compulsory Health Insurance Databases

Janez Svoljšak, Irma Dovžan
Health Insurance Institute of Slovenia

Abstract. The compulsory health insurance databases represent fundamental infrastructure to the implementation of the Health Insurance Institute of Slovenia (HIIS) operations, i.e. for its effective performance in all the fields of its business. This paper presents the legal bases of the database management, the logocal database structure, the supply of data from various data sources, and the role of databases as the primary source of supply for the data collections kept by other institutions in Slovenia.

1. The health insurance institute of Slovenia (HIIS) primary business

The HIIS primary business activity is compulsory health insurance, which provides to the persons affiliated and fulfilling all the obligatory conditions, with social security in the events of disease, injury, birth giving or death.

To this end, the HIIS is, by statute, the manager of compulsory health insurance databases, which keep data on insured persons affiliated in compulsory health insurance, and data on their employers, who are, by statute, authorised and responsible for the registering of persons into insurance and of settling the insurance contributions. The databases' purposes are :

- They enable, at any moment, the examination whether a particular insured person fulfils the obligatory conditions to be entitled particular rights deriving from compulsory health insurance.
- They facilitate the preparation of statistical data serving as the basis for the formulation and implementation of the health care and health insurance policies in Slovenia.

1.1 Insured Persons

The HIIS keeps the following data on insured persons:

General personal details : family name and first name, date of birth, nationality, citizenship status in Slovenia, address of permanent or temporary residence as appropriate, validity of residence visa for foreigners

Data on the dates, forms and conditions of affiliation in compulsory health insurance : date of commencement or termination of insurance, insurance status, validity of temporary working permit in the cases of foreigners, validity of certificate of school attendance, ...

- *Data on the obligor* for the registering into insurance and for the settling of compulsory health insurance contribution

Insured persons fall into two categories:

- **Insurees**

  This category comprises those insured persons that are actual holders of compulsory health insurance. They are affiliated in health insurance on the bases of applicable

conditions (status of employee in R Slovenia, carrying out individual economic or professional activity in Slovenia, receiving various financial compensations or allowances in Slovenia, ...).
For the duration of affiliation of an insured person of this category in insurance, the respective contribution obligor is paying insurance contribution for the person; such contributions make the compulsory health insurance funds.

- **Family members**
  This category comprises those insured persons who are affiliated in insurance through their holders of compulsory health insurance (insurees), subject to conditions provided in the law . Entitlement to such a status covers spouses, children, step children, grand children etc. For the duration of affiliation of an insured person of this category in insurance, no specific compulsory health insurance contribution is paid.

1.2 Obligors

The contribution obligors can be either physical persons or legal entities.
Their role is dual:

- Submission of applications for the registering of insured persons into and out of compulsory health insurance, and applications for any modifications during the affiliation in insurance.
- Settling of compulsory health insurance contributions during the insured persons (insurees) affiliation in insurance.

The HIIS keeps the following data on obligors:

General details of legal entities :type of organisation, title, activity according to SKD classification, date of entry into and erasure from the court register, business address, ... or, *general details of physical persons* :family name, first name, date of birth, date of death, citizenship, address of permanent or temporary residence, validity of residence visa in the cases of foreigners, ...

Specific data on obligors :date of commencement and expiration of the obligation of the payment of compulsory health insurance contribution, date of registering out of insurance, obligor's tax number, ...

2. Compulsory health insurance (CHI) register logical scheme

2.1 Breakdown of Insured Persons

An insured person may enter compulsory health insurance either as an insuree or as a family member of an insuree, who, in such a case, is called the insurance holder.
Basically, the compulsory health insurance is a relation between the insured person and the contribution obligor,
or between the family member and the insuree covered by a valid compulsory health insurance.
Based on this relation, an insured person enters compulsory health insurance.
The particularity of this rule lies in the fact that a family member enjoys valid compulsory health insurance subject to the validity of compulsory health insurance of his/her insurance holder (insuree).

In a schematic form:

Insured person = insuree

has M / *belongs 1*

compulsory insurance = relation between insuree and contribution obligor

belongs 1 / *has M*

contribution obligor

Insured person = family member

has 1 / *belongs 1*

family relation

belongs 1 / *has M*

insuree

has M / *belongs 1*

compulsory insurance = relation between insuree and contribution obligor

belongs 1 / *has M*

contribution obligor

2.2 Breakdown of Contribution Obligors

Pursuant the Law on Health Care and Health Insurance, the contribution obligors may be physical persons
or business enterprises
In view of data to be kept on a contribution obligor (= title of the obligor) by the HIIS, the obligors are categorised in the following manner:
- the data of either a person or an organisation (i.e. any type of entity other than person).
- the specific obligor data regardless of the obligor type.

A person or organisation may turn up in several instances as a contribution obligor. Thus, a borough may be a contribution obligor for:
- the employees in borough administration, and
- the persons without any personal income.

3. Implementation of the CHI registers

Based on the logical scheme and on the accessibility of data from official registers, we defined the CHI relational database:

Data collection – table	Role in the logical scheme	Official register	Role in the implementation
PERSONS	Insured persons (insurees + family members), Obligors (persons)	CRP	Infrastructure
ORGANISATIONS	Obligors (persons)	PRS	Infrastructure
ADDRESSES	Addresses of persons + addresses of organisations	CRP, PRS, RTE	Infrastructure
OBLIGORS	Obligors	HIIS	CHI
COMPULSORY HEALTH INSURANCE	Relation between the insured person and the obligor	HIIS	CHI
FAMILY MEMBERS	Relation between the insuree and the family member	HIIS	CHI

Every person or organisation has at least one address.
If an organisation appears in CHI, it can only appear as a contribution obligor.
Contribution obligor may be either a person or an organisation.
In CHI, a person may appear as a contribution obligor and/or insured person.
If appearing as an insured person, it may be either an insuree or a family member.

4. Supply of data to compulsory health insurance databases

4.1 Data Capture in HIIS

The compulsory health insurance databases are primarily kept by the officers in the registering service in the HIIS regional units and branch offices, by entering of data from the statutorily prescribed forms and public documents applied by the obligors' in regulating the insured persons' insurance. After being successfully verified, any such modification becomes accessible to all other information technology supported HIIS business sectors that utilise the integrally interlinked compulsory health insurance databases.

The major information technology supported procedures carried out by the registering service officers in day-to-day maintenance of compulsory health insurance databases:

- **Maintenance of data on business entities**
- **Maintenance of data on physical persons**
- **Maintenance of data on contribution obligors**
- **Maintenance of data on insurees**
- **Maintenance of data on family members**

4.2 Supply of Databases from Other Official National Registers

HIIS also updates its compulsory health insurance databases, on the basis of statutorily provided legal bases, from several other official national registers.

Central register of population : The collection of data on persons having permanent residence in R Slovenia. This database is kept by the Ministry of Internal Affairs. Reported on a monthly basis.

Business register of RS : The collection of data on all business entities having their business seat in R Slovenia. Its manager is SURS. Reported on a monthly basis.

Register of territorial units : The collection of data on all territorial units of R Slovenia (boroughs, towns, villages, streets). Its manager is SURS. Reported on a monthly basis.

5. Reporting of data to external institutions

Under the auspices of the Ministry of Work, Family and Social Affairs, a project of rationalisation of reporting and gathering of identical data for the purposes of keeping and maintaining of data collections on insured persons and employees has been under way for several years. This project enrols:

the Health Insurance Institute of Slovenia;
the Pension and Invalidity Insurance Institute of Slovenia;
the Employment Institute of Slovenia, and
The Office of Statistics of Slovenia (SURS).

Multipurpose application of identical data gathered and captured only in one instance, implies rationalisation for the data providers (insurance contribution obligors, employers) in their carrying out of obligations, as well as rationalisation on the part of data collection managers, who require such data in their operation:

- The entry of data on registering in / registering out / modifications of insured persons and employees is carried out applying *common M forms*.
- In the formulation of the contents of the M forms, *unified methodological principles and standards* have been agreed, with due consideration of all specific requirements of individual data collection management institutions.
- *Common methodological bases* have been published, providing instructions for the completion of forms, unified statistical standards and the list of mandatory data in registering into insurance and registering of employment.
- Data capture from the M forms under information technology support is carried out in the HIIS.
- The data so captured are reported, under corresponding agreements and contracts, to the following institutions:

  ⇒ **Office of Statistics of RS :** Pursuant to the Law on National Statistics, this office is the statutory manager of the Statistical Register of all occupationally active population. It gathers data for the purposes of statistical research in the field of work, monitors the status of employment from the viewpoint of demographic research by fields.

  ⇒ **The Pension and Invalidity Insurance Institute of Slovenia :** Pursuant to the Law on Central Registers, this Institute is the statutory manager of the Central Register of persons affiliated in pension and invalidity insurance. It gathers data on pension and invalidity insurees and on the contribution obligors, for the purposes of procedures of implementing the rights derived from pension and invalidity insurance.

  ⇒ **The Employment Institute of Slovenia :** Pursuant to the Law on Employment and Insurance for the Case of Unemployment, this Institute is the statutory manager of the data collection for the purposes of monitoring the evolution of employment and unemployed persons by sectors.

  ⇒ **Tax Administration of Slovenia :** In accordance with the Law on Tax Service, this Administration is the statutory manager of the tax obligor database. It gathers data for the purposes of supervision of accounting, settling and recovery of compulsory health insurance contributions and of other statutorily provided contributions and duties.

6. The primary chi registers - its role as the HIIS infrastructure

Under the primary CHI registers, the following data collections are assigned infrastructural character:
- ORGANISATIONS
- PERSONS
- ADDRESSES.

The primary CHI register serves as the basis for:
<u>a) the insured persons' implementation of rights derived from CHI:</u>

- accounting and disbursement of compensations and allowances;
- approval and registering of technical aids;
- processing by medical boards;
- absence from work

b) register of the partnerial service provider segment under the health insurance and health care system and of related business sectors:
- health care service providers
- physicians

c) CHI register and register of the service providers together provide the complete data infrastructure for IHIS's primary business activity.

7. Conclusion

The HIIS primary mission is the provision of compulsory health insurance in the sense of providing the population the basic social security in the events of disease, injury, or birth giving. In information technology support to implementing this mission, a major role is assigned to the compulsory health insurance registers including their infrastructure.

This support has been implemented by the HIIS so as to ensure equal availability, applicability, currency and uniqueness of these data to all business sectors within HIIS.

The above facts demonstrate the CHI database as the primary and indispensable data basis for the entirety of the HIIS operations.

References

[1] Zakon o zdravstvenem varstvu in zavarovanju (Law on Health Care and Health Insurance), 3/96

[2] Metodolo{ko gradivo I (Methodologic bases I), 1/87, reprint with amendments, 11/98

[3] Reporting of data for the purposes of establishing and keeping of the central register of the pension and invalidity insurance, of the central register of health insurance, and of the record of entering employment status (M-1, M-2, M-1A, M-3, M-3A, M-D^)

[4] ZZZS, Pravila obveznega zdravstvenega zavarovanja s pojasnili in izvedbenimi navodili (Regulations on compulsory health insurance, complete with clarifications and instructions on implementation), 9/95

[5] ZZZS, Informacijski model, a`urna verzija repozitorija CASE orodja (Information model, current version of the CASE tool repository)

Medical Informatics Europe '99
P. Kokol et al. (Eds.)
IOS Press, 1999

Database for gynecological laparoscopy

Elena BERNAD
University Clinic of Obstetrics and Gynecology "Bega", Timisoara
Sandor BERNAD
"Politehnica" University, Department of Hydraulic Machinery, Timisoara
Ioan MUNTEANU
University Clinic of Obstetrics and Gynecology "Bega", Timisoara

Abstract. Laparoscopy is a wonderful tool for performing gynecologic surgery. Whether or not laparoscopic surgery is advisable to diagnose or treat a particular gynecologic problem requires a careful consultation with an experienced gynecologist, who can help the patient weight the pros and cons of laparoscopy versus other options. For the management of this kind of surgical intervention we realise a computer based patient record.

1. Introduction

Nowadays most clinicians are still working with the paper records without being convinced that the electronic patient record (EPR) offers more advantages. More publications in medical informatics emphasize the (dis)advantages of a paper-based record compared to the EPR [1, 2]. The conclusion is that the paper-based record offers various disadvantages compared to the functionality of the EPR.

Because the "electronic patient record" should be used to describe a mechanism for storing patient data that facilitates solving recognized healthcare problem [3]; we create an EPR for gynecological laparoscopic surgery. The benefits of an EPR are well known - such as an integrated view of patient data, access to knowledge resources, proactive influence on physician order entry and clinician data capture, integrated communications support, and clinical decision support.

2. Medical informations

Laparoscopy is a procedure that involves insertion of a narrow telescope-like instrument through a small incision in the belly button. This allows visualization of the abdominal and pelvic organs including the area of the uterus, fallopian tubes and ovaries.

When compared to open surgery (surgery via big incision, usually 5-7 inches long), laparoscopic surgery offers patients many benefits including:

- less post-operative pain
- shorter hospital stay (ranges from few hours to 48 hours instead of 3-7 days)
- faster return to normal activities (1-2 weeks instead of 4-6 weeks)
- more cosmetic (small scars if any)

The decision to perform a laparoscopic procedure is a very individual issue that requires close consultation between the patient and her physician. Laparoscopy is almost always an "outpatient" procedure, meaning patients feel well enough to go home the same evening as their surgery.

Indications for gynecologic laparoscopy include the following:

- pelvic pain
- infertility endometriosis
- tubal ligation (tying tubes)
- tubal (ectopic) pregnancies
- pelvic inflammatory disease
- repairing damaged fallopian tubes
- lysis of adhesions (removing scar tissue)
- laparoscopic assisted vaginal hysterectomy
- removal of ovarian cysts or the entire ovary
- evaluation and removal lymph nodes
- diagnosis and treatment of some uterine anomalies
- destroying or removing some uterine fibroid tumors

Because of the cost and invasive nature of laparoscopy it should not be the first procedure or diagnosis test performed as part of the couple infertility diagnostic evaluation. In general, semen analysis, hysterosalpingogram and documentation of ovulation should be assessed prior to consideration of laparoscopy. For example, if the woman has a clear ovulation problem or her male partner has a severe sperm defect then it is unlikely that laparoscopy will provide additional useful information that will help them to conceive.

Complications associated with laparoscopy include the possibility of damage to other structures in the pelvs such as the bladder, ureter, bowel and blood vessels. Unexpected open surgery (larger incision) is always a possibility, but is very uncommon. Any surgery can have an anesthesia-related complication or be associated with post-operative infection, such as a skin infection at an incision site. Fortunately, all of these complications are very unusual when laparoscopy is expertly performed on young, healthy women.

In our clinic, we use the laparoscopy more as a step from in vitro fertilization (IVF) program. IVF involves taking eggs from the woman, fertilizing them in the laboratory with her partner's sperm and transferring the resulting embryos back to her uterus (usually 2 or 3) days later. IVF can be used as an effective treatment for infertility of all causes except for women with infertility caused by an anatomic problem with the uterus, such as severe intrauterine adhesions.

Every laparoscopy is finished with a laparoscopy report which describe the status of the internal genital organs. This report together with the film of the operation is added at another investigation maked by the patient in the FIV program.

3. Structure and functionality

The application was structured in three parts:

1. the first part contain general data about the patient

2. the second part contains the results of the laboratories, clinical and paraclinical examinations
3. the third part describe the surgical intervention and the postoperator evolution of the patient

The general data are provided from the patient paper record. The data resulted from different examination, laboratories or other paraclinical respective investigations are provided from the respective department.

Each laparoscopic intervention is recorded on the videotape - figure 1. From here, we include in the application just the principal parts of the surgical intervention as animation.

So, the user can see just the surgical procedures as movie in the application. If he want to see the complete operation, he searches the videotape. Therefore the application contain a location of the surgical intervention on the videotape.

With GYN-LAP the gynecologist can make different reports. The physician can query the database to make statistics [4].

4. Actual state

Today, the database contains the data with the patients, which made laparoscopic operations from 1996 to 1998. Each of them was introduced from the paper-based patient records. Because of the well-known disavantages of the paper-based record, from 1999, the data are stored directly on the PC.

5. Security problems

We try to prevent of the unauthorised disclosure of information, to prevent of unauthorised modification of information and to prevent of unauthorised withholding of information or resources in order to have accurate patient data. Therefore the data are introduced by a single person who is authorised to do it. The access is permited just after a password. The other users has just the possibility to read the data, but no possibility to modify it [5].

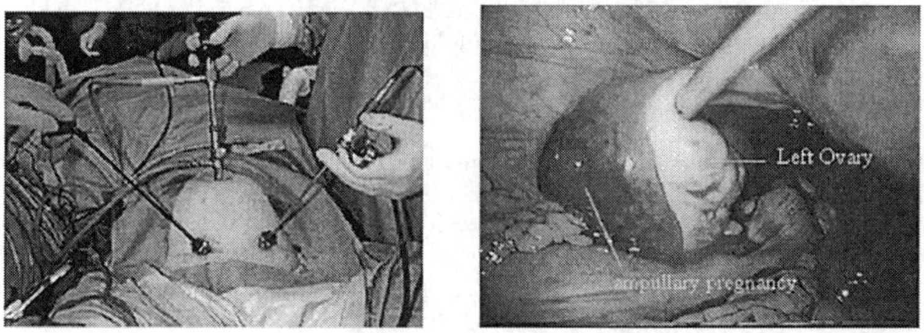

Figure 1 - Imaging from laparoscopy

6. Implementation

The application has a friendly interface. To implement it, we used Microsoft Visual Basic and Microsoft Access. The movies which were introduced in the database are "avi" files. To run it we used the Media Clip application. For a better management of the laparoscopy images including in the database, the movies are saved on compact disks.

To run the application it is necessary less a Pentium PC 200MHz, 64M RAM with CD-ROM.

7. Future intent

Because of the more types of data which provide from more sources, we intend to realise another application where:

- the demographic data will be introduced on the administration;
- the results of the examinations will be written by the physician who examinated the patient;
- laboratories and different paraclinical examinations will be complete by respective departamentes;
- the description of the surgical intervention and the postoperation evolution of the patient will be written by the surgeon;
- the nurses will complete the nurses notes.

In the near future, we intend to realize a little information system, which will connect the examinationroom [6], the laboratory, and the ultrasonography with the surgicalroom. Thus, the data will be introduced more rapidly, and it will be up to date in every moment.

References

[1] RS Dick, EB Steen, The computer based patient record. An essential technology for healthcare, Washington DC: National Academy Press,1991

[2] P. W. Moorman, A. M. van Ginneken, P.D. Siersema, J. van der Lei, J.H. van Bemmel, Evaluation of reporting based on descriptional knowledge, Yearbook of Medical Informatics (Eds. Jan H. van Bemmel, Alexa T. McCray), Schattauer, 1996

[3] D. Pitty, C. Gordon, P. Reeves, A. Capey, P. Vieyra, T. Rickards, The place of SGML and HTML in Building Electronic Patient Records, Proceeding of Medical Informatics Europe, (Eds. C. Pappas, N. Maglaveras, J-R. Scherrer), IOS Press, 1997

[4] S. I. Chowdhury, Computer-based support for Knowledge Extraction from Clinical Database, Linkoping, 1990

[5] Albert Bakker, Security in perspective; luxury or must?, CD with Proceedings of The 9th World Congress on Medical Informatics, IOS Press, eds. B. Cesnik, A.T. McCray, J.-R. Scherrer, 1998

[6] G. L. Solomon, M. Dechter, Are patients pleased with the computer use in the examination room?, Yearbook of Medical Informatics (Eds. Jan H. van Bemmel, Alexa T. McCray), Schattauer, 1996

Medical Informatics Europe '99
P. Kokol et al. (Eds.)
IOS Press, 1999

Application Report: Preliminary Evaluation of the T-IDDM Project in Pavia

R. Bellazzi, A. Riva, S. Montani, C. Larizza, M. Bestazza, S. Fiocchi[1], G. d'Annunzio [1], R. Lorini[2], M. Stefanelli
Dipartimento di Informatica e Sistemistica, Universita' di Pavia, Italy
[1] Clinica Pediatrica, IRCCS Policlinico S. Matteo, Pavia, Italy
[2] Dipartimento di Pediatria, Universita' di Genova, Istituto G. Gaslini, Genova, Italy

We present the preliminary results of the verification phase of the EU funded T-IDDM [1,2] (Telematic Management of Insulin Dependent Diabetes Mellitus) project, collected at the Pediatric Department of Policlinico S. Matteo Hospital in Pavia.
The T-IDDM architecture is composed by two main elements: a Patient Unit (PU), devoted to collecting data and to providing suggestions to patients, and a Medical Unit (MU), that supports physicians in the overall patient management process. The two units are connected through a telecommunication system, that allows the patients to send their home monitoring data, and the physicians to revise and send back the therapeutic protocol in the light of the collected information; moreover patients and physicians may rely on an e-mailing system to maintain a continuous interaction and to better manage the monitoring task. The MU provides physicians with a collection of Web-based services, such as data management and retrieval, decision support, and communication. Each PU is a PC-based software, running at the patient's house, and interfaced with commercial instrumentation for Blood glucose Level readings.
In the implementation of the T-IDDM architecture we developed in Pavia, the PU is connected to the hospital through standard Public Switched Telephone Lines, while the distributed services of the MU are accessible over the Local Area Network of the Policlinico S. Matteo hospital. In particular, all patients' data are stored in an Oracle™ data-base, residing at the hospital EDP, while the intelligent data analysis and the decision support tools run on a workstation at the Scientific Direction. The communication among the elements of this distributed system, as well as with the PU, relies on **lispweb** [1], an HTML/HTTP server written in Common Lisp. All services are routinely accessed from the Pediatric Clinic Department.
The T-IDDM verification phase started at the Pavia site in the period April-June 1998, and currently involves 4 pediatric patients, 2 diabetologists, 2 physicians under training programs on pediatrics, 1 nurse and 1 dietician.
The project has been evaluated by the ethical committee of the Policlinico S. Matteo Hospital, and a detailed consensus has been signed by the involved patients.

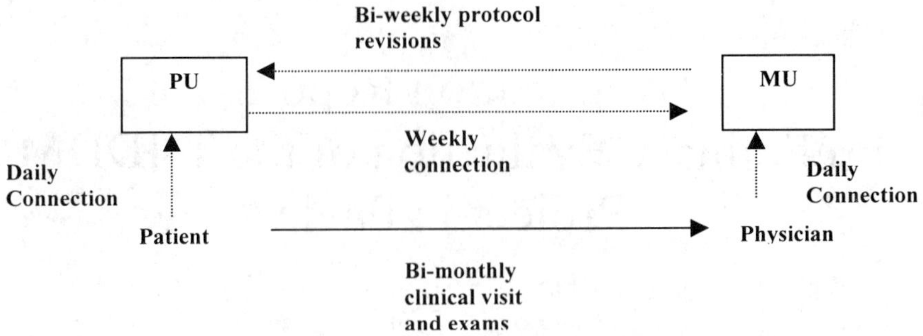

The protocol applied during this first evaluation phase id described in the figure above. Moreover, other information where collected in these months, such as the frequency of the data flow, the frequency of ambulatory visits, and the impact on the physicians workflow is being carefully analyzed. Moreover, the usability of the interfaces, and the usefulness of the collection of decision support tools is under consideration.

The preliminary results obtained up to March 1999 at the Pavia center are shown in the Table below:

Parameters of the period June-March 1999	
Follow up days	270
Distance between consecutive data communications	4-7 days
Number of messages sent by physicians	23-39
Number of messages sent by patients	28-44
Number of BGL per patient per day	1.44-3
Average HbA1c modification	-066 (sd 0.7)
Number of protocol changes	4-7
Schedule	
Physician consultation	Daily
Patient consultation	Daily

Although the small number of patients does not allow to obtain statistically significant results, there are several interesting issues that arise from the collected data. First, the high frequency of logging on the system, and the high number of messages exchanged between patients an physicians demonstrates that both patients and physicians have found helpful to rely on the system's functionality, and that the system is quite easy to use, having a sufficiently user-friendly interface; a quantitative evaluation of these indicators will be provided through the examination of some usability questionnaires that have been distributed to patients and physicians. The weekly schedule has been nearly maintained, as well as the required BGL measurements per day.

Moreover, the average number of protocol changes has been nearly doubled with respect to clinical practice; when working without the system support, the physician just evaluates the patient's condition on the visit day, while T-IDDM permits him to verify the metabolic state more frequently. In such a way, if a problem arises, the patient does not have to wait, as the physician is immediately able to make a therapy revision to cope with it.

We believe that such an increased frequency in therapy adjustments has led to a reduction of the mean HbA1c level in the patients under monitoring: helped by the system, physicians have been able to better and sooner understand the patients' peculiar needs, and to define insulin treatments properly tailored on the specific situation under examination.

Finally, it is of interest to consider the data coming from one patient in a greater detail. The following table shows the Blood Glucose Level descriptive statistics calculated over two different periods, one at the beginning of the verification, and the other at the end. It is easy to see how the use of the system improves not only mean and median, but also the standard deviation, that is known to be an important risk factor in patient's treatment.

	Breakfast		Lunch		Dinner	
	1/4/1998 30/6/1998	**1/12/1998 28/2/1999**	**1/4/1998 30/6/1998**	**1/12/1998 28/2/1999**	**1/4/1998 30/6/1998**	**1/12/1998 28/2/1999**
Mean	186	184	165	156	167	159
Median	200	184	152	143	162	141
SD	55	60	65	59	69	70
Min	72	62	63	56	61	52
Max	345	304	355	287	322	389

References

[1] Riva A, Bellazzi R, Stefanelli M. A Web-Based System for the Intelligent Management of Diabetic Patients. MD Computing. 1997; 14:360--364.

[2] Bellazzi R, Cobelli C, Gomez E. and Stefanelli M. The T-IDDM project: Telematic management of Insulin Dependent Diabetes Mellitus, Health Telematics '95, (M. Bracale, F. Denoth eds.); 1995: 271—276

Medical Informatics Europe '99
P. Kokol et al. (Eds.)
IOS Press, 1999

Lesson learnt from a halt of the hospital information system

M.C.Mazzoleni *, P. Baiardi *, I.Giorgi **
**Medical Informatics Unit, **Psycology Unit - S.Maugeri Foundation, IRCCS – Pavia, Italy*

Abstract. The present paper deals with an experience of blackout of the hospital information system at our Medical Centre, trying to evaluate the impact on internal users (physicians, nurses, clerks) and patients population. Limited inconveniences have occurred to out-patients in terms of delay in collecting medical reports after diagnostic test execution. As regards direct users, impact was evaluated through a structured interview. Administrative personnel, that have been using computer-based system for at least ten years, have not declared particular inconveniences, accepting the overtime or the extra-work as simply unavoidable. On the contrary, health-care personnel reported a heavy negative impact of the system failure on their activity. After a great effort to achieve the system acceptance and direct physicians usage, the blackout of the system has pointed out that the situation has changed since a few years ago: now the HIS, and particularly its clinical core, is considered mission critical.

1. Introduction

The present paper deals with an experience of blackout of the hospital information system (HIS) at our Medical Centre, trying to evaluate the impact on internal users and patients population.

An integrated patient-centered HIS [1,2] has been developed by the medical informatics unit, and it is in use since 5 years ago. Starting from a system mainly aimed at billing, it now consists of a network of 130 windows PC clients connected to a database server, and manages information for administrative and clinical purposes (typically EPR). In particular physicians direct usage has been achieved in clinical units.

2. The fact

On a Friday afternoon, August 28th, the system stopped running with a database message "primary and mirror chunks are bad". A hour has been spent trying to reboot the system and to understand the reasons for the failure. Then the hardware supplier technical assistance service was contacted, under a 5-days office hours contract for database engine software maintenance. On Monday evening, after a long series of contacts with both hardware and database suppliers shifting the responsibility on to one another, the problem (caused by a conflict between Unix resources management and the DBMS) was identified and removed.

No serious halt has ever occurred since the installation of the first core of the system. So, no direct experience was available.

Being the HIS (with the exception of laboratories systems and booking system) developed inside the medical centre, we have the control of software. Support is needed as regards systemistic knowledge, this the reason for the database engine maintenance contract.
As regards hardware, the database server (HP D350) is equipped with the classical redundancy devices (disk mirroring, independent disk controllers, double LAN interface, etc). No hardware support contract is active, having been chosen a on demand intervention.
As regards data every morning an automatic procedure backs up the database and can restore the situation with a controlled loss of data. We decided not to restore the back copy until it had to be was absolutely necessary (and it was not necessary).

3. Actions taken regarding continuity/recovery

Some subsystems didn't need any intervention: laboratory systems are running on departmental hardware interfaced to the HIS in order to achieve functional independence from the central system. The same for booking procedure that, at present, supports only the radiology service activity.
For others subsystems, a procedure has been preventively identified to face a system halt: this is the case of registration and billing for out-patients for which a server, usually used for software development, was identified as possible alternate system and hence maintained updated , in terms of database structure and billing rules. Client PC workstation had simply to switch the database, with a minimum effort.
In all the other cases traditional information flow based on paper document has been restored: in-patients administrative admittance documentation was manually handled on original paper form, and it was used to perform the input when the system started again. For in-patients, requests to services and labs for tests had to be performed using predefined available paper form. No support was provided to nurses for labels production and worksheet for samples, diets and so on.
The available paper medical record – printout of the electronic medical record - that still continues to be the only legal document and whose presence is mandatory , was the clinical information support. Updates of the medical records, hand-written during the system halt, had to be entered into the system off-line by physicians.
The use of standard WP products was proposed to services and out-patient departments in order to supply the medical report. Anyway re-input - or at least "cut and paste"- of the data would have been necessary in order to preserve both clinical information completeness in the EPR, and quantification of activities for administrative purpose. While out-patients departments have accepted the solution of WP usage and subsequent re-writing, Radiology and nuclear medicine medical reports input have been delayed (with a few exceptions).

4. The impact on patients

No queue at the out-patients counter windows occurred, due to the fact that the halt occurred at afternoon, and most of the ambulatory activity is performed in the morning. For a limited number of patients payments have been delayed to the time when they came back to collect medical report. No problem for the execution of tests or visits. The day after, cash functionality was restored. About 50 out-patients collected their radiology and nuclear medicine medical reports with an average delay of two days.
As regards in-patients, the necessity of hand-writing the admittance documentation has slightly prolonged the patient (or a relative) stay at the admittance office, even if data for

frequently re-admitted patients were not completely collected, being they available at the restart of the system. No interaction with the patients occurs at discharge, since billing is performed once a month at fixed date. The unavailability of some medical reports had no impact on the length of staying: in a 230 bed hospital in absence of the written medical report, information about the result of a diagnostic test is quite easily available from the physician who have performed it. Some problems have occurred about the timeliness of supplying clinical discharge documentation.
After all, inconveniences have been limited.

5. The impact on the users

Server switching, together with available software to ensure a controlled merge of administrative data, have maintained the inconveniences for users of the out-patient administrative area within reasonable limits. In-patients administrative data input as regards admissions and discharges has entailed a 2 hours overtime work of a clerk. Due to the interruption of interfacement to the HIS (and in particular to the demographic information of in-patients), laboratories personnel had to spent about 3 hours to verify patient identification for a correct import of results into the HIS. It didn't involve overtime.
All the above-mentioned personnel have been using computer based systems for at least ten years. They have not declared particular inconveniences, accepting the overtime or the extra work as simply unavoidable.
On the contrary, health-care personnel reported a heavy negative impact of the system failure on their activity.
Through a structured interview, users (all the physicians and nurses-in-chief on duty in that period, and 50% of the total number of nurses) have declared the extent of inconvenience induced by the unavailability of the system, using a four point scale (values: 1.not at all; 2. a little; 3.quite; 4. a lot). Most of them (72%) answered "quite" or "a lot". A figure of 98% of the interviewed users have realized that the system was down, confirming a broad usage of the system.
Considering the emotional reaction (1. indifference;2. worry;3. irritation; 4. other), nurses (the system helps them in many boring manual procedure, aimed at the management of the patient during the hospitalization) seem to be more worried (65%) than physicians, who are mainly (74%) irritated by the unavailability of the system. Only 6 people over 96 were indifferent. Considering the 40 physicians taking care of in-patients, they globally had to manage in the traditional manual way 78 new admittances, 68 discharges, 67 day-hospital encounters, with a mean of 197 hospitalized patients. To ensure information completeness, a posteriori clinical data input is mandatory. The average workload in that period of late summer was not so heavy, and 65% of physicians declared not to feel excessively overburdened by re-writing the collected data into the system.
So, what are the reasons for the complaints? When considering unavailability of functionalities, most of the physicians (85%) ranked the lack of historical data inspection support higher than any other (many of our patients are chronic), followed at a small distance by the lack of support in providing exhaustive organized documentation (considered an important added value to the specialist-general practitioner communication) on the stay of patient, the results of all the tests performed, and the therapeutic indications.

6. Discussion

When a system halt occurs, generally the main worry is how to reduce inconveniences to the public, to prevent long queues and waiting times. The loss of corporate image that derives can cause also long term damage, especially in a medium size city, where, as it is in our case, the market of qualified medical services is competitive.

When thinking to the possibility of a system failure, we as developers and managers of the system itself, have privileged the continuity of administrative functionalities and the reduction of the impact onto the out-patient population. Such a decision implies a discrimination between what is critical and what is optional.

After a great effort to achieve the system acceptance, direct physicians usage, completeness and recording timeliness of information, have we ourselves under-evaluated the importance of clinical information availability? Being still far from a paperless situation (as regards medical record the present legislation doesn't permit it), information are, more or less easily and quickly, available also without the system.

What happened was typically the temporary suspension of a service, not a disaster with loss of data. The reaction of both people who usually benefit from clinical information availability and the management reveals inconvenience, worry and irritation, but we have not interpreted the temporary halt as a real serious problem. Have the traditional roles (informaticians as supporters, and health-care personnel as the ones to be convinced of the opportunity and necessity of information system) been exchanged?

Our feeling is that now the experimental phase of clinical information system introduction can be considered concluded, and the system is a tool the users perceive as useful in daily activity and they are not willing to give it up.

This one has been the first halt occurred, and 30% of the users have modified –even if not in a drastic way- their opinion about system reliability. Other similar events could lead to an irreversible abandoning of the system. Being the clinical encounter a primary source of information useful to both physicians and the hospital managers, the halt of the system, even if occurred in a not particularly critic moment, has shown good reasons to review not only the maintenance contract policy (80% of hospitals in our region have similar 5-days contract, but the most important problem is the quality of technical support), the procedures and resources to face similar situation, but also the central role played by the HIS.

The blackout of the system has pointed out that situation has changed since a few years ago: now the HIS is considered mission critical. This local scenario is also supported by the fact that our regional governmental body takes now into account the presence of a HIS as a qualifying element for health-care institutions.

References

[1] Mazzoleni M.C., et al.. Spreading the clinical information system: which users are satisfied? In Proceedings of Medical Informatics Europe '97. IOS Press pag.162 –167.

[2] Mazzoleni MC, Baiardi P. et al. Physicians Usage and Acceptance of a Clinical Information System - Proceedings MEDINFO'98

Medical Informatics Europe '99
P. Kokol et al. (Eds.)
IOS Press, 1999

Selection of Hospital Information Systems: User Participation

Jürgen Stausberg
Institute for Medical Informatics, Biometry and Epidemiology, Medical Faculty, University of Essen, Hufelandstr. 55, 45122 Essen, Germany

Abstract. Motivated by economic and quality management issues, many hospitals strive for the introduction of information systems into the clinical environment. To introduce the most suitable software product, a systematic selection procedure is required involving all affected staff. The paper describes a methodology that guides the clinical users to an objective motivated decision. This semi-formal methodology is necessary in view of missing standard models for the description of hospital information systems and leads to high acceptance in practical use. The methodology consists of structured product demonstrations with a quantitative assessment, benefit-value-analyses based on step weights for the functions needed, and test installations. Prerequisite of this procedure was the definition of objectives and priorities in a standard catalog that was used as reference in the whole project. Selecting a software product following this systematic procedure establishes a sound basis for a successful application in the clinical environment.

1 Introduction

Selecting software products for the clinical environment requires a description of the functionality needed. But this is quite a difficult problem. There are not any evaluated models or standards available to describe the tasks and functions of the clinical parts of a hospital information system for a call for tender. Currently presented models are lacking in dynamic elements [1] or granularity [2]. In this situation a semi-formal methodology of selecting a software product ought to be accepted. One important characteristic of this methodology should be the involvement of the affected users. Physicians, nurses and medical assistants are the only persons who are able to compensate the missing formal models through their knowledge about clinical processes and resource allocation. A second important reason for the close integration of clinical users during a selection procedure is the acceptance of the later introduced product. The introduction of software for planning and resource allocation will change the present processes. In the sense of process optimization this is to some extent a desired outcome. But we have to accept that software products currently available require the adaptation of users and processes to the behavior implemented. Thus the users should gain the feeling that it is their product and they had been responsible for the decision on procurement.

The presented project within the university clinic of Essen used a semi-formal methodology for the integration of clinical users during the selection procedure of surgical parts of the hospital information system. The surgical parts will be connected with other parts (central patient database, lab, billing, etc.) by standard communication protocols (Health Level 7) and a communication server. In the following the methodology will be described and results from the project will be reported.

2 Methods

On behalf of the director of administration the project was launched in November 1997. The objectives were to define a standard catalog for a common information system of all surgical departments within the university clinic of Essen and to select a commercial software product. Corresponding to the importance of user involvement the project team includes one responsible physician from every surgical department, one representative from the head nurse, members of the works council, the data protection registrar, representatives from the central computer unit, and the sub-departments of reimbursement, controlling and cost accounting. The project leader was specialist in medical informatics.

Within two meetings a standard catalog could be developed providing three levels of details. The first level of priorities was proposed for the agreement between the involved user groups and was derived from strategical aims of the clinic. The second level provides a functional overview. It was addressed to be the relevant one for the assessment of commercial software products through clinical staff. This level should also be used for the acceptance of the purchased product. Level three provides the finest granularity of the catalog with a detailed listing of technical and functional features. It should assist medical informatics staff by remembering all relevant aspects of the system. The functional features of the third level were bases for two benefit-value-analyses. The benefit-value-analyses combine two figures for calculation. The first figure describes weights for the variations of one feature and the second step weights for feature groups.

To reduce the number of potential products to a number small enough for a detailed analysis, a structured and moderated presentation was carried out. Each vendor was requested to use the real product for its presentation and to follow along a predefined sequence of tasks. The duration of one presentation was 90 minutes including questions from the auditorium. An assessment form was handed out to each surgical department as well as to the representative of the head nurse. They were asked to score the products using school marks for the 8 functional groups defined in level 2 of the standard catalog. In addition a general mark was permitted. The average for the 8 specific marks was calculated. This average and the general mark were weighted to 50 % per form. The condensed marks were used to rank the software products within one department. Last the average rang was calculated. The best products of the presentations were installed in a computer lab for 3 months. During the first 6 weeks every employee of the involved departments has the opportunity of testing the products. In the last 6 weeks a subgroup of the project team evaluated specific functions in view of level 1 of the standard catalog.

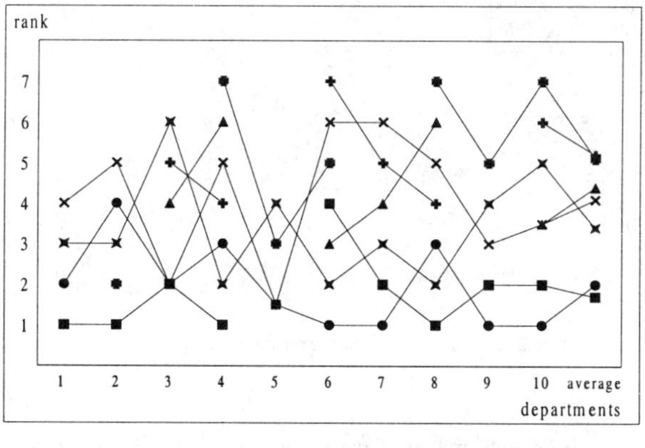

Figure 1: Ranks of the 7 software products.

3 Results

Part one of the standard catalog[1] defines 6 priorities with an ordering oriented to the importance for the selection procedure. The second level defines 8 functional groups with 32 subheadings. The requirement profile consists in its hierarchical functional part of 327 leafs. The tree is build up from the two steps of the functional overview. In addition the requirement profile lists 87 technical characteristics of the system looked for.

A pre-selection of relevant software products was based on a detailed market analysis (cf. http://www.uni-essen.de/~tmi030/ak_chirurgie/) provided by the working group surgery of the German Association of Medical Informatics, Biometry and Epidemiology (GMDS).

Seven vendors presented their products in the structured and moderated demonstration. The presentations took place in spring 1998. Only two departments did not attend these appointments. Ten from 13 assessment forms were received after the presentations. The results from the calculation according to the algorithm introduced above are shown in figure 1. This method splits the 7 products in two halves with 2 products at the top: product A, presented in the figures by circles, and product B, presented in the figures by squares. Every department ranked either A, B, or both at the top; both products were exclusively ranked at the top four times. As conclusion from this assessment, the further evaluation concentrated on the products A and B.

These vendors were asked for information on their products, dissemination, company, and prizes. The first benefit-value-analysis was calculated for the over all functionality as described by the vendors in the requirement profile. The second analysis calculates the values for the characteristics proven with the test installations based on the same step weights[2]. The benefit-value-analyses (cf. figure 2) clarified the strengths and weaknesses of both products and made some impressions reliable and transparent.

Information solely from the benefit-value-analyses or from the test installations was not sufficient enough for a decision. Thus in the end the selection was based on two major criteria. First product A shows slightly advantages concerning priority one, documentation of all relevant legislative, internal and medical data. Second the majority of the departments preferred this product through its capability of representing a detailed and high tailored medical documentation. Costs for the products were estimated and compared but there was no relevant difference. The other user groups agreed because the methods demonstrated no counter argument. A recommendation could be reached in a consensus at a final meeting.

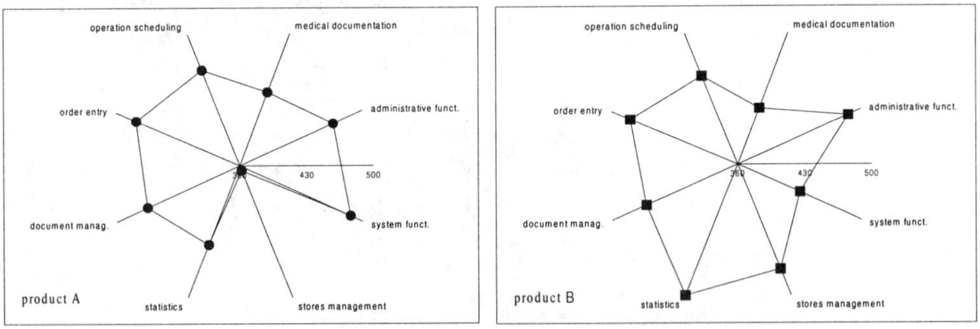

Figure 2: Star plots representing the over all functionality.

[1] The catalog is available in German from http://www.uni-essen.de/~tmi030/ak_chirurgie/info/auswahl.htm.
[2] The detailed step weights are available from the author.

4 Discussion

Papers on this topic are rare. A search in MEDLINE from 1990 up to now for the terms "purchase hospital" and "selection" in connection with "hospital information system" or "information system" found zero papers. "Procurement" and "purchase" are not available as catchword. In the indexes of the proceedings from AMIA Annual Fall Symposium (1995-1998) and MEDINFO (1995/1998) one paper was found with the catchword "procurement decisions" [3], which discusses this topic regarding general practitioners. A manually performed search in the above-mentioned proceedings as well as MIE (1994–1998) receives two further references. The first presents results from a project on laboratory systems [4]. The second reports the changes in time of physician involvement and emphasizes the importance of user participation [5]. It will be necessary for the next future to increase research on methods that further improve the results of selection procedures. This will support the successfully introduction of software products in the clinical environment.

The presented project demonstrates that clinical staff is very competent in assessing potential software solutions for their daily work if there is a clear selection methodology behind. Moderated and structured presentations can be highly recommended to decrease the number of products for a detailed analysis. The ranking method had broken the products down into two groups with a significant distance. Through the quantitative approach unobjective discussions could be avoided. The availability of the products primarily selected in a test installation was widely accepted and intensively used. Especially nurses were highly motivated in testing the products concerning their concrete working conditions. The whole time a computer specialist was available assisting the users, because detailed knowledge about the products was necessary for these tests. As predicted in part one of the standard catalog the decision was based on the assessment of the products in view of the priorities. Without this clear and predefined selection of criteria, a ranking of the products based on the requirement profile alone had not been possible. The analyses from the requirement profiles were successfully transmitted to the users with the presented star plots avoiding confusion through the masses of information.

It is obvious that the decision for a product is not the end of introducing an information system in health care. The next important task includes the definition of "Who does What at Which time with the selected product and What are the data dealt with". But we are confident in having high acceptance and good will of the clinical users as well as the most suitable product for our needs through the selection procedure presented in this paper.

References

[1] A. Winter and R. Haux, A Three-Level Graph-Based Model for the Management of Hospital Information Systems, *Methods of Information in Medicine* 34 (1995) 378-396.

[2] European Committee for Standardisation (CEN), Medical Informatics – Healthcare Information Systems Architecture Part 1 (HISA). Healthcare Middleware Layer. prENV. Brussels, 1997.

[3] S. Kay, An Easier Route for Choosing Appropriate Health Care Technology? In: R. M. Gardner (ed.), Nineteenth Annual Symposium on Computer Applications in Medical Care. ISBN: 1 56053 123 1. Hanley & Belfus, Philadelphia, 1995, p. 959.

[4] T. Rosenal et al., Procurement of Information System Effectively (POISE): Using the New UK Guidelines to Purchase an Integrated Clinical Laboratory System. In: R. Greeens et al (eds.), Proceedings of the Eighth World Congress on Medical Informatics. ISBN: 0 9697414 1 3. North-Holland, Amsterdam, 1995, pp. 549-553.

[5] S. Wakefield et al., Physician Involvement in Hospital Information System Selection: A Success Story. In: R. Greeens et al (eds.), Proceedings of the Eighth World Congress on Medical Informatics. ISBN: 0 9697414 1 3. North-Holland, Amsterdam, 1995, pp. 554-558.

Medical Informatics Europe '99
P. Kokol et al. (Eds.)
IOS Press, 1999

The use of the Balanced ScoreCard (BSC) in the Model for Investment and Evaluation of Medical Information Systems.

Karsten Ulrik Niss (kun@v-chi.dk)
Virtual Centre for Health Informatics (V-CHI), Aalborg University, Fredrik Bajersvej 7D-2, DK 9220 Aalborg East, Denmark

Abstract. This paper describes the use of the Balanced ScoreCard (BSC) in the MIEMIS meso-model (Model for Investment and Evaluation of Medical Information Systems). The scope of the MIEMIS model is to integrate the evaluation process into the whole lifecycle of an information system using both a prospective and a retrospective approach.
We conclude, that the MIEMIS-model has benefited from implementing the BSC into the model due to the fact, that the BSC can support the project management work. This approach helps ensuring, that the new information systems are fulfilled according to the plan and with a balance between the four perspectives (financial, customer/user, internal, and innovation/learning perspective) to avoid that the financial aspect is the driving force in developing and implementing a new information system, for example.

1. Introduction

The scope of the MIEMIS project is to develop a Model for Investment and Evaluation of Medical Information Systems - the MIEMIS model. The philosophy is to move from a traditional independent evaluation process to an integrated approach, where the evaluation process is integrated into the lifecycle of an information system with identifiable elements each characterised by a set of well defined prerequisites. In the dimension of generality the model is divided into three layers - the macro or high level model, the meso or intermediate level model, and the micro or detailed level model [1,2]. This paper focuses on the meso layer of the model.

The background of the work is the fact that many projects in the health care sector have failed in the past due to mainly three reasons [3]:

1. Technical shortcomings
2. Project management shortcomings
3. Organisational shortcomings

We have constructed a model that helps managing reasons 2 and 3 leaving the managing of technical shortcomings to other approaches. Of course there are still problems with the technical issues, but compared to earlier the technical issues are not the most important areas any more.

2. The MIEMIS-model

The scope of MIEMIS (Model for Investment and Evaluation of Medical Information Systems) can be divided into a prospective and a retrospective part. The prospective part should develop a better methodology for ensuring that the expectations from a medical information system are fulfilled during the implementation. The retrospective part should ensure that not only systems with a short financial pay-back time are evaluated positively, but also systems with a large impact on elements like quality, interpersonal relations, job motivation / job enhancement and other issues, that are difficult to measure in figures [4].

The MIEMIS-model has three levels: macro, meso and micro. Moving from macro to micro is a process where macro is described in mostly theoretical oriented and micro mostly empirically oriented, whereas the meso model is a combination of theory and empirical methods.

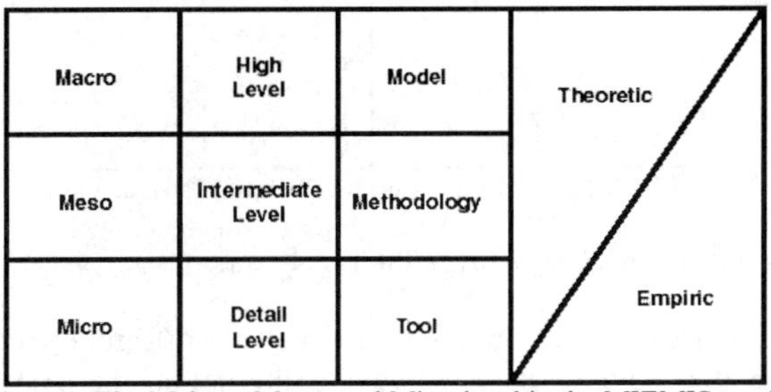

Figure1: The Makro-, Meso- and Microlevel in the MIEMIS-model.

2.1. The Macro level

The macro level is the high level in the model. This level gives an overview of the MIEMIS-model, and shows how the individual elements of the model are related to each other.

2.2. The Meso level

The meso level is the more detailed level, where methodology transforms theory into useful procedures for implementing information systems. The meso level specifies metrics, costs and benefits for the new information system.

2.3. The Micro level

The micro level is the lowest level in the MIEMIS-model and it fully describes tools for all the details in the MIEMIS-model. The tools will be defined so that they can be used directly in the empirical settings where the new information system will be developed and implemented.

3. The MIEMIS meso model for the Benefit Management Process

The MIEMIS meso model for the Benefit Management Process - in the following referred to as the meso model - is a three-dimensional model. The first dimension covers seven phases in the information system lifecycle from idea through strategy/planning, context definition, content definition, application development, system implementation to use and maintenance. The second dimension is related to each phase in the information system's lifecycle and covers process, technology, people, skills & competencies, organisation and culture. Moreover, we have included a review part that is a method to ensure the quality and content of each phase in the lifecycle, and to ensure the integration of the seven phases. The third dimension is inspired from Kaplan and Norton and their Balanced ScoreCard (BSC) and is the topic of this paper [5,6].

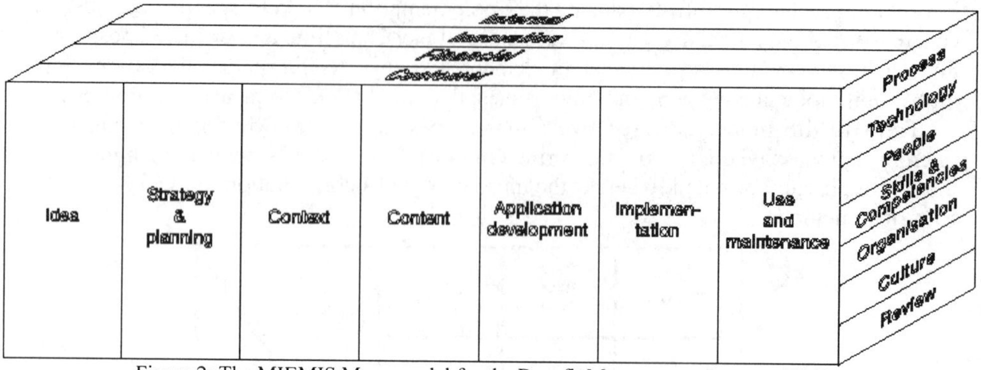

Figure 2: The MIEMIS Meso-model for the Benefit Management Process (BMP).

3.1. Definition of the Balanced ScoreCard (BSC)

According to Kaplan the BSC is organised around four different perspectives - the financial perspective, the customer perspective, the internal business perspective and the innovation and learning perspective. The term 'balanced' indicates the balance to be achieved between short- and long-term goals, between financial and non-financial measures of performance, between lagging and leading indicators and between external and internal performance perspectives [6]. By using the four different perspectives in the BSC and balancing them to each other the above mentioned balanced should be achieved.

3.2. Use of the Balanced ScoreCard in the meso model

The MIEMIS-model uses the BSC in the project management process during the seven phases in the information system lifecycle and to ensure the balance between the four perspectives. In relation to the management process an important aspect is to include the different user-groups in the development of the contents of the four perspectives. In that way the BSC form the common basis of the whole information system lifecycle because nearly every person who participate in the project during the information system lifecycle will know the content of the BSC and during the formulation of the contents he or she has at some level committed him or her to the content of the BSC. In that way the BSC will be a tool to ensure that the participants in the project have a common understanding of the objectives of the information system.

We also use the BSC as an active part in the meso model. The first outcome is during the formulation of the vision and idea of the information system, which could be more precisely defined if the BSC is completed and updated during the information system life cycle using the feedback coming during the fulfilment of the phases in the lifecycle. At the same time the BSC will be a tool to ensure that the visions and ideas are fulfilled during the system life cycle because the visions and ideas are clearly formulated and communicated to the involved persons and therefore they could have a better understanding of the visions and ideas.

According to statements mentioned above the BSC can be used in the project management process to plan and to determine goals and to focus on those parts, which are under the estimated level - or maybe ignored. Another approach could be to check the measures in the BSC and to list the degree of fulfilment for each measure. The project management approach can be different, but at least two main approaches can be used:

- focus on the measures with the lowest degree of fulfilment
- focus on the measures which are fulfilled or almost fulfilled

Normally we would prefer the first approach, but in some cases the latter would be preferred, e.g. if it is impossible to find a pattern in those measures that are not fulfilled or if it is of minor importance for the fulfilment of the information system project. Figure 3 shows an example of the information that a project manager can get from the BSC. In this example the score for the financial and for the innovation and learning perspective are much higher than for the two others, and therefore the project manager has do decide what to do. In this way he can use this simple graph in his management work, and as a visualisation tool for the workgroups in the project.

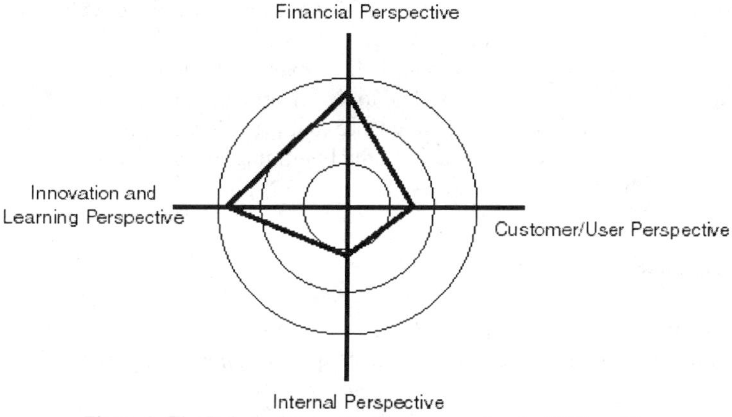

Figure 3: The Balanced ScoreCard - an example of a BSC-profile.

The feedback to the different workgroups will be a way to optimise the outcome of their work and to give them an opportunity to learn from their previous work to become better to do their job in the future. It is important that the project manager motivate the different workgroups to learn from their former work - not only to change the outcome of their work (single-loop learning), but also to change their way of working (double-loop learning) [7,8].

3.3. The benefits from the use of the Balanced ScoreCard

The use of the BSC in the meso-model will result in a reasonable tool which can form the basis for improving the quality of work in all the phases of the information system lifecycle and as an input to improve the implementation of the learning organisation and the double-loop learning concepts. The scope and content of an information system is normally justified during the development and implementation phases due to change in the surroundings or in the users awareness about the context and content of the information system. Several projects have shown that the traditional project management methods have difficulties in handling these adjustments. We claim that the BSC will be a useful part of the project management process and will give the project manager a dynamic and event driven tool to optimise the benefit from the information system and to show the consequences even in a changing environment. Balance is the keyword in this process, because without a balance between the financial perspective, the customer perspective, the internal business perspective and the innovation and learning perspective it will be difficult to achieve the maximum benefit from an information system.

4. Conclusion

Finally we can conclude that the MIEMIS-model have benefited from implementing the BSC into the meso-model. We use the ideas in the BSC to develop and implement an information system to ensure, that the processes regarding the new information systems are fulfilled according to the plan and with a balance between the four perspectives to avoid that for example the financial aspect are the driving force in developing and implementing a new information system.

5. Future work

The future work on the MIEMIS-model is concentrated on the development of content and tools in the macro model, and to implement additional tools for project management. The three dimensions in the meso model will be extracted into concrete tools for every combination of the three dimensions. The tools for project management will be integrated into all levels of the MIEMIS-model to ensure that the information system is fulfilled according to the user expectation stated at the beginning of the information system lifecycle and updated during the lifecycles.

6. Practical use

In the forthcoming months the MIEMIS-model will be tested on the implementation of an electronic nursing patient record at three hospitals in the county of Northern Jutland.

Acknowledgements

This project is supported financially by Kommunedata A/S and the County of Northern Jutland, Denmark.

References

[1] K. Niss and G. Reinbacher, MIEMIS macro-model - a high level Model for Investment and Evaluation of Medical Information Systems. TEHRE 98. 1998.

[2] D. Remenyi *et al.*, Achieving Maximum Value from Information Systems - a Process Approach. Chichester: John Wiley & Sons Ltd., 1997.

[3] N. Lorenzi and R. Riley, Organizational Aspects of Health Informatics - Managing Technological Change. New York: Springer-Verlag, 1995.

[4] K. Niss and G. Reinbacher, MIEMIS - Model for Investment and Evaluation of Medical Information Systems. In B. Cesnik *et al.*, MEDINFO 98. 1998 Aug 19; Amsterdam: IOS Press; 1998; 888 p. Studies in Health Technology and Informatics.

[5] R. Kaplan and D. Norton, The Balanced Scorecard - Measures That Drive Performance. Harward Business Review. Boston: HBR Publications, 1992; (January-February 1992). 71-79.

[6] R. Kaplan and D. Norton, The Balanced Scorecard: Sådan bygges bro mellem vision, værdier og strategier. 1 ed. København: Børsens Forlag A/S, 1998 (in Danish).

[7] D. Kolb, Experimental Learning - Experience as the Source of Learning and Development. New Jersey: Prentice Hall, 1984.

[8] C. Argyris C and D. Schön, Organizational Learning II. Addison Wesley, 1996.

Medical Informatics Europe '99
P. Kokol et al. (Eds.)
IOS Press, 1999

HIS Purchase Project: Preliminary Report

M. Madjaric, Ph.D., Leodolter W., Ph.D., Leitner H., Ph.D., Gell G., Ph.D.
Krankenanstaltenges.m.b.H, IT Department, Graz, Austria
Department for Medical Informatics, Statistics and Documentation, Graz, Austria

Abstract. The KAGes (Krankenanstaltenges.m.b.H) is a company, owned by the state of Styria in Austria, which operates 20 hospitals with about 8.000 beds and 14.000 employees, serving a population of ca. 1.2 million people. KAGes is on its way to purchase a new hospital information system (HIS) for it's hospitals.. Within the strategic IT plan and the "System Structure New" (SSN) project a methodology was developed, for making an effective HIS purchase. Several steps of this project are described in the paper: request for product information, evaluation of vendor proposals, product presentations, test site evaluation, reference site visits and selection of vendor finalists. The authors present the internal project management methodology, including the structure of the project team, project information management through intranet, criteria for different steps of the evaluation and evaluation site organization. Four major HIS vendors with leading HIS products qualified for this stage of the project (evaluation site). About 60 teams with 400 members (end users and IT-experts) have assessed all the products installed, during one or more, repeated, test sessions. The decision on which new HIS to purchase will be based on the recommendations derived from this evaluation. Two pilot installations (one general hospital and one teaching hospital department) are planned for implementation in the year 1999/2000 and subsequent roll-out (including substitution of the legacy system) is scheduled until the year 2003.

1. Introduction

The SSN project is aimed at defining the future structure of information systems in KAGes, together with its joint venture partner – the Faculty of Medicine of the University of Graz. Consequently this development emphasizes IT support for medicine, nursing and research. It is based on KAGes strategic information management plan, that suggests the implementation of standard software systems, rather then new developments. Within the SSN project standard software in the HIS field is defined as follows:

- substantial market presence (especially in German language areas)
- positive references (especially in complex hospital institutions and teaching hospitals)
- modern technology implemented
- originating from major producer/vendor

The project officially started in spring 1998 with a kick-off meeting, where the project work plan was accepted.

2. Project highlights

The selection of the new information system that involves, at the end, almost 10.000 end users and links 20 hospitals is a strategic decision and a major investment. Therefore the project analyses the global HIS market and involves the broadest possible user representation. The first step in the project was a marketplace screening (a European request for information about products and related services), that yielded 15 bids. After preliminary meetings conducted through the project "core"

team 6 vendors that fitted our strategic constraints ("standard software") were selected. These vendors were invited to perform product presentations based upon representative procedures from our functional requirements.
Within the project structure three functional task force groups were defined for basic systems, standard subsystems, and for scientific and special subsystems.
All of these three groups together form the so called "integration project team". The group heads and deputies form the so-called "core project team".

2.1. Functional requirements

Based on our experiences in developing specifications for new and modified information systems in the medical field, we did not design detailed system requirements. Instead, we defined a systematic list of the processes, that should be supported by an information system. This list has the following structure: core processes (e.g.: ancillary services), process fields (e.g.: medical chemical labs), processess (e.g.: communication of findings) and sub-process or function (e.g.: presentation of cumulative findings).
Due to this approach we avoided huge expenditures for the development of detailed requirements (that always turn out to be incomplete in production!) and gave to the vendors enough information about the systems functions that should be implemented. Supplementary to this "end users functionality" our functional requirements encompass some standard electronic data processing (EDP)-features, such as data protection, communication standards etc., as well as the general quality issues, such as functionality, applicability, reliability, performance and maintainability.
To obtain comparable results during the product presentation, we also developed two "sample" medical processes: Angina Pectoris. and Oncological Surgery. These two "sample" processes showed the behavior of the products at work and were substantially used to select four finalists for a further phase of assessment.

2.2. Assessment criteria

This selection procedure was based upon criteria that were defined in advance by the integration project group and are derived from our strategic definition of "standard software":

Vendor and bid:
- Size
- Reputation
- References
- Bid quality

Bid scope and qualifications:
- Project management
- Implementation in production (incl. legacy systems)
- User and EDP-personnel training and support
- Product maintenance

Product - general:
- Technical state-of-the-art
- Compatibility to EDP-standards
- Flexibility
- General quality criteria
- Standard interfaces
- System components availability
- Data protection

Product - functionality
- (according to functional requirements)

According to the evaluation of the integration project team the steering committee decided to keep the following four products (and vendors) for final evaluation (alphabetically ordered):

- HNA-Millennium (Siemens/Systema), USA
- IS-H/IS-H*Med (EDVg), Austria/Germany
- Orbis/ClinicWare (GWI), Germany

- PATIDOK (PCS), Austria

2.3. Evaluation site organization

According to accessible sources, this part of our project methodology seems to be unprecedented in HIS purchase procedures on this scale. All 4 qualified vendors installed their systems in SSN project rooms, with 3-5 workstations, 2-3 printers and all supplementary peripheral devices (scanners, digital cameras, bar code devices, voice recording facilities, etc). All the systems installed were to be fully functional for production and remain, for three months (February to April 1999), at the disposition of assessment teams and other KAGes visitors. KAGes will reimburse the vendors (whose bid will not be accepted) the evaluation site expenditures, given the test-system functionality.

The vendors had to provide: hardware installation, pre-installation of software, local users support, remote support for KAGes EDP-personnel, system modifications through customization and system de-installation.

KAGes provides an infrastructure with one evaluation site co-ordinator (general organization, co-ordination, infrastructure issues, communication), four evaluation site organizers - "product sponsors" (thorough training in products assessed, customization evaluation, contact persons for expertise with vendors, product reviewers) and contact persons for specific issues (subsystem connecting, network infrastructure, legacy issues).

The assessment procedure is performed through assessment teams, representing different professions (doctors, nurses, secretaries, EDP-experts etc.) and medical specialities. Every team is obliged to assess and review all four sites, usually within two days. If some major problems, missing or inappropriately customized functions are noticed, the team may repeat the site inspection after the deficiency was fixed through vendor support. The team should plan their visit in advance and use evaluation plans with functional specifications, sample processes, real medical records and real nursing documentation for the evaluation process, recording their results with standardised assessment forms with the following evaliuation criteria:

- functionality
- flexibility
- user friendliness
- support (at the test site)
- general issues (such as: data protection, performance, system stability etc.)

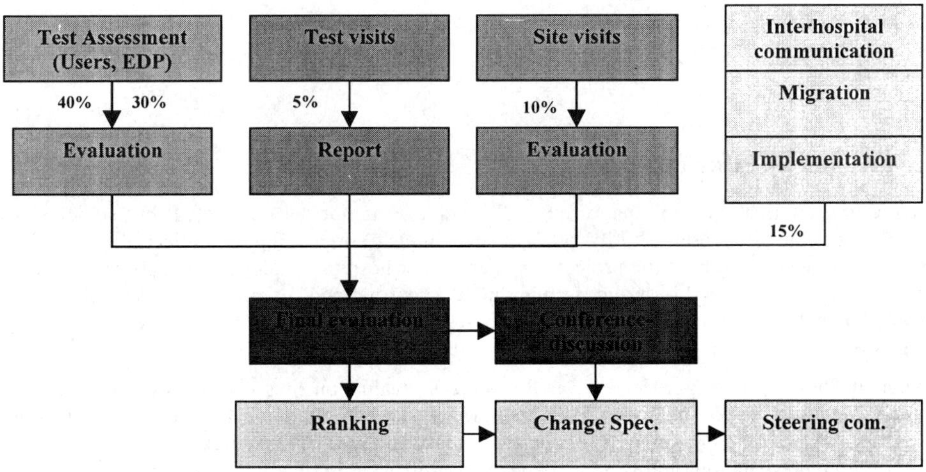

Fig 1: Assessment flow

The condensed product assessments were the basis for the final evaluation meeting (whole integration project team and assessment team heads), a two-day conference at the end of April 1999 where the final expert recommendation ti the steering commitee for the best products were formulated.

2.4. Documentation and communication: intranet-based project library

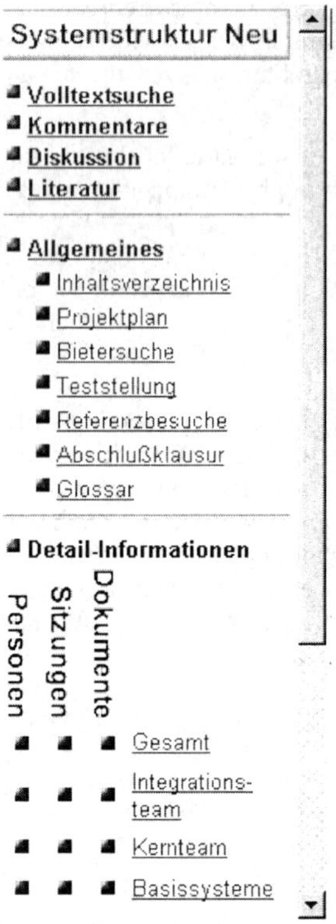

Fig. 2: Navigation frame for intranet presentation of SSN project library

A project of this scale cannot be successfully performed without proper documentation and communication. Duc to the fact, that KAGes infrastructure allows the corporate-wide access to the Intranet services (LAN and WAN), an SSN-Project intranet-site was developed. All employees of KAGes and Faculty of Medicine that have access to the network can browse all relevant documents and other project information. This Intranet site is organized in a similar manner to the project itself (see fig 2).

It has been proved, during numerous project meetings, that applying this technology in combination with LCD-projection for broader auditorium improves the conference efficiency substantially, due to momentary accessibility to relevant documents and its presentation to all discussion participants. The accessibility of several hundreds of documents is especially improved through the introduction of web site search features (with natural text search syntax).

3. Preliminary experiences

At the time of finalizing this paper our SSN project was not yet completed, but some relevant experiences could be presented. First of all, the technique of organizing the project library proved to be of major benefit for both the project teams and other hospital employees that are to be informed about project contents and it's progress, avoiding the "paper-flood" usually related to projects of this scale. About 150 of site visitors monthly approve this preliminary appraisal of the intranet project library.

Secondly, the very new approach used in this project - evaluation sites - is a major challenge to both vendors and KAGes. We decided to give the priority to the evaluation sites in preference to vendor presentations and vendor site visits for numerous reasons. Some of them are:

- both presentations and vendor site visits are restricted in time
- there is little chance to show flexibility features of the product
- there is no possibility to appoint numerous assessment teams

- customization in other hospitals is fitted to local needs

there is no possibility to enter and browse the data without interfering with actual production.

Of course, our approach of evaluation sites also brings some risks, especially in high expenditures for both parties.

The experiences concerning the products are also very indicative:

- none of the HIS products inspected complies fully with our definition of "standard software"
- all of the products are in "development", "integration" or “translation” phase
- the products aimed primarily to medical documentation have to be coupled to some administrative system, without clear solution of integration issues
- integration of system components is based exclusively on data level; user interface and functional integration are yet to be solved
- on preliminary inspection all of the products showed major problems e.g.: lack of on-line help, lack of user guidance and straightforward navigation, complex customizing, errors by referential integrity, poor coverage of hospital data protection requirements etc.

All of the systems offered in our project show absolutely the same strategic architectural concept: they are highly customizable. The systems usually use classical programming (3- or 4GL) of HIS administrative part and widely flexible design of medical documentation and presentation features through customizing. During first inspections we detected following problems in this field:

- a considerable part of classical programming has been shifted to customizing (parameters); the tools used in classical programming languages (formal checks, x-references) are not used in the parameterized part of "development", so customizing errors (especially due to lack of referential integrity) are detected as late as in the HIS production;
- the customizing tools often do not provide a user friendly development environment (no assistants, on-line help, tutorials or samples)
- with the customizing approach the investor actually buys the "HIS development tool" and has to adapt the standard or "base line" hospital system to local needs
- all products offer the use of user-defined documents, additional data structures and reports; their functionality however is in some instances very poor and the possibility of implementation is to be tested in detail

In addition to the evaluation of the test installations, selected sites with installed and operational HIS from the four vendors have been visited to answer questions that naturally can't be inspected through evaluation sites: overall performance in production, system stability, support quality and costs. General conclusion after this vendor site visits is, that the end users get less that the system could offer - due to expensive customization.
Differences in evaluation are significant through the project phases:

	vendor ranking after:		
vendor	bid, hearing	presen-tation	test site
A	3	1	4
B	8		
C	1	2	3
D	4		
E	5	3	1
F	7	4	
G	9		
H	1	5	2
I	6	6	

Our comment of this outcome is, that both vendor hearings and presentations suffer from the substantial credibility deficit. We believe that the basis for such a major decision could be gained only through extensive evaluation in production-like environment (test site or a pilot installation).

This evaluation of vendor test sites was accepted through the project steering comitee and two vendors were invited to the contract negotiations. KAGes intent to conduct the contract negotiations within seven weeks, aiming to get detailed bids from two vendor finalists and to issue the letter of intent for implementing two pilot installations and further planning of roll-out for other KAGes hospitals. The major issues for the contract negotiations are:

- extending the existing users' requirements through:
  - repairing the major product definiciencies recorded during the evaluation of test sites
  - implementing some excellent features of products not qualified for the final round
  - defining so called far-reaching "paper-less" hospital (that includes also the substantial reduction of telephone communication) as general system requirement to be achieved
- defining of so called "exclusion list" of deliverables, that are not covered through the bid
- vendor linkage to the the system's success (license, implementing and maintaining fees depending on users' acceptance and the depth of the system usage).

4. Outlook

- Condensing the results of the evaluation of the test installations and the findings of the visits to operational HIS-sites the integration team will produce a technical report with a ranking and a list of highlights and deficiencies of the different products
- This report serves as the basis for the selection of probably two companies for technical and commercial negotations for a contract, including a list of change specifications etc.
- The product chosen will be implemented in two pilot institutions of KAGes until mid 2000; these pilots are not to be considered as the beta-test installations, but as the first phase of the roll-out. However, if the system or the support is found to be inadequate, there is an option to step back from the contract.
- Roll-out in about 20 KAGes hospitals is planned until year 2003-2004; after completing the pilot phase further change specification will be made aimed to fix the problems detected as well as to implement new technologies.

References

[1] Barber, B, A.R. Bakker, S. Bengtsson (edt.): Caring for Health Care Information: Safety, Security and Secrecy; Elsevier 1993
[2] Bemmel van, J.H., M.A. Musen (edt.): "Handbook of Medical Informatics", Springer Verlag, Houten/Diegem 1997
[3] CHIM: Guide to Making Effective H.I.S. Purchase Decisions, Ann Arbor, Michigan USA, 1991
[4] Denert, E: Software engineeering; Springer Verlag, Berlin, 1992
[5] Marciniak, J.J.: Encyclopedia of SW engineering; John Wiley & Sons, Inc., New York, USA, 1994
[6] GMDS: Arbeitsgruppe Klinische Arbeitsplatzsysteme; www.med.uni-muenchen.de/gmds/kas/
[7] Tan, J.K.H.: Health Management Information Systems; Aspen Publishers, Inc., Gaithersburg, USA, 1995

Medical Informatics Europe '99
P. Kokol et al. (Eds.)
IOS Press, 1999

The Survey of Healthcare Software in Yugoslavia

Dragana Grbic[1], Snezana Simic[2], Jelena Marinkovic[2], Nikola Kocev[2], Borislava Matijevic[3]
[1]*Institute of Public Health Pancevo, Pasterova 2, 26 000 Pancevo, Yugoslavia*
[2]Institute *of Social Medicine, Statistics and Health Research, School of Medicine Belgrade, University, Dr Subotica 15, 11000 Belgrade, Yugoslavia*
[3]*Institute of Public Health Pancevo, Pasterova 2, 26 000 Pancevo, Yugoslavia*

Abstract. The aim of this study is to identify vendors of software packages applicable to health care system as well as to evaluate software packages offered to the health sector by a variety of sources, namely state owned software development companies, privately operated software development companies as well as sole traders. The approach undertaken was to preselect the potential suppliers via an initial targeted interview. Subsequently a questionnaire, consisting of 23 questions, was addressed to the selected vendors and suppliers. The response rate to the questionnaire was 58%. Investigation of 113 has revealed the non government software suppliers clearly lead in copyright ownership, IBM compatible personal computers were the platform of choice whereas majority of code was written utilising languages capable of supporting relational data base queries. The final outcome of the above study is a database of software packages and applications available to the health sector offering the health professionals and institutions guide lines and support in developing information systems, relevant subsystems and modules.

1. Introduction

Evaluation of health care software packages and applications from usability perspective had been neglected in preference to technical and functional issue [1]. Although the new fourth generation software has enormously eased the burden of computing for medical users, they have also created a confusing, difficult problem in software evaluation and selection because of: 1. huge number of available software packages, 2. the rapid technological change in the software technology, 3. the lack of appropriate technical expertise among medical staff, 4. the lack of applicable evaluation paradigms, and 5. dependency on the appropriateness of the design tools. [2]. The emergence of significant number of software packages applicable to health care system in the Yugoslav market enforces a need for a thorough and systematic approach to their evaluation. *The goals of this investigation are 1. To survey the software applications on offer from software development companies and individuals; 2. To evaluate and classify the software applications on offer; and 3. To create a unique database of software applications offered to the Yugoslav health care system with the view to assisting in fulfilling it's information technology requirements.*

2. Method

A cross sectional approach was adopted in evaluating and quantifying the software applications on offer during 1996 and 1997 from private and state operated companies as well as individual software developers. Utilising a set of criteria, published in Journal of Computers in Biology and Medicine Pergamon Press 1994, [3] an investigation and evaluation of software application in health sector on offer in Yugoslavia was commenced.

Both formal and informal sources of information relating to the vendors were canvassed since, at the start of the survey there was not a single definitive source of information identifying the software and information technology development companies and individuals. The companies were initially interviewed by telephone with ten general questions dealing with the nature and activities of the companies. The contact information on individuals identified to be active in providing software to the market did not always allow a direct telephone contact precluding the initial telephone interview. All of them identified as manufacturers, or vendors of licensed software for the health sector were presented with a questionnaire specifically addressing the software products on offer. The analysis of data obtained during the company interviews and responses to the questionnaires by both companies and individuals have resulted in formation of a registrar of software manufacturers and a registrar of manufacturers of public domain medical software. Only 47 companies and individuals involved in health care software responded with 113 questionnaires identifying their products. The questionnaire, which was used as a instrument of investigation to identify and evaluate the software applications, consists of 23 questions, providing details of individual software applications; product name, copy right ownership, authorship, type of software, level of collaboration with the health industry during the design and the writing process, potential end users of software, hardware platform used to develop the application, programming language, operating systems and hardware platform required for proper operation of the software, availability of software, requisite end user training, availability of source code, provision of on line help and documentation, version and release of software, place of utilising of software packages, familiarisation with software, adaptability of the application, price and a short description of the application. Response rate to the questionnaire was 58 %.

3. Results

Analysis of data pertaining to the physical attributes of the software companies indicates that more than two thirds (71%) of them are located in within the administrative centre of Yugoslavia, that is Belgrade metropolitan area. The remaining companies are to be found in Novi Sad, Nis, Pristina, Podgorica, Kragujevac, Valjevo, Subotica and Kraljevo, which are high urban cities in Yugoslavia. ANOVA highlights a statistically significant difference between the geographical location of the company headquarters, and the presence of software manufacturing companies is proportionally larger in Belgrade than in other areas ($F = 46.902$; $p<0.01$). The 83 respondent companies employ from one to forty employees in the development of software for the health market and more than half of the company's employ more than five employees. There is statistically significant difference amongst the software companies with respect to the number of employs. Companies which manufacture software for the health industry employ a greater number of software experts than companies manufacturing software for other applications (Man Whitney test $Z=2.012$; $p<0.05$). Although majority of respondents (97.8% of them) was clearly orientated towards the IBM compatible hardware, other platform was also represented: RISC based machines (12.1%), mini computers (9.9%), and main frame computers (11.0%).

Analysis of answers indicates that 87.6% of the health care software are application packages and 108 of them had specified the copyright ownership. Significantly it was noted private companies were represented in 53.7% of the responses, whereas the remaining response were representative of state companies, foreign representatives and individual traders ($F=27.24$; $p<0.01$). The descriptions of 111 software packages reveal that the IBM compatible platform represents more than three-quarters (77.5%) of specified hardware.

Health care software packages were developed under a broad range of development tools. From the analysis of 99 submitted package descriptions it was noted that 25 different programming languages were utilised. The most significant group of programming languages (63.6% of respondents) is those, which support work with relational databases. Analysis of operating systems information shows that from a field of 112 responses more than a half (59.8%) will operate in both single and multi-user environment, 25.0% require single user OS and 15.2% require multi-user OS exclusively ($F =25.6$; $p<0.01$).

With the view to evaluating the software packages it was necessary to establish a number of modalities with respect to the sphere of activity, job definition and type of institution in

which the software user is engaged. Hence 112 packages were evaluated in terms of potential use and 92 in terms of actual use. The sphere of activity based analysis of the packages indicates majority of users (79.3%) are engaged in health and medicine related activities. The second, job category, relates to the sorts of jobs that the user is engaged in. It was established that 68.1% of software packages are used in support of maintenance of medical records and documentation as well as appointment scheduling. Statistical analysis of software packages based on job definition indicates that packages aimed at supporting medical records and documentation are more prevalent rather than packages used in administrative work ($F=33.20$; $p<0.01$). The third category relates to the institutions, which employ the end users. It was established from the analysis of end user reference lists from 87 software packages, that 31% are employed in hospitals and 29.9% in primary health care institutions, encompassing the majority with respect to the remaining health institutions (institutes of public health, pharmacies, etc.). Analysis of software packages based on end user employer indicates that there is statistical significant difference between hospitals and health centres, which is almost the same, comparing to all other types of health institutions where the usage is relatively rare ($F=8.93$; $p<0.01$).
Software packages were investigated in terms of how well they were marketed. The criteria were existence of demo versions, product presentation, through a trial offer and/or a combination of the above. Analysis of 101 responses indicates future end users may familiarise themselves with the software package via a product presentation in 47.5% of cases, this being the most common form of introduction of products.
Analysis and evaluation of respondent's health care software packages has resulted in a recommendation for a model of a database presenting the salient features of software applications in health market.

4. Discussion

Cross sectional study has offered a relatively straightforward method of attaining the aims of the research with the exception of difficulties associated with locating of a single published source of manufacturers and suppliers of information technology in Yugoslavia. It is obvious that the fundamental marketing strategies are dysfunctional in this market place since the questionnaire had met with approximately 50% response rate. The use of a questionnaire to define and describe a software package in health sector as a basis to evaluate a software application is limited by the inability of achieve the necessary level of appreciation which can only be achieved in a hands on environment. Brender [4] has, in describing new trends and methodologies in assessment and evaluating software solutions in health care field, highlighted that in addition to quantity performance, accuracy, response time, economics and satisfaction of use and a plethora of other attributes, it is important to be able to evaluate the ergonomics of the solution.
Analysis of software manufacturers specific to the health sector reveals a very high concentration of companies in Belgrade. They are very good supplied and have the most competitive market in Yugoslavia and although limited to Serbia, this trend is indicative of a large number of health institutions (in Belgrade). Prior research dating to 1994 had shown that the Belgrade based health institutions relied on software tools than their counterparts in central Serbia [5]. Evaluation and analysis of technological attributes of software packages offered to the health sector has highlighted facts which support trend in the development of information technology in health sector during the course of the eighties and partially nineties [6]. Common to many published models of software evaluation and at the same time (simultaneously) of greatest importance to health sector professionals, future users of software packages, is the evaluation and classification of software applications with respect to the individual aspects and characteristics of work processes in health sector [4]. Previous surveys of applied information technology in health institutions of Serbia in 1994 point to an overwhelming bias in favour of administrative function [5]. However, 79.3% of applications surveyed in this research were employed in a narrow medical sphere. It is now quite probable that the specialised administrative applications have developed into a broader based product encompassing the tasks of generating and maintaining medical records and appointments. This current research has identified influx of information technology into primary health care level, with the aim of improving efficiency, lowering of

costs and enhancing of provided care [7], so between end users 23.9% of software packages are now utilised in health centres.
The possibility of familiarisation with an application is an instrument used in sales and marketing of software applications. In literature on sales and marketing of software attributes particular significance was given to the advertising and promotional aspects of the marketing effort [8]. This is not the case in health care market in Yugoslavia; because only one fifth of surveyed software packages could be trial as demo version.
The recommended model of the database on software applications in health industry in Yugoslavia formulated by this study shows similarities to the model developed by Pincireli [9] and his study of software applications in health industry. Unlike the Pincireli model, this model does not specify determinants of software quality, however the current set of parameters would meet the primary needs of interested buyers by providing fundamental information on the characteristics of the software package applicable to health care system. The next step would be, taking into consideration the mutual goals and aspirations of both the end users and software manufacturers towards quality software.

5. Conclusions

Investigations of software available to the health sector by software development companies and individuals as well as software vendors are concentrated in Belgrade. Evaluation of general characteristics of applicable software to the health sector identifies private companies as leading owners of copyright whereas the software is the result of collaborative effort between two or more authors or software experts. Evaluation of technical characteristics of software applications in health industry showed that the IBM compatible personal computer is the most often specified platform and languages are capable of supporting relational databases. The suppliers of software applications port their products to a variety of operating systems. Evaluation of salient user orientated attributes of software offered to the health care system indicates that the end users are most often supported in maintenance of health and medical records and documentation as well as maintenance of appointments records. Future users of software applications in health industry wishing to either purchase or develop new software solutions required by their respective organisations, may query the data base in order to become familiar with fundamental attributes of software applications on offer to the health care in the Yugoslav market.

References

[1] J. C. Lowery, J. B. Martin, Evaluation of Healthcare from a Usability Perspective, Journal of Medical Systems 14 (1-2) (1990) 17-29.
[2] P. Kokol, A New Microcomputer Software System Evaluation Paradigm: The Medical Perspective, Journal of Medical Systems 15 (4) (1991) 269-275.
[3] Software Survey Section. Computers in Biology and Medicine - An International Journal 24 (5) (1994), pp 1-4.
[4] J. Brender, Assessment of IT - Based Solutions in Healthcare: Trends in Today's Practice and Justification of Tomorrow's Approach. MIE '97, IOS Press, Amsterdam, 1997, pp. 730-735.
[5] S. Simic, J. Marinkovic, S. Stanojevic i saradnici, Analiza stanja informaticke tehnologije u zdravstvenim ustanovama Srbije, Srpski arhiv 123 (2) (1995) 5-8.
[6] F. M. Frankenfeld, Trends in computer hardware and software, American Journal of Pharmacy in Hospitals 50 (4) (1993) 707-711.
[7] J. G. Anderson, C. E. Aydin, S. J. Jay, Evaluating Health Care Information Systems. Sage Publications Thousand Oaks, London, New Delhi, 1994.
[8] Vella, P. Phillips, Department of Computing The University of Luton, Obezbedjenje kvaliteta softvera, Seminar, Beograd, decembar, 1996.
[9] F. Pincireli, C. Combi, G. Pozzi, A Database schema for public-domain medical software, Computers in Biology and Medicine 24 (4) (1994) 243-254.

Medical Informatics Europe '99
P. Kokol et al. (Eds.)
IOS Press, 1999

Developing a Health Care Information System for Scotland

M. Howard WILLIAMS[a], Gavin VENTERS[b], George VENTERS[c] and David MARWICK[a]
[a] *Heriot-Watt University, Edinburgh, Scotland*
[b] *Information and Statistics Division, CSA, Edinburgh, Scotland*
[c] *Lanarkshire Health Board, Hamilton, Scotland*

Abstract. The rapid development and uptake of Internet technology has created opportunities for large-scale information networks to replace paper-based information sources. In order to obtain the maximum benefits for patients and medical practitioners it is important that health care providers work together to produce an integrated information service. However, the task of bringing together a large number of different information providers to create a huge structured pool of information covering a wide range of topics with appropriate quality assurance is non-trivial. This paper describes an approach being used to create healthcare information systems in a set of co-operative healthcare information networks in Europe, and specifically in Scotland.

1. Introduction

The Internet has transformed our notions of information provision within society. Many healthcare organisations are already making information available to the public, patients or medical practitioners through the Web [1] and a much greater number are likely to do so in the future. Although information aimed at the medical practitioner is not generally intended for patients, much of it is publicly available and there is no necessity to prevent patients from accessing it. Even where information is sensitive, appropriate password protection and encryption is often sufficient protection for it. Only in the case of patient-related data does the problem of security become a serious issue and the suitability of the Internet is in question.

Thus most major health care organisations are likely to establish Web sites over the next few years to provide information both to patients and medical practitioners. However, one problem with this is the difficulty that faces users in finding the information they require. The huge size and anarchical organisation of information on the Internet means that users can be overloaded with information as hundreds or even thousands of responses are found for individual search queries. In addition, the fact that anyone can establish a web site means that a high proportion of information can be of questionable quality [2]. This difficulty of finding relevant and reliable information in an ever-growing information pool when one does not know where to look detracts from the potential usefulness of this powerful tool.

For this reason the idea of a Co-operative or Community Healthcare Information Network (CHIN) has evolved [3, 4]. One objective of a CHIN is to co-ordinate the efforts of different healthcare information providers and impose some structure on their contributions. This makes it easier to group together sets of information from different providers (to simplify the task of finding information) and to make best use of linkages between information sets).

This paper describes the approach which has been developed as part of the CHIN project - a European funded project aimed at developing Co-operative Healthcare Information Networks in different European countries, exploiting the commonalities between different implementations and interlinking the resulting systems to produce an international CHIN.

2. Scottish Health on the Web

As part of the CHIN project an information network is being developed for Scotland which will co-ordinate the efforts of a range of different healthcare providers. This has been given the title Scottish Health On the Web (SHOW). The overall goal is the creation of a virtual health care library for Scotland that will enable patients to take a more active role in their own health care and provide support for professionals in a variety of ways. The current thrust of activity is aimed at involving all the key health care providers in Scotland and changing their approach to information dissemination to a strategy focused on Web-based tools. After this the content available on the network will expand steadily and become the major source of health care information in Scotland.

Most health care institutions produce a range of paper-based documents aimed at patients. This information may vary from simple patient handbook information to more detailed advice on screening on different medical conditions and their treatment, on particular surgical operations, on support groups, and so on. The problem for a patient is not merely to lay hands on such documents, but to know that they exist and where they can be found. By bringing them all together into a single virtual health care library, one creates a huge source of information that is accessible from any part of the country. Thus all the information which any patient in Scotland may require should be accessible in this information pool. An additional benefit is that institutions can easily learn from each other and are motivated to improve the information sets that they want to target at patients.

From the point of view of medical practitioners this virtual library of healthcare information also includes information aimed primarily at the professional. Hospitals already provide information directed at general practitioners, including information on changes to existing services or the introduction of new ones, laboratory handbooks, etc. Organisations focusing on specific health care problems (e.g. e-coli, cancer, heart disease, etc.) provide information targeted at the professional. Even the Management Executive of the NHS in Scotland needs a rapid channel of communication by which to reach health care professionals.

3. Main Information Providers

The vast majority of healthcare organisations which are contributing to SHOW (or who will do so in the future) are providers of healthcare services and their entries reflect this by presenting some or all of the following [5]:

- Information on services available
- Information on how to access the services
- Guidance on the use of services
- Statistics on the performance of services
- Information on the cost of services
- Information on the usage of services.

The service providers are currently grouped into four categories:

(1) Regional health authorities (or health boards).
(2) Hospitals.

(3) Primary care providers (including general practitioners, healthcare clinics and specialists practitioners).
(4) Other organisations providing "infrastructural" support to the health service, such as parts of the CSA (e.g. Information and Statistics Division).

In addition to these a small set of organisations are responsible for educational material. This material can be grouped into three categories:
(1) Public Health Education. The purpose of this is to provide the general public with information to enable them to preserve their health (through healthy eating, exercise, etc.) or to understand the risks and problems associated with smoking, drug taking, AIDS, etc.
(2) Patient Education. This covers information on specific medical conditions and their treatment.
(3) Professional Education. Currently this is focused on the publication of clinical guidelines.

4. Creating Individual Entries

From the set of information providers, three types were identified which have enough in common to make the development of generic information structures desirable. These were hospitals, health boards and general practices. Although there are many differences between hospitals, different staff, different departments, different services, etc., there is also much in common. The same is true of general practices. Thus it is possible to develop tools to aid in creating these entries.

Through consultation with information providers, a set of guidelines has been developed which provides recommendations on site structure and navigation, page layout, use of colour, typefaces and legibility of information, response times, etc. Other guidelines include basic HCI recommendations and performance considerations, such as the limited use of graphics and limiting "key" graphic files to <30KB, limitations on the use of more sophisticated features of sites to facilitate support by "naive" providers and to enable sites to be maintained with minimal technical expertise, the avoidance of features which are not supported by both Netscape and Internet Explorer, etc. Using these guidelines and the specific requirements of the information providers, a set of reference sites was created.

These reference sites were then used to develop templates that can be used to support more general implementation by other providers within a region. A frame-based approach is followed with page content contained in the right-hand frame and navigation features in the left-hand toolbar frame. This allows the structure of a site to be stored in one place (the navigation frame) with the page content (optionally) free of any programming or control structures. This eases the task of site development as site developers can concentrate on the provision of content for the content pages without the need for much expertise. The JavaScript content of the toolbar frame has also been designed to be easily configurable by non-expert users.

The JavaScript templates have been used to develop a tool that generates an information site automatically. The tool takes the form of a "wizard" that guides the user through different stages and enables him/her to customise an information site according to the particular needs for the organisation concerned. Thus instead of setting up an information site from scratch by creating different content pages each time, pages that are common for the particular type of site (hospital or general practice) need only be customised according to the specific needs of the site. The user starts by selecting which type of site to generate and then selects which of the "standard" pages to include in the new site. The individual pages are linked together by the wizard and the user can then view the result and customise individual pages as required. The application has been designed to be portable and has been tested on a range of different systems, including Macintosh, PC and Sun.

5. Conclusion

The development of a health care information network as the prime means of distributing general information on health care to both patients and medical practitioners will transform the dissemination of health care information for the future. Maximum benefit can be achieved if different information providers work together to produce an integrated information service. As such the Co-operative or Community Healthcare Information Network (CHIN) will have a significant impact on the way in which healthcare information is distributed in the future.

In Scotland an information network called SHOW (Scottish Health On the Web) has the support of the Management Executive of the NHS in Scotland (see Scottish Health Service White Paper [6]). Currently, of the 15 health boards in Scotland, all but four have developed or are developing SHOW sites. Of the 47 hospital trusts in Scotland, more than half have live SHOW sites or are preparing them. All of the HQ organisations of the NHS in Scotland have SHOW sites which are live or in preparation. In all 74 organisations now have live SHOW sites while a further 23 have sites under review awaiting release.

In addition to providing information on health care services in Scotland, the network provides a natural repository for a wide range of reference material such as guidelines for medical professionals, laboratory handbooks, blood transfusion information, etc. The usefulness of the system is enhanced by the integration of links to database systems. By linking these systems into the network in a seamless fashion, the basic information provision is greatly enhanced. Databases such as the support group database (HEBS), statistical databases (ISD), publication databases, etc. are currently available without the user being aware of any database interface. Others, such as the Travax database of health care information for travellers, are available to a restricted set of users who have password access.

The rate of access has grown steadily since SHOW became live and currently the hit rate is over 24,000 page hits per day. At this stage a major problem lies in building up content in a structured form as rapidly as possible. Tools have been developed to aid in this task.

Acknowledgements

This work was funded as part of the CHIN project under the Framework IV Telematics programme of the European Union and the authors acknowledge this support. They also thank other partners of the CHIN project and the many organisations contributing to SHOW.

References

[1] F. Norman, Organising medical networked information (OMNI), Med Inform (Lond), 23(1): 43-51 (1998).

[2] P. Impicciatore, C. Pandolfini, N. Casella and M. Bonati, Reliability of health information for the public on the world wide web: systematic survey of advice on managing fever in children at home, BMJ, 314:1875 (1997).

[3] M.H. Williams, G.G. Venters and G.A. Venters, Towards co-operative health information networks, Proc. 7th Int IMEKO Conference, MBB95 (1995), pp 273-277.

[4] A.J. Weser, L. Kleinholz, P.O. Soderstrom, P. Eklund, G. De Moor, M.H. Williams, G. Venters and B. Mahr, Co-operative Health Information Networks, MIE (1996).

[5] G.A. Venters, M.H. Williams and G.G. Venters, The SHOW Approach to Internet delivery of healthcare information, Proc. of Current Perspectives in Healthcare Computing 1998, Harrogate, eds. B.Richards and H.Wood, BJHC Ltd., Surrey, 214-221 (1998).

[6] Scottish Office, Designed to Care: Renewing the National Health Service in Scotland. Scottish Office White Paper, 1997.

Medical Informatics Europe '99
P. Kokol et al. (Eds.)
IOS Press, 1999

Paediatric case-mix of the Lorraine regional database in 1994 and 1995

P.Gillois H.Garin F.Kohler
Laboratory SPIEAO Faculty of medicine Nancy I, BP184 F54550 Vandœuvre - France

Abstract. In the region, there is a need to predict the necessary number of paediatric beds. Paediatric discharge data from the 1994-95 Lorraine regional database of Anonymous Discharge Summaries (ADS) are used for this study. We analyse the concentration and specialisation of the hospital activity types and we estimate the numbers of paediatric beds needed for the year 2 000. For the same percentage of the case-mix by hospital group, concentration of the activity is more important in the small District General Hospital (DGH) than in the Teaching Hospital (TH). In the most important Medical Diagnosis Categories (MDC), the case-mix variation by age class can't be characterised inside of the MDC group. The different methods we use to estimate the need of paediatric beds, give similar estimations for the year 2 000.

1 Introduction

The French Diagnosis Related Groups (DRG) originate from Fetter's DRG [1] and have been introduced in the eighties to face the financial crisis. Their use has been instituted to implement a medicalised control of hospital expenditures. DRG have been conceived and adapted to describe short hospital length of stays in France and are now used as a basis of classification of hospital stays in the French Health Care Management Information System [2-3]. The use of medical information in the budgetary allocation has entailed the making of a regional database [4]. Access was given to the data by the GRAIH[1] in the French East region named Lorraine. The aims of this study are to analyse the concentration and specialisation of the medical activity in the different hospital groups and to estimate the need of paediatric beds in the region for the year 2000. The regional database used in this study excludes independent clinics (private clinics) and independent maternity units.

2 Material and method

2.1 Data used

Patient hospital short stay data from the 1994-95 Lorraine regional database of Anonymous Discharge Summaries (ADS) were used for this study. Only hospitals with more than 100 short stay beds participated in the constitution of this database. ADS include informations on hospital type, obtained according to its activity in terms of number of annual stays and the juridical entity (public, PHPHC[2]), patient's sex and age, patient's characteristics in terms of principal diagnosis, major diagnosis categories (MDC), DRG and medical or surgical type of the latter. Version 2.3 of the French DRG classification was used for both years [5]. Age was truncated at 18 years, to follow the age cut-off determined by the DRG

[1] Regional Health Care Management Information Group
[2] Private Hospitals participating in the Public Health Care

classification. Our choice of age classification in groups of children aged less than 16, 12, 3 years and 3 months was dictated by paediatric service definitions, puberty age (age limit for specific interventions such as respiratory airways endoscopy and the age entry for nursery school), infancy and age at the second medical certificate, respectively. Age was thus grouped into 6 categories.
Groups of diseases were determined from the data available, by subdividing the MDC into medical and surgical sub-categories: under a given MDC, stays can be classified into medical or surgical DRGs. Thus, 44 groups designated as MDCms are obtained by eliminating the 24th CM (hospitalisations shorter than one day) and the non-existent medical or surgical sub-categories. From the aggregate levels, an intermediate cut-off point between that determined by MDC (too unrefined) and that determined by DRG (too accurate) was identified to obtain sufficient size within each cell of the contingency table by MDCms.
In accordance with GRAIH of Lorraine, and in order to preserve the anonymity of the hospitals, the study cannot identify any isolated hospital. Roundups that we have undertaken summarise principles of these used in the cost scale of 1995 [6]. We have thus created four groups of public hospitals according to their size and a group corresponding to private hospitals participating in the public health service. The latter group contains a mix of characteristics due to the size of different hospitals, their degree of specialisation and their method of working (specific health insurance of the mining region). The first group includes district general hospitals (DGH) which are not teaching hospital (TH) with more than 14 000 in-patients per year, the second between 7 000 and 14 000 (including the regional public maternity hospital) and the third less than 7 000. The fourth consists of the private hospitals participating in the public health service (PHPHC) as well as the only Lorraine cancer centre. The last group is made up of the teaching hospitals of the region.

2.2 *Statistical analysis*

The statistical analysis includes three points:
-Analysis of the regional database of Lorraine in 1994-95 by age class.
-Analysis of concentration of the activity and specialisation of hospital groups.
-Estimation of the number of beds for paediatric activity in the Lorraine region for year 2 000.
Data analysis was made with SAS Software.

3 Results

The Lorraine two-year database included 855 636 hospitals admissions and with the previous selection, we obtained 131 570 stays (15.4% of the total database). The 1994's ADS represent 50.9% of the paediatric regional biennial database. Teaching hospitals have taken care of 37% of the paediatric stays and 45.6% of traditional stays are equally divided among highly busy and moderately busy DGH. PHPHC carry out only 13.2% and the less busy DGH 4.2% of paediatric ADS for patient under than 18 years. Most in-patients have stayed in only one medical unit inside the hospital (89.7% of stays). Male paediatric cases are the majority (54.4% of stays). Without taking into account the 25 266 normal newborns, mean age equals 6 years and 9 months and standard deviation is 6. The medical characteristic of the DRG is predominant with 81.2% of ADS. Traditional stays have on average 0.7 diagnoses associated (the standard deviation is 1.2) and 1.3 act by ADS (the standard deviation is 2.1). Stays are equally distributed across months.

3.1 *Analysis of in-patients by age class*

By analysing the part of each MDCms in the case-mix by age class, in decreasing frequency order, we can notice that:
- MDC 15 (newborn illnesses and neonatal period) is the most frequent, with more than the quarter of the stays. It is especially true for patients under 1 year for whom it represents

47% to 84% (with the normal newborn) of the case-mix of the age class. We have to moderate these results, due to the non-substantial proportion of normal newborn: 25 266 stays in the class [0-90 days].

- Medical MDC 06 (gastro-enterology) is frequent whatever the age. Rate by age class fluctuated from 3.1% to 16.4% with the peak in the class 1-3 years. Surgical MDC 06, ranking 8th by decreasing value of case-mix, is found mainly in children over 3 years, with rate fluctuating from 6.2% to 8.5%.

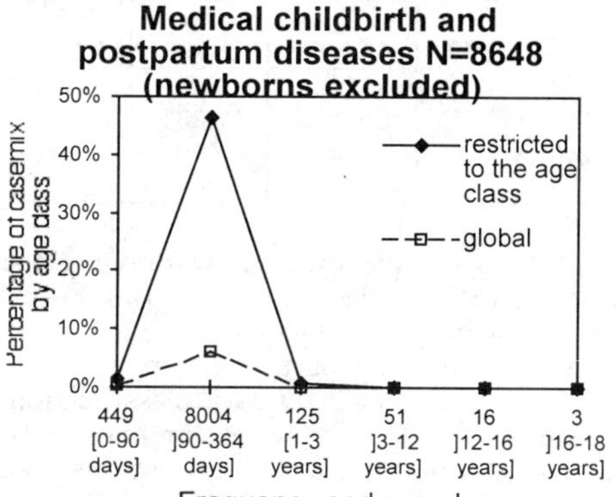

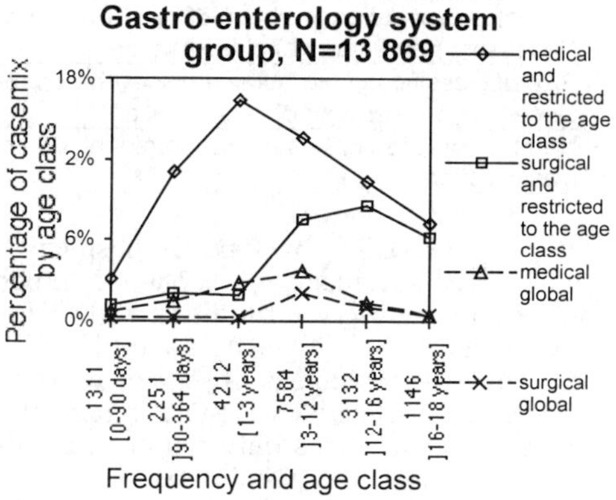

Figures 1 & 2 : Distribution of frequencies by age class for each class and globally

The peak of 47% in the age class [90-364 days] represents only 6 % of the global case-mix. The twelve most important medical and surgical MDC, are displayed in table 2 with for each age class and for each medical or surgical MDC, the number of stay and the relative frequency code. By increasing order the codes are: very seldom (VS) for less than 1% in the age class, from 1 to 5% seldom (S), from 5 to 10% frequent (F), from 10 to 40% more frequent (MF) and more than 40% the most frequent (TMF).

Table 2

Age classes **Size and frequency code restricted to the age class**	**[0-90 days]**	**]90-364 days]**	**[1-3 years]**	**]3-12 years]**	**]12-16 years]**	**]16-18 years]**
Medical nervous system group	VS	S	MF	MF	F	F
Medical childbirth and postpartum disease	S	TMF	VS	VS	VS	VS
Medical respiratory system group	S	MF	MF	S	S	S
Other medical health factors	S	F	S	S	S	S
Medical skin and breast group	VS	VS	S	S	F	F
Pathological pregnancy	VS	VS	VS	VS	S	MF
Gastro-enterology system group						
Medical	S	MF	MF	MF	MF	F
Surgical	S	S	S	F	F	F
Ears Nose Throat group						
Medical	VS	VS	S	MF	S	S
Surgical	S	F	MF	F	F	F
Muscular skeletal system group						
Medical	VS	S	S	F	F	F
Surgical	VS	VS	S	F	MF	MF

The other MDCms are barely constitutive of the case-mix by age class, they do not represent more than 17% of the total case-mix.

3.2 Case-mix and concentration indicators

If we focused on the distribution of the MDC, to obtain 50% of the case-mix, 3 MDC are sufficient (13% MDC): neonatalogy, gastro-enterology and Ears Nose Throat system group while the first 8 MDC by decreasing order of frequencies represent 80% of the case-mix: rhumato-orthopedics, neurology, pneumology, dermatology and other causes of health care utilisation.

Table 1

Frequencies	MDC	MDCms	DRG	MD
Size of classification to obtain **50% of the case-mix**	3	5	10	41
Necessary percentage of classification	13,04%	11,36%	2,44%	1,14%
Size of classification to obtain **80% of the case-mix**	8	11	46	294
Necessary percentage of classification	34,78%	25,00%	11,22%	8,16%
Number of possibilities in the regional database by classification	23	44	410	3 602

By filing the DRG by type of hospital, by decreasing frequency and by drawing the cumulative percentage, we obtain 5 progression curves for the case-mix. The fastest progression is observed for the small DGH, while for teaching hospitals the slope is slower. The medium DGH, large DGH and PHPHC seem to have similar progression curves.
The same progression is observed by using MDC, MDCms and MD as a classification. Concentration of activity is more important in the small DGH that in the teaching hospitals. The small DGH treats only a limited number of DRGs while the teaching hospitals take care of almost the whole existent DRG. That is in disagreement with the usual specialisation notion of the teaching hospitals with the highest speed progression of indicator for the small DGH, supposed to be general hospitals.

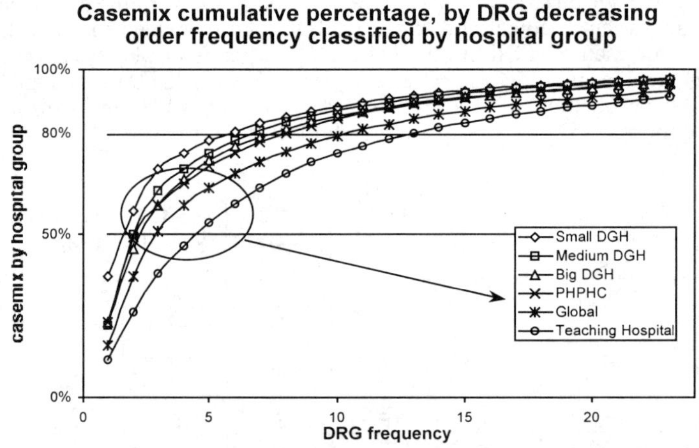

Figure 3

3.3 Lorraine region demographic simulation of beds number

In 1995, the Lorraine region was constituted by 2 311 263 residents. The French demographic projection named OMPHALE provided by INSEE[3], shows for the year 2000, a raise of the total population of + 0.21% (4 931 residents) for all ages. Moreover, for the less than 18 years, their proportion should decrease by -3.86% (less 22 789 residents) to become lower than the quarter of the total population. Only classes of age less than 1 year and more than 16 years sustain a raise. The other age class all decrease, ranking from -0.14% for the 11 years to -13.65% for the class 6 years.

[3] Statistic and Economic Study National Institute

This total decrease of the paediatric population should have an incidence on the estimated number of beds needed in year 2000. To appreciate this influence, we calculated for each age the regional case-mix. This case-mix, associated to national lengths of stay, enabled us to calculate annual occupation duration times taking into account the occupation official rate (0.85). We obtain thus a number of theoretical beds for the year 1995, that is 1 042 beds. By applying fluctuations by age of the population to the case-mix by age of 1995, we obtain a sum of lengths of stay and thus a number of estimated beds for the year 2000, which is 1 024 beds.

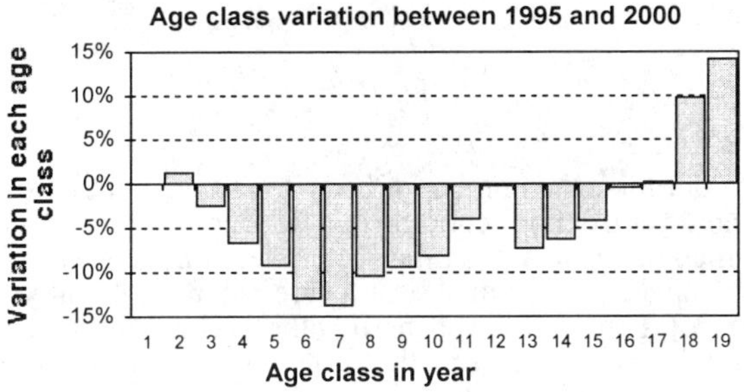

Figure 4

The case-mix being regarded as constant by age unit, the number of beds calculated on national length of stay applied to the regional case-mix of 1995 shows a weak decline of approximately 18 beds. By using lengths of stay observed in the Lorraine region to calculate the number of beds, we obtain 1 016 beds for 1995. Compared to 1 024 estimated beds for the year 2000, the region requires a raise of the number of paediatric beds of + 8 beds.

4 Discussion

This study confirms the well-known paediatric situation for hospital morbidity for specific diagnosis groups and by age classification. The structural effect of these different types of hospitals is found inverted in comparison with the missions of the hospitals.
Moreover the French administrative cut-off of 16 years for paediatric departments is not well reflected in this database, as the diagnosis and DRGs globally are the same for patients aged 16 to 18 years. This cut-off should be adjusted.
Without any possibility of linkage between admissions, analyses of health care pathway and medical economic plan are tricky, more particularly when excluding the 24th CM (hospitalisations shorter than one day). In the private medical structure this linking is operational and enables to check the health care pathways.
The evolution of the French classification for the 15th MDC is more pertinent for the medium-term medical economic plan and in particular for the perinatal period. The five DRGs including newborn with problems are taking into account neither birth weight, nor discharge mode. The new classification deserves better attention of these issues.
Similarly, severity of illness at admissions is not adequately taken into account [7-9]. This problem should result in an evolution of these DRGs into Homogenous Stay Groups which would include indicators of coverage complexity, as can be seen in geriatric care, and means of linking several stays for one patient.
The specialisation notion, based on the case-mix cumulative percentage as specialisation and concentration indicator, was the opposite of the usual notion. The small DGHs require less DRGs with higher concentration activity than TH, the latter having lower indicator for a given same case-mix.
It should be noted that the calculation of the number of regional Lorraine beds is based on the following hypothesis:
-the case-mix remains constant from 1995 to 2000 by age groups. This is to say that the incidence of illness, medical practice in terms of access to hospital and medical financial

health care coverage, and hence length of stay in hospital, will remain the same in 1995 and 2000.
-the national lengths of stay observed come from the 1995 scale of cost and are therefore not necessarily representative of all hospitals in the region.
-the lengths of stay observed are used for the calculation of the number of beds in our second hypothesis, but the same quality requirements apply.
The quality of health care is not tackled, only some statistical references independent of the quality of care are. For these one thousand paediatric beds, they are not prejudging of health care efficiency.

5 Conclusion

Faced with a tendency to optimise the number of beds due to the population decline, factors such as social poverty could artificially conceal this decline, and, therefore should not be ignored [10]. Different methods result in similar estimated numbers of beds, which shows the need for an original database for regional health care planning. Finally this study can be carried out in other area of France, as well as in other geographic sectors like sanitary sectors, health care pool, life pool (defined by the access behaviour on postal or commercial services), or labour pool inside another area.

References

[1] Fetter R., Shi, Y.-S., Freeman J.-L. et al.. Casemix definition by Diagnosis related groups. *Med Care*, 1980; 18 : 1-53
[2] Guide méthodologique de production des résumés de sortie du PMSI. Paris: Direction des Journaux Officiels. 1994. (Bulletin Officiel N° spécial 94-6).
[3] Phelan PD, Baxter K, Bishop J, Hudson I, Hindle D Do diagnosis related groups separate the case-mix of a specialist children's hospital and a paediatric unit in a general hospital? *J Paediatr Child Health* 1993 Aug;29(4):266-269
[4] Fetter R. B. DRG refinement. Implication for Europe. *PCSE Conference*. Stockholm, Suède. Juin 1988.
[5] Manuel des Groupes Homogènes de Malades. Paris. Direction des Journaux Officiels. 1994. (Bulletin Officiel N° spécial 94-2 bis).
[6] Graih Circulaire DH/PMSI 45 du 9 juillet 1991.
[7] Bulletin Officiel. n° 95 - 5 bis. L'échelle nationale des coûts relatifs par groupes homogènes de malades. Direction des Journaux Officiels.
[8] Phelan PD Are casemix developments meeting the needs of paediatrics?*Med J Aust* 1994 Sep 5;161 Suppl:S26-S29
[9] Hanson RM, Phythian MA, Jarvis JB, Stewart C The true cost of treating children. *Med J Aust* 1998 Oct 19;169 Suppl:S39-41
[10] Vergnenegre A, Bisser S, Sagnes-Raffy C, Sene E, Bonnaud F Explanatory factors of length of stay at the diagnosis-related group 129:common pneumonia and pleurisy, aged over 69 and/or associated co-morbidities *Rev Pneumol Clin* 1996;52(4):245-252

Medical Informatics Europe '99
P. Kokol et al. (Eds.)
IOS Press, 1999

Introduction of a new Hospital Information System at the Innsbruck University Hospital

Verena Callegari*, Karl Peter Pfeiffer*, Georg Lechleitner**
* *University of Innsbruck, Department of Biostatistics and Documentation*
** *TILAK Gmbh, Innsbruck*

Abstract. The aim of the introduction of an advanced hospital information system at the Innsbruck University Hospital is mainly to support the care process and to improve quality and efficiency of care. These requirements entail changes in the clinical processes and many obstacles with respect to the organization have to be considered. The article gives an overview of the goals, organization and problems of the introduction which is still in the planning phase.

1. Project Introduction

1.1. Goals

In the past few years complaints and new requirements showed that the existing IT-environment at the Innsbruck University Hospital is no longer sufficient. Single departments started to install proprietary systems. The result is a heterogeneity of systems which have to be integrated for a hospitalwide use of patient data. The new system should provide functions for documentation, communication, presentation, evaluation, quality assurance and decision support.

Further reasons for the introduction of a new system are listed below:
Accessibility and management of the paper-based medical record is problematic. The goal is an electronic patient record who allows immediate access and a clear view to all relevant patient data no matter where these data come from. An important step will be the integration of inpatient and outpatient data since these data are separated in the Innsbruck University Hospital for administrative reasons now.

The procedure of ordering and resulting at the moment takes a lot of time to wait for someone who picks up the orders and the results. Many phone calls are made to specify the orders and to find out the stage of the processing. In the new system it must be possible to enter an order directly into the computer where it will immediately show up at the ancillary site. The processing can be tracked by giving status reports like „specimen arrived“, „in process“, etc.

One of the high priority goals is a scheduling system where patients can be scheduled for more than one examinations at different sites at the hospital. This process should be supported automatically by the system.

Since the introduction of a new hospital financing system in Austria the importance of electronic capturing of patient data is growing. The inpatient encounters are no longer charged by length of stay, but by service and diagnosis. For this purpose a data set with the most important patient data, as patient demographic data, organizational data and medical data, has to be captured. Therefore flexible forms for structured electronic data entry will be necessary to facilitate this process.

Furthermore standardization and optimization of the care process should be managed by the new system.

1.2. Environment - TILAK Organization and Innsbruck University Hospital

TILAK is a holding company, responsible for the management of 4 hospitals. The biggest is the University Hospital in Innsbruck - around 1600 beds, compared with a total of around 2400. The new system will be introduced in all TILAK hospitals, the start will take place in Innsbruck. Innsbruck University Hospital delivers care for around 61.700 inpatients and 275.000 outpatients per year. The requirements of an University Hospital exceeds the ones for a „normal" hospital. Features like flexible medical documentation possibilities for clinical trials are necessary as well.

1.3. The existing IT-technology

The current central patient information system is a ASCII-format oriented system for patient registration and a few medical documentation possibilities. Viewing results from the laboratory system and entering diagnoses and services are examples of the functionality. All outpatient clinics and all wards are integrated in this system, with a total of 500 workstations and 2.200 users at the moment.
Furthermore some departmental systems and clinical support systems are integrated via the communication server „Cloverleaf". There are standardized HL-7 interfaces as well as proprietary interfaces.

2. Organization of the Implementation

2.1. The Decision-Making Process

Beside the requirements defined above the search for a suitable product was performed by the following criteria. The system was expected to be
- highly integrated
- Windows based
- clinical oriented
- suitable for science and research with tools for quality assurance, data analysis and presentation.

Further requirements were a well structured, flexible database with a modern database management and the expectation of a continuos development of the system.

After an international search for hospital information systems the decision for Cerner Corp., Kansas City, MO, was made. This company developed a system called HNA-Millenium which focuses on the care process rather than on the administrative and billing process.

Before starting the implementation a group of software specialists has been established in Austria. This group has been trained on the system to serve as consultants for the this project and further projects in Europe.

2.2. Where to start – Pilots and Rollout

Two reasons prevent the simultaneous introduction of the whole planned functionality at all departments: The size of the hospital and the immense cultural change that will accompany change-over. Therefore the decision was made to split the functionality and implement it in four stages depending on the priority and complexity and to start the implementation at two pilot clinics which will be followed by the other departments during a rollout-phase. This means the implementation of stage 1 will be carried out at the pilots and then be extended on the other departments. Then stage 2 will start at the pilots etc.

The pilots were chosen because of the high motivation and a high level of structuring at these departments. It might be easier to implement the system and collect experiences there first before rolling out to more complex departments.
One of the pilots already uses a departmental system which is not ready for the Y2K problem. This means that there's a deadline for the basic functionality of the old system - December 1999.

2.3. Functionality

At the first stage the existing functions of the old system should be implemented in the new system to guarantee a continuous transition. These functions will mainly be administrative ones, e.g. patient management. It is necessary to implement interfaces to the old system, because this system will remain the registration system which assigns the unique patient and encounter identification numbers.

HL-7 interfaces to subsystems which are important for the department (e.g. radiology, laboratory) will be set up for the inbound of information. Thus results from these ancillary sites will be routed directly into the new system. At the first stage it will not yet be possible to set up an order via an HL-7 interface. A basic communication system will be introduced for the users of the system as well as scheduling functions for the outpatient clinics.

The coding of diagnoses and procedures is necessary for the billing process as described above and should therefore be integrated in the new system from the beginning.

The composition and storage of patient oriented clinical documents e.g. discharge summaries within the system will also be implemented at the first stage.

An important prerequisite for a continuous transition is the data transition from the old system to the new one.

Advanced functionality as ordering/resulting, additional interfaces to important subsystems, implementation of standards for treatment and nursing, proactive functions, decision support up to an integrated case management will be introduced at the following stages.

2.4. Prototype

Since there was no German demonstration material available the decision was made to develop an prototype of the Orthopedic Department which is one of the pilots. Real doctors' names, real patients, local facilities, German expressions, forms and user interfaces should be the environment of a real world scenario to give an impression how the system will look like and how processes could be carried out in the future. The design of the prototype was also a chance for the implementation team to get known to the system, its constraints and possibilities.

2.5. Process Redesign

The organizational changes which accompany the introduction of a new system have to be considered. Processes have to be redesigned to reach optimal support by the system.

The system itself is based on a workflow management where tasks can be defined. These tasks are listed in personal or common task-lists. Clinical documentation such as forms for structured data entry are integrated in these tasks and can be accessed during the processing of the task. Thus the user is supported through integrated documentation in the task. The importance of the connection between process management and document management was shown also by [1].

The reengineering of processes is part of the implementation strategy suggested by the Cerner Corp. This implementation strategy is called "Designer's workbench". There tools for the implementation especially for the process reengineering can be found.

First step is a current state analysis to inquiry the clinical processes as they are carried out now and the constraints given by the organization. An example for a constraint in the described environment is the lack of mobile computers. There won't be any mobile computers available - at least at the beginning- , so data captured on the bedside will be written down on paper and afterwards transcribed into the system.

Processes are visualized by the use of flowcharts which makes it easier to find bottlenecks and possibilities for improvement.

The next step is to analyze these processes in view of these constraints and the system's possibilities and to reengineer them. An important consideration is to include clinicians in the planning of these processes. Accordance has to be reached to assure acceptance.

An example of a process which will change substantially is the ordering and resulting process. Changing this process to an order process in the system disturbance will be reduced, the communication will be faster and a tracking of the stage of the order can be done easily.

The reengineering will be necessary not only for the first stage but also for the next three phases which will entail even bigger changes.

3. Experiences and Considerations

3.1. Current status

The Current State Analysis is nearly finished for the pilots (May 1999). The main processes have been analyzed in detail with the help of physicians, nurses and secretaries. Teams have been formed who are familiar with these processes.

The next step is to analyze the processes in view of potential benefits which can be gained through the use of the new system. These teams will differ from the former teams, because in this team stakeholders will be included to make the conversion easier.

The aim is to define standard processes which will be the basis for all departments.

3.2. Expected problems and challenges

The step by step introduction of the system means there has to be a parallel execution of the old and the new system which will force the staff to do some of the work in one system and some in a different system. The desired benefits will not be obvious until overall integration is reached.

The users' acceptance of the system and the change management are challenges, but there are many obstacles. There are high expectations that have to be met which might end up in disillusion and demotivation, especially in the early phase where only a small part of the whole functionality is available.

Associated with the problem described above is the security concept. Security can be defined by different levels as department, role of the care provider, etc. At the moment there are several task which are legally restricted to physicians, but in real life are done by nurses. A system will only allow authorized users to have access to some applications, tasks or data which might cause problems concerning the acceptance.

An other critical point is the scheduling of the training on the system, because of the large numbers of users. Therefore a training concept has to be developed.

The HNA-Millenium has been developed for the American health system mainly hence some effort will be necessary to adjust health system specific issues.

Today many documents consist of unstructured information mainly. To structure as much information as possible is a necessary prerequisite for analysis, scientific reasons, quality assurance and for the development of standards for treatment and nursing. A major part of the documentation considerations will be the design of forms for structured data entry.

Although the aim is the electronic capturing and storing of all patient data (see [2] for the requirements of an CPR) it will not be possible to integrate all documents in the system. Some of the remaining paper documents could be scanned, e.g. results from external sites. Still there are some documents that cannot be replaced via electronic documents because of legal reasons. The patient's compliance if he needs a surgical procedure e.g. has to be signed by hand and stored. There's no legal possibility to forego a handwritten signature yet.

There are lots of catalogues which have to be maintained and updated regularly. These catalogues are partly national catalogues partly local catalogues. A synchronizing concept has to be developed to synchronize these catalogues for the old and the new system.

References

[1] J.Bergmann, O.J.Bott, K.Dresing, D.P.Pretschner, K.-M.Stürmer. Spezifikationen der Anforderungen an das Dokumentationssystem einer klinischen Abteilung am Beispiel einer Klinik für Unfall-, Plastische un Wiederherstellungschirurgie, Methoden der Medizinischen Informatik, Biometrie und Epidemiologie in der modernen Informationsgesellschaft, pp 98-102, 1998.

[2] Jeffrey S. Rose. Clinical Information System and Computerized Patient Record Principles – Functions – Prototype, Toward An Electronic Patient Record ´96. Proceedings Volume One, pp 6-14, 1996.

Medical Informatics Europe '99
P. Kokol et al. (Eds.)
IOS Press, 1999

The Health Management Information System of Romania

Dan D. Farcas, Dr.math.
Bucharest, Ministry of Health

Abstract. In Romania a Health Management Information System (HMIS) project is in progress. The project covers the main activities of the Ministry of Health (MoH), of the 42 District Health Authorities and more than 250 other health care units. The first applications will be implemented at the middle of 1999. The paper shows the context of the HMIS among other Health Information Systems in Romania, its main parts and some organizational issues of the HMIS project, achievements and difficulties encountered.

1. The Romanian health information systems

In the Romanian health care system there are a great number of organizations and structures, and the relations between them are quite complex. Each of these organizations has its own specific information system, with a different degree of IT involved. These health information systems can be classified in the following five groups:

- **The Health Management Information System (HMIS)**, with its components: Ministry of Health, Center for Computing, Health Statistics and Medical Documentation (CCHSMD), District Public Health Authorities, etc.
- **Health care units information systems:** hospitals, other units with beds, polyclinics, dispensaries, ambulance stations, blood harvesting and transfusion centers, forensic medicine laboratories, drug warehouses and pharmacies, etc.
- **Health Insurance Information Systems (HIIS):** The National Health Insurance System (central, district and offices), Other State Health Insurance Systems (army, transports etc.), Private Health Insurance. (*note*: *they are scheduled to start their activity in 1999 or later*);
- **Information Systems of Health Research and Education:** The Academy of Medical Sciences, Health Research and Development Organizations, Medical and Pharmaceutical Universities, other health education organizations, Health Information and Documentation Centers,
- **Information Systems of other health care organizations:** The College of Physicians, The College of Pharmacists, health care professional associations etc.

2. The HMIS project

In Romania a 18 million USD World Bank loan Project is now in progress, for an integrated Health Information System, covering only a part of the systems above: the main part of HMIS and some functions of the activities of the health care units (Fig. 1). Also some of the functions included in this project could be useful for the future National Health Insurance System.

The Health Management Information Systems was structured in the following three **levels**:

1. **Central:** Ministry of Health, CCHSMD,
2. **District:** District Public Health Authority Neamt (pilot district), Other District Health Authorities and of Municipality Bucharest, Public Health Inspectors and of Municipality Bucharest,
3. **Local:** Hospital, Policlinic, dispensary, rural health centers, District ambulance stations, Blood collecting and preservation centers.

The present phase of this project started in 1995, with a technical specification. A bid was organized in 1996 for a turn-key solution. Due mainly to the frequent changes in the leadership of the Ministry of Health, the winner was announced only in July 1997 and the contract was signed only in February 1998 with Sema Group France, as integrator, having as subcontractors: Digital (now Compaq), SAP, etc. and using licenses from Comshare, CHU Grenoble, Hematos etc. It is expected that the system will start to be functional in the middle of the year 1999. For the application software, the system will be build by multiplying of some standard structures, adapted to the specificity of each customer. To keep the coherence of the whole system, all modifications in the programs will be performed only from one point: the Center for Computing, Health Statistics and Medical Documentation, which is the "competence center" of the future system.

Besides hardware and communication, the main subsystems and modules and the main application software provided by this project are: resources management, medical data management, ambulance, blood donors, reporting system and decision support, document management. The medical applications as well as the resources management for health care units are implemented in only one **pilot** district (Neamt). The decision support is provided for the Ministry of Health and for the 42 District Health Authorities, and the document management only for MoH. In the following, these subsystems will be briefly described.

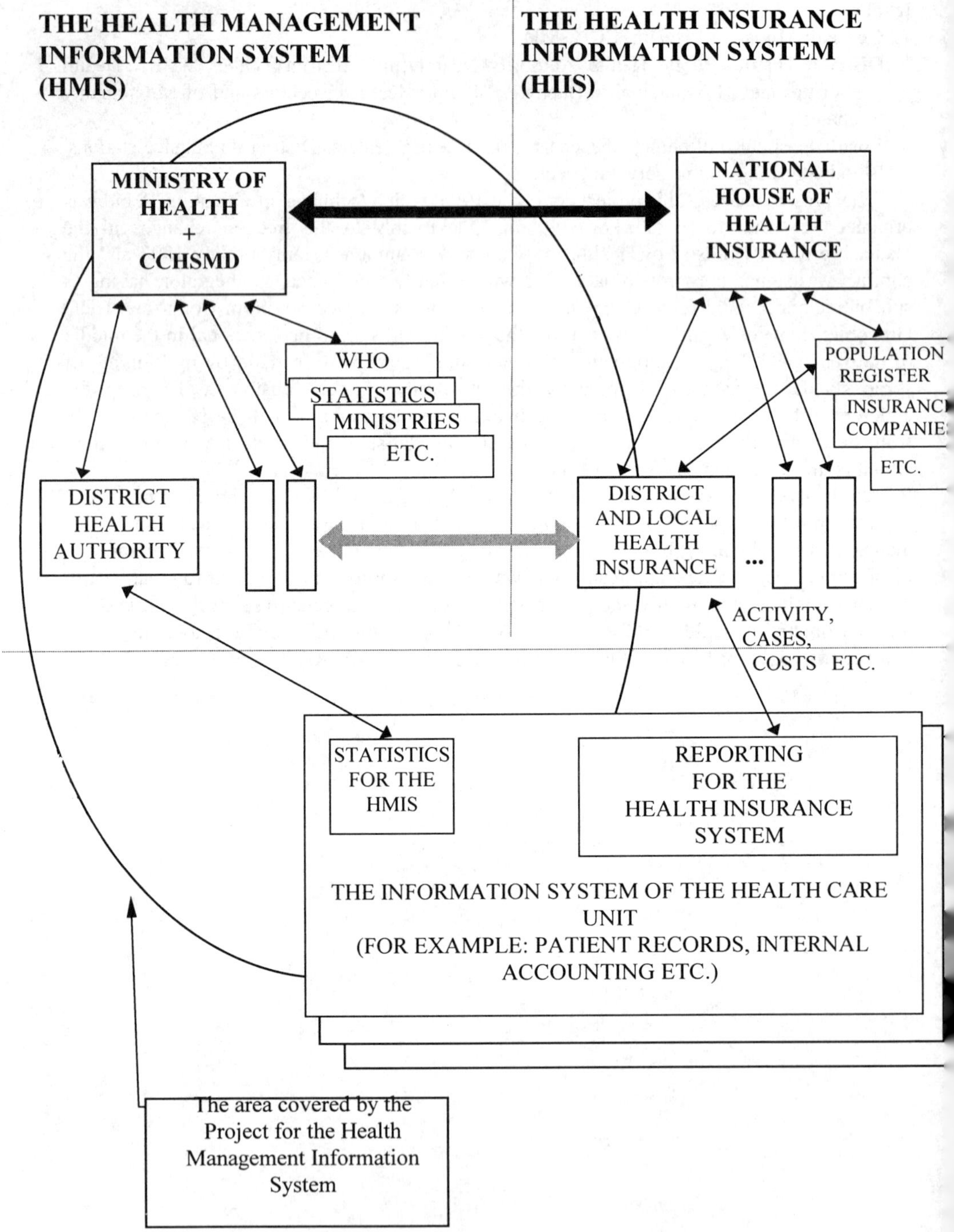

Fig. 1 **Scheme of the area covered by the world bank project for the Romanian health management information system**

2.1. hardware and communication

The contract included **goods:** hardware, WAN communication hardware, standard software, application software (including guarantee), recovery solution, consumable, as well as **services:** standard hardware and software installation, application software installation, WAN communication services, project management and training. Finally a number of some 230 servers and more than 900 PC-s were installed in 320 different places in all the 42 districts of Romania. The communications at the first two levels is done using the X25 standard through permanent lines. The connections between District Health Authorities and health care units are by dial up phone line. Inside the system an *intranet* system is used. All users have access to the *internet* including *e-mail*. A *firewall* will protect the sensitive data; however, a great amount of statistical health data will be accessible soon, through *internet*, as well as a web page of MoH. Some of this data can be used by the HSI/HFA programs distributed by WHO Europe.

2.2 resources management

For resources management the integrator company chose the SAP solution with the R/3 package, covering the accountability, budget, equipment, supplies, drugs, personnel, costs. In the first step a *pilot* system will be developed for the Neamt district health authority and the main subordinated health care units: hospitals, ambulance, blood transfusion. In a further step, if the solution will be appropriate, the roll-out of this system is expected to all districts and main health units. The R/3 is in process to be installed in the Ministry of Health too, and it is expected to control the expenses covered by the national health budget.

2.3 medical data management

For the management of *health care units* and for medical patient records the solution of the *Grenoble University Hospital Center* (CHU) was adapted to the conditions of Romanian hospitals, polyclinics, dispensaries etc. The patient record is comprehensive and flexible. It is initiated at the reception desk, and filled with data about investigation, diagnosis, medical acts, drugs, health conditions etc. There is a short, statistical, patient record too. Health documents could be edited (e.g. for family doctors). The patients are identified by a unique ID number (13 digits), already in use for the whole population of Romania. The coding are ICD-10 and other recommended by WHO. Bed management and other administrative modules are included too. The reporting interfaces from the health care units to the health insurance and the district authorities are coherent.

2.4 ambulance / emergency

A small application is installed in 34 district ambulance stations (in the other 8 a different system is already in use). The programs ensure the follow-up of the ambulances, calls, transportation, a short patient record, compatible with CHU, report generation and export of data for statistics.

2.5 blood donors

A pilot application, using "Hematos" software is installed in the Neamt district transfusion center. It controls the donors, their health status, the blood and blood products, including quality check, the use of the blood at the receiver and the possible accidents, identifying the source of them. In future the application is intended to be extended to the other district transfusion centers of Romania.

2.6 reporting system and decision support

The decision support system is using the data from all the applications above, as well as from external sources (health statistics, other applications, from National Statistical Office, WHO etc.) through the *external data* module. The programs of the *Exchange* module introduce all these data in an *Oracle* data base. The data will be filtered, integrated and transferred to a the decision support system organized with the *Comshare* software (Fig. 2). This product has a multidimensional database (organized in 6 "domains", containing 29 "cubes", each of them with several indicators), user-friendly interfaces (graphics, maps, statistical tools), facilities to define complex indicators, as well as reporting and export facilities toward current software as *Word* or *Excel*. This product is in process to be installed in the MoH and the 42 District Health Authorities. In the MoH will be also installed the *TeamLinks* product for document management.

3. Achievements and failures

For the Romanian Health System 1998 and 1999 was a period of great transitions. The District Health Authorities were restructured and split in two parts: one of them included in the health insurance system, the other part was unified with the District Public Health Inspectorates. Among other troubles, this produced changes in the rooms scheduled for installing the equipment. A new administrative district was also organized. Many laws, regulations and hierarchical command lines were changed. A completely new payment system for medical staff will be established in 1999, based on the regulations of the future Health Insurance Houses. All this process is not yet finished.

During 1995-1998 the leadership of the Ministry of Health and of CCHSMD was changed frequently. As well was changed the project manager, mainly to increase the involvement of the MoH in the project. These changes and the fact that the job descriptions of the participants to the management team were not always very well defined, produced delays and some discontinuities in achievements. Incoherence in legislation gave some delays in payment procedures

In the Ministry of Health and in the District Health Authorities some resistance to the changes was recorded, mainly in places where some old IT solutions were used. The result was also a delay in implementing the applications.

Because of the great time gap between the bidding and the delivery, the hardware and software was several times updated. For each site were established: acceptance committees, drafts of the rooms, forms filled with information about existing facilities. The data obtained was periodically verified and updated. Some problems arose because of the lack of direct telephone lines.

An estimated number of 2000 users have to be trained in the next year. Therefore four training centers were organized in four corners of the country. In the first step, only two of them were functional. More than 25 *training* courses were organized, starting with September 1998, in Bucharest and Neamt district, for over 400 persons, mainly trainers for the future courses. Some problems were given by the travel and accommodation expenses, not provided in the budget, and with a "brain drain" of IT and public health specialists to other areas (even after they finished the courses), owing to the low salaries in the health administration. Many specialists moved to the new health insurance houses, where the salaries are higher than in the state administration.

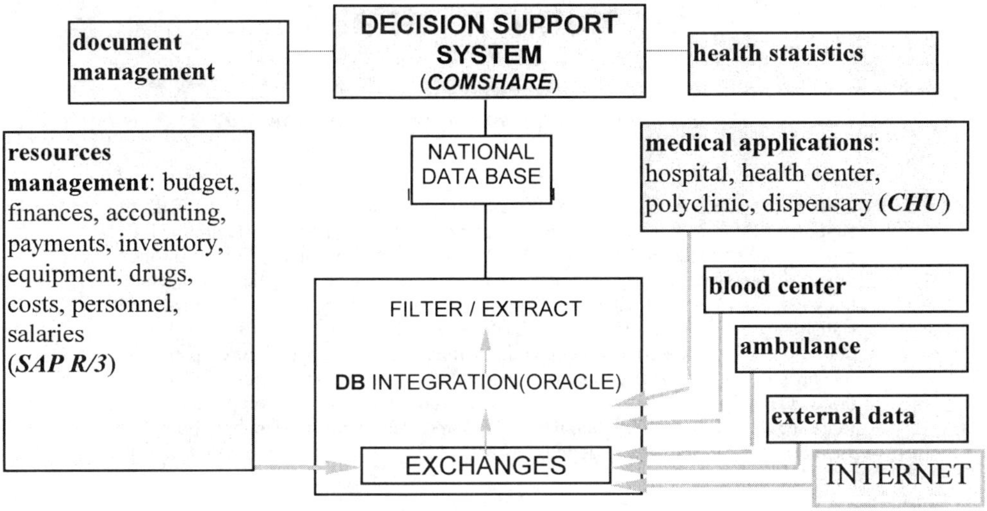

Fig. 2 **The main data flow from the applications to the decision support system**

Some functions of the new information system as the payment of the general practitioners are expected to migrate to the future *Health Insurance Information System (HIIS)*. However, the whole HIIS will be a completely new system, with its own coherence. A close cooperation with the Center for Computing, Health Statistics and Medical Documentation is highly advisable, but was not yet agreed.

A general evaluation of the project outputs, as well as of the efficiency of the solutions is expected at the beginning of the year 2000. A new project is expected for the roll-out of the accepted applications, in all districts, as well as in hospitals, blood transfusion centers etc., and for new solutions in the areas not properly covered. The financing of this new project is not yet established. Some functions could be accomplished by the CCHSMD team.

NOTE: The author is former director and deputy director of the Center for Computing, Health Statistics and Medical Documentation (CCHSMD) of the Romanian Ministry of Health, the organization responsible for the project, and he is actually chief of the health information research service in CCHSMD. The author is also full member of the Romanian Academy of Medical Sciences, president of its IT Committee, and vice-president of the Romanian Society for Health Informatics. He was involved from the beginning in the management of this project and is still part of it.

Medical Informatics Europe '99
P. Kokol et al. (Eds.)
IOS Press, 1999

National Information System on Hospital Treatment

Gorazd Raič
Public Health Institute of the Republic of Slovenia

Abstract: National information system on hospital treatment (HOSTREAT) supports health management system applied by the Ministry of Health and its professional services at the Public Health Institute of Slovenia. The main project objective was data quality, having in mind advanced analytical methods such as knowledge discovery in databases. The step was a huge one, as the related national statistics rests on every single hospital event, called an episode. By the project definition, an episode covers therapeutic treatment of *one* sick or injured person in *one* hospital within *one* health service specialty. So, many problems arose within the three years of project phases. Much research work was to be done on programming tools and the information system itself. This paper deals with five strategic problems and corresponding corrective actions.

1. Strategic Problems and/or Project Objectives

1.1 Ignoring the Multi-discipline Nature of Informatics

The problem above shows up especially in medical informatics. Why?

In the therapeutic sphere, medical doctors traditionally retain all the authority and responsibility. Spreading out from the consulting room, a medical person is encountered with other domains which should be accordingly managed by other professionals. That is easy to say, but difficult to consider if management policy is inclined to discrimination.

Moreover, the two areas require extremely distinct ways of professional mentality. Namely, the medical area arises from *stochastic* system while the informaticians solve problems by most acute *deterministic* methods.

1.2 Omitting the Feasibility Study (regarding the database)

The planned health care analysis is not based on the hospital episode, mentioned in the abstract. The project concentrates rather on the concept of hospitalization, which covers therapeutic treatment of *one* sick or injured person in *one* hospital, causing one or more episodes. So, an episode is more or less an ambitious means to reach a higher level of data analysis to come.

In the preliminary phase, the *hospital admission key* was made up of a single datafield (called »the ordinal case number«) defined deep in manuals as the *ordinal hospitalization number*. But, apparently a little ease in the end-user training (rather: in naming the key datafield) caused much redundant work and research. We must bear in mind that many of the 324.000 collected records were not keyed as expected: end-users assigned a new ordinal case number to each patient move within hospital. There was no way to reject the received records, so a substitute key was needed to preserve the future information.

1.3 Data Extent and Structure

The project recognizes seven hospitalization areas: hospital treatment due to *diseases, injuries, poisoning, rehabilitation, birth, sterilization, fetal death*. The same structure of primary key is assigned to all hospitalization areas, while the episode attributes differ to some extent according to each hospitalization type. A typical record gives such parameters:

Record:	#key segments:	#attributes	#total fields	#verification cases
ADMISSION	12	13	25	54
EPISODE	8	11	19	40
	20	24	**44**	**94**

At present, data are collected by 28 hospitals and 18 rehabilitation centers, producing around 324.000 medical events. Medical records come in from seven hospitalization areas in 83 input files. Each file in the data entry process occupies four states, thus yielding 332 different file names at least twice a year.

1.4 Non-relational Working Files (aggregated episode records)

The traditional way of further national health care analysis is rather through classical statistics programs (such as SPSS) – *not depending directly on relational database*. The purpose of aggregating records is to form four basic *linear files*, suitable for classic statistical analysis:

+ episodes, aggregated into one record for each hospitalization
+ grouping the sets of hospitalization episodes according to:
  specialty, main diagnose and both (specialty & main diagnose)

Data processing related to aggregation of episode records (or splitting the hospitalizations) is quite demanding. It takes around 80 hours of computer work, done through the batch file of 42 application calls, calling 12 distinct computer programs.

1.5 Implementing Knowledge Discovery in Databases (KDD)

Some modern methods are making their way in the analytical world as a supplement to standard statistics. The project team attended a preliminary workshop (performed by the Institute Jožef Stefan from Ljubljana), dealing with the »analysis of medical records by machine learning methods«. The focus of the workshop was pointed at knowledge discovery in databases. The proposed methods operated on the HOSTREAT subsystem, presenting hospital treatment of injured persons, which makes around 9% of the total database size.

2. Methods and Results

2.1 Improving the Teamwork in the Multi-dicipline Environment

The project had just one preliminary step, where the only output was the so-called »minimal data set«. This data set included data dictionary and medical requests related to semantic consistency of attributes. Therefore, at least a formal study of information output, a feasibility study and database design were left for further consideration. So, the project implementation started with database design and proceeded with computer programming. Unfortunately, the feasibility study was neglected in full, thus causing four program versions before the system could be put in operation.

Table 1. The functional project structure within the »wide« implementation phase

#	FUNCTION	EDUCATION & SKILLS
1	Project Management	Organization and Informatics (Communication Officer)
2	Database Administration & Programming	Organization and Informatics (System Analyst & Designer)
3	Data Semantics & System Evaluation	Public Health Specialist (diseases)
4	Data Semantics & System Evaluation	Public Health Specialist (injuries, poisoining, rehabilitation)
5	Data Semantics & System Evaluation	Public Health Specialist (obstetrics)

For the first time, the project was implemented solely by the staff within the Institute. (There was no »outsourcing«). Such approach enabled a less formal communication, giving opportunity for a valuable feed-back to recognize the complementary professional areas.

2.2 Implementing the Concatenated Primary Key to Work-around the Semantic Faults

Due to irrational data privacy&security reasons, the patient identification number was not to be entered in patient records (practiced in 1997). So, some other significant data domains were selected to define a unique record of hospital admission.

Table 2. The Episode Primary Key, Reflecting the Hospital Admission in *input data*

A. HOSPITALIZATION AREA	...derived from the input file name
B. HOSPITAL ADMISSION	Data collection year Hospital standard code Patient birthdate Patient municipality **Hospital admission date** ***Hospital admission clock-time*** (*)
C. HOSPITAL EPISODE	Episode start-date Episode end-date *Episode ordinal number* (**) Medical department type

(*) applied only **to distinguish actual or »false« twins**
(**) used only **to differentiate more actual episodes on one day**

But, unfortunately, the key above was not a satisfactory solution in subsequent steps, as

- hospital admission date was not entered as supposed: end-users usually mistook it for the episode start date
- hospital admission clocktime was entered only in ≈10% records (coming from injuries/poisoning), so the primary key was not unique in cases of true or false twins.

So, in the forthcoming *working files,* Hospital admission date & clock-time were to be ignored and replaced by the *computed* Hospitalization ordinal number. The key structure in section B was reconfigured in this way:

Table 3. The Episode Primary Key, Reflecting the Hospital Admission in *working files*

B1. HOSPITALIZED PERSON KEY	Data collection year Hospital standard code Patient birthdate **Patient sex** Patient municipality
B2. HOSPITALIZATION SPLIT KEY	***Hospitalization ordinal number*** **Medical specialty code** **Main diagnose**

Thus, a new hospitalization would take place under two disjunctive (OR) conditions:

- whenever a new hospitalized person key (B1)comes in
- if the time sequence of episodes within one hospitalized person is discontinued (the start date of the next episode is not equal to the end date of the previous episode)

However, the third version of the auxiliary admission key is not theoretically unique, too. Database distortions are scarcely *but* possible in two cases:

- a record of a hospitalized person might be missing, thus rendering two distinct hospitalizations
- hospitalized person key may represent two (or more) actual patients in the same **hospital**, provided that they have the same **birthdate, sex** and are registered in the same **municipality** (Such cases are called true or false twins).

Other information subsystems are designed to check the occurrence of twins, so the key structure above sufficiently serves the purpose so far.

The remaining key segments, being Medical specialty code and Main diagnose, are designed to split the hospitalization into hospitalization segments.

2.3 *Typified File Names and Automated Data Verification*

In order to keep surveyance, the input file names were given the following structure:

XXYZZZZZ.QQQ

XX	data collection year (last two digits)
Y	data collection period (semester, year)
ZZZZZ	hospital/rehabilitation center code
.	the prescribed delimiter
QQQ	hospitalization domain code

Much attention was drawn and paid to data verification and data storage.The filename keeps its original name while entering several verification phases, changing only its directory.

Table 4. Typified Filenames and Directories as a Measure to Keep Surveyance

Directory:	State of file:	Application:
HOSTREAT\ENTRY	Input text file	
		QQQ_BASE
	Relational database:	
HOSTREAT\ADMISSION	Admission records (master)	
HOSTREAT\EPISODE	Episode records (related)	
		QQQ_B
HOSTREAT	Control list (TXT)	
		QQQ_E
	Relational database:	
HOSTREAT\ADMISSION	Corrected admission records	
HOSTREAT\EPISODE	Corrected episode records	
		QQQ_PRIN
HOSTREAT	Database report (TXT)	

(QQQ is the symbol to be replaced by the hospitalization area)

The table reveals both ways of error identification and correction:
- QQQ_B: a batch program, rendering a list of errors/warnings identified by the computer program
- QQQ_E: an interactive program, enabling the end users to detect/correct errors during on-line data entry or later

Each datafield undergoes two verifications on average. Such a strict, consistent and unexpected control caused some frustrating experience. Let us draw attention to the data quality gradation during the test operation. The sample refers to one hospital:

Table 5. Data quality gradation during the »shakedown« test

	#admissions	#pages	*#errors/admission*
Fist trial:			10.5
Quarter	19.874	4774	6.90
Semester	41.148	1228	0.40
Year	72.259	499	***0.08***

2.4 *Promoting Automated Standard Output Tables*

Many public health reports appear standard, especially those in statistical annuals. The consuming overall aggregation of episode records and, what is more, the unreliable manual conversion from one tool to another, can be avoided by special application programs, fit to produce standard spredsheets. So far, nine standard reports have been worked out.

The output record of a typical standard report, based upon aggregated episodes from all hospitalization domains, is given below:

Table 6. A simple standard report based upon aggregated episode records

Hospital code (primary key)	# hospitalization # lenght of stay average length of stay # surgical operation # death # autopsy

#... »total number of...«

2.5 *Some Observations Regarding KDD, supported by decision trees (systems C4.5 & M5) and decision rules (system CN2)*

- *Occurrence of partial tautology*
  results from transitive dependence due to aggregated hospitalization records and/or supplemental datafields. In fact, they bring forth a violation of Codd's normal form, which is not the case with relational database. Two examples:

Diagnose	-	diagnose category (ICD10 block, chapter)
Hospital department type	-	medical specialty

- *Misuse of leading questions*
  Example: »What are the reasons for external cause of injuries?«
  Causes and effects are beyond the scope of a database. Databases express the state of a system rather than the process itself. The question should be put in a **static** mode: »Relation between the external cause of injuries and other selected factors?«
- *The absence of holistic survey*
  Decision trees are not clear enough when dealing with complex results. The psychologic theory of cognition recommends the so-called magic numbers 4&7. The optimal number of hierarchic levels is up to four while the optimum number of members within each level is up to seven. Further, decision trees ignore the relations within a narrow subsystem.

3. Conclusion

There are two global kinds of manuals, one of them giving technical support (answering the question HOW). The other manual type is the *procedure prescription*, pointing out the authority and the responsibility (answering the questions WHAT, WHO, WHEN and sometimes HOW MANY). In future, more attention should be paid to procedure manuals in order to maintain greater technical discipline when the system is put in operation.

We are aware that data quality cannot be obtained just by strict controls. A well motivated team will certainly give further results. Moreover, a record can be logically consistent while its contents do not reflect the actual situation.

Setting up large information systems is always an act of probability. Mistakes are expected, arising from ill-defined data set and data procedures. These spring up not until the implementation phase. Professional skills and education do not suffice to pave the way. A proper management policy and personality profile of project teams is needed, indeed.

References

[1] Inštitut za varovanje zdravja RS:
Zdravstveni informacijski sistem bolnišničnih obravnav, Metodološka navodila, 1996

[2] Sašo Džeroski, Blaž Zupan: Analiza medicinskih podatkov z metodami strojnega učenja
Poročilo iz delavnice, Inštitut Jožef Stefan, 15.-16. julij 1998

[3] Ryszard S. Michalski, Ivan Bratko, Miroslav Kubat: MACHINE LEARNING and DATA MINING
John Wiley & Sons ltd., 1998

[4] Gorazd Raič: Preverjanje in shranjevanje zapisov v zdravstvenem informacijskem sistemu »BOLOB«
Mednarodna multi-konferenca INFORMACIJSKA DRUŽBA – IS'98, Ljubljana, 6.-9. oktober 1998

Medical Informatics Europe '99
P. Kokol et al. (Eds.)
IOS Press, 1999

An IT awareness programme for the health sector in Ireland

Jane Grimson, Michael Flahive, *Centre for Health Informatics, Trinity College Dublin*
William Grimson, *Dept. of Electrical Engineering, Dublin Institute of Technology*
Rory O'Moore, John Nolan, *Central Pathology Laboratory, St. James's Hospital, Dublin*
Geoff Chadwick, *Royal College of Physicians of Ireland*
Email: jane.grimson@tcd.ie or chi@cs.tcd.ie

Abstract. This paper describes an Awareness Programme delivered throughout Ireland which aims to increase the level of understanding of healthcare professionals as to the benefits of Information and Communications Technology (ICT) and of emerging trends in Health Informatics in Europe. The programme examines the use of ICT across the whole health sector – primary, secondary and tertiary. It has been delivered at over 30 centres to more than 1500 health professionals.

1. Introduction

In 1990 the Committee of Ministers of the Council of Europe issued Recommendation No. R (90) 21, which recommended *inter alia* that governments of member states "*... ensure that, as soon as possible, those staff involved in health care receive appropriate, multidisciplinary training, both theoretical and practical, for health information systems within an overall public context;*" [1]

In response to this, the Centre for Health Informatics, a multidisciplinary, inter-faculty unit established in 1991, at Trinity College Dublin, has developed a programme to raise awareness of Information and Communications Technology among health professionals in Ireland. The programme is funded by the European Social Fund and the Irish Department of Health and Children, in association with the Department of Enterprise and Employment. Ireland, like many other countries in Europe and elsewhere, is in general not as advanced in the application of Information and Communications Technology (ICT) in the healthcare sector compared to other industries, and the level awareness among healthcare professionals needs to be addressed. As the emphasis switches from the use of ICT to support administration to supporting clinical computing, the need to involve the users, the healthcare professionals, directly, becomes crucial to delivering the benefits promised by ICT [2,3,4,5]. It is the users who should drive the exploitation of the technology and determine how it should be used in the delivery of healthcare. However, if users are to get involved then they need to understand both the potential benefits and the potential risks associated with the technology. It is these issues which are addressed in the Awareness Programme.

The objectives of the Programme can be summarised as follows:

- to examine the use of information and communications technology for healthcare professionals
- to increase awareness, understanding and utilisation – identify barriers, resistance and apprehensions

- to encourage exploitation of technology to support cost-effective and seamless healthcare
- to enhance the visibility of the many success stories in Ireland and elsewhere.

The Programme takes the form of a Symposium which has been delivered in centres throughout Ireland and is aimed at all health professionals (General Practitioners, hospital doctors, nurses, pharmacists, diagnostic service personnel, administrators, etc.). The Programme makes extensive use of state-of-the-art multimedia technology and should help to empower users to make informed technological choices and to actively participate in the exploitation of ICT in the health sector.

2. Overview of the Programme

Health Informatics is a multidisciplinary field and the design and implementation team consisted of clinicians from various specialties and backgrounds, computer scientists and engineers, graphical designers and experts in multimedia. The Symposium is divided into 4 parts:

- Presentation of a typical scenario of a patient's encounter with the health system illustrating the proliferation and duplication of information in the absence of integrated ICT systems
- Illustration of how ICT can help to enable more efficient and effective delivery of healthcare at primary, secondary and tertiary levels
- Discussion of the wider issues and developments, including, for example, Inter- and IntraNet, Electronic Healthcare Records, security and confidentiality, and ending with some examples of best practice from across Europe and elsewhere
- Question and answer session.

The Symposium is generally delivered by a clinician supported by multimedia presentation material and takes approximately one hour followed by an additional 30 minutes of discussion.

2.1 Part 1 – scenario development

The aim of the Programme is not to *teach* ICT to health professionals, but rather to show how it can be usefully applied at a practical level. It was decided therefore to motivate the Programme through the use of a typical scenario of a patient and their encounter with various levels of the healthcare system. This scenario is presented mainly in the form of a video. The patient selected was a middle-aged male who visits his GP for the first time in almost 10 years complaining of an aching sensation in his chest. Following examination, the GP decides to order an ECG and fasting blood tests to be performed in the local hospital.

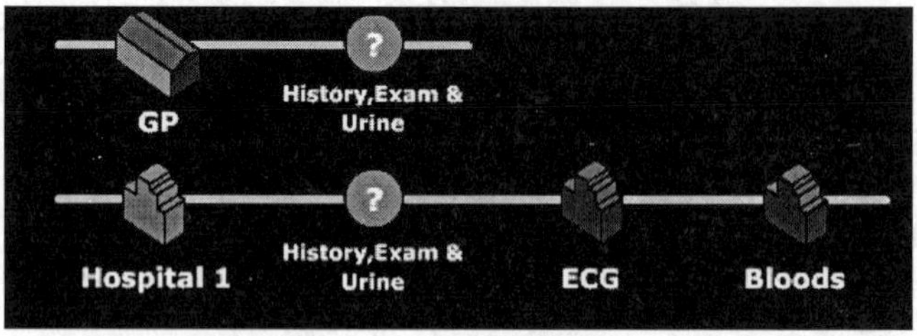

Figure 1 GP and Outpatient Records

The patient attends the outpatient department of his local hospital where the tests are carried out and the results posted to the GP, arriving some days later. The GP suspects that the patient has diabetes and refers him to the diabetes clinic at the local hospital for investigation. At this point, two non-communicating, independent records have been created, with some of the information duplicated in both, as shown in Figure 1. The scenario then moves on to the patient's visit to the diabetes clinic where yet more investigations, including an exercise ECG, are carried out. A separate specialist diabetes chart is created, thus further fragmenting the patient record. The patient is then referred to the cardiologist where yet another record, the cardiac record is established, and an angiogram is performed. It is decided that bypass surgery is required. At this stage, the patient has acquired two more independent, non-communicating records. However, before the surgery can be scheduled the patient suffers an acute heart attack and is admitted to a different hospital for emergency surgery, which requires the patient's cardiology record in the first hospital to be sent by courier to the second hospital. He recovers and is eventually sent home. Thus at the end of the presentation of the scenario, at least 8 separate, independent, non-communicating records have been created: there is considerable duplication in these records as shown in see Figure 2.

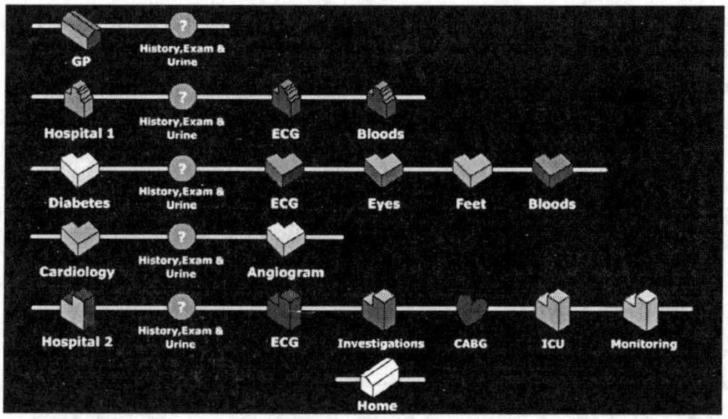

Figure 2 Final set of records

2.2 Part 2 – how ICT can help

The second part of the Symposium revisits the scenario showing where ICT can help and support the healthcare delivery process in primary care, in the hospitals and at tertiary level. Ireland does not currently have a unique patient identifier for all citizens and the problems which this causes in terms of duplication of information and communication difficulties are highlighted. The emphasis throughout this section and indeed throughout the Symposium as a whole is on ICT enabling and facilitating the healthcare delivery process. The focus is very much on what is routinely available and can be achieved with today's technology. Healthcare is an information intensive industry generating enormous volumes of information every day in hospitals, GP surgeries, clinics and laboratories. Yet much of this data continues to be processed manually in spite of decades of experience in the successful application of ICT In other information intensive industries such as banking and insurance. The message that is reinforced in this part of the Programme is that ICT can help.

2.3 Part 3 – some key issues and trends

The third section focuses on the broader issues with the strong underlying theme that the appropriate use of ICT in health should free-up health professionals to do the things that they are good at, namely, patient care. Computers are good at computing and this is what they should do. Even the most sophisticated decision support system is not intended to replace clinical expertise, experience and judgement. Central to the use of ICT in health is the ability it provides to communicate information reliably and efficiently ensuring that the right information is available in the right format in the right place and at the right time. At the heart of modern telecommunications today is the Internet so the Inter- and Intra-net and Web are explained with illustrations from the best – and the 'not so good' – web sites. The increasing availability of information to patients and the consequences of this in the context of a global health market are discussed.

A major focus of this section is on the Electronic Healthcare Record (EHCR). Ireland has virtually no EHCR systems and certainly there is no obvious awareness of the impact which the EHCR is likely to have in the future. Extensive use is made of visual images to illustrate the concepts as shown in Figure 3. The closely related issues of security, confidentiality and integrity of healthcare data are introduced within the context of national and EU legislation [6,7]. The fact that security is not simply a technical issue and that the technology exists today to guarantee secure transmission of data (e.g. as used in e-commerce) is emphasised. The importance of standards in the healthcare sector such as those emanating from CEN TC/251 (ENV12967-1 Health Information Systems Architecture, ENV12265 Electronic Healthcare Record Architecture) is stressed, as without these, the electronic sharing of information between systems and users is virtually impossible. The Synapses project which is concerned with the development of a standard to facilititate sharing of healthcare records and related healthcare data is used as an example [8,9]. Finally the formal part of the Symposium concludes with a presentation of examples of best practice in the use of ICT in health from Ireland and Europe with reference made to the EHTO Observatory [10].

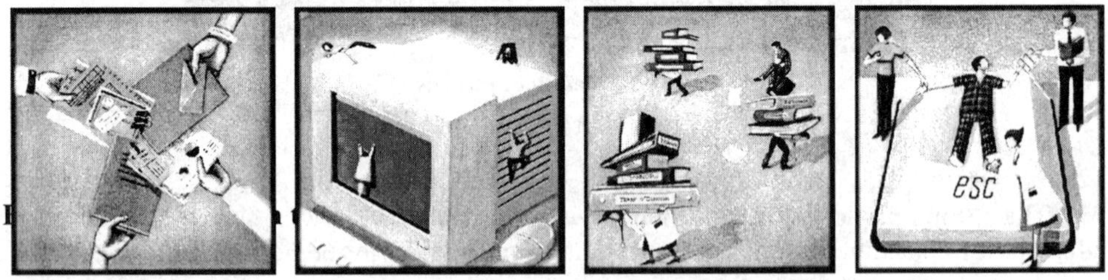

Figure 3 Sample images from the Programme

3. Evaluation and Conclusions

To date the Symposium has been delivered at over 30 different centres throughout the country to almost 1500 healthcare professionals. The response has been very positive. It is clear that there is a growing appreciation of the importance of ICT in health coupled with a strong desire for education and training in Health Informatics. Attendees are provided with supporting documentation including a CD which covers most of the material presented in the Symposium, and information about "leading edge projects". The Centre also maintains a web site which provides further information about Health Informatics generally [11].

The developers of the Programme recognise the importance of “follow-up”. Raising awareness and increasing expectations require further actions to be taken both in terms of general education and training in health informatics, and also in terms of promoting the development of a national strategy in the area, with particular reference to the movement towards EHCRs. Thus the Centre, in addition to delivering the symposia, organised a major seminar addressed by experts from across Europe on *Increasing the benefits of Information and Communications Technology in Healthcare.* The Centre also runs a part-time Diploma/MSc in Health Informatics aimed at both IT and healthcare professionals, and which has a truly interdisciplinary flavour. Plans are underway to develop a distance learning version of the Diploma delivered using the latest educational technology on the web [11]. The potential of ICT in a citizen-centered world to improve both the quality and cost-effectiveness of healthcare is enormous. The Awareness Programme has sought to release some of this potential through the empowerment of healthcare professionals in driving the exploitation of the technology.

Acknowledgements

The authors are grateful for the financial assistance of the European Social Fund and Department of Health and Children and for the guidance of the Department of Enterprise and Employment in developing and delivering the Programme. Many people contributed to the Programme and the authors would particularly like to acknowledge the work of Colum Foley and Sean Murphy on the multimedia design side, and Paula Hicks on the organisational and logistical side.

References

[1] Hasman A, Albert A, Wainright P, Klar R, Sosa M, (Eds), *Education and Training in Health Informatics in Europe*, IOS Press, 1995.

[2] Curtis AC, *Multi-facility integration: an approach to synchronised electronic medical records in a decentralized health care systems*, Procs. MEDINFO 1992, 138-143

[3] Van de Welde A, van der Werff A, Kilsdonk A, Damon W, Hubert M, *Towards a European framework referernce model and architecture for the development of open hospital information systems*, Procs. MEDINFO 92, 188-193.

[4] Slack VW, Bleich HL, *Barriers to clinical computing in American hospitals*, Procs. MEDINFO 92, 178-181.

[5] Bleich H, *Why good hospitals get bad computing,* Procs. MEDINFO 98, IOS Press, 1998, 969-972.

[6] Seismed Consortium (Eds), *Data security for health care*, Vols 31-33, IOS Press, 1996.

[7] Barber B (Ed), *Towards security in medical, telematics,* in *Studies in Health Technology and Informatics,* Vol. 27, IOS Press, 1995

[8] Grimson W, Berry D, Grimson J, Stephens G, Felton E, Given P and O'Moore R, *Federated healthcare record server - the Synapses paradigm*, International Journal of Medical Informatics, Vol 52, 1998, pp3-27.

[9] Grimson J, Grimson W, Berry D, Stephens G, Felton E, Kalra D, Toussaint Pand Weier OW, A CORBA-based integration of distributed electronic healthcare records using the Synapses approach, IEEE Transactions on Information Technology in Biomedicine, Sept 1998, Vol2, No 3, 124-138

[10] http://www.ehto.be/

[11] http://www.cs.tcd.ie/chi

Medical Informatics Europe '99
P. Kokol et al. (Eds.)
IOS Press, 1999

Slovenian national health insurance card: The next step

T.Kalin, (1) G.Kandus, (1) D.Trcek, (2,1) B.Zupan, (1)
(1) "J.Stefan" Institute, Ljubljana, Slovenia
(2) Faculty of Computer and Information Sciences, University of Ljubljana, Slovenia

Abstract. The Slovenian national health insurance company started a full-scale deployment of the insurance smart card that is at the present used for insurance data and identification purpose only. There is ample capacity on the cards that were selected, to contain much more data than needed for the purely administrative and charging purposes. There are plans to include some basic medical information, donor information, etc. On the other hand, there are no firm plans to use the security infrastructure and the extensive network, connecting the insurance company with the more than 200 self service terminals positioned at the medical facilities through the country to build an integrated medical information system that would be very beneficial to the patients and the medical community. This paper is proposing some possible future developments and further discusses on the security issues involved with such countrywide medical information system.

1. Introduction

Despite their broader name, the Health Cards were initially introduced in the various European countries mostly as Health Insurance Cards, and even within this scope mainly for the identification purposes. It was soon realised that the potentials of the Card are far broader, and the plans were initiated to extend the information on the Card with a basic set of medical data. France, Spain and Germany, for example, seem now to be the countries that went farthest in this respect [1].

Like other European countries, Slovenia is undergoing a similar scenario. Within the first phase of the introduction of the Card by the Slovenia national health insurance, the Card carries only insurance-specific information [2]. Possible extensions with a limited and basic set of medical data are planned, but have not yet been executed. Despite the promise for any user or provider of health services, the problem for a further extension of the Card's functionality is to identify *who* is going to coordinate and supervise such extensions and *how* will they be implemented. Namely, the Slovenia national health insurance, who is the main investor and developer of the information system that will use the Card as its primary information holder, is not (and should not be) responsible for any medical data. Instead, the Card and the project by the Slovenian national health insurance must therefore be recognised as a spark to boost the collaborative and systemised way to introduce health and medical informatics throughout the health institutions in Slovenia, but the main coordinator has to be found elsewhere.

At present, full deployment of the Health (insurance) Card is on its way. The contracts for deliveries of the equipment: card readers, self-service terminals, networking equipment, server computers and smart cards themselves are in the phase of negotiations, or delivery.

The communication subsystem will be composed at first of 120 POP's (Points of Presence) placed in all medical establishments that serve more than 300 patients per day. A POP consists of a communication router running the TCP/IP communication protocol, connected to the central site at the National health insurance company, either via leased line, or through the Slovenian public administrative network, operated by the Governmental office for informatics. Self-service terminals are connected at 80 sites directly to the routers, and to the existing or new local area networks at 40 locations. The network is supposed to have a large degree of redundancy and operate on 24 * 365 basis.

The purpose of the self-service terminals is to enable the patients to regularly (once every three months) the insurance information on their smart cards. Thus, for every patient using the terminal, an access has to be made to the central data base of the National health insurance company and to the insurance companies involved in the market of additional medical insurance. All transactions will be routed to the appropriate data base by a "transaction server system" composed of a fault tolerance twin system at the central location.

A patient with a valid insurance information will be able to use the medical service after presenting her/his Card to the administrative or medical staff of the medical facility. To be able to access the administrative and medical information on the Card, two additional security precautions are implemented, in the form of a Professional Card with a accompanying PIN code that have to be inserted in the card reader at the same time, and entered by the authorised member of staff.

It is very easy to observe that an extensive network is used at this time only for the validation and updating of the medical insurance information, which is consequently used off-line. The network using internet technology will be present in the lobbies of all significant medical facilities in Slovenia with routers ready for connection of additional 80 local area networks and the existing LAN's capable of supporting more computers than just few self-service terminals.

One could envisage a much wider use of computer/network supported work by the medical professionals as well as by the administrative staff in the medical care, including:

- transfer of all administrative accounting information from the medical entities to the insurance companies. (At present 60 % of all accounting information is transferred electronically to the National insurance company, daily through the dial-up connections. It is obvious that this application is a natural candidate to be integrated as soon as possible.),
- establishment of the "Slovenian Medical Intranet", for communication and information dissemination among the Slovenian medical community,
- e-mail servers, list servers for the "Medical Intranet",
- WWW servers established by different medical and governmental authorities for the use of the professionals,
- other possible new applications,
- and finally, using all necessary security precautions (e.g. Firewalls) establishment of a gateway to the global Internet.

It is clear, that the communication network will have to be expanded and upgraded as soon as the new services will be introduced, but the kernel has been planted and should be utilised to its full potential.

2. Possible future developments

Before proposing a possible direction for further development in the medical information system triggered by the potentials of the Healt Card system under deployment, one should note that Slovenia is overall relatively well-developed country in terms of medical and health informatics. As stated in [3], the health institutions are reasonably well equipped with personal computers, and there is an undergoing development present to introduce networks that link computers within institutions and provide connection to the Internet. However, the problem in Slovenia is that the medical and health information systems may be well developed within selected institutions or even within certain regions, while the level of countrywide integration is weak. Institutions use different standards, implementations of Electronic Patient Record are mutually incompatible, or the systems are based on outdated technology that does not allow further integration or extension without a substantial re-engineering. There are trends to unify the data formats across the country – for example, An Institute of Public Health of Republic of Slovenia requires the same hospitalisation report format for all Slovenian hospitals – but the unification takes place at reporting level rather than at the level of physical organisation of the data bases.

For the country of only two million people, there is therefore an imperative to create a common health information system that allows seamless integration of all specialised institutions. It is the existence of the Health Insurance Card that can provide the common ground for such countrywide development. For the Card to improve its usefulness beyond mere insurance identification purposes, we propose the following scenario:

1. The card has to be first recognised as a potential identification media for countrywide health and medical information system under development.
2. The Slovene Ministry of Health has to form a Consortium (or some other specialised body) to control and supervise the development and extensions of the Card, specifically by:
   - setting the standards to be used by the card (by adopting the safety, health and medical data standards of EU),
   - setting the guidelines how some independent institution can use the card and extend its functionality (registering, standards required, technical information),
   - resolving security-based questions.
3. Most importantly, the Consortium has to be involved in the motion by Slovenia to revise and develop a country-wide medical and health information system that will be build around a commonly accepted and standardised Electronic Patient Record. It would be naive to expect that the Card will resolve any of the major issues in such development. Instead, the Card can be regarded as a starting point and a lowest common denominator in the system. Slovenia must not afford the development of the parallel health information systems, where the Card would be present at one but absent in the other one.

Such potential co-emergence of the Card, unified health information system and Electronic Patient Record can of course provide grounds for many services that else generally stem from the invocation of information technology in medicine and health care. From the patient's point of view, this should ultimately lead to better health care provision, faster services, and easier access to private data (where granted). From the point of view of health care providers, such development should give grounds to better organise the whole health care system, make required patient data more accurate and available on time, and finally, support the decision making process both at levels of referring physician and specialists. By providing a unique identification across different information systems, the Card should also enable institution-based and countrywide data warehousing. This should further enable outcomes analysis, a task that is almost impossible to achieve in present diverse and non-standard system, but can itself potentially lead to substantial improvements in quality and costs.

3. Security considerations for the future development

Using open global public networks for digital exchange of every kind of data is a definite choice for the future. This is the case in all sectors, ranging from financial to medical sector. However, a vital point of such approaches is protection of data, which should especially be emphasized in the medical and health-related sectors.

The Slovenian health insurance card project has considered security issues from the early stages. As the project officially started back in 1996, it was obvious that it had to rely on technology that was not only available, but also acceptable in terms of investments. Besides, the lack of some other supporting systems (i.e. security infrastructure) made symmetric key based cards and related solutions the most cost - benefit choice. On the communications level the project decided for a TCP/IP approach. Besides the general openness of such approach (TCP/IP is the mainstream technology in this field), this assured a possibility of incorporation of new security standards and technologies in the future. However, by that time some specific measures had to be taken to make the piloting project operational.

As the technological progress in this field is enormous, steps to be followed regarding security are the following. On the level of smart cards, symmetric-cryptography architecture could stay in place, as it is cheap and fast. However, it is limited to a small scale and a relatively closed environment. Depending on a need for integration with a general Slovene medical information system and its integration with similar systems in Europe, asymmetric technology might turn out to be the way to go. More specifically, to minimize costs and assure openness, JAVA based smart cards have to be considered seriously, as their prices are coming in the range of acceptable expenses. Besides, JAVA means an open standard on a smart card level, which can be of a general purpose (not limited only to health insurance data) and which allows more flexibility in subsequent redesign of information system.

On the transport level, a network is to be expanded. An integration of health insurance network with a medical information system should be done. The best option to be followed in this area is IPSec [4], which enables an itroduction of virtual private networks (VPNs) over public networks. Additional support of SSL, developed by Netscape, which is a de facto standard, should also be considered.These technologies assure appropriate security services for protection of sensitive medical and medical related data. Besides, they are expected to be widely available that is already the case with SSL, which is incorporated in every WWW browser. This would enable use of the Slovene health information infrastructure for general purposes: from electronic exchange of prescriptions to making appointments for examinations at specialists. Thus every taxpayer would be able (according to his / her access rights, identified via smart card) to securely use any service from anywhere, even from a home PC.

The important points that should be considered in the future design of a nation wide health services information network (where health project card should present only a staring point) are:

- the establishment of a system of certification authorities, which is needed for support of public key technology in line with X.509v3 and related standards [X509]. It requires proper legislative steps and operational steps (accreditation of a particular provider).
- a problem of a lack of international health sector related general specifications. These should cover interactions of players (sequences of steps), flows of documents (sequences of exchanged documents), the structure of these documents (EDI) and cryptographic services (primitives) implemented in each step. This all is vitally for a successfully implemented security in a nation wide system.
- a sufficient legislation framework for use of digital signatures and medical records.
- a coordination between Ministry of health and Ministry of social affairs.

4. Conclusion

It is clear that a lot of political determination and extensive coordination between various players in Slovenia will be absolutely necessary to establish a framework upon which to build an integrated national medical information system. Participation in international activities and projects will be of paramount importance. This will not be an instant process, but nevertheless, one should not wait and should start making the necessary first steps that will to a great extent fairly soon generate benefits for the medical professionals and for the patients.

References

[1] Health Cards '97. L. van den Broek and AJ Sikkel (eds.). IOS Press, 1997.
[2] B Kramberger, M Toth, M Sušelj: Introducing the card technology in the Slovene health care system. In (L. van den Broek, AJ Sikkel, eds.) Health Cards '97. pages 60-66. IOS Press, 1997.
[3] G Cerkvenik and M. Premik: State-of-the-art of the Slovenian Medical Informatics. *Informatica Medica Slovenica*, 19-22 (5), 1998.
[4] Kent S., Atkinson R., Security Architecture for the Internet Protocol, IETF RFC 2401, november 1998.
[5] ITU-T Q15/7, Final Text of Draft Amendments DAM 4 to ISO/IEC 9594-2, DAM 2 to ISO/IEC 9594-6, DAM 1 to ISO/IEC 9594-7, and DAM 1 to ISO/IEC 9594-8 on Certificate Extensions, Geneva, April 1996.

Medical Informatics Europe '99
P. Kokol et al. (Eds.)
IOS Press, 1999

Transformation of the Process of Administrative Patient Management

Milan ČRV
University Medical Center Ljubljana, Information Center, SI-1525 Ljubljana, Slovenia

Abstract. The risks involved with performing a process tranformation project are significant. The success rate can be improved if a formal process with concrete guidance is used. This paper introduces an object-oriented approach to process transformation and information system development. The proposed approach affords adequate freedom, encourages innovative thinking and points the way to the desired goals. Its main aim is to combine different activities into a uniform process with the use of object-oriented modelling.

1. Introduction

A holistic approach to process transformation in any company entails systematic redesign and continuous improvement of processes. This is a long-term activity, where initial success provides no guarantee for success at a later stage. The most common reasons why process transformation does not achieve the desired goals are:

- Unfamiliarity with the technical and social aspects of the transformation process.
- Lack of human and financial resources.
- Misconceptions about the role of information technology. Its great strength lies in enabling the company to adopt a different, more successful way of work, rather than in automating the existing processes [1].
- Lack of appropriate technological support and a chaotic approach to the transformation process.

2. Background

University Medical Center is the largest general hospital in Slovenia. The hospital has more than 40 wards on several locations and treats nearly 90.000 inpatients per year. The performing of the proces of administrative patient management is highly centralized. The implementation of new communications technology and shared computing resources enables to adopt a more successful way of work.

3. Method

The process of transformation must be looked upon as a continuous repetition of cycles from the foundation of the company until it ceases to exist. The most common sources of dissatisfaction with the existing way of work are its ineffectiveness, often connected with a poor quality of results, inefficiency, and inadequate flexibility [2]. The proposed approach represents a general framework for implementation of the transformation process and recommends the use of several well-known and verified techniques.

The main phases of a process cycle are: *Preparation of the environment, Process analysis and transformation*, *Reorganization*, and *Implementation of the new process*. A directive for change implementation, which may already contain proposals for improvement, is needed to start the cycle. The starting point for each new phase is the outcome of the preceding phases. Aside from the basic connections, feedback connections are also present between individual phases of the process cycle, since newly acquired knowledge and solutions may affect also the outcome of earlier phases.

3.1. *Preparation of the environment*

For the implementation of changes and undertaking of new responsibilities, an environment must be created within the company that will be receptive to changes and willing to support their implementation. This is especially difficult in a public institution, where the absence of competition, lack of strategic planning, and normative organization create barriers that are difficult to overcome. Consequently, the initiative for transformation in public institutions rarely comes from the management. Problems due to the existing way of work are experienced mainly by employees responsible for operative tasks, and they are most frequently the source of initiatives for technological and organizational improvements. The creation of an environment receptive to change includes:

- Identifying the core processes and selecting the process to redesign.
- Developing a vision of the new process in keeping with the strategic orientation of the company, the available technology, human resources and current organization.
- Securing the management's support for the implementation of changes.
- Drawing up the organization of the project and appointing process redesign teams.
- Identifying risk factors.

3.2. *Process analysis and transformation*

The core phase of the process cycle is analysis and transformation of the selected process. A feature common to both activities is process modelling, which in the phase of transformation, extends to encompass also analysis, designing and implementation of the information system. In order to facilitate reuse of the results of activities conducted in previous phases or process cycles, it is advisable to adopt a unified modelling approach, using the same or comparable techniques. In accordance with the process of standardization in the field of object-oriented system analysis and design, the use of techniques employed by the Unified Modeling Language [3] is recommended.

3.2.1. Analysis of the existing process

Knowledge of the existing way of work is prerequisite to successful transformation of the selected process. The content and scope of analysis of the existing process depend on the targets of the process cycle. For describing the flow of events triggered by a specific external actor that is connected with the process, use cases are employed [4]. The analysis usually comprises:

- Evaluation of the existing use cases with the aid of carefully selected criteria.
- A critical survey of the event flow for individual use cases, to determine the possibilities for integration or elimination of individual activities.
- Appraisal of possibilities for short-term improvement.
- Analysis of the available human resources and information technology.

3.2.2. Process transformation

A model of the future process is a convenient way of designing the future way of work. The limits of the process as well as the external actors that are connected with it, use it, trigger certain actions or receive its results should be clearly defined. The way of carrying out the process should be presented as the outcome of interaction between objects directly involved in the process. This is followed by the procurement of an adequate information system to support the new process.

A use case diagram shows the structure of a process. However, for analysing the sequence of actions, a sequence diagram is more suitable. It shows objects, actors and exchange of messages in the same sequence as is described in individual use cases. The diagram can be supplemented with text to describe in detail each step of the use case under consideration. From a sequence diagram it is impossible to figure out which activities are carried out simultaneously. Therefore it is more advisable to use an activity diagram, which is very suitable for modelling parallel activities and describing the workflow across several use cases [5]. Activity diagrams describe very accurately the behaviour of a system, but they do not show as clearly who is responsible for individual tasks. This shortcoming can be overcome by arranging the activities in vertical zones, so that activities connected with a specific object occur in the same zone. In the activity of process transformation special attention must be devoted to:

- Substitution of linear performance of activities with a parallel scheme, which appreciably reduces the process cycle time.
- Horizontal compression of work, whereby several specialized tasks are combined into a single activity, to be performed by an individual or a group.
- Vertical compression of work, whereby the employees carrying out operative tasks are authorized to make their own decisions. Simultaneous vertical and horizontal compression of work is an efficient way to reduce delays and lower overhead costs.
- Accurate registration of data at the time of their occurrence to ensure that the management support information is the result of performance of the process rather than of additional activities.

3.2.3. Information system support

The collaboration of information technology experts in the process redesign team and the use of appropriate techniques for the presentation of various models make it possible to reuse the results of process modelling in developing the information system [6]. The transformation of the process model into the object model of the information system is a repetitive activity. Feedback connections often develop between the models, and the process model may have to be adjusted as a result of additional findings. The information from the process model is usually inadequate for the development of the definitive information system model. Detailed analysis of individual use cases often results in the introduction of additional objects, mostly related to special features of the implementation environment.

Obviously, the development of a new information system is not the only way of procuring adequate information system support for the new process. There are two other options:

- To purchase a commercially available information system.
- To adjust the existing information system to the new process. This is the most common solution, especially when only minor changes have been made.

3.3. Reorganization

A new way of work often requires certain changes in the organizational structure, the management system and the values and beliefs of the employees. The existing organizational structure and management system must be revised and adjusted to meet the requirements of the new process. The process owner, who is responsible for the entire process, and the process teams, which carry it out, are the core of the new process organization. Changes in organizational structure are mirrored in altered responsibilities of the employees participating in the transformed processes. Their new responsibilities must be defined and they must receive appropriate training, so that they can carry out their new tasks.

3.4. Implementation of the new process

Efficient implementation of the new process is a critical stage in every process transformation cycle. Before the full-scale implementation of the new way of work, it is very helpful to test it on a smaller scale, in the form of a pilot project. The disadvantage of conducting a pilot project is that it causes a delay. However, encouraging results of the trial are of help in overcoming the resistance to change normally present within the company.

Efforts to maintain the results achieved with the new way of work in the initial phase of its implementation and to introduce further improvements should become part of the daily routine. Study and understanding of the reasons for success of the new way of work on the one hand and its shortcomings on the other should form the basis for starting a new process transformation cycle. This may be aimed at consolidating the results of the previous cycle. If the object of the previous cycle was a subprocess, the next cycle can focus on the process as a whole.

4. Results

The process of administrative management of patients can be described with three use cases: *Patient admission and discharge*, *Ordering laboratory investigations and receiving results* , *Registration and billing of services*. The above use cases may be connected with each other. So an association exists between the use case *Patient admission and discharge* and the use case *Ordering laboratory investigations and receiving results*, which allows the functionality of the former use case to be extended, under certain conditions, by the latter. Outside the process are the actors *Patient* and *Payer* that are connected with the process.

The number of functional units participating in the new process model has been reduced on the basis of analysis of the existing way of work, its shortcomings and general recommendations for more efficient performance of clerical tasks for the patient. The tasks formerly performed by the admission office and the invoicing department have been taken over by the ward. In the new process of administrative patient management, the nurses and clerks within each ward have much broader responsibilities compared to the previous process.

The information system has been adjusted with special attention to the interface between untouched legacy and the new part of the system. The pilot project has been succesfully finished. The new process of administrative patient management is now in the phase of full-scale implementation.

5. Conclusion

A formalized approach with appropriate techniques is a valuable tool in the demanding activity of process transformation. The main advantages of a proposed approach are the following:

- It takes into account both technical and social aspects of process transformation.
- A unified process modelling techniques facilitate communication among experts in different fields and contribute to better results.
- Active involvement of information system designers in the transformation team shortens the time required for the development of a suitable information system.
- Various models developed during the transformation process may be reused in further cycles.

References

[1] M. Hammer and J. Champy, Reengineering the Corporation: A Manifesto for Business Revolution. HarperCollins Publishers, New York, 1993.

[2] W. Winslow, Strategic Business Tranformation: Achieving Strategic Objectives Through Business Re-engineering. McGraw-Hill Publishing Company, London, 1996.

[3] G. Booch, J. Rumbaugh and I. Jacobson, Unified Modeling Language: User Guide. Addison-Wesley Longman, Reading, 1998.

[4] I. Jacobson *et al.*, Object-Oriented Software Engineering: A Use Case Driven Approach. Addison-Wesley Publishing Company, Wokingham, 1995.

[5] M. Fowler and K. Scott, UML Distilled: Applying the Standard Object Modeling Language. Addison-Wesley Longman, Reading, 1997.

[6] I. Jacobson, M. Ericsson and A. Jacobson, The Object Advantage: Business Process Reengineering with Object Technology. Addison-Wesley Publishing Company, Wokingham, 1995.

Medical Informatics Europe '99
P. Kokol et al. (Eds.)
IOS Press, 1999

National Health Care Providers' Database (NHCPD) of Slovenia – Information technology solution for health care planning and management

Tit Albreht[a], Mojca Paulin[b]
[a]*Institute of Public Health of the Republic of Slovenia, Ljubljana, Slovenia*
[b]*Health Insurance Institute of Slovenia, Ljubljana, Slovenia*

Abstract. Introduction: The article describes the possibilities of planning of the health care providers' network enabled by the use of information technology. The cornerstone of such planning is the development and establishment of a quality database on health care providers, health care professionals and their employment statuses.

Material and methods: Based on the analysis of information needs, a new database was developed for various users in health care delivery as well as for those in health insurance. The method of information engineering was used in the standard four steps of the information system construction, while the whole project was run in accordance with the principles of two internationally approved project management methods. Special attention was dedicated to a careful analysis of the users' requirements and we believe the latter to be fulfilled to a very large degree.

Results: The new NHCPD is a relational database which is set up in two important state institutions, the National Institute of Public Health and the Health Insurance Institute of Slovenia. The former is responsible for updating the database, while the latter is responsible for the technological side as well as for the implementation of data security and protection. NHCPD will be inter linked with several other existing applications in the area of health care, public health and health insurance. Several important state institutions and professional chambers are users of the database in question, thus integrating various aspects of the health care system in Slovenia.

Conclusions: The setting up of a completely revised health care providers' database in Slovenia is an important step in the development of a uniform and integrated information system that would support top decision-making processes at the national level.

1. Introduction

Slovenia is a relatively small country with 2 million inhabitants but with a fairly long-standing tradition in health care and its delivery. The backbone of health care providers' network as we know it now has been developed over the past 35 years, especially at the primary level. Still, recently, two processes brought about major changes. Firstly, independence declared in 1991 and internationally recognised in 1992. Secondly, Slovenia entered an economic and political transition while still being part of Yugoslavia. Both of these intense processes have triggered the need for good information that could represent a management tool.

Before 1996 data collection on health care providers was not very reliable, resulting in certain dubious summarised data which could not be used by health care managers and planners efficiently. Data was inaccurate, often delayed, data collection was decentralised, etc., there was rarely a real up-to-date insight in the situation. Of course, the new database did not arise from the very roots since the previous database was already computer supported. That solution was, unfortunately, to a great degree already superseded by current trends. So, technology was also part of the requirements presented to the project group.

Due to the clearly structured three levelled system of health care in Slovenia, it is necessary to have a good overview of the organisation and manpower at the national level. Primary, secondary and tertiary level of health care bear different roles in providing health care to the population and good coverage is essential. It needs to be stressed that re-establishment of private practice [1] also introduced some challenges to the ways we used to follow health care. Regular follow-up of the network is necessary for reasons that are essentially twofold. Firstly, concessions for private practice are issued on the basis of the stability of system for which updated data are needed, secondly, any changes should not affect the availability (geographical or financial) of the health care services. Shared responsibilities of the state and of municipalities determine also the needs and the requirements of the database users. Those will be discussed in more detail under 'Materials and methods'. Reporting of data goes directly from health care providers via regional Institutes of Public Health, respecting the multi-levelled structure of health care.

Based on such basic outline and requirements, interests were identified within the Public Health system as co-ordinated by the National Institute of Public Health of the Republic of Slovenia as well as by the Health Insurance Institute of Slovenia. A common project group was formed with clearly defined tasks. Methods of jointly adopted project management were used in order to facilitate good performance of the individual tasks. As shown from the results such a type of co-operation resulted in a very positive outcome after a dynamic and fruitful co-operation.

2. Materials and methods

2.1. Outlines and goals

Outlines for the re-engineering of the NHCPD:

- different users' requirements
- taking into account the experience and data from the existing database
- system changes in the organisation of health care (see also Introduction)

Goals of the new NHCPD were essentially:

- facilitated analyses of data on health care providers and health care professionals
- improved management and planning of the health care network

2.2. Methodology of database development

In developing our health care providers' database, we chose the method of information engineering [2]. Information engineering is a set of tools and techniques for planning, analysis, design and construction of information systems. The individual phases are time-dependent and follow in a sequence from top to bottom.

In the planning phase [3], stress was on developing the strategy of an information system that would support guidelines, goals and plans in health care delivery. In that phase, based on identified strategic information needs and requirements, we developed a raw business model that contains descriptions, requirements of functions, processes, organisation, groups of entities and their relationships.

In the analysis phase [4], we gathered and analysed users' requirements. In the health care system, we identified all potential users and their information needs. We developed a precise data model and a process model. Products were presented in the form of models that allow for easy communication between users and informaticians and among informaticians themselves. The data model [5] was described with the standard tool: E-R (Entity-Relationship Diagram). Elements of the E-R diagram are entities and attributes and relationships between entities. The process model was described with the standard DFD (Data Flow Diagram) and a decomposition diagram. Elements of DFD are processes, external agents, data stores and data flows.

Products of the analysis phase are: process model and process definitions, data model with defined entities, defined relationships between entities and defined attributes, matrix entities-processes, matrix processes-events and the conceptual design of the future information system: database concept, dependency diagram of transactions, matrix triggers-transactions, definition of codes.

The next phase was system design. On the basis of data model, process model and the conceptual model we prepared a specification of requirements for information technology. We prepared software architecture, defined programmes and modules. Data model was used for the formation of a relational database. In this phase, we prepared a dialogue for the communications between the user and the computer. This phase already depends on information technology. And finally, construction phase was the last phase of development of the database during which we established a relational database, produced software and tested altogether.

The finalised software (application) was included in the existing health information system. Data already in use were verified, made up-to-date and corrected and finally, loaded to the new database. We defined and composed all the relevant codes, prepared instructions and documentation for users and trained them for the work with the new application.

With the development of the health providers' database we used two standards for project management. One was used with the design of the new database [6] and the other [7] for the management of the entire project. A project definition was prepared with aims and deadlines, as well as the overall plan of the project. A project board composed of the managers of the main participating institutes as well as of the representatives of the key users and end users. Organisation of the project was set up together with the reporting lines and problem-solving mechanisms. Users took part in all phases of the project.

At our work, we used CASE Tool (Computer Aided System Engineering) which offers computer support to the life cycle of the development of information systems by phase [8].

We used CASE ADW© by KnowledgeWare. The tool builds its own encyclopaedia, knowledge database, based on the inputs and definitions. It provides for the accuracy, consistency and completeness of design. We designed data and process models, drew graphs and matrices and the complete project documentation. CASE tool was of great assistance in the analysis phase at modelling and in the design phase at the logical and physical design of the database.

2.3. Users' requirements

The project group identified several groups of key users of the NHCPD. We list them as follows together with their specific requirements and roles.

- Ministry of Health: needs data on health care providers regarding their structure, geographical locations, facilities, as well as data on health care professionals. The

Ministry is responsible for the health care network as well as for ensuring equity of the citizens in view of the availability and accessibility of the health care services. The Ministry is also, by Law of Health Services [1], responsible for the keeping of several registries, among them are: registry of medical doctors and of dentists, registry of private health care practitioners, registry of doctors in speciality training.

- National Institute of Public Health requires data on health care network for the needs of health care planning, overview of the distribution and the network of health care facilities, manpower planning, etc. The Institute is responsible also as the issuer of the unique health care professionals' codes. It assists the Ministry in preparing the National Health Plan. One of the main Institute's tasks and products in the field of Social Medicine is the Health Statistics Annual. Data on health care providers' network and health care personnel are one of the most important in that respect. The Institute also requires data on health care providers in order to fulfil the country's responsibilities versus the World Health Organisation in preparing the indicators related to the physical extent and functioning of the health care services. It works closely with Regional Institutes of Public Health that have similar responsibilities as the National one, just limited to the regional level. They perform an important task in co-ordinating the work in the Public Health area in its broader sense.
- Health Insurance Institute of Slovenia is the only insurer for the compulsory health care [8] insurer and the main insurer for the voluntary health care insurance. They are contracting services with individual providers which in turn can be public institutions such as health care centres or hospitals or, on the other hand, private practitioners. Quality data on the facilities and regularly updated registries of key health care professionals (medical doctors, dentists, pharmacists) are required by the Health Insurance Institute.
- The Medical Chamber of Slovenia holds responsibilities in the field of licensing, postgraduate training, continuous medical education and quality registries of medical doctors and dentists.
- The Pharmacists' Chamber of Slovenia has similar responsibilities and tasks, certainly referring only to the network of pharmacies and the personnel employed in them.
- Other potential users: Statistical Office of the Republic of Slovenia, Nursing Chamber of Slovenia, etc.

3. Results

3.1. Management and use of the Health Care Providers' Database

Management and use of the Health Care Providers' Database was architecturally set up in the two state institutes. The physical part of the database was done in the Health Insurance Institute of Slovenia, while managing it was enabled through a direct communication from the National Institute of Public Health. A DB2 database was set up in MVS operating system on the IBM HOST computer of the Health Insurance Institute of Slovenia. A direct communication link has been established between the Health Insurance Institute of Slovenia and National Institute of Public Health as well as direct links between individual regional Institutes of Public Health and Health Insurance Institute of Slovenia. The updating of NHCPD is run centrally at the National Institute of Public Health. An organisational procedure was established for the registration of health care personnel and providers and for the registration and maintenance of the employment statuses of health care professionals.

The use of the database is two-tiered: it serves as the reference base for computer supported operative work at the HIIS. On the other hand, translated as Data Warehouse [9] at the National Institute of Public Health it is used for the analyses and planning of the health care network in Slovenia. For the latter purposes the data warehouse will be run in Paradox© v.7.0 by Borland™ and statistically processed by SPSS© statistical package.

Within the Health Insurance Institute of Slovenia the following applications use NHCPD [10]: Contracts with providers, The Choice of Personal Physician, Analysis of drug prescriptions, Issues of personal use prescriptions, Health Insurance Expenditures, Health commissions, etc. It is expected that a very important project in the area of health insurance, Health Insurance Card project and especially its segment, Health Professional's Card, will largely rely on the data from the NHCPD.

3.2. Advances in data collection, processing and analyses

A large step forward had been made in establishing a communication network between the National and Regional Institutes of Public Health and connecting them to the information system of the Health Insurance Institute of Slovenia. By doing that, we are now able to have quick on-line queries and data analyses done in a very short time. The same is true with respect to the updating of data, especially in the present quickly changing environment.

For the purposes of data protection and security a contract was signed between the National Institute of Public Health and the Health Insurance Institute of Slovenia in order to establish such mechanisms for the safe keeping of data that would enable a high level of data protection and security.

Already in 1997, the new database enabled the National Institute of Public Health to prepare quality analyses of the health care providers' network and of the health care personnel, with a stress on detailed data about medical doctors and dentists and the relevant specialists of the two professionals.(see Table 1).

4. Discussion

We managed to fulfil requirements of various users of data on health care network and health care professionals with a single application. Several users use the same data set, thus facilitating the identification of errors and also, through a single solution, significantly reducing costs of maintaining several separated databases. Certainly the process of establishing clear definitions and finding appropriate solutions was not an easy one. It was actually a major external dependency causing a significant delay on the project (about 6 months).

Certainly, our project initiated several secondary projects, some of them also dealing with data protection and security. NHCPD is a source of many personal data on key health care professionals and as such is particularly vulnerable. Special solutions needed to be developed for a secure and protected access that will protect the interests of all parties involved.

Finally, one needs to stress the fact that complete legal framework for the database is to be defined within the Law on Databases in Health Care which is to be adopted by the National Parliament, hopefully by the end of 1997.

The National Institute of Public Health which is responsible for regularly updated information about health care providers and health care professionals will be able to produce statistical analyses and offer support to end users in a more efficient way.

All potential users of such data will be able to take advantage of quickly delivered information that will also be of a higher quality.

5. Conclusion

National Health Care Providers' Database is a part of the Uniform Health information system that we are trying to design and develop with joint efforts of various institutions interested. The key roles in the project described were played by the National Institute of Public Health and by the Health Insurance Institute of Slovenia.

We believe that the new database will offer quality data on health care providers and health care professionals thus enabling the most responsible state institutions as well as health care professionals' chambers for their functions.

We see a broader informatics support for health care management and planning, especially through quality information about health facilities, health equipment and appliances, etc. a necessary step in the future.

References

[1] Zakon o zdravstveni dejavnosti (Law on Health Care Activities). *Uradni list Republike Slovenije(Official Gazette of the Republic of Slovenia)* 1992: II(9): 590-601.
[2] Martin J. *Information Engineering*. Prentice Hall, Englewood Cliffs, New Jersey, 1989.
[3] *ADW/Planning Workstation Workshop, Issue 2.0.* KnowledgeWare Inc.
[4] *ADW/Analysis Workstation Workshop, Issue 2.0.* KnowledgeWare Inc.
[5] Batini C, Ceri S, Navathe SB. *Conceptual Database Design.* The Benjamin/Cummings Publishing Company Inc., 1992.
[6] *Project Management Life Cycle.* Ernst&Young International Ltd., 1992.
[7] *PRINCE Introduction Guide, Version 1.0,* NCC Blackwell Ltd., Oxford, UK, 1990.
[8] Zakon o zdravstvenem varstvu in zdravstvenem zavarovanju (Law on Health Care and Health Insurance). *Uradni list Republike Slovenije (Official Gazette of the Republic of Slovenia)* 1992: II(9): 577-590.
[9] Vidette Poe. *Building a Data Warehouse.* John Wiley & Sons, USA, 1996.
[10]*Projektna naloga ZZZS: Integralni model informacijskega sistema ZZZS.* Ljubljana, 1993.

Medical Informatics Europe '99
P. Kokol et al. (Eds.)
IOS Press, 1999

A Unified Model to Support an Information Intensive Health Care Environment

Claire BURDIS[1], Barry EAGLESTONE[2], Paula PROCTER[3]
[1] *Bassetlaw Hospital and Community Services NHS Trust, Worksop, UK*
[2] *Department of Information Studies, University of Sheffield, Sheffield, UK*
[3] *School of Nursing and Midwifery, University of Sheffield, Sheffield, UK*

Abstract. The two parts of this paper respectively analyses the mismatch between current systems and practice in health care, and present an outline design for enhanced Integrated Care Pathways (ICP) knowledge and information management based upon mature ICT technologies.

1. The Mismatch Between Systems and Practice

Central to healthcare is the patient. The next most important group comprises the information management advocates for patients and their relatives, i.e., the nursing team.

Registered nurses (RN) must spend three years or more in full-time education to gain the required knowledge which fits them for practice. Where further education and training have taken place, nurses become advanced practitioners with increased knowledge, skills and expertise. Why then are RNs treated as novices and offered mechanised systems of paper based processes that are flawed from the outset?

The main role of nursing is that of communicator. Nurses act as the information advocate for patients and communicate patient care to other nurses, medical and allied staff. Nurses must be given opportunity to assume self-identity, as Gidden states [5]: "A person with a reasonably stable sense of self-identity has a feeling of biographical continuity which she is able to grasp reflexively and, to a greater degree, communicate to other people." What is needed are Information Systems (ISs) that recognises registered (expert/master) nursing knowledge and freely permits communication for the benefit of patient care. "Information shared and communicated to other health care professionals will allow new views and relationships to evolve where multiprofessional care and patient involvement will become increasingly commonplace, leading to better patient care." [1]

In reality, delivery of care by RNs is the conscious design of interventions, based upon often unconscious assessment and matching of nursing, medical and societal knowledge. In observation, RNs plan prospectively but often record care retrospectively. These interventions can be nursing activities, but could be used by all those interacting with the patient. Medical diagnosis, if known, activates evidence set(s) which are defaults associated with the interventions. If the medical diagnosis is unknown, recorded interventions retain validity and so we envisage a computer link to a "problem base". Evidence as defaults recognises the importance of supporting activity and for adding to the body of evidence supporting practice. Opportunity must be present to highlight additions specific to the patient, also adding to the body of knowledge that is evidence based practice. There is a knowledge need for seamless inclusion of information to and from the general practitioner (GP) in the case of secondary (or tertiary) care. In community care, there is a knowledge need for inclusion of secondary care information to the GPs. We therefore envisage a non-segmented IS in which the RN enters the interventions, the medical practitioner enters the medical diagnosis and the computer system links the two "knowledge bases" (Figure 1).

Interventions and medical diagnosis are linked through an IS. Problem(s) can then be identified from stored knowledge, thus adding the final dimension to the building of evidence based practice. Outcomes are developed from changes to interventions and medical diagnostic record.

Through recording interventions, the 'active' part of the system, clinical coding, workload data, skill-mix and costing information can be generated from everyday activities. Medical diagnosis can provide a link between direct medical input and a structure of coding classification without need for administrative secondary input. Nursing can act as the generator of patient information without detriment to care, through reduced administrative data collection. Responsibility for practice is maintained through unique identity and password use of the system by the multidisciplinary team. Care progression can be monitored from recording when care has been given. Management can view activity levels of service provision, and interlinkage with support services, such as transport, meal provision can be directed from the interventions. Printouts can be selected to fit need, for example, if one RN is handing over to another RN the intervention printout may be selected. If an RN is supervising a student, the full process-orientated record may be requested, showing problem(s), evidence set(s), intervention(s) and outcome(s). If a multidisciplinary case conference occurs, then all progression information can be included.

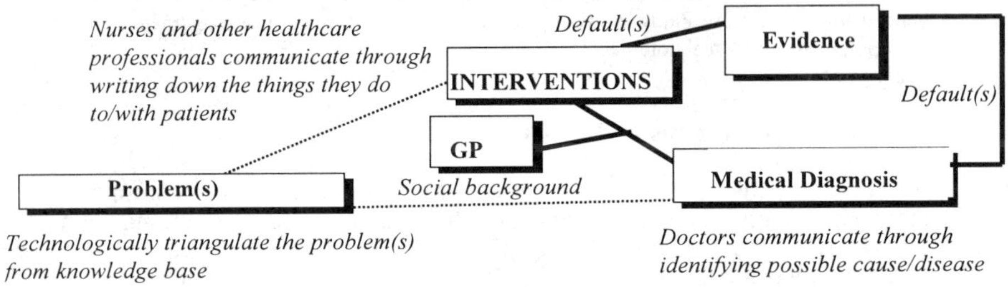

Figure 1: Intervention-based care delivery

Students of nursing (or other disciplines) have available to them, through mirrored educational computerised systems, actual practice records giving them not only information on interventions set against outcomes for quality of care determination, but also a live data set of healthcare today. It is envisaged that such information access will reduce the theory-practice gap significantly and ensure that nurses and other healthcare professionals are prepared to understand their identity in the health care society and improve the activity of patient care. "...the promise of the information age has not been realized in health-care because of the technical short-sightedness of closed systems and socio-political boundaries that inhibit collaboration and data sharing." [2]

2. An Infrastructure for Enhanced ICP Knowledge and Information Management

Preliminary IS modelling of the use of ICP knowledge within primary health care (Figure 2) was motivated, in particular, by our desire to seek an infrastrcture in which the triangulation in Figure 1 can be supported. Our aim was therefore to abstract out intrinsic processes and information, from aspects which are simply a consequence of the systems currently in operation and which cause the current mismatch between systems and practice.

Figure 2. depicts abstract repositories for: knowledge about "best practice" treatment, in the form of ICPs; operational data about treatment of patients, including prescribed ICPs, interventions and outcomes; and historical experience that (potentially) exists in the form accumulated and aggregated operational data. The information flow is an idealised feed back loop. Healthcare knowledge on which treatment is based is constantly updated on the basis of historical knowledge about treatments, interventions and outcomes. "Best practice" knowledge (ICP knowledge base) is applied to prescribe appropriate care for patient conditions, in the form of ICPs; data about patients' conditions, prescribed treatment, care interventions and outcomes are recorded (ICP Patient database) during ICP administered;

and the feedback loop is completed by collecting together patient data (ICP data warehouse) and inferring new "best practice" knowledge from evidence provided by the patient data.

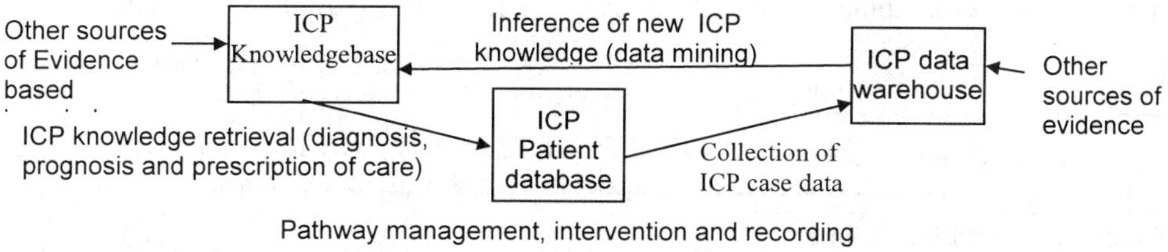

Figure 2: A high-level abstract model of ICP-related information flow

This model suggest use of established ICTs (Figure 3). Relational databases can be used to implement "ICP Patient Database". "ICP Data Warehouse" can be implemented as a data warehouse, using data mining techniques to derive new knowledge based on treatments, interventions and outcomes which diverge from the expected norm. "ICP Knowledge base" can be implemented using relational database technology, as collections of facts and constraints about hypothetical patients and treatments. There is also potential for artificial intelligence solutions, such as deductive databases, for automated reasoning relating to diagnosis, prognosis and prescription. An intranet can provide communications infrastructure necessary for seamless integration of the system across healthcare and professional boundaries, for example, through point-of-care data capture and access. The servers, ICP-KB, ICP-DB and ICP-DWH, respectively manage the knowledge base, database and data warehouse components in Figure 2. The client applications maintain and utilise information and knowledge represented in these repositories. ICP-KBA and IPC-Consultant respectively supports administration of knowledge in ICP-KB and retrieval, into ICP-KB, of ICPs for specific patient conditions. ICP-Manager supports administering IPCs (in ICP-DB) and capture of data generated. ICP-Miner implements data warehousing and mining functions to maintain ICP-DWH and derive evidence-based IPC knowledge.

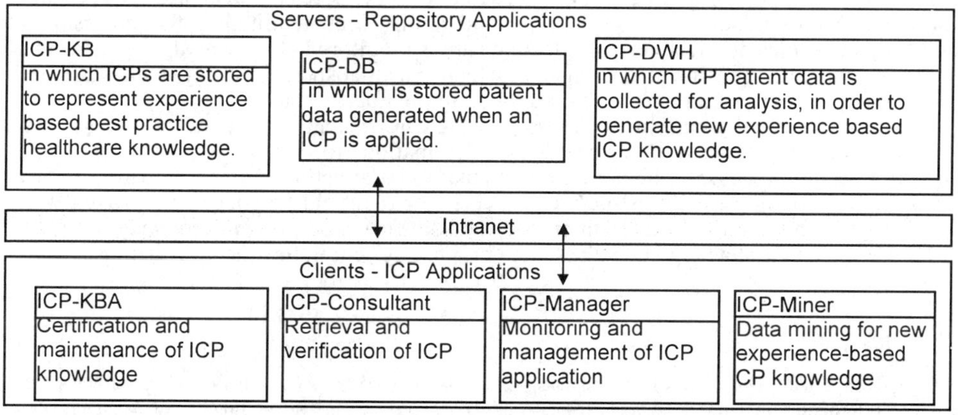

Figure 3: ICP Information Management System Architecture

We also note that modelling patients and treatments is a special case of the general problem of modelling histories of artefacts. We therefore propose using the GENREG data model [4] for representing ICP data. GENREG is a temporal model developed and implemented using relational database technology at the National Museum of Denmark to represent historic and administrative information about the museum's artefacts. GENREG can represent ICP information as graphs in which nodes represent patient data, and edges are labelled with descriptions of events that associate them (Figure 4).

This simple representation of information as data is surprisingly powerful and expressive, since artefacts may be connected by multiple edges, each labelled with the same or different events. This feature can be used to represent and access patient or care information in all of the contexts within which it occurs, for example, to record alternative diagnoses and prognoses or to evaluate alternative treatment pathways. This representation also supports manipulating and combining pathways, for example, for treatment of multiple conditions.

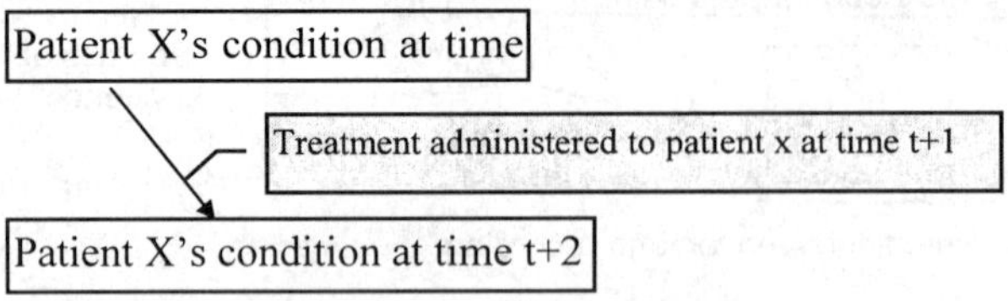

Figure 4: GENREG representation of Patient Data

The data structure depicted represents a step in the progress of an ICP. The white boxes (artefacts) represent details of the patient before and alter treatment. The shaded box (event) represents the intervening treatment event, prescribed by the ICP.

To the best of our knowledge, no one has yet looked at supporting what actually happens in the clinical setting. Projects to transcribe structures which have worked in other areas to the health care domain have largely failed. The majority of work in the field has been in the USA. Only small systems are currently available in the UK, which may help to design and analyse variances from paper-based ICPs. None currently allow recording of progress on the ICP, though HBOC are writing a system (MRPC module of DMNWSE) to do this.

3. Conclusions

In the UK, the White Paper, "The New NHS: Modern and Dependable" [3] has set many challenges and introduced and developed concepts which will affect how the health service functions. Two main themes can be linked to this paper: modernising information management and technology and its use within healthcare; and the establishment and delivery of proven clinically effective care. "Information for Health" [6] clearly focuses on delivering information to healthcare professionals to support day to day clinical practices. Co-ordinated patient care is one of the primary objectives of the strategy. Also, technological support of care delivery is needed to provide access to evidence bases in order for clinicians to update their knowledge and skills; thus facilitating the provision of clinically effective care. Delivery of effective care is monitored closely by the department of health in the form of clinical governance, which places responsibility of quality and safe practice not just onto chief executives, but onto all members of staff.

We have identified a current weakness in healthcare systems, i.e., conflict with practice. An IS modelling approach revealed an information feedback loop and associated repositories and processes which are fundamental to administration of healthcare. We have proposed a technological infrastructure, which implements this model using proven ICTs. This system can reduce conflict with practice and advance exchange of knowledge.

Future work is to develop and validate the propose system in healthcare situations.

References

[1] K. Calman, The Role of Informatics in the Future NHS, In: C Dollery and J Williams (eds) Informatics in Undergraduate Medical and Dental Education, Royal Society of Medicine Press Limited, London, 1996, p5

[2] P. Degoulet, F-C. Jean, C. Safran, Multimedia Workstations: Electronic Assistants for Health-Care Professionals, In: J. H. van Bemmel and A. T. McCray (eds), Yearbook of Medical Informatics 1996, Integration of Information for Patient Care, Schattauer Verlagsgesellschaft mbH, Stuttgart, 1996, p65

[3] Department of Health, The New NHS: Modern and Dependable, DoH Publications, Wetherby, 1997.

[4] B. Eaglestone, R. Holton, L. Rold, A Historical Data Model Based on Event Graphs, 7th International Conference on Database and Expert Systems Applications (DEXA'96), Zurich, September, 1996, Lecture Notes in Computer Science 1134, Springer, 1996, pp 254-263.

[5] A. Giddens, Modernity and self-identity, Polity Press, Oxford, 1995, p54.

[6] NHS Executive, Information for Health, DoH Publications, Wetherby, 1998

Medical Informatics Europe '99
P. Kokol et al. (Eds.)
IOS Press, 1999

Human aspects of medical computer application

Dr. Geza Lakner <glakner@hiete.hu>
Haynal Imre University of Health Sciences,
1st Department of Medicine — Department of Medical Informatics ,
Budapest, Hungary (H-1389 Budapest P.O.B. 112)

Abstract. Most of the research activities in the field of medical informatics are directed toward technological-technical problems. Human factors of computer use are often a neglected topic. Even the application of the tiniest microcomputer embedded in a medical diagnostic equipment may pose user acceptance and motivation problems but to mention larger scale hospital information systems. In this paper the author presents some aspects of the human-computer interaction problems in a medicinal computer application setting.

1. Introduction

Users of medical informatics solutions form a very heterogenous population. In some cases even non-professionals use such systems, e.g. hospital/polyclinic-based in-house information systems for patients or community health care information networks. The professional user group may contain technicians, financial clerks, receptionists, nurses or doctors : people with different expectations, different comprehension, different task completion approach. These users are heterogenous also in psychological terms: overt or less evident personality factors are apparent in terms of introversion/extroversion inner/outer motivation sensing/acting personality types etc.

2. User acceptance

The user may ask such questions when confronted with a new software system:

- What can I accomplish with the software package ?
- May me or technical problems cause faults with data loss ?
- How can I recover from an error ?
- How easily is the software to comprehend ?
- Will this new environment make my work more efficient ?
- Can I customize the program and import data from my previous system ?

The software quality measures are based upon such questions - psychological observations, the well-known six-domain ISO 9126 standard features a way to express metrics about

- functionality
- reliability
- usability
- efficiency
- maintainability
- portability.

Moreover, specific expectations of medical systems are communicated via the forthcoming CEN-standards like the HIF (Healthcare Information Framework) or HISA (Healthcare Information Systems Architecture). While the ISO and CEN standards provide an abstract way determining the criteria, the roots of these standards systems lie in complex user expectations. On the other hand it is questionable whether between user-initiated expectations and the features presented in these standards the distance would not increase with each technological revision.

3. User interface vs. functionality

The user acceptance of a sofware greatly depends on the user interface. Ease of handling may win over richness of functionality. It is a commonplace that 90% percent of users use regularly the 10% of functions of an application software. Almost invisible, abstract assets of a system - like security policies - are not the mostly appreciated parts for an average user. The neat visual appearance with simple, straightforward operation on the "good" side and sparky protuberations of the UI on the "bad" side are jousting in each new software development.

It is very difficult to specify what would be the users' real, *sui generis* expectations in a non-industrialized setting, without the “pushing” effect of the software industry.

What could be the requirements of an "ideal" UI ?

· functions are plausible and correspond well to real world terms

· cohesiveness

· graphical : the optical appearance of an interface element is uniform throughout the environment

· semantical : the same element / action does not have different meanings or effects in the same or different context

· syntactical : the syntax of the commnd should not change in the program environment

Perception of a good software may be attributed to both functionality and a well-designed interface. Users with different technical knowledge judge differently on software quality: a workspace cluttered with toolbars satisfies a power user but confuses a novice user with limited abilities; on the functions side limited system functionality , with inherent simplicity captivates the ordinary user while annoys an advanced one. Customization of the visible side of functionality i.e. hiding / revealing menu or toolbar fragments is essential for a software developed for a wider range of users. Judicious use of the *metaphor approach* in UI design (i.e. arrangement and behavior of graphical elements simulates the real world: ward or office-like items on the desktop etc.) definitively increases user confidence.

4. Computing environments

4.1. General computing tasks

Everyday operating system-related activities like copying or moving files, new directory creation or folder navigation seem to be difficult to deal with. Deletion of unused files and archiving is not a problem - only a few of the medicinal users do like that, - the huge hard disk capacity covers the flaws. System security is the weakest part of user activities: logging on with a collegue’s identification code, leaving the terminal logged-in while leaving the room even for longer time periods are daily events.

4.2. General office work

The difference in office automation package skills comes whether the actual person is involved in scientific research activities or not. "Purely" patient managing doctors stick with a word processor and basic touch-typing knowledge without relevant text formatting or structuring abilities. On the next level the user applies predefined templates. Doctors with report-generating obligations (scientists, contractual workers for pharmaceutical industries) go further : they work with efficient direct text formatting, sometimes use styles to automate the process. Document organization and outlining (e.g. index generation, figure numbering) are often beyond this level.

4.3. Internet activities

The confrontation with Web-browsing and e-mail is surprisingly positive. The browsers have an intuitive and simple user interface. The users mostly lack to exploit the convenience of bookmarking - they type the URL repeatedly again and again.

Sending and receiving e-mail does not pose problems to medical computer users. Attaching files may be a more difficult task. Compressed transfer of attachment files are avoided (similar ideological and skill-"hiatus" like archiving). The author had not encountered with anyone using automated mail filtering : manual selection of mail messages is almost exclusive.

The average user does not even know about newsgroups, despite the integrated newsreader in the WWW-browser. File downloads occur within the browser. (Note: it is a shame for the leading browser developers that retry-resume features are no implemented although many freeware ftp-clients offer "disconnection-proof" file downloading feature).

4.4. Document reading

In the life of a medical doctor studying-reading has a continous role. Beyond printed , paper-based information electronic media - multimedia, hypermedia - fight their way to acceptance.

Hypermedia can be interpreted as structured, “entry level" information systems. Even simple computer-based books (e-books) offer certain advantages over printouts: easy reproduceability (within legal copyright frames), searchability and some customizability of the user interface (i.e. changing display fonts, draft/page WYSIWYG view, individual keyborad code bindings etc.) . The Internet has achieved a lot in this area: the standard World Wide Web representation of documents via HTML offers more flexibility than “serial” formatted or non-formatted text. HTML with recent extensions enables embedding of feature-rich multimedia into web pages: still pictures, sound, 2D movies or even 3D virtual world walkthroughs.

Hypermedia versus serial text - people's opinion is not equivocal. Although hypertext is more structured, navigating back and forth via hyperlinks e.g. between a Table of Contents page and section body text may be cumbersome when the reader wants to read the whole article. Multi-level hyperlinking in a hypertext document can be more disastrous because today's browsers offer only one-dimensional navigation: they feature only back-and-forth movements. Reliable tree-like representation of WWW sites would be beneficial.

4.5. Professional (hospital, outpatient etc.) information systems

Professional computer systems form the “compulsory” side of the medical human-computer interaction. Being used during most of the office hours the staff should be - by virtue - very familiar with them. Many users meet with computers only by the application of such information systems. Today’s HISs are tailored for everyday use in the healthcare , in contrast with legacy systems of the past decades - in the latter case general (mostly business) applications with minor modifications were advertised as patient management systems.

The acceptance of HISs (or any professional information system) poses the question of motivation: is the right way to assimilate the new working environment with external psychosocial drive ? Will the user be satisfied with promises of enhanced productivity - and will fulfill the increase in performance from an internal psychological drive, being truly motivated ?

From a certain view HISs are dead end for learning general computer skills:

· These systems are not built for creativity: they are surely concise , but even customization for personal needs may be a neglected or unexploited feature.

· Many comprehensive HISs do not run on "PC" platform They represent a "closed world" offering no bridges to everyday personal computing.

5. Conclusion

The obvious paradoxon of the complex medical thinking and the generally apparent inability to communicate with computers seems overt.

Medical problem solving is a multithreaded, non-deterministic process involving the manipulation of huge , loosely-structured information. The key to understand this discrepancy may be the *fuzziness* of medical thinking. A decisive milestone of artificial intelligence would be the adequate modeling of the abstraction process (in fact this discovery would be an infinitesimal side-effect of the solution of the general thinking-puzzle).

The medical application of ergonomics - beside infrastructural (workplace organisational and hardware) issues relies on software design. The software industry should prepare more user friendly programs to eliminate the gap between customer electronics and computing.

Although the highly appreciated GUI conformance (X-Windows or Microsoft Windows or whatever windowing environment) in the business scenario is a premiere issue, medical systems may (and they do) have distinct, genuine interface philosophy.

The thoughts of years long in-house and external consultations, teaching among medical doctor collegues are presented below:

- Knowledge or skill is not necessarily age-related : young doctors may be "rookies" while senior researchers may be more knowledgeable in computer application.
- Doctors without research activities are less experienced computer users than scientists.
- Professional systems need more training time than just the usual few (4-6 hours) agreed in informatics development contracts.
- Nursing informatics is often a neglected area: nurses and paramedics are less susceptible to the advantages of computer systems (either professionnal systems or home office automation)

Abbreviations

UI	User interface
GUI	graphical user interface
OS	operating system
HCI	human-computer interaction
HIS	hospital information system

References

[1] H. Ledgard, Andrew Singer, John Whiteside : Directions in Human Factors for Interactive Systems ; Springer Verlag 1981

[2] A.V. Salvemini: Improving the Human-Computer Interface : A Human Factors Engineering Approach; M.D. Computing Vol.15 No.5 1998, p. 311

[3] M. Berg: Medical Work and the Computer-Based Patient Record : A Sociological Perspective; Methods of Information in Medicine 1998 : 37: p294-301

[4] M. Giardina (ed.): Interactive Multimedia Learning Environments; Springer Verlag 1992

[5] B. Schneiderman : Software Psychology; Winthrop Publ. 1980

Medical Informatics Europe '99
P. Kokol et al. (Eds.)
IOS Press, 1999

An Architecture for Bridging between Research and Practical Use in Health Informatics

Stig Kjær ANDERSEN[1,4], Christian NØHR[1,4] , Knut BERNSTEIN[3,4], and Søren VINGTOFT[2,4]
1: Aalborg University, Denmark, www.auc.dk
2: Danish Centre for Health Telematics, Denmark, www.cfst.dk
3: Danish Institute for Health Services Research and Development, Denmark. www.dsi.dk,
4: Virtual Centre of Health Informatics, Denmark, www.v-chi.dk

Abstract. Health informatics is a true interdisciplinary research discipline combining computer engineering, health science and fields dealing with organisation and communication issues. Much of the research published within the area has a common goal: to develop optimal information systems for better access to relevant data, information, and knowledge in the health care sector. As a respond to existing discontinuity between research and practical use, we present an architecture for an interdisciplinary virtual organisation promoting synergy across health informatics environments including research, industry, clinical, and educational settings. A set of key lessons learned from a practical implementation of the architecture are reported

1. Background

The efficiency of the interfaces between health informatics researchers, producers of health care information technology, practical users, and professional education in health informatics is an important parameter for successful use of IT in the health care sector. Researchers need inspiration from the problems identified during the development and use of health informatics systems. In order to optimise the use of IT in the health care sector, it is mandatory for providers to use the insights and understanding created by researchers. In the fast moving area of health informatics it is necessary to ensure dynamics in the professional training by close relation to both research and the practical use. Based on these facts we have created a personal network bridging the four groups by promoting a mutual professional grounded interaction between the identified actors..

2. Approach

We have established a set of goals, created an architecture for a framework, identified a set of tasks and services, and implemented the concept. We followed two interacting tracks in order to bridge. The first track was to create an interdisciplinary environment promoting synergy across health informatics projects. This was implemented by creating the Virtual Centre for Health Informatics (V-CHI) as an *umbrella organisation*. The second track was to disseminate research results through carrying out a university level educational programme for health care professionals.

3. Setting the goals

We are creating an interdisciplinary environment - a forum where researchers, professional users and producers of health care information technology are closely related on a personal level as well as on an organisational level. Therefore we need a mutual understanding of common goals. We must be aware that individual partners in an interdisciplinary environment can have conflicting goals at the operational level, i.e. a research partner has research goals and a commercial partner has commercial goals.

Generally, we have to ensure the rational use of information technology within the health care sector and to contribute to an optimisation of resources. To meet these aims, planning and the ability to intertwine prospective conflicting goals are necessary qualities. We also aim to improve the competitive power of the national health informatics industry. Such improvements require increased access to knowledge and well-educated human resources.

We expect that a rational use of information technology within the health care sector will free human resources that can be used for quality improvement of care and treatment. We expect that information technology will make it easier to compare treatments across place and time, providing new insight and knowledge for increased quality of care and treatment.

The basic idea is that both the research goals and the commercial goals can be achieved through an interdisciplinary framework [1] that promotes and supports health scientific projects containing substantial elements of health informatics.

4. The architecture of the framework

The framework support can be either administrative/financial or in the form of medical professional skills. By creating channels for sharing results from project to project, a constructive synergy between the projects is stimulated. Projects are thus part of an overall competence development that generates knowledge and results for future education. The supportive framework can also contribute to more effective management tools within the project organisations themselves.

Project participants in cross-disciplinary projects have anchor points in different types of environments such as research, industry, clinic or education. The main agendas for the two ways communication between any two environments are identified in fig. 1 e.g. scientific understanding between research and clinical environments, quality of labour between industry and educational environments. The task of the *umbrella organisation* is to mediate a 4-way communication between the different types of environment.

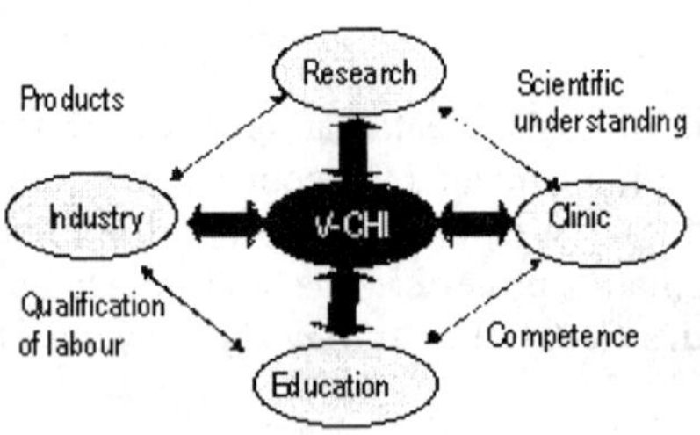

Fig. 1: V-CHI as a mediator between research, Clinic, Education and Industry

Implementation of these ideas is carried out through the creation of the Virtual Centre for Health Informatics (V-CHI). V-CHI is a co-operation between professional groups at Danish universities, the Danish health care sector and industry. The founding partners represent a wide range of organisations: 1) Universities: Aalborg University, the three faculties of Humanities, Social Sciences and Engineering and Science, and the University of Aarhus, Faculty of Health Science. 2) R&D organisations: DSI - Danish Institute for Health Services Research and Development, Copenhagen, and Danish Centre for Health Telematics, Odense. 3) Health care providers: The Counties of Aarhus and North Jutland, and Aalborg Hospital. Industry participates through a network of Commercial Affiliates.

The organisational basis is created through a network where co-operation and interdisciplinarity are given a favourable environment. This is realised and legalised through a mutually binding co-operation agreement between the partners, now running in its fourth year. The *partners* work through local organisations with individual health informatics activities. An *appointed board* charts the course of V-CHI activities. Each initial partner is represented by decision-makers on the board. V-CHI activities are managed and coordinated by *a secretariat* headed by a managing director.

We try to reach the goals through supporting project-oriented work, which means that persons from different environments cooperate to solve a specific problem. V-CHI maintains an information technology expertise in order to support the projects. This is done partly by the appointment of competent staff, and partly by utilisation of expertise from the partners. V-CHI creates and maintains cooperation with partners and relevant external organisations by means of agreements at managerial levels. V-CHI promotes cross-organisational project cooperation.

A project is carried out by one or more partners. Each project has specific health scientific goals with essential elements of health informatics. Professional cooperation is organised through these projects with V-CHI providing different services to the projects in return for contributions to secure overall goals. The exact conditions are specified in project contracts. The projects are classified according to different criteria such as scientific focus, the extent of V-CHI involvement, etc.

5. The Health Information Education Programme

An educational programme for health care professionals was created to qualify its students to play an active role in the development and implementation of health information systems. The educational track is implemented through an Open University programme in health informatics at the Masters level [2,3] at Aalborg University, Denmark. Up to now 50 have graduated as Masters. Through this initiative we hopefully contribute to a development where medical professionals are *mastering* IT instead of being mastered *by* IT. The strength of the programme is that the V-CHI connection means that the programme is continuously updated on the basis of results achieved in the projects. On the other hand, the experience which the Masters students acquire through their own projects also continuously contributes to the build up of the knowledge base of the total V-CHI network.

6. Commercial Affiliates

When bridging the gap between research and commercial partners, a platform for communication is needed. We have chosen to form the *V-CHI Commercial Affiliates*, a co-operation between 35 companies in Denmark and other interested parties. The *Commercial*

Affiliates network provides a platform for communication and cooperation between industry, the health care sector and research centres, as well as opportunities for informal relationships allowing the exchange of knowledge between academia and industry.

To support the interaction, we initiate newsletters, workshops and seminars on health informatics subjects such as standardisation, interfaces, integration, project life cycles etc. Moreover, it is possible for companies to participate in research projects and thereby be part of the latest research and development.

7. Competence and Activities

The gap between research and practical use of health informatics is bridged by activities building up overall competence. Since V-CHI is an umbrella organisation, its competence is embedded in the participants. V-CHI is working towards its goals through a set of activities and services offered to the participants. First of all the activities include participation in health informatics projects, performing basic strategic research and applied science, and development and presentation of knowledge. Health informatics focal points and competence building activities are shaping the V-CHI profile:

Decision support systems and their implementation in the health care sector. The interplay between change in the organisational structure of the health care sector and the development of information technology: And finally, the interplay between the interpersonal and the technological communication processes in the health care sector.

National and international R&D projects: Project participation is an important element in developing competence. Experience from the V-CHI partners' participation in projects is that the interaction between projects should be supported by both formal and informal activities. Formal activities include meetings, debates, newsletters, a joint website, etc., while informal gatherings create a comfortable social atmosphere for exchange of ideas and contacts.

Diversity is a key objective in order to promote optimal cross-fertilisation. The projects represent different health informatics research themes ranging from IT and organisational issues in the health sector to frontline technological projects. The following list of project examples shows the diversity in competence[4]:

Electronic Patient Record (EPR) Observatory (funded by the Danish Ministry of Health): On the basis of a national strategy for development and dissemination of EPR, the project is initiating a nation-wide coordination and consensus-based development of EPR at 11 different sites. Special focus is on benefits of EPR, integration of EPR systems with other relevant information systems, impact on health care organisations and security issues.

SIOL (Health Care Professionals, Information Technology and Organisational Learning) (funded by the Danish Research Council): The objectives for the project are twofold: (1) to analyse if and how the concept of organisational learning can support the changes needed within hospitals and other health care sectors, and (2) to analyse if and to what extent information technology can support the creation and maintenance of the learning organisation

TANDEM (partially funded by the EU Leonardo programme). The project focuses on giving the chronic disease patient, the core care health professionals, and auxiliary care health professionals skills and competencies in the use of information technology to promote more team-based and network-oriented management of chronic diseases. The patient is empowered to take more control of his / her own illness. The TANDEM model and pilot methods are being tested in relation to diabetes.

MIEMIS (Model for Investment and Evaluation of Medical Information Systems). (Funded by regional funds and industry) : The project develops a dynamic methodology for ensuring that the expectations to a medical information system are fed into the implementation process. The methodology will also handle the impact of factors as quality, interpersonal relations and job motivation / job enhancement on the implementation of medical information systems.

HC-REMA (Health Care Resource Management) (funded by the EU Telematics Applications programme): The project aims to provide different types of health care professionals with a set of tools for building decision support systems for resource management optimisation and quality control of health care policies in selected areas, such as instrumentation purchase, therapy assessment and trial and screening scheduling.

PatMan (Patient Management Workflow System)(funded by the EU Telematics Applications programme): The PatMan project aims to promote effective and efficient health care delivery by helping physicians to cope with both medical and organisational aspects during patient management.

Virtual Brain (national research funding and private funds): The Virtual Brain project aims at developing a computer-based neurosurgery simulator. The system is intended for use in both the education of neurosurgeons and for pre-operative planning for trained surgeons. The project also encompasses an activity to develop a 3D localization system for use during stereo tactic surgery.

MedCom - The Danish Health Care Network (funded by health care authorities, industry and health professional organisations): MedCom develops the EDI standards for communication of the most frequent cross sectorial health care messages, i.e. referral and discharge letters, request and results, prescriptions, reimbursement etc. Currently more than 1 million messages are exchanged each month.[5]

CoCo - Coordination and Continuity in Primary Health Care . (Funded by the EU Telematics Applications programme): The project is establishing regional health care networks in 14 European regions. CoCo has developed the standards needed for EDI and multimedia communication. The results also include extensive guidelines for implementation and organisational change as well as computer tools for EDIFACT standard development and testing

Precisely because of the diversity in project subjects, the V-CHI framework provides a forum not only for the exchange of new insights and knowledge between the projects but also a forum for mutual inspiration and synergy.

Experiences The initiative “Virtual Centre for Health Informatics” has been in operation since 1996 and the Open Education in Health Informatics since 1994. The first Masters of Information Technology in Health Informatics graduated in 1998.

Through these two tracks for filling the gap, e.g. the V-CHI network and the Masters level educational programme, we have identified a set of key prerequisites for increasing the success rate for coherence and continuity between R&D, dissemination and practical use of health informatics.

8. The key lessons

In health informatics projects it is mandatory to create an interdisciplinary understanding and acceptance that successful implementation is not only a technical matter but also requires the necessary interplay of organisation, person, and system.

Projects must acknowledge that health informatics R&D is interdisciplinary, and hence that the measure of quality needs to be based on traditions in the basic disciplines that health informatics is built on.

Given the rapid developments in the health informatics field, it is crucial that there be a learning relationship between educational health informatics programmes, health informatics research and practical applications of research results.

The gap between research and the practical use of health informatics is between different cultures. The initiative described here cannot totally fill the gap, but we have gained valuable experience with ways to bridge the gap: by developing a common language and understanding of theoretical and practical health informatics issues, by creating an appreciation of mutual interdependence between researchers and practioners, and by developing channels for cross-disciplinary co-operation.

Coordinates: Virtual Centre for Health Informatics (V-CHI), Fredrik Bajers Vej 7 D2, 9220 Aalborg East, Denmark, Tel: +45 96 35 88 09. Fax: +45 98 15 40 08..
e-mail: info@v-chi.dk Homepage: www.v-chi.dk

References

[1] Hultengren, E.Health informatics and the Humanities. Proc. The 9th World Congress on Medical Informatics, Seoul, August 18-22, 19981

[2] Nøhr C, Bygholm A, and Hejlesen O, 1998. Strategic planning of the Master Programme in Health Informatics at Aalborg University: targeting and updating the programme to meet explicit customer demands. In International Journal of Medical Informatics 50 (1998) pp. 207 – 213. 1

[3] Andersen, S.K., Andreassen, S., Bygholm, A., Hejlesen, O.K., and Nøhr, C., 1996. The Education in Medical Informatics at Aalborg University. In 1996 IMIA Yearbook of Medical Informatics. Schattauer (eds. Bemmel and McCray) pp. 111-115.

[4] V-CHI Website: ULR=http://www.v-chi.dk

[5] Bernstein K, Bjerregaard Jensen H. A National Strategy for Harmonisation of Health Care Applications. Results: A Danish Health Care Network in two years. In: Waegemann C P (editor). Proceedings of Towards an electronic patient record '97. Medical records institute 1997.

Medical Informatics Europe '99
P. Kokol et al. (Eds.)
IOS Press, 1999

The bridge between administrative and clinical information system

F. Borst, Cl. Bréant, D. Campi, S. Momjian, Ph. Rossier, G. Thurler, Cl. Revillard, R. Baud
Division d'informatique médicale - Hôpitaux universitaires de Genève
1211 Geneva 14 - Switzerland

Abstract. On one side, physicians are asked to record administrative information, such as activity measurement, case-mix of their specialty, billing, for statistical, legal or reimbursement purposes ; and on the other side, they need to gather detailed information about their own patients in terms of clinical evolution, for the day-to-day care of the patients or for clinical research purposes.
Many other actors are also involved with these processes, both on the administrative side, such as registration officers, administrators and on the clinical side, nurses and other care providers. Applications have been developed within hospital information systems for capturing and disseminating information according to these specific actors and dedicated purposes. But more and more appears the need to integrate these data for insuring the coherence of information and avoiding redundancy of data capture. How to conciliate these objectives?
We describe the Geneva's approach for integrating the administrative and the clinical systems.

1. Introduction: what are the needs of a Hospital Information System ?

A hospital information system is logically a link between each patient element (administrative data, reports, lab results, images,...) and physically a network between machines and applications. A patient in a (teaching) hospital is geographically split, between its bed, the labs, the radiology department, or between hospitals and general practitioners, and split along the time. The link provided by the hospital information system is thus mandatory for putting together the scattered parts of the patient and providing a homogenous view.

The information handled within a hospital has to fulfil three types of needs: around patient care, for administrative purposes and towards an "across-patient" view.

1.1 Patient care

The first need represents the patient dimension. The care provider needs information about the patient ("how is my patient") : a view to the patient history, the medical reports (discharge letters, specialists and radiology reports, etc.), the laboratory results, the list of performed radiology examinations, operating room reports, the images, etc. Patients are considered one by one, during one hospital stay or along successive readmissions and ambulatory visits.

At the patient care level, major efforts are dedicated for data capture, in terms of performance (speed) and ergonomy of the man-machine interface.

The geographic view of the patient is itself more and more enlarged, with several aspects:

intrainstitutional, between several departments, such as medicine, surgery, radiology, or hospital and ambulatory care

extrainstitutional, including the General Practitioner or home care

extraregional, towards network of care.

Actors involved at this level are physicians, nurses, physiotherapists, etc., all people directly involved with the direct care of the patient.

1.2 Administrative purposes

The second set of needs may be defined as administrative, including activity measurement, statistics, billing and reimbursement. This category could also includes the need of optimizing a resource (i.e. reservation of an operating room) or ordering a resource (i.e. a laboratory request or a drug prescription order).

1.3 Several patients: the "across-patients" view

For taking his decisions about one patient, the physician needs also information about other patients. He requires information about the literature ("what does say the literature"), i.e. an access to MEDLINE for providing the bio-medical references. He may also require information about previously known similar patients "are there other patients who are similar to my patient?". In other words, if the Electronic Patient Record is primarily designed for being used patient by patient, i.e. for helping to take decisions about the patient in front of the physician, it should also participate to the elaboration of a more general medical knowledge, for treating other patients: "How the knowledge of one treated patient can be used for treating other patients?".

This "across-patient" view can be used at several levels:

at a demographic level (number of treated patients, age and sex of patients)

at rough diagnostic level (i.e. evolution of cardiovascular disease as reason of death)

or at a more clinical level (including details on severity of the disease, evolution of clinical findings and patient's outcome).

At the first two levels decisions are taken, maybe in terms of regional healthcare planning, or for creating a new hospital specialty. The clinical level is almost never used beyond the research purposes of one medical specialty.

2. Problems and issues around the Hospital Information System

The applications of a Hospital Information System may by viewed around several aspects, which raise specific questions.

2.1 Space view

Should the patient record be specific to a medical specialty or should it cover the intrainstitutional, extrainstitutional and extraregional views? At the beginning, administrative systems are more or less unique within a hospital, whereas clinical systems are dedicated. Physicians of one given specialty have the need to gather their own data, without the necessity to communicate data between departments. They often build their own database with their own vocabulary. After a few years come several problems such as archiving and security, and the need of getting the patient identification record from the central administrative system or the need of getting an access to laboratory data. Later comes the need of getting clinical information from other departments (such as a patient going from a surgical department to a radiological examination or to a gastro-enterological examination, or for the child going from obstetrics to the pediatrics department). If these records should communicate, what are their specific parts and their shared parts? [1, 2].

It is the role of a medical informatics department to ensure a transversal view among departments. This need of a transversal medical record is even increased by ambulatory care, where all action around a patient (from investigation planning to diagnostic, therapeutics and further treatment planning) is to be performed during the reduced time of the encounter [3].

Clinical data are the most expensive to capture, because they are provided by physicians who have almost no time for doing it. The transversal view of these data is furthermore most important for avoiding redundancy of data capture, i.e. insure reuse of data.

2.2 Time view

How large should be the time vision of the patient:

how long should be watched the patient evolution and outcome: up to the hospital discharge or wider ? (We measured in Geneva canton hospital that among all patient treated during 1997 in hospital and ambulatory care, 18% were hospitalized once only ; all other had been seen several times in ambulatory or hospital care)

should we be able to read the medical records 10 years later ?

should we be able to keep a history of the evolution of a hospital (such as the creation of new structural entity, or the date of emergence of a new surgical technique that will undoubtedly modify the practice and the statistics)

what happens with the history of medical statistics when a new classification appears (which recently happens in Switzerland with ICD-10 ?)

Time also interferes with data capture, which can takes place:

before an event : for operation room reservation, for medication ordering or lab request

when the event takes place : admission of a patient, vital sign capture

or after the event : discharge letter, specialist report, statistical medical summary.

These implications are most important on the design of applications.

2.3 Level of detail view

How detailed should be the patient view? A formerly seen, the "across-patient" view can be built at several levels, demographic, diagnostic or clinical level. Up to now, healthcare planning decisions have been taken with information coming from the first two levels, but how far can we imagine that detailed clinical data could intervene in these decisions, specially when speaking of comparisons of patients between hospitals?

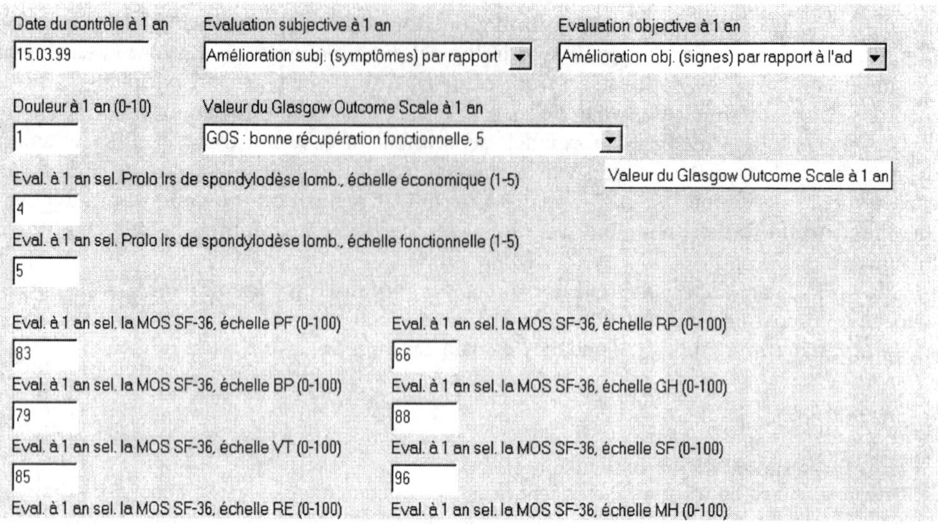

Figure 1: example screen of "detailed clinical data" application for neurosurgery

3. Geneva's approach as example of solution

Applications have been in Geneva historically mainly developed around actors and purposes. Nurses capture transfer and discharge information for activity measurement and communication purposes; physicians capture medical summaries for statistical purposes or they capture clinical data for research purposes; secretaries capture medical reports for patient documentation and communication purposes; financial employees capture acts information for billing purposes, etc.

DIOGENE Hospital Information System applications cover almost all hospital activities [4]. Each application is running on a transactional basis, i.e. they act as a natural way of communication between hospital actors:

ADT (Admission-Discharge-Transfer) is directly performed by the nurse when announcing a patient movement from the ward;

laboratory request is performed by physicians or nurses from the ward workstation;

UNILAB (UNIX-LABoratory) application handles the specimen from its arrival in the laboratory up to the edition of the result in the patient ward unit, even if the patient has been transferred;

an operating room procedure can be planned in advance throughout a dedicated application, PROGOP;

Pharmacy is directly ordered by the nurses, ward by ward. Individual drug prescription is under development;

Personnel is managed on a central application by each of the nine administratively independent units of the hospital.

Statistics on Intranet In order to constantly improve the quality of the HIS data, an immediate feedback is provided to the hospital actors be giving them statistics on a private hospital Intranet network. Statistics are available on an annual, monthly and even daily basis, about ADT, outpatient clinics, laboratory consumption, etc.

UNIDOC, containing the patient reports (discharge letters, surgical reports, specialists and radiology reports, admission notes, etc); Reports are dictated as usual by the physicians and typed by the secretaries [5].

Medical encoding in Geneva is directly performed by physicians, throughout a dedicated application called MODCOD, using a special tool for browsing the classifications, LUCID. Once entered, such a summary can be edited for being sent to the family physician, after appropriate signatures by the intern and the resident. The complete encoded history of the previous stays is available when a patient is readmitted, providing thus immediate and valuable information [6].

"Detailed clinical data": going further towards measuring quality of care requires more specific protocols for a given disease (cf fig. 1). Specialties have developed their own databases for capturing such detailed information. "Detailed clinical data" is an integrated application for capturing this information specifically to each department and also insuring a transversal view, i.e. sharing data between them.

OSIRIS, an image viewer, with an access to the PACS images (Picture Archival and Communication System).

3.1 Geneva's projects for communication between applications

Integration of these distributed applications has been developed in several directions. First, "integrators" have been developed, i.e. applications integrating data coming from several scattered sources. Such integrators are:

Archimed ; all patient applications save their related data within a common application called ARCHIMED ("ARCHIves MEDicales"). This application gathers all the DIOGENE patient-related data, beyond the actual archival process of each application (including pointers to texts and images). This powerful application allows to find "all facts of a given patient" and to retrieve "all patients matching to a given profile." [7]

Domed provides to physicians a common interface to the patient's documents (Unidoc reports, MODCOD summaries, histological reports and structured data coming from Archimed: patient trajectory, laboratory results, performed radiology examinations, histological summaries, etc). This application is mostly welcome among physicians.

Secondly, links between medical applications capturing data are under development. Data captured by physicians may be classified in three categories:

structured clinical data, such as "weight", or "temperature", or "Glasgow coma score", or "type of diabetic retinopathy"

diagnoses and therapeutics codes, corresponding to an internationally recognized classifications, such as ICD-10 or ICD-9-CM. These codes are able to generate a medical summary and statistics of the service, maybe based on AP-DRGs

free text, usually typed by secretaries as complete reports, but sometimes typed by physicians themselves as a short comment or conclusion of a visit.

These data are up to now captured in Geneva by three distinct applications: "Detailed clinical data", MODCOD and UNIDOC. But physicians ask more and more to record documents containing these three types of data altogether. The first idea was to build a new application integrating these functionalities. But each application contains specificities and is relatively complex. UNIDOC contains a sophisticated system for structuring texts into paragraphs, allowing to share paragraphs between documents, to build standardized texts for each medical specialties and to facilitate word indexation for free text retrieval. MODCOD contains mechanisms for checking the exhaustivity of summary, i.e. a mapping between the dates of the administrative hospital stays and the dates of the coded summaries, which mechanism being able to generate lists of un-encoded stays. The decision was then taken to keep the specificity of applications and to build communication mechanisms between them.

4. Conclusion

Applications within a hospital information system have multiple purposes and are used by multiple actors. Physicians themselves use applications dedicated to administrative purposes on one side and to clinical purposes on the other side. Having the intent to maintain the coherence of data and to avoid redundancy of data capture, tools for integrating these views are described. Furthermore, knowing that the patient's view becomes more and more wide across time and space (from the unique hospitalization to healthcare network), communication of detailed structured clinical information becomes more and more useful.

References

[1] Zeng Q, Cimino JJ. Linking a clinical system to heterogeneous information resources. Proc AMIA Annu Fall Symp (United States), 1997, 553-7 .

[2] Einbinder LH; Remz JB; Cochran D. Mapping clinical scenarios to functional requirements: a tool for evaluating clinical information systems. Proc AMIA Annu Fall Symp (United States), 1996, 747-51.

[3] Rappaport SH. Supporting the "clinic without walls" with an event-directed messaging system integrated into an electronic medical record. Proc AMIA Annu Fall Symp (United States), 1996, 648-52

[4] Scherrer JR, Baud RH, Hochstrasser D, Ratib O. A integrated hospital information system in Geneva. *MD Computing* 1990 ; 7 (2) : 81-9.

[5] Tange HJ, Hasman A, De Vries Robbe PF, Schouten HC. Medical narratives in electronic records. *Int J Med Inform* 1997;46:7-29

[6] Borst F, Griesser V, Rossier P, Bourdilloud R, Scherrer JR. Fifteen Years of Medical Encoding in the Diogene HIS. In MEDINFO'95, Proceedings of the Eighth World Congress on Medical Informatics, Vancouver, Greenes, Peterson, Protti (eds), Healthcare Computing & Communications Canada (Publ Comp), Edmonton 1995, 43-46.

[7] Thurler G. et al, "Archimed: An Open Network of Normalized Integrated Information Systems", to be published in Meth Inf Med.

Medical Informatics Europe '99
P. Kokol et al. (Eds.)
IOS Press, 1999

Research needs and priorities in Health Informatics – early results of a Delphi Study

Jytte BRENDER[1], Peter McNAIR[2], Christian NØHR[1]
1) Aalborg University, Virtual-Centre for Health Informatics, Fredrik Bajers Vej 7D, DK-9220 Aalborg East, Denmark; jytte.brender@v-chi.dk.
2) Hvidovre Hospital, Dept. of Clinical Biochemistry, Kettegaard Allé 30, DK-2650 Hvidovre, Denmark; peter.mcnair@dadlnet.dk.

Abstract. A four-phased Delphi study has been performed on the topic of "research needs and priorities to implement the Information Society within Healthcare". This contribution presents the outcome of the first three phases. The biggest surprises are that 'Telemedicine' is relatively lower ranked than expected, and that 'Business Process Re-engineering' is the highest ranking topic, as judged from the number of issues and barriers raised by the expert panel.

1. Introduction

Ever increasing options for diagnosis and treatment are available. One can get spare parts for replacement of even unthinkable body parts. The option for personal insight into one's physical body and its prognosis goes almost infinite with the gene-technology and genomics. The information technology can send a man to the moon and can nurse a nuclear power plant, etc. The Information Society is here and glues it all together for the individual client and/or server (respectively the patient in spe and the health care staff). The political demand for effectiveness and efficiency is increasing, as is the population's demand for insight, service and influence on one's own situation. However, as compared with other domains healthcare has not yet exploited the advances of Information Technology and Telecommunication. In view of the revolutionary effect of the photocopying machine from invented to handle a simple duplication task till today's revolution of administration and case management, the Information Technology may also imply a completely new world, the Information Society.

The Health Informatics[1] literature includes a number of recent contributions by highly esteemed researchers on future research needs and priorities, both for the domain as a whole and for individual sub-domains, see e.g. [1-13][2] - just to mention some highlights. The huge technological potential and the fast evolution means that we can not afford (economically, organisationally, ethical) investment failures. So, to support prioritisation of research initiatives one needs to balance individual perspectives on the subject against each other, rather than adopting the (subjective) viewpoints within the literature. Thus, the scope of the present investigation was defined as "the aim is to achieve a 'kind of' map (a rich picture) of the needs and priorities within Health Informatics research for the next decade".

A Delphi approach was selected. Delphi is a consensus method [14-16], at which a central team interrogates with a panel of experts on a predefined topic, and at which the experts

---

1) We let this term be synonymous with Health / Medical Informatics & Telecommunication in a broad sense.

2) … plus all the commentaries on [5].

comment on each other's contributions and/or adjust their own contribution in an iterative process controlled by the core team. The Delphi approach has proven to be effective in exploring future trends and forming a basis for strategic planning. The participants are all experts in a domain and have the ability to extrapolate trends and events within their domain. Brought together in the Delphi phases they adjust and inspire each other.

2. Method

The methodological aspects, options, perils and pitfalls within a Delphi investigation are excellently described in [14-18]. A Delphi investigation is normally starting with an open question, which at some point in the process is converted into a questionnaire to achieve (semi-)quantitative answers on the original qualitative statements. We chose a four-phased approach, as outlined in Table I. When writing this, the study is in the middle of its fourth phase: the questionnaire developed has been distributed to the panel.

Table I: The contents of the selected four phases.

Phase	Phase contents
1	Brainstorming phase: Elicitation of research items from the expert panel on the basis of the open question *"What research questions would you intuitively point at as the ones which should be emphasised within the next 5-10 years as the most important in addressing the Information Society in health care?"* A small scenario related with the Information Society was used to focus the mind-set of the respondents, but to avoid a bias no example was given.
2	Evaluation phase: Mutual commenting is applied to get constructive and critical feedback, thereby extending the original views and facilitating revision. As our information need is of a qualitative nature there is no need to have everyone comment every other expert's contribution. So, to minimise the burden on the panel and to avoid the effect of duplicates, the contributions were grouped. The grouped material was personalised for each member in a way that he/she received the contributions from Phase 1 only of his/her fellow group members. The material was made anonymous by coding and removal of potential identifiable information, and subsequently harmonised with respect to layout. For each research issue a pre-cooked list of questions (with options for free text commenting) were inserted, related to the respondent's expertise on the specific topic, the relevance/usefulness of the topic, specific constraints and aspects of feasibility of the topic.
3	Feedback phase: Submission of comments received within the second phase to the individual contributors with insertion of all feedback, including insertions into the original text. The main purpose of this phase was to allow for clarification or extension of the original contributions.
4	Questionnaire phase: Submission of a questionnaire prepared on the basis of the original contributions and all the comments. As we are looking for a rich picture of the future rather than a quantitative statement on priorities, it will suffice with one interrogation on the questionnaire.

The entire communication with the experts was performed through e-mail as recommended by [18]. It was accomplished in a bilateral fashion to maintain anonymity within the panel of experts. There has been no explicit deadline, but the response was pushed implicitly through the accompanying letter and reminders. The philosophy was that for busy people it is in general not a matter of 'deadlines', but of priority.

To get a broad representation, we defined the following characteristics of the candidates:

- the experts' should posses a visionary capability and insight into the Health Informatics domain as a whole, as well as a broad research-profile,
- the panel as a whole should cover the main elements within a model of factors that forms or influences the future research (market forces, the political arena, application research, basic research and meta-assessments),

- the panel of experts should cover a broad range of sub-domains within Health Informatics[3],

Candidate panel experts were identified on the basis of literature reviews on the topic or on our personal knowledge. The list was supplemented with experts from domains outside our personal area of expertise by recommendation according to the same criteria. Fulfilment of all combinations within the above list of criteria would require a huge expert panel. We therefore made the best compromise realistic to accomplish the study scope. The handicap with these criteria is that only V.I.P.s are candidate members of the panel, which may make it difficult to get fast and efficient feedback, or even to get feedback.

The leading principle for grouping of experts within Phase 2 was (1) to separate 'similars' (e.g. 2 experts contributing with the issue 'telemedicine') to minimise a bias in the prioritisation and commenting, (2) to keep all contributions of a given expert in one group to ease the processing, and (3) to make the groups as homogeneous (parallel in contents) as possible.

3. Results

Out of 55 calls for participation, 25 submitted contributions. These experts represent Australia (1), Brazil (1), Canada (1), Europe (Scandinavia 3, Anglo-Saxon/Celtic countries 5, Central-Europe 6, Southern Europe 2), South Africa (1) and USA (5).

The experts were grouped during Phase 2 into 5 groups according to the above mentioned principles. Eighteen responded on the call for comments. This input was fed back individually to the contributor with an option to make corrections accordingly. Three contributors were explicitly addressed with specific questions for clarification, like non-common abbreviations or concepts.

One the basis of the original contributions and all comments, a list of research needs was prepared by cumulating thc individual contributions, sorting into main topics and then by cutting and pasting the original texts, followed by a merge of duplicates or almost duplicates. Compound contributions were separated into singular issues and integrated. Depending on the nature of the individual comments from Phase 2, these were incorporated either as new independent research issues or integrated within or extending the existing issues. Subsequently, the entire material was edited and harmonised with respect to appearance and language, but not the semantics. Finally, the text was structured into the following parts for each main topic: a) a short description of a scenario or vision of what might come, based on contributions of a more argumenting or descriptive type of the issues and questions raised, b) a list of research items, and c) a list of potential barriers.

The outcome was a total of 110 research items and 58 supplementary barriers divided on 14 topics, see Table II, of which one is concerned only with the nature of Health Informatics. None of the contributions received a unanimous opinion of "already existing/has been solved" or "not particularly relevant or useful" by the group members, and hence, none of the contributions was cut. Some of the comments received within the second phase also addressed the issue of whether this or that belongs to the core of Health Informatics; however, no contribution was deleted for that reason - again because of lack of unanimity.

The mere distribution on these main topics constitutes a simple measure of priorities, as it reflects the main concerns present in the expert panel.

---

3) The nursing (informatics) area is rather extensively dealt with within the literature of Delphi investigations on priorities and needs, and hence this area is downsized as an explicit target within the present study.

Table II: The distribution of research issues and potential barriers on the identified main topics.

Main Topic	Research issues identified No.	Example	Potential barriers suggested No.	Example
Business Process Re-engineering[4]	17	Research on the extent to which injection of Information Technology into the environment actually changes the way that health care is delivered (and not just automate what is currently being done).	13	… or are the health professionals motivated to become part of such a change?
Electronic Patient Record and connected inter-operating systems	15	Research on the infrastructural support to share the contexts of the care episodes among clinicians.	5	… or are the 'people issues' (like motivation and compliance with common definitions, etc.) vital to the success of such an electronic patient record project, and does the success have little to do with the technical implementation?
Management, policy and financial aspects	7	Development of methods and tools of information processing for up-to-date and comprehensive reporting on public health status.	9	… or is it a question of pragmatic decisions rather than a core Health Informatics research area?
Quality of life & compensat-ing physical handicaps & bioengineering	11	Research on measures of well being.	3	… or is the economics of compen-sation of physical handicaps by informatics and bio-engineering completely out of range?
Evidence-based Medicine & Clinical Guidelines	9	Research on medical decision-making and representation of medical treatment plans	4	… or is it a matter of seeking ISO certification or accreditation, and to take this from the macro level to the micro level of care given to individual patients?
Utility of Deci-sion Support / Knowledge-based Systems	10	Research on the context for application of decision-support systems, i.e. how to integrate knowledge-based decision support into the clinical process, so that it turns into clinically useful and operational systems, - i.e. the whole field of <u>decision support</u>.	2	… or are knowledge-based systems mainly relevant for continuous education rather than as clinical (etc.) decision support?
Knowledge extraction from clinical data and free text	7	Development of system wide intelligent systems that are self learning, i.e. research regarding data warehousing and data mining (machine learning from clinical data and information).	4	… or is data dredging as a "re-search" method a basic fallacy, because of the quality of data in Electronic Patient Record Systems?
Education	7	Research on how to obtain a virtual world for consultance at diagnosis and treatment in general. We can not all be super-experts and as the volume of knowledge and technological options for diagnosis and treatment increase ongoing we need ongoing support.	4	… or is the distance learning simply a matter of using the web technology as it is now?
Telemedicine	5	Research on operational costs	5	…or s it a matter of the remuneration issues?
The Informed Patient	7	Research on issues within patients' access to their own patient record in particular and to medical knowledge in general, such as how to overcome the many legal, cultural, linguistic and ethical challenges?	1	… or is this perspective simply economically unreachable?

[4] This concept is used here (and below) in its broadest sense as covering all types of approaches and methods for managing organisational change.

Legal, ethical and security issues	4	Research on the trade-off between the harms of security breaches vs. harms of security measures, … among others also balanced against the need to obtain timely access to data for treatment purposes and to do research on patient outcomes and epidemiology	3	… or are the mentioned legal / ethical issues of a size that will hamper exploitation of the involved technological options?
Information and cognition	6	Research on how alternative formats for clinical information (text, structured text, tables, graphs, time lines, pictograms...) on paper or computer screen influence the ease with which clinicians find and interpret it.	1	… or can image analysis improve clinical decisions or are images just pretty pictures for software demos/journal articles?
Point-of-Care technology	5	Research on a standard for informatics around POC ('Point Of Care') analysers.	1	… or is this something we can expect solved by the suppliers of laboratory equipment?
Nature of Medical/Health Informatics	0	(none)	3	… or will people originating from the 'computing' and the 'healthcare' sides develop the same skills and knowledge after a while?

4. Discussion

The sorting of research issues into main topics and the 'how and what to merge' are based on a judgement of contents and relations, which inevitably are subjective by nature. Nevertheless, the contrast on number of issues raised for the different main topics is marked. Let's point out a couple of interesting aspects.

The biggest surprise was the relatively low ranking of 'Telemedicine' as compared to the explosion of activities in this field (see [12,13]) and a political interest on the subject as e.g. emphasised within the past EU 4th Framework Programme for R&D in Europe.

Another big surprise was the top ranking of 'Business Process Re-engineering' issues (BPR). Except from [2,6] and partly [9,11] - the papers cited in the Introduction ([1-13]) only emphasise this topic marginally, and many of them don't even mention the need for basic organisational change to accompany the application of IT-systems within healthcare. To some extent, this may be explained by differences in the perception of what Health Informatics is, as also reflected in the discussions by e.g. [3-5,9]. We agree with [3] and numerous others that Health Informatics is a multidisciplinary domain, and it must be self-contained in the sense that skills needed to accomplish the process of IT development/application has to be an integrated part of the Health Informatics domain. Insertion of any new technology into an organisation imposes significant changes into its structure or work processes (or other aspects) [19], so the active management of change has to be on the list of issues within Health Informatics.

It was no surprise when counting conference headings during the last couple of years that Electronic Patient Records (or similar advanced connected inter-operating systems) would be high ranked.

Moreover, Evidence-based Medicine (and clinical protocols) is on the same level as the issue of decision-support systems & knowledge-based systems in ranking (when knowledge elicitation is kept separate), in agreement with the main line within the literature cited above. The lack of success of decision support was reflected within the needs raised, as the development of such systems was not raised, whereas the integration of decision support within the clinical processes was, i.e. a BPR issue.

We would say – as [2,6] - that the organisational (and hence Business-Process Re-engineering) aspects are the most important new aspects on the agenda of tomorrow, and recognised as such by interpretation of the early Delphi study results. This conclusion is in contrast to the conclusion of [1] that the challenges identified are the ones already under way. The outcome of the last phase of this study, however, will show whether the preliminary conclusions are in agreement with the general opinion of the experts.

Acknowledgement

We would like to give a very special thanks to the experts involved for their kindness and willingness throughout. However, as the study is ongoing, we will keep the panel of experts anonymous here.

References

[1] Sittig DF. Grand Challenges in Medical Informatics? JAMIA 1994;**1**:412-413.
[2] Riley RT. Organizational Issues in Health Informatics: The Challenges We Face. In: Greenes RA, et al., eds. Proceedings of the MEDINFO 95. Edmonton:Healthcare Computing & Communications Canada Inc. 1995, pp. 1570-1574.
[3] Degoulet P, Fieschi M. Critical dimensions in medical informatics. Int J Med Inform 1997;**44**:21-26.
[4] Gell G. The internal challenges of medical informatics. Int J Med Inform 1997;**44**:67-74.
[5] Haux R. Aims and tasks of medical informatics. Int J Med Inform 1997;**44**:9-20.
[6] Lorenzi N, Riley RT, Blyth AJC, Southon G, Dixon BJ. Antecedents of the People and Organizational Aspects of Medical Informatics: Review of the Literature. JAMIA 1997;**4(2)**:79-93.
[7] Moehr JR. Grand Challenges in health informatics, An information systems perspective commentary on Haux. Int J Med Inform 1997;**44**:27-37.
[8] Saba VK. A Look at nursing informatics. Int J Med Inform 1997;**44**:57-60.
[9] Moehr JR. Informatics in the Service of Health, a Look to the Future. Meth Inform Med 1998;**37**:165-170.
[10] Rindfleisch TC. (Bio)Medical Informatics in the Next Decade. JAMIA 1998;**5(5)**:416-420.
[11] Rindfleisch TC, Brutlag DL. Directions for Clinical Research and Genomic Research into the Next Decade: Implications for Informatics. JAMIA 1998;**5(5)**:404-411.
[12] Taylor P. A survey of research in telemedicine. 1:Telemedicine systems. J Telemed Telecare 1998;**4**:1-17.
[13] Taylor P. A survey of research in telemedicine. 2:Telemedicine services. J Telemed Telecare 1998;**4**:63-71.
[14] Linstone HA, Turoff M. The Delphi Method, Techniques and Applications. Reading, Massachusets: Addison-Wesley Publishing Company. 1975.
[15] Crisp J, Pelletier D, Duffield C, Adams A, Nagy S. The Delphi Method? Nursing Research 1997;**46(2)**:116-118.
[16] Adler M, Ziglio E. Gazing into the Oracle, The Delphi Method and its Application to Social Policy and Public Health. London: Jessical Kingsley Publishers. 1996.
[17] Dalkey NC. The Delphi Method: An Experimental Study of Group Opinion, Prepared for United States Air Force Project Rand. Santa Monica, CA: Rand. 1969.
[18] Kreiner K, Nielsen A. Erhvervsbyggeriets fremtid – en delphi undersøgelse. Lyngby:Danmarks Tekniske Højskole. 1975. (in Danish)
[19] Müller J, Kjaer-Rasmussen J and Nohr C: Proactive Technology Assessment as a Tool in HIS Development. In: Barber B, Cao D, Qin D, Wagner G, eds. Proceedings of the MEDINFO 89 Conference. Amsterdam :Elsevier Science Publishers B.V. 1989, pp. 308-311.

Success Factors of Hospital Information System Implementation: What must go right?

Vesna Prijatelj
Information Centre, University Medical Centre, Zaloška 2, 1000 Ljubljana, Slovenia

Abstract. Health care institutions are considering a variety of information technologies in the hope of increasing efficiency, reducing cost, re-engineering work processes, and improving quality of care. When we talk about any information system implementation, we need to keep in mind that there are actually three phases to such a project: pre-implementation, implementation and post-implementation. The aim of our contribution is to present the realities of successful implementation and our experience with such project.

Keywords: information system, implementation, success factors

1. Introduction

The Ljubljana University Medical Centre (UMC) is the largest public health centre in Slovenia. With its 3,200 hospital beds, an average of 120,000 days of hospital medical care annually, and with 800,000 examinations in outpatient departments and ambulatory care, it is also one of the larger public health centres in Europe. Information technology support in the UMC is organised by the Information Centre, serving the hospital, ambulatory, laboratory, pharmacy, as well as general management departments. In the course of developing and implementing hospital information systems over six year period we have identified a critical success factors of such projects. We realize there may be others, but in our experience, these seem to be most crucial. As Oscar Wilde once said, ''Experience is the name we give to our mistakes'.

A critical success factors were defined as 'what must go right' to achieve successful results. Our organisation has found that there are actually three phases to such a project: pre-implementation, implementation and post-implementation. While we pay close attention to the implementation process, we often overlook the critical needs that exist before and after the implementation itself.

2. Pre-implementation

Vision

Every successful implementation begins with a clear vision of the business and its future Who are we? What do we want to become? And what do we need to get us there [3,7]? This vision needs to be clearly communicated to, and understood by, all levels of the organization; for it is within this context that the processes of needs definition, system selection and implementation must occur. The new system effort should facilitate support of a better way of doing business and patient care. Vision leads to a definition of the mission, and the mission to strategy; the new system must be capable of supporting this strategy.

A clear definition of expectations and deliverables from the new system must be developed. The definition of deliverables should not only include the end objectives (in terms of data quality, time improved, paperless etc.), but also milestone expectations at various points in the implementation process to ensure the process is on track [4].

Business and requirements needs analysis

The next step is to carefully conduct a business and requirements needs analysis. This step is of extreme importance. In too many cases, an information system is developed or purchased to achieve vague and somewhat idealistic goals that cannot possibly be accurately measured. An example of this type of goal would be to "reduce papers or time improvement." What exactly does that phrase mean? Reduce what papers, improve which time? All papers? After you identify what papers you are going to reduce, by how much are you going to reduce it? Why? What is the anticipated return on investment?

The business and requirements needs analysis provides an organization with measurable, concrete results that can be used to determine the progress of the implementation and to see if the implementation should be undertaken at all. A business needs analysis is a careful, step-by-step examination of how our business functions. It includes the collection of data from a variety of areas within an organization [5]. The results of the business needs analysis are a solid assessment for identification of opportunities for improvement.

Project leader

Perhaps one of the most critical determinants of success lies in the selection of the right project leader. The project leader must come from within the organization. The ideal project leader is a senior manager who has a working knowledge of all aspects of the business, and good people skills to interface with the entire user community; delegation of the role to a junior person in the organization diminishes its perceived importance to both management and the user community. To ensure that continuity in the project is maintained, it is also imperative that the project leader be assured of a permanent position in the organization once the project is considered to be complete; but at the same time, he or she should recognize that ongoing demands will occur to help resolve issues which arise with the system after implementation.

3. Implementation

Implementation team

Choosing team members is never easy, it often involves political, professional and personal issues. Teams with negativity, interpersonal conflicts and hidden agendas do not achieve successful implementations. Team members must be people who directly affect daily operations and who understand the benefits of an hospital information system.

Team members must have the responsibility and authority to "make it happen." If they do not, the implementation will fail. Some teams falter because they do not have the authority to mandate new processes or procedures. Each team member needs to be responsible for specific tasks. A key element in team planning and team development is identifying the role each member will play. A simple way to do this is to establish team member "job descriptions." The description should be composed of the overall goal of the team and the tasks each member needs to perform to achieve team goals. Members must be held accountable for their assigned tasks. The job description should be reviewed weekly to monitor progress and to identify potential problems.

Once the team is formed and functioning, it must avoid working in secrecy. The team must communicate continually and accurately to the rest of the organization. Every user in the organization must be continually informed of the progress and requirements of the implementation. The team can be sure that bad news and setbacks will travel far and wide. The trick of the job is to make sure good news and accomplishments travel just as far. One way to do this is to document and distribute time and money savings as soon as they occur. When savings are documented and distributed quickly, the momentum will help keep the organization excited about the implementation and encourage the team in difficult times.

One of mistake is to make one person responsible for an entire implementation. When one person is responsible, there is only one person to blame or one person to locate when things aren't going well. However, our experience has shown that one person cannot successfully implement a system. Only a team can accomplish a successful implementation.

Users Understand and Use the System

Documented procedures are essential to the smooth start-up and continuation of a new system. The procedures are crucial to the users, and need to define, in detail, the processes and steps required of each user role.

Depending on the user's level of computer knowledge and experience, the use of a new system can be most frustrating. An introductory course on system use would include keyboard skills, screen navigation and software help functions. Education of users in health care principles is crucial to their gaining confidence, knowledge and understanding of the reasons behind the implementation; why the use of the hospital information system is important; and how to perform their day-to-day job functions. It is important to convey the fact that with HIS is possible to health care processes improved, not simply automated of old and possibly inefficient processes.

The aim of HIS is to support the processes, not control them. It can provide some aspects of logical and context data but there should be a strong focus on the individual responsibility for data quality. Problems with user's use of the system can be rooted in lack of understanding and ease of use.

Post-implementation

Too often we expect users to be able to use the new system effectively based on relatively short time education period; but this is like expecting someone to learn to drive a car by reading the owner's manual. Much of the learning process actually occurs through hands-on use of the system in normal operating circumstances. Many of the dysfunctional issues which will plague a system tend to arise after the new system is in place; yet, it is often in this last phase that we are the most lax in pursuing the implementation to completion. There exists an ongoing need for a designated person to continue to interface personally with all system users and monitor the usage and problems involved in the new system. Often, issues will arise which were not anticipated or identified in the phases of requirement analysis. As a new problem is encountered, and a new solution developed, it is imperative that the circumstances be documented and communicated to all system users in similar roles.

Finally, there must be an ongoing post-implementation training program in place. This program should not only be oriented toward new users, but also to the provision of "refresher" courses for existing system users. In the spirit of quality circles, there should also be periodic meetings of systems users to identify and review issues and problems which have arisen and encourage interchange of experience gained through acquired familiarity with the system.

4. Conclusion

Unsuccessful HIS implementation occurs when a health care organization focuses on the technical aspects of an HIS project while ignoring the importance of people, processes and data. Technical training alone does not result in implementation success. When implementing an HIS, we are changing the practices and procedures of our organizations. We must teach people how to handle the change and adapt to the new procedures. If the project leaders and members of implementation team can frame the change in comfortable, easily recognized word, the mysterious new computer system becomes a little easier to understand. Focus on benefits to the health care process and not on the hardware and software that makes it possible.

References

[1] AE. Caldas, Success Factors in the implementation of Patient Care Information Systems. Proceedings: Toward an Electronic Patient Record, 1995, pp. 8-13

[2] YM. Chae *et al.*, Measuring the success of implementation of information system for health center. Medinfo, 1995, (2):1549-52

[3] TH. Devenport, Process Innovation: Reengineering Work Through Information Technology. Boston. Massachusetts: Harvard Business School Press, 1993, pp. 336

[4] A. Harrison, Bussiness Processes: Their Nature and Properties. Examing Bussiness Process Re-engineering, Current Perspectives and Research Directions. Edited by G. Burke and J. Peppard. London: Kogan page Ltd., 1995, pp. 60-69

[5] K. Marek *et al.*, Implementation of a Clinical Information System in Nurse-Managed Care. *Canadian Journal of Nursing Research*, 1998, 30(1):37-44

[6] G. Pare and JJ. Elam, Understanding the Dynamics of Information Technology Implementation: A Study of Clinical Information Systems. Medinfo, 1995, (8):544

[7] GH. Watson, Bussiness Systems Engineering: Managing Breakthrough Changes for Productivity and Profit. New York: John Wiley & Sons, 1994, pp. 287

[8] ST. Young and JS. Chang, Implementation of a Patient-centred and Physician-oriented Healthcare Information System. Medical Informatics, 1997, 22(3): 207-214,

Telemedicine and Telematics

Medical Informatics Europe '99
P. Kokol et al. (Eds.)
IOS Press, 1999

The Community Social Alarm Service as a Primary Health Care Service

Drago Rudel[a,b], Marjan Premik[a], Nina Licer[c]
[a] *University of Ljubljana, Faculty of Medicine, Institute of Social Medicine, Ljubljana*
[b] *MKS Electronic Systems, Ljubljana, Slovenia (drago.rudel@mf.uni-lj.si)*
[c] *Community Social Alarm Centre, Home for Elderly, Ljubljana, Slovenia*

Abstract. The history of calls to the community social alarm centre in Ljubljana and the service subscribers' records were analysed with the aim of finding out how the service helps in emergencies when calls related to health problems are received. The network, being a pilot project in Slovenia, was established in 1992 primarily to offer social services to elderly and disabled people living in their own home environments. The article highlights the role of the network in solving the medical problems of the users of the system. Among the 18,500 calls received in four years at the centre, 395 (2.1%) of them were health-related. An additional 24 emergency calls (0.2%) were received from non-subscribers to the centre using an "ordinary" telephone. Although the absolute number of health-related calls is low, the network plays an important role in preventive primary health care aimed at the observed population groups. The network meets most of the specific technical and organisational requirements for a community health care emergency call system. From a telematic point of view it is important that a telematic device - an emergency call unit - has entered an elderly or disabled person's home and been well accepted.

Keywords: primary health care, elderly, community social alarm, telematics

1. Introduction

Slovenia is a central European country with a population of 2 million and has undergone political, economic and demographic transitions which have accentuated the social and health problems of elderly and disabled people most of all. Although the demographic pointers show a tremendous increase in the number of over-65-year-olds, funds for the preferable institutional care have not been adjusted accordingly. Consequently, non-institutional care, being considered a reasonable and affordable alternative solution, becomes increasingly important, although the government does not regularly support it. Long-term experience in some developed European countries shows that a care network based on telematic applications (e.g. community social alarms) can significantly improve home-based care efficiency in terms of quality, quantity and co-ordination. Permanent help encourages frail people to stay in their environment as long as possible instead of being institutionalised.

The first community social alarm service was introduced in Ljubljana, the capital of Slovenia, in 1992 [1,2]. A combined telephone-alarm unit, the *Lifeline* telephone (*Tunstall Group, Whitley Bridge, Surrey, UK*), is installed at the resident's home and linked to a public telephone network [3,4]. Pressing a button on a small body-worn radio transmitter can activate the unit. This enables two-way hands-free speech communication from a distance of a few metres. The telephones are monitored 24 hours a day by a community social alarm control centre which has full details of each caller, provided by clients when they subscribe to the control centre. These details are automatically displayed as soon as a call is received. Following a call, the control centre staff can send whatever help is needed. On separate telephone lines operators contact service providers and accept phone calls from citizens using an "ordinary telephone".

Social alarm centres are not just an emergency back-up service but also a 24-hour help-line and reassurance service [5]. They manage a database of clients and service providers, and co-ordinate help services. Because they have adequate information on the help needed, control centres can assist in designing comprehensive primary care arrangements at the local level and contribute to the efficiency of primary health care on a nation-wide basis.

The *Lifeline* network represents a telematic application within a social care environment. The application is considered a social innovation in our society. Neither its impact on health care service provision nor its outcome has yet been investigated. It is the aim of this article to highlight the role of the community social alarm network in solving the medical problems of the users of the system.

2. Methods

This study covers:

a) the experimental implementation of telematic technology designed primarily for solving social problems in order to achieve the broader aims of primary health care;
b) a descriptive analysis of:
    - the tasks of the control centre operator
    - the actions and measures of the control centre operator upon receiving an emergency health-related call
    - links to a public emergency health service - ambulance;
c) a quantitative analysis of the user's population group;
d) a quantitative analysis of calls to the control centre.

3. Results

Community social alarm network

The community social alarm service covers an area of 280,000 inhabitants in the capital city and is a pilot application in Slovenia. Over the five-year period there has been a total of 160 users of the community social alarm network linked to the control centre. The number of subscribed clients has been limited to the number of available call units and varies around the 100 mark on average. The units are leased from the centre on a revolving system - a returned unit is passed to the first candidate on a waiting list.

Users

The average age of the subscribed client to the community control centre is 85 years: 20% are over 80 years old and 9% over 90. A total of 88% of them are women. The user-population structure is similar to that in an average residential home in Slovenia. Clients suffer from almost identical health problems to their institutionalised colleagues: 39.9% heart, 7.1% stroke, 6% diabetes, 3.3% locomotion, 2.1% cancer and 41% grouped problems.

Tasks of control centre operator

The operator's tasks could be grouped into:

- consulting - chat, preventive advice (dos and don'ts);
- mediating

- call for medical intervention - doctor on duty contacts the client directly by phone;
- call for ambulance - rescue service;
- call for nursing care service;

• co-ordination - harmonisation of activities performed by different service providers and carers;
• monitoring - service providers, clients (taking pills on time, reminding clients not to forget, reminding them how to use alarm button, etc.).

Actions and measures of control centre operator

When a call is received from a *Lifeline* alarm unit, an operator on duty tries to establish conversation with a caller already recognised by a receiving device. If it is established, the operator asks the caller about his/her requirements or tries to find out the reason(s) for the call. If the operator concludes that medical help might be needed, he/she contacts a medical doctor on duty at a public medical intervention centre by using a separate telephone line. If conversation with the client is not possible, the operator uses the client's computerised record and follows instructions there. They could be also to contact an emergency service immediately. When waiting for an ambulance, the operator stays online to the caller, encouraging and advising him/her until the service (doctor) arrives.

Calls to the control centre

In Table 1 the type and number of calls received by the community control centre from 1992 to Dec 1998 is presented. Calls were made by subscribed clients having *Lifeline* call units and by non-subscribed citizens using an "ordinary telephone".

Table 1: Statistics of calls to the Ljubljana social alarm control centre in 1992-1998.

Calls made by alarm units			Calls made by "ordinary telephones"		
Reason for call	**No. of calls**	**%**	**Reason for call**	**No. of calls**	**%**
info, advice, chat	13.553	51.0	advice, chat	2.135	10.6
technical tests of the operation of the system	8.553	32.2	info on services, service orders	14.302	70.9
emergency	666	2.5	emergency	26	0.1
demonstrations	385	1.5	other	3.706	18.4
positive social control	3.392	12.8			
TOTAL:	**26.549**	**100**	**TOTAL:**	**20.169**	**100**

Links with public emergency health service - ambulance

Medical doctors on duty at the Ljubljana public health emergency centre process an operator's call from the community control centre in the same way as all other requests for their intervention. They appreciate that information on a client, given by the operator, is comprehensive. This is possible as the centre keeps computerised records, which also contains data on the client's health status and current therapy. Such information is helpful to the doctor in making decisions.

4. Discussion

Health problems among elderly and disabled people living alone in their home environments are complex - a holistic approach is required for their efficient solution. The co-ordination of medical, social and other services being part of primary health care in a community is of great importance to them as end-users. In Slovenia, medical and social sectors are separated both administratively and organisationally, which affects primary health care efficiency. New telematic applications like the presented *Lifeline* community alarm network enable co-ordination of medical, social and other services in a community and provide a chance to link those sectors at a local level. Furthermore, they advance solutions related to the co-ordination and harmonisation of activities performed by medical and social workers and a number of informal carers. The network could be considered as an important step towards realisation of political declarations of equity in primary health care.

The *Lifeline* community social alarm system is considered a social innovation in Slovene society [1,2,5]. Although the network is still small in size and is slow in its growth it meets most of the specific technical and organisational requirements which are characteristic of health care emergency call systems. The network was established primarily to offer social services, but its functioning is important for an integrated approach to preventive and curative solutions to primary health care problems targeting elderly and disabled people in their home environments.

The percentage of health-related calls to the community control centre (2.5 %) is low but it indicates the importance of the community alarm system for preventive primary health care. The number of calls is much higher than in countries, which have been using similar telecommunication emergency call systems for decades (e.g. UK). This could be explained primarily by differences between the population groups using the system. Call units in Ljubljana are mostly used by people facing major health problems and by those who have already experienced falls or a heart attack [5]. The average age of our clients is high (85 years old), so the units are implemented more as a curative than a preventive measure what is the case in UK. Statistics shows a decline in number of health-related calls, which may be due to the familiarisation process (between a user and a device). It is encouraging that the control centre has also been alerted by citizens who are not subscribers to the system (0.1 % of calls). An "open telephone line" significantly increases the number of potential users of the network services.

From the telematic point of view it is important that a telematic device such as the *Lifeline* emergency call unit enters the home of an elderly or disabled person. Once there it could be implemented in different ways to increase the resident's independence and safety level. For the user it is important that there is just one simple button to be pressed enabling him/her access to all the various primary health care services organised, monitored and co-ordinated by the community alarm control centre.

These findings impose an obligation on the national health authorities to support the dissemination of the system throughout the country. The application itself enjoys a good reputation among strategic planners but has also triggered some negative intentions e.g. to run a parallel “healthcare network” targeting the same population. The idea should be justified.

References

[1] Rudel, D., Premik, M., Hojnik-Zupanc, I.: Caring Network Based on Community Social Alarm Centres in Slovenia: A Country in Transition, In:MEDINFO' 95 Proc. R.A.Greenes et al. eds, 1995 IMIA, 1503-5.

[2] Premik M, Rudel D. Community Social Alarm Network in Slovenia, Centr.Eur.J Hlth **4**,1996;4:223-5.

[3] Harbert WB. Community Alarms - Improving the Care of Elderly and Handicapped People. In: Proc. 4th Inter.Conf. - SYSTED 1991, Barcelona, 1991.

[4] Robinson B. Lifeline Services - An Industry Still Defending Its Own Identity.Ageing Internat.1991;42-7.

[5] Hojnik-Zupanc I, Licer N, Hlebec V. Community Alarm System as a Social Innovation to the Slovenian Society (in Slovene). Zdrav Var 1996; **35**: 289-94.

[6] Jones D. Health maintenance for the frail elderly. In: Oxford Textbook of Public Health, Second edition, Vol.3 Application in Public Health, Holland W. Detels R.Knox G. eds. Oxford University Press 1991; 107-23.

Medical Informatics Europe '99
P. Kokol et al. (Eds.)
IOS Press, 1999

Psychiatry By Videophone: A Trial Service In North West England

C R May, N T Ellis, T Atkinson, L Gask, F Mair, C Smith
Correspondence: Dr C R May, School of Primary Care, University of Manchester, Rusholme Health Centre, Walmer Street, Manchester, M14 5NP, United Kingdom

Abstract. In this paper we report on the use of a video link between two general practices and a hospital based mental health team in North West England to provide a trial telepsychiatry service for individuals with depression and anxiety related disorders. Patients (n=16) took part in an evaluation of the service by both structured questionnaire and semi-structured interview. The results of the evaluation study suggest that patients may be highly critical of telemedicine systems and that they do so not simply on the grounds of the technical quality of video links, but also because the remote link increases the difficulty that the patient faces in expressing deep seated emotional and existential problems. It is not, therefore, simply a matter of technical quality in the link, but also a question of the quality of interpersonal relations perceived by the patient.

1. Introduction

New technologies for telecommunications apparently offer clinicians an enormous range of opportunities for developing remote doctor-patient interaction [1]. The use of interactive video, especially, seems to promise the possibility that geographical inequalities of service provision and access might be minimised. Certainly there is a growing technical and clinical literature that is founded on this kind of assumption. The promise that new technologies offer in this regard is not new: indeed, clinicians have been working on developing telecommunications-based medicine since the 1870s [2] However, the tremendous advances made in video-conferencing and store-forward data transmission technology in the past two decades have made telemedicine a real and practical possibility.

In this paper we describe some results from an evaluation study of a telepsychiatry service in North West England. Interactive video seems to be uniquely suited to psychiatry, since the latter depends primarily on the doctor seeing and speaking with the patient rather than on an examination of vital signs. The problems that are encountered by medical or surgical specialties—in collecting and transmitting a range of data about the physical state of the patient while simultaneously engaging in verbal interaction are absent from such an encounter [3]. The existing literature on remote doctor-patient interaction in psychiatry is encouraging, since it seems to suggest a high degree of acceptability and efficacy of these consultations in the view of both clinicians and patients [4].

In normal circumstances people with minor mental health problems who need specialist help—for example, with anxiety or depression—are referred by their general practitioner to a mental health team based in a nearby hospital. This may involve the patient in a considerable waiting time, followed by a visit to an outpatient clinic that may be a source of considerable disturbance or anxiety to them. In the present study, patients presenting at two general practitioners' surgeries in North West England which referred to the same mental health team were offered an appointment with a psychiatrist by video link.

2. The Study

2.1 *Service and evaluation methodology*

The project reported provided a trial service by videophone for psychiatric consultations between two general practice surgeries in North West England and their local Mental Health Team. Patients (n= 16) suffering anxiety and depression related disorders (n=6 males, mean age 47; and 10 females, mean age 32) were referred by general practitioners for remote assessment or management by a psychiatrist. One patient did not attend for an initial consult using the system. Subsequently, 10 of these patients used the system for follow up interviews with the psychiatrist. No patient waited more than 7 days to be seen via the videophone link, whereas the normal wait to see a community psychiatric nurse was 12 days, and to see a consultant psychiatrist 26 days. The videophone link was set up in a quiet room away from other public areas of the general practitioners surgery. On arrival the patient was shown to the room and then left alone to speak to the psychiatrist. No member of the surgery staff or evaluation team sat in with the patient. The psychiatrist's videophone link was set up in an office at the mental health team's building some miles away.

Evaluation was conducted using both structured questionnaires and semi-structured interviews. The latter were tape-recorded and transcribed and subsequently subjected to a conventional model of qualitative analysis of natural language data [6]. Appropriate research ethics committee approval was obtained and all patients provided properly informed consent: all patients (n=15) agreed to take part in the evaluation and were interviewed after using the videophone link. All clinicians involved in the provision of psychiatric services to this population were also interviewed.

2.2 *Technical description of the videophone system*

The service reported in this paper was based on two British Telecom VS1 videophone units, connected by standard British Telecom ISDN2 lines. This unit was selected because it was by far the simplest videophone unit available to us, which could be used with a minimum of training by both clinicians and patients alike. It was also highly portable, and this meant it could be moved between sites without specialist technical support and assistance. In these respects, the VS1 was superior to existing PC based systems, which while much cheaper were less portable and more demanding of specialist technical support. It also had the advantage of being very obviously a telephone with a video screen, rather than a computer with a video-camera attached: this, we felt, had certain advantages when offering a service to people with mental health problems, who were already highly anxious. The videophone also has the advantage of being difficult to interfere with its configuration. There is no keyboard that might accidentally or deliberately be interfered with by users. Even so, the VS1 unit used in conjunction with ISDN2 poses a number of problems. It has a relatively slow and jumpy picture, and the picture quality itself is often poor. It emphasises both frame tension (uncertainty about who is outside the field of vision defined by the LCD display); and gaze disjunction (neither participant in the exchange actually makes eye contact because they are observing each other on screen, rather than looking directly at the video camera). These have been established as key problems in doctor-patient interaction by interactive video [5]. During the life of the trial service it was intended that the videophone service should be available for 75.5 hours. In fact, nine hours were lost because of user error or service withdrawal.

3. Responses To The Video Link

Patients who used the videophone link seemed to express a degree of satisfaction with the service they received. The system was certainly acceptable to them. The advantage of qualitative research techniques, in this context, however, is that it is possible to develop a picture of patients' experiences in some depth. In this context two kinds of technical objection to the videophone link emerged. The first of these related to the way in which the videophone itself affected the conduct of interactions.

> "There was a time lapse I noticed, which I found disconcerting sometimes—because you both want to say something and then you both stop—you don't know who's going to carry on, so you wait for a time lapse, [but] I got used to that..."

In this context the delay that arises from a relatively low speed connection affected the conduct of *verbal* interaction. Both clinician and patient found themselves speaking at the same time and initially it was difficult for both to engage in a fluid conversation. The important implication of this for the psychiatrist was that it was difficult to develop a picture of how the patient verbalised their feelings and problems. But it also meant that the psychiatrist had to adjust his consultation style to fit the technology rather than the patient.

> "Because of the gap and the pause, you have to be just a little bit ahead of the game. So if you want to interrupt somebody, you have to time it a little bit different."

The second kind of objection that patients offered to the videophone link was one which relates to the problems that are involved in using a relatively poor quality picture. Neither patient nor clinician could necessarily *see* the other with the degree of detail that they regarded as necessary.

> "The thing that came over to me was that you don't sort of interact in a face to face way because it's difficult to pick up expression, facial expressions—as to whether he [the psychiatrist] was pleased with what he was saying, or whether he understood what I meant."

But these objections came together in a more fundamental way. Indeed, we might see them more usefully not as criticisms of the technology itself, but rather as indicators of a troubling interactional problem for the patient using such a system. The patients who used the videophone link had to find a way to convey some deeper aspect of their *self* through it to the doctor. It was apparent that their difficulties in doing this were the source of their dissatisfaction.

> "It was very difficult to show emotion, hear or see emotion, obviously, on the screen. So you tended to hold back a little bit that way...."

Or, in another case:

> "You feel stupid. You feel like you're talking to yourself really. I felt just like I was talking to the telly."

Patients who used this system were not, of course, simply trying to convey a set of neutral facts about their condition to the psychiatrist. They were also trying to convey some sense of the character of their lives, and the *emotional reality* of their circumstances to him. In this sense, they were following a wider pattern of learned behaviours that circulate in our society about how to convey the experience of illness to the doctor [7]. Anxiety and depression are, at one level, experiences of highly extended and abnormal emotion. In therapeutic terms, the psychiatrist then faced the problem of how to deal with these extended emotions in a context in which he was both physically, and emotionally, remote. For example:

> "I think, what has been difficult for those people who have found it difficult is that they [did so] because they seemed to be aroused and anxious. When you are with someone face to face for an hour, most people settle by the end of the hour, they would feel more relaxed—I would be able to help them feel more relaxed. But on occasion it has been difficult in these conditions."

This was not simply a matter of helping the patient to 'relax' into a technological 'fix'. It had important therapeutic implications because much of the verbal doctor-patient interaction in psychiatry is not simply about establishing the nature of the patient's disorder, but developing interactional strategies to ameliorate and mitigate this.

> "But I think.... What has been clear to me is that when, in a case of addressing people's problems using say, for example, behavioural techniques for anxiety problems, I would normally run through with them the principles of behavioural techniques and demonstrate some techniques to them, that's actually quite difficult when you are not face to face."

The critical points that both patients and clinicians made about the videophone system are important in understanding the limitations of such a system in clinical practice at a time when proponents of telemedicine are pressing for greater investment in remote service provision [8]. However, it is important to also note that for some patients, this system seemed to pose relatively greater perceived benefits. Some patients found it 'far easier to tell him things I wanted to say'— in one case precisely *because* the patient could not see the doctor's facial expression clearly. One patient in particular, who was dealing with a crisis of sexual identity amongst other things, was glad of the distance that was inherent in the system.

4. Conclusion

Much debate about telemedicine has assumed that once the question of the technical standard of data transmission is resolved, then consultations will follow in a form that replicates that of the normative face-to-face consultation [9]. In part, this may be because evaluation studies have employed one-dimensional measures of acceptability and utility. This study suggests that patients' and clinicians' perceptions of the acceptability of telemedicine systems are the product of a range of factors that are not necessarily amenable to such measures. In particular, we have noted that criticisms of the technological quality of telemedicine systems may mask a more fundamental problem: that the quality of human interaction that is maintained through a video link may not be sufficient to achieve a genuinely therapeutic result.

Acknowledgements

We thank both the patients and the clinicians who took part in this project for their time and candour. We are grateful to colleagues in the NW Telemedicine Evaluation Consortium, notably Dr Aneez Esmail, Professor Martin Roland and Professor Christopher Griffiths for their helpful comments on the design of this study. We also thank Allison Burgess for her secretarial support throughout the study. This study was funded by the NHSE NW Region R&D Directorate, whose support is gratefully acknowledged.

References

[1] Wootton, R. Telemedicine in the National Health Service *JRSM.* 1998: V91:12 pp614-621
[2] Reiser, SJ. *Medicine and the Reign of Technology.* Cambridge, Cambridge University Press (1978).
[3] Mair F, Whitten P, May C, Doolittle G. Patient perceptions and satisfaction with a telemedicine specialty clinic: results from a qualitative study. *Telemedicine and Telecare* submitted
[4] McLaren P. et al An Evaluation of the Use of Interactive Television in an Acute Psychiatric Service *Journal of Telemedicine and Telecare* 1995 4: 2 pp 79-85
[5] Mair F, Whitten P, Allen A. Interpersonal and organisational issues in telemedicine. *Health and Social Care in the Community* 1997; 5: 55-59
[6] May C. The preparation and analysis of qualitative data. In Roe B and Webb C (eds) *Research and Development in Clinical Nursing Practice* London, Whurr (1998)
[7] Good BG. *Medicine, Rationality and Experience: An Anthropological Perspective* London, Cambridge University Press (1994)
[8] NHSE. *Information for health: an information strategy for the modern NHS 1998-2005.* London, NHSE. 1998
[9] Harrison R.M. Clayton W. Wallace P. Is there a role for telemedicine in an urban environment? *Journal of Telemedicine and Telecare* 1997 pp15-17

Medical Informatics Europe '99
P. Kokol et al. (Eds.)
IOS Press, 1999

Telepathology and Imaging Spectroscopy as a New Modality in Histopathology

Sandor G. VARI, MD
VariMed, Szalanci u 5, H-1124 Budapest XII, Hungary
Gerhard MÜLLER Dr. h.c. Dr.-Ing
Laser-und Medizin Technologie, gGmbH, Berlin, Krahmerstr 6-10, 12207Berlin Germany
Jeremy M. LERNER
LightForm Inc. 601 Route 206, Suite 26-479, Belle Meade New Jersey 08502, USA
Rolf-Dieter NABER
Tritech GmbH, Hubert-Netzer-Weg 2/1, 88316 Isny im Allgäu, Germany

Abstract. Telemedicine started in the late 1950's by transmitting data on patients' pulse and heart rates. In the 1980's it expanded to radiology and orthopedics. The technology is now expanding to other specialties that can digitally gather patient data. Telepathology comprises the transmission of microscopic images via telecommunication network. Image compression and multiplexing technologies enabled high-resolution telepathology as well as real-time video consultations over international telephone lines. Organ transplantation has become a viable treatment and offers new life to an increasing number of patients suffering from chronic end stage diseases and from irreversible organ failure. Rejection is still a major problem in kidney, liver, and heart transplantation. To gain further insight into the complex interactions within the components of the immune system, it has become increasingly necessary to develop rapid and simple methods to monitor the status of the immune system in patients. Clinical signs suggest organ rejection and abnormal laboratory test results, but only histological signs on biopsy specimens are adequately specific. The financial cost of organ transplant makes it imperative to develop tools for the early identification and treatment of organ rejection. An increasingly sensitive and accurate way of localizing key structures and abnormalities is through spectroscopy of either H&E stained samples or with a fluorescent tag (fluorophore) or by relying on natural fluorescence. The system is based on a unique Prism and Mirror Imaging Spectroscopy System ("PARISS ™"), spectrometer originally designed and implemented for remote Earth monitoring from space and aircraft and astronomical imaging spectroscopy. Compact and lightweight both the mirror and prism are presently constructed in inexpensive glass but can also be injection molded in plastic. Any number of vendors anywhere in the world can produce all parts of the assembly. This greatly enhances the chances of future commercial viability. The Interactive Histopathology Consultation Network INTERPATH (PL961121) project integrated of remote control imaging microscopy system, imaging spectroscopy, and communication networks called SPECTROMIC. This telepethology unit will be a useful tool in the Regional and International Integrated Telemedicine Network for Medical Assistance in End Stage Diseases and Organ Transplant, RETRANSPLANT HC 4028 (HC) & IN 4028 (HC).

1. Introduction

Quality improvement and standardization of diagnosis in histopathology and cytology are important for the future of the discipline. Nominal scale diagnoses dominate the practice and their standardization depends on relevant and reproducibly identifiable criteria as well as on communication of these among pathologists. Telepathology, i.e. the transmission of adequately detailed color images of microscopic fields over the telephone network is now a realistic possibility [1,2]. Telecommunication links available inexpensive worldwide in the form of the public telephone net, with the restriction of a limited channel capacity. The restrictions imposed by the application of the telephone net (preferentially the ISDN service) are investigated by Schwarzmann et al and strategies outlined to overcome these restrictions [3,4]. Working at the microscope in the framework of the pathology laboratory daily routine was thus improved for quality of decision-making, management of medical information [1].

Multi-spectral imaging (MSI), developed by NASA for planetary probes and remote sensing, has recently come into wide use for earth studies. It is used for oceanography, geology, climatology and environmental studies. It is also used commercially, with applications in agriculture, process control and graphics. All of these applications rely upon the unique combination of imaging and spectral analysis that MSI supplies. Although most of the digital imaging techniques developed for monochrome microscopy work well with color images, there are a few considerations specific to the analysis of multispectral imagery. The method consists of the determination of spectral characteristics of different elements of interest. These include obtaining a properly balanced multicolor digital image, specifying the color components of the image, and multispectral imaging yields functional maps, showing *what* and *where* biological molecules are located within a structure. Histopathologists recognize the need for more accurate, automated data analysis to enable better decision making. The use of the Prism and Mirror Imaging Spectroscopy System ("PARISS ™"), as an imaging spectrograph will go a long way to adding the extra degrees of freedom necessary for complete spectral object identification. The workstation of the pathologist in the year 2000 could be the combination of a microscope, a HD-TV-camera, imaging spectroscopy and a personal computer.

2. Materials and Methods

The telepathology imaging spectroscopy (TISP) system will add a new feature to the integrated microscopy workstation. The system consists of at least two main parts:

The PARISS spectrograph is based on an imaging spectrometer originally designed for Remote Earth Monitoring and Astronomy and is currently in use for both applications in military and civilian environments. The original spectrograph was patented

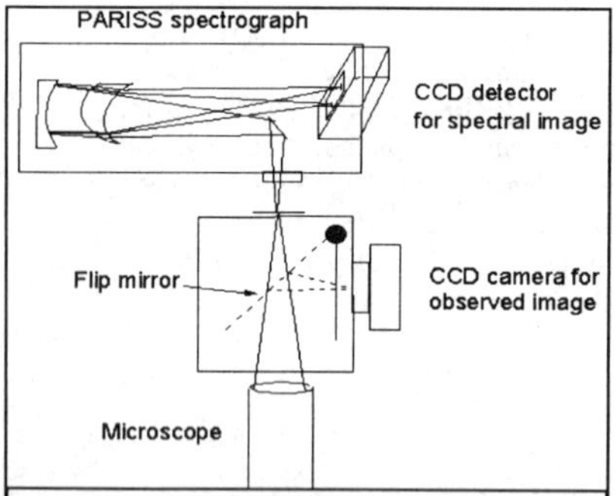

Figure 1. Schematic of PARISS Imaging Spectrometer

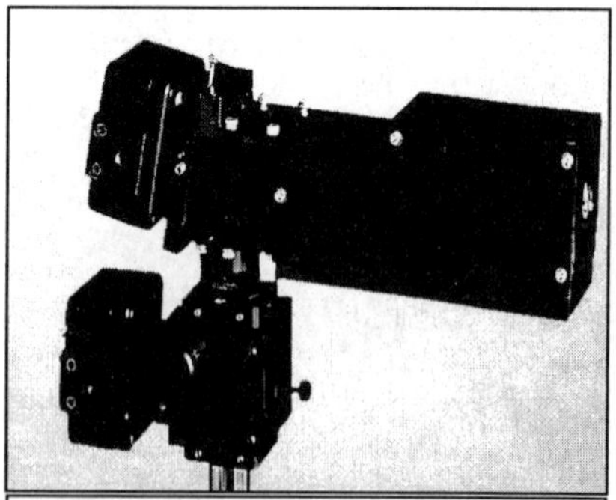

Figure 2. PARISS mounted on an epi-fluorescence microscope

by The Aerospace Corporation (TAC) for use in the infrared from 3 to 15μm. LightForm acquired the rights to the patent and redesigned the optics for use from 360 to 800nm. The acronym "PARISS" is derived from "Prism and Mirror Imaging Spectroscopy System". It was the goal of the investigators to demonstrate that the device, with an origin in a military environment, could be of value in the life sciences. The system works by accepting an image projected by a microscope that presents a particular field containing "objects" onto the entrance slit of the PARISS spectrometer. A slice of image passes through the slit and strikes the first curved surface of the prism, is refracted, strikes the second surface, and exits to strike the spherical mirror. The light then returns through the prism to be focused onto the CCD matrix array, wavelength dispersed (see ***Figure 1***). Over 80% to 90% of all light, over the entire wavelength range, is transmitted through the system. The system uses a prism made of inexpensive flint glass, as illustrated in ***Figure 1 & 2***, but the support and body of the unit will be in either cast aluminum, or ribbed metal plate for enhanced rigidity. The optical system was fully ray-traced and performance was found to meet or exceed expectations. ***Figure 2*** shows the finished PARISS assembly on a microscope. The system generates spectrally and spatially resolved topographical maps of histopathology samples and will recognize natural fluorescence of a formalin fixed H&E stained tissue sample, a frozen sample, immunofluorescence of immunoglobulin deposits that have been fluorescence tagged of allografts with manifesting organ rejection. The PARISS spectrograph receives light projected by the microscope objective onto its entrance slit. The spectrum is wavelength dispersed onto a CCD detector. The data is sent to a trained Hybrid Neural Network (HNN) that automatically classifies each object in terms of characteristic spectral features (CSF) and paints the results in false colours to a computer screen superimposed onto a white light image. The HNN provides the intelligence to automate the processing of these multi-spectral images (MIS) and performs non-linear transformations providing the sophisticated deconvolution and correlation routines needed to handle real-life-convoluted samples.

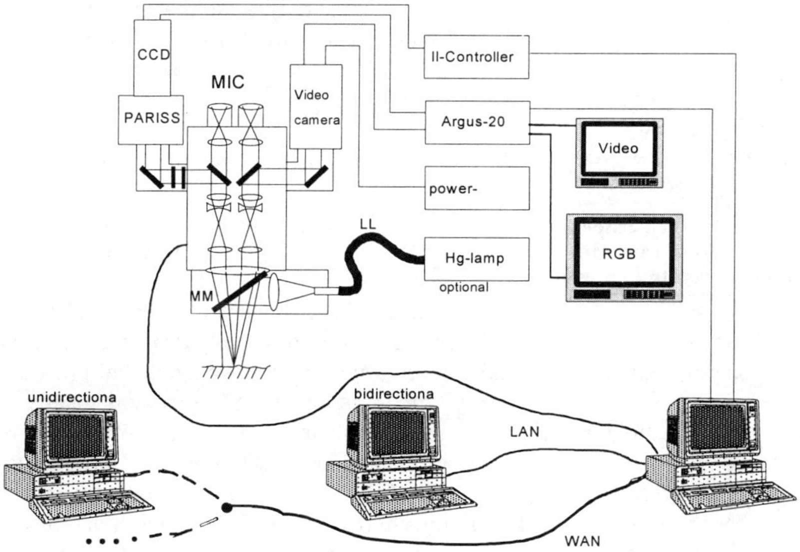

Figure 3: Technical setup of the TELEPATH microscope workstation. MIC = microscope, LAN = local area network based on optical fiber system, WAN = wide area network based on ISDN telecommunication network, LL = liquid light guide (if necessary), MM = movable diachronic mirror, MCP = multi channel plate

For the local area network preferable to use an optical fiber network with Novell multi-user software connected to a bare fiber-AUI converter and an Ethernet AUI Interface. So on this way a high-speed data transfer achievable, and in the other direction, a remote control of the microscope workstation could be performed. In ***Figure 3*** a wide area network demonstrated. A high speed active ISDN PC-card embedded in a special mailbox software delivers a fast image transfer to a workstation in a foreign country.

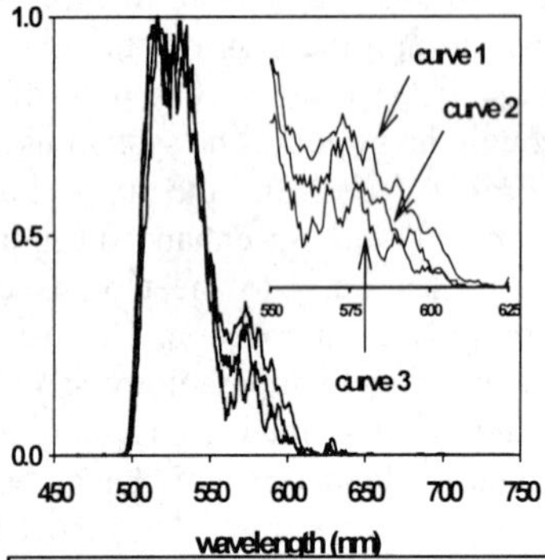

Figure 4: Comparison of spectral features, immunofluorescence stained for IgA, IgG and IgM.

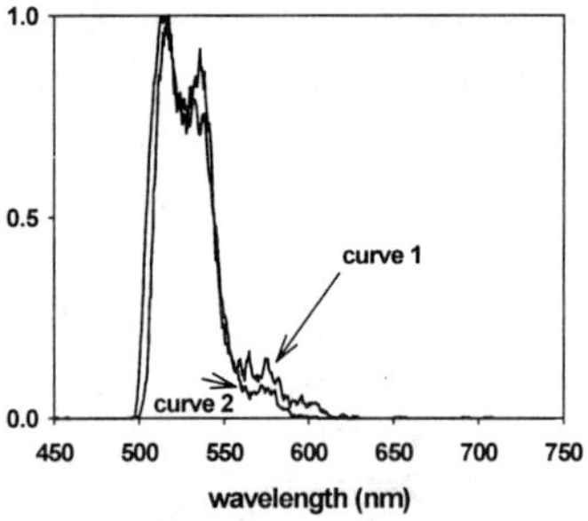

Figure 5: Comparison of spectra from transplant biopsies negative for humoral

3. Results of Kidney and Heart Biopsies

System operating parameters

The microscope objective: 40X. Entrance slit to the spectrometer: 50 µm. Average acquisition time of spectra: 9 Sec. Average acquisition time of Observed image:1 Sec. Number of objects per acquisition: 240. Size of each object: 0.5 µm by 2.5 µm. Spectral range per acquisition: 400 to 800nm. Number of Renal disease patients: 7. Number of repeat tests per slide: 6. The excitation wavelength was 405nm and spectra were acquired through a long pass filter that allowed all light of greater than 470nm to pass, and blocked the excitation wavelength and all wavelengths shorter than 470nm.

Figure 4 shows clear differentiation between the spectra of immunofluorescence staining for IgA, IgM and IgG in the spectral region from 550nm to 650nm. Curve 1: Patient with chronic diabetic nephropathy and glomerulosclerosis. Stained for IgA.

Curve 2: Patient with chronic diabetic nephropathy and glomerulosclerosis. Stained for IgG.

Curve 3: Patient with chronic diabetic nephropathy and glomerulosclerosis. Stained for IgM.

In the heart transplant Non-rejection pathology is frequently seen post transplant to include ischemia or catacholamine effects, interstitial fibrosis, myocardial calcification, and cyclosporine-associated endocardial infiltrates called the Quilty effect. It is therefore very important to be able to automatically diagnose evidence of immunosuppressive disorders even if there is no evidence of cellular rejection. The International Society of Heart Transplantation (ISHT) provides criteria to enable grading of heart rejection ranging from Grade 0 to +4. ***Figure 5*** shows two spectra from two patients, both negative for humoral rejection with an ISHT Grade 0 and also negative for Quilty effect. Both were of right ventricular septal endocardial biopsies of heart transplant patients. The slides were stained with FITC conjugated antisera to immunoglobulins, the third component of complement and fibrinogen. Both spectra are fundamentally the same. Curve 1: Negative Quilty effect, negative rejection, ISHT Grade 0. Curve 2: Negative Quilty effect, negative rejection, ISHT Grade 0. This example provides a good indication that spectra are consistent between patients with similar findings. Identification and differentiation between patients with and without the Quilty effect.

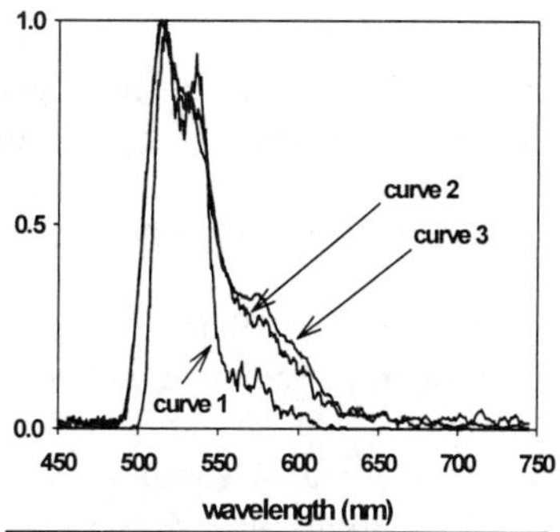

Figure 6: Comparison of transplant biopsies with and without Quilty effects.

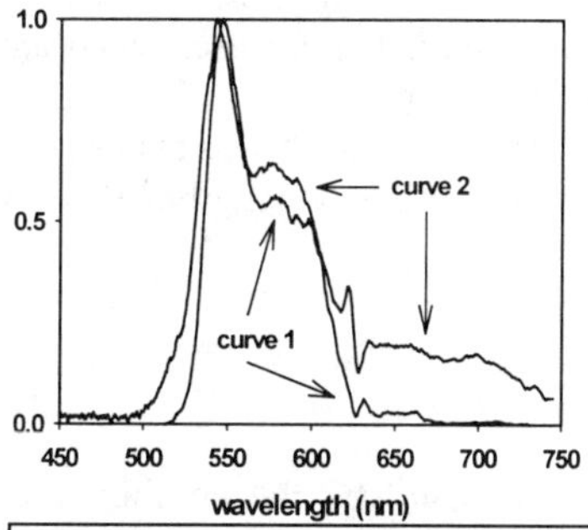

Figure 7: Comparison of spectra from normal aorta wall and aorta showing degeneration.

Figure 6 shows that the spectra for patients with the Quilty effect, curves 2 and 3, are very similar, even though one is negative and the other positive for rejection. Both are different from the spectrum of the patient negative for both rejection and Quilty effect. This is a good example of how the fluorescent spectral envelope can change as a function of cellular condition and would not be detected with single filter observation. Curve 1: Negative Quilty effect, negative rejection, ISHT Grade 0. Curve 2: Positive Quilty effect, negative rejection, ISHT Grade 0. Curve 3: Positive Quilty effect, positive for cellular rejection, ISHT Grade 1A.

Figure 7 shows Marfan's Syndrome: aorta stained with Hematoxylin and Eosin (H&E). The samples were examined under the epi-fluorescent microscope excited at 436nm. There was a strong blue-green fluorescence. The spectral features shown in Figure 7 clearly differentiate between a normal aorta wall and an aorta showing degeneration. Curve 1: Normal aorta wall. Curve 2: Degenerating aorta wall.

4. Neural Network development

During the initial part of the project there was insufficient data to train a Supervised Neural Network. It was therefore decided to implement an Unsupervised Neural Network that was designed to self-train on subtle differences between spectral signatures. This approach proved highly successful. The Windows 95 platform caused many memory management problems that reduced the number of spectral objects that could be processed simultaneously from 240 to about 100. These issues will be resolved with the possibility either of changing the existing code to Windows NT or converting to LabVIEW code written for the Windows NT environment. Pathologists are used to viewing slides through a microscope with excellent optics. They observe high resolution images with a large field of view. The Phase I camera was a low cost 8-bit black and white model with 177K pixels made by Electrim Corporation of Princeton, NJ. Although this camera was very effective, it is also low resolution. Future PARISS systems will be equipped with a higher resolution (higher pixel density) color CCD manufactured by Eastman Kodak Corporation. We believe that many pathologists and researchers will consider the improved resolution and performance to be worth the additional cost.

5. Discussion

The use of image transmission in pathology - telepathology - is applied mainly three purposes:

1. To enable rapid diagnosis of frozen sections prepared by technician in a operating theater lacking present of expert pathologist, using spectroscopic imaging method integrated into a remote imaging microscope.
2. To establish on-line consultation with experts throughout Europe, on difficult and rare cases of histopathology / cytopathology.
3. To join the European telecommunication systems via Euro-ISDN connection in order to ensure more tasks, as diagnostic standardization, quality assurance and education programs.

In general the results were most encouraging even with low signal strength. It would appear that the technique is robust. There were strong indications that it is possible to differentiate between acute and chronic renal transplant rejection and differentiate cyclosporine toxicity. It appears that the wavelength range from 550 to 650nm shows the greatest change as a function of abnormality. This is evident in Figures 4 through 7. A comparison of Figures 4 and 5 clearly shows that there are differences in the shape of the spectral envelope depending on the target feature. Even though fluroresceinated antisera specific to IgA, IgM or IgG all are usually observed by eye with the same filter set, the PARISS system reveals that the total envelopes of each are different. It was also shown that the presence of the Quilty effect and cyclosporine toxicity also have a tangible effect on the spectral envelope emitted by the stained organ.

6. Conclusion

The workstation of the pathologist in the year 2000 could be the combination of a microscope, a HD-TV-camera, elector-optics for imaging spectroscopy and a personal computer with many software's allowing treatment and transmission of numerous pictures. Archival immunofluorescence-stained renal and heart transplant samples were investigated and weak fluorescence acquired. The slide specimens under study had already been subject to fluorescence investigation and many samples were already substantially photo-bleached. In spite of this, spectral acquisitions were surprisingly sensitive given the weak signals. In the Countries of Central and Eastern Europe (CEEC), an integrated network would significantly reduce the cost of histopathology and record management. For small hospitals with limited availability of local pathology services and for hospitals with a deficiency of specialists, telepathology may be a worthwhile substitute. The system can be expanded to include interactive audiovisual technology in continuing medical education and training, to video conferencing.

References

[1] **Brugal** G, IMPACT, Integrating Microscopy for Pathology Activities and Computer Technology. New Communications Age, M.F. Laires et al. (Eds.) IOS Press, 304-312, 1995.

[2] **Busch** C. Department of Pathology, Telepathology in Sweden. A national study including all histopathology and cytology laboratories. Zentralblatt fur Pathologie. 138(6):429-30, 1992 Dec.

[3] **Kayser** K. Drlicek M. Rahn W. Department of Pathology, Thoraxklinik, Heidelberg, Germany. Aids of telepathology in intra-operative histomorphological tumor diagnosis and classification. In Vivo. 7(4):395-8, 1993.

[4] **Schwarzmann** P. Telemicroscopy. Design considerations for a key tool in telepathology. Zentralblatt fur Pathologie. 138(6):383-7, 1992.

Transtelephonic ECG in Slovenia

Vojka Gorjup, MD; Anja Jazbec, MD; Borut Geršak, MD, PhD
Clinical Center Ljubljana, Zaloska 7, 1525 Ljubljana, Slovenia

Abstract. Transtelephonic ECG has been introduced in Slovenia in 1996. It has been operating on a regular basis since September 1997. Users of the system are health institutions and patients with CV diseases. They use portable 12- channel ECG weighing less then 200 grams. Diagnostic center is located in medical ICU in Clinical Center Ljubljana. In the first 20 months of regular operation we have received 852 calls, 450 of them being diagnostic. The most common reasons for calling were: ischaemic chest pain, atypical chest pain, palpitations and dyspnoea. Most common diagnoses made on the basis of history and ECG were: AMI, angina pectoris, paroxysmal tachycardias and atypical chest pain. In 186 cases the cardiologist's advice sufficed, 171 patients were reffered to the ER, 142 immediately and 29 only if suggested therapy hadn't been successful. To 82 patients new medication or chenged dosage of previous medication was suggested. With the intent to evaluate accuracy of the diagnoses made on the basis of history and transtelephonic ECG evaluation we followed up the patients who were sent to ER in Ljubljana upon our cardiologists' advice. On the basis of preliminary results we can conclude that TTE is as diagnostic as the conventional ECG and its' use shortens time from onset of symptoms to initiation of treatment, it lowers disability and mortality due to CV diseases and improves cost benefit.

1. Introduction

Transtelephonic ECG (TTE) has been introduced in the USA in the late sixties. In Slovenia TTE began to operate on the regular basis in spring 1997. It is our first step into one of the youngest branches of medicine – telemedicine. Our TTE system is divided into two large groups called Telelink and Mobilink. Patients with cardiovascular (CV) diseases and different health institutions like emergency outpatient clinics, old age homes and health resorts use Telelink. Mobilink includes people at high risk for CV diseases. ECG is recorded by a portable device [2,3,4] weighing 180 g, measuring 120 x 60 x 25 mm. It is world's first all - 12 – channel ECG. There is also special type of ECG device, which operates on a principle of a Holter monitor; it can memorize 30 sec before and 30 sec after the event. To record an ECG three self-adhesive electrodes are needed. They are connected with a device, which is placed in three different positions on patient's chest. It takes about one minute to record an ECG. Upon joining the system a user is instructed how to record an ECG, he or she is assigned an ID number and a reference ECG is recorded and stored in the computer. In a period without symptoms every user has an opportunity to send test ECGs. With that we try to limit sending of low quality recordings. In a Diagnostic center, located in medical ICU of Clinical Center Ljubljana, a nurse answers a call and stores a recording in the computer. Cardiologist then takes history, evaluates ECG and immediately gives advice to the patient. Diagnostic center has 24 – hours coverage with nurses and cardiologists.

2. Methods

It is a retrospective study of twenty months experience with TTE in Slovenia.

3. Results

In the period between September 1, 1997 and April 30, 1999 we received 852 calls. Out of that 450 were diagnostic (sent because of different symptoms), 223 of low quality and 179 reference and test ECGs.

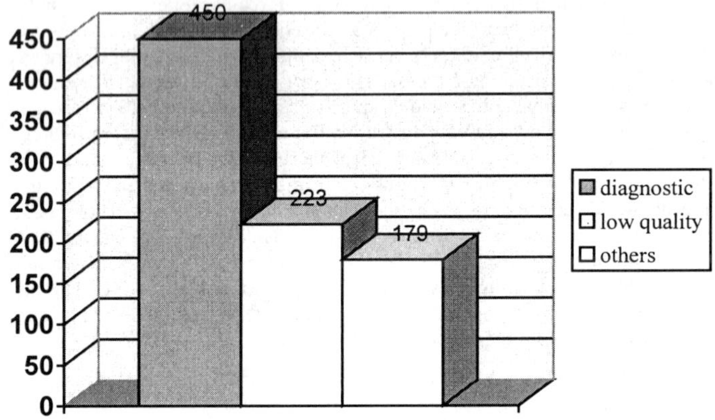

Figure 1. Call types: diagnostic – ECGs sent because of different symptoms; low quality – technical quality too low for evaluation; others – reference ECGs and tests

Private users sent 218 and health institutions 634 recordings.

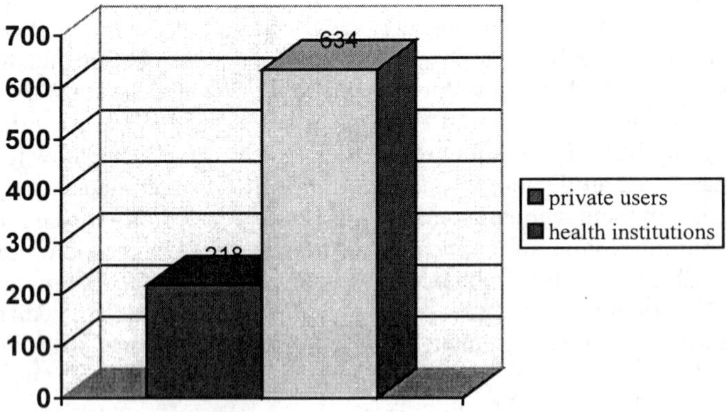

Figure 2. ECGs according to the sender: private users; health institutions.

Reasons for sending diagnostic ECGs were: ischaemic chest pain (32%), atypical chest pain (20%), palpitations (12%), dyspnoe (8%), syndrome GMAS and its equivalents (1%). 27% of ECGs were sent for other reasons.

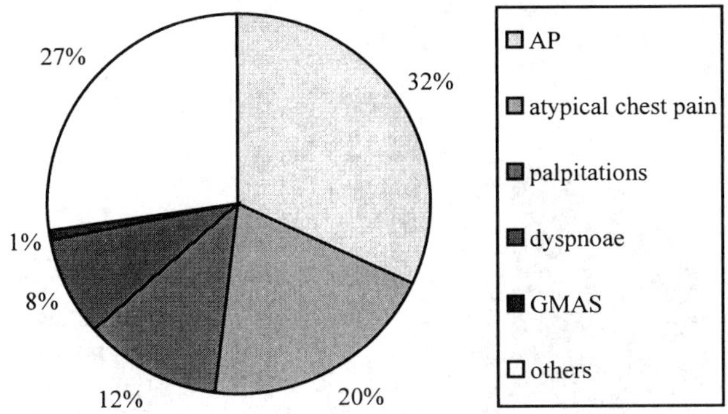

Figure 3: Reasons for sending ECGs: AP – angina pectoris, atypical chest pain – nonischaemic pain, palpitations, dyspnoea, GMAS – syndrome GMAS and its equivalents, others.

On the base of patient's history and ECG 25 acute myocardial infarctions, 131 anginas, 35 paroxysmal tachycardias, 4 GMAS syndromes and 2 pericarditides were diagnosed. 88 patients had unischaemic chest pain. The rest had less relevant diagnoses.

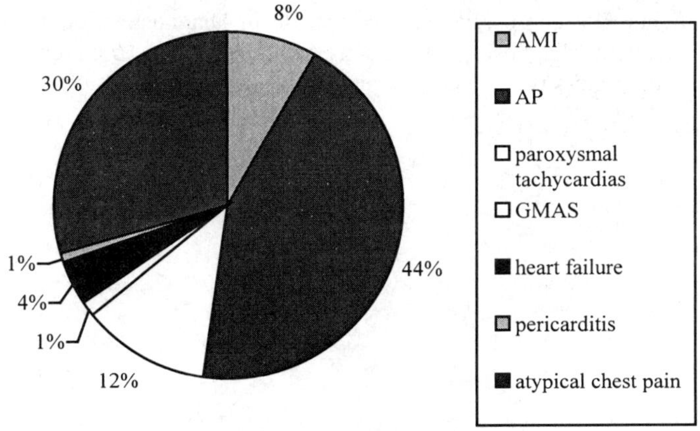

Figure 4: Most frequent diagnoses made on the basis of patient's history and ECG evaluation: AMI – acute myocardial infarction, AP – angina pectoris, paroxysmal tachycardias, GMAS – syndrome GMAS and its equivalents, heart failure, pericarditis, atypical chest pain.

In 184 cases only advice sufficed and changes in persisting medication or new medication was suggested to 82 patients. 171 patients were sent to ER, 142 immediately and 29 only if suggested therapy hadn't been successful. In two cases cardiologist guided general practitioner (GP) through CPR.

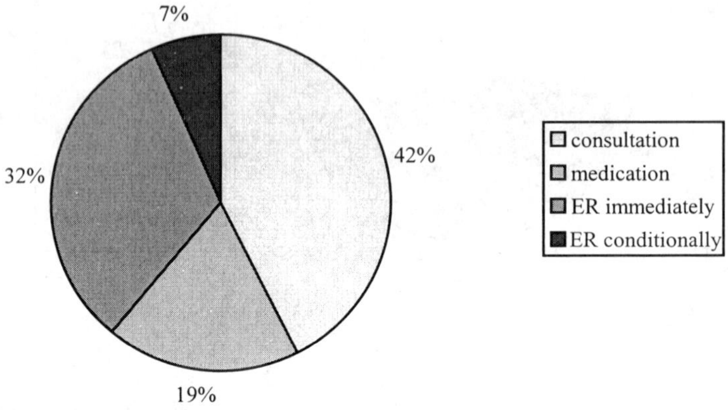

Figure 5. Doctors' measures: consultation – consultation only, medication – changed dosage of old medication or new medication advised, ER immediately – patient immediately referred to ER, ER conditionally – patient referred to ER only if suggested medication hadn't been successful, CPR – help in cardiopulmonary resuscitation.

To estimate the accuracy of the system we followed up the patients who were sent to ERs all over Slovenia. In twenty months there was 172 of these patients. We successfully followed up 66 patients. We compared diagnoses made in Diagnostic Center with those made in ERs. In 50 patients diagnoses were exactly the same and in 16 patients they were different. Severity of the illness was never underestimated.

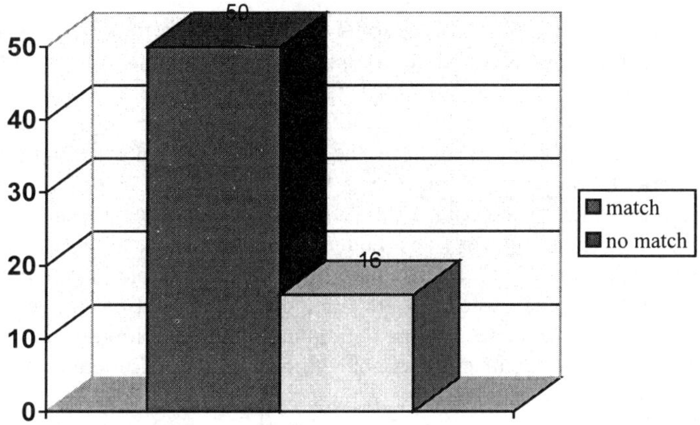

Figure 6. Diagnose matching

4. Discussion

Out of all 852 recordings 223 were of too low quality to be evaluated. The main reasons for that were low quality telephone lines on which we have no influence and unskilled senders. That indicates the need for better education of system users. We had no problems in receiving the ECGs. Personnel answering the calls are skilled enough and cardiologists were always available. In the beginning call reports were sometimes incomplete.

A significant majority of ECGs was sent from old age homes and emergency outpatients' clinics. In these cases TTE served as important help to GPs who are less skilled in ECG interpretation. GPs also had immediate opportunity to consult a specialist. Two most frequent reasons for sending diagnostic ECGs were chest pain and palpitations. These are also the most frequent reasons for patients to come to medical ERs in our country. In 6.5% of patients potentially life-threatening conditions (acute myocardial infarction, syndrome GMAS) were diagnosed. We can assume that these patients arrived to the ERs sooner, which shortened the time from onset of symptoms to treatment. They were also better monitored during the transportation than the others were. CV diseases are the main reason for mortality in Slovenia (7903 deaths in 1996, all deaths 18620). As the time to treatment is crucial for outcome we can conclude that an immediate consultation with a specialist and a quick correct diagnosis can lower mortality from CV diseases. In 3% of patients paroxysmal tachycardias were seen in ECGs most of them atrial fibrillations. With the use of TTE these patients more likely arrived to cardiologist within 48 hours, so the need for long-term anticoagulation was avoided. Almost two fifths of sent ECGs were normal. Most of these patients only got advice so they didn't need to visit the doctor. This certainly unburdens ERs.

5. Conclusions

Comparing to the rest of the world [1] our system has been operating for a relatively short period of time so our conclusions are made on small number of calls. In spite of that we think that TTE is as accurate as conventional one [4]. The most important achievement is shortening of time from onset of symptoms to the adequate treatment. This is of most importance in urgent cases such as acute coronary syndrome and rhythm disturbances. In countries where TTE is more widespread it replaced frequent visits of cardiologist following the implantation of a pacemaker [5]. In Slovenia we expect that to happen in the near future. One of the advances brought by the system is also unburdening the ERs as to a great deal of patients only advice suffices. With our future work we will get more information about prevalence and course of CV diseases in Slovene population. We will try to prove that use of TTE can improve cost benefit in treating patients with CV diseases and we would like to make it affordable to as many people as possible. Transmission of ECG signal through cellular phone system offers immediate consultation between cardiologist and a GP on a house call. Information technology and developing on line computer communication between medical staff is one of the main assignments of World Health Organization for the next millenium.

References

[1] Gonzalez-Espino JF, Nolasco RR, Miranda JAA et al. La electrocardiografia transtelefonica en Mexico. Reporte de los primeros 3434 casos. Arch Inst Cardiol Mex 1995; 65: 207-15.

[2] Roth A, Bloch Y, Villa Y, Schlesinger Z, Laniado S, Kaplinsky E. The CB-12L: A new device for transtelephonic transmission of a 12-lead electrocardiogram. Pacing Clin Electrophisiol 1997; 20: 2243-7.

[3] Reifart N, Weil HJ, Goehring S, Dietl J. Verlaesslichkeit eines neuen 12-kanal-EKG mit telefonischer Uebertragung. Dtsch Med Wochenschr 1997; 122: 1137-40.

[4] Bernard P, Chaitman BR, Scholl JM, Val PG, Chabot M. Comparative diagnostic performance of the Telemed computer ECG program. J Electrocardiol 1983; 16: 97-103.

[5] Weber H, Kiss H, Joskowitz G, Pfundner P, et al. Wertigkeit der EKG-Telefon-Telemetrie in der Erfassung symptomatischer Herzrhythmus-Stoerungen. Klin Wochenschr 1984; 62: 689-97.

Southern Health Board – Advanced Telematic / Telemedicine in Healthcare Services in the South West of Ireland

Ms. U.M. O'Sullivan, *IT/EU Projects Manager, Southern Health Board, Wilton Road, Cork, Ireland*
Mr. Jack Somers, *Management Services Officer, Southern Health Board, Wilton Road, Cork, Ireland*

Abstract. The Southern Health Board has been involved in Telematic Healthcare services for the past number of years. Our involvement in a number of EU funded projects has given us extensive experience and expertise in this area. The primary focus of our telematic applications is optimising health services delivery with a particular emphasis towards people who are isolated due to social and physical boundaries and limitations.

Our main projects are:-

NIVEMES (Network of Integrated Vertical Medical Services) includes the exchange of medical information between urban centres and isolated communities including those at sea, rural, elderly and disabled persons.

RISE (Remote Information Services for the Elderly) focuses on the enhanced healthcare services of the elderly and disabled through the use of telemedical applications.

HEALTHLINE To strengthen the successful outcome of Telehealth implementation by specific projects in the EU by providing the expert Training and Information dissemination services to providers, beneficiaries and the general public, using the Telehealth systems and infrastructure applied by those projects

KATE (Killarney & Telecom Éireann) the SHB in conjunction with the Information Age Town Project in Killarney are working towards benefiting the local community through the innovative use of Information and Communication Technologies.

TASTE (Technology Assessment in Telemedicine) An EU funded trans-national initiative aimed at developing a methodology for assessing medical technology, particularly in the area of Neurosurgery.

FECV (Forward Emergency Control Vehicle) An European Space Agency project through which we are developing an advance communications vehicle for major emergence/event management through Satellite linkage to SHB systems.

The increasing cost of the delivery of healthcare is a major concern for all governments within the EU. The spiraling cost of the hospital sector is a common policy problem and one of the difficulties of effecting major change. Almost every country in Europe is struggling to reshape its hospital services, particularly in the large cities where medical science has far outreached hospital buildings that are inappropriate, inefficient or in the wrong location.

The hospital networks of the future will have fewer beds than those of today, as lengths of hospital stay reduce and ambulatory surgery increases. The big breakthroughs in diseases like cancer will only happen if governments can draw together the many threads that make up their health services and encourage them to work together.Over the next decade, we believe that a small number of European centres will emerge as pre-eminent in these highly specialised fields and as a consequence attract patients from across the community as well as professionals for training. The quality of healthcare and equity of access remains a huge challenge in all countries. Quality varies enormously. Clinical audit systems are developing well and they will throw light on poor or inadequate performance.

How Information Technology and Telecommunications respond to these challenges will play a significant role in achieving the new models of healthcare required. In the hospital hence the increasing development of digital information and media for diagnostic and therapeutic care has led to increasing demands for systems that can store and manage this information. This is a considerable advance on the existing traditional Hospital Information Systems.

Through a number of Projects both EU funded and of our own initiative the Southern Health Board is addressing these challenges. We have been involved in Telematic Healthcare services for the past number of years. The primary focus of our telematic applications is optimising health services delivery with a particular emphasis towards people who are isolated due to social and physical boundaries and limitations.

1. Description of the Irish Environment

The Southern Health Board area of healthcare responsibility is the South West Region of Ireland incorporating the counties of Cork and Kerry. With an overall population of 546,400 in the region, it is perhaps the most varied of areas encompassing populous urban areas such as Cork City with approximately 250,000 citizens, average size towns of population 5,000 to 15,000, small rural villages and islands with residents of between 50 and 300 people.

The area is a major tourist attraction due to the scenic farmlands and river valleys which contrast with the wild sandstone hills of the south west, and above all there is the magnificent coastline scooped and fretted by the Atlantic into great bays and secret coves strewn with rocky headlands. These aesthetic delights are in themselves some of the contributory factors to the isolation of some of the population of the region. The Ring of Kerry for example is unequalled as a place of great beauty and the hair-raising cliff edge roads add to its mystic. However it is not appreciated when the journey is a medical emergency or a trip for neo-foetal monitoring in the middle of winter.

Provision of Acute Hospital care in the region is based at two primary centres, Cork University Hospital a high-tech Class One Trauma Centre and Tralee General Hospital where we have Regional Specialist Services, supported by two smaller general Hospitals at Bantry and Mallow. There is also a network of 21 Community Hospitals which provide locally based health support services to the community.

Of the 546,400 citizens in the region, the majority of the population are entitled by virtue of Government Tax deductions from wages to subsidised healthcare and a smaller number have private medical insurance. In the region 183,000 people are entitled to free medical care due to age, health or economic circumstances. These people are assigned to a local GP for primary care and a capitation fee is paid to the GP under the National General Medical

Payments System. This category of patient forms a General Medical System [GMS] panel at the GP Surgery.

Attendance at hospital clinics are by appointment and usually the patients have to travel from the remote rural areas to the central hospitals for specialised diagnositc services such as X-Ray, Ultrasound and dermatological assessment. Accident and emergencies are dealt with by the A&E departments at the hospitals with patients being transferred by air or land ambulance services. In more remote locations initial assistance is given to the patient by locally based General Practitioners [GPs] or Public Health Nurses [PHNs]. Examples of this are outlined further in this chapter.

Developments through NIVEMES of GP linkages, HIS integration and the continuing development of medical device interfaces, have presented opportunities to complement and expand emerging technologies and to translate these technologies into achievable service initiatives. For example, the use of the electronic patient record and the integration of medical devices have led to the development of Virtual Patient Clinics focussed on the elderly in the succeeding and complementary project (RISE) . Amongst many tangibles in relation to services, the NIVEMES project has developed a number of added value aspects to the System. In particular the facility to Electronically 'Tag' messages ensures greater security of the confidential patient record. Clear identification of Sender, Recipient, etc., gives accountable audibility of the transaction.

Prior to this, when x-rays or ultrasound images were physically posted between sites, once the film left the remote site it was dependent on providence and goodwill in almost equal measure to arrive at its intended destination. Prior to the advent of NIVEMES the only reliable way to have the x-ray diagnostically evaluated at the central hospital was to send the patient to that central hospital for their x-ray in the first place. Through the use of NIVEMES System this unreliable method is no longer necessary and the efficiency leads not only to cost savings [far fewer repeat events due to misplaced film] but also to more timely diagnosis, immediate integration of the event into the patients record and far less inconvenience to the patient as a person.

The NIVEMES System is also an important improvement at a time when the International Shipping Industry is rapid adopting new standards and technologies for communication between ships and shore e.g. GMDSS. Extending the scope of NIVEMES services is in line with increased flexibility demands, and will most certainly provide for the long-term survival of marine and island communications systems like NIVEMES that are based on the use of digital equipment.

2. Caherciveen Community Hospital

Located 2 hours from Cork and 1 hour from Tralee, Caherciveen Community Hospital is the first hospital built specifically as a community Telemedicine mode. Therefore NIVEMES in particular, and other Telemedicine and ICT initiatives had a particularly important role to play in its establishment and development and are integral to its sustainability. The main user group of this hospital are the elderly but the availability of Telematics e.g. Transmittable Ultra Sounds and X-Rays at local level will be of benefit to the local population as a whole [8731 (1530 aged 65+)].

Prior to the launch of Telemedical Services at the purpose built unit in Caherciveen Community Hospital, people had to travel to Tralee for routine X-rays, post-operative monitoring, ECGs, ultra sounds in addition to general specialist clinics.

For example Neo-foetal monitoring could only be done at Tralee General Hospital [40 miles away over mountainous terrain], a deterring journey for 'mothers to be', X-rays meant a trip over the same terrain and then a comparatively long wait for results. In fact on the day of the Official Opening an ambulance arrived at the hospital to take two elderly patients to Tralee General Hospital for X-rays and was told that they were not needed as the patients, both in their 70s, had been X-rayed in Caherviveen. The hospital has a high nationwide profile as it is situated in the constituency of the Irish Minister for Justice, Equality and Law Reform John O'Donoghue T.D.

3. KATE

KATE (Killarney & Telecom Éireann) the SHB in conjunction with the Information Age Town Project in Killarney are working towards benefiting the local community through the innovative use of Information and Communication echnologies. The synergy created by the RISE and KATE Projects has resulted in the establishment at Killarney of the first Virtual Out Patient Clinic. We are making Killarney a Virtual Co-ordination Centre (V.C.C.). This will enable the provision of seamless, co-ordinated, shared healthcare and community services for everybody living in the Killarney district using modern Information & Communication Technologies (ICTs).

Through these ICTs we plan to introduce at Southern Health Board sites and at strategic publicly accessible points e.g. Cyber Café, facilities for Tele-Access to the Board's services. We envisage that the bulk of this traffic will be local but provision will also be made for transfer of the caller to more definitive services available only at Tralee or Cork. As technology develops these initial tele-services may be upgraded to multi-media services.

Another innovative area using ICTs is the integration of General Practitioners (GPs) into the Southern Health Board system. This provides for easier booking of clinic appointments, tests etc., and the more efficient dissemination of patients' results back to their local GP.

The V.C.C. is being augmented by the implementation of Ireland's first 'Virtual Out-patient Centre for the Elderly', where elderly people in Killarney are able to 'virtually attend' specialist clinics in Tralee and Cork whilst still physically in Killarney. In essence this will bring specialist care to Killarney instead of people always having to travel to Cork and Tralee.

During the development use is being made of ICT Services and equipment such as multi-media, health telematics, smart cards, alarm systems and portable computers for the provision of an integrated suite of services including:-

- Telemedicine
- Homecare Support
- Teleservices such as Entertainment, Human Communication and Special Interest Groups support.

4. FECV – Forward Emergency Control Vehicle

In April 1982, in a report advocating the use of satellite communications in emergencies, Jerry FREIBAUM of NASA Headquarters stated, "The unpredictability of locations and time of need mandates that the communications system must be able to operate anywhere at any time. Similarly, because human survival and property damage are directly affected by response time, high degrees of mobility, reliability and availability must be inherent to the system. This equates to a requirement to operate despite breakdowns of terrestrial systems due to weather, explosions and saturated 'phone systems".

The FECV is specifically designed to meet the needs of "high degrees of mobility, reliability and availability" in a way that is "affordable" in all economies. In particular, it addresses the demands for rapid deployment and intervention in the "Golden Hour"; the first 60 minutes of any major emergency/disaster in which medical treatment is most critical to the preservation of life and limb. The design of the FECV results from the Southern Health Board's own extensive experience of major emergency and disaster management and its own initial familiarisation with both the supply and demand sides of the market for such vehicles. Similar vehicles currently available are mostly designed for military use and are, therefore, too expensive, too large and too sophisticated for most healthcare and other relevant organisations. In contrast, the FECV combines an optimum level of technological sophistication with low cost. The FECV is also significant in its integration of terrestrial and satellite communications. This combination enables the establishment of communications immediately upon arrival on-site and before SatComs can be established. Thus, maximum advantage is taken of the Golden Hour.

5. Training

To successfully implement all of the above, in addition to non-telematic changes in work patterns and processes, we had to undertake a major training initiative. The challenges that telematic applications presented in terms of Training had to be recognised and addressed. An essential aspect of finding the optimum training plan was taking account of the opinion of those who are trained and their managers. The comprehensive and detailed Software Manual is suitable only for indepth application training over an extended period of time or for use as reference material in a non-emergency situation. Given that the majority of End-users are located at remote sites or on board ship the training for these persons had to be equally remotely accessible. It must also be remembered that these personnel, who in the majority are neither medically or IT qualified, will most likely be using the systems 'under pressure' in a stressful emergency situation.

To address this problem with alternative training delivery mechanisms, we needed to develop an approach to 'remote training'. This remote training can be used to supplement an existing channel (e.g. providing "real person" question and answer support to compliment a CBT application) or as a stand-alone alternative. In some cases a complete introduction to ICTs was necessary such as basic PC use.Training in the actual use of some some of the devices or their adaptations for use with telematic systems also had to be organised, planned and delivered. It was necessary to consider not only the initial contact training but also the on-going support which the user will require over the longer term. This will apply not only to difficulties which may arise and to software developments but also in the event of additional devices being integrated into the systems.

The telematic system however is more than Software. Its real strength and usefulness is in the range of services it facilitates, aimed at a number of target groups such as Hospitals, Insurance Organisations, Maritime Industry e.t.c. All these users need to be instructed on the best possible way of running the services, in order to acquire not only a cost efficient installation but also the best possible management of the system.

6. Conclusion

The changing demographics of the population in Europe with an ever increasing elderly population will present new and difficult challenges to healthcare providers. The requirement to maintain and support the elderly in their own communities is critical to the provision of these services. The important questions of equity of access will also pose major questions for governments. The social policy of supporting rural development cannot be taken in isolation from the provision of healthcare services.

It is clear that one of the newest and most innovative mechanisms in support of new models of healthcare delivery is Telemedicine. Apart from the important aspect of medical care delivery which has been demonstrated in telematic projects, the development of systems based on digital acquisition of medical data will play a key role in the move towards the measurement of clinical outcomes and evidence based medicine.

The constantly evolving I.C.T. area is presenting the system designers with new affordable technologies. The liberalisation of the Telecommunications Industries have compressed distances and time. The opening of gateways to globally accepted and standardised E-mail systems will mean great savings and added flexibility for telehealth systems.

Now that, through telematic R&D projects, such those we've just skimmed through, telemedicine has matured in effectiveness and efficiency with concrete medical impact, it is important and timely to ask whether telemedicine may have a role in developing countries.

Developing countries face particular problems in the provision of medical services, which relate to the lack of capital, facilities and systems. Roads and transportation are inadequate and difficulties in transporting patients are often encountered. For countries with limited medical expertise or resources, telecommunications can provide a solution to some of these problems. The continued development of telematic systems as a compressed global network for text and multimedia communication has the potential to influence and shape new models of healthcare delivery globally and we for one [sic] can't wait to be part of it.

Or visit our website www.shb.ie

Medical Informatics Europe '99
P. Kokol et al. (Eds.)
IOS Press, 1999

Using IP-videoconferencing systems in a Surgery Consulting

Nina HALÍN* and Pekka LOULA*, Pekka JAATINEN**, Pertti AARNIO***
**Tampere University of Technology, Pori*
Science Park 3 (P.O. Box 30) FIN-28601 Pori, FINLAND
***Noormarkku, Health Care Center, FIN-29600, Noormarkku, FINLAND*
****Satakunta Central Hospital, FIN-28100, Pori, FINLAND*

Abstract. In this paper we describe how to use IP-videoconferencing systems in medical surgery consulting. We started to think about how we could use special doctor's services without patients having to travel a long way. The answer to this question is that the information goes from one place to another, not the patient. First we had a pilot project, where we used the 3xISDN transmission rate and now we are using ATM. We have here in Satakunta a local area network between our Satakunta Central Hospital and the Health Care Center in Noormarkku and Kankaanpää, so we have very good environment to do this kind of research. Our network is quite fast, we can use the 10 Mbps bitrate and in this network there are no other activities in this moment, so there are not any interferences. There is a surgery specialist in the hospital and a doctor in the health care center with a patient. The specialist looks at the monitor, where there is a videopicture of the patient from the health care center. Then the specialist makes the treatment plan for the patient.

1. Introduction

Telemedical practical research have been done by The Health Informatics Center of Excellence in Satakunta (HC-ICE). In this consortium there are three different parties. They are Satakunta's healthcare department, Pori School of Technology and Economics and Pori Telephone Company. The aim of the project is to develop telemedicine services for health care centers [1]. Telemedicine services include teleradiology[2], telepathology, tele-endoscopy and teleultrasound medical examinations and laboratory-medical referral-opinion.

The development of those activities which support the use of information technology in health care is important for the project. The project will be implemented in co-operation with other information network projects in order to find synergy between them. We have four medical projects. These are surgery consultation services to health care centers, evaluation of radiology services [3], citizens' and experts' information services using various transfer media and web based clinical information sending- and storing server service. This paper treats the surgery consultation service for health care centers.

In the first surgery consulting pilot project we used ISDN *(Integrated Services Digital Network)*-video conferencing systems. The outcome of the pilot project was that the end users, doctors and patients were very satisfied with the technical reliability of the system [4]. We utilized Picture Tel videoconferencing systems with document cameras. In this project we had 50 surgery patients from two health care centers. The surgery specialist was in the Satakunta Central Hospital and the Health Care Center doctors were with the patients in the health care centers.

Because we got good results from the first project and Pori Telephone Company built a fast and modern local area network, we decided to test surgery consulting by IP-based videoconferencing systems. With this pilot we wanted to find a good, low-priced desktop videoconferencing system which is also easy to use. With this kind of system we can give the same expert services to all patients in spite of were they live and in which hospital the specialist works.

2. Methods

The ISDN-conferencing systems and services use the H.320 standard that enables transmission speeds 384 kbps. This speed is enough to get a good quality picture, but these systems for clinical use are quite expensive. And these new desktop videoconferencing systems that utilize TCP/IP - protocol are less costly but require high bandwidth. This standard H.323 enables transmission speeds of up to 768 kbit/s. Videoconferencing is highly valued because it enables businesses of all kinds to conduct diversified, visual communication over distances that otherwise could only be bridged by time-consuming travel.

In this project we used the virtual local area network, that Pori Telephone Company has built. This local area network is a secure private virtual network. The 10 Mbps transmission rate is used between the hospital and the health care center. At this moment there are no other activities in this network, so there are no interferences. The connection between the partners are based on PVCs (*Permanent Virtual Connection*) and the information rate varies from 2 Mbps to 10 Mbps. The protocol used is TCP/IP and the LANs are connected virtually. In figure 1 we represent our consulting technical setup and the architecture of the IP (*Internet Protocol*) over ATM *(Asynchronous Transfer Mode)* area network in Satakunta.

For both Satakunta Central Hospital and the Health Care Center in Noormarkku the desktop videoconferencing system is provided by Sony Trinicom. This videoconferencing system contains a videoconferencing card, a small colour videocamera with microphone and datasoftware for the program and it uses the TCP/IP-protocol.

In this surgery project we had 50 patients. The surgeon was in Satakunta Hospital and the patients were with an other doctor in the Health Care Center of Noormarkku. The surgeon saw the picture of the patient on the PC screen. The general picture was shown with the smaller camera, which was placed over the monitor.

The document camera (EV-450 AF PAL) was used to look at the patient from further off. The document camera contained a good zoom lens, a base light possibility, and a possibility to turn the camera. It was good also, when the patient was on the examination table and the surgeon wanted to get an exact picture. We also showed paper documents and X-ray pictures with the document camera.

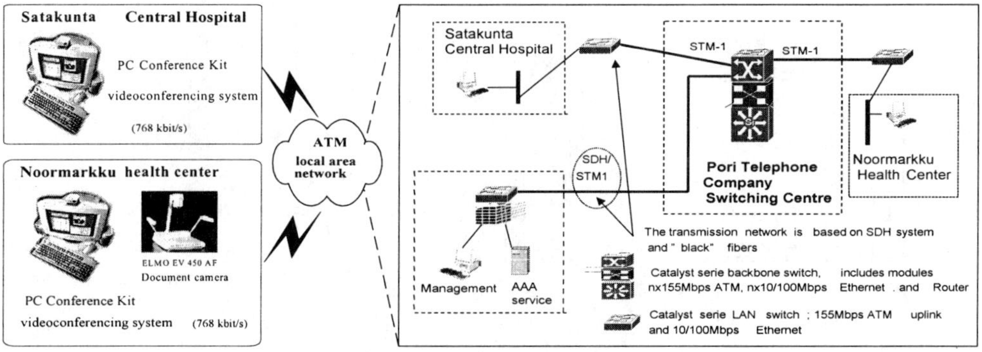

Figure 1. Technical setup

3. Results

In the surgical consultations the doctor in the health care center interviewed and examined the patient in front of the videocamera, as the surgeon watched the PC-monitor in Satakunta Central Hospital. The study material consisted of 50 surgical patients. 23 of them were men and 27 of them were women. The men were aged between 12 and 80 and the women were aged between 15 and 90. The data was collected from questionnaires filled out by the doctors and the patients.

Figures two and three we represent the average answers five technical questions, such as "How well could you present your problems in teleconsultation compared with a visit to the doctor?" Figure two shows that the patients' opinion of the technical suitability of the teleconsultation was superior in 21 % and good in 54 % of the cases. Figure three shows that the doctors' opinions were that in 65 % of the cases the technical suitability of the teleconsultation was superior and in 29 % it was good.

Figure four shows the average answers to the questions regarding satisfaction and reliability. For example " The treatment plans made in teleconsultation were as reliable as if they had been made in hospital". Forty-four out of 50 patients (60 % completely agreed and 28 % agreed) thought that the decisions concerning their problems were as reliable as in face-to-face contact and only three % of the patients thought that the decisions might have been unreliable and two patients didn't say their opinion. Figure five shows the average of the doctors' opinions of satisfaction with teleconsultation. In 75 % of cases the health care center doctor thought that the teleconsultation was very reliable compared with a visit to the outpatient clinic at the hospital, and in 22 % of the cases satisfactorily reliable.

Then we presented the patients with different kind of statements dealing with how much the technique disturbed the consulting, such as " The technique got so much attention, that my problems were in secondary place". 59 % of the patients thought that it didn't disturb at all and 19 % thought that it maybe disturbed a little. A few patients thought that the technique disturbed the consulting too much. This is shown in figure six. The doctors thought that the technique didn't disturb the consulting in none of the cases. These doctors' opinions are represented in figure seven.

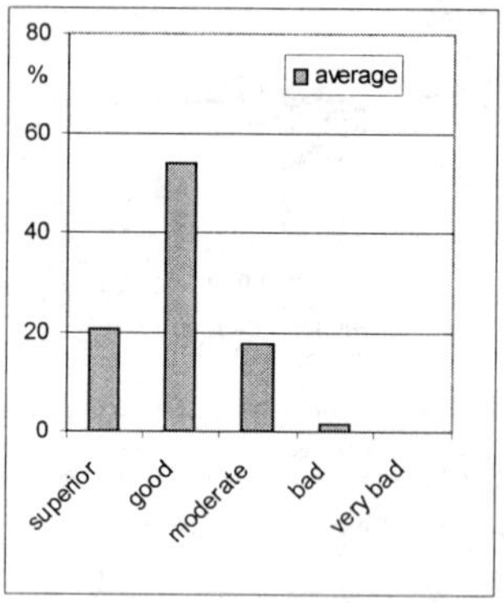

Figure 2. The patients' opinions of technical suitability of the teleconsultation

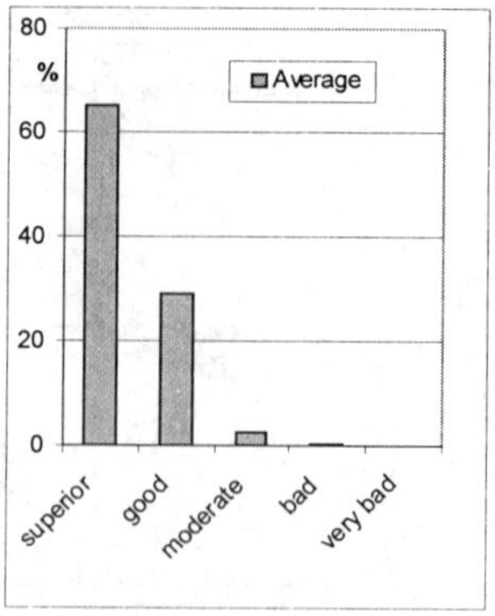

Figure 3. The doctors' opinions of the technical suitability of teleconsultation

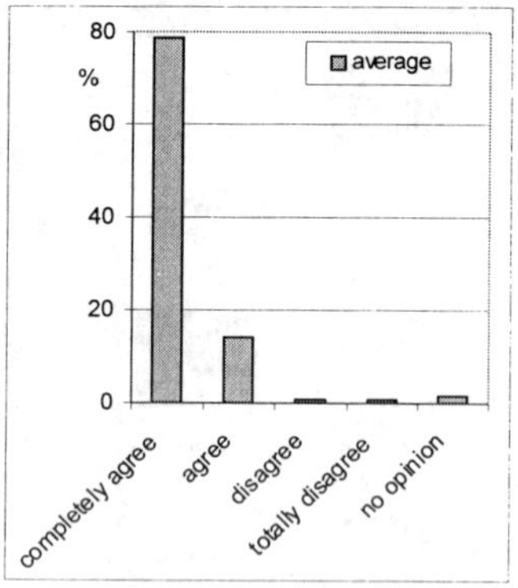

Figure 4. The patients' satisfaction regarding teleconsultation

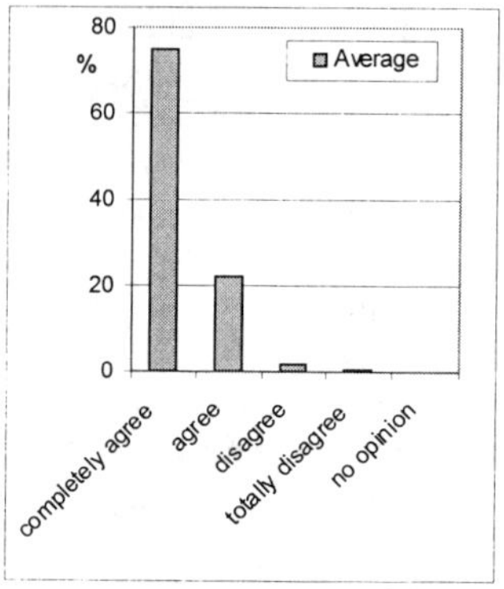

Figure 5. The doctors' satisfaction regarding teleconsultation

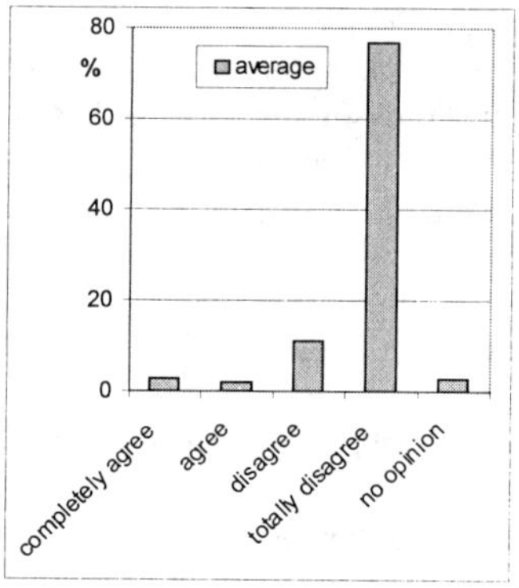

Figure 6. The patients' thoughts the disturbing aspects of the technique

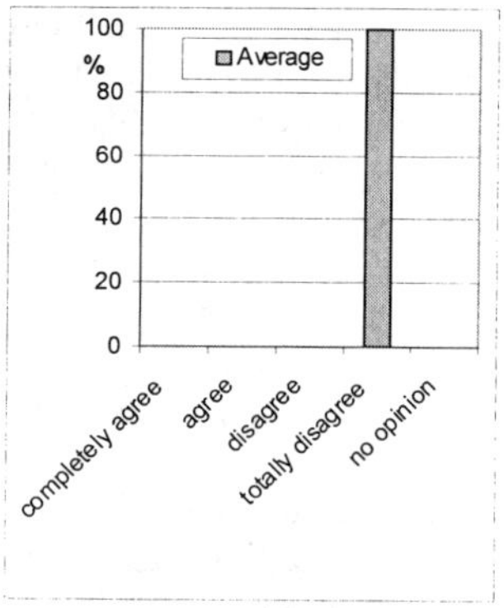

Figure 7. The doctors thoughts of the disturbing aspects of the technique

4. Discussion

First we had some problems with sound. We used in the first instance the microphone of the small camera. If the patient and the doctor were far away from the camera, the doctors and the patients didn't hear each other well. We also had problems with the sound, if more than one person talked at the same time. We resolved this problem using the callport. The callport is a machine which includes loudspeakers and microphone in the same device. With the callport we got a good sound quality. But it is quite an expensive way to do it. We have to study if it is possible to reach the same quality with using a soundcard and a cheaper microphone. We have tested some but we haven't found a good system yet.

Another thing which we have to test, is to make a videoconferencing between H.320 and H.323 systems using a gateway. We have to learn if these different systems are negotiating with each other. If they do, there are more possibilities to extend videoconsulting to many other health care centers. And of course we have to study how the multipoint videoconsulting suits the medical consulting.

Technically the videoconferencing system functioned reliably, and the quality of the video picture was good. Nearly all patients would have been saved from travelling to a face-to-face appointment, because they got a detiled treatment plan during the videoconsultation. The doctors were satisfied with the reliability of the medical treatment plans in teleconsultation.

We can conclude that surgical consultations are reliable in a teleconferencing system, and that the patients were satisfied with the new method.

References

[1] Loula P., Jaakkola H., Rantanen P. Re-engineering of the public health care services - using telemedicine application. The proceeding of PICMET'97. Portland, Oregon - USA, 27-31.7.1997, pp 755-759

[2] Loula P., Rauhala E., Erkinjuntti M., Räty E., Hirvonen K., Häkkinen V. Distributed clinical neurophysiology. Journal of Telemedicine and telecare, 1997; 3: 89-95

[3] Lamminen H., Nevalainen J., Alho A., Lindholm T.S., Tallroth K., Lepistö J. Experimental telemedicine in orthopedics. Journal of Telemedicine and Telecare 1996;2; 170-173

[4] Aarnio P. Surgical consultations with a teleconferencing system, Wootton R. (ed.) European Telemedicine 1998/99. Kensington Publication , pp 97-98

Medical Informatics Europe '99
P. Kokol et al. (Eds.)
IOS Press, 1999

Teleconsultation for Endoscopic Diagnosis of Gastrointestinal Diseases - Concepts and Architecture of the Service ENDOTEL

Thomas Balbach[1], Helmut Sußmann[1], Thorsten Jansen[1], Hans-Dieter Allescher[2], Alexander Horsch[1]
[1] *Institut für Medizinische Statistik und Epidemiologie*
[2] *II. Medizinische Klinik*
Klinikum rechts der Isar der Technischen Universität München
Ismaninger Str. 22, 81675 München
Email: balbach@imse.med.tu-muenchen.de

Abstract. This paper introduces ENDOTEL as a new project in telemedicine, aiming to reduce local disadvantages in medical health care in rural areas. The progressing specialization in medicine results in a concentration of experts in few medical centers and to deficits of expert knowledge in rural areas, which remain as a domain of unspecialized physicians. ENDOTEL expands the conventional synchronous telemedical communication, which usually means videoconference, by an asynchronous multimedia communication and its resulting advantages. ENDOTEL breaks up with the need that participants have to be present simultaneously.

1. Introduction

1.1 Sponsor and long-term targets

ENDOTEL is one of several projects within the program BAYERN-ONLINE II, a telecommunication initiative of the Bavarian state government, Germany, in cooperation with the European Community, whose target is the acceleration and expansion of the application of modern telecommunication methods in Bavaria. Within this program ENDOTEL serves to promote rural areas by intensifying the use of telecommunication technologies in medicine. ENDOTEL aims to reduce location disadvantages in health care in these regions and to achieve a closer binding to the centers of dense medical development. ENDOTEL is scheduled for a period of two years starting in January 1999.

1.2 Today's situation

In rural areas there is, in common, a lack of medical experts which are concentrated in medical centers. The patient often gets examined by an unspecialized physician. In case of an ambiguous diagnosis the patient has to be sent to an expert in a medical center for further diagnosis and, depending on the results, for adequate treatment. This transportation means inconvenience for the patient, costs for the medical care system and in most cases a repeated examination by the expert. Finally the whole procedure of patient transportation and repeated examination may have been unnecessary if the expert could have been consulted before.

Up to now, before sending a patient to a specialist, the physician consults this specialist by phone to explain his current findings, discuss them and ask for a second opinion. As a specialist in a medical center is busy in clinical workflow and not sitting at a hotline, he may be on ward, doing an examination or an operation, not being able or having time to respond to the phonecall of his colleague. So either several phone calls are necessary to contact the specialist directly or a third person gets involved to act as intermediary with a loss of information. This situation is unsatisfying especially in case of endoscopy, where no videos or hardcopies can be exchanged at the phone to discuss them. These media can only be sent by mail. The specialist hasn't got all information to make a diagnosis and decide about further examinations and the treatment, so he must see the patient for himself and in general examinations already done are repeated.

1.3 Reasons and benefits

In consideration of the difficulties mentioned above ENDOTEL can simplify the interaction between physician and specialist within the field of gastroenterology. ENDOTEL will offer synchronous and asynchronous communication with easy exchange of written text, pictures, videos and sound. By means of asynchronous communication participants can work independent on a case. The specialist can be provided with all information needed to decide whether a transportation to his clinic is necessary. In case of a synchronous communication via videoconference a consulted specialist can directly influence an ongoing examination.

Therefore many transports of patients from rural areas to medical centers can be avoided meaning less inconvenience for the patient, less costs for the medical care system and saving of time for all participants [1]. With ENDOTEL there will be less unnecessary examinations for the patient. Generally rural areas will be promoted by means of location independent access to medical competence, cooperation between physicians and specialists will be strengthened and the transfer of medical knowledge from centers to periphery intensified. The service can easily be extended to other domains like e.g. neurology or dermatology where diagnosis is based on medical imaging.

2. Architecture

2.1 Participants and responsibilities

The participants in the ENDOTEL project are not only specialists in medical centers and physicians in rural areas, but also intermediate small clinics of the appropriate counties.

- Department of Medical Statistics of the Technical University of Munich
- II. Medical Clinic of the Technical University of Munich
- Telecenter Telehaus Stamsried
- Three Hospitals and nine doctor's offices.

2.2 Design and technologies

The ENDOTEL project will be implemented as an online service and has a client/server architecture. The server at the telecenter in Stamsried consists of two subsystems, an Apache WWW server and an Oracle database server. The server is connected through a 2 Mbit/s network to the Technical University of Munich. The WWW clients of the participating hospitals and physicians have a 128 Kbit/s ISDN connection, except the hospital of Cham, which is connected through a 2 Mbit/s network with the server.

2.3 Services offered

- Teleconsulting and telediagnostic service - Target 1 is the clarification of difficult cases before briefing or transfer of patients and thus to avoid multiple investigations and transport costs as well as inconvenience for the patients.
- Endoscopic information system (EIS) - Target 2 is the supply of general accessible and constantly updated therapy standards in a digital form in the Internet for the acceleration of knowledge transfer [2].
- Use of the EIS in education - Target 3 is the use of the service in education i.e. for lectures, courses and self-instruction.

3. The process of consultation

The physicians, who participate on ENDOTEL, are free to use the system whenever need for consultation arises. The following process describes consultation using the ENDOTEL system. The involved physicians can be sender (Inquiry Sender IS) or addressee of inquiries (Inquiry Addressee IA). *Figure 1* shows sending of inquiries and responding according with step 5 to 9.

First step, but – of course - not supported by the ENDOTEL application:
(1) Endoscopic or sonographic examination of the patient by physician;
The next steps are supported by the ENDOTEL application: (2) Physician digitizes the relevant data material (endoscopic and/or sonographical video, x-rays, laboratory findings); (3) Physician formulates an inquiry with a description of the problem either using a text processor, a voice recognition system or generating an audio file (voice clip); (4) Physician chooses addressee from list; (5) Physician (sender) transmits data material to the database located at Telezentrum Stamsried (the system informs the addressee) (6); Addressee looks at the data material; (7) Addressee formulates a response; (8) Addressee transmits his response to the database located at Telezentrum Stamsried (the system informs sender of inquiry); (9) Physician (sender) reads response

Necessary condition for the acceptance of this proceeding is an as possible as user-friendly application. This should enable even physicians inexpierienced with computers to use the ENDOTEL service.

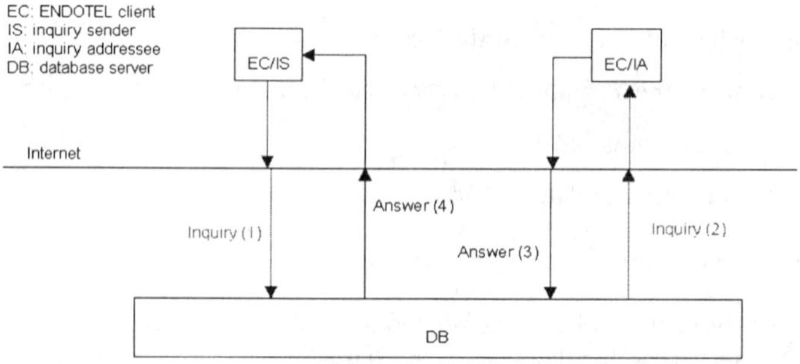

Figure 1: *Sending of inquiries and responding*

4. System development process

An object–oriented analysis and design method is used to engineer the ENDOTEL system, the Unified Modeling Language (UML) [3,4]. During requirement acquisition in December 1998 the consultation process has been analyzed. The next step will be to visit the ENDOTEL participants to talk about their expectations and requirements by means of use-case-diagrams, activity diagrams and class diagrams, which are part of the UML. These models proved to be valuable for the understanding of the system to build. We are going to put much emphasis on this requirements engineering task, because only a system that meets the expectations of the doctors will be used in clinical routine. On the basis of the specified functions required by the doctors, the system will be designed. For the design task we are going to use – in addition to the diagrams mentioned above – state, collaboration, sequence, component and deployment diagrams. We hope that object orientation and the UML will help us to design a system that meets the high expectations of our medical partners.

5. Discussion and conclusions

Under common effort of developers and users a telemedicine service will be established, not only to increase the importance of rural areas but also to bring benefit to the patient. ENDOTEL can help to decrease costs for the medical health care system in Germany and improve communication between physicians and medical specialists. The concept is also an approach to canalize the large number of various inquiries to these experts.

Acknowledgements

The authors thank Mr. Ellwanger from the Telehaus Stamsried for the helpful support of the project. Fabian Sturm from the ENDOTEL team deserves our special thanks for his excellent and engaged work.

References

[1] Roland Berger & Partner GmbH: Telematik im Gesundheitswesen - Perspektiven der Telemedizin in Deutschland. Study by order of the German Ministery of Research and the German Ministery of Health, August 1997.
[2] Sancho JJ, Oliveri NC, Faba G, Campos M, Sanz F, De Dombal FT: ELCANO: European and Latin-American Countries Associated for a Networked database of Outstanding guidelines in unusual clinical cases. MIE'96, 103-107
[3] Grady Booch, Ivar Jacobsen, Jim Rumbaugh, et al.: The Unified Modeling Language User Guide, Addison-Wesley
Pub Co, 1998.
[4] Martin Fowler, Kendall Scott: UML konzentriert: die neue Standard-Objektmodelierungssprache anwenden, Addison Wesley Longman, 1997.

Medical Informatics Europe '99
P. Kokol et al. (Eds.)
IOS Press, 1999

Electronic consultations and referrals in Kymenlaakso Hospital District

Erkki Läike[1], Timo Koivu[2], Riitta Järvinen[2], Aarni Ahtola[3]
[1]Kymenlaakso Central Hospital, FIN 48210 Kotka, Finland
[2]Kymenlaakso Hospital District, FIN48210 Kotka, Finland
[3]Kymenlaakso Polytechnic, FIN 48210 Kotka, Finland

Abstract. The meaning of this paper is to introduce the medical network which has been taken to Kymenlaakso Hospital District and the primary experiences in utilizing. Actual numeral results are not ready because of short time. First results will be ready in August 1999.

1. Introduction

Kymenlaakso Hospital District is one of the 18 hospital districts in Finland, locating in South-East Finland and it has a population of 190000. There is two general and two psychiatric hospitals for special care and 11 primary care health centers. Hospital district has ca 150 physicians and primary care ca 150. Hospital district has yearly about 220 000 visits in special care of which 15% are primary visits, number of referrals is 20000. Emergy care visits are about 15000. Continuous increasing of visits has made necessary to find ways of decreasing these visits. Lack of flexible method of communication was one of the main causes why primary care doctors had always sent patients to hospitals when a specialist consultation was needed. On the other hand for the same reason after treatment could not be at local health centers.

To find and create a new method a projectgroup was appointed. This group of medical and data specialist began working at the beginning of 1998. Working was carried out so that practical use of new system could begin in April 1999.

2. Technical solutions

Choosing the technical solutions main inportance was to use as far as possible those means that already existed. Dataconnections are handled via Internet and the program is running in Windows NT server. Workstations are PC.s with Windows 95, 98 or NT using normal browsers as MS Explorer or Netscape. User ID and dataencryption is made by SecGO Crypto IP® (Instrumentointi Oy/Special Systems Divison), picture 1. KONSU® program (Compaq Computer / Datawell Oy) has been developed in connection with our projectgroup. Integration to other datasystems has been carried out with HL7 by DataGate®. System infrastructure is presented in picture 2.

Medical network is running separately and independently from all local systems but is integrated and makes possible to get a sight to data in other organisations.

Medical network in Kymenlaakso Hospital Disctrict consist now

- Electronic consultation and referral service
- Means to follow the whole chain of careprocess
- Support of decision making (statistics, reports etc)

3. Beginning of utilization

Technical solutions had been made but the utilization required careful defining of judiciary because similar systems was not been used before. Judiciary facts has been solved with authorities and written approval of every patient is needed.

To get system usable more than 200 physicians had to be trained in technical use of the system and motivating in the new concept. One physician-trainee was hired for 3 months fulltime training which was carried out in small groups (max 4 at the same time).

Using of system was gradual but was carried through in one month and now all units are using it.

4. Discussion

The final goal is to get better quality and economy having right patient in right place at right time. It is too early to say anything about that in our system. We are having a research with Health Care Department of Kymenlaakso Polythechnic. The situation before new system has been defined paying attention to viewpoint of the patients and the organisations. Follow up will be done and first results will be seen during next months. Final results will be seen much later.

We have had in Finland no other as covering system as ours. Because of different organisation models and working habits international results are not always to be transferred analogous to our healthcaresystem

There has been one larger trial in Finland. Peijas-Rekola Hospital in Vantaa has had electonic consultations between one specialty (medicin) and one health care center. They have experienced that the number of referrals will decrease and consultations will increase. Also they have found that expenses in total can be decreased. This trial has also showed very good satisfaction of both patients and physicians. [1]

5. Future

Development in practise and program will continue. Especially the utilization of structured referrals when possible and transferring other forms of data (pictures, x-rays etc) are coming in near future. Use of the network in standardizing care of special diseases has been began. We are also waiting that in long term the knowledge of primary care physicians will increase and need to consult or send patients to special care will decrease. Aftertreatment can be carried out more in local health centers and the patients do not have to travel.

References

[1] Harno Kari, Finnish Medical Journal 1998:16:1691

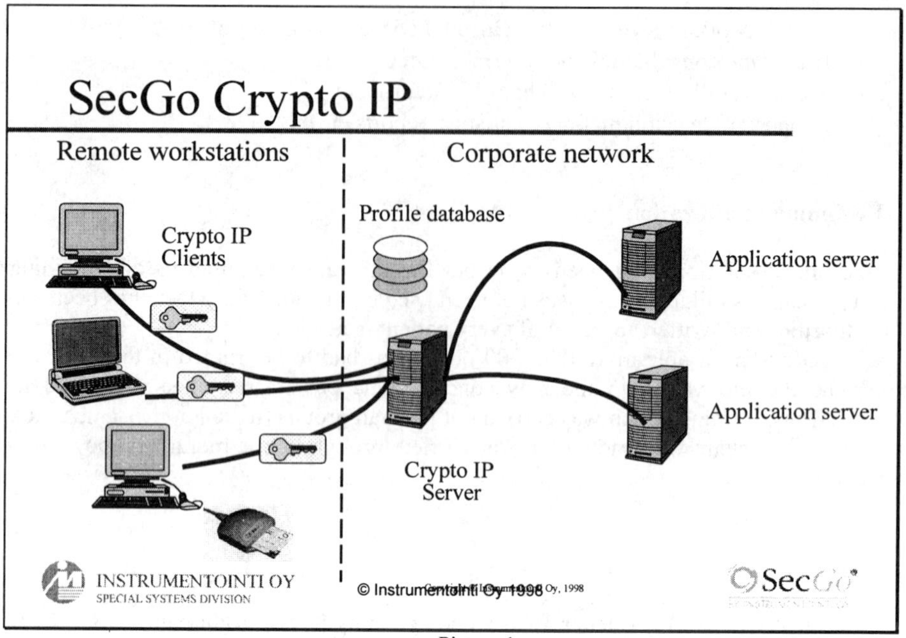

Picture 1

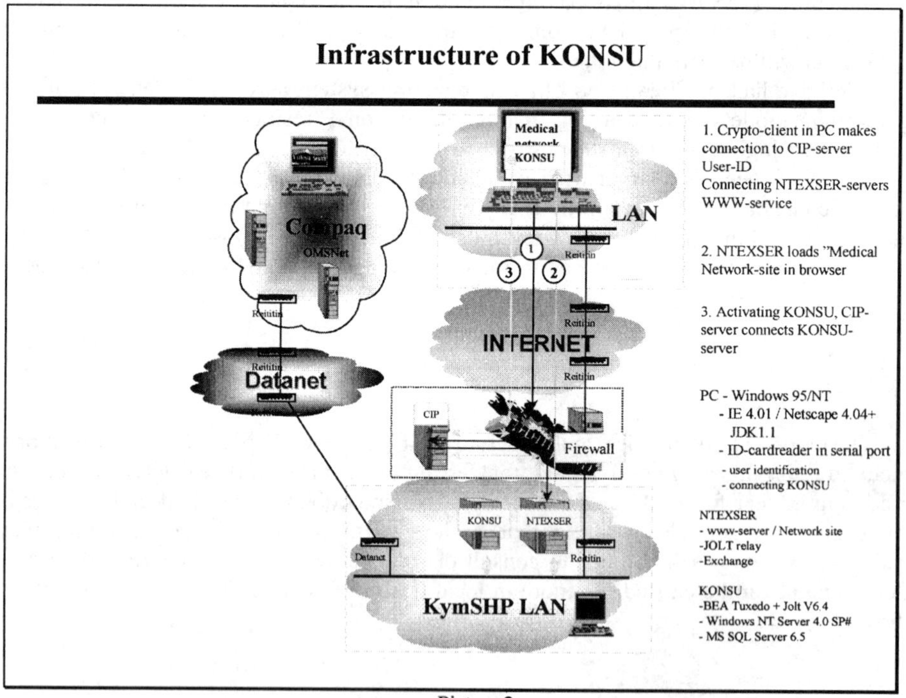

Picture 2

Medical Informatics Europe '99
P. Kokol et al. (Eds.)
IOS Press, 1999

The Hip Status: A Telemedical Application

Dragica SMRKE[1], Gregor CERKVENIK[1],
Dunja PIŠKUR-KOSMAČ[3], Vlado STANKOVSKI[1]
[1]Department of Surgery, University Medical Centre, Zaloška 7, SI-1000 Ljubljana, Slovenia; [2]Ministry of Health, Štefanova 5, SI-1000 Ljubljana, Slovenia

Abstract. Biomedical informatics and biomedical engineering are interdisciplinary sciences that are growing fast and have a significant impact on healhcare delivery. The University Medical Centre in Ljubljana and the Medical Faculty through its institutes have initiated the building of their own telemedicine systems. These systems concern only the medical informatics field. However, in this work a telemedical application that uses a combination of biomedical engineering methods and methods of biomedical informatics is presented. This telemedical application was built at the Department of Surgery and it was named "The Hip Status Application". Its aims are to provide services of preventive medicine and health promotion for people with potential problems with the hip-joint, guidance for people that have already underwent an operation of implantation of hip endoprosthesis, or have in any other way affected hip-joints, remote system consultation for diagnostic purposes, etc. The application is still under evaluation, and it is meant as a start of a new era of engineering-powered telemedical applications at the Department of Surgery following the trends in the most developed countries of the World.

1. Introduction

Health care can be understood as a full spectrum from prevention through medical treatment (diagnosis and treatment) to rehabilitation. Biomedical informatics and biomedical engineering are interdisciplinary sciences that are growing fast and have a significant impact on healthcare delivery. Both disciplines have applications in health care, and ultimate goal to enable the healthcare professionals to improve the quality and efficiency of care delivery.

Biomedical engineering applies engineering methods, science and technology to problems in medicine and biology. It integrates engineering, physical and mathematical sciences, biomedical sciences and clinical applications. The results are advances in medicine, such as the artificial heart, pacemakers, medical imaging techniques, lasers, prosthetic implants, such as hip endoprostheses of various types, life support systems, and devices that help the disabled people to integrate in the society. The term biomedical engineering includes a number of disciplines such as biomechanics, biomaterials, biosensors, physiologic modelling, simulation and control, biomedical instrumentation, medical and biologic analysis, rehabilitation engineering, prosthetic devices and artificial organs, medical informatics, medical imaging, biotechnology, clinical engineering, biologic effects of electromagnetic fields and genetic engineering.

The medical informatics comprises of the theoretical and practical aspects of information processing and communication, based on knowledge and experience derived from processes in medicine and healthcare. Examples of well-established methods and applications are biosignal and images analysis and processing, image guided surgery, clinical data management and decision support systems, hospital information systems, computer-based patient records and many others. Among methods that still need to be accepted are the expert systems of the second generation (machine learning systems) emerging from the need to aid the decision making process. The scope of medical informatics can be even broader to include the aspect of communication and »telecare« with the topics such as teleconsultation, telemonitoring, telesurgery, emergency telemedicine services, regional helathcare networks, etc.

An important trend is a move towards more involvement of patient or citizen in receiving information, in decision making and in responsibility for own health. The prime feature of this trend to shift from healthcare-institution centred care to the citizen-centred care is the emphasis on continuity of care from prevention to rehabilitation. This vision can be achieved through shared care which builds on health telematics networks and services, linking hospitals, laboratories, pharmacies, primary care and social centres offering to individuals a "virtual healthcare centre". Furthermore, this vision implies provision of health services to homes with new innovative services such as personal health monitoring and support systems and user-friendly information systems for supporting health education and awareness. These new innovative systems will require the integration of the new advanced sensors and micro systems with information systems and electronic health records that will be accessible, secure and highly usable in a multilingual environment.

The University Medical Centre in Ljubljana and the Medical Faculty through its institutes have initiated the building of their own telemedicine systems. These systems concern only the medical informatics field. However, in this work a telemedical application that uses a combination of biomedical engineering methods and methods of biomedical informatics is presented. This telemedical application was built at the Department of Surgery and it was named "The Hip Status Application". Its aims are to provide services of preventive medicine and health promotion for people with potential problems with the hip-joint, guidance for people that have already underwent an operation of implantation of hip endoprosthesis, or have in any other way affected hip-joints, remote system consultation for diagnostic purposes, etc. The application is still under evaluation, and it is meant as a start of a new era of engineering-powered telemedical applications at the Department of Surgery following the trends in the most developed countries of the World.

2. The Hip Status Application

The hip status application is a screen-based questionnaire which can include any queries likely to feature in a typical follow-up consultation. The screens are configured so that information can be included into a database in a most efficient manner, encoding the information in a numerical array which becomes a descriptor of patient condition.

A protocol for evaluation of the status of the hip [1, 2], including clinical and radiographic aspects has been recently developed. The data which are collected enable determination of the values of different standard hip scores such as Larson hip score, Harris hip score, Merle d'Aubigne and Postel hip score and Kavanagh hip score. In order to unify the hip evaluation and enable comparison between different analyses, this protocol is recommended by »Hip Society«, »Societe Internationale de Chirurgie Orthopedique et de Traumatologie« (SICOT) and »The American Academy of Orthopaedic Surgeons«.

The conventional scores rely upon a summation individual features, weighted according to their assumed importance, to give a single figure description of performance. Whilst this single score may be useful to understand how a prosthetic device is performing in general, it is not able to indicate the full details of a particular condition. The Hip Status Application collects all relevant data for future calculations.

An important feature is that the structure of the evaluation is not fixed but can vary at the discretion of those oranising a follow-up. There are various »standard« assessments collected in a library of assessment definitions. These may either be used directly or modified to suit the normal follow-up practice at a particular clinic.

In a case when someone is remotely using the application stickers containing this numerical description of outcome can be included into the patient's clinical notes where they form a shorthand alternative to the written clinical document. A clinician can become adept at identifying numerical patterns which indicate concern.

The clinical information is also collected in a computer database and can be recalled to show how the treatment of a particular patient is performing. Furthermore, because of the consistency of the follow-up, powerful statistical applications and machine learning applications may be used. The average scores of a group of patients who receive a particular treatment can give an appreciation of the efficacy of that treatment. A deviant numerical pattern may indicate cases where a close future scrutiny is warranted. The correlation of the clinical scores with success or failure may define numerical patterns which are indicative of outcome. In each case the Hip status application may be used to assist clinical decision making [6, 12, 13].

Furthermore, data about the biomechanical status of the hip may also be collected [3-5, 7-11]. Digitised standard antero-posterior radiographs are used for this purpose. On the bases of the radiographs the geometry of the hip and the pelvis is calculated and predictions are being made on the basis of already existing models. These data are also included in the database to evaluate the influence of the biomechanical status of the hip on the long-term outcome after hip arthroplasty.

3. Discussion

The Hip Status Application combines methods, which are known from the biomedical informatics field and methods, which are known from the biomedical engineering field. The common goal of both fields is the efficiency of health care delivery, so, it is not surprising that they can be combined well together.

In other countries, telemedicine services are currently employed to support various aspects of healthcare delivery, such as remote (physician-to-physician or physician-to-patient) consultation for diagnostic purposes; remote guidance in the performance of variety of therapeutic and surgical procedures, thus making expertise available at remote sites (e.g. site of an accident, geographically isolated areas, on board ships and planes, sea-plants battlefields, hazardous environments, space stations, etc); global access to educational material and statistical information; and remote use of distributed medical information processing facilities. Furthermore, telemedicine also supports continuity of care, making the electronic healthcare record of a patients readily, timely and transparently available wherever and whenever needed.

The application is still under evaluation, and it is meant as a beginning of new era of telemedical applications at the Department of Surgery.

References

[1] R. Beden and D. Smrke, Računalniški sistem za oceno zdravstveno-epidemiološkega statusa pacienta ob poškodbi kolka: preliminarni rezulatati. In: Zajc B, ed. Zbornik 7. elektrotehniške in računalniške konference, zvezek B; 1998 sep 24-26; Portorož. Ljubljana: Slovenska sekcija IEEE, 1998; 319-22.

[2] R. Beden and D. Smrke, Statistična obdelava zdravstveno-epidemiološkega statusa poškodovancev ob zlomu stegneničnega vratu. *Inform Med Slov Print ed* 1998; 5 (1-2): 9-12.

[3] D. Smrke, A. Iglič, V. Kralj-Iglič and J. Prinčič, A possible mechanism of loosening of total hip endoprosthesis in acetabular region. In: Miklavčič D, Bajd T, Stanič U, eds. Proceedings of the 9th International Conference on Mechanics in Medicine and Biology; 1996 Jun 30-Jul 4; Ljubljana. Ljubljana: Slovenian Society of Medical and Biological Engineering, 1996; 587-9.

[4] D. Smrke, B. Kersnič, V. Stankovski, V. Kralj-Iglič, A. Iglič and J. Prinčič, Influence of the bipolar hip prosthesis neck length on the radial stress in the hip joint. Proceedings of the 3rd World Congress of Biomechanics (Abstract Book), Sapporo, Japan. 1998; FC 5-1.

[5] D. Smrke, A. Iglič, V. Kralj-Iglič and J. Prinčič, Stress distribution in the hip joint after implantation of the bipolar hip endoprosthesis. In: Abstract book of the 6th International Congress of the Hungarian Society of Traumatology. Budapest, 1997:177.

[6] D. Smrke, J. Demšar, I. Bratko, B. Kersnič and V. Stankovski, Analiza implantacij kolčnih endoprotez z regresijskimi drevesi. Inform Med Slov Print ed 1998; 5 (1-2): 111-6.

[7] V. Stankovski, V. Kralj-Iglič, B. Kersnič, D. Smrke and A. Iglič, Object oriented approach to determination of biomechanical parameters of the hip-joint. In: Power H, Brebbia CA, Kenny J, eds. Simulations in Biomedicine IV, Computational Mechanics Publications, Southampton, Boston, Cromwell Press, Wiltshire (UK), 1997; 237-46.

[8] V. Stankovski, A. Iglič, V. Kralj-Iglič, B. Kersnič and D. Smrke, Determination of the stress distribution in the hip-joint contact surface. In: Zajc B, ed. Zbornik 6. elektrotehniške in računalniške konference, zvezek B; 1997 sep 25-27; Portorož. Ljubljana: Slovenska sekcija IEEE, 1997; 355-8.

[9] V. Stankovski, D. Smrke, B. Kersnič, V. Kralj-Iglič and A. Iglič, Computer system for evaluation of possible migration of acetabular and femoral components of bipolar endoprosthesis. Proceedings of the 3rd World Congress of Biomechanics (Abstract Book), Sapporo, Japan. 1998; FC 19-2.

[10] V. Stankovski, A. Iglič, V. Kralj-Iglič, D. Smrke and B. Kersnič, Vis et pressus in coxa Simulator.In: Proceedings of the VIII Mediterranean Conference on Medical and Biological Engineering and Computing, MEDICON'98, CD-ROM; full-length paper - 6 pages and Book of Abstracts, 1998; 196.

[11] V. Stankovski, B. Kersnič, D. Smrke, A. Iglič and V. Kralj-Iglič, Difference in size of hip-joint weight bearing area in male and female population. In: Ashton-Miller JA, ed. Proceedings of the 10th International Conference on Mechanics in Medicine and Biology; 1998 Mar 2-5; Waikiki USA. Waikiki: Pacific Centre of Thermal-Fluids Engineering (PCTFE), 1998; 248-50.

[12] L. Todorovski and D. Smrke, Analiza pojava bolečine v spodnjem udu pri bolnikih z vstavljeno kolčno endoprotezo. In: Zajc B, ed. Zbornik 7. elektrotehniške in računalniške konference, zvezek B; 1998 sep 24-26; Portorož. Ljubljana: Slovenska sekcija IEEE, 1998; 117-20.

[13] L. Todorovski, D. Smrke, V. Stankovski and B. Kersnič, Vstavitev kolčne endoproteze in pojav bolečine v spodnjem udu. Inform Med Slov Print ed 1998; 5 (1-2): 129-33.

The Telemedicine and Second Medical Opinion

Borut Gersak, MD, PhD; Vojka Gorjup, MD; Anja Jazbec, MD
University Medical Center Ljubljana, Zaloska 7, 1525 Ljubljana, Slovenia

Abstract. Telemedicine is declared as delivery of care to patients anywhere in the world by combining communications technology, with medical expertise.
The well established applications of telemedicine are in the field of teleradiology, pathology, cardiology. In some cases video-conferencing (VC) may be applied.
Second medical opinion is an important additional viewpoint on the patient diagnosis and treatment. The established network of consultant hospitals and worldwide Second opinion centers enable a fast (24 – 72 hours response) second medical opinion consultation service with the telemedicine application. The consultant hospitals at present time are: UCSF – San Franscisco, Stanford Medical Center, Bowman Gray School of Medicine, The Brigham Radiology Foundation , Emory University Hospital, University of Pennsylvania Medical Center. The second opinion centers are located worldwide, just to mention some of them: London, Budapest, Ljubljana, Tel Aviv, Bombay, Athens, Milano, Seoul.

1. Introduction

Second Opinion Consultation service in Slovenia started to operate on regular basis in May 1998. It was established in a response to the need of second opinion consultation. With it our patients have the opportunity too get second opinion on their disease from several best hospitals in the world. At present the following hospitals are included into the system: UCSF – San Franscisco, Stanford Medical Center, Bowman Gray School of Medicine, The Brigham Radiology Foundation , Emory University Hospital and University of Pennsylvania Medical Center. Second opinion consultation can be obtained on all fields of medicine from surgery to internal medicine, radiology, pathology, oncology... The system is sponsored by three big Slovenian companies (a bank, an insurance company and company which provides cell phone services). A second opinion request can be made by a patient or by a health institution where he is treated.

2. Methods

This is a retrospective analysis of one year experience with second opinion consultation service in Slovenia.

3. Results

In the first year of operation we proceded 58 requests for second opinion consultation (three patients needed consultation from two clinicians), 28 patients were female and 30 male. Patients' age varied from 17 months to 72 years, average age being 40 years. In 22 patients our only request was clinical consultation , in 37 we also needed radiology consultation and in 2 cases pathology slides were sent to USA for pathology consultation. In a complicated cardiology case of a young athlete with dilative cardiomyopathy a video conference was organised to provide a direct communication with the consulting specialist. Internal medicine consultations were the most prevalent (15), followed by the surgery (12), neurology (10), oncology (7), pediatrics (5), orthopedy (4), ENT (3), ophthalmology (2) and gynecology (2). In internal medicine field cardiology consultations were most frequent and in surgery they were neurosurgery. Average time from completed request for second opinion consultation to sending the request was less than 24 hours. Average waiting time for the complete consultation was 12 days, waiting time for radiology consultation only was always shorter, it was around three days. In almost all cases diagnoses are the same as in primary opinion, but treatments differ from time to time.

4. Discussion

When we started with second opinion consultation service we had relatively small number of patients probably due to the fact that patients weren't well enough informed about the new possibilities. Now the number of consultations is gradualy increasing, the current rate is around six per month. Besides from the patients the increasing number of consultation requests is received from the doctors who are treating patients with complicated diseases. We are very pleased with high rate of diagnose matching. In most cases when suggested therapy differs from the primary one our doctors accept the advice and very rarely our intervention is needed.

5. Conclusions

From responses which we get from our patients and doctors we can conclude that second opinion service is a valuable addition to better health care especially for complicated cases. With that our knowledge on rare and difficult cases is expanding and we can offer better care to present and future patients and we do all that with the help of telemedicine which offers us the opportunity to be in permanent contact with the best hospitals in the world.

Medical Informatics Europe '99
P. Kokol et al. (Eds.)
IOS Press, 1999

Computerised System for the Networking of Health Services
(Proposed solution for the informational support of the Health Insurance Law in Romania.)

M. Teseleanu, V. Afteni, M. Sucholotiuc, L. Stefan, I. Dobre
Institute for Computers ITC S.A .- 167 Calea Floreasca, sector 2, 72321 Bucharest, Romania

Abstract. The integration of health services in the health insurance system can only be performed by using an advanced informational system, due to the large volume of documents needed for the payment of medical services by the health insurance firms.
To better facilitate the access to the medical databases throughout the country is it necessary that the different application and their respective supports are able to communicate with each other.
Every component of the health system (doctors' offices, clinics, hospitals, pharmacies, county health insurance offices) consist of a local LAN/WAN network according to the individual computer capabilities.
These networks are connecting through the Internet which can be describe as a network of networks that permits long range communication.

The data on the health of every citizen, gathered in a database from the interaction between patients and the health services (physicians, specialist, hospitals, pharmacies, etc.), is necessary both to the individual patients as is to the management of the health services offered to the public.

The access to this database will allow for a higher quality of health care, through an efficient evaluation of the living condition and general health of the population, better epidemic control as well as throughout the integration of the health services in the health insurance network.

To better facilitate the access to the medical databases throughout the country is it necessary that the different application and their respective supports are able to communicate with each other.

Every component of the health system (doctors' offices, clinics, hospitals, pharmacies, county health insurance offices) consist of a local LAN/WAN network according to the individual computer capabilities.

These networks are connecting through the Internet which can be describe as a network of networks that permits long range communication.

The greatest advantage of the Internet when working with a large database is that any updating made by an individual through the network is immediately accessible to everybody; also the data can be protected by encryption during the transmission.

1. Health data

Entry data referring to the initial state of the patient are introduce by the family doctor and further updated by the other health services (clinics, specialists, pharmacies, etc.) where the patient is sent by his/her doctor. This data is a duplicated exactly in the main database at CNAS (The National Health Insurance Office).

2. Access to the database

Accessing the database at CNAS by any doctor is possible by using the patient's access code, which is read from the patient's smart card (SC). The SC contains data about the patient's health insurance status and the access is restricted according to the clearance of the person accessing the database. The clearance of the person's right to accessing the database is read of his/her own personal SC. Access to the database in an emergency situation, when the patient does not have his/her SC, is provided using his/her personal code from the Population Database, for access to medical information of strict necessity through the Internet (simple or encrypted e-mail). Any access to the CNAS Database is made through the Internet.

3. Services payment

Payment claims to the CAS are made through HTML forms filled in by the provider of medical services. The CAS consults the patient database to check if the medical services mentioned in the HTML form were actually provided, and to check if the procedures used were compliant with the diagnostic according to the 'Therapeutic Guide of Romanian Medical Practitioners'. If the treatment is approved, the CAS sends a transfer order to the bank, which transfers the funds into the provider's account. These transfers to and from the bank are also done through the Internet.

4. Collection of health insurance fees

Collection of the health insurance fees is obligatory and contractual. Institutions send to the CAS the list of persons for whom the fees were paid, through HTML forms mentioning the total amount, at the same time that a payment order is sent to the bank for that same amount. The bank transfers the funds from the institution's account to the CAS account. Banking services are provided through the Internet. Individuals pay their fees directly to the CAS. The date until which the insured person has the right to health services, is then updated on the person's SC.

To provide a person with access to health services regardless of the location of the providers of those services, health smart cards will be used. The data stored on the SC are useful to the patients and they must give their consent to the storing of their medical data. If doctor-patient privileges are going to be respected, the patients will allow their medical data to be stored, they will believe in the benefits this system will bring, and the development of this technology will be a success. It is known that the patient is the weakest link in the chain of the health insurance system, and, because of that, all the steps leading to the establishing of this system in Romania must be accompanied by the use of protocols meant to protect the interests of the patients when dealing with the informational system.

The introducing of the SC into the health system will allow:

1) patient's mobility between different health services providers
2) rapid patient's identification and less paper forms traffic
3) off-line access to urgent medical data
4) the confidentiality of medical data

SCs and networking are two complementary technologies that, when use together, can better the quality and efficiency of the health system, two necessary requirements of the modern society.

5. System overview

The integration of health services in the health insurance system can only be performed by using an advanced informational system, due to the large volume of documents needed for the payment of medical services by the health insurance firms.

I) The document route for the payment of services provided by medical practitioners

a) medical cabinet
- filling in of medical records
- payment orders (based on consultations, treatments, drugs, etc. matter of diagnostic) to the CAS

ATTENTION! The same forms can be filled in by pharmacies, hospitals, specialists, etc., who provided services and demand payment from the CAS.

a) The Health Insurance Office (the CAS)
- verifying the appropriateness of the medical services provided
- sending the order to the bank to pay the provider of medical services

b) The bank (the Ministry of Finance)
- receives the payment order from the CAS
- transfers the money into the medical services provider's account

II) The documents route for the collection of health insurance fees from the population by the CAS

a) the institution or private citizen
- documents notifying the CAS of the payment of health insurance fees
- payment orders to the bank for the CAS

b) the CAS
- the daily updating of the database to include the most recent fee payments from the population and verifying the correctness of the payments

c) the bank
- receiving payment orders from the institutions
- transferring the money into the CAS account

6. The characteristics of the core elements - extract from the Health Insurance Law

The **CNAS**: The new health protection system of the population in Romania is made up of the social health insurance services. Social health insurance is obligatory, and is provided by the payment of fees by the insured. The administration of the health insurance fund is taken care of by the National House of Health Insurance (CNAS), by the county health insurance offices, and by the Bucharest health insurance office. The insured status is received from the moment when the contract between the citizen and the CAS is signed and is kept as long as the contract is respected. The contract is drafted by the CNAS and by the National Medical Doctors Association of Romania (CMR), with the consent of the Ministry of Health (MS). The contract draft regards mainly the conditions of health services, specifically the list of services and drugs provided to the insured, the criteria and payment modes of health services and the ways of payment and documents necessary for this purpose.

The **CMR**: The Medical Doctors Association of Romania has the following obligations: the creation of therapeutic patterns, the accreditation of medical personnel and medical institutions, and to see to it that there are enough medical services providers throughout the territory. The CMR will have branches in every county, as will the Pharmacists Association (CF), who will represent the interests of the pharmacists.

The relationships between the CAS and the medical services providers (physicians and medical staff, medical cabinets and institutions of diagnostic and treatment, hospitals and other medical institutions) are established and regulated by a legal contact between the two.

The **MS**: The Health Ministry (MS) drafts, implements, and co-ordinates the public health programs, with the purpose of achieving certain national health goals, with the participation of all the institutions responsible for the implementation of the national health policies. These goals are established in collaboration with the CNAS, the CMR, and University hospitals, research institutions, non-governmental organisations, syndicates, etc.

This application simulates the data flow inside the health system, and it was created using Visual Basic 4.0 for the access to the database through a network. It is made up of several programs that use a network-distributed database.

These programs are:

- the CAS interface;
- the interface for the family doctor's office;
- the interface for the pharmacy.

These interfaces are user friendly and easy to learn.

Each program uses a local database that can also be found in the general CAS database.

This demonstration will be ran using Windows NT 4.0 network managed by the integrated BackOffice Small Business Server software package. This package will allow for communication services between the users of the same network, as well as between them and the external network (the Internet), easy administration of the network and easy administration of the Internet connection.

Medical Informatics Europe '99
P. Kokol et al. (Eds.)
IOS Press, 1999

End-user point of view to establish real-time broadband ATM connection over Europe

Pekka LOULA, Timo LUMMEVAARA*, Jouni ILOLA**, Pertti AARNIO**
Tampere University of Technology, Pori
P.O. Box 30, Fin-28601 Pori, Finland
**Pori telephone company*
***Satakunta central hospital*

Abstract. There have so far been few discussions about how the international broadband services will be created in practice. In this paper we concentrate on two separate international telemedicine trials in which Satakunta Central Hospital took part in the HIM project. In these trials we tested real-time video consultation over the international point-to-point ATM network connection between hospitals in Finland, Portugal and Germany. The quality of the consultations were clinically first-rate in both trials. The technological lesson learned from these trials was valuable for the operators in establishing broadband connections in Europe. The network connection was analysed based on transmission capabilities of the network connection.

1. Introduction

Some of the European countries, such as Finland and Sweden have enjoyed free competition of the telecommunication services. The prices of the telephone calls in Finland have been among the cheapest in the world. Now we live in a time when the liberalisation of the telecommunications sector is starting in the rest of Europe [1]. Nowadays teleoperators work within a geographically limited area providing services locally. In the near future the alliances and mergers will play a major role in tele-business in Europe.

Telemedicine is assumed to be one of the promising application areas utilising high-speed networks [2,3]. The availability of high-speed wide-area networks facilitates a range of new services in health care. The performance of videoconferences combined with software for computer-supported co-operative work make possible better diagnosis of digital medical images [4]. Continuing education benefits from telemedicine providing methods for better patient care [5]. Life-long learning is part of normal working routine in modern medicine. Video consultation and conferencing provide the possibility to participate in far-site education programs, especially in rural areas [6]. At the same time the service providers are looking for a killer application which will be the final breakthrough in applying broadband services. One of the possible killer applications is video-on-demand service. Unfortunately, the technology needed behind the service is still rather expensive. Although the compression methods and user access techniques, i.e. digital subscriber line based modems are very competitive, the capacity of media servers and number of subscriber lines at the near-end of the server should be better. Other possible application areas are TCP/IP (Transmission Control Protocol/Internet Protocol) based broadband services, e.g. voice-over-internet and H.323 standard based desktop videoconferencing seem to be the technology which the industry relies on.

This paper reports experiences from establishing international broadband telemedicine services at Health Care Informatics Centre of Excellence (HC-ICE) in Satakunta, Finland. Especially, the paper exposes the practical technical problems and solutions related to creating telemedical services in the future.

2. Methods

The HIM (High-Performance Information infrastructure in Medicine) project of the European Commission (N°B3014) which concentrated on evaluating international medical trials in Europe. The main goal of the project was to study the use of high speed connections like ATM (Asynchronous Transfer Mode) in an international setting for medical data interchange. The HIM project has been running since 1994. During the last phase of the HIM project several ATM- based clinical trials were performed [7].

The required network connection was provided by the JAMES (Joint ATM Experiment on European Services) consortium, which is a collaborative project between 18 European network operators. In the HIM project the information transmission rate varied from 2 Mbps to 155 Mbps (figure 1). Finland took part in two international trials at the end of 1996 between Pori and Porto and at the beginning of 1997 between Pori and Mainz. The consultation settings between the partners are shown in Figure 2. The videoconferencing system environment was very similar at each site.

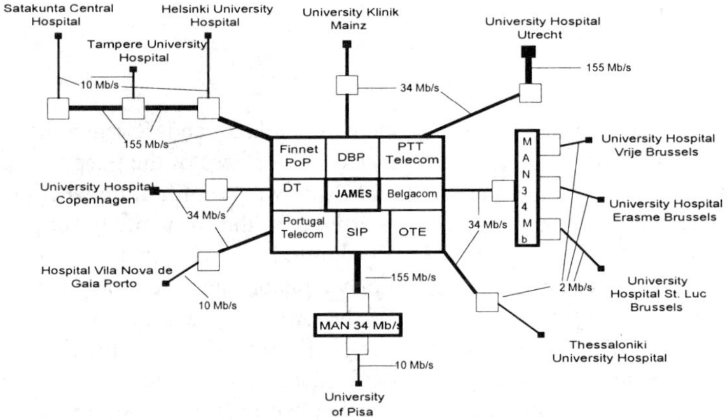

Figure 1. The hospitals and their transmission rate of ATM connection involved in the HIM project.

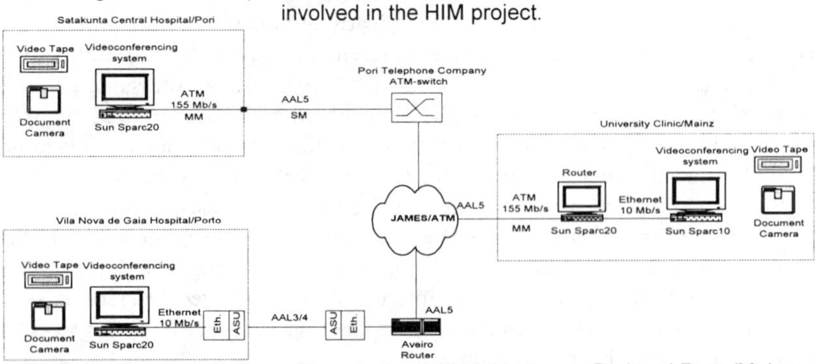

Figure 2. The consultation settings in the HIM trial between Pori and Porto/Mainz. The operators with JAMES accepted a peak rate level of 19300 cells per second in both directions (send/receive) at their nodes.

The responsible partner *at the Pori site was Satakunta Central Hospital.* At the Pori site the workstation (Sun Microsystems) with Solaris 2.4 operating system was equipped with a 155 Mbps multimode network adapter (Efficient Network Inc.). The workstation was directly connected to a Fore ATM switch in the Pori telephone company using a permanent virtual connection (PVC). In the network adapter the ATM channel was allocated to ensure a constant bit rate (CBR) of 7 Mbps. Because of the distance of 5 km from Satakunta Central Hospital to the operator the use of a multimode / singlemode fiber optical converter was required at the hospital. The responsible partner *at the Porto site was Central Hospital de Vila Nova de Gaia.* At the Porto site the workstation (Sun Microsystems) was equipped with 10 Mbps Ethernet adapter (Sun) and the SunOs 4.1 operating system. The responsible partner *at the Mainz site was Mainz University Clinic.* At the Mainz site there was a router (Sun Microsystems) that was equipped with a 155 Mbps multimode network adapter (Efficient Network Inc.) and it was connected through Ethernet (10 Mbps) with another workstation (Sun Microsystems). The Ethernet workstation was running SunOs 4.1.

Communique! 4.1.0 (InSoft Inc.) was chosen for the desktop conferencing application. It supported the UNIX desktop and provided transparent video compression and network interoperability for open conferencing. It also integrated real-time digital video technology with fully interactive, real-time collaborative tools, such as application sharing, shared white board, chat, audio, text and graphics tools. The conferencing workstations in Pori, Porto and Mainz contained a high quality Sun Microsystems SBus video card (Parallax Graphics, PowerVideo™). The video card supports high performance video with full motion live video display at 60 fields/seconds (30 frames/second) for NTSC or 50 fields/s (25 frame/second) for PAL or SECAM, 24-bit full motion colour video and full resolution live video display at 640x480 pixels for NTSC or 768x576 for PAL or SECAM. As external devices each site had a videotape recorder and a document camera for showing medical videos and documents.

The communication protocol between the sites was Classical IP. The information over the international ATM network was delivered in AAL5 (ATM Adaption Layer) cells. Both Pori and Mainz were transmitting AAL5 cells from their local area networks. At Porto there was an Ethernet-Ethernet router connected to an ASU (Acquisition and Synchronisation Unit) that converted the IP packets to AAL3/4 cells. In Aveiro these AAL3/4 cells were converted back to IP packets to allow a connection to a router (Cisco). The router converted IP packets into AAL5 cells, which was required by the JAMES ATM connection.

3. Results

The first HIM trial in Satakunta Central Hospital started 18th of November 1996 with Hospital Vila Nova de Gaia in Porto. During the first two days we had a lot of problems in establishing the PVC connection. The operators between Belgium and Helsinki had configuration differences and at the Pori site the workstation was not able to get any TCP/IP based connections. After the changes of the ATM interface card configurations in Pori the connection was confirmed by using Ping, Telnet and Ftp software. The transmission rate using those programs was very poor, for example ftp used only 51 Kbps when putting files from Porto to Pori. We also had some problems using videoconferencing. Although Pori was able to see pictures from Porto, the Porto site was not able to see video images from Pori.

On the third day Porto was sending a full sized video window with 2500 Kbytes/second and a 1/16 video window with 800 Kbytes/second, but there were still problems in providing a continuous video conference. There were differences between outgoing/incoming cell rates: 7000/2000 cells/second in Porto and 2000/4000 cells/second in Pori. There were a lot of dropped cells when the transmission rate was higher. Both sites asked the operators (Porto/Portugal Telecom and Pori/Finnet) to check the cell rates at each node of the JAMES network. The study revealed that the established connection was able to transmit only 19300 cells/second (approx. 8 Mbps). Therefore, the transmission rate was decreased from 10 Mbps to 7 Mbps at the Pori site. After the configuration the quality of the videoconference was technically suitable for medical consultation.

On the 21st of November 1996 medical doctors from Vila Nova de Gaia Hospital began to show some intravascular ultrasound and echocardiography examples from video tape and some real time coronary angiographies from the cath lab to medical doctors in Satakunta Central Hospital. They discussed the quality of the images and made some diagnoses based on them. The specialist in Satakunta, Dr Jouko Remes was surprised by the quality of the picture when he saw the real time angiography signal from Porto. The resolution and overall quality were excellent, the frame rate was between 25-30 frames/second, the data flow was smooth and there was no jitter in the picture. In our knowledge this trial was the first international ATM connection through Europe which was clinically accepted by the doctors for the real-time diagnosis. Earlier trials in HIM were made by using Microsoft NT workstations and software compression methods, and therefore they suffered of jittering and the frame rate was not adequate. During the trial (12 days) there were many discussions with doctors about telemedicine and common interest over the videoconference.

On the 28th we had two real cases of coronary angioplasty with diagnostic quality. The two cardiologists from both hospitals talked about all these images and commented on them. On the last day there were some technical problems between the operators in Germany and Sweden. After the delay Pori sent video images of a vascular anastomotic technique from video tape. The quality was not as good as during the previous days, because the video window size (full size) was too large for that kind of images. The quality of the image improved very much with the medium size window. The presentation was commented on by two cardiac surgeons, one in Pori and the other in Porto. The consultation was technically successful and the quality of the picture and sound was good.

The second HIM trial from Satakunta Central Hospital was arranged with Mainz University Clinic at the beginning of 1997. Both sites had experience about the HIM trial and the general preparations went quite easily. At the Pori site the videoconferencing system was moved to the Hospital's videoconferencing room so that we had a possibility to receive a live analogy video signal to the conferencing system from the operating theatre via a video matrix.

After technical preparations the JAMES ATM connection was successfully established and tested on the 15th of January. There was a conventional videoconference with the medical doctors about the forthcoming program. On the next day there were a few problems with the communication software when Mainz was sending video images from their video recorder. After the problem was corrected a doctor from Pori made an ultrasound examination of a new-born which was sent through in real-time and there was some discussion about these images.

On the following day the Pori site sent a live real-time picture from the operating theatre. The surgery was made by Dr. Pertti Aarnio who introduced a new clip-technique for blood vessel operations. The image quality was very

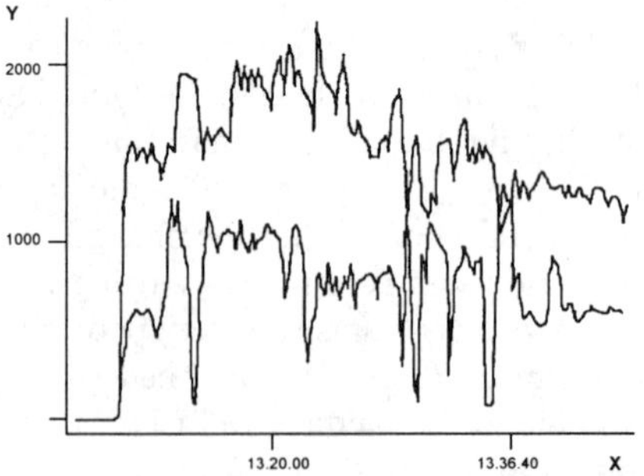

Figure 3. The performance of the applications (hardware/software) used in the HIM trial between Pori and Mainz. The graph plots the transmission rate in Kbits/s (Y-axis) versus the measurement time (X-axis).

good during the operation but the sound was poor because it was sent by a phone to the microphone connected to the videoconference and there was a lot of echo from the operating room. After the surgery the operating doctor talked about the operation and also showed documents and a video concerning the new equipment used (VCS clips).

The highest transmission speed of the connection from Pori to Mainz was 3,5 Mbps and the lowest speed was 40 Kbps. Figure 3 shows the average transmission rate that was measured from the ATM switch in Pori telephone company on 17th of January. The upper curve displays the cell rate of incoming cells from the workstation in Satakunta Central Hospital and the lower one displays the cell rate of incoming cells from Mainz over the JAMES cloud. The difference between these two cell rates during the videoconference was due to different video window sizes that were used in Pori and Mainz.

4. Discussion

In inspecting the real-time telemedical trials from the end-user point of view, we notice that the technological knowledge required is overwhelming for most clinicians. The end-user should be familiar with the telecommunication protocols and desktop standards.

The quality of the digital video signal is directly related to the compression and display hardware on the card. Some video cards, such as the SunVideo™ card which uses CellB compression and the maximum motion speed for high resolution window (640x480) of 10 frame/second, produce a different level of video quality than others, such as those from Parallax which use JPEG compression and the maximum motion speed for high resolution window of 30 frame/second. Such compression techniques as JPEG are needed to obtain high quality video signals for medical diagnosis in real-time consultation that was demonstrated in the HIM. The disadvantages of JPEG compression are that it requires more network bandwidth and consumes more system resources to decode than for example CellB. A reference of a SunVideo card and CellB based videoconferencing over ATM network is the distributed clinical neurophysiology which has been set up in Satakunta Central Hospital [8]. In this case the shared EEG review application was the main property of the system and the video link was used for discussion purposes between the specialists.

There are several obstacles which prevent or slow down the establishing of European wide telemedical consultation services. The security aspects of the tele-link and possible differences in legislation between European countries should be clarified. The price of the broadband connection with a quaranteed bandwidth is still definitely too high. Especially when the end-user asks the consultation service which is based on continuous real-time connection. In order to prepare the broadband link across Europe a lot of prior preparation and configuration work needs to be done. Our trial showed clearly that it will take a couple of days from a team of technical experts to succeed in forming a multinational link across Europe. For example in the Pori-Porto trial there were over 20 routers which were manually routed by the teleoperators in different countries. The co-operation with the operators should be flexible.

An important issue in ATM technology is the debate concerning whether the service should be based on Permanent Virtual Circuits (PVCs) or Switched Virtual Circuits (SVCs). PVCs are virtual circuit connections between two locations that remain permanently set up and SVCs are virtual circuit connections that get set up and discarded (switched) based upon whether data is actually being sent. PVCs require a one-time initial set-up between the switch and the router, but become inconvenient and costly in networks requiring any-to-any connectivity (the number of PVCs required is proportional to n-1 where n is the number of sites in the network). The benefit of SVCs is that the virtual circuits are only established based upon data demand. Therefore, the number of virtual circuits is proportional to the number of actual conversations between sites rather than the number of sites. SVCs are preferred in networks that require any-to-any connectivity and dynamic VC set-up, whereas PVCs are better for partially meshed networks designed to mimic leased-line topologies.

CBR guarantees a minimum transmission rate and is suited for services which require a continuous data flow between the applications, i.e. audio or video consultations. Of course it is the most costly service. Unspecified bit rate (UBR) and variable bit rate (VBR) services are more suited for applications which do not need continued data flow, e.g. e-mail type applications, or applications which are based on streamed inputs e.g. internet radios.

Another interesting question is how the international broadband connections will be connected to the local extranet services. Locally, Satakunta Central Hospital uses IP over ATM technology for IP-videoconferencing between primary health care and secondary health care. It connects the major local health care organisations in Satakunta with a link of from 2 Mbps to 155 Mbps. The local area networks connected to the ATM backbone as a virtual local-area network (VLAN) are based on ethernet and fast ethernet. It is estimated by industry experts that fast / gigabit ethernet will dominate the LAN solution and ATM will govern the wide area network [9].

Desktop conferencing requires desktop conferencing software and real multimedia PC equipment, i.e camera, speakers and microphone. Compared to ISDN based video conferencing the costs are reasonable. For example Microsoft Corp's NetMeeting software is freely downloadable. It is however, necessary to remember that for medical diagnostics the video camera should not be the cheapest one. Already conferencing with ISDN video conference studios, multipoint conferencing and multicasting over internet is possible [10].

This type of unique European wide high-speed network trial showed that telemedicine based services can be provided across Europe even when the demand for the service by the users is the most demanding. That kind of services may be real-time interactive teaching, patient consultation in difficult cases, and even consultation during operation if an unexpected finding occurs. The quality of video images was clinically acceptable and the clinicians were very satisfied. The price of international ATM connection is still rather high, but hopefully in the near future the prices of high-speed connections established by new innovative technologies will be reasonable.

References

[1] P. Sandler, Recent developments in telecommunications policy in the European Union. *IEEE Communications Magazine* 1997;35:42-48

[2] BKT. Ho, RK. Taira, RJ. Steckel, H. Kangarloo, Technical considerations in planning a distributed teleradiology system. *Telemedicine Journal* 1995;1:53-65

[3] A. Mark, MD. Goldberg, J. Samuel, III. Dwyer, Telemammography: Implemention issues. *Telemedicine Journal* 1995;1:215-226

[4] M. Eichelber, AJ. Hewett, P. Jensc, RETAIN -an ATM pilot project for applications in health care. *Journal of Telemedicine and Telecare* 1996;2:13-16

[5] H. Lamminen, J. Nevalainen, A. Alho, TS. Lindholm, Tallroth, J. Lepistö, Experimental telemedicine in orthopaedics. *Journal of Telemedicine and Telecare* 1996;2:170-173

[6] JA. Schnepf, DHC. Du, ER. Ritenour, JA. Fahrmann, Building future medical education enviroments over ATM Networks. *Communications of the ACM* 1995;38:54-69

[7] E. Neri, JP. Thiran, D. Caramella, C. Petri, C. Bartolozzi, B. Piscaglia, B. Macq, T. Duprez, G. Cosnard, B. Maldague, Interactive DICOM image transmission ,and telediagnosis over the European ATM network. *IEEE Transactions on Information Technology in Biomedicine* 1998;2:35-38.

[8] P. Loula, E. Rauhala, M. Erkinjuntti, E. Räty, K. Hirvonen, V. Häkkinen, Distributed clinical neurophysiology. *Journal of Telemedicine and Telecare* 1997;3:89-95

[9] D. Clark, Are ATM, Gigabit ethernet ready for prime Time? *Computer* 1998;31:11-13

[10] A. Dutta-Roy, Virtual meetings with desktop conferencing. *IEEE Spectrum* 1998; 35: 47-56.

Medical Informatics Europe '99
P. Kokol et al. (Eds.)
IOS Press, 1999

Real-time Medical Applications and Telecommunications

Miroslav Štravs, dipl.ing.
Smart Com d.o.o., Brnčičeva 45, 1000 Ljubljana, Slovenija

Abstract. Telecommunications play an important role in telemedicine. Many forms of telecommunication services based on different telecommunication technologies are developed for various needs. The paper deals with complex real-time applications which demand high telecommunication requirements. At the beginning, medical applications are categorised and real-time applications qualified as multimedia applications. Requirements for multimedia elements are listed separately. Later on, short introduction of related telecommunication protocols is given. Real-time medical applications can show their ability in case of guaranteed quality of services delivered by telecommunication network as it is explained in the end.
Key words: ATM (Asynchronous Transfer Mode), Internet protocol, telemedicine

1. Introduction

There are two kinds of telemedicine applications [1]. One of them is ''store and forward'' type. This type combines a knowledge of medicine as a primary involved science which needs data for its practice, with medical informatics that deals with storage and processing of medical data, and telecommunications that allow distribution and provide integration of medical information systems.

The second type of telemedicine applications is ''real-time'' type. The nature of the application is such that no real-time storage and processing of data are required although some of the obtained data can be stored and post-processed. The multimedia medical data are transported via telecommunication system between two or more locations to provide collaborative work for participants.

The paper deals with the second type of applications that require a unique approach in designing telecommunication services and networks.

2. Common requirements

The ''store and forward'' type of telemedicine uses telecommunication facilities for transport of all kind of data. Most medical data can be identified as character type:

- general data about the person
- patient's history and results of physical examination
- laboratory findings
- admission form and letter of dismissal
- prescriptions and so forth

There are other types of data that are generated at more detailed patient examination. These data are generated by medical instruments and are in the form of still medical image, short video, and sound or telemetry data. The size of data is such that data can be stored and archived in electronic form.

Transportation of such data between medical databases or database and desktop of practitioner in electronic form is generally not complex and can be realised by conventional data telecommunication networks. Internet protocol is universal and that is why it is more and more popular while ftp service over internet is probably the most used way of transportation of medical data.

Telecommunication requirements in such cases are not high:

- There is no transport bandwidth reservation on links shared by more virtual channels
- There is no special requirement for a transition delay. The data need to be transported in a reasonable period.
- There is no requirement for delay variation.
- If implemented protocols of upper OSI telecommunication layers in a terminal equipment deal with corrections which occur in network, there are even no high requirements for reliable communication channel with very low bit error rate.

Because of the low level of requirements, users are not concerned about the quality of telecommunication service types. They are satisfied with best-effort telecommunication service. The mentioned are typical parameters that become important at implementation of ''real time'' medical applications.

3. Real-time applications

There are special medical activities that require simultaneous communication between two or more participants:

- emergency medicine
- consultation to medical specialists
- intra-operative surgical consultation
- medical education etc.

Typically, 'real-time' applications are used when immediate action is important for saving lives and/or providing large economical benefits. It is a combination of live picture transfer and real-time data transfer. Real-time applications can be understood as multimedia applications. Better results are achieved when interactive communication (voice and video) is provided. All participants share the same medical data in form of image, sound or other forms. Medical data should be in a condition that allows best quality of medical decisions. Medical data can be obtained from various sources:

- pre-prepared and obtained from medical information system
- live generated by peripheral medical equipment

4. Definition of real-time

Telecommunications activity transforms a source signal to a form which is suitable for digital transport. Most of data that are analogue become digitised and eventually compressed at the transmitting side then telecommunication network introduces additional distortions and analogue signal is recovered at receiving side. Participants involved in real-time communications do not want to feel the distance and beside distortions can introduce additional barrier to their communications. A telecommunication network needs to provide them the simultaneous communication.

Generally, the exchanged information is one of multimedia type: telemetry data, images, speech, video etc. The most critical elements are speech and video that provide virtual presence. The basic requirement for voice communication is the delay between microphone and speaker that needs to be less then 300 ms, bandwidth requirements are low, typically 64 kbit/s. Requirements drastically change when voice channel is used for transfer of high quality sound (e.g. heart beat).

The quality of real-time video is difficult to measure but no one would be satisfied with more then 1s of delay and a quality that is provided with the channel capacity less then 384 kbit/s. There are several modalities of video transport specified that accommodate transport to certain transport protocols and available media.

Other data used at real-time communication such as image (x-ray image, CTI, MRI etc.), telemetry data (ECG, vital signs, various evoked signals etc.) are shared by participants. Data which origin at the location of one of the participants or is already stored in database, need to be transported in seconds to terminals used by other participants. The visual information can be presented in many ways (selected, zoomed, rotated and so forth) and all participants need to share the same view. Commands demanded by one of the participants need to be executed on all terminals immediately.

5. A data telecommunication perspective

OSI system defined for telecommunication purposes describes seven telecommunication layers. The first one is physical layer that accommodates data to specific telecommunication media. There are many media used on the access network and others used in the core. Their availability and reliability differ and the capacity of media depends on the current status of technology.

The second layer called data-link layer is more complex and defines the segments of data that are transferred or switched over the network. There are several functions that are implemented in the layer: error detection and correction, flow control, network problem notification etc. Nowadays frame relay and ATM are the most known protocol on data-link layer. They are connection oriented protocols, this means the direction of data flow is predefined. Specific features of data flow are guaranteed by the network.

The next is the network layer that deals with a route for data over the network. In general there are three kinds of route establishment over packets network:

- The simplest is PVC (Permanent Virtual Circuits).
- More complicated are SVC (Switched Virtual Circuits) that can be compared to POTS (Plain Old Telephone Service). Both of them are connection oriented.
- The third one is datagram type that is connectionless oriented. Internet protocol is a member of the third group.

Internet protocol has become so popular because of the features that distinguish it from other protocols which are its simplicity, robustness and spread. But in real world it has some disadvantages that we all face with daily:

- uncertainty of transfer
- a lack of security integrated
- no privacy and/or ability to create virtual private networks
- no manageability
- difficulties at billing issues

There are upper layer protocols that are implemented in terminal equipment. Some of them are not implemented everywhere. Transport Control Protocol TCP which is known by its combination to Internet protocol sits on the fourth layer called transport layer.

Seventh layer is the application layer and supports telecommunication elements directly used by application (e.g. ftp, telnet).

6. Relation between Internet protocol and lower layer protocols

The future belongs to the Internet protocol and this was recognised by medical standardisation bodies as well. For example, DICOM standard [2] tends to be open to various telecommunication protocols but TCP/IP was chosen as a special pair of protocols. It is similar else where. Transport of voice over IP is becoming reality even out of labs. New compression techniques, fast Intranet links and especially affordable price of communication boost its use. Similar has happened to transportation of video signal over Internet what is defined by ITU-T H.323. Internet protocol is driven by both users and industry.

Telecom operators' main orientation is quality of service delivered to customers. They have forced development of telecom oriented multimedia protocol, cell based ATM. This provides broadband capacities, guaranteed quality of service (QoS), VPNs, interworking with existing telecom protocols such as wideband frame relay and narowband ISDN, further on, it is manageable, with billing issues are almost solved. But all numbered features lead to its complexity and make it cheapless.

A reader probably noticed that both modern protocols origins at different worlds and most of telecommunication users would like to combine the benefits of both. Internet provides them common telecommunication interface to broad range of applications, ATM provides that different applications requirements are mapped into different telecommunication service.

7. Quality of service

Telecommunication networks based on statistical multiplexing technologies show their quality under traffic load. Services delivered to a customer should not be affected by services delivered to other customers.

For instance, an urgent patient transportation to hospital by ambulance should not be affected by traffic jam on roads and streets. Light and sound signals are used to notify drivers to release a traffic lane. The same philosophy can be mirrored to telecommunication networks. Possible congestion in telecommunication networks should not affect telemedicine applications. Even more, network resources and bandwidth capacities on links should be released in case of emergency medical action. Some emergency features are already implemented in POTS and GSM networks.

The reader can now understand why no telecommunication protocol is unique to ATM. Frame Relay which is another statistical multiplexing method was developed as a step toward ATM. It provides Class of Service parameters. Traffic belonging to one class of service will take priority over traffic of another class of service. The network does not provide a constant quality of service and it varies over the time.

ATM has introduced the ability of delivering multiple form of traffic successfully under traffic load. Several traffic types were defined for different services:

- Constant Bit Rate (CBR) for application that require fixed bandwidth and synchronisation (e.g. real-time video)
- Real-time Variable Bit Rate (rt-VBR) for applications that do not require fixed bandwidth but synchronisation is required (e.g. compressed real-time video)
- non Real-time Variable Bit Rate (nrt-VBR) for applications that do not require fixed bandwidth nor synchronisation (e.g. internet traffic)
- Available Bit Rate (ABR) occupies vacant bandwidth and is used for applications that do not require fixed bandwidth nor synchronisation
- Unspecified Bit Rate (UBR) occupies vacant bandwidth and no delivery is guaranteed

Requirements for the traffic types are defined by traffic parameters: cell delay, cell delay variations, peak cell rate, sustainable cell rate and others. Some of them are used for set up values related to amount of transferred data, others are time related parameters.

Similar activities have been started in organisations which provide regulative documents for frame relay protocol. New technology of voice transport over frame relay requires quality of service. That is why two new classes have been introduced by standards: real-time 1 and best-effort.

8. Internet and ATM as matching technologies

There have been many initiatives in last years that were trying to provide optimal interworking between the described protocols [3]. The most useful interface for delivering Internet traffic to any kind of transport network is Ethernet (ordinary 10 Mbit/s or fast Ethernet or giga Ethernet). That is why transport of Internet traffic started as simple bridging, no routing capabilities were integrated in the network.

More complex solutions have also appeared that are focused on integration of more benefits that both protocols contribute to partnership. The first larger innovation was Multiprotocol over ATM (MPOA) that had been designed for Local Area Networks. Later on the same vendor has introduced new improvements in Carrier Scale Internetworking (CSI) which is designed for Wide Area Networks. There are other initiatives like Multiprotocol Label Switching (MPLS). Both mentioned solutions are not focused on ATM and Internet merely, they combine other data-link layers like Frame Relay and Point-to-Point Protocol (PPP).

9. Conclusion

There are other building blocks of telecommunication system that contribute to quality of service. I need to mention at least the telecommunication network management systems which provide troubles recognition, fast reactions to network problems, service (Carrier Scale Routing) developing and establishing and a lot of business functions.

Telecommunication networks and services are expensive. The costs are even higher if telecommunication networks and services are not designed carefully. A telecommunication network must be a tool like medical instruments or informatics system to medical specialists who use it. Practitioners should know how telecommunication systems react to their telecommunication needs, but details have to be covered by telecommunication specialists.

References

[1] ITU-D: Telemedicine and developing countries; Document 2/155 (Rev.2)-E, 5 August 1997

[2] National Electrical Manufacturers Association: Digital Imaging and Communications in Medicine; Part 1: Introduction and overview, PS 3.1-1998

[3] Malcolm Duckett: The IP/ATM Controversy – Redressing the Balance; Conference: IP & ATM Architectures for next Generation Internet and Broadband

Medical Informatics Europe '99
P. Kokol et al. (Eds.)
IOS Press, 1999

Barriers for dissemination of a National Health Care Data Network A list of recommendations for better dissemination

Ib Johansen, MI.[1], Lone Kaalund Thiel, MI.[2]
1. Danish Centre for HealthTelematics, Heden 18, 5000 Odense C
2. IT – Health Care, County of Northern Jutland, Hobrovej 42D, 8000 Aalborg

Abstract. Establishment of a Danish Nation-wide Health Care Data Network for exchange of health care related information using standardised EDIFACT messages is agreed between the Danish Government, the Hospital Owners and the GPs organisations.
The aim is, within year 2000 in the MedCom project, to reach a level of 66% of all messages between the secondary and primary health sector must be send electronically using EDIFACT.
There are many barriers for reaching this goal, and to reveal this barriers an investigation was done, and a list of recommendations are set up.
The investigation was based upon literature, interviews and most important a questionnaire among 200 GPs and specialists all over the country.
After 6 months where the recommendations have been handled there is seen an increase in communicated messages on 40%, and from January 1999 more than 1.1 mill messages are exchanged each month.

1. Background

The use of IT-systems within the Health sector has been very common during the last 20 years. Mainly to handle administrative tasks, but also Laboratory Information Systems (LIS), Radiology systems and recently EPR. In the primary health sector, i.e. are many GPs and Pharmacies using electronic systems to day.

All this systems are stand-alone and normally not interconnected. In Denmark a great effort to interconnect these systems has been done during the last 6-7 years. The interconnection is not directly, but data is transferred using standardised EDIFACT messages. A national strategy to use these messages is set up and agreed between hospital owners, the Government and all SW vendors. MedCom manages the strategy: The Danish Health Care Data Network.

The goal is that at least 66% = 23 mill/year of all messages between primary and secondary sector must be transferred electronically, using EDIFACT within year 2000.
The messages are amongst others: discharge letters, laboratory results from all type of laboratory x-ray reports, referrals, reimbursements and prescriptions.

To reach this goal it is a must, that the sender and the receiver has electronic system i.e. GP - Electronic Patient Records (EPR) and a mailbox system to handle EDIFACT messages.

Today 95% of all laboratories has got LIS, 80% of all hospitals has got PAS and x-ray systems which can handle EDIFACT. 75% of all GPs has EPR but only 50% have established a mailbox for EDIFACT communication.

All GP-EPR systems can handle the MedCom EDIFACT messages.
To reach the goal it is important that more GPs invests in a mailbox and the EDIFACT software, but also that the use of GP-EPR increases.

2. Benefits

There are many benefits when using standardised EDIFACT i.e.

- No waiting time - results ready when needed
- No retyping of data – higher quality – reuse of data
- Cheaper than normal mail
- Results and information ready in patients record when needed

But why don't all GPs use EDIFACT then. Some of the negative things might be, but are never investigated:

- Electronic mailbox cost money
- Not all hospitals can send EDIFACT
- Still many local codes
- EDIFACT are difficult for the suppliers and training is needed

3. Barriers – an investigation

To reach the goal of at least 66% of all messages are transferred using EDIFACT and to find out what could be done to raise the level of EDIFACT use by GPs an investigation was done.

The hypothesis was:

1. The GPs age is relevant for the change to new technology. Younger GPs are more ready for computers than older ones.
2. The number of GPs in group practice are significant for the use of computers
3. The economy plays a big role for buying IT.
4. Users are afraid of the technology
5. Routines and workflow are preferred to be unchanged
6. Marketing of GP EPR not good
7. The EDIFACT possibilities in some counties are not satisfactory.

200 GPs (10% of all Danish GPs) was asked in a questionnaire about the hypothesis.

4. The conclusions was

- That the age of the GP is very relevant for the use of computers.
  In the age above 50 years there is a much lesser use IT than below 50. Remarkably was that all GPs younger than 40 years are using computers in their clinic.
- Money plays a role. Start using IT is dependant of the economy in the clinic, but when the investment was done, the additional cost for using EDIFACT was negligible.

- The size of the clinic. In group practice with 2 or more GPs the use of IT and EDIFACT are most common. The investment can be shared between all. One-man clinics are using EDIFACT remarkably lesser than group practices.

- The number of different EDIFACT messages from the hospitals was too low. If there is nothing or very little to communicate, why then invest in EDIFACT communication module.
- The marketing efforts from the GP SW vendors are not sufficient. More training courses and information relevant for the staff in GP clinics are really needed.
- Semantic problems. The information in the EDIFACT messages are not tuned to computers, but still like paper-based information. Too much irrelevant information.
- Everybody is ready to change workflow and routines.

5. Recommendations

The conclusions led to the following recommendations to increase the use of EDIFACT in GP clinics:

1. All hospitals, Labs, x-ray departments and Pharmacies must offer EDIFACT communication from all departments and wards within year 2000.
2. Refund of part of the investment when establishing EDIFACT communication in GP clinics.
3. More information from SW suppliers and MedCom directed to non- –EDIFACT users, supplemented with training courses.
4. The EDIFACT messages must be adjusted to electronic medium
5. Obligatory use of EDIFACT for reimbursement.

6. Results

Information from SW suppliers by direct mail to non-EDIFACT users and training courses from MedCom where the advantages are discussed has been established.

A direct contact and visit to each county and lab for discussing and planning start of using EDIFACT has been performed.

The price for sending EDIFACT Reimbursement is reduced to the same price as sending a letter.

A group of professionals has been established to make recommendations for relevant content of EDIFACT documents.

A booklet: Better starting with GP-EPR and electronic communication is published.
And the number of messages are increased 40% during the intervention period, and the number of EDIFACT GPs are increased by 19% which means an increase from 50% to 69% in January 1999.

Medical Informatics Europe '99
P. Kokol et al. (Eds.)
IOS Press, 1999

Regional Health Care Networks

Morten Bruun-Rasmussen[1], Knut Bernstein[1], Sandor Vari[2], Bostjan Bercic[3]
[1]*Danish Centre for Health Telematics, Heden 18, 5000 Odense C, Denmark*
Phone +45 66 13 30 66, Fax +45 66 13 50 66. mbr@health-telematics.dk
[2]*VariMed, Szalanci u 5, H-1124 Budapest XJJ, Hungary*
Phone +36 1 212 5636
[3]*INFONET, Planina 3, 4000 Kranj, Slovenia*
Phone +386 64 331 131

1. Summary

Communication cross primary and secondary care, between organisations or between different types of professionals causes special problems. The communication often implies exchange of data between different computer systems. The INCO-COPERNICUS[1] project PRIMACOM (**PRIMA**ry **C**are **P**hysician's **COM**munication Network) demonstrates how such communication can be established in regions in Hungary and Slovenia. PRIMACOM is building on European messaging standards for EDI (Electronic Data Interchange) with practical experience from the Danish MedCom project. The paper points out the need for standardising health care messages and via the Danish MedCom project documents the return of investment.

2. Introduction

In modern health care, services are characterised by a high level of specialisation and division of labour. Without this specialisation it would not be possible to apply advanced technique and the many distinct functions provided by home care, consultants, laboratories, etc. At the same time, the patient requires a coherent service and expects the health care professionals involved having access to all relevant information. The authorities demand efficiency and quality in treatment, care and rehabilitation and the health care professionals want to deliver an esteemed and cost-effective service.

On average each hour of consultation with the general practitioner (GP) results in more than one message to another part of the health care sector. This generates a large flow of routine messages, such as prescriptions, referrals, examinations, discharge letters and laboratory results. When adding to the reimbursement communications (which makes up about one-third of the medical messages) the total number of messages exceeds the communication in the financial sector.

The cost of communication is equal to 1-2 % of the total health expenditures[2].
Because of the specialisation and division of labour, there is a need for extensive communication between the participants involved in the health care sector, i.e. communication of everyday routine messages such as prescriptions, referrals, discharge letters and laboratory results.

The PRIMACOM project addresses these challenges of the fragmented health care sector by using the experience from previous National and European projects by adaptation and implementation of UN/EDIFACT (United Nations/Electronic Data Interchange for Administration, Commerce and Trade) standards. The IT-systems are integrated by building Regional Health Care Network. It is important to mention that the regional Health Care Network is logical network integrated through EDI standards. The physical networks can be built in many different ways, depending on local conditions. In some regions they use modem and normal telephone lines, X.25, X.400 and even the Internet can be used for transferring the data depending of the level of security.

Once the Regional Health Care Network has been established, the communication will be of such size that operations and further developments are expected to continue under normal commercial conditions.

3. The Technology

The participants have computer systems from many different vendors, but the Regional Health Care Network together with the developed UN/EDIFACT standards makes electronic communication between the systems possible. The systems used by the different health care participants can exchange structured information and not only e-mails with free text. Thus, the data entered in the senders system can be "understood" and reused in the receivers system.

The basic idea of PRIMACOM is to send structured electronic messages from one computer to another computer. This means that data entered once can be re-used elsewhere in the sector. To make this EDI (Electronic Data Interchange) work, standards for the communications format are needed. PRIMACOM will start with the implementation of the most needed communication link, the discharge letter. This is an achievable goal with a large impact and a success in one area will pave the way for later extensions.

After having tested the transfer of discharge letters in Hungary and Slovenia the system providers and users will be familiar with the technique, and it will be easier to extend to other messages i.e. laboratory results and referrals.

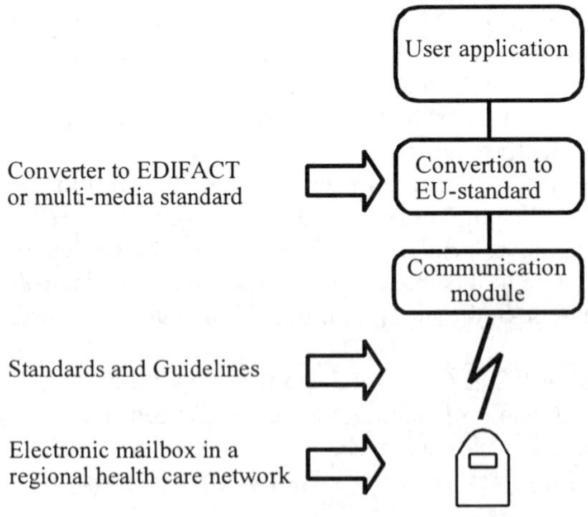

Figure 1 – The basic technology used in PRIMACOM

PRIMACOM is not inventing new technology, but is building on existing application, the most appropriate infrastructure in the specific situation, the European standardisation work and well-known mailbox technique to exchange data between the partners.

4. Standardisation

Standard messages are necessary to make large-scale communication from "all to all" in health care possible. Only if international standards are present and stable, market for integration can be developed. Therefore, several national and international organisations have been working with standardisation not only in the health care but also in trade, finance and commerce. In all these areas the UN/EDIFACT-syntax are used for interchange of structured data.

However, standardisation on this level is only the first step. Like in all other standardisation issues, the standardisation process is a dialectic process between general theoretically developed frameworks and practical work in pilot implementations. Only during practical testing, it is possible to develop real, functioning communication standards.

Today the European standardisation bodies have produced pre-standards and working documents for the classical messages in heath care. These standards are in nature broad, maximum frameworks using a pan-European generic terminology and are the first (but necessary) step towards European standards. In real implementation a much more precise description is needed using national terms and reducing the very complex European pre-standards. This precision and simplification can only be made during real implementation in pilot projects. In this process a consensus data list (CDL) showing exactly what part of the pre-standard are actually used in each pilot.

In the PRIMACOM project, a narrow EDIFACT and CDL for discharge letters have been made for the pilots and have been adjusted to specific needs in Hungary and Slovenia.

This paper has mainly focused on the specific syntax – EDIFACT – for electronic data interchange (EDI). However, EDI can take place using other syntaxes and communications technologies. Regardless of which syntax is used, the core of the standardisation process, i.e. the consensus process and the harmonisation of terminology and concepts, can not be avoided.

5. MedCom - the Danish Health Care Network

In recent years IT systems have been widely introduced into the Danish health care sector and IT systems are now used for the most common tasks in most hospitals, medical practices and pharmacies.

The spread of electronic patient record systems in general practice is Denmark started in spring 1983 and experienced explosive growth in 1994-95, following a slow development phase lasting 10 years. This course of developments is typical of many IT-systems in the health care sector. The development of electronic communication has probably been an important factor for the rapid growth of the patient record systems in general practices. The Danish Centre for Health Telematics has been a driving force in the dissemination of cross-sector electronic communication in Denmark through its co-ordination of regional and national programmes and European projects.

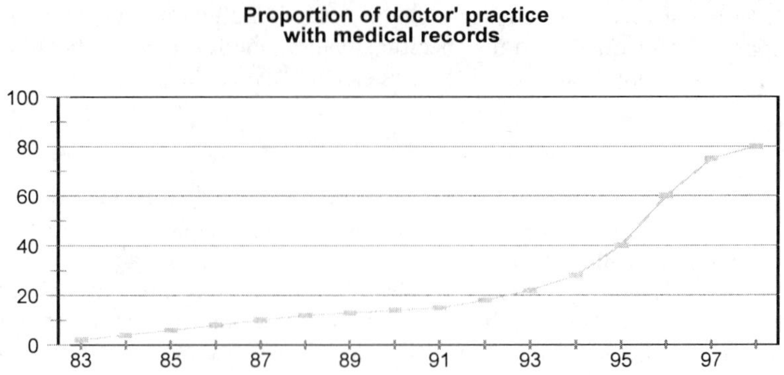

Figure 2 – The development in medical records, 1983-1998.

The Danish Centre for Health Telematics was established in December 1994 based on an initiative from the County of Funen. Three project groups under the same management are sharing facilities in the centre, all having implementation of Electronic Health Care Networks as the focal point. The three project groups are the regional networks FynCom, the national network MedCom and European projects working with standardisation and network in Europe. Furthermore, the centre provides Consultancy as well as project-support concerning Telematics in the health care sector.

The objectives of the centre are:

- to strengthen the quality, service and coherence in the health care sector by establishing electronic communication between parties in the health care sector,
- to utilise the centre's expertise to boos the commercial use of EDI in the health case sector in the County of Funen, in Denmark and internationally,
- to maintain and develop the expertise and jobs on Funen within the electronic communication in the health care sector.

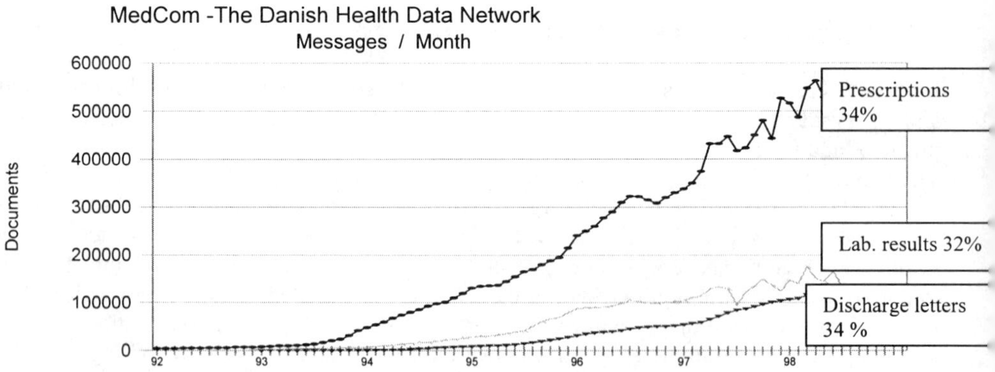

Figure 3. Messages per month in the National MedCom project. In total, approximately 1 million messages are exchanged per month.

The purpose of MedCom is to establish a nation-wide Danish health and social care data network. The most frequent types of health care messages are covered, based upon international EDIFACT-messages. Solutions using Internet, i.e. a combination of EDI and Internet, are also implemented. Today 35% of the prescriptions, laboratory results and discharge letters are sent through the network. The goal of the project is to increase this to 66% in year 2000, to extend the use of to other messages and to explore the use of Internet[3].

The project facilitates a standardised, open market for electronic communication (EDI). The individual SW-supplier develops and markets systems with communication capabilities. As a part of the project, pilot projects are being launched country wide, involving all Danish counties and more than 30 SW-suppliers for the health care sector.

The National Board of Health, the Danish county association and the Danish Telecom Company has made the financing of MedCom. The total investment in MedCom is DKK. 50 mill over five years and the direct saving in year 2000 are estimated to DKK. 250 mill per year.

6. PRIMACOM contractors and associated contractors:

DK	Danish Centre for Health Telematics.
	RAMBOLL Informatics.
H	VariMed.
	FADAM – Family Doctors Association of Miskolc.
	Semmelweis Hospital.
SI	FAGOR –Family Doctors Association of Kranjska Gora.
	INFONET.
I	TSD-Projects Srl.

References

[1] [1] INCO-COPERNICUS Information package, Co-operation with third countries and international organisations, European Commission DGs XII, III XIII,XVII, Second edition 1997/98.

[2] [2] Jensen H.B. The missing Link. May 1994.

[3] [3] MedCom – the Danish Health Care Network towards the year 2000. March 1998.09.04

[4] [4] Bangeman, M. Recommendations to the European Council. Europe and the global information society. The European Commission 1994.

Medical Informatics Europe '99
P. Kokol et al. (Eds.)
IOS Press, 1999

Teleradiology as a seed of the Regional Health Care Intranet in a rural region in Spain

Juan Pablo de Castro, Roberto Hornero, Alonso Alonso, Begoña Medina, Rafael Mompó, Evaristo Abril, Miguel López
E.T.S.I. Telecomunicación. University of Vallodolid- 47011 Spain

Abstract. Castilla y León is a rural region with a very sparse population of about 2,560,000 habitants. Special health care challenges appear due to this region's very aged population and large dimensions. A theoretical model of services of Telemedicine is proposed and an experimental teleradiology trial is carried out between a rural Health Care Centre and its Reference Hospital to make easier the planning of future projects. The total number of studies was increased due to availability of specialised support and higher skills of physicians, but the percentage of studies consulted to specialists diminished. Continuing education through physicians communication was hightly improved.

1. Introduction

With an extension of 94.224 squared kilometres Castilla y León is the biggest Autonomous Community of Spain and of the European Union. Its population of about 2,560,000 makes its density rather low: 27.1 inhabitants per squared kilometre, only the third of the population density of Spain that is nearly 77 which also is lower than the mean density of Europe. Not only its mean density is low, but also with 97,9% of the villages having a population of less than 5,000 inhabitants, this region has a great dispersion. [1]

Moreover, there is a very aged and rural population that increases the need of health care. The rural dwellers often have the sensation of being discriminated, causing a lack of social cohesion. [2]

The Regional Government and local telecommunications operators are considering a regional Intranet as the solution of supporting a variety of services including Telemedicine. Our work is intended to be the theoretical approximation to a future global system and to estimate the technical and functional requirements of such an Intranet. Based on the local Health Care System activity we can help the planning of new services with a-priori realistic information that nowadays is not available.

2. Methods

In order to arrange the aforementioned information in a useful way, we have formed a space of services and infrastructures that comprises both the medical services and technical requirements points of view. By crossing the categories we have formed a grid of cells that forms our model for Telemedicine services parameterisation.

Both the medical areas of actuation and technical categories were discussed and defined in several round tables with politicians, health care system managers, and technicians according to the current state and needs of the region.

The data types were classified by technical requirements as:

- *Laboratory reports or analytics.* This is treated separately because it is a very critical information item in the diagnostic chain, so it was considered to be treated with priority.
- *Clinical and management data.* This includes medical reports and other information atoms of day to day health care system's function. It carries the information from which clinical records are made of, and provides the physicians with the best information available for making their diagnostic.

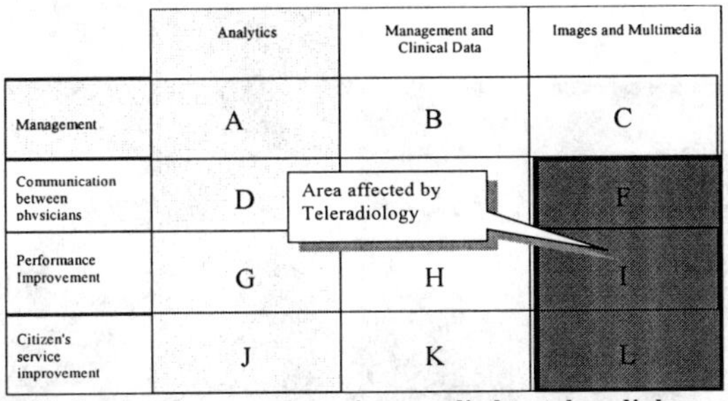

Fig. 1: Model of infrastructures and services applied to teleradiology applications.

- *Images and Multimedia.* This type of information is the most exigent type of data. Although videoconferencing is the preferred way of interaction, it is not an essential part of Telemedicine; this is why roughly 60% of Telemedicine projects uses store and forward systems. [3] Imaging techniques are the principal diagnostic tool of modern medical practice and it generates the greater part of the information.

The medical services categories are:

- *Management.* This is the information needed by managers to drive the sanitary units and regional health plans.
- *Information provision and communication between physicians.* This includes the services aimed to make information available to physicians in the form of clinical data about patients, interaction with colleagues, continued training, etc.
- *Service improvement for the citizens.* These applications are intended to make available new services for patients or to improve those that are already working but are very limited or inefficient.

A representation of the aforementioned model is shown in Fig.1 with the areas affected by teleradiology remarked as an example.

Each cell formed is suitable to be studied in terms of transmission and storage requirements, benefits and costs. As similar applications require similar resources, anyone interested in implanting a telemedicine project in Castilla y León can find this model useful as a source of realistic measures. This information is not available by today. It is necessary a first step like this study to facilitate the planning of future projects.

Several simplifications and assumptions are needed to obtain useful results. Per example, the way a hypothetical service will perform or the acceptance it will have between the users is an unknown difficult to estimate before the real system is tested. The future ratio between digitised images to conventional ones and the pattern of consultations are other sources of uncertainty in estimates.

3. Teleradiology trial

In order to test real world applications a teleradiology experiment was under trial from January 1998 and it continues by today. Initial use of the system is represented in figure 3, in the second year the consults rate is almost one per day.

It connects a small rural health care centre with its reference hospital 50-km away. The platform is composed by a pair of UNIX workstations linked by a basic ISDN line. As the primary care centre has no digital radiology equipment, it was equipped with a laser scanner (LUMISCAN 75) that is able to digitise the conventional radiograph with the quality and fidelity required. A large plate is transformed in a digital image of 2500 by 2000 pixels with 12 bits of contrast resolution with an optical density of 0.001 OD LSB.

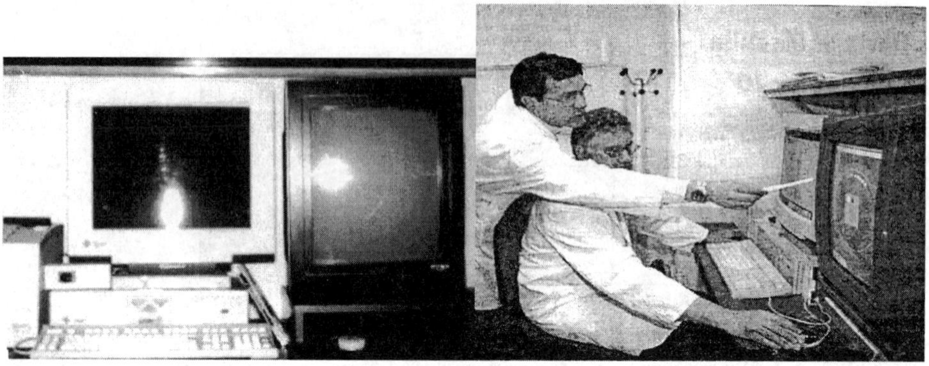

Fig. 2: Teleradiology workstation with high resolution monitor and radiologists at work.

The radiologist's workstation has a pair of high-resolution and high-contrast monitors (MEGASCAN UHR 4820-P with DOME video controller) that are able of displaying 2000 by 2500 pixels images with an higher luminosity than conventional computer monitors. (See figure 2) [4]

The human resources involved in the trial comprise two radiologists at the hospital, eleven general practitioners at the rural centre of health care, and an engineer for supporting and maintaining the equipment.

Each film is digitised and sent by the practitioners in a few minutes. After a lossless compression, it is transmitted in about 10 minutes. When the radiologist receives the message in his mailbox, he informs the case and reply with the answer. If necessary, a collaborative session for shared consultation is established between both then radiologist and the general practitioner.

More than 75% of the studies are of thoratic radiographs, which are the most exigent modalities of radiology (except mamography). This type of imaging requires a resolution of 2000x2000, which matches a radiological resolution of four pairs of lines in each millimetre. Although there are other imaging modalities less exigent, they are not useful to rural areas because such equipment is often confined to specialised centres like hospitals, and not rural health centres. (US, CT, MR, etc.) [5, 6]

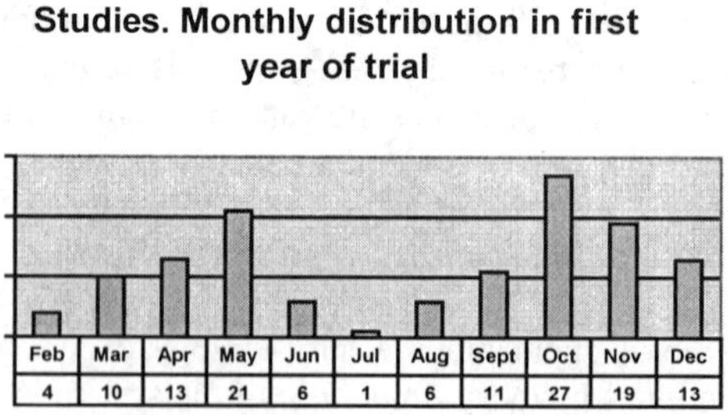

Fig.3: Studies transmitted with the system during the first year.

4. Results and conclusions

In the course of the trial, some conclusions was learned:

- The number of radiology studies made in the rural centre grew by 17%, from nearly 3200 to 3800 per year. Physicians remark two important reasons: the availability of an easily accessible specialised support and the great improvement of formation acquired by the general practitioners due to interaction with specialists.
- In spite of the increase of radiograph generation, the percentage of images that needs to be consulted with teleradiology diminished as the experience of physicians increased. (This is especially true in tuberculosis control that is the most difficult and frequent diagnostic task in this rural area.)
- The opinion of specialists about image quality of the system is that specific monitors are required only in a very small fraction of the cases. For non-radiologists' work is enough with a lower resolution image and conventional monitors, but always with the radiologist's report attached.
- A few urgent cases where treated with the aid of this teleradiology system, showing that the better communication between primary and specialised health care the better the service received by patients. Some urgent transportation where avoided and some special cases where treated much faster than with traditional clinical protocols.
- In the organisational side, the physicians ask for a re-estructuration of clinical protocols more oriented to information flow instead of current static procedure lists.

The aim of this experiment and further projects is to improve physician's communication and implication of patients in their own health care by means of an easy access to health care system and information.

The current political and strategic circumstances are important for the deployment of telemedicine in Castilla y León, because both deregulation of telecommunications and shift of responsibilities in health care from the central to the regional autonomous government are happening. The imminent shift of health care management responsibilities to the Junta de Castilla y León (regional government) makes the current moment a good one to test new processes and technologies to improve the health care system in this region. Taking advantage of this propitious background to introduce changes in a wide range of institutions, the regional Intranet is being planned as a solution to the region's challenges by supporting a variety of services including telemedicine.

References

[1] Consejería de Economía y Hacienda: *Anuario estadístico de Castilla y León*, Junta de Castilla y León, 1996, Valladolid, Spain

[2] Jeremy Holland (CEST): *Telemedicina: cumplimiento de la promesa* The IPTS Report, IPTS - JRC, pp 28, September 1997, Sevilla, Spain

[3] Randy Barrett: *Telemedicine on the rise on the Internet* Interactive Week, Interactive Enterprises Inc, Inter@ctive Week, May 12, 1997, EEUU

[4] Brent K.Stewart, Denise R. Aberle, M. Ines Boechat, Zoran Barbaric, Ricky K. Taira, James W. Sayre, Samuel J. Dwyer III: *Clinical utilization of grayscale workstations* IEEE Engineering in Medicine and Biology, IEEE, March 1993, EEUU

[5] D.F.Leotta, Y.Kim: *Requirements for picture archiving and communications* IEEE Engineering in Medicine and Biology, IEEE, March 1993, EEUU

[6] Seong K.Mun, Matthew Freedman, Rajiv Kapur: *Image management and communications for radiology* IEEE Engineering in Medicine and Biology, IEEE, March 1993, EEUU

Medical Informatics Europe '99
P. Kokol et al. (Eds.)
IOS Press, 1999

Teledermatology - UK Experience of Setting up an Integrated Teledermatology Service

M Clarke, R W Jones, D Lioupis, S George*, D Cairns*
Brunel University, Uxbridge, UK
**Amersham General Hospital, Amersham, UK*

Abstract. Telemedicine has traditionally been seen as an all or nothing solution to the problem of providing medical service to remote communities. In the UK, however, the majority of the population lives within easy travelling distance of medical service, and it is inappropriate to apply telemedicine for the same reasons and in the same way. We describe an alternative approach, where telemedicine is used to complement the existing clinical infrastructure of the outreach clinic and hospital visit, and the patient may opt to have any follow up appointments by video conference. We also describe the concept of the virtual consultation that we have developed to support our work.

1. Introduction

Telemedicine has traditionally been seen as an all or nothing solution to the problem of providing medical service to remote communities. In the UK, however, the majority of the population lives within easy travelling distance of medical service, and it is inappropriate to apply telemedicine for the same reasons and in the same way. A new role must be found. This leads to the conclusion that telemedicine should be integrated within a range of options that are offered to patients for their convenience.

Telemedicine projects are comparatively widespread, with numerous examples of its application in many areas of medicine. Dermatology has been shown to adapt well to telemedicine, and has been particularly popular. Many studies have shown that the rates of correct diagnosis and decisions for appropriate treatment plan are similar to face to face consultation [1, 2, 3, 4], even using low cost video conferencing equipment and standard ISDN-2 data rates of 128 kbps [5]. Others have also shown that the technique is well accepted by both patient and doctor [6, 7, 8]. Its use in a remote environment, where it can remove the need for any face to face contact, is not doubted [9, 10]. Video conferencing has been shown to be critical to the success of teledermatology and the success rates for correct diagnosis can be improved to 95%, compared to 80% for simple store and forward methods using electronic reports incorporating digital images [11, 12].

2. The Project

2.1. Clinical Methods

Outreach clinics in a general practice surgery are currently given by a consultant dermatologist once a month, patients normally being referred to the clinic by the GP. In the clinic, patients would be given a treatment plan, but may also be required to attend the hospital clinic for treatment or investigation. In general, these patients require a subsequent follow up consultation, which currently takes place at an outpatient clinic in the hospital, as this is where the clinical information of any hospital procedures on a patient is held. Although the hospital is not a great distance, it can be an inconvenient journey, and it is stressful. We have chosen to integrate telemedicine into the current service by offering the patients the option of having their follow up consultation using virtual consultation. A doctor or nurse will be present with the patient at the remote site, figure 1.

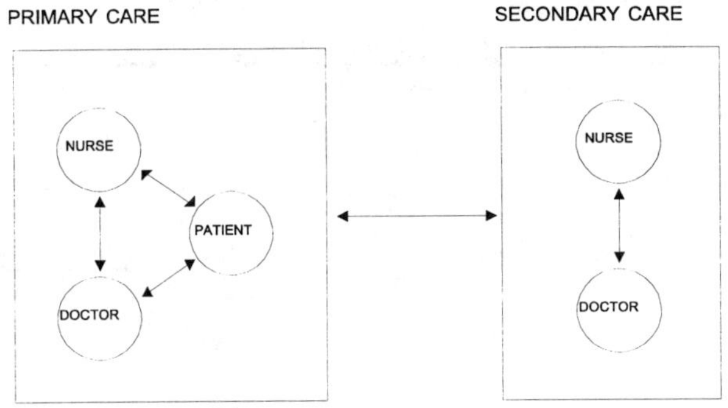

Figure 1. The Virtual Consultation

2.2. Virtual Consultation

The face to face consultation in dermatology will often involve all five physical senses, and frequently the sixth, intuition. The virtual consultation must be able to provide a communication channel for each of these, if the same success as the face to face consultation is to be achieved. We have used low cost video conferencing to give sight and sound, and augment this by using still digital pictures to provide high definition views. Video is interactive, and affords the opportunity to question the patient and elicit vital information that may help lead to a correct diagnosis, a significant advantage over any store and forward technique. During the consultation, the patient is accompanied by a medically trained person, figure 2, who can be the "hands and nose" of the consultant and can also operate the camera to achieve an optimum view or angle to aid diagnosis. However, they may have a significantly more important role, that of an advocate for the patient during the consultation.

2.3. Communications Infrastructure

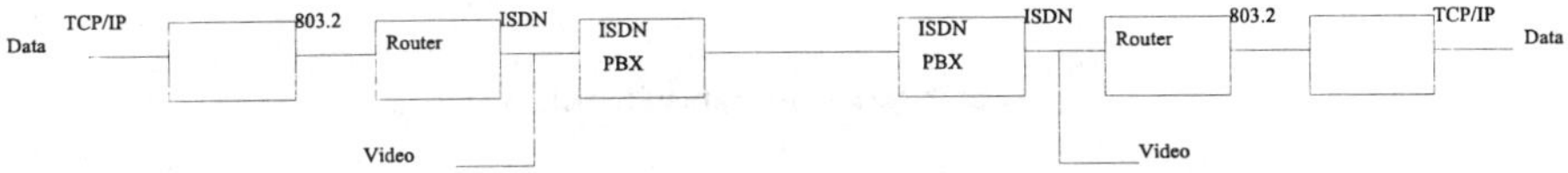

Figure 2. Network Infrastructure

The system, figure 2, is currently built on the use of ISDN basic rate for its communications infrastructure. This supports both TCP/IP for data transfer outside of video conferencing sessions using ISDN routers, and the H320 protocol for video conferencing. We may investigate using TCP/IP to carry video. Although this would degrade the service due to the packet overhead that is incurred and the possibility of excess traffic, it would give greater flexibility in distribution of the video stream within each site on the local area network. Data transfer may also be accomplished within a video conference using the T120 tools, which also support application sharing. This latter facility is particularly useful as it can allow access to information stored remotely by running an application on the remote system to access that information. Data transfer can be of high resolution images taken by digital camera or scanner, and by disabling the video stream, the full 128 kbps is available, which allows moderate sized images to be transferred in seconds.

2.4. Assessment Methods

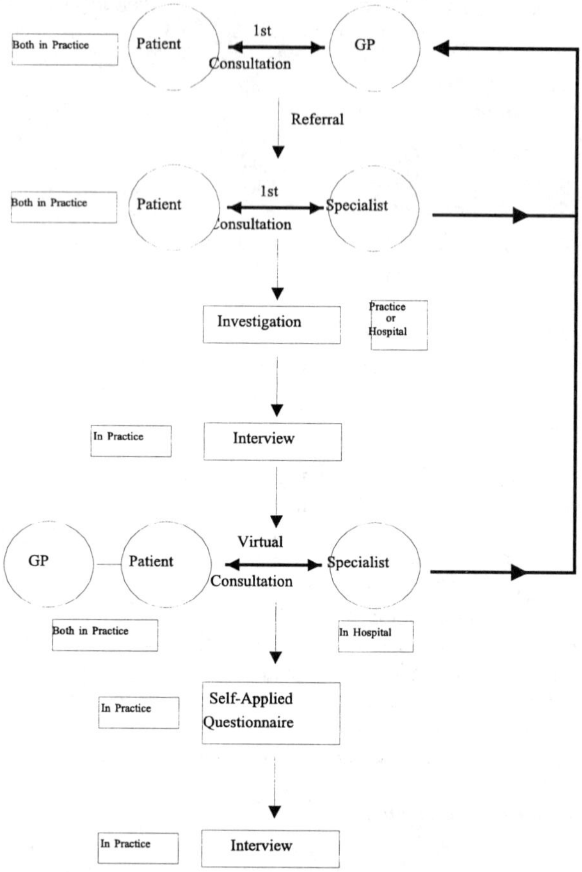

Figure 3. Determining Patient Satisfaction

The purpose of the study is to assess patient satisfaction with telemedicine as an alternative to the more usual hospital visit. We are using a combination of self-applied questionnaires and recorded interviews to determine the perception of patient in terms of their satisfaction with the process and with the outcome of the consultation. We are also interviewing the patients in advance of their virtual consultation to try to assess the preconceptions that the patients take with them to a medical consultation and how this may influence their perception of the virtual consultation.

3. Discussion

It is too early to discuss the final results of the work in this paper, and we can only present the system design and our expectations at this stage. Our aim is to investigate how such a service could be integrated into an existing service to improve the patient experience, both in terms of the perception of the consultation and the impact of advocacy on the consultation process. Others have reported their observation of advocacy in the consultation [7], but we are not aware of any detailed study into this phenomenon.

Our concepts are being extended to support the outreach clinics of other areas of medicine, including cardiology and general surgery.

4. Conclusion

Telemedicine clearly has an increasingly important role to play in numerous application areas. We hope to show that its role should not simply be restricted to the all or nothing solution of communication to remote areas and that it has value as one of a number of services available to patients. Early results indicate that patients like its convenience and that having a familiar doctor or nurse familiar makes the consultation more attractive and improves the quality of outcome.

Acknowledgements

The AIDMAN Project is funded by the Commission of the European Communities Directorate General XIII – Contract TEN 45593 (FS).

References

[1] Gilmour E, et al, Comparison of teleconsultations and face-to-face consultations: preliminary results of a United Kingdom multicentre teledermatology study, *British Journal of Dermatology*, **139** (1):81-7, 1998 Jul.

[2] Loane MA, et al, Diagnostic accuracy and clinical management by realtime teledermatology. Results from the Northern Ireland arms of the UK Multicentre Teledermatology Trial, *Journal of Telemedicine & Telecare*, **4** (2):95-100, 1998.

[3] Lowitt MH, et al, Teledermatology and in-person examinations: a comparison of patient and physician perceptions and diagnostic agreement, *Archives of Dermatology*, **134** (4):471-6, 1998 Apr.

[4] Lesher JL Jr, et al, Telemedicine evaluation of cutaneous diseases: a blinded comparative study, *Journal of the American Academy of Dermatology*, **38** (1):27-31, 1998 Jan.

[5] Tsuchiya H, Telemedicine using a desktop conference system (Phoenix) in Kyushu, Japan, *Telemedicine Journal*, **4** (1):43-8, 1998 Spring.

[6] Freeman K, Groves-Phillips S, Lewis L, Telemedicine and Education, *World Congress on Telemedicine*, Nov 1995 pp188.

[7] Freeman K, Wynn-Jones J, Groves-Phillips S, Lewis L, Teleconsulting - a practical account of pitfalls, problems and promise, experience from the TEAM project group, *Journal of Telemedicine & Telecare*, **2** Suppl 1:11-13, 1996.

[8] Low S J, Lewis L, Goldberg B, Transforming the Patient Experience Through Telemedicine, **HC '96** Harrogate.

[9] Oakley AM, Duffill MB, Reeve P, Practising dermatology via telemedicine, *New Zealand Medical Journal*, **111** (1071):296-9, 1998 Aug 14.

[10] Jones DH, et al, Teledermatology in the Highlands of Scotland, *Journal of Telemedicine & Telecare*, **2** Suppl 1:7-9, 1996.

[11] Zelickson BD, Homan L, Teledermatology in the nursing home, *Archives of Dermatology*, **133** (2):171-4, 1997 Feb.

[12] Kvedar JC, et al, The substitution of digital images for dermatologic physical examination, *Archives of Dermatology*, **133** (2):161-7, 1997 Feb.

Medical Informatics Europe '99
P. Kokol et al. (Eds.)
IOS Press, 1999

Third Generation Electronic Pharmacy Communications

Recommendations Based On Ten Years' Experience

Karin Demkjær, Ib Johansen and Knut Bernstein
Danish Centre for Health Telematics, Heden 18, 5000 Odense C, Denmark

Abstract: The number of electronic prescriptions in Denmark is increasing and almost 600,000 electronic prescriptions are now sent every month. There is therefore a strong interest in directly reusing the data entered in the medical practitioner systems in the pharmacy systems. It has therefore been decided to introduce a shared data foundation in all medical practitioner and pharmacy systems in Denmark in conjunction with the introduction of the new MEDPRE electronic prescription standard. Parallel to the standardisation work, concrete guidelines have been prepared for the individual EDP (Electronic Data Processing) systems to ensure rapid, problem-free prescription communication. The aim in the longer term [1] is for 95% of all EDIFACT prescriptions to reach the receiving pharmacy no more than 20 minutes after being sent from a medical practice.

1. Introduction

Electronic prescription communication [2] started in Denmark at the beginning of the 90s with the "Amager trial". Data from the doctor's EDP system was transferred directly to a pharmacy system, which in turn used the data for direct reordering from the wholesaler. A national EDIFACT standard for prescriptions (RECEPT) was developed. This standard was later extended and all medical practitioner and pharmacy EDP systems were required to be subjected to the Danish National Board of Health's approval procedure. The international EDIFACT message MEDPRE (MEDical PREscription) has now replaced RECEPT, which, in spite of many years' faithful service, has shown itself to be unsatisfactory in certain essential areas. The guidelines for mapping and data content for the system houses were insufficient and unclear.

The MEDPRE project aims to design, implement, test and spread the use of the new MEDPRE electronic prescription standard for all the EDP systems of doctors and pharmacies in Denmark. A prerequisite for MEDPRE's improving the data content in prescriptions is the simultaneous implementation of a shared data foundation. [3]

The Danish National Board of Health, the Danish Pharmaceutical Association and the Danish Medical Association support the implementation of the new prescription message based on MEDPRE. In connection with this process, one working group has formulated requirements for the implementation of MEDPRE, while another working group has been engaged in co-ordinating the existing medicinal databases.

The CEN/TC 251 standardisation organisation has prepared a number of syntax-independent standards for medicinal communication. These are being implemented as EDIFACT messages in collaboration with EBES/EEG9. MEDPRE has been developed under the auspices of EBES/EEG9. [4]

2. Implementation of a shared data foundation and simultaneous updating in the medical practitioner and pharmacy systems

Before the start of the project, it was found that a large percentage of all EDIFACT prescriptions caused problems due to uncertain identification, as the product number and medicinal name did not concur. This problem, as well as a desire for improved possibilities for the automatic production of labels at the pharmacy, could only be solved by all parties using a common database that was updated in a uniform fashion and that contained codes for texts to as great an extent as possible. Parallel to the implementation of MEDPRE, it is therefore the objective to create practical (including financial) opportunities for updating the common data foundation among medical practitioners, so that the despatching parties have access to the same data foundation as the pharmacies.

If a doctor's system despatches EDIFACT prescriptions, its medical databases are to be updated using a new version of the data foundation (usually once every fortnight in accordance with given deadlines). There are no requirements regarding updating deadlines if the system does not despatch EDIFACT prescriptions, but the user saves both himself and the pharmacy the trouble of making contact for clarification purposes if the database is regularly updated. A questionnaire study [5] performed among all doctors with EDIFACT communication has shown that only a third of doctors currently update every fortnight and that over half of the medical practices update their data foundation every third month or even more seldom.

Updating occurs in different ways. Almost 60% currently update using floppy disks supplied by an EDP system supplier. This will be changed in line with the MEDPRE project's requirement for updating once every fortnight. Approx. one third can at present retrieve data from a BBS and a number of medical practitioner systems can also download the data foundation from the Internet.

One of the MEDPRE project's goals is for 80-90% of the text in despatched EDIFACT prescriptions to be sent in coded form. This covers dosage and indication texts. This requires that the texts match the needs. The plan is thus to analyse the prescriptions sent to one or several pharmacies in order to catch frequently recurring non-coded texts and then to encode these texts.

The medical practitioner's system must support the option of choosing between proposed dosage texts and proposed indications that are medicine-specific. The system house or the users must not enter other coded texts for a given medicine.

It is a natural idea that, instead of entering free text, it should be possible to retrieve an already existent text from the database's tables covering all dosage texts and indications. It is important to note, however, that in functional terms this will be a free text, the code should not be used. The pharmacy's check of the prescription must find instances in which the code does not belong to the data foundation's codes for texts for the relevant medicine.

The implementation of coded proposed texts in the data foundation will also introduce a new style for these texts, as the texts are formulated so that they can be transferred directly to the label on the medicine (this will not just be an option, it will be mandatory). This poses greater requirements to the users, who must be aware that free texts are also transferred directly to the label.

3. Recommendations for an optimal medical practitioner system/pharmacy system and flow of prescriptions

Parallel to the MEDPRE project, all the prior procedures in the medical practitioner systems, on-call doctor systems and pharmacy systems have been analysed (the DUR report concerning the ultra-fast prescription).

3.1 Method

A number of interviews and visits to users and software suppliers have been made, and information on experiences and proposals for improvements has been collected. In order further to clarify issues relating to medical practitioners' use of EDIFACT prescriptions and communication of these, questionnaires have been sent to all medical practices with a location number.

The questionnaire was sent to 1,172 medical practices and replies from 792 practices (equivalent to just over 67%) were received. The number of doctors in the practices that have responded amounts to almost 73% of doctors with electronic addresses.

Likewise, a questionnaire was sent to all pharmacies regarding their use of EDIFACT prescriptions. The questionnaire was sent to 335 pharmacy units, of which 258 (77%) have replied. The answers were received in the period November 1997 – January 1998. On the basis of this information and the conclusions in Dan Net's analysis of the tele-infrastructure in the health sector [6], detailed guidelines and proposed improvements have been prepared for each system supplier.

The final goal for these guidelines is to provide the basis for uniform procedures for doctors and pharmacies, so that the goals of fast prescription communication can be achieved. These goals are specified as follows:

1. 95% of all EDIFACT prescriptions reaching the pharmacy no more than 20 minutes after being sent from a medical practice.
2. 95% of all EDIFACT prescriptions reaching the pharmacy no more than 5 minutes after being sent from an emergency medical service.

3.2 Functional requirements for a medical practice system

The report first describes the optimal system for a medical practice seen in relation to prescription communication. Some of the recommendations for the optimal system for a medical practice are described below. The medical practice system should be a true multi-tasking system (e.g. Windows 95/NT), so that communication can run in the background. All medical practices should have an ISDN modem and ISDN connection.

The main recommendations for an optimal system for a medical practice are given below:

- The common data foundation should be updated once every fortnight in the system's background, so that the medical practice does not have to remember to do this.
- All the pharmacy's electronic addresses should be updated in the system.
- Prescriptions should be despatched automatically. At suitable intervals (depending on the number of doctors in the practice), the system should check whether there is anything to despatch.
- An electronic receipt should be issued for the receipt of a prescription.
- In the event of an error in the call-up to the VANS (value added network services), the system should automatically call up three times until the transmission is correctly sent/received.

- It should be possible to investigate the cause of significant communication problems through a communications menu. This menu should list possible errors in the communication system (e.g. no contact to modem, no dial tone, VANS busy, lack of connection, wrong baud rate, error in transmission).
- All prescriptions generated by a medical practice should automatically be ready for transmission. The doctor should be made aware via his screen of any prescriptions generated by a secretary that are awaiting approval in good time before the next call up to the VANS.
- Prescriptions should be created in a journal system, where it should be possible to see which medicines have previously been prescribed to the patient.
- If a whole prescription or a single medicine is deleted during the approval procedure, this should be automatically deleted in the patient's journal. This will avoid a number of misunderstandings between the doctor, pharmacy and patient (most often the "abuser").
- It should not be possible to re-prescribe a fixed medicine that has been removed from the common data foundation since the last prescription.
- PUSH technology should be used for the reception of EDIFACT prescriptions so that the pharmacies receive the prescriptions on an on-going basis.

3.3 Processing an EDIFACT prescription at the pharmacy

When the prescription is processed, the data is automatically displayed on the screen for approval. Changes can be made during the procedure as required (parallel imports, delivery, etc.). Prescriptions that have not been created using a coded dosage or indication that complies with the MEDPRE standard are highlighted when displayed. The pharmacy can thus see which prescriptions require a special pharmacist check.

3.4 The present transmission pattern

There are not many medical practices with a communications set-up that automatically calls up a VANS at regular intervals. Approx. 50% transmit only once to three times a day, or not at all. The timing of the different medical practices' call-ups also coincide (when telephone consultation is finished and around lunchtime). It is desirable that this should be changed so that there is a more even distribution of the receipt of prescriptions at the pharmacies. An even flow of received prescriptions at the pharmacies will allow them to prepare the medicine so that it is ready to be delivered to the patients when they ask for it. It is clearly apparent from the free-text answers to the questionnaire that the doctors and patients desire this.

4. Conclusion

The implementation of electronic prescriptions depends to a high degree on the implementation of a common data foundation among all the involved parties and the simultaneous introduction of the new MEDPRE standard for prescriptions. In addition, a number of functional requirements relating to the medical practitioner system must be fulfilled. The DUR report recommends the appearance that an optimal medical practitioner system should have.

The description of the optimal system has been received positively by the suppliers, several of whom have announced that they will make program changes in line with the DUR project's recommendations. Following the program changes, an intensive effort in the areas of training and information for users must be made. One medicinal supplier has developed and installed a prototype of an "optimal" system, seen from the aspect of prescription communication. This has halved the average time from when a secretary-generated prescription is written until it is approved and forwarded to the VANS. One doctor has also installed an ISDN connection. According to the doctor, this connection is much faster than an ordinary telephone connection.

As the flow of prescriptions, in line with the recommendations of the DUR project, becomes better distributed over the doctors' consultation time, and the MEDPRE prescription standard and the common data foundation are implemented, with a consequent more error-free use of data in the pharmacies, it will be possible for all the pharmacies to process prescriptions before these are asked for by the customers/patients.

References

[1] [1]MedCom – the Danish health care data network towards the year 2000. MedCom publication. March 1998.

[2] Jensen et al. MEDPRE – den nye EDIFACT recept (MEDPRE – the new EDIFACT prescription). Farmaci no. 9, 1998 (in Danish).

[3] [3] Testprocedure ved implementering af MEDPRE (Test procedure in the implementation of MEDPRE). The Danish National Board of Health. April 1998 (in Danish).

[4] [4] Meddelelses-implementering-vejledning til MEDPRE-meddelelser (Message implementation guidelines for MEDPRE messages). The Danish National Board of Health. June 1997(in Danish).

[5] [5] DUR rapporten (DUR report). MedCom publication. May 1998 (in Danish).

[6] [6] Analyse af teleinfrastrukturen i sundhedssektoren (Analysis of the tele-infrastructure in the health sector). Dan Net A/S. February 1998 (in Danish).

Medical Informatics Europe '99
P. Kokol et al. (Eds.)
IOS Press, 1999

Telemedicine in the Malaysian Multimedia Super Corridor: Towards Personalised Lifetime Health Plans

Syed Sibte Raza ABIDI & Zaharin YUSOFF
Health Informatics Research Group, School of Computer Sciences,
Universiti Sains Malaysia, 11800 Penang, Malaysia.

Abstract. The Malaysian Telemedicine initiative advocates a paradigm shift in healthcare delivery patterns by way of implementing a person-centred and wellness-focused healthcare system. This paper introduces the Malaysian Telemedicine vision, its functionality and associated operational conditions. In particular, we focus on the conceptualisation of one key Telemedicine component i.e. the *Lifetime Health Plan (LHP)* system—a distributed multi-module application for the periodic monitoring and generation of health-care advisories for all Malaysians. In line with the LHP project, we present an innovative healthcare delivery info-structure—*LifePlan*—that aims to provide life-long, pro-active, personalised, wellness-oriented healthcare services to assist individuals to manage and interpret their health needs. Functionally, *LifePlan* based healthcare services are delivered over the WWW, packaged as *Personalised Lifetime Health Plans* that allow individuals to both monitor their health status and to guide them in healthcare planning.

1. Introduction

The Malaysian *Multimedia Super Corridor* (MSC) [1] is a large-scale Information Technology (IT) infrastructure and services project initiated by the Malaysian government. The MSC-based Telemedicine initiative takes a holistic view of healthcare, thereby promoting a person-centred and wellness-focused healthcare system that aims to deliver hitherto remote 'information-centred' healthcare services at the individual, family and community-level. The label "Tele-Health" is perhaps a more appropriate description of the MSC Telemedicine initiative [2] [3].

The MSC Telemedicine initiative, in particular the *Lifetime Health Plan (LHP)* pilot project, provides the best opportunity to promote a paradigm shift vis-à-vis a shift of primary focus towards the health information and maintenance needs of the consumers of healthcare services rather than its providers. The LHP project proposes an 'innovative' healthcare system that emphasises wellness maintenance (as opposed to illness management) and re-asserts the role of the individual in maintaining his or her health, on a continuous 'life-long' basis.

In this paper, we will give a brief overview of the *Lifetime Health Plan (LHP)* [4] pilot project. We will present an innovative healthcare delivery info-structure, called *LifePlan* [5], [6], [7], that aims to meet the charted objectives of the LHP Project.

2. The MSC-Telemedicine Based Lifetime Health Plan Project: An Overview

The MSC Telemedicine model encompass four key pilot projects: (1) *Customised/Personalised Health Information and Education*, (2) *Continuing Medical*

Education, (3) *Teleconsultation* and (4) *Lifetime Health Plan (LHP)*. The remainder of this paper specifically concentrates on fleshing out the LHP component of the MSC-Telemedicine project.

The LHP is probably the most unique and yet complex of all the Telemedicine pilot projects. Key feature of the LHP system is its person-centred implementation, ensuring a lifelong continuity between episodic contacts with healthcare service providers (throughout the nation). A systematic, consistent and temporally relevant summary of an individual's Electronic Medical Record (EMR) will manifest as the *Lifetime Health Record (LHR)*—which is to be used to formulate prospective *Personalised Lifetime Health Plans (PLHP)* that cater for both wellness preservation and illness treatment. In summary, the LHP project will provide the healthcare infrastructure to deliver PLHPs directly via the WWW to individuals or alternatively via primary healthcare providers. The LHP project is designed as a suite of integrated application systems, divided into three basic components on the basis of their intended functionality: (1) *Clinical Support Systems;* (2) *Healthcare Information Management and Support Services (HIMSS);* and (3) The *PLHP system* for the generation and delivery of lifelong healthcare plans—PLHPs—pro-actively customised to meet each individual's specific health needs.

The major role of the PLHP system is to generate individual PLHPs tailored to specific wellness and illness requirements of individuals. Once generated, the PLHPs will be stored in the LHP repository, and will be frequently referenced by their 'owners'. A typical PLHP will integrate all existing medical records (the past), with all recommended healthcare plans assigned by various healthcare providers (the future). The emergent PLHP, is intended to be easily understood by individuals, thereby placing them in a much better position to make well-informed health-related choices. More so, the PLHP will dynamically adjust itself with respect to changes in an individual's state of health.

3. Functional Description of LifePlan

LifePlan is a sophisticated healthcare deleivery info-structure that aims to provide life-long, pro-active, personalised healthcare services to assist individuals to manage and interpret their health needs based on their health history. Put simply, LifePlan will act as an agent representing and guarding the person's health-related interests and concerns, enabling a continuum of care for the individual. LifePlan will maintain comprehensive, cumulative, correct, coherent and changing *Personalised Lifetime Health Plans (PLHP)* – personalised healthcare plans that 'intelligently' integrate existing illness records (the past health perspective) with wellness plans (the future health perspective) to guide the individual in healthcare planning. The value-added component of LIfePlan is that the PLHP will dynamically adjust itself with respect to changes in an individual's state of health. LifePlan will empower individuals to take responsibility for and an active role in *monitoring* and *maintaining* their own (and their family's) health status. This will be achieved by providing an Internet based health monitoring and recording system through which individuals will be able to monitor their own and their family's health status [8].

In IT terms, LifePlan is an amalgamation of diverse computer technologies—Artificial Intelligence [9] [10], Multimedia [11], Internet and Databases—and is realised by a systematic integration of various task-specific modules. A fusion of technology, role transformation and behavioural change is the distinguishing facet of LifePlan [12].

Figure 1 below describes the overall healthcare delivery system pertaining to LifePlan in more detail and charts our methodology behind the design of LifePlan. Note that the health management team (Mgt. Team) depicted on the left hand side of the Figure 1 reflects two critical changes to the current healthcare models: (1) The individual becomes an integral part of this team and assumes 'ownership' for their wellbeing; and (2) Health management occurs in the community, with the primary care provider assuming a 'wellness' focus and new responsibility as 'gatekeeper' to the healthcare delivery system.

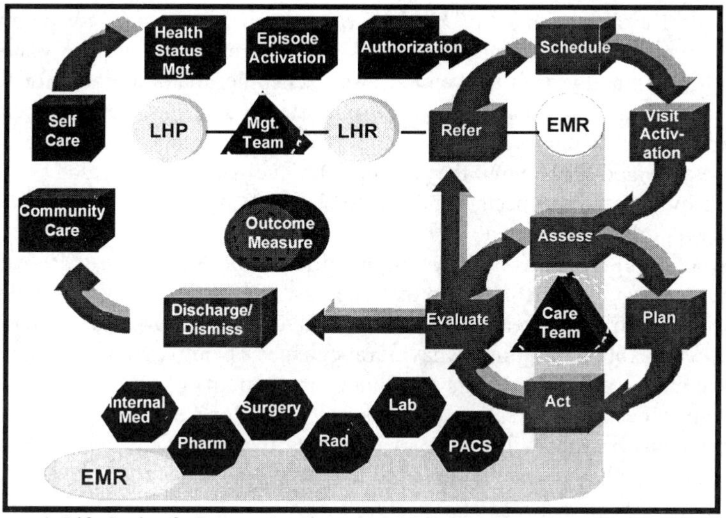

Figure 1: Life Cycle of a Persons Involvement with the Healthcare Management System.

Figure 1 provides an overview of the life cycle of an individual's involvement within the healthcare management system. Each box in the diagram represents a major process or workflow element that can be further described as a number of discrete activities depending on the specific environment (e.g. care setting, level of automation, etc.). Community and "wellness" related processes are depicted in the left half of Figure 1. It is here that an individual spends most of his/her life. Whilst, care delivery processes are depicted in the right half of the Figure 1. We explain below the lifecycle of an individual within the proposed healthcare management system, which in turn also illustrates our methodology behind the design of LifePlan.

- Overall the individual may be considered to be in a steady state under *self-care* with *health status* monitoring as frequently as required. From time to time the person will need to be a consumer of healthcare services and so an episode of care will begin.
- Depending on health system access and usage privileges, some *authorisation* is required before or concurrently with presentation to a care setting.
- At the beginning of an episode of care provision, the person may be *scheduled* or placed on a waiting list. Once the patient is ready to be seen, a formal *visit or encounter* is activated.
- At this point, the core *iterative* clinical process begins with *an assessment*, a phase of data gathering that will allow a decision to be made which usually includes past and most recent history, as well as examination. Once a decision is made, there is a (treatment) *plan* of action.
- Once these *actions* are carried out and recorded, an *evaluation* is made, and the patient may go through the cycle again, be scheduled for another encounter, or be *discharged* from that encounter.
- Here the consumer re-enters the community and depending on the nature of the episode may return to the *self-care/health status monitoring steady* state, or may require a period of *community based care delivery.*

4. Principal Role of *LifePlan*: An Overview

The principal role of LifePlan is to generate individual PLHPs tailored to the 'owner's' specific health status and to deliver it via the Internet either through PCs or Tele-Services. A PLHP comprises a merged set of *Health Expectations* and *Health Tips* (shown in Figure 2). Health expectations are evidence based health events that require planning. They include such items as the routine immunisation schedule, mammograms for females over 45, a new Health Risk Appraisal to be performed, etc. All of these health expectations have the following characteristics:

- Once activated (see below) they are for a uniquely identified person
- Time by which the expectation needs to be satisfied
- The event that is expected
- The action(s)—such as notification of Primary Care Provider (PCP), rescheduling *n* times, etc.—to be performed on the "success" or "failure" of event satisfaction.

Health tips are lifestyle recommendations that do not occur at a particular time but suggest (or even exhort) on-going behavioural changes. Compared to a health expectation, an individual can revert to old habits and "undo" the benefits of the health tip. By contrast, once a health expectation is satisfied, it cannot be undone and the benefits remain. For example, a tetanus booster will reduce or eliminate the risk of tetanus for 5-10 years, but stopping smoking only reduces the risk until the individual starts smoking again.

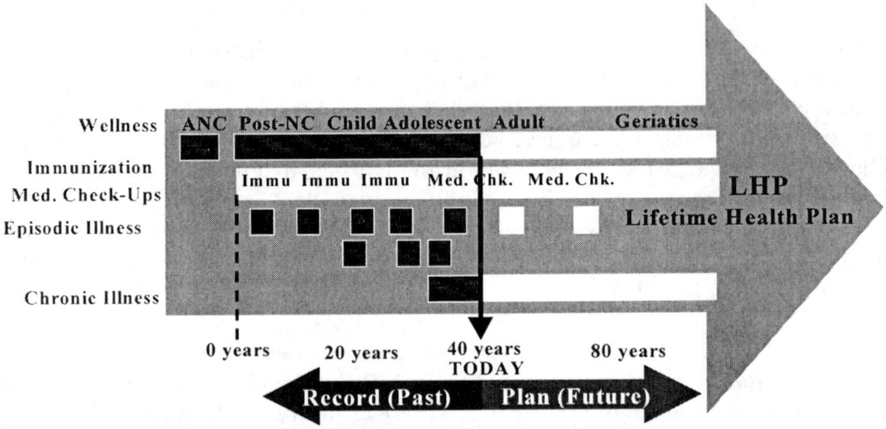

Figure 2: An overview of a typical Personalised Lifetime Health Plan. The boxes will be filled with both wellness and illness related information.

Automation of LifePlan translates into two activities - PLHP Generation and PLHP Delivery. The former involves periodic generation of comprehensive and specific PLHPs. The latter involves global access to the generated PLHP, via a 'live electronic consultation session'—that entails the generation of 'dynamic' Web-based questionnaires—in a timely manner as the individual moves through life. Figure 3 shows the infrastructure for implementing these two activities. Next, we briefly elaborate the modules responsible for PLHP Generation and Delivery.

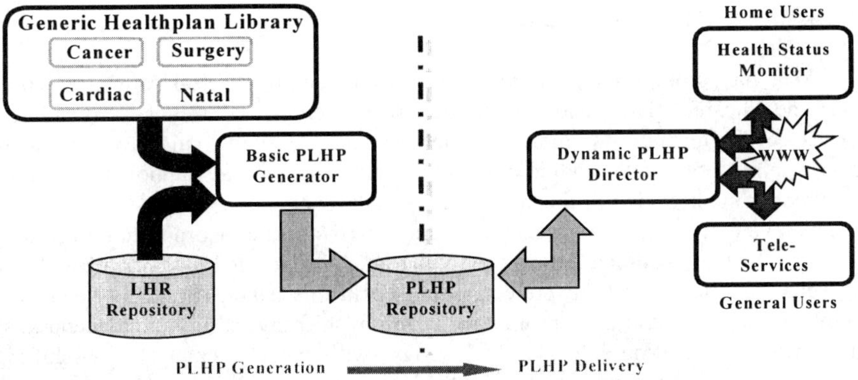

Figure 3: The PLHP infrastructure. Illustrating modules involved in the Generation and Delivery of PLHPs.

4.1. PLHP Generation

The PLHP Generation activity is implemented in terms of two main modules:

Generic Healthcare Plans Repository (GHPR): GHPR is an electronic archive to store a suite of generic healthcare plans. Each generic healthcare plan will be wellness oriented and will incorporate specialised guidelines, procedures, milestones, observations, advice, treatment and test schedules.

Basic PLHP Generator (BPG): The BPG is the core engine responsible for the autonomous and 'intelligent' generation of 'basic' PLHPs—a basic PLHP reflects the various health aspects of the individual that need to be addressed by the individual—that is deemed as being complete, consistent, satisfying multiple constraints and operable. BPG works in concert with the LHR repository, GHPR and/or a healthcare professional. Note that BPG is activated whenever a new PLHP needs to be generated.

4.2. PLHP Delivery

PLHP delivery is achieved by the implementation of the following modules:

Dynamic PLHP Director (DPD): The Dynamic PLHP Director (DPD) is the core 'intelligent' engine responsible for the dynamic and automated customisation of PLHP's based on the individual's most recent health status. DPD will direct all user-PLHP transactions via a web-based virtual 'consultation session', during which it will inquire (using electronic questionnaires) about the current health status of an individual based on his/her existing PLHP. Based on the individual's response, DPD will dynamically customise the PLHP, i.e. it will generate relevant questions either to clarify previous responses or to explore a suspected abnormality in the individual's health profile.

Functionally, DPD is the server side of the PLHP delivery infrastructure; for delivery purposes it interfaces with the PLHP delivery media, i.e. the Health Status Monitor and Tele-Services. Furthermore, DPD also supports the application middleware—a toolset for defining object relationships, configuring user preferences and security profiles for PLHP delivery purposes.

Health Status Monitor (HSM): HSM is a self-contained home-based health maintenance application that can be used by individuals to monitor their personal health status.

Tele-Services: Tele-Services refer to a confluence of PLHP delivery mediums, notably public multi-purpose kiosks, email and telephone. Individuals who do not have PC facilities are intended to use Tele-Services for all interactions with LifePlan.

5. Discussion & Concluding Remarks

Malaysia has proposed an enterprising and challenging 'Tele-Healthcare' vision for national healthcare. The vision is in line with international trends in healthcare and advances in IT technology, more so the systematic amalgamation of an innovative healthcare philosophy with leading edge Information Technology support have realised an all-encompassing, holistic healthcare model for Malaysia [1].

We believe that an investment in healthcare in terms of the incorporation of information technology must be accompanied by the right strategy to provide long-term benefits . The MSC-Telemedicine based LHP project, discussed in this paper, should be seen as a bold and novel initiative that aims to promote a paradigm shift towards a 'person-centred system of healthcare'. Cutting-edge IT technology will be the catalyst for shifting the responsibility of health management from the healthcare provider to 'informed' individuals. For maximum effectiveness, the 'Tele-Healthcare' vision will feature informed, health conscious and empowered individuals that are capable of choosing optimum lifestyle and health management options resulting in a sustained state of self-wellness. For added value, these wellness maintenance services will (a) pro-actively reach out to individuals, (b) be seamless in implementation, (c) continuous in presence, and (d) tailored to the individual's and community's requirements [13] [14].

To meet the objectives set forth by the LHP project, we have presented *LifePlan*—a healthcare delivery infra- and info-structure that successfully enables a continuum of care. The LifePlan infra- and info-structures are currently translated into technical deliverables, with completion of the entire solution being targeted for the year 2001.

References

[1] The Multimedia Super Corridor. URL: www.mdc.com.my, 1997.

[2] S.S.R. Abidi, A. Goh & Z. Yusoff, Telemedicine and Medical Informatics in the Multimedia Super Corridor: The Malaysian Vision. *9th World Congress on Medical Informatics (MedInfo'98)*, Seoul. (1998).

[3] S.S.R. Abidi & Z. Yusoff, Tele-Healthcare: 'Virtual' yet Efficacious Healthcare in a Wired World, *4th International Conference on Communications and Computer Networks (SEACOM'98)*, Penang, (1998).

[4] Government of Malaysia CRFP Telemedicine Flagship Application: Lifetime Health Plan. (1997)

[5] J.E. Larsson & B. Hayes-Roth, Guardian: An Intelligent Autonomous Agent for Medical Monitoring and Diagnosis. *IEEE Intelligent Systems*, Jan/Feb, (1998).

[6] B. Hayes-Roth, *Guardian:* A Prototype Intelligent Agent for Intensive-Care Monitoring. *Artificial Intelligence in Medicine*, 4 (2) (1992) 165-185.

[7] M.S. Turtle, Bringing Knowledge to the Point of Care. *Proceeding of Healthcare Information Management Systems Society (HIMSS) Annual Meeting*, Texas (1995).

[8] S.S.R. Abidi, A WWW Based Tele-Healthcare Information and Diagnostic Environment. *International Conference on Multimedia and Information Technology*, Kuala Lumpur, (1998).

[9] E. Keravnou et al (Eds), Artificial Intelligence in Medicine, Lecture Notes in Artificial Intelligence 1211. Springer-Verlag, New York (1997).

[10] E. Rogers, AI and the Changing Face of Healthcare. *IEEE Intelligent Systems,* Jan/Feb (1998).

[11] J. Wennberg, Shared Decision Making and Multimedia. Health and the New Media: Technologies Transforming Personal and Public Health, Linda M. Harris (ed.), NJ:Lawrence Erlbaum Associates, Inc., (1995).

[12] B. Hayes-Roth & J.E. Larsson, A Domain-Specific Software Architecture for a Class of Intelligent Patient Monitoring Agents. *Journal of Experimental & Theoretical Artificial Intelligence,* 8 (2) (1996).

[13] M. Moore, Elements of Success in Telemedicine Projects. Report of a Research Grant from AT&T, Graduate School of Library and Information Science, University of Texas at Austin (1993).

[14] J. Flower, The Future of Healthcare. *Encyclopaedia of the Future*, Macmillan & Co. (1995).

Security

Medical Informatics Europe '99
P. Kokol et al. (Eds.)
IOS Press, 1999

Communication Security in Open Health Care Networks

Bernd BLOBEL, Peter PHAROW, Kjeld ENGEL, Volker SPIEGEL, Rolf KROHN
University of Magdeburg, Leipziger Str. 44, D-39120 Magdeburg, Germany

Abstract. Fulfilling the shared care paradigm, health care networks providing open systems' interoperability in health care are needed. Such communicating and co-operating health information systems, dealing with sensitive personal medical information across organisational, regional, national or even international boundaries, require appropriate security solutions. Based on the generic security model, within the European MEDSEC project an open approach for secure EDI like HL7, EDIFACT, XDT or XML has been developed. The consideration includes both securing the message in an unsecure network and the transport of the unprotected information via secure channels (SSL, TLS etc.). Regarding EDI, an open and widely usable security solution has been specified and practically implemented for the examples of secure mailing and secure file transfer (FTP) via wrapping the sensitive information expressed by the corresponding protocols. The results are currently prepared for standardisation.

1. Introduction

Meeting the challenge of efficient and high quality health services, the health care systems of developed countries are changing to health networks corresponding the shared care paradigm. Shared care is defined as "a continuous and co-ordinated activity of different persons in different institutions under employment of different methods at different times in order to be able to help patients optimally with respect to their medical, psychological and social being" [2]. Such shared care networks must be supported by interoperable information systems, i.e. the distributed co-operating information systems involved into the shared care association are increasingly communicating. To enable communication between applications independent of their environment, the operating systems of the computers included into the network as well as the communication interfaces of the applications and communication protocols must be standardised and implemented. In general, the communication may be provided in two different ways: connection-oriented and connection-less. Other terms to describe the differences are synchronous and asynchronous communication or channel-oriented and message-oriented communication. The current paper is especially dealing with EDI (Electronic Data Interchange) communication, but also other protocols will be mentioned.

Important examples for communication protocols standardising syntax and semantics of communication interfaces are the EDI protocols HL7, EDIFACT, xDT and, in the future, XML. EDIFACT and xDT enable interorganisational data exchanges, whereas HL7 was originally developed for the internal communication of hospitals. xDT is a set of German standards dealing with communication between doctor's office systems as well as between them and other providers. The paper is based upon the research of the authors and their development results within the MEDSEC project, which is funded by the European

Commission, DG III, as part of the ISIS Programme (Information Society Initiatives for Standards).

2. HL7 in Distributed Health Information Systems

HL7 (Health Level 7) enables communication between any systems independently of their architecture and hardware basis. This is achieved by standardising the syntax and semantics of exchanged messages. HL7 interfaces realise the request/service procedure in the sense of sending and receiving these messages, including the transformation from the proprietary format to the standardised format and vice versa. The communication is managed by communication servers or by a standardised middleware architecture, which both are not part of the HL7 communication standard.

The basic principle of HL7 is a *point-to-point information interchange paradigm* (1:1 or 1:n in the case of broadcast). Communication is controlled either by *trigger events* (in the case of trigger event paradigm of process coupling, *unsolicited* or real time) or by *query/response interchange* (in the case of query/response paradigm of retrospective interchange or *solicited*). Therefore, HL7 enables to manage concurrent processes and non-concurrent interchange of messages. Using unique object identifier, the messages can be arranged within a given time. HL7 provides both basic and enhanced acknowledgement paradigms.

HL7 is widely introduced in the US healthcare sector and increasingly used in countries externally to the US like Australia, Canada, Finland, Germany, Japan, The Netherlands. The successful dissemination of HL7 will be promoted by the harmonisation of the different healthcare information interchange protocols performed by the Joint Working Group for Common Data Model (JWG-CDM) and chaired by IEEE. The objective of JWG-CDM is to develop object-oriented models and specifications that are needed to support a generic messaging standard. In addition, interfaces to standard middleware architectures like ASN.1, CORBA, and OLE/COM/DCOM will soon be realised. Industry driven working groups like the HP-promoted AndoverGroup focus on JWG-CDM compliant products, starting with HL7 related procedures and followed by CORBA integration.

EDIFACT (Electronic Data Interchange for Administration, Commerce and Transport) is the European pendant of HL7, but is actually not achieving a similar significance in healthcare.

The current HL7 version (V.2.3.1) contains *common specifications* (common rules, formats, control segments, queries, encoding rules and master index files) and *chapter-specific specifications* (trigger events, messages as well as segments and fields). The variable length delimited ASCII messages produced from the abstract message definition by standardised encoding rules are human-readable. HL7 functional areas include typical healthcare (clinical) domains as, e.g., *ADT*, *Registration*, *Orders*, *Results*, *Financial*, *Non-ASCII character sets*, *Query language support*, *Medical documents (Medical Records)*, *Clinical trials*, *Immunisation reporting*, *Adverse drug*, *Reactions*, *Scheduling*, *Referrals*, *Problems and goals,* as well as *Master files*.

Preparing the HL7 version 3, the HL7 community starts *object-oriented modelling* of processes and the related EDI. In this context, the specification of the HL7 communication standard consists of:

- *common specifications* (common rules, formats, control segments, queries, encoding rules, master index files),
- *the HL7 reference model*,

- *chapter-specific specifications* (information model, interaction model, hierarchical message description), and
- *implementable message specifications.*

In addition to the information model and interaction model mentioned above, the following message development components are defined in HL7 version 3:

- *transaction scope,*
- *use case model,*
- *messaging (sub-)model.*

A detailed discussion of middleware approaches realising interoperable health information systems as well as an extended list of references may be found in (Blobel and Holena, 1997).

3. EDI Security Requirements

Especially in the healthcare domain, communication and co-operation between providers within an organisation and particularly between different organisations require extended security services to respond to the security requirements in health information systems.

In the EDI environment the threat model consists of at least two principals that are authorised to perform message transmissions to each other using several communication protocols over various infrastructures. Threats are active user (attacker) interactions causing the vulnerability of the systems. According to the security policy, threats, vulnerabilities and accepted risks require the fulfilment of the security requirements by appropriate security services. The following consideration is based on the common security model distinguishing the concepts of communication security and application security. The first concept is controlled rather globally, whereas the latter is put more locally. Each of these concepts defines a set of security services, which are provided by sets of security mechanisms based on security algorithms applied to data. The different levels of granularity allow views of different groups of users (medical users, system administrators, implementers) within the same specification framework. Additionally, for implementation purposes the protocol-services-mechanisms relationships looking for standards and products have to be considered.

An unauthorised principal may try to attack the communication system using passive (as monitoring, listening and sniffing of data system exploration, traffic analysis) or active (as creation, insertion, deletion and replay of data) techniques. For example, this may enable the intruder to perform masquerading. A short summary of threats and security services is given in table 1.

Table 1: Threats and Security Services

Threats	Security Services
masquerading (unauthorised use of authorised services)	principal identification and authentication
data manipulation	integrity
concealment or manipulation of data origin	accountability in the sense of non-repudiation of origin
repudiation of receipt	accountability in the sense of non-repudiation of receipt
disclosure of data	confidentiality

4. Security Model for EDI Communications

Regarding the security of health information systems, internal security services provided by the communicating and co-operating information systems as well as the communication infrastructure can be distinguished from external security services provided by Trusted Third Parties (TTP) (Blobel et al., 1998a,b). Based on the Generic Security Model published, e.g., in (Blobel, 1996; Blobel et al., 1997), the security services for EDI communications needed are mentioned in figure 1 (written in black characters). The internal security services needed are strong authentication, integrity, confidentiality as well as non-repudiation of origin and receipt.

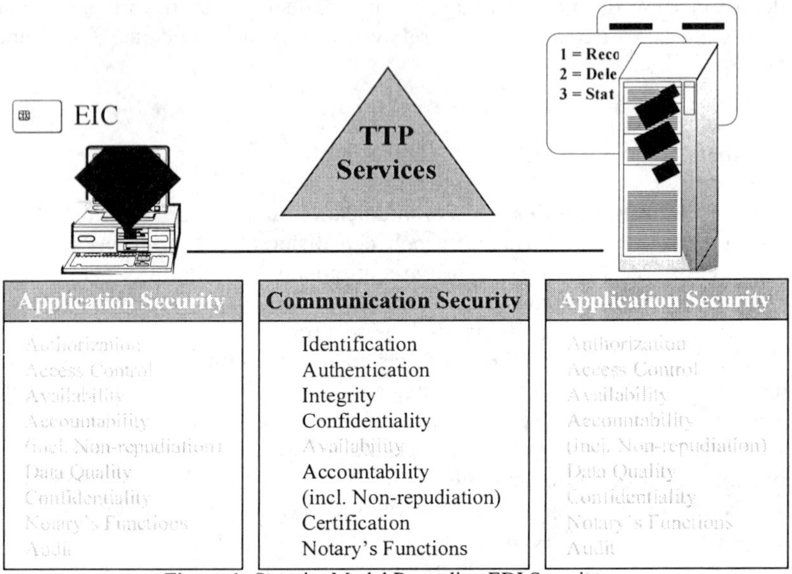

Figure 1: Security Model Regarding EDI Security

5. Protocol Relationships of Security Services

To realise secure distributed health information systems, different protocols enable security services on different levels of the ISO OSI model of open systems intercommunication as shown in table 2.

The general solution for EDI security including the HL7 communications standard is based on two types of security services sets providing strong authentication, integrity check, confidentiality of messages transferred and non-repudiation of both origin and receipt. On the ISO OSI model application layer, the first set realises end-to-end message security by wrapping the data presented in a standardised format, e.g. HL7, EDIFACT, XML, MIME (figure 2) using security mechanisms like digital signature or encryption. Secure email via S/MIME, PEM or PGP/MIME, but also sFTP, MOSS, PKCS#7 and the Internet-tool-based SHTTP are well-known representatives for secure messaging. The second set of system-to-system security services establishes a kind of "secure channel" on the ISO OSI transport layer transparently to the user (for example used in the CORBA Security Specification for security unaware applications, [OMG, 1997]). Examples of that solution are SSL and TLS, IPv6, and SOCKS, but also tunnel protocols like PPTP operating on the data link layer, have to be mentioned.

Table 2: Placement of Security Services

Security Services / OSI Layers	Confidentiality	Integrity	Entity Authentication	Data Origin Authentication	Non-Repudiation of Origin	Non-Repudiation of Receipt
Data Link	SILS/SDE, PPTP[1], L2TP	SILS/SDE, L2TP	PPTP, L2TP, L2F	SILS/SDE, L2TP	–	–
Network	IPSEC, NLSP	IPSEC, NLSP	IPSEC, NLSP	IPSEC, NLSP	–	–
Transport	SOCKS, TLSP, SSL, TLS, PCT, SSH	SOCKS, TLSP, SSL, TLS, PCT, SSH	SOCKS, TLSP, SSL, TLS, PCT, SSH	TLSP	–	–
Application	SHTTP, SPKM, MHS, MSP, PEM, SFTP, PGP/MIME, MOSS, S/MIME, PKCS#7	SHTTP, SPKM, MHS, MSP, PEM, SFTP, PGP/MIME, MOSS, S/MIME, PKCS#7	SHTTP[2], SPKM, SFTP	SHTTP, SPKM, MHS, MSP, PEM, SFTP, PGP/MIME, MOSS, S/MIME, PKCS#7	SHTTP, SPKM, MHS, MSP, PEM, SFTP, S/MIME, ESS	SPKM, MHS, MSP, SFTP, S/MIME, ESS

Regarding the implementation of secure EDI using different transport protocols, the handling of control data and application data must be considered separately. These details have been specified in the corresponding MEDSEC project deliverables (Blobel et al., 1998a,b).

Figure 2 demonstrates a secure EDI communication solution based on the secure message paradigm. Using a communication server and a XML-like tag-length-value format to exchange security protocol details, the different applications enabled for one of the standard protocols may transparently communicate with a second application enabled for another one, mediated by the communication server which transforms not only message syntax and semantics but also the protocols used. By such a way, security policy issues may be negotiated.

In the case of secure channels, security services are provided transparently to the communicating and co-operating principals who haven't to be security-aware (figure 3). Therefore in the CORBA security specification, secure channelling is favoured.

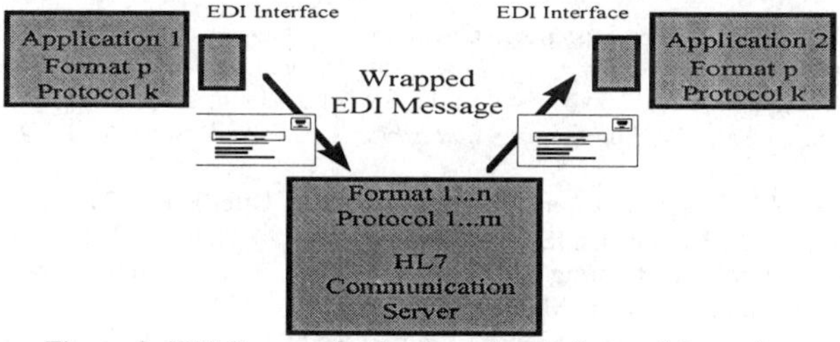

Figure 2: EDI Communication Security via Secure Messaging

---

[1] PPTP does not address any security issues in the current version, but end-to-end security is addressed by PPP which is tunnelled by PPTP through an IP network.

[2] Only the client is authenticated to the server by showing that he is able to apply message enhancement according to the security requirements of the server.

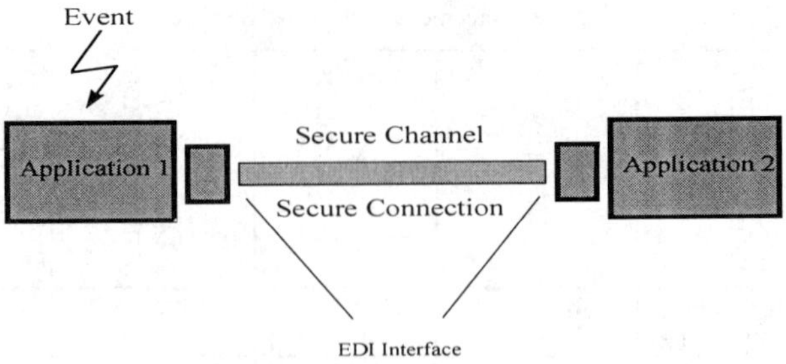

Figure 3: Secure Channel

6. Conclusions

Especially in the healthcare domain, communication and co-operation between providers within an organisation and among different organisations requires extended security services. Based on a general security model, the corresponding services for provision of both the communication security and the application security have been specified. To facilitate communication and co-operation between different systems, open security mechanisms must be realised. Therefore, open protocols which are based on standards have been specified and implemented considering secure FTP with S/MIME and PKCS protocols as well as secure mailing on the message security level and SSL or TLS on the channel security level alike.

The work presented is part of the MEDSEC project which was launched within the European Union ISIS (Information Society Initiatives for Standards) Programme. The deliverables are also defining the draft for the HL7 Security Service Framework. The solution was successfully demonstrated at different places and is used in routine within the regional Cancer Registry Magdeburg/Saxony-Anhalt. Thereby, also the independence of message exchange formats, transport protocols and cryptographic algorithms/protocols was practically tested.

Acknowledgement

The authors are in dept to the European Commission and to the Ministry of Education and Science of the German Federal State Saxony-Anhalt for funding. They like to thank the HL7 community in USA and Germany as well as the partners of the MEDSEC project.

References

[1] Blobel, B. (1996) Clinical Record Systems in Oncology. Experiences and Developments on Cancer Registries in Eastern Germany, in *Preproceedings of the International Workshop "Personal Information - Security, Engineering and Ethics"* pp 37-54, Cambridge, 21-22 June, 1996, also published in *Personal Medical Information - Security, Engineering, and Ethics* (edr. R.Anderson), pp 39-56. Spinger, Berlin 1997.

[2] Blobel B, Bleumer G, Müller A, Louwerse K, Flikkenschild E, Ottes F. (1997) Current Security Issues Faced by Health Care Establishments. ISHTAR Project HC 1028, Deliverable 09 (Fin), February 1997.

[3] Blobel B, Holena M. (1997) Comparing middleware concepts for advanced healthcare system architectures. *International* Journal of Medical Informatics 46 (1997): 69–85.

[4] Blobel B, Roger-France F. Healthcare Security View Based on the Security Services Concept. ISHTAR Project HC 1028, Deliverable, August 1998.

[5] Blobel B, Spiegel V, Krohn R, Pharow P, Engel K. (1998) Standard Guide for EDI (HL7) Communication Security (Draft). ISIS MEDSEC Project, Deliverable 30, August 1998.

[6] Blobel B, Spiegel V, Krohn R, Pharow P, Engel K. (1998) Standard Guide for Implementing EDI (HL7) Communication Security (Draft). ISIS MEDSEC Project, Deliverable 31, August 1998.

Medical Informatics Europe '99
P. Kokol et al. (Eds.)
IOS Press, 1999

Can a database be anonymous?

Catherine QUANTIN [1], François-André ALLAERT [1,2], Philippe d'ATHIS [1], Liliane DUSSERRE [1]
1 – Dijon University Hospital, Medical Informatics Department, Dijon, France
2 – W2 "data security" European Federation of Medical Informatics

Abstract. Sensitive data are most often indirectly identifiable and so need to be rendered anonymous in order to ensure privacy. Statistical methods to provide anonymity require data perturbation and so generate data processing difficulties. Encryption methods, while preserving confidentiality, do not require data modification.

1. Introduction

In the last decade, the demand has increased considerably for microdata sets *"i.e. data sets containing data on individual respondents..."* [1] and for detailed information such as, for statistical studies, large multidimensional tables. However, both tables and *"microdata sets lead to considerable problems when trying to protect the privacy of the respondents"* [2].

The European directive 95/46/CE, from the European parliament and the Council on the protection of individuals, about processing and circulation of personal data, defines "personal data" by "*any information relating to an identified or identifiable natural person ; an identifiable person is one who can be identified, directly or indirectly, in particular, by reference to an identification number or to one or more factors specific to his physical, mental, economic, cultural or social identity"*. With this definition, the elements identifying a person are quite varied and have different discriminant powers : for instance, the birth date is much more discriminant than the sex. Moreover, the preambles 14 to 17 of the Directive extend this definition to data issued by techniques *"used to capture, transmit, manipulate, record, store it or communicate sound and image data relating to natural persons"* so that, from the legal point of view, it appears often difficult to recognize personal data.

Sweeney [3] stresses that *"de-identifying data"* i.e. removing or replacing variables that directly identify an individual (such as name and address, called direct identifiers) does not guarantee anonymity because *"The term anonymous implies that the data cannot be linked to identify any individual"*. So, the data are not anonymous if a combination of variables allows a one-to-one relationship with the corresponding individuals in a public nominative register. These variables, even if they are not direct identifiers, are said "sensitive" because they allow identifying individuals for which sensitive information may be revealed.

This paper aims at showing how the statistical point of view on identification meets the legal one, and the limits - and the dangers - of the techniques used to provide anonymity.

2. "Indirectly identifiable" information from the statistical point of view

The statistical problem is to estimate the probability of identity disclosure through data linking, which implies the possibility to know all the public (or private) files that can provide linkage with the identity of the individuals. In the USA, *"Population registers, such as local census data, voter registration lists, city directories, motor vehicle agencies, tax assessors, real estate agencies and the World Wide Web, are publicly available and often include a postal code and birth date along with the accompanying name and address"* [3] : they are maintained by federal agencies and protected by a complex web of federal statutes [4]. Similar files, particularly for commercial purposes, are used in Europe where the legislation on data protection is more restrictive.

The next point is to define a threshold for the risk of identifying a person [5] under which anonymity could be admitted.

The USA Social Security Administration, recognizing that unique combinations of characteristics can be linked with other data sources, defined as a rule that the data must contain at least 5 individuals with the same combination of characteristics. In fact, the risk to be identified could depend on this number of individuals matching the same characteristics not only in the file to be released, but also within the other sources used for re-identification. Greenberg and Voshell [6], for example, showed on files from different geographic regions a relationship between the percent of individuals with a unique combination of characteristic values and the size of the region. That is why statisticians [7] suggested basing the threshold computation on the percentage of identifications obtained from linkage attempts between the data to be released and a nominative public register.

More precisely, statistical reasoning [8] about disclosure is based on the a priori probability for an individual, whose characteristics are in a file, to be identified. In an earlier paper, Biggeri and Zanella [9] considered the hypothesis that all individuals had the same a priori probability, which they split into three factors : a) probability, for an individual in the file to protect, to appear either in a public nominative file or in data collected for illegitimate purposes (intruder's file) ; b) probability, for such an individual, to have common data with the intruder's file and c) probability, for such an identifiable individual, to be the object of a disclosure attempt.

A new difficulty for determining the threshold is then to define a level of information privacy : *"disclosure takes place if publication of statistical data makes it possible to determine the identity of even a single individual"* [6], because the damage caused to an individual by revealing sensitive information will not be reduced by a low probability of disclosure. Conversely, for the community, a given individual's interest should not interfere with the possible benefit of data processing for epidemiological research, for example.

As a solution, statisticians proposed to estimate the risk of disclosure not as an average risk for a file but separately for each individual : the principle is to take into account the characteristics of the individuals and to determine the frequency of each combination of values of the sensitive variables. So, Franconi and Benedetti [7] estimate an individual probability (which may vary between individuals) : they count the individuals corresponding with each combination of values of the sensitive variables, then group the combinations according to the number h of individuals they identify. This locates easily identifiable combinations since the risk of identifying an individual decreases when the corresponding h value increases : a birth year and the name of a small city may be associated to $h = 1$ individual only, while a birth year and the name of a big city may be associated to $h = 5$ individuals, so that the risk of disclosure is obviously higher in the first case. Reasoning this way, Biggeri and Zanella [9] have only considered the simplest case of combinations each describing a unique individual ($h = 1$).

Sweeney [3] also stressed that the threshold should take into account the degree of anonymity required for the released data : for example, medical databases may contain more sensitive information than databases dealt with by travel agencies. Supposing that valuable data (e.g. medical data) will merit more effort (visiting or phoning the individuals, direct mailing) for identification, the threshold should be decreased to render these efforts useless.

3. Statistical methods to provide anonymity

Statisticians focused on aggregation of individuals in a data file by enforcing them to share the same characteristics, through data perturbation such as *"changing singletons to median values, inserting complementary records, generalising codes, swapping entries, scrambling records, suppressing information"* [3] : for examples, to reduce a birth date into the year, to remove either the age or the full record of a centenarian ...

For generalising codes, controlled rounding (i.e. replacing the true value by an appropriately rounded value) has been the most studied method [10,11,12]. Other authors proposed to mask microdata by adding noise, generated by bootstrapping from the original empirical distribution of the data [13].

Sweeney [3] introduced the Scrub System, for removing or *"scrubbing"* identifying information in text documents [14], and the Datafly System, devoted to field-structured records [15], where the user must specify a level of anonymity for each variable field : this level is a number between 0 and 1 determining the minimum bin size for the field, so that every value in the field occuring less than this minimum bin size is recoded (for example birth date is recoded in months or years), or even removed, if after this generalisation the bin size still does not meet the requirement.

The other approach proposed by Statistics Netherlands [16] is considered as the most usable confidentiality software in the European Community : like the Datafly system, the program μ-Argus generalises values or even removes outlier information in order to achieve a minimal bin size requirement but, unlike Datafly, does not suppress entire records.

The problem then is to evaluate the effect of these modifications on the data processing and the resulting statistical biases. More generally, it raises the question of the loss of quality that we can accept in exchange for anonymity.

4. What loss of data quality can we accept in exchange for anonymity ?

Data perturbation, being not obtained at random, implies a statistical bias. Moreover, removing or substituting outlier values may strongly affect mean and standard deviation or hide rare events, such as serious complications whose consequences upon the studied disease may be ignored.

Cox demonstrated [17] for two-dimensional tables that, among the different methods for data suppression or perturbation, only controlled rounding met the objectives of unbiasedness and reduced data distortion, but this technique appears too complex for higher dimensional tables [14 ,18]. Fuller proposed to reduce biases by treating as a measurement error [18] the masking error due to data perturbation. Some statisticians [19] proposed algorithms minimising the information loss due to data perturbations or suppressions. But many methodological problems must be solved before applying these techniques appropriately.

Anonymous data, by definition, prevent any possibility to find the original document, e.g. a medical record, for checking : this implies a strict validation of all data recorded in the base before providing anonymity whereas, in practice, it is rare to eliminate all errors before processing.

Another problem appears with research in evidence based medicine, where data perturbation disagrees with auditability and the " Good clinical practices " which state that the database used for the statistical analysis must reproduce exactly the medical files. It is moreover unacceptable that data perturbation could lead to unfair assessments by choosing the method to provide anonymity which insures the "best" results.

5. Conclusion

Statistical methods for anonymity, implying data perturbation and thereby loss of data quality, make appealing the methods proposed by computer scientists [20] to achieve data protection through security systems based on user identification, passwords, cryptology, output control, operating system safeguards and review of both job requests and outputs [21]. In particular, computer scientists have focused on restrictions [22] concerning sequential queries to a database.

Although the idea of using cryptology in communication to maintain good levels of security and privacy is not new [23], encryption techniques are under-utilised in official statistics, likely due to legal restrictions. For example, the French legislation concerning encryption has only been recently updated in order to simplify the use of encryption techniques for personal data security.

An extreme solution could be to systematically demand, through legislation, encryption of all data, and not some as suggested by Dalenius [24], without specifying any degree of anonymity : this would suppress the problem to define *"indirectly identifiable"* information and would facilitate recognition of the sender of a file and record matching while preserving confidentiality [25], which would be very useful for multi-centre studies. Moreover, encryption could be performed at the data capture to reinforce security. However, to ensure data privacy, data processing requiring decryption resulting in *"nominative or indirectly nominative"* data should be placed under the responsibility of a certified authority.

References

[1] de Waal A.G. and Willenborg L.C.R.J. Global Recoding and Local Suppression in Microdata Sets. Statistics Netherlands, Department of Statistical Methods. 12th International Symposium on Methodology Issues: From data to information, Statistics Canada, Ottawa, 1-3 November, 1995.

[2] Willenborg L.C.R.J., de Wall A.G. and Keller W.J. Some Methodological Issues in Statistical Disclosure Control. Statistics Netherlands, Department of Statistical Methods. Second Cathy Marsh Memorial Seminar, november 7th, London, 1995.

[3] Sweeney L. Three Computational Systems for Disclosing Medical Data in the Year 1999.MEDINFO 98, IMIA, B. Cesnik, A. McCray, J.-R. Scherrer (Eds). IOS Press, Amsterdam, 1998, 1124-1129.

[4] Cecil, J.S., Confidentiality Legislation and the United States Federal Statistical System, *Journal of Official Statistics*, **9** (2) 519-535.

[5] Duncan G.T. " Inferential Disclosure-Limited Microdata Dissemination, " Proceedings of the Section on Survey Research Methods, American Statistical Association, Alexandria, VA, 1990, pp. 440-445.

[6] Greenberg B. and Voshell L. Relating Risk of Disclosure for Microdata and Geographic Area Size. Proceedings of the Section on Survey Research Methods, American Statistical Association, Alexandria, VA, 1990, pp. 450-455.

[7] Franconi L., Benedetti R. Some Aspects of Disclosure Avoidance in Complex Microdata Files. http://europa.eu.int/en/comm/eurostat/research/publications/ros/a3.htm.

[8] Willenborg L.C.R.J. Remarks on Disclosure Control of Microdata. Statistica Neerlandica, 1992, **46** (1).

[9] Biggeri L., Zannella F. Release of microdata and statistical disclosure control in the new national system

of Italy : main problems, some technical solutions, experiments. Proceedings of the 48th ISI session, 1991, Cairo.

[10] Causey B., Cox L.H. end Ernst .R., Application fo Transportation Theory to Statistical Problems, *Journal of the American Statistical Association*, 1985, **80**, 392, 903-909.

[11] Cox L.H., A Constructive Procedure For Unviased Controlled Rounding, *Journal of the American Statistical Association*, June 1987, **82**, 520-524.

[12] Dalenius T., A Simple Procedure for Controlled Rounding, *Statistisk Tidskrift*, 1981, **3**, 202-208.

[13] Bowden R.J. and Sim A.B., The Privacy Bootstrap, *Journal of Business and Economic Statistics*, 1992, **10**, (3), 337-345.

[14] Sweeney L. Replacing personally-identifying information in medical records, the Scrub system. Proceedings, American Medical Informatics Association. Washington: Hanley & Belfus, 1996.

[15] Sweeney L. Guaranteeing anonymity when sharing medical data, the datafly system. Proceedings, American Medical Informatics Association. Nashville : Hanley & Belfus, Inc, 1997.

[16] Hundepool A. and Willenborg L. μ and τ-argus : software for statistical disclosure control. Third International Seminar on Statistical Confidentiality. Bled: 1996.

[17] Cox L.H. Disclosure Control Methods for Frequency Count Data. Presented at the Census Advisory Committee Meeting of the American Statistical Association, Bureau of the Census, 1984.

[18] Fuller W.A., Masking Procedures for Disclosure Limitation, *Journal of Official Statistics*, 1991, **9** (2), 383-406.

[19] Cox L.H., Suppression Methodology and Statistical Disclosure Control, *Journal of the American Statistical Association*, 1980, **75**, 377-385.

[20] Keller-McNulty S. and Unger E., Database Systems : Inferential Security, *Journal of Official Statistics*, 1993, **9** (2), 475-499.

[21] Cigrang M. and Rainwater L. Balancing Data Access and Data Protection : the Luxembourg Income Study Experience. Proceedings of the Statistical Computing Section. American Statistical Association, Alexandria, 1990, VA, 24-26.

[22] Adam N.R. and Wortmann J.C., Security-control Methods for Statistical Databases: A comparative Study, *ACM Computing Surveys*, 1989, **21** (4), 515-556.

[23] Denning D.E. Cryptography and Data Security, Addison-Wesley, Reading, MA 1982.

[24] Dalenius T., Finding a Needle in a Haystack or Identifying Anonymous Census Records, *Journal of Official Statistics*, 1986, **2**, 329-336.

[25] Kardaun J.W.P.F. and Willenborg L.C.R.J.. Cryptological Applications in Official Statistics. Statistics Netherlands, Department of Statistical Methods, Seminar on New Techniques and Technologies for Statistics, Bonn, November 20-22, 1995.

Medical Informatics Europe '99
P. Kokol et al. (Eds.)
IOS Press, 1999

A Secure Web-based Interface to Maternity Records with Decision Support

M. Howard WILLIAMS[a], Olive LIEW[a], Ken BODDY[b], Athanasios VARIAS[a] and Mairin EYDMANN[b]
[a]*Department of Computing & Elec. Eng., Heriot-Watt University, Edinburgh, UK*
[b]*Department of Obstetrics, University of Edinburgh, Edinburgh, UK*

Abstract. The recent developments in Web technology now make it easy to create user-friendly interfaces to databases and link them to the Internet or to local Intranets. With the acceptance of this new approach one can take advantage of the opportunity to use this development to incorporate additional knowledge into the interface. Not only can this provide a more supportive interface, but it can also create the opportunity for sharing and comparing such knowledge in the future. This paper describes how this has been used to develop an interface to a database of maternity case records which incorporates a knowledge base of rules relating to care plan protocols and uses this to provide decision support to the carer. The issue of security is a serious problem and some aspects of the measures taken are discussed.

1. Introduction

The recent dramatic growth in use of the Internet has led to radical changes in the approach to distributed provision and access to information [1,2]. One consequence of this has been a concerted move by database vendors to provide the means to connect their systems to the Internet and access them via Web browsers. With the current tools for preparing and presenting information on the Web, users can develop user friendly interfaces to databases. The tools make it possible to produce high quality pages (including images, graphics, animations, etc.) accessed via a Web browser in the same way as other Web documents.

At the same time this new technology has created an opportunity to build up medical knowledge by associating it with databases in a similar way. This can be used directly by the interfaces to databases or exchanged with other users or programs. This opens up new opportunities for sharing and comparing knowledge with obvious benefits in the long term.

This paper is concerned with the application of this approach to maternity case records. At the Simpson Memorial Maternity Pavilion (SMMP) in Edinburgh, a paper-based record known as a Riskcard has been in use to record information relevant to the progress of a pregnancy. On first registration, information on the past history and current state is recorded together with administrative details. At regular intervals during the course of the pregnancy the card is updated to take account of changes arising during the course of the pregnancy.

By using Web technology to provide access to an underlying database, an electronic equivalent of the Riskcard has been created which is familiar to existing users. This is easy to use and can be accessed remotely thereby enabling the information to be accessed within the central hospital, from outlying clinics and even from a client's home. In developing such a solution advantage has been taken of the opportunity to incorporate a rule-based component to support the user. One serious problem encountered relates to the issue of security.

This paper describes the overall approach used and some aspects of the measures taken to ensure a reasonable level of security.

2. Web-Based Interfaces

The development of a Web-based interface using HTML pages that can be accessed using a standard Web browser provides a simple and effective means for non-expert users to communicate with a database. With careful design an interface can be rapidly created that is easy to learn and easy to use. However, this simple approach can have serious consequences for security. First, traffic across the Internet is vulnerable to eavesdropping. Even within a closed Intranet the problem of eavesdropping exists. Secondly, by linking to such a network one opens up the possibility that unauthorised persons may gain access to the database either directly (bypassing the interface) or indirectly (e.g. via the interface).

An initial prototype was developed using JavaScript enhanced HTML pages provided by Microsoft's DbWeb, an Internet Database Connector (IDC) which allows a Web page to access any ODBC (Open Database Connectivity) compliant Database Management System. This worked by taking user input from HTML forms, generating SQL queries to the database and then formatting the results for HTML forms.

However, this suffered from both types of security problem mentioned. In particular since HTTP is a stateless protocol, maintaining a user's session information in a secure way is a non-trivial problem. More serious though are weaknesses in the DbWeb software, which allow unauthorised users to bypass the login procedure and gain direct access to non-initial HTML pages in the interface. Another problem arises from direct access to DbWeb itself without going through the interface at all.

In the light of this experience a secure approach was sought based on Java. This has advantages in terms of security and portability. To link to the underlying database, JDBC™ (Java DataBase Connectivity) is used. This consists of a set of classes and interfaces written in Java which provide a standard API for writing database applications. From this, using a JDBC-ODBC bridge, it is possible to link to any ODBC compliant database. Hence an SQL statement can be sent to almost any relational database.

The Java application was written as a set of Java servlets. Servlets are similar to applets except that where applets are executed on the client machine, servlets are executed on the server. They serve the same function as CGI scripts although they provide a number of advantages over current CGI architectures.

The architecture adopted follows a three-tier approach. The user accesses the system via HTML documents at the client side. They send requests to the servlets, which access the database via the JDBC link and from the results generate HTML files which are returned to the client.

An important aspect of security lies in the user session management. For this purpose a proprietary sessions protocol has been employed rather than the simple HTTP sessions model. In the current model the underlying relational database system is used to store data on the users presently using the system, including the IP address of the computer from which the user has logged in, when he/she last accessed the session, etc. From this, the system will ensure that the same user cannot log in for more than one session concurrently. One may place constraints on which computer any particular user may use to log in to the system. A time-out period is specified and if any active sessions are inactive for a period exceeding this maximum idling time, they are automatically logged out.

To protect against eavesdropping, SSL (Secure Sockets Layer) is used. The SSL protocol runs below HTTP and provides the capabilities of server authentication (which allows a user to confirm a server's identity), client authentication (which allows a server to confirm a user's identity) and encrypted connection (which ensures that information between client and server is encrypted by the sending software and decrypted by the receiver).

3. Care Plans

One important facet of the treatment of maternity cases at the SMMP is the formalisation of a set of protocols for identifying any potential risks and recommending actions to minimise potential negative consequences that might result. These protocols have been adopted as a means of ensuring that standard practices are followed by carers [3,4].

When the client first registers, the basic information (including information on past obstetric history, current state and administrative details) are recorded. At this stage the protocols are used to determine an initial care plan for her. On each subsequent occasion when a carer sees her and records information on the visit, the protocols are again applied to determine any additional care actions that may have become advisable. This is also recorded on the Riskcard.

In automating the maternity record system, one problem that arises is that of dealing with the care plan. In the manual system the protocols are an established set of rules which are applied with appropriate interpretation by the carer. The resulting care actions are recorded on the Riskcard. The electronic record could handle the care plan in an identical fashion, with the carer continuing to interpret the protocols appropriately and entering the care actions as text strings in the client's record.

However, the move to a user-friendly Web-based interface to an electronic maternity record provides an opportunity to improve the system further by incorporating the protocols into the interface to provide support to the user by generating the care plan automatically. In doing so the move needs to be treated as a logical progression that does not take away from the carer's responsibilities but aids the carer in ensuring consistent treatment of clients.

In adapting the rules for use within the interface, some aspects of interpretation need to be identified and formalised. For example, actions such as "Chiorionic Villus Sampling (CVS) at 10.5-11 weeks" need to be adapted if the patient is a late booker who only registers after 11 weeks. Standardisation of action primitives and grouping of these primitives appropriately within rules is also required.

In order to handle the rules efficiently, both elementary conditions and actions are represented using simple numeric codes. These are mapped into appropriate strings for output. However, this form of internal representation is essential since, when a care plan is generated, a number of actions may result which need to be stored in the maternity record and referenced at a later stage. Furthermore, different rules may be invoked with the same resulting action and, when this occurs, duplicate actions need to be removed.

The interface operates in such a way that, whenever a record is inserted or updated, the new information is checked and if any of the rules are satisfied, the corresponding actions are added to the care plan. These are stored as a set of codes within the record and displayed as appropriate strings. In addition to recording actions recommended, the system also keeps track of which actions have been completed, when the database was notified of this and who recorded the fact. This necessitates additional fields in the record but provides a more complete account of the client's history. Figure 1 shows a typical screen produced by the interface for a case where some actions have been completed.

Another important facet of the system is to allow it to change with time without affecting the historical record of past client data. Thus to allow the protocols themselves to change with time, the rule base is maintained as a separate component from the interface and can be updated from time to time as required via another simple Web-based interface. Although new protocols may be inserted and existing ones updated or deleted, basic actions may not be changed. If a new primitive action is required, it can be added to the list but the existing actions and their corresponding codes may not be changed or deleted as this may affect both existing clients and historical records.

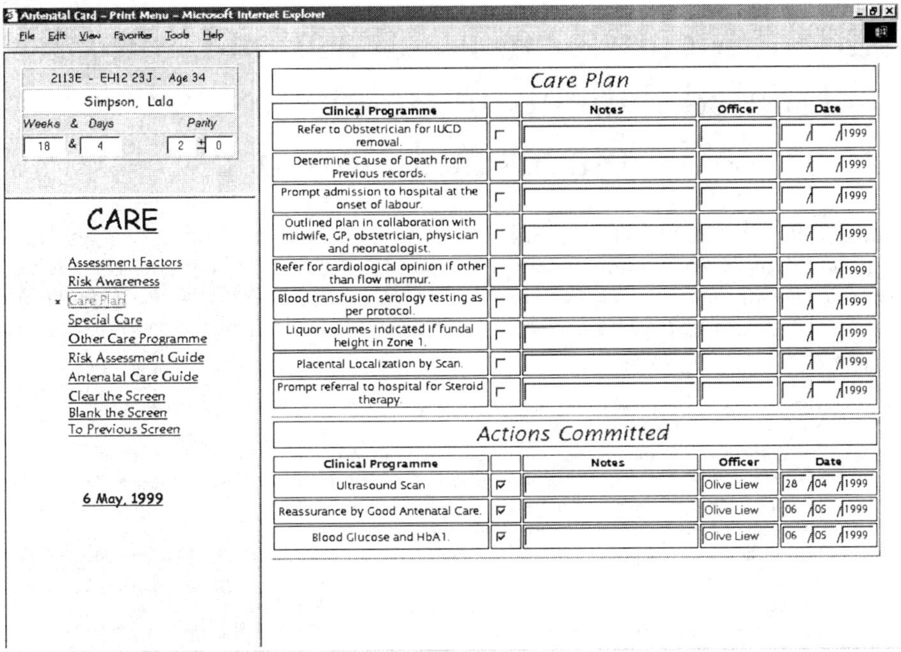

Fig. 1. Example of care plan

4. Conclusion

Web-based technology is now at a stage that it can be used to create user-friendly interfaces to medical databases and make them accessible from wherever they are needed. However, problems of security remain even if they are used within a closed intranet. An approach is described which has been implemented as a prototype for a maternity database.

This new technology provides an opportunity to formalise the relevant medical knowledge as a set of protocols and incorporate it into the system to provide support to users. This has been used to generate care plans automatically for the maternity database. It also provides a first step towards being able to compare alternative sets of protocols from different sources.

Acknowledgements

This work is funded under the Framework IV Telematics programme of the European Union as part of the CHIN and HERMES projects and the authors acknowledge this support.

References

[1] Williams, M.H., Venters, G.G. and Venters, G.A., ' Towards co-operative health information networks', Proc. 7th Int IMEKO Conference, MBB95 (1995), pp 273-277.

[2] Weser, A.J., Kleinholz, L., Soderstrom, P.O., Eklund, P., De Moor, G., Williams, M.H., Venters, G. and Mahr, B., 'Co-operative Health Information Networks', MIE (1996).

[3] Boddy, K., Parboosingh, I.J.T. and Shepherd, W.C., 'A schematic approach to prenatal care', booklet, Lothian Health Board, 1988.

[4] Boddy, K., 'The Sighthill maternity team, the way ahead', Scottish Medicine, 192,

Medical Informatics Europe '99
P. Kokol et al. (Eds.)
IOS Press, 1999

Personal Identifying Number as a Unique Patient Identifier in Database on Clinically Treated Patients in Belgrade: Its Use, Advantages and Drawbacks

Anka Saulic[1], Jelena Marinkovic[2], Snezana Simic[2], Nikola Kocev[2], Nenad Marjanovic[1]
[1]*Institute of Public Health of Belgrade, 29. Novembra 54a, 11000 Belgrade, Yugoslavia*
[2]*Institute of Social Medicine, Statistics and Health Research, Medical Faculty, University of Belgrade, Dr Jovana Subotica 19, 11000 Belgrade, Yugoslavia*

Abstract. Database on clinically treated patients in Belgrade served as an example for analysis of possibilities for the use of Personal Identifying Number (PIN) as an Unique Patient Identifier. In the first part of the paper we analyzed filling up of the fields which contained data on PIN within complete databases in 1981, 1991 and 1996. Filling up of PIN was significantly changed in the three observed years: it was 18% in 1981; 68% in 1991, and 56% in 1996 respectively. Analysis of interactions among the chosen factors (type of hospital, demographic and social characteristics of patients, length of stay in hospital, manner of treatment, main diagnosis, treatment outcome) and measuring time, showed a different degree of statistical significance. In the second part of our paper we analyzed the unexpected decrease in filling up of PIN in 1996 (as compared to 1991) ussing the method of logistic regression, on 1% samples from the databases for the two respective years. On the basis of obtained models of filling up of UPI data, taken as dependent variable and the above factors (predictors) we analyzed the advantages and drawbacks of UPI application as an unique patient identifier.

1. Introduction

Identification of patients represents an important daily activity within the process of health care and one of the essential functions of health care information system. It is performed momentarily, at the time when a patient contacts the system of health care, in all sites where medical services are offered, or at these where an exchange of patient information among variuos participants in the process of health care is performed. Since one patient may have multiple contacts with providers of health care, in different sites, levels and at different times, it is desirable that identification of patients is performed throughout the system of health care in an unanimous manner, through an unique patient identifier [1,2].

Database on clinically treated patients in Belgrade is a part of the health statistics information system. The data are collected through individual statistical reports – Hospital Discharge Reports (in accordance with the relevant legislation).Computer processing of those data started in 1979 and has been performing ever since. Greatest part of data input and processing has been centralised and performed by the Institute of Public Health of Belgrade. Personal Identifying Number (PIN) is a part of gathering of identification data about a patient who is hospitaly treated. It represents a sole item which enables unique identification and connection of files within a base, related to a single patient. PIN belongs to a group of identifiers based on unchangable features of each person (date of birth, sex) and is given at birth, under a regulated scheme (numeric,13 digits) by the state authorities (on the basis of the law passed in 1976). It is written down in all identification documents of a person.

2. Aims

The aim of the paper is to analyze filling up of fieds which contain data on personal identiying number (PIN) within the database on clinically treated patients in Belgrade.

3. Methods

Databases for 1981, 1991 and 1996 were analyzed. The use of PIN in 1981 was still in the early stages and it was mainly applied in state-governed institutions. In 1991 it was extensively used, in various systems, social and administrative services. The 1996 database was the last one to be processed in the similar manner as in the year before; new software and hardware solutions have been applied since 1997. Observation units were data files, concerning events of hospitalisation. Response variable was filling-up of fields of PIN in a file. The analysis had been going on in two stages.

In the first stage a two-factor ANOVA with repeated measures was used for analysis. Dependent variable was defined as repeated measuring in all three observed years. Factors, or independent variables, whose impact was analyzed were: type of hospital, patient`s age, patient`s sex, duration of hospital treatment, surgical vs. non-surgical type of treatment, treatment outcome and type of insurance.

In the second stage we analyzed 1% systematic samples taken from databases for 1991 and 1996. In the study we applied logistic regression, an adaptive non-linear statistical learning method [4]. Observation units had remained the same. The dependent variable (FULPIN) was defined as dichotomous one, with possible values: 0 = PIN field is not filled with data, and 1 = PIN field is filled. Independent variables (predictors) were defined in two ways: dichotomous (dummy) variables and categorical variables with several levels. Dichotomous variables were: type of hospital (HOSP1, HOSP2, HOSP3 - clinical hospital; HOSP4 - specialised hospital; HOSP5 - rehabilitation center); type of ward (WARD1 - internal; WARD2 - obstetrics and gynecology; WARD3 - pediatrics; WARD4 - surgical; WARD5 - rehabilitation), patient`s sex (SEX); type of insurance (INSUR1 - employed; INSUR2 - family member of employed person; INSUR3 - retired person and family member; INSUR4 - farmer and family member; INSUR5, INSUR6 - other insured person; INSUR7 - uninsured person), participation in treatment expenses (PINSUR); patient`s profession (PROF1 - farmer; PROF2 - industrial worker; PROF3 - service worker; PROF4 - protection and military personel; PROF5 - management and administration; PROF6 - expert; PROF7 - other; PROF8 - supported person; PROF9 - retired); surgeries performed (SURG); group of IX International Classification of Diseases for the main cause of hospitalisation (ICD1, ICD2,...,ICD17); presence of co-morbidity (CMORB); treatment outcome (REZ1 - discharged; REZ2 - transferred to another hospital; REZ3 - deceased). Possible values were: 0 = does not belong to and 1 = belongs to the defined group. Categorical variables were: patient`s age (AGE, with possible values: 1 = <1 year; 2 = 1-6 years; 3 = 7-14 years; 4 = 15-19 years; 5 = 20- 44 years; 6 = 45-64 years; 6 = >64 years), length of hospitalisation (LENGTH: 1 = 1-7 days; 2 = 8-14 days; 3 = 15-30 days; 4 = >30 days). For each variable, included in the equation of logistic regression we calculated:

partial regression coefficient - B; standard error of the coefficient B - SE B; estimated probability that the model is adequate - p (Chi-square test, degree of freedom = 1); relative risk - rr = exp(B) and confidence interval (95%) for the relative risk - CI.

4. Results and Discussion

The number of events of hospital treatment has not significantly changed during the observation period: in 1981 it was 233812, in 1991: 252265 and in 1996: 249911. The average filling-up of fields was 18.03% in 1981, 67.66% in 1991 and 55.90% in 1996. For all factors in our analysis, filling-up of PIN demonstrated statistically significant changes in the three observed years. In relation to 1981 highly significant increase of filling-up ($p<0.01$) was observed in 1991 and 1996, while 1996 was marked by a significant decrease in relation to 1991 ($p<0.05$). Interaction of observed factors and time (i.e. the years in wich measurements were performed) was not statistically significant for the following factors: type of hospital, patient`s sex, duration of hospital treatment, surgical vs. non-surgical type of treatment and treatment outcome. Analysis of the interaction of the factor “patient`s age” and the years in which measurements were performed showed statistically significant differences in the dynamics of filling-up of PIN by certain age groups of patients. Differences found in age groups: 45-64 and >64 were not statistically significant. Those groups had best filling-up in all three observed years (1981: 32.64% and 71.28%; 1991: 71.94% and 73.55%; 1996: 62.22% and 58.28%, respectively). Other age groups shoved highly statistically significant changes ($p<0.01$), with greatest changes of filling-up beeing observed in the youngest age groups: >1 year and 1-6 years (1981: 0.72% and 0.60%; 1991: 19.53% and 53.72%; 1996: 10.80% and 37.90%, respectively). The analysis of the interaction of the factor "type of insurance" and the years in which measurements were performed did show statistically significant differences ($p<0.05$) in the dynamics of filling-up of PIN in the two groups of the insured: "retired persons and their family members" and "employed persons and their family members" (1981: 97.92% and 7.50%; 1991: 74.86% and 74.22%; 1996: 63.32% and 66.09%, respectively.

The logistic regression analysis was first done on the comprehensive database for the two years. The resulting logistic regression model confirmed our previous findings, i.e. that there is a very significant multiple correlation between described independent variables and the respective year (time of measurement). In order to exclude this factor`s influence on the analysis of fillig-up of the fields which contain data on PIN (FULPIN variable), further analysis was performed independently for each respective year. Resulting logistic regression models are presented in tables 1 and 2. Independent variables are presented in the order of their entrance into the regression equation.

LOGISTIC REGRESSION MODEL FOR VARIABLE FULPIN IN 1991.

Table 1

No	Predictor variable	B	SE B	p	rr	95% CI for rr	
						Lower limit	Upper limit
1	PINSUR	-0.589	0.112	0.000	0.204	0.164	0.254
2	PROF8	-0.410	0.129	0.002	0.664	0.515	0.854
3	ICD17	-0.906	0.196	0.000	0.404	0.275	0.594
4	WARD2	1.078	0.312	0.001	2.939	1.595	5.415
5	WARD5	0.917	0.340	0.007	2.502	1.285	4.871
6	ICD11	-0.124	0.333	0.001	0.325	0.169	0.624
7	INSUR4	-0.766	0.195	0.000	0.465	0.317	0.682
8	ICD6	-0.822	0.211	0.000	0.439	0.291	0.664
9	WARD3	-0.640	0.186	0.001	0.528	0.366	0.760
10	REZ1	0.552	0.205	0.007	1.736	1.161	2.595
11	ICD5	-0.663	0.242	0.006	0.516	0.321	0.829
12	PROF7	-0.486	0.200	0.016	0.615	0.415	0.912
13	LENGTH	0.125	0.545	0.023	1.133	1.018	1.261
14	SURG	0.252	0.117	0.031	1.287	1.023	1.620
15	INSUR6	-0.395	0.200	0.048	0.673	0.455	0.997
16	CONSTANT	2.524	0.250	0.000			

In the 1991 model the analysis included 2248 out of the total of 2523 observation units. Sensitivity of the chosen model was estimated on the basis of the ratio between the number of correctly estimated values, obtained by application of the model, and the real, observed values of FULPIN variable. Correct estimation was done on 75.3% of the variable values. The final list of predictors contains 15 variables, out of which 5 show a positive correlation with the dependent variable and the remaining 10 - a negative one. Patients treated in obstetrics and gynecology wards (WARD2) had the greatest relative risk for the PIN data to be filled.

In the 1996 model, 2302 observation units out of the total of 2555 were included in the analysis. Correct estimation was done on 65.6% of the FULPIN variable values. The final list of predictors contains 8 predictors, out of wich 4 show a positive correlation with the dependent variable, and 4 - a negative one. The patients whose main cause of hospitalisation belonged to the 4th group of ICD-IX (blood related deseases), had the greatest relative risk for the PIN data to be filled.

LOGISTIC REGRESSION MODEL FOR VARIABLE FULPIN IN 1996.

Table 2

No	Predictor variable	B	SE B	p	rr	95% CI for rr	
						Lower limit	Upper limit
1	PINSUR	-0.872	0.094	0.000	0.418	0.348	0.503
2	WARD3	-1.004	0.159	0.000	0.366	0.268	0.500
3	INSUR1	0.446	0.108	0.000	1.563	1.265	1.930
4	INSUR6	-0.545	0.135	0.000	0.580	0.445	0.755
5	SURG	0.421	0.096	0.000	1.524	1.265	1.836
6	ICD17	-0.418	0.182	0.022	0.659	0.461	0.941
7	ICD4	0.984	0.493	0.046	2.674	1.018	7.028
8	REZ2	0.631	0.324	0.051	1.880	0.996	3.547
9	CONSTANT	1.429	0.143	0.000			

5. Conclusions

PIN represents the only part of the set of identification data on a person, that enables unique identification of a patient and connection of the data on various episodes of one`s hospital treatments in the database on clinically treated patients in Belgrade. The use of PIN in the database has significantly increased in the observed period, as expected. The decrease in filling-up of the PIN fields in 1996 database is rather unfavorable and it makes the use of PIN as unique patient identifier more difficult. We applied the statistical learning method of logistic regression to predict filling up of the PIN data. The obtained models of logistic regression proved to be highly sensitive and able to improve our knowledge related to the problem. They should serve as the basis for creating measures through which we may improve the process of PIN data filling up in the groups of patients who belong to the predictor variables.

Conceptual and operational characteristics of PIN do satisfy a majority of criteria necessary for its application within the whole health care system. Its basic advantages are broad distribution, widespread use and existence of the infrastructure necessary for the allocation and application of the PIN itself. However, its basic drawback is insuficient confidentiality of data. Its basic structure allows the data on the patient`s age, sex and allocation site to be traced, so it is not sufficiently protected from unauthorised misuse. Confidentiality and safety of data within the health care system are the prerogative of their collection [5,6]. The present form of PIN is not suitable for the application within the health care system. It should be modified by some of the encryption technics and made safer in order to be used as an unique patient identifier.

References

[1] I.A. Solomon, Analysis of Unique Patient Identifier Options, Final Report. US Department of Health and Human services. November 1997.

[2] C.L. Murray *et al.*, Healthcare Delivery Reorganisation Innovative Outcome: Universal Computerised Patient Identification, *Medinfo* **2** (1995) 1637.

[3] L.I. Iezzoni, Assessing Quality Using Administrative Data, *Annals of Internal Medicine* **270** (1993) 666-674.

[4] M. Ennis *et al.*, A Comparison of Statistical Learning Methods on the GUSTO Database, *Statist. Med.* **17** (1998) 2501-2508.

[5] O. Lawrence and J.D. Gostin, Privacy and Security of Personal Information in a New Healthcare System, *JAMA* **270** (1993) 2487-2492.

[6] M. Acherman *et al.*, Standards for Medical Identifiers, Codes and Messages Needed to Create an Effitient Computer-stored Medical Record, *Journal of American Medical Informatics Assotiation* **1** (1994) 1-7.

Medical Informatics Europe '99
P. Kokol et al. (Eds.)
IOS Press, 1999

Experiences with a new Security Standard for Healthcare Information Systems

Kees Louwerse, Margot van Ditmarsch, Erik Flikkenschild
Leiden University Medical Centre (LUMC)
Central Information Processing Department (CDIV)
P.O. Box 9600, NL 2300 RC Leiden

Abstract. This article describes the results of the implementation and demonstration of the Standard CEN ENV 12924 (Security Categorisation and Protection of Health Care Information Systems), that was performed as part of the ISIS/MEDSEC project of the EU. The categorisation scheme given in the standard was followed through for almost all information systems or sub-systems in the Leiden University Medical Centre. The status of the security measures was evaluated for ten systems; further implementation plans were then drawn up for these systems, and partly effectuated. Findings are reported, both on the present security level, and on the applicability of the standard (which in general was found to be very positive). In the course of this work, use was made of a database support tool, developed in an earlier EU project (SEISMED).

1. Introduction

Information systems nowadays play a very important role in patient care, and malfunctioning of these systems may become outright dangerous to the patient. Nevertheless, in many cases not enough attention is paid to the security of these systems. In recent years, several tools have become available which should help improve this situation.

One of the results of the working programme of CEN/TC251 (Medical Informatics) was the standard for Security Categorisation and Protection for Healthcare Information Systems, which was formally adopted in 1997 by CEN as a pre-standard (CEN ENV 12924 [1]). As part of the MEDSEC project [2] (which forms part of the ISIS programme of the European Union), a first demonstration and implementation effort was performed in Leiden.

This standard contains a security categorisation model for information systems in health care, distinguishing six categories, plus some refinements. For each category it specifies the required protection measures. The project task consisted of demonstrating and implementing (as far as possible within a limited period) the standard in a real life situation, and providing feedback on these results to the CEN organisation. An overview is presented here.

2. CEN ENV 12924

The standard provides a method for categorising Health Care Information Systems according to their security requirements. Taking into account the different aspects of Integrity, Availability and Confidentiality, six categories are distinguished. For each category a comprehensive set of protection measures is specified.

Apart from these 6 categories, the standard also allows for different environmental and connectivity factors (6 classes for physical environment, 3 classes for physical connectivity, and again 3 classes for the logical connectivity).

3. Categorisation

To perform the categorisation, a series of interviews was held with the managers of all concerned sub-systems (this involved at least the technical manager, but quite often also his counterpart on the user side). About 30 persons have been interviewed, giving information about 91 sub-systems of the central Hospital Information System and 21 other systems.

A summary of the results is given in the table below.

Table 1 - Security categories

category	availability	confidentiality	integrity	number of systems HIS	other
I	non-critical	sensitive	non-critical	1	8
II	non-critical	sensitive	critical	7	4
III	critical	sensitive	critical	2	3
IV	non-critical	very sensitive	non-critical	12	1
V	non-critical	very sensitive	critical	19	1
VI	critical	very sensitive	critical	22	0
none	..	non-sensitive	..	26	4

The systems, for which the category is indicated as 'none', are the ones in which no confidential data are handled. For non-HIS systems the sample is not complete.

This categorisation exercise led to the conclusion that the categories are relevant, and sufficiently varied for the purpose; the categorisation scheme can well be used in practice.

Some suggestions for improvement were made, like adding an extra category (confidentiality non-sensitive, critical for the other aspects) with a corresponding protection profile, and improving the definitions of some of the terms used in the standard.

Our experience indicates, that the necessary information for the categorisation step can be easily obtained in the course of a brief interview with the responsible person(s).

4. Selection of sub-systems for further investigation

From the complete set of systems, a selection of 10 was made, for which the (present and future) applicability of the standard was investigated in detail. In making this selection, we tried to obtain a representative cross-section of the types of system in use in the Centre.

5. Detailed examination of the selected (sub)-systems

Using the standard, an inventory of the present situation with respect to information security was made for all the selected systems. A further series of interviews were held with the responsible system managers. During these interviews, the recommendations given in the standard were discussed, and the current status for the actual system was recorded. For the status, one of the following indications was used: high priority / include in this year's plan / include in next year's plan / still under discussion / partially implemented / already (fully) implemented / accept the level of risk / not applicable (for specified reasons).

6. Bookkeeping with the SIDERO model

For each system, a detailed report on the results has been written, including:

- an implementation plan to make the system compliant with the standard, as far as is considered necessary, and
- an analysis of the suitability of the standard for this type of system.

The implementation plans have been initiated or even (partly) effected, as far as time and required effort allowed.

In order to facilitate bookkeeping of the findings and results, these were recorded in the measuring instrument SIDERO [3]. This is essentially a database model for security guidelines and measures, which was developed during an earlier EU project (SEISMED [4]).

This tool was adapted for the present purpose by adding the recommendations from the standard as a table to this database. For each system, a quantitative description was produced of the current protection status, as compared to the standard. The database provided an easy means of producing reviews, e.g. for each status separately. These reports were discussed in detail with the responsible system managers, and on the basis of this discussion, action plans were produced, indicating the time scale on which appropriate measures would be effected, or in some cases, explaining e.g. that a certain measure would not be applicable in our case.

7. Examination on how well the standard is adhered to at present

On the basis of the examinations, we could form a good picture of the present security situation for the various sub-systems. Details were collected in separate (confidential) internal reports for each system.

Briefly summarised, the results can be given as follows:

- the standard does provide an sufficiently complete set of measures for the systems considered; only a few relevant measures were found which could not be fitted within the context of the standard;
- for the systems considered, a significant part of the requirements from the standard had been fulfilled, some would be implemented in the near future; but of coursc, some work remains to be done;
- in several cases, a requirement could not be realised within the technical scope of the present system; weak points in the protection usually were concerned with:
  - access control (usually only a password mechanism is available; procedures for managing and using passwords are improving, but are still relatively poor);
  - logging facilities (usually mainly aimed at recovery, and not providing sufficient facilities for tracing what has happened);
  - protection procedures, (non) use of encryption; and
  - back-up provisions;
- there were many examples, where facilities offered by suppliers in their products are not sufficient at present to enable the users to conform to the standard;
- in a few cases, the requirements from the standard are considered as being too strict.

In general, it was found that the protection level of the centralised systems was reasonably close to the prescribed situation, although there were some clear exceptions, as mentioned above.

For the various departmental systems, we have encountered different situations, but in general the protection level was significantly lower than for the centralised systems.

On the whole, however, all persons interviewed agreed that the level indicated by the standard was appropriate, and should be taken as the target.

8. Conclusions

Our overall conclusion is that the standard CEN ENV 12924 provides a very useful instrument for evaluating and improving the security situation in Health Care Information Systems. Although it should not be considered as a substitute for a formal Risk Analysis, it may well serve as a tool for a first evaluation of the information security status of health care environments, and indicate where improvements are most urgently needed and effective. It can also highlight the places, where a more thorough Risk Analysis would be mandatory.

Some suggestions have been made for amendments in a few of the recommendations in the ENV; e.g.: inclusion of a seventh information category (confidentiality non-sensitive, but critical for the other aspects) would provide a more complete picture.

The effort within the MEDSEC project has been limited to experiences within one hospital in the Netherlands (with some additional work at a major German hospital). It would be worthwhile setting up a broader evaluation of the standard to verify the present findings, also taking into account some other categories of health care institutions. In our opinion, after such a further verification, this document should be recommended to serve as a basis guideline for information systems security in European health care.

The practical use of the standard is simplified significantly by the use of a bookkeeping tool (like we have used SIDERO).

Available information systems from vendors usually do not offer sufficient functionality to implement all requirements from the standard. Wide acceptation of the standard, preferably made mandatory by national regulations, would increase the possibility of getting such features realised in future versions.

References

[1] CEN ENV 12924 (Security Categorisation and Protection of Health Care Information Systems); CEN, Brussels, 1997

[2] MEDSEC (Health Care Security and Privacy in the Information Society): European Commission ISIS Programme; deliverable 27: Demonstration Results for the standard CEN ENV 12924
More details about the ISIS programme can be found at http://www.ispo.cec.be/isis/

[3] SIDERO: E.L.A. Flikkenschild and C.P. Louwerse, The Implementation of Security in the Health Care information Systems, closing the gap between theory and practice. In: R.A. Greenes et al. (ed.): Proceedings MEDINFO '95 (Vancouver), ISBN: 0-9697414-1-3. North Holland, Amsterdam, 1995, pp. 648-651.

[4] SEISMED consortium: Data Security for Health Care (handbook; 3 vols.), ISBN 90 5199 263 7. IOS Press, Amsterdam, 1996.
The SEISMED project (Secure Environment for Information Systems in MEDicine) was initiated in 1992 within the context of the AIM-programme (Advanced Informatics in Medicine) of the European Commission. One of it's important products was this set of three handbooks, providing guidelines for several aspects of information security in Health Care Information Systems.

Medical Informatics Europe '99
P. Kokol et al. (Eds.)
IOS Press, 1999

Authorisation & Security aspects in the Middleware-based healthcare information system

Jose Andany[1] - Christer Bjorkendal[2] - Fabrizio Massimo Ferrara[3]
Jean-Raoul Scherrer[4] - Stéphane Spahni[1]

[1] Medical informatics division, University Hospitals of Geneva, 24 rue Micheli-du-Crest, 1211 Geneva 14, Switzerland
[2] Enator Medical, Margaretavagen 1, 22100 SE, Lund, Sweden
[3] GESI Gestione Sistemi per l'Informatica srl & Consorzio EDITH - Via Rodi, 32 - 00195 Roma, Italy
[4] Health On the Net foundation, Medical informatics division, University Hospitals of Geneva, 24 rue Micheli-du-Crest, 1211 Geneva 14, Switzerland

Abstract: The integration and evolution of existing systems represents one of the most urgent priorities of health care information systems in order to allow the whole organisation to meet the increasing clinical organisational and managerial needs. The CEN ENV 12967-1 'Healthcare Information Systems Architecture'(HISA) standard defines an architectural approach based on a middleware of business-specific common services, enabling all parts of the local and geographical system to operate on the common information heritage of the organisation and on exploiting a set of common business-oriented functionality.
After an overview on the key aspects of HISA, this paper discusses the positioning of the authorisation and security aspects in the overall architecture. A global security framework is finally proposed.

1 THE MIDDLEWARE-BASED ARCHITECTURAL APPROACH

Figure 1 shows the layered structure formalised by the CEN ENV 12967-1 standard 'Healthcare Information Systems architecture'.

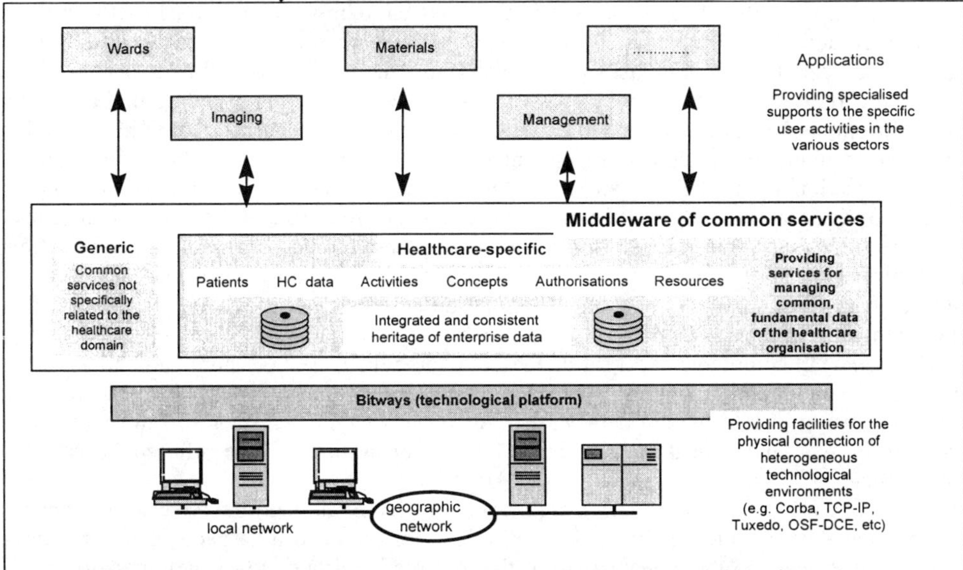

Figure 1. The 3-layers structure of the CEN architecture of health care information systems

- *The Applications* layer consists of a set of components responsible for interacting with the users, providing a specialised support to the various activities carried out in the various sectors of the health care organisation.
- *The Middleware* layer provides a set of services which support the whole system with respect to the management of those common data and procedures of paramount relevance for the whole organisation..
- *The Bitways* layer represents the technological platform, providing facilities enabling the various modules of the information system to interact through common mechanisms, hiding the diverse technologies adopted for their implementation and the mutual location over the (distributed) environment.

Through its services for the definition and management of the information common to the whole organisation, the middleware represents both the key element for ensuring the openness and modularity of the information system, and an operational infrastructure suitable for the integration of legacy systems and for the development of new modules.
By extending the scope of its services, also specific business procedures (e.g. admitting patients, making requests for services, managing complete healthcare records, etc.) may become common facilities of the information system, directly exploitable by the various applications with major benefits in terms of overall consistency and reduction of development/maintenance costs.

2 AUTHORISATION VS. SECURITY

The term ‘security’ is frequently used to generically refer to all aspects relating to the identification, authorisation and validation of one agent (either individual or software process) in the information system. Approaching them all together in one unique term (or component of the information system) is risky with respect to the final results. An incremental methodological approach -as recommended by the Open Distributed Processing (ODP) and HISA-based on different levels of abstraction is therefore beneficial for simplifying the whole matter.
We can first of all identify a set of requirements related to how the individual users carry on their daily activities. Such aspects formalise the rules according to which each user is authorised to perform certain tasks (e.g. registering a diagnosis), as well as to access / manipulate certain data, both clinical and administrative (e.g. the results of some laboratory tests for one patient, the salary of other employees, etc.). Such issues are completely independent from any technological or implementation aspect of the system; they just relate to the organisation and to the laws and procedures which are in force in that place or country. The identification of a clear and common set of terms of reference on how to formalise and manage such aspects represents thus a fundamental pre-requisite for any implementation initiative. This set of requirements and the formalisation of a comprehensive, technological independent, framework for their description and management can be more properly referred to with the term ‘*Authorisation*’.
A *different* (but complementary) set of requirements relates to the secure authentication of the agents (i.e. individuals and software processes) performing the tasks, to the reliable communication of information between two agents and to the archiving of information according to legal and ethical requirements. This set of aspects will be referred to with the term ‘*Security*’.
In the three-layer model of the HISA architecture, different classes of services (and of components) are responsible for the Authorisation and for the Security aspects. The formalisation of the model and the management of the information related to the authorisation rules and criteria is under the responsibility of the healthcare-specific services of the middleware. The mechanisms, tools and technologies according to which the security requirements are

implemented are under the responsibility of the 'bitways' layer of the architecture. Obviously, generic services are employed by the middleware and by the applications to operate according to the security requirements imposed in the specific organisation.
It may be stressed that, while a generic model and a common set of services can be identified for the management of the authorisation aspects throughout all information systems, it is very difficult to define a unique and standard set of security technologies to be implemented in all healthcare information systems of all European countries due to the diversities in the rules, budget, cultural characteristics of the various organisations,. Moreover, the rapid evolution of the techniques should be taken in account. An open environment, therefore, should conform to the following fundamental rules:

- To provide a common framework and a common set of services for allowing all applications and components to retrieve the authorisation aspects of the organisation and to operate accordingly;
- To foresee a set of 'sockets' in the physical implementation, allowing to simply plug-in additional components and services responsible for providing specific security features.

3 AUTHORISATION ASPECTS IN HISA AND IN THE DHE

3.1 CURRENT FEATURES OF HISA

Besides the need for supporting the diversification of roles and responsibilities, additional critical aspects can be identified in the healthcare scenario due to the particular type of information which is managed, implying also ethical and legal aspects. Moreover, moving from country to country or from one healthcare centre to another, different levels of authorisation may be applied to similar types of users.
The Authorisation Common Services in the middleware layer of HISA aim at supporting this specific need, by providing:

- a comprehensive and consistent repository where those responsible in the organisation may define the rules according to which the users may execute the functions provided by the system;
- a standard mechanism according to which the rest of the system may check whether one user is allowed to perform the activities they are requesting.

Each component may be described in terms of a set of controlled functionalities, whose invocation and manipulation by external agents is subject to specific authorisations. For each component, a set of authorisation profiles are defined, usually reflecting the jobs and responsibilities in the organisational area where the system is operating. Each profile may operate with a set of functionalities, according to one set of conditions such as:

- the working ways, which define whether the profile is allowed to access that element by adding new data or reading, updating, or deleting existing data;
- the time frame, which permits the specification of the temporal limits of the authorisation, through a start and end time every day;
- the workstations, which specify a list of workstations or nodes of the information system from which the agent is allowed to interact with the object.

Data being maintained through these services is schematised in Figure 2.

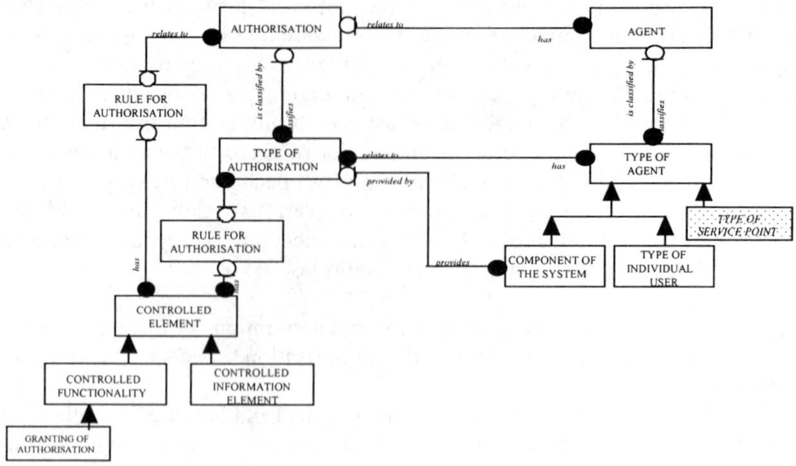

Figure 2: The Data model of the middleware Authorisation Common services

An *Agent* is an individual user or a software component authorised to interact with the information system, while the *Controlled element* represents an element for which authorisation mechanisms are defined. The general procedures according to which the agents may operate are formalised through the '*Type of Authorisation*' and the '*Rules for Authorisation*'. Each agent inherits the authorisations defined for his/her class (i.e. type of agent). Should some particular cases occur (e.g. vacancy, temporary substitution, etc.) individual authorisations overriding the generic values may be formalised. The HISA implementation "Distributed Healthcare Environment"(DHE) fully implements such model.

3.2 ENVISAGEABLE EXTENSIONS TO THE STANDARD

The need for a homogeneous set of components, supporting the specific need for authorisation has dramatically increased during the last decade. The development has changed from proprietary legacy systems, usually running on mainframes to distributed applications running in local environments. A common situation today is that a hospital is supported by different vendors providing different applications not able to fully communicate one with each other.

If on the other hand we look on authorisations from the health care organisation point of view we need to have a flexible model due to the fact that organisations change constantly and that a user could adopt different roles. The combination of user and role is time related which means that when working nightshift, the user may have one authorisation profile but when working dayshift another one is used.

Another most important issue today is how to improve the quality of care by using IT without interfering with respect of the patient privacy. To let the physicians have more adequate information on the patient you need to have something like a "virtual electronic health care record", able to keep track of all the activities belonging to one patient regardless of where and by whom they have been performed. With such approach we need to have a kind of generic model for authorisation in order to specify a unique global authorisation that can be executed on different organisations. The authorisation model, which already exist in the specification of HISA, needs to be extended to have a more accurate control, adapted to its purpose.

Based on the conceptual model for security and authorisation described in HISA three components, integrated in the DHE, are planned or under construction. These should be seen as middleware components with open interfaces as shown in figure 3.

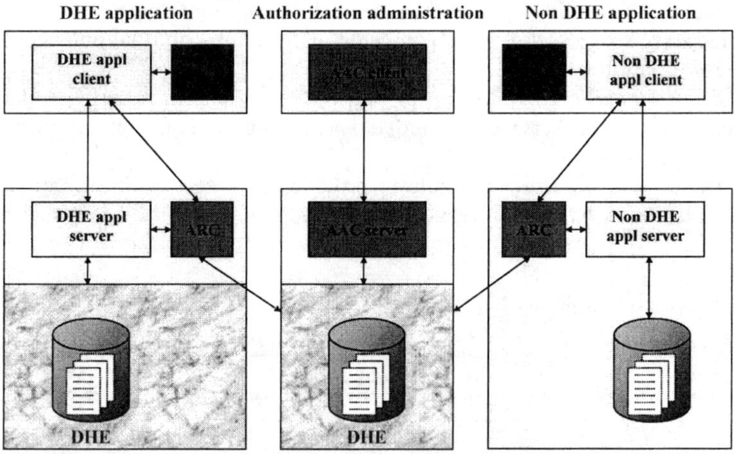

Figure 3: The authorisation components

- *Authorisation Administration Component* (AAC) is a client-server module for the authorisations administration.
- *Authorisation Runtime Component* (ARC) provides a client or a server component with the users authorisations in a standard structured record.
- *Login and Session Component* (LSC) provides the ability of sharing a common session between different applications for different environment.

Two additional components are also provided:

- *Authorisation eXchange Component* (AXC) provides facilities for import/export authorisations data to / from some other system in a standardised XML format.
- *Dynamic Authorisation Rules Component* (DARC) generates automatically authorisation depending on certain rules and regulations.

The need for restrictive authorisation is going to dramatically increase over the next couple of years as the physicians demand more and more patient related information. From the European market point of view there is already today a defined need for such functionality, especially from the Nordic countries but also for the European market in general. Therefor we consider these components most valuable for the European Health Care Sectors.

4 SECURITY ISSUES

In the physical implementation of the DHE, several security features are implemented, as it is briefly schematised in the following.

- *Encryption/decryption* modules based on private and public keys may be activated on both the client and the server side.
- *Digital signature* may be added when validating or entering health data. A function can validate the authenticity of the signature.
- *Certification* of the user activities is provided for auditing and/or legal purposes as a log of all interactions occurred which is signed and encrypted by the user.

Those features could collaborate together with the authorisations in an extension of HISA based on the following security principles:

- *The secure extranet principle* specifies that the treatment of a user request cannot be affected by any other system than those handling the request. It implies that the systems implied have to be securely authenticated and are the only that can access the key to exploit the information.
- *The systematic computation of the authorisation rules* certifies that *any* request addressed to *any* of its services is validated according to the actual authorisation rules before being processed.
- *The a posteriori proof* is able to provide the necessary information to verify that the above principles have been respected within the execution of any of the received requests.

Those principles can be implemented within the standard architecture as in figure 4.

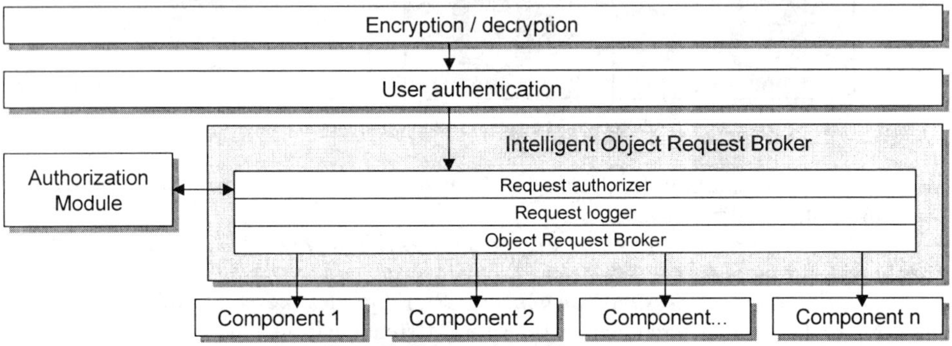

Figure 4: The security architecture

In this approach the broker guaranties to each component that any request it receives is authorised and logged in accordance to the organisation security rules. The information carried by the extranet is encrypted and the user is clearly authenticated. Only the request authoriser, logger and /or the authorisation modules have to be customised according to the rules of a specific organisation.

In such architecture, the universality of the middleware's components is easier to reach. The framework for the collaboration between these new components and the existing ones is clearly defined in order to reduce their interdependency and the service duplication. The three proposed services can be considered as generic components as their behaviour is independent of a specific business area such as health care.

REFERENCES

[1] CEN/TC251 ENV 12967-1 'Health care Information Systems Architecture'
[2] CEN/TC251 ENV12265 'Electronic Health care Record Architecture'
[3] The DHE middleware: - Information view, Functional view and API's – SPRI 1998
[4] S. Spahni - J.R. Scherrer - D. Sauquet - P.A. Sottile. 'Consensual trends for optimising the constitution of middleware', SYNAPSES project, Telematics Application Programme of the Commission of the European Communities, project No. HC1046 published in SIGCOMM Computer Communication Review, vol–28, no 5, 1998, pp 76-90.

Biomedical Processing, Data Analysis and Image Processing

Medical Informatics Europe '99
P. Kokol et al. (Eds.)
IOS Press, 1999

Bias in meta-analysis and funnel plot asymmetry

Milicic Biljana [a], Marinkovic Jelena [b], Jeremic Branislav [c], Radotic Milorad [a]
[a] *Department of Statistics, Medical Faculty, Kragujuevac, P.O. Box 124; Svetozara Markovica 69. 34000 Kragujevac, Yugoslavia, tel: (381) (34) 335 572; fax: 335 321*
[b] *Insitute of Social Medicine, statistics and Health Research, Medical Faculty, Belgrade, Dr Subotica 15 "Silos", 11000 Belgrade, Yugoslavia*
[c] *Department of Oncology, University Hospital, Kragujevac, Zmaj Jovina b.b. 34000 Kragujevac, Yugoslavia*

Abstract. International experiences reveal the important role played by scientific research and systematic study a problems, in effectively tackling change in the health sector. Meta-analysis was introduced to address the problem of synthesizing the large quanty of information on a particular subject. It is viewed, only as a step in the process of developing better tools to quantify information across studies.
The selection of trials for inclusion in a meta-analysis may be biased if selection is restricted to published trials, to trials published in English language journals, to trials published in prestigious journals or to trials cited by other authors.
Funnel plot is graphical display of sample size plotted against effect size for the studies included in a meta-analysis, which can be used to investigate bias. When all the studies have been located, the distribution of points should resemble a funnel. If there are gaps in the funnel shape it indicates that some studies may have not been published or located.
In evaluating bias, we use meta-analysis studies about radiotherapy alone versus combined radiotherapy and chemotherapy in stages IIIa and IIIb non-small cell lung cancer.
A simple analysis of funnel plots provides useful test for the likely presence of bias in meta-analyses, but as the capacity to detect bias will be limited when meta-analyses are based on a limited number of small trials the results from such analyses should be treated with considerable caution.

1. Introduction

Evidence Based Medicine is the conscientious, explicit and judicious use of current best evidence in making decisions about the care of individual patients. The practice of evidence based medicine means integrating individual clinical experts with the best available external clinical evidence from systematic research.

When a doctor is pondering what is the best cours of treatment for an uncommon disease or a biomedical researcher is launching a new project this person would review current literature for relevant citation on the subject of interest. The search of literature database is an efficient way to begin the assembly of relevant information from vast volume of biomedical publication.

Papers that summarise other papers are systematic reviews and meta-analyses. Systematic rewiev is an overview of primary studies that used explicit and reproduciable methods. Meta-analysis in clinical research is based on simple principles: systematically searching and when possible quantitavely combining results of all studies that addressed a similar research question. A good meta-analysis is often easier for the non-statistician to understand then the stack of primary research papers from which it was derived [1].

The selection of trials for inclusion in a meta-analysis may be biased if selection is restricted to published trials (publication bias), to trials published in English language journals (language bias), to trials published in prestigious journals or to trials cited by other authors such as in review articles (reference bias). Furthermore, even if all relevant trials are eventually published, the selection of trials may still be biased if it is restricted to trials that are published early [2]. The findings of some meta-analyses have letter been contradicted by large randomised controlled trials.

Although several ways of examing the potential impact of publication bias on the results of systematic review have been described, all of them are problematic. There is growing concesus that the only satisfactory way to address this bias is through prospective registration of trials. Nonetheless, reviewers may want to consider using a "funnel plot" to look for publication bias if there is a sufficient number of studies. This can be done by plotting the study weight (one divided by variance of the odds ratio) or sample size (on the "y" axis) against the odds ratios (on the "x" axis). Typically this will give the appearance of a funnel with larger studies (with greater weights) at the top in the middle and smaller studies spread out at the bottom. A gap at the bottom of the funnel on the right side (assuming smaller odds ratios (less than one) represent beneficial effects) indicates that small "positive studies" were identified wheras equal numbers of small studies in the opposite direction were not. In the absence of bias the plot will resemble a symetrical inverted funnel. If there is bias, funnel plots will often be skewed and asymetrical.

Through visual examination funnel plots have been interpreted differently by different observes. We want systematically examined symmetry or asymmetry of funnel plot because that we measured funnel plot asymmetry numerically [3].

2. Material and methods

We used a linear regression approach to measure funnel plot asymmetry on the natural logaritham scale of the odds ratio. The standard normal deviate (SND; the odds ratio divided by its standard error) is regressed against the estimates precision (the inverse of the standard error). Regression equation:

$$SND=a+b\text{x}precison$$

Small trials will be close to zero on both axis. First, precision depends largely on simple size and because that small trials will be close to zero on the x axis. In other hand small trials may produce an odds ratio that differs from unity, but because the standard error will be large, the resulting standard normal deviate will again be close to zero. Large studies will produce precise estimates and, if the treatment is effective, standard normal deviates is also large. Situation corresponds to a symmetrical funnel plot will be when the points from homogeneous set of trials not distorted by selection bias will thus scatter about a line that runs through the origin at standard normal deviate zero (a=0), with the slope b indicating the size and direction of effect.

If there is asymmetry, the regression line will not run through the origin. The intercept a provides a measure of asymmetry. When the larger its deviation from zero the more pronounced the asymmetry. If the smaller studies show big protective effects, they will force regression line below the origin on the logarithmic scale. Smaller studies show more pronounced beneficial effects than larger studies when we have negative value of intercept a.

Power of study including in meta-analysis, in some situations is gained by weighting the analysis by the inverse of variance of the effect estimate.

The test for funnel plot asymmetry in contrast to the overall test of heterogeneity, provides a more powerful test in this situation. However any analysis any analysis of heterogeneity depends on the number of trials included in meta-analysis which is generally small, and this limits the statistical power of test. Because that, we based evidence of asymmetry on $p<0.1$ and we present intercept with 90% confidence interval [3].

We use meta-analysis studies about radiotherapy alone versus combined radiotherapy and chemotherapy in stages IIIa and IIIb non-small cell lung cancer and single agent chemotherapy versus combination chemotherapy in advanced non-small lung cancer. The bibliographic search for published reports meta-analysis was made using MEDLINE database in all languages, covering period from 1993 to 1998.

3. Results

We examined bias in three meta-analysis about therapy in stages IIIa and IIIb non-small cell lung cancer. In that study an adaption of method Mantel and Haenszel was applied to estimate and pool odds ratios (ORs) of death. Values of OR less than unity indicated beter overall survival with chemotherapy/radiotherapy than with radiotherapy alone. Tabele 1 show results of analysis of funnel plot asymmetry. One out of three meta-analyses showed significant ($p<0.1$) funnel plot asymmetry. In two meta-analyses funnel plot don't show statistical significant.

Tabela 1 Analysis of funnel plot asymmetry

Meta-analysis	No of trials	Linear regresion analysis	
		Intercept (90% CI)	P value
Milicic B. [4]	8	2.769 (-1.233-6.770)	0.141
Marino P. [5]	12	2.741 (-1.287-6.769)	0.126
Marino P. [6]	9	-9.650 (-17.779-(-1.521))	0.026

Pooled OR in one of them was 1.05 (CI=0.7-1.5), while other gave pooled OR value about 0.84 (CI=0.68-1.04). Study with significant funnel plot asymmetry gave value of poolrd OR 0.8 and its 95% confidence interval 0.6-1.0 thus favoring combination chemotherapy. In that meta-analysis larger study had OR less or equal unity, while smaller show OR larger than unity. OR discordance between small and large study include in this meta-analysis was consequence of a large study showing more beneficial effects of use combination, rather than single agent chemotherapy in advanced non-small cell lung cancer than small study.

4. Discussion

International experiences reveal the important role played by scientific research and systematic study a problems, in effectively tackling change in the health sector. Meta-analysis was introduced to address the problem of synthesizing the large quanty of information on a particular subject [7]. It is viewed, only as a step in the process of developing better tools to quantify information across studies. It has been suggested that investigators should combine quantitative and qualitative review data to enable practioners to apply results to individual patients or program problems. In this way researches can investigate issues that are important, but difficult to quantify. Non-quantitative information, such as expert opinion and anecdotal evidence, does have a significant impact on policy.

Finally, one must be concerned that although, even the best meta-analysis may represent all available trials and relevant studies, it may not represent clinical practice because, of the nature of how and where research is conducted.

The validity of meta-analysis depends on complete sampling of all the studies performed on a particular topic. Validity can be preserved if representative sampling of studies is obtained, but any incomplete sampling is a potentially biased one [8].

Sources of bias and funnel plots asymmetry

Selection bias

- Publication bias
- Location biases:
  -English language bias
  -Citation bias
  -Multiple publication bias

True heterogeneity

- Size of effect differs according to study size:
  -Intensity of intervention
  -Differences in underlying risk

Data irregularities

- Poor methodological design of small studies
- Inadequate analysis
- Fraud

Artefactual

- Choice of effect measure

Chance

The selection of trials for inclusion in a meta-analysis may be biased if selection is restricted to published trials, to trials published in English language journals, to trials published in prestigious journals or to trials cited by other authors. It is the tendency of studies which report statisticly significant results to be published. Publication bias is a form of selection bias. This will lead to a biased review but can be minimised by using a comprehensive search and unbiased processes for choosing studies for inclusion [9]. Multiple publications bias occurs when studies whose results are published in series of articles are more likely to be sampled than those published only once [10]. There is systematic differences between studies included in meta-analysis and the studies which were missed which relating to the study results.

In the language of meta-analysis, homogeneity means that the results of each individual trial are mathematically compatible with the results of any of the others. Statistical heterogeneity is a mathematical exercise and is the job of the statistician, but explaining this heterogeneity (looking for, and accounting for, clinical heterogeneity) is an interpretive exercise and requires imagination, common sense, and hands-on clinical or research experience. Critical examination for the presence of publication and related biases must therefore become an essential part of meta-analytic studies and systematic reviews. The findings presented here indicate that a simple graphical and statistical method is useful for this purpose.

Another source of funnel plot asymmetry arises from differences in methodological quality. If study results are weighted for quality in the analysis a bias in scoring study quality may have real impact on meta-analysis results. Smaller studies are on average conducted and analysed with less methodological rigour then larger studies. Trials of lower quality also tend to show larger effects [11]. The degree of symmetry found in a funnel plot may depend on the statistic used to measure effect. Odds ratios overestimate the relative reduction, or increase, in risk if the event rate is high [12]. This can lead to funnel plot asymmetry if the smaller trials were consistently conducted in patients at higher risk. Similarly, if events accrue at a constant rate, relative risks will move towards unity with increasing length of follow up. In large trials, follow up is often longer than in small studies.

The trials included in meta-analysis may not estimate the same underlying effect of the intervention, and such heterogeneity between results may lead to asymmetry in funnel plots.

Some interventions may have been implemented less thoroughly in larger trials, thus explaining the more positive results in smaller trials. Small trials are generally conducted before larger trials are established. In the intervening years, control treatments may have improved or changed in a way that could reduce the efficacy of the experimental treatment [13].

Finally, an asymmetrical funnel plot may arise by chance.

5. Conclusions

Meta-analysis has made and continues to make major contributions to medical research, clinical decision making, and standards of research reportage. Aggregation of data from multiple trials should enhance the precision and accuracy of any pooled result. But combining data requires a leap of faith: it presumes that the differences among studies are primarly due to chance. In fact, differences in the direction or size of treatment effects may be caused by other factors including subtle differences in treatments, populations outcome measures, study design and study quality. Thus meta-analysis may generate misleading results by ignoring meaningful heterogeneity among studies entrenching the biases in individual studies, and introducing further biases through the process of finding studies and selecting results to be pooled.

If the sensitivity analysis that are done do not materially change the results, it strengt hens the confidence that can be placed in them. If the results change in a way that might lead to different conclusions, this indicates a need for greater caution in interpreting the results and drawing conclusions. It might also enable reviewers to clarify the source of exsiting contraversis about the effectiveness of an intervention, or lead reviewers to hypothesise potentially important factors that might be related to the effectiveness of the intervention and warrant further investigation.

The possibility that the study selection was affected by publication bias can be investigated in the data analysis. Funnel plots show the distribution of effect sizes according to sample size: it is to be expected that the points will full a funnels shape, there being more variability in reported affect sizes for smaller studies. Large gaps in the funnel indicate a group of possibly “missing” publications. These omissions are usually small studies showing no effect and are unilikely to be missing at random. Statistical methods are available to investigate how serios publication bias would have to be to change the review’s overall conclusion. The technique discussed here should contribute to this goal, providing reproducible measure for the likely presence, or apparent absence of such biases.

Meta-analysis cannot tell clinicians how to treat an individual patient but it can provide information that helps decision making.

References

[1] Greenhalgh T. Papers that summarise other papers (systematic reviews and meta-analyses). BMJ 1997:315, pp 672-675.
[2] Stern J.M., Simes J.R. Publication bias: evidence of delayed publication ina a cohort study of clinical research projects. BMJ 1997:315, pp 640-645.
[3] Egger M., Smith G.D., Schneider M., Minder C. Bias in meta-analysis detected by a simple, graphical test. BMJ 1997:315, pp 629-634.
[4] Milicic B., Mrainkovic J., Jeremic B., Radotiv M., Arsenijevic N. Radiotherapy alone versus combined radiotherapy and chemotherapy in stages IIIA and IIIb non-small cell lung cancer: meta-analysis study. 9 th World Congress on Medical Informatics. Medinf' 98. IOS Press, 1998 Amsterdam; pp: 885.
[5] Marino P., Preatoni A., Cantoni A. Randomized trials of radiotherapy alone versus combined chemotherapy and radiotherapy in stages IIIa and IIIb nonsmall cell lung cancer. A meta-analysis. Cancer 1995: 76, pp: 593-60.
[6] Marino P., Preatoni A., Cantoni A., Buccheri G. Single agent chemotherapy versus combination chemotherapy in advanced non-small cell lung cancer: a quality and meta-analysis study. Lung Cancer 1995: 13, pp: 1-12.
[7] Stephan B., Tacher M.D. Meta-analysis. A quantitative approach to research integration. JAMA 1988: 259, pp: 1685-9.
[8] Framer M.R., Reynolds J.M., Moor R.A., McQuay H.J. Impact of covert duplicate publication on meta-analysis: a case study. BMJ 1997:315, pp 635-640.
[9] Gotzche P.C. Reference bias in reports of drug trials. BMJ 1987: 295, 654-6.
[10] Felson D.T. Bias in meta-analytic research. J Clin Epidemiol 1992:vol 45 No8, pp: 885-892.
[11] Villar J., Piaggio G., Carroli G., Donner A. Factors affecting the comparability of meta-analysis and largest trials results in perinatology. J Clin Epidemiol 1997: 50, pp: 997-1002.
[12] Schulz K.F., Chalmers I., Hayes R.J., Altman D.G., Empirical evidence of bias. Dimensions of methodological quality associated with estimates of treatment effects in controlled trials. JAMA 1995: 273, pp: 408-12.
[13] Altman D.G. The scandal of poor medical research. BMJ 1994:308, pp:283-4.

Medical Informatics Europe '99
P. Kokol et al. (Eds.)
IOS Press, 1999

Developing shared understanding through simulation

Nicholas HARDIKER RGN BSc MSc, Stephen KAY BSc MSc PhD MBCS
Medical Informatics Group, Department of Computer Science,
University of Manchester, Manchester M13 9PL, UK

Abstract. In this article relevant key findings of a review of selected published work are used to provide a foundation for a new approach to developing a shared understanding of aspects of health care delivery. The new approach makes use of simulation models. It is hoped that this approach will provide support for improved decision-making and for the development of more appropriate enabling tools.

1. Introduction

This article presents a case for using simulation models to represent processes within the health sector (unlike much simulation, the approach to modelling is directed more toward soft qualitative analysis than harder quantitative analysis). It describes how these models have been used interactively with 'owner', 'actors' and 'customers' [1] to facilitate the development of a shared understanding with the analyst of the problem domain. Other related work in the health sector can be found in the educational domain [2, 3]. The factors which differentiate our approach from similar previous approaches include the use of discrete event simulation models as the focus of interaction rather than more overtly qualitative models such as those used in the application of Wolstenholme's 'Systems Thinking' [4], and the inclusion of the analyst in the interaction. While we accept that 'analyst' might (and perhaps should) also play the role of 'owner' or 'actor', the main motivation behind our work is to bridge the gap between analyst and user. We believe that our approach goes some way towards achieving this end.

2. Operational Research in the health sector

Over the past two decades, a variety of aspects of health care delivery have been examined under the banner of 'Operational Research'. Research has been diverse, ranging from medical record storage [5] to the optimal allocation of staff [7]. A major motivation for the research has been to provide support for decision making. A variety of solutions have been proposed. Butler *et al.* argue that such variety is necessary [6].

2.1. Supporting decision-making

Butler *et al.* present a hierarchical view of hospital planning with four distinct levels and suggest that the particular level at which a decision is being taken dictates the particular approach which should be used to aid the decision-making process. They define these levels as:

1. Strategy formation, product planning and long-term capacity planning;
2. Facilities planning and fixed capacity allocation;
3. Aggregate operations planning and demand management; and,
4. Systems or procedures for detailed execution of plans.

This hierarchy may be viewed as a continuum with strategic decision-making at one end, through tactical decision-making, to operational decision-making at the opposite end (see Figure 1). Operational decision-making activities such as those concerning the detailed execution of plans imply a highly dynamic world. On the other hand, strategic decision-making activities such as strategy formation, product planning and long term capacity planning imply a relatively slow-moving world. The number of variables to consider decreases as we move along the continuum from operational decision-making to strategic decision-making. However, the significance of each variable increases as we move in the same direction as a result of increasing aggregation. Thus according to Butler *et al.* it would be possible to place the different approaches which should be used to aid decision-making on this continuum according to their ability to handle change, number of variables and significance of variables. For example, a flip chart might be used for strategy formation; a simple spreadsheet for fixed capacity allocation; a deterministic model for aggregate operations planning; and simulation for procedures for the detailed execution of plans.

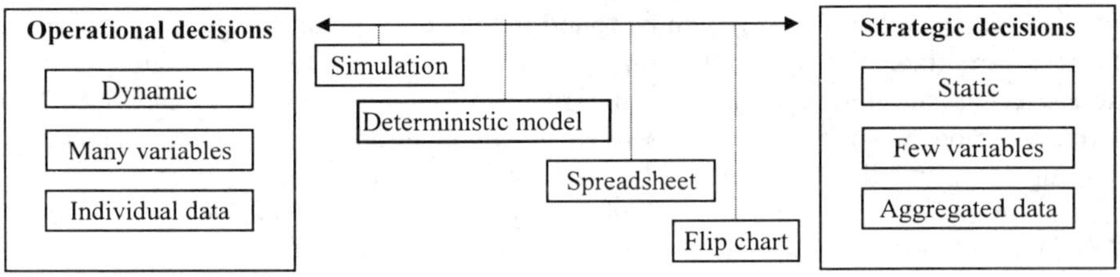

Figure 1: Multi-level model of decisions and decision aids, adapted from Butler et al. [6]

The multi-level model of decisions and associated decision aids presented above would appear to contradict the suggestion made nearly 20 years ago by Boldy *et al.* that "...simulation is becoming increasingly used in strategic planning" [8]. The development of the model with the suggestion that simulation is best suited to operational decision-making, is perhaps an indication that the increase in use of simulation at a strategic level has not maintained the momentum anticipated in the 1970's. This view is reflected in published accounts of simulation projects, which tend to be confined to more tactical or operational decision-making activities [9, 10].

2.2. Indications for using simulation approaches

Variability and uncertainty are key factors in selecting simulation over other approaches [11], or where there is a need to assess the impact of change dynamically [12]. Among other things, simulation models can use distribution data independently of the model structure;

they allow the imposition of constraints; take account of appropriate attributes for individual entities; and use any appropriate time units [13].

The increasing complexity of the health care environment and health care organisations coupled with the rate of change that characterises the early 1990s have contributed to the increasing importance of simulation [2]. In certain situations it is no longer possible to solve problems analytically. For example, a deterministic model using averages is inappropriate for determining factors such as available bed space, arrival rates of patients and length of stay patterns. A stochastic model is needed due to the dynamics of the system [14]. These views would appear to validate the Butler *et al.* model in that simulation is seen as more appropriate in uncertain and changing environments i.e. towards the operational decision-making end of the continuum.

The confinement of simulation to tactical and operational decision-making is not in itself a guarantee of success. In addition to complex and uncertain nature of the problem domain, there is the model itself to consider. According to Huang *et al.* a model should be "both valid (i.e. it is a sufficiently accurate representation of the system under study) and credible (i.e. the user finds it useful and is willing to use it as an aid in his or her decision making). But a model cannot accurately simulate every aspect of a complex system. Hence a model is valid if it can sufficiently accurately simulate the impact of various factors of concern on the key performance indicators of the system." [10].

The successful implementation of simulation projects depends on factors such as: whether decision making is inevitable, the timing of the project and the close involvement within the project of the health organisation [15]. Other non-technical factors must also be taken into account. The culture of the health sector is traditionally not oriented to quantitative methods; nor is it oriented to planning [16]. The primary concern of the majority of health sector employees is in the care of individuals. There is little incentive for greater efficiency. Over recent years in the UK, a range of political initiatives such as the Resource Management Initiative have attempted to introduce a business approach to clinical practice. A major effect of such initiatives has been a marked delineation between clinical practice and health service management. The divisions between clinicians and managers and lack of mutual understanding have caused tension. This has resulted in a tightening of professional boundaries, with clinicians refocusing attention onto the needs of individuals rather than onto the efficiency of the service, and managers attempting to introduce measures to increase efficiency with little regard for the needs of individuals. It has also resulted in a degradation of the decision-making hierarchy.

2.3. Qualitative modelling

Recently there has been a general movement in strategic analysis toward recognising the need for rigorous ideas for knowledge capture and communication of mental perceptions based on modelling methods i.e. modelling as learning. For example, Wolstenholme presents an application of system dynamics in community care as a framework for strategic debate [4]. A revised framework for System Dynamics, which Wolstenholme calls 'Systems Thinking' combines knowledge acquisition and qualitative and quantitative modelling, supported by microworlds and archetypes to aid dissemination of insights. The emphasis of the Wolstenholme study is on using qualitative models interactively with different groups of participants in the problem domain. The use of qualitative models seeks to assist in the development of a shared understanding of how culture, power and politics combine to affect the behaviour of a process when subjected to externally superimposed changes in responsibility.

3. A foundation for a new approach

A number of key themes emerge from the discussion above:

- Health care is a rapidly changing and complex environment with much variability and uncertainty
- There is a limit to the cognitive ability of the human brain to process multi-variate problems
- The use of simulation can facilitate an improvement in systemic understanding
- Simulation approaches are best-suited to operational decision-making
- A simulation model must be a sufficiently accurate and focused representation of the domain in question
- Users must be willing to use a simulation model and find it useful for decision-making

In addition, the timing of simulation projects must be appropriate and users should be in a position to implement change at a time when change is possible. Moreover, the provision of health care is increasingly viewed as collaboration between health care disciplines. More recently this collaboration has started to include different agencies including Voluntary Organisations, Social Services, Housing, etc. Thus it is very important that organisational boundaries should be represented explicitly to facilitate the study of the influence of culture, power, and politics.

It is clear that simulation approaches have a useful role to play, particularly at an operational level. At such a level within health care, the focus is on the shared care of individuals. Any understanding of activities at this level can only be derived from an examination, with users, of key indicators of qualitative aspects of patient care. Thus, in modelling these activities and examining the resulting models with users, there should be an emphasis on qualitative elements. Dynamic display facilitates visualisation of the underlying model. More importantly perhaps it affords the possibility of seeing beyond quantitative elements by showing patterns traced by recognisable artefacts in familiar situations.

This represents a shift in emphasis. The main motivation behind modelling is not to optimise existing processes; nor is it to plan resources for the future. Rather it is to communicate and influence the present. Although the resulting model represents day-to-day operational activities, the utility of that model goes far beyond the operational level. It provides an operational view of the world, which will be used to enhance the interaction between user and analyst and to promote dialogue between different levels of decision making

4. Implementing the framework

The new approach described above has been used as part of a project to Assist Process Performance and Utilisation through Simulation (the APPUS project). The focus of the project is upon facilitating better communication between users (clinical and non-clinical) and analysts within a community health care setting. Case studies were used to introduce simulation models and process models to non-computer scientists from a Community Health care Trust with the aim of understanding how they might help to elicit system requirements through dialogue (the focus of this article is on simulation models only).

The use of case studies permitted access to a relatively small but important group of healthcare professionals to engage with actual problem scenarios in their work situations while enabling the researchers to consider the communication offered by the simulation models in workshop settings.

A discrete event simulation product, WITNESS, was used to develop simulation models of key processes. It is important to note that APPUS used only the dynamic, visualisation aspects of WITNESS. The reason for this was that the main interest was in the behaviour of and interactions between individual entities rather than in aggregations. Our application of simulation to health care does not have the usual emphasis upon optimisation and efficiency but with the effectiveness of care delivery. Pitt [17], in a related study, emphasised the characteristics of the entity (i.e. the patient) to facilitate the capture of the situation's statistics, whereas in APPUS the primary concern was with the interaction between the entities (staff, patients and others). It was necessary therefore to use only a subset of the WITNESS product. Indeed, one of the objectives of APPUS was to compare the effectiveness of this form of visualisation for the dynamics of interaction with static paper-based process models [18].

5. Results and discussion

The case study approach within a workshop setting was found to be a pragmatic vehicle for studying how simulation models can be used. It managed to provide a focus for the attendees and, without exception, the conclusion was that it was both enjoyable and useful. Given the past track record of technical innovation and adoption in the Trust, this in itself was a remarkable finding. One manager is on record (unsolicited) as saying that in the 3 years since he had been at the Trust, no other way had so successfully facilitated communication across the professional boundaries. This was a testament both to the particular technique and to the workshop setting that allowed groups to participate in communication of their work processes. One certainty was that the use of scenarios was found to be valuable as a means of articulating process.

As the case studies unfolded, so it became clear that small scenarios provided the best return. The developer could model these very quickly with little time required by the customer. Once produced, however, they could be used and reused for gathering new requirements. Such scenarios may have even greater potential for reflective practice and training where, like requirements elicitation, someone within the Trust has to explain to an outsider (or newcomer or other professional) what the work is like from their perspective. The clinical scenarios, in particular, permitted the non-clinical managers to appreciate the intricate working structures and processes of the staff they were expected to support and manage. All the scenarios were found to be additional sources of knowledge that could facilitate organisational and possibly clinical change. It is also clear that at least for the initial requirements exercise, it is not necessary to engage in substantial, detailed, timings to develop the simulation models. The users fill in the gaps and 'assume' that the model is accurate unless it does something that is anomalous. The attendees volunteer timings for the interactions and consequently the timing aspects can be regarded as a refinement rather than a pre-requisite to the model.

In summary, APPUS has confirmed our view that the use of simulation models can facilitate the development in users of a deeper understanding of relevant aspects of their work; an understanding which is shared by the analyst.

In this way, such an approach might provide support for the development of systems that better fit with working practice. A follow on project seeks to contribute more appropriate enabling tools.

Acknowledgements

The work embodied in this article was carried out as part of the (Assisting Process Performance and Utilisation through Simulation) APPUS project (EPSRC Grant GR/L/15043). WITNESS is a product of the LANNER Group, which has also supported the project. The project team would like to thank all of those people at Mancunian Community Health NHS Trust who gave their time and effort to the project.

References

[1] Checkland, P., *Soft systems methodology in action.* 1990, Chichester: Wiley.
[2] NHS ME IMG, *HERMES - Hospital Environment Resource Management Education Simulator.* 1992, London: HMSO.
[3] Kirkup, B. *et al.*, *Numberside 2.* NHS Management Executive News, 1992, **54**: 6-7.
[4] Wolstenholme, E., *A case study in community care using systems thinking.* Journal of the Operational Research Society, 1993. **44**(9): p. 925-934.
[5] Nimmo, A., *A model for medical record storage.* Journal of the Operational Research Society, 1983. **34**(5): p. 391-399.
[6] Butler, T., K. Karwan, and J. Sweigart, *Multi-level strategic evaluation of hospital plans and decisions.* Journal of the Operational Research Society, 1992. **43**(7): p. 665-675.
[7] Vassilacopoulos, G., *Allocating doctors to shifts in an accident and emergency department.* Journal of the Operational Research Society, 1985. **36**(6): p. 517-523.
[8] Boldy, D. and D. Clayden, *Operational research projects in health and welfare services in the United Kingdom and Ireland.* Journal of the Operational Research Society, 1979. **30**: p. 505-511.
[9] Weiss, E. and J. McClain, *Administrative days in acute care facilities: a queuing-analytic approach.* Operations Research, 1987. **35**(1): p. 35-44.
[10] Huang, X.-M., C. Taylor, and I. Stewart, *Computer simulation of an A&E department.* OR Insight, 1995. **8**(2): p. 18-23.
[11] Babes, M. and G. Sarma, *Out-patient queues at the Ibn-Rochd health centre.* Journal of the Operational Research Society, 1991. **42**(10): p. 845-855.
[12] Hannan, E., *A Markov sensitivity model for examining the impact of cost allocations in hospitals.* Journal of the Operational Research Society, 1984. **35**(2): p. 117-129.
[13] Davies, R., *An assessment of models of a health system.* Journal of the Operational Research Society, 1985. **36**(8): p. 679-687.
[14] Grove, D. and D. Hewitt, *A hospital capacity planning model.* OR Insight, 1995. **8**(2): p. 12-15.
[15] Tunnicliffe Wilson, J., *Implementation of computer simulation projects in health care.* Journal of the Operational Research Society, 1981. **32**: p. 825-832.
[16] Clayden, D., *Unpredictable change?* OR Insight, 1995. **8**(2): p. 2-4.
[17] Pitt, M.A. *A generalised simulation system to support strategic resource planning in healthcare.* in *1997 Winter Simulation Conference.* 1997. Atlanta: WSC.
[18] Kay, S., *et al. Process Modelling and Simulation for Managing Clinical Care in the Community.* in *AMIA'98.* 1998. Orlando, FL: Hanley & Belfus, Inc.

Medical Informatics Europe '99
P. Kokol et al. (Eds.)
IOS Press, 1999

Data integration to assist gastric emptying data analysis

M. Giacomini[1,2], C. Ruggiero[1,2], P. Borro[3], C. Mansi[3]
[1]*DIST - Dept. of Communication Computer and System Sciences, University of Genova, Via Opera Pia 13, 16145 Genova – Italy. E-mail: giacomin@dist.unige.it*
[2]*DIST laboratory, Advanced Biotechnology Center - ABC, Genova - Italy*
[3]*Department of Internal Medicine, Gastroenterology Unit, University of Genova - Italy*

Abstract. The diagnosis of dyspepsia is very difficult because the symptoms are clinically aspecific and the gastric emptying time tests are of complex interpretation. An integrated and automated analysis of clinical and instrumental data may improve the diagnostic process. We present a system to collect data on dyspeptic patient from different sources which has been set up to assist the clinician in the diagnosis of dyspepsia. The data base integrates a wide set of symptoms with data coming from laboratory tests. Moreover, we assess the feasibility of classifying gastric emptying profiles using both octanoid acid excretion data and electrogastrography.

1. Introduction

Dyspepsia is a common condition characterised mainly by pain or epigastric discomfort and frequently associated with delayed gastric emptying. The diagnosis is very difficult because the symptoms are clinically aspecific and the gastric emptying time tests are of complex interpretation. An integrated and automated analysis of clinical and instrumental data may improve diagnostic process. We present a database which has been set up to assist the clinician in the diagnosis of dyspepsia. The data base integrates a wide set of symptoms with data coming from laboratory tests. The data base has also been used to assess the feasibility of the classification of data on gastric emptying time, using artificial neural networks.

2. Methods

SVGAS is a system developed based on a relational database which can easily interface with other programs which produce raw laboratory data .The data structure has been designed using the mixed approach [1]. The main entities of the data base are: patient, examination and test, closely connected (fig. 1 shows the level 0 of the Entity-Relational diagram of the data base). Patient data can be recorded without duplication, independently of the number of examinations and tests which are stored. In the same way general test data are recorded only once, without any duplication for each specific test performed. Tables to record anamnestic information (smoke, alchool, etc.) and specific symptoms information (epigastric/retrosternal pain or discomfort, postprandial fullness, bloating, early satiety, postprandial nausea, belching after meals, postprandial vomiting, anorexia) are present in the database. These tables are directly linked to the corresponding patient records.

Test entity has been subdivided into three specific entities to retain the differences in methods. We consider above all two experimental methods: ^{13}C-octanoic acid breath test [2], and electrogastrogram [3]; but for some cases we recorded also data from scintigraphy [4].

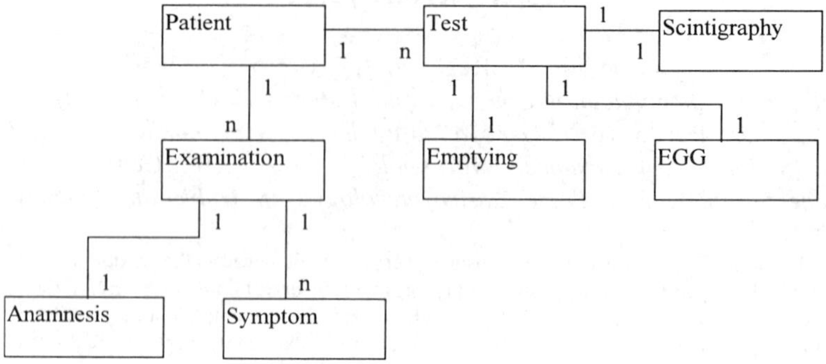

Fig.1 E-R level 0

^{13}C-octanoic acid breath test is a reliable tool for measuring gastric emptying. It is based on the administration of a substrate with a functional group containing ^{13}C which is the stable isotope of carbon. The functional group is enzymatically cleaved during the passage in the gastrointestinal tract, further metabolized by liver to $^{13}CO_2$ which mixes with the blood "bicarbonate pool" and finally expired in the breath. Therefore, $^{13}CO_2$ excretion reflects gastric emptying rate.

Electrogastrography (EGG) records gastric electric activity by means of electrodes attached to the abdominal surface, similar to electrocardiographic recording. The origin of the electric activity from the stomach has been confirmed in animal models and humans. Simultaneous myoelectric recordings with electrodes implanted in the gastric mucosa and placed on the abdomen have shown that EGG signal shows an underlying slow wave frequency [5]. Recently, EGG was used to examine the pathophysiology of upper gastroinestianl symptoms.

The three methods mainly differ, from a computer science point of view, for the inter sample interval, breath test and scintigraphy use inter sample time interval of 10 - 30 minutes; while electrogastrogram uses a inter sample time interval of 0.25 seconds. So the amount of data to be recorded for each test and the mathematical methods used for their analysis are significatively different.

The test tables contain quality control information for each test performed. The data tables are linked to both the test table (to allow the follow up of the patient) and external data analysis programs.The database is integrated with a series of automatic procedures to perform controlled data insertion and assisted data consultation. Specifically, some procedures to automate data insertion from laboratory instruments are present.

Patient insertion is a manual operation performed by the clinician, just after patient examination, in order to store reliable clinical data. The test data insertion is performed in a semiautomatic way: technicians only have to select the test type and the specific work list, locate the directory of the communication files and supervise the validation control and data interpretation procedures. Fig. 2 shows the data flow diagram of this operation.

The data is protected by a set of access password to identify the authorised user with a compulsory login procedure.

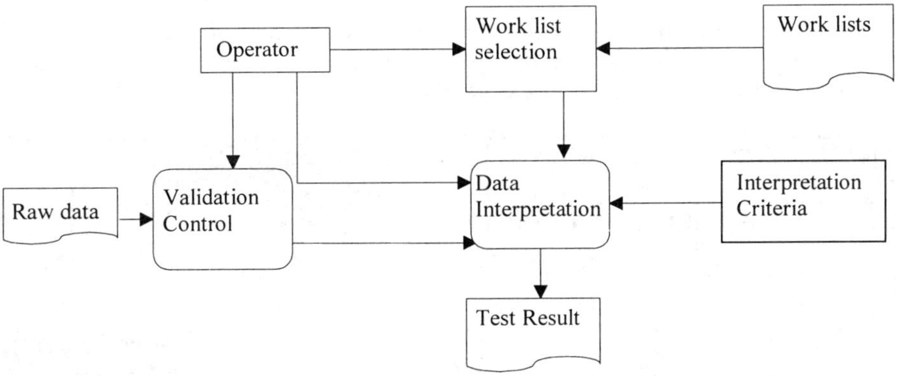

Fig. 2 DFD diagram of result insertion

3. Results

The data base is now being validated at the Gastroenterology Unit of the Department of Internal Medicine of the University of Genova, and is mainly used by internists in training without any specific experience in computer science, who have been given only a short presentation of the system and of its main opportunities. In the first three validation months, they have inserted, without any particular difficulty, data on 66 subjects. We have performed a preliminary study on these data to assess the feasibility of using artificial neural networks to classify, in an objective way, data obtained from acid octanoic excretion.

According to Ghoos's classical parameter [2] the 66 subjects were divided into 5 categories: 21 normal subjects, 8 accelerated subjects (A), 11 subjects with low level slowness (L); 8 subjects with medium level slowness (M); 18 subjects with severe slowness (S).

21 healthy volunteers and 45 dyspeptic patients (25 F, 20 M, mean age 41 years) were studied. Measurement of gastric emptying time was performed by ^{13}C-octanoic ac. breath test. Breath samples were collected before and every 15 minutes for 4 hours after a standard test meal with 100 mg ^{13}C-octanoic ac. (Cortex Italia, Milan, Italy) incorporated into egg yolk and analysed by isotope ratio mass spectrometer (AP 2003, UK). On the basis of T1/2 parameter of gastric emptying according to Ghoss et al. [2], all subjects were subdivided in the following subgoups: normal (N - 70±20), accelerated (A - < -2SD), slightly delayed (L - >2 SD), mild delayed (M - >4 SD), severe delayed (S - >6 SD).

The parameters indicated by Ghoos et al. [2] and the sequence of data coming from the octanoic acid excretion test have been appropriately normalised for each subject and given as input to an unsupervised neural network. The network used for this study is based on the Kohonen algorithm [6] with an output organised in a 9x9 matrix, implemented within a Matlab 4.3 environment, running on a Pentium PC. Fig. 3 shows the results obtained with this preliminary study. As it can be noted in fig. 3, all cells assigned to the categories are grouped in well distinguishable and ordered sectors of the output map. All subjects, except one, have been classified in the correct category. The only subject classified in the wrong category is one of the medium group, which has been classified together with subjects of the low level group.

We are also performing another feasibility study on the applicability of supervised neural networks in order to clear electrogastrographical signal from electrical noise and other external artefacts. We used input signals recorded on 10 healthy subjects about 30,000 samples long, in which 40% of samples were classified as noise by expert gastroenterologists. Of these signals 5 were used in the learning set and 5 in the test set. We used a input window of 100 samples for a network structure of 100 input neurons, 50 hidden neurons and 2 output neurons. The agreement between the network and expert interpretation was 96% in signals of the learning set and 90% in the test set signals.

A1-A2-A3	A4-A5	N1-N3	N4-N6-N11	N21	L6	L3-L5	L9-L10-M1	
A6	A7-A8	N9	N12-N14	N20	L4-L7		M4	M7
N2	N5	N15	N18			M6		
N8-N10	N16	N17		M3		M8	S3	S6
N13	N19	L1	L8	M5	S1		S7-S9	
	L11	M2			S8	S12	S14	S15
L2						S13		
			S5	S10-S11				
		S2-S4		S16		S17		S18

Fig. 3 Output Kohonen map: A, accelerated subjects ; N, normal subjects ♡; L, slightly delayed subjects ♡; M mild delayed subjects ♡; S severe delayed subjects ♡.

4. Discussion and conclusions

The validation phase, carried out at the Gastroenterology unit of the Department of Internal Medicine, has been successfully completed, specially referring to use by gastroenterologists, who appreciated above all its user-friendly features. The preliminary results of the feasibility trials suggest that neural networks can improve the analysis of breath test data and allow a better discrimination among different groups of patients. However, further work is necessary before making methods based on neural networks become suitable for the clinical practice.

References

[1] C. Batini, S. Ceri, S.B. Navathe: *Conceptual database design*, Redwood City, (CA – USA): The Benjamin Cummings Publishing Company, Inc, 1992

[2] Y.F. Ghoos, B.D. Maes, B.J. Geypens, G. Mys, M.I. Hiele, P.J. Rutgeerts, G. Vantrappen: "Measurement of Gastric Emptying Rate of Solids by Means of a Carbon-Labeled Octanic Acid Breath Test", Gastroenterology, vol. 104, pp. 1640-1647.

[3] J.D.Z. Chen, R.W. McCallum: "Electrogastrographic parameters and their clinical significance", in *Electrogastrography: Principles and applications*, J.D.Z. Chen, R.W. McCallum (eds), New-York, Raven Press, 1994, pp. 45-73.

[4] C. Scarpignato: "Gastric emptying measurement in man", in *Clinical Investigation of Gastric Function*, C. Scarpignato, G. Bianco Porro (eds), Basel, Karger, 1990, pp. 198-246.

[5] B.O. Familoni: "Validity of the cutaneous electrogastrogram", in *Electrogastrography: Principles and applications*, J.D.Z. Chen, R.W. McCallum (eds), New-York, Raven Press, 1994, pp. 103-125.

[6] T. Kohonen: *Self Organisation and Associative Memory*. Springer-Verlag 1990.

Medical Informatics Europe '99
P. Kokol et al. (Eds.)
IOS Press, 1999

Three-dimensional ROIs in Brain PET

Jouni Mykkänen[†], Martti Juhola[†] and Ulla Ruotsalainen[‡]
[†]*Department of Computer Science, University of Tampere,*
P.O.Box 607 FIN-33101 Tampere, Finland, e-mail: jm@cs.uta.fi
[‡]*Turku PET Centre, University of Turku, Finland*

Abstract. A semi-automatic system for determining volumes of interest (VOI) from positron emission tomography (PET) scans of brain is described. The VOIs surface extraction is based on user selectable threshold and three-dimensional target flood-fill. Contrast to anatomical volume detection approaches, volumes are determined from functional PET images and the obtained objects are checked against anatomical images. The developed VOI program was evaluated with brain FDOPA-PET studies where the striatum was the object. The results were comparable to entirely manual method and the target extraction time is reduced to about one third of manual method.

Keywords: volume of interest, region of interest, positron emission tomography

1 Introduction

Positron emission tomography (PET) images are analysed by drawing region of interest (ROI) from an image and calculating results by using these ROIs. A set of ROIs describing the same object in a volume space constructs a volume of interest (VOI). This can be used to calculate average radioactivity concentration in a homogeneous functional or anatomic structure.

A ROI can be determined by manually drawing areas point by point and plane by plane on the image. Points are connected (in order) by lines to obtain a closed region. With PET images, this manual approach has been reasonable because of the irregularity of target objects, noisy data and relatively low resolution. The anatomic accuracy of a manually drawn region is likely to decrease when the number of subjects and planes grows. Results are also sensitive to the analyser. Relatively more time is spent to the laborious manual drawing task instead of analysing results and making judgments.

Image processing techniques can offer tools for automating parts of this demanding process of outlining objects from medical images. With studies in literature (shortly reviewed in [1]), the time used for target extraction is reduced significantly and the reproducibility of results is superior compared to the results of manual segmentation.

2 Concept to determine volume of interest

The spatial distribution of tissue radioactivity concentration is registered by a PET-scanner and the acquired data is stored to a sinogram. Images are reconstructed from the sinogram. The developed program determines a VOI from the image with the aid of user. The VOI is written out to a file. Average radioactive concentration of a target object is determined from the image by using the obtained VOI. Figure 1 shows the schema of the whole analysis process including data acquisition.

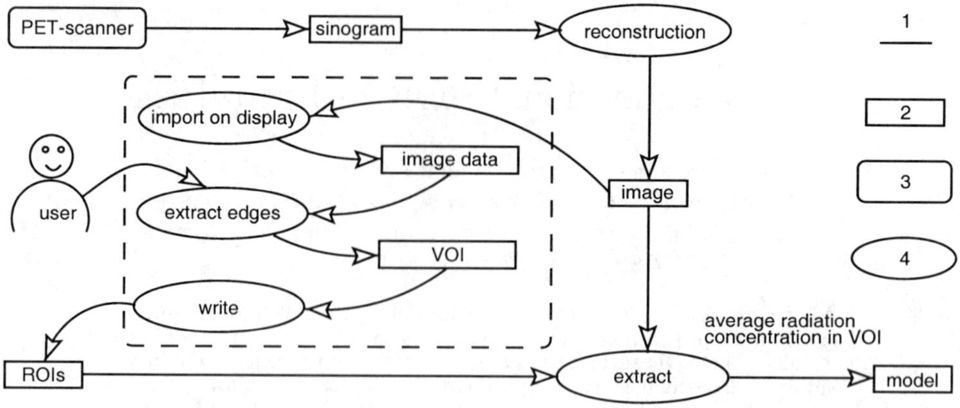

Figure 1: Schema of the analysis process and the data flow. Symbols: 1 data flow and direction, 2 data, 3 active process producing data and 4 action. The dotted box outlines the developed program tasks in the whole analysis process.

The original image is a three-dimensional stack of planes representing spatial distribution of radioactive concentration. The threshold image represents the original image in binary form and it is split to left and right thresholds. The threshold values are set by user. Surface extraction of the functional structure will be done by referring to the threshold image. The user selects a start pixel inside of the functional structure.

A standard flood-fill (region growing) algorithm is used from the start pixel to generate marked image for extracting the surface of object. The surface is described by a set of boundaries on the three-dimensional image. A boundary is extracted from flood-filled image by following the edge on plane by Algorithm 2. All distinguishable boundaries are seeked, extracted and stored as described in Algorithm 1.

Algorithm 1 Find projections of VOI on planes

Set thresholds, select start pixel p_0, and flood-fill object starting from p_0.
for all (marked) planes **do**
  scan all p_i:s from the marked image to find coordinates of projected VOI
  if p_i marked **then**
    Trace boundary by Algorithm 2 and mark traced boundary
  end if
end for
Store obtained projections of VOI.

Algorithm 2 Trace boundary

Get direction d and pixel p_i and set last direction $d' \neq d$.
repeat
  if $d \neq d'$ and $p_j \notin$ boundary b **then**
    add p_j to b, update p_j according to d and d according to neighbourhood pixels of p_j. {Boundary tracing is done counter-clockwise by keeping in pixels on the left-hand side.}
  else
    update p_j according to d
  end if
until $p_j = p_i$ or maximum number of pixels exceed

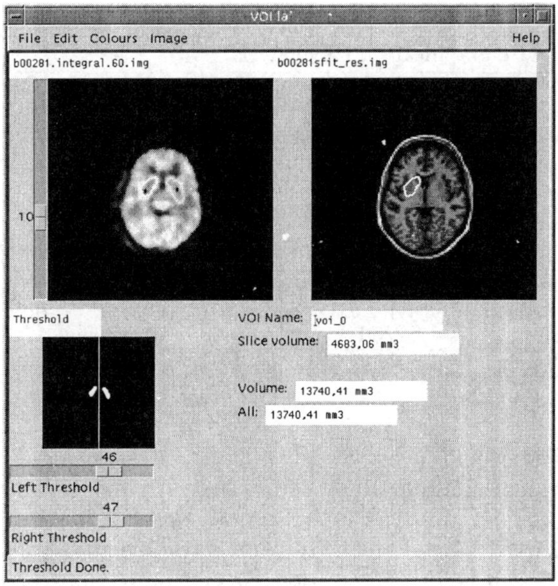

Figure 2: User interface. The upper left image is a user selected plane (transaxial slice) from a three-dimensional image. A vertical slider on the left hand side is used for plane selection. The slider also shows the number of the current plane. The lower image shows the corresponding thresholded version of the current plane. User may select some other plane to view by dragging the slider. The horizontal sliders at bottom are used to adjust threshold levels. The upper right image is optional and is used for verifying results by displaying corresponding ROIs on it. On the lower right part, the current VOI information is shown.

3 Implementation

The program [1] window, shown in the Figure 2, is split to three main parts, menu bar, the data display area and status bar. The data display area includes name of an image file, plane view to an image, vertical slider to select a plane, a plane view to a threshold image, two horizontal sliders to select the threshold values and selected information about the currently defined VOI. Optionally, it is possible to show a second image. The program was implemented by using Sun's Workshop, X11R5, Motif libraries and C/C++ -compiler. The hardware used for development is Sun Ultra 2 with Solaris 2.x.

4 Experiments and results

Experiments of the described concept was carried out in the Turku PET-Centre, Finland. The program was applied to five FDOPA-PET studies and one phantom study. The PET scans were made with ECAT 931/08-12 (CTI/Siemens, Knoxville, USA) scanner. It produces fifteen planes per scan. Magnetic resonance images were obtained with 1.5 T Magneton (Siemens, Erlangen, Germany) PET and MR scans were coregistered by using AMIR [2] method. The phantom PET scan was made with GE Advance (GE, Milwaukee, USA) scanner, which produces 35 planes per scan. The images, except phantom, were reconstructed with a new iterative median root prior (MRP) [3] method. With specific tracer, FDOPA (Fluoro dopa) study has high contrast against background and the visible functional structures can be seen clearly. For example, the

Table 1: Experiments with median root prior (MRP) reconstructed images. Ki is influx constant determined with graphical Patlak analysis.

patient	average Ki value for striatum, $*10^{-2}$ manual ROI method	semi-automatic VOI method	difference VOI-ROI	VOI/ROI volume, cm^3 manual ROI method	semi-automatic VOI method
1	1.04	1.32	+0.28	7.8	29.8
2	1.35	1.25	-0.10	9.3	25.1
3	1.12	1.10	-0.02	11.0	21.5
4	1.05	1.29	+0.24	9.0	14.5
5	0.91	1.04	+0.13	10.0	13.1
average	1.05	1.20	+0.15	9.4	20.8
	average activity, kBq/cm^3 true	VOI	VOI-true	volume, cm^3 true	VOI method
phantom	39.5	24.3	-15.2	24.3	23.9

striatum consisting of caudatus and putamen is such a target and it was studied.

With the traditional method, all ROIs are drawn manually on the MR image by using CTI Imagetool program. The ROI positions were evaluated by displaying ROIs on the corresponding PET planes. In VOI method, VOIs were determined from the PET images as described here. The positions of VOI projections were displayed on the corresponding MR images. ROIs and projections are saved for analysis.

Table 1 represents results of analysis and the target object volumes by using the traditional method and VOI method. The time used for extracting VOIs takes about 5-10 minutes per image with manual drawing (ROI), and about 2-3 minutes per image with program (VOI). The volume of phantom striatum is determined by using program and the manual value is the true filled value.

5 Discussion

The volume obtained from VOI method is about three times the corresponding manually determined volume. The manual method boundaries were determined only from two representative planes from the image, while the semi-automatic method finds a true three-dimensional objects from the image causing the difference in volume. Greater volume increases the accuracy of determination of activity concentration. Our tests show about one third time reduction for object extraction, but it is likely to be much better when there are more planes than with the test set of images. Results are reproducible. The simple segmentation method applied is obviously a limitation of the program. It can find the striatum, but cannot split it to its parts. Splitting can be done manually. Automated separation may require a prior knowledge of the structure. With precautions, applying advanced three-dimensional segmentation methods with prior knowledge is certainly interesting topic for further investigation in brain PET.

References

[1] J. Mykkänen, M. Juhola, and U. Ruotsalainen. Three-dimensional ROIs in brain PET. Technical Report A-1999-6, Dept. of Computer Science, University of Tampere, 1999.

[2] B. A. Ardekani. *Fusion of anatomical and functional images of the brain.* PhD thesis, University of Technology, Sydney, 1995.

[3] S. Alenius and U. Ruotsalainen. Bayesian image reconstruction for emission tomography based on median root prior. *European Journal of Nuclear Medicine*, 24(3):258–265, 1997.

Medical Informatics Europe '99
P. Kokol et al. (Eds.)
IOS Press, 1999

A computerised study on the results of In-Vitro-Fertilisation

Cadman J, [a] Richards B, [a] D'Souza S, [b] Lieberman B A, [c] Buck P, [d] Rivlin E [e]

a. *Medical Informatics Department, UMIST, Manchester, UK*
b. *Department of Child Health, St Mary's Hospital, Manchester, UK*
c. *IVF Unit, St Mary's Hospital, Manchester, UK*
d. *Department of Obstetrics, St Mary's Hospital, Manchester, UK*
e. *Department of Clinical Psychology, Winnicott Centre, UK*

Abstract. This project has been concerned with the comparison of children born as a result of fresh embryo transfer (IVF) with children conceived and born via the natural process. The former included children who were the single outcome of the birth (singletons) and children who were the result of a multiple birth (eg twins, triplets). A computer database was established into which was put 23 items of data on each child, making a total of 12788 items overall. There were 278 "normally conceived" children (controls), 150 IVF Singletons, and 128 children from multiple births. The results show interesting differences in the gestational age at birth, the birth weight, the mode of delivery and the degrees of birth abnormalities and malformations.

1 Introduction

The occurrence of multiple births (twins, triplets, quads) is now more common than it used to be [1]. This is no doubt due to the fact that modern techniques of In-Vitro-Fertilisation (IVF) and embryo-transfer often produce multiple births. In fact the number of multiple births resulting from such procedures greatly exceeds that of the "normal" population. [2]. The reason for this is that, with fresh embryo transfer, *three* embryos are transplanted into the mother's womb, the expectation being that at least one of them will survive. This was done in our cohort. The result was that, in a total cohort of 278 children born via IVF, there were 150 singletons, 100 twins, 24 triplets and 4 quadruplets. These infants were followed-up over a period of four years from birth. A cohort of "control" children, born at term, approximately 40 weeks were chosen on the basis of being matched for age, sex, and social class. Both groups were assessed for neonatal conditions, minor congenital anomalies, and major congenital malformations.

2 Methods

A database was set up into which all 23 variables for each patient were put. Various statistical tests, (eg Chi-squared, t-test, Fisher's Exact Test) were carried out as appropriate.

The assessments were carried out over a four-year period after birth. These included a clinical history, a general medical examination, and a developmental assessment. All minor abnormalities and major malformations were recorded as were any significant events occurring during the pregnancies. Major congenital malformations were considered as being those which would cause functional or social impairment. Standard assessments of disability were used [3] and the Developmental Quotient was obtained also.

3 Results

In the IVF, the ratio of boys to girls was 1.03 to 1. Of course it was the same in the Controls since these latter were matched for sex. It is known that the ratio of boys to girls is higher in pre-term (premature) babies than those delivered at term, ie after 37 weeks gestation. See Table 1.

Table 1: The sex ratios in the three cohorts

	IVF						Controls	
	Singleton (N=150)		Multiple births (N=128)		Total (N=278)		(N=278)	
Boys	80	53.3%	61	47.7%	141	50.7%	141	50.7%
Girls	70	46.7%	67	52.3%	137	49.3%	137	49.3%
Total	150	100%	128	100%	278	100%	278	100%

In the IVF Group 46% of the children were from multiple births. Not unexpectedly there was a statistically significant difference in the mean gestational age both between the IVF Singleton births and the IVF Multiple births ($p<0.001$) and between the IVF Singleton birth and the Controls ($p<0.00001$). A paired t-test was used for this latter. See Table 2.

Table 2: Gestational Age in the three cohorts

		IVF						Controls	
		Singleton (N=150)		Multiple births (N=128)		Total (N=278)		(N=278)	
Mean±SD Gest.age(wk)		38.41±2.51		35.24±3.06		36.95±3.19		39.45±1.25	
	≥37	127	84.7%	54	42.2%	181	67.3%	278	100%
	32-36	19	12.7%	57	44.5%	76	27.3%	0	0.0%
	<32	4	2.7%	17	13.3%	21	7.6%	0	0.0%

A similar comparison was made in respect of birthweight. The results were, for singletons versus multiples, ($p<0.001$) and for IVF singletons versus Controls, $p<10^{-7}$. See Table 3.

Table 3: Birthweights in three cohorts

	IVF						Controls	
	Singleton (N=150)		Multiple births (N=128)		Total (N=278)		(N=278)	
Mean±SD Birth wt(gm)	3016.3±641.6		2078.6±612.7		2584±783.2		3379.8±428.3	
≥2500	128	85.3%	30	23.4%	158	56.8%	276	99.3%
1500-2500	17	11.3%	73	57.0%	90	32.4%	2	0.7%
1000-1500	4	2.7%	23	18.0%	27	9.7%	0	0.0%
1000-1500	1	0.7%	2	1.6%	3	1.1%	0	0.0%
Totals	150	100%	128	100%	278	100%	278	100%

Fortunately there were very few anomalies or malformations in any of the three Groups. The results are shown in Table 4. There were no differences between the Groups when compared for minor anomalies: in fact the numbers were very small. However, for the major malformations, there were none in the controls and a total of 7 in the IVF Groups, See Table 4.

Table 4: Congenital anomalies and malformation

	IVF			Controls
	Singleton (N=150)	Multiple births (N=128)	Total (N=278)	(N=278)
With minor congenital anomalies	5 (3.3%)	5 (3.9%)	10 (3.6%)	7 (2.5%)
With major congenital malformations	5 (3.3%)	2 (1.6%)	7 (2.5%)	0 (0.0%)

4 Conclusion

The computer has proved a valuable aid in this investigation. Not only has it stored the data and produced the tables but it has carried out the statistical analyses using in-house designed software.

Clinically, the conclusions must be that the IVF treatment produces significantly more multiple births than in the Controls, and these multiples are born, on average, prematurely. The mean birthweight of IVF singletons (3016 gm) was significantly lighter (by approximately 400 gm) than the Control singletons (3400 gm). The former thereby encounter all the problems associated with pre-term delivery. Thus 45% of the IVF babies had noteworthy neonatal problems as compared with only 7.6% in the Controls. Further, 39.9% of the IVF Group were delivered by Caesarean Section (C.S.) compared with only 6.8% in the Controls: and within the IVF Group itself, 55.5% of the multips were delivered by C.S. as compared with only 26.7% of the singletons. Also 26% of IVF singletons were born by C.S. but only 9% of the Control singletons. In terms of disabilities after birth, one Control child had a conductive hearing loss, whereas 4 multips had mild disabilities and 2 had moderate disabilities. There were no reports of severe disabilities and no chromosomal abnormalities were detected. Overall, 2.1% of the IVF Group and 0.4% of the Control Group had mild disabilities. These included squint, conductive hearing loss, feeding difficulties, and sleep disorders, all of which were resolved shortly after being reported.

The overall conclusions must be that the practice of implanting three embryos into the mother has definite drawbacks for the off-spring. Implanting a lower number reduces the chances of success, as can be seen in the above figures. Thus of 278 implantations only 128 (46%) resulted in a multiple birth: conversely in 54% of the cases, implanting three embryos resulted in only one baby being born. One might hope that a happy mean could be found. Maybe the technique suggested by Staessen [4] might prove advantageous, as might the technique of implanting only *two* embryos.

References

[1] Botting B. J., MacDonald Davies I., Macfarlane A.J. Recent trends in the incidence of multiple births and associated mortality. Arch Dis Child 1987: **62**: 941-50

[2] Dunn A, Macfarlane A. Recent trends in the incidence of multiple births and associated mortality in England and Wales. Arch Dis Child 1996; **75**: F10- 19.

[3] Cooke R.W.I. Factors affecting survival and outcome at 3 years in extremely pre-term infants. Arch Dis Child 1994; **71**: F28-31

[4] Staessen C, Janssenswillen C, Van E, Abbeel D, Devroey P. Avoidance of triplet pregnancies by elective transfer of two good quality embryos. Hum Reprod 1993; 8: 1650-3

Medical Informatics Europe '99
P. Kokol et al. (Eds.)
IOS Press, 1999

Uniforming of outpatient health care statistics

Mitja Rogač, M.Sc., dipl.ing. (Math.)
Daša Moravec Berger, M.Sc., MD
Public Health Institute of the Republic of Slovenia, Trubarjeva 2, Ljubljana

Abstract. In the process of developing the health care information system, the Public Health Institute of the Republic of Slovenia harmonised the outpatient health care statistics at the national level. This paper presents the goals, contents, methodology and a brief analysis of the new data structure. The main functions of the ZUBSTAT computer program, user training methods, and planned further activities in this field are described.

1. Introduction

With the aim of improving the existing data reporting method at the national level in the field of outpatient health care statistics [1], the Public Health Institute of the Republic of Slovenia (PHIRS) has created a new uniform record structure for reporting data on attendances and referrals as well as the established diseases and conditions in outpatient health care activities.

Outpatient health care activities are performed in health care centres, specialist outpatient offices in hospitals, and private practices. There are more than 1000 such health care providers in Slovenia. During their work with patients, health care personnel enters the required data into computers.

At mid-year and at year's end, health care providers are obliged to prepare the required data structure on the basis of their daily entered records, according to the instructions of PHIRS, and send them to their regional Health Care Institute (HCI) by the prescribed deadline. There are nine regional HCIs in Slovenia: in Ljubljana, Kranj, Nova Gorica, Koper, Novo Mesto, Celje, Ravne, Maribor and Murska Sobota. Regional HCIs collect data from the health care providers in their region, check them using the ZUBSTAT program and, if errors are found, send them back to the originating provider with a list of errors.

This new method of data reporting was introduced in the following basic health care activities [2]:

- General practice
- General practice - prevention
- Occupational medicine
- School health care - curative
- School health care - prevention (regular check-ups)
- Pediatric health care - curative
- Pediatric health care - prevention (consultancies)
- Developmental (pediatric) outpatient facilities
- Women's health care (Gynaecology and obstetrics)
- Women's health care - (consultancies for pregnant women)
- Women's health care - (consultancies for contraceptive practices)
- Specialist outpatient health care: by medical specialty

Data reporting using the new computerised method according to the instructions of the Ministry of Health, was introduced on 1 January 1997.

2. Goals of uniforming data reporting methods

PHIRS has decided on a new, uniform record structure for reporting data on outpatient health care statistics at the national level [3], on the assumption that the set of data entered by health care personnel on a daily basis remains unchanged.

The objectives of this new reporting structure are as follows:

- Uniforming of methods for data reporting on attendances and referrals, as well as those on diseases and conditions from basic and specialist health care.
- Data reporting using the new three-digit municipal codes, in effect since 1 January 1997.
- Monitoring of patient structure by municipality of residence for each health care centre, i.e. patient gravitation towards health care centres (which is enabled by the new reporting structure of data on attendances and referrals).
- Data reporting by more detailed age groups and by sex.
- Collection of data on diagnoses by the tenth revision of the International Classification of Diseases (ICD-10), which has been used in the field of health care statistics since 1 January 1997.
- More detailed definitions and standards for data collected.
- Separate collection of data on "diagnoses upon the first attendance" and "final diagnoses".
- Checking of data with regard to valid code schemes and logical associations between data.
- Higher quality of output data given an unchanged amount of input data.

3. Contents of the new data structure

In connection with diseases and conditions in outpatient health care activities at the national level, PHIRS collects and monitors the following data [4]:

- Designation for the reporting period
- Health-care provider's municipal code
- Health care provider's code
- Designation of the provider's basic activity
- Code of the provider's health care service
- Code of the provider's location
- Designation of the type of diagnosis (diagnosis upon the first attendance or final diagnosis)
- Diagnosis code (ICD-10)
- External cause designation (ICD-10)
- Disease group designation (special morbidity list according to ICD-10)
- Number of patients by age group and sex
- Number of patients by health insurance category
- Number of patients with work-related injuries
- Number of pregnant women grouped by duration of pregnancy

The key attribute is "Diagnosis Code" (ICD-10), to which all other attributes are associated. Each attribute has its own definition of content and reference to the corresponding code table, which has been harmonised at the national level.

Patient age groups have been determined as follows:

01.	from 0.00 to 2.99 months	pre-school children
02.	from 3.00 to 5.99 months	
03.	from 6.00 to 11.99 months	
04.	from 1.00 to 3.99 years	
05.	from 4.00 to 6.99 years	
06.	from 7.00 to 9.99 years	school children
07.	from 10.00 to 14.99 years	
08.	from 15.00 to 19.99 years	
09.	from 20.00 to 29.99 years	adults
10.	from 30.00 to 39.99 years	
11.	from 40.00 to 49.99 years	
12.	from 50.00 to 59.99 years	

13. from 60.00 to 64.99 years
14. from 65 years onward

In connection with attendances and referrals, PHIRS collects and monitors the following data:

- Designation for the reporting period
- Health-care provider's municipal code
- Health care provider's code
- Designation of the provider's basic activity
- Code of the provider's health care service
- Code of the provider's location
- Designation of the type of attendance
- Municipal code of the patient's residence
- Number of patients by age group and sex
- Number of patients by health insurance category
- Number of pregnant women grouped by duration of pregnancy
- Number of patients referred to the hospital
- Number of patients referred to a specialist

The key attribute here is "Designation of the Type of Attendance", to which all other attributes are associated. In this case as well, each attribute has its own definition of content and reference to the corresponding code table, which has been harmonised at the national level.

The types of attendances are divided into the following classes:

100 - Curative attendances, first
200 - Curative attendances, repeated
300 - Preventive attendances in the pre-school period
400 - Preventive attendances of schoolchildren, youth and students
500 - Preventive attendances of women
600 - Preventive attendances of adults and the active population
900 - Preventive attendances of sportsmen, draftees, amateur drivers, other preventive activities and other services

4. ZUBSTAT program

PHIRS has prepared a specification for this program, while the software company Vizija d.o.o. of Celje has produced the ZUBSTAT program for the collection, checking and merging of outpatient health care statistics. The program operates on a graphical Windows 98 platform and is intended for PHIRS, HCIs and all providers engaging in outpatient health care activities, including outpatient specialist health care in hospitals.

The program enables the following:

- Checking of input data with respect to code schemes in use at the national level, and checking for logical association between data. For each basic activity, the checking function also prepares sums by type of attendance and by type of diagnosis.
- Merging of input data into a common database.
- Review and correction of data in the database in connection with all corresponding code schemes.
- Preparation of printouts from the database. Some basic printouts are defined:
  - List of providers owing data;
  - List of providers which have already sent the data;
  - List of attendances and referrals by designation of the basic activity for each individual provider, or for each individual region;
  - List of diseases and conditions by designation of the basic activity for each individual provider, or for each individual region;

  The program also contains a generator of printouts which allows the creation of optional printouts from the database.
- Preparation of output data from the database in ASCII format, merged at the level of the health care organisation, for reporting data to the regional or national level, or for processing with the use of other software tools.

5. Initial user training

The initial user training was conducted at two levels. At the first level, PHIRS introduced the ZUBSTAT program to HCI personnel, providing them with appropriate methodological materials. A presentation of these materials and a course on the program's use were organised.

At the second level, HCIs informed all public and private health care providers in their regions of the overhaul of outpatient health care statistics in Slovenia. If problems appear or questions arise, health care providers can first consult their HCI; if this does not suffice, they may contact PHIRS directly. PHIRS collects all comments and questions from health care providers and addresses them at joint meetings with HCIs.

6. Discussion and conclusions

The uniform record structure for reporting data on attendances and referrals, as well as data on diseases and conditions, has provided several pieces of information to be accessible at the national level:

- Data on diagnoses are now reported at a level of detail comprising all of the categories and subcategories of ICD-10 in use, whereas before they were merged into inexact groups.
- Data on age are now reported at a level of detail comprising the prescribed age groups, while before separate groups existed only for pre-school and school-age children and adults.
- Data on sex are now reported.
- Data on the municipality of the patient's permanent residence are now reported.

But analysis of data reported in the new manner also showed that:

- The reported data are incomplete, since certain providers failed to send them to the national level.

  The degree of completeness of data reporting from primary health care activities for 1997 was satisfactory. At the level of secondary health care, data reporting was very incomplete as many providers failed to report their data. The greatest amount of unreported data is from specialist outpatient offices in certain hospitals. In the overall report for Slovenia for 1997, almost half of the data from specialist outpatient offices are missing.
- Incorrect content of reported data

  A test analysis of data from 1997 showed very different percentages of final diagnoses for the same selected diagnosis among individual providers (many of them actually did not even record a single final diagnosis).

If health care providers took into account the present definitions of the terms "diagnosis upon the first attendance" (reason for the first attendance) and "final diagnosis" (the established diagnosis), the final diagnoses (diagnosis type 2) should include the total number of actually established and reported diagnoses, while diagnoses upon the first attendance (diagnosis type 1) should include that percentage of final diagnoses which were reliably established upon the first attendance. Diagnoses upon the first attendance should also include all those which could not be proven during further diagnostic procedures and were therefore refuted, and all other reasons for the attendance.

Theoretically, one would expect that the percentage of final diagnoses established correctly upon the first attendance would be similar for a certain disease, and a certain type of health care activity, in the majority of providers.

However, a test analysis of the total number of patients with a diagnosis of *herpes zoster* made by general practitioners has shown that quite the opposite is the case. In the majority of health care providers, the number of diagnoses upon the first attendance that were the same as the final diagnoses was very small and there were great differences in this respect between individual health care providers.

Possible explanations:

- When registering the diagnosis upon the first attendance, the majority of health care providers did not enter the data under both types of diagnosis.
- Upon the first examination, the doctor suspects a diagnosis and enters it into an ICD-10

group, although he is actually supposed to enter it only when the disease is proven.

- The definitions of the terms "diagnosis upon the first attendance" and "final diagnosis" are not sufficiently clear.
- Errors in programs which prepare data for reporting.

7. Further activities planned

The uniform data structure was introduced in order to improve the quality of data in the field of outpatient health care statistics. Naturally, data quality does not depend merely on the procedures used to collect and check data, but also on professional and conscientious initial data entries by health care providers. The motivation of health care providers to make correct entries of data will need to be improved through improvement of methodological instructions and additional analyses of data on morbidity in the population and gravitation of the populus to health care institutions.

In a similar manner, PHIRS plans to harmonise the methods for collection of data on personnel and hours worked in outpatient health care at the national level.

References

[1] Ministrstvo za zdravstvo, Konceptualni okviri nadaljnjega razvoja zdravstvenega informacijskega sistema v Republiki Sloveniji. Ljubljana, 1992.

[2] WHO, Elements of the Role of Informatics in the Health for All Policy of the World Health Organisation. Copenhagen, 1994.

[3] Inštitut za varovanje zdravja RS, Projekt Elementi enotnosti zdravstvenega informacijskega sistema v Republiki Sloveniji. II. fazno poročilo, Ljubljana, 1994.

[4] Inštitut za varovanje zdravja RS, Zunajbolnišnična zdravstvena statistika. Metodološko gradivo, Ljubljana, 1998.

Medical Informatics Europe '99
P. Kokol et al. (Eds.)
IOS Press, 1999

Application Of Space Technologies For Valuation Of A Stress Level

Oleg Yu. MAYOROV[1] and Roman M. BAEVSKY[2]
[1] *Kharkiv Medical Academy of Postgraduate Education,*
[2]*Institute of Biomedical Problems, Moscow, Russia*
P.O.BOX 7313, Kharkiv 310 002, Ukraine. E-mail: uacm@kharkov.com

Abstract: The adaptation of large long-term experience of application Heat Rate Variability in space biology and medicine and medical researches is represented. The description of the new approaches is given which are fixed in a basis of diagnostic computer systems "NeuroReserchers™ 5.0" (or System of Computer Vegetology "CardioTensionTest™ 5.0" as module in the frame of "NeuroReserchers™ 5.0") and "Varicard". These systems for thorough clinical and experimental scientific investigations and experimental investigations (for specialists of R&D institutes, doctors of functional diagnosis rooms of hospitals possessing clinical bases of R&D institute and medical university chairs, during clinical and preclinical testing of drugs, medical and biological R&D institutes carrying out Nneurophysiological investigations in the field of labour medicine and sport medicine, development of infantile nervous system, medical education establishments.

1. Introduction

At the boundary of XX and XXI Centuries the significance of emotional stress on health of the people is promptly increased. In this connection the necessity in simple for realisation, scientific based methods of a quantitative evaluation of power of systems regulation of an organism increases. There is a necessity because of objective quantitative measurements of a level of emotional stress and reserves of regulation cardio-vessels systems regulation in time to apply the reasonable methods of treatment and preventive maintenance of stress-genesis diseases, to predict outcomes myocardial infarction or origin " of sudden death " on a hum noise of complete well-being.

The problem of valuation of a stress level of the space crewmembers has arisen from the most first steps of cosmonautics development. It solution was connected to development of the concept about cardiovascular system as an indicator of adaptive reactions whole body.

Since the 60-th years during the first human flights in space was developed the technology of researches, based on the heart rate variability analysis and valuation on these data of a autonomic system state and activity of subcortical centres, connected with psycho-emotional excitation and increasing the energo-metabolic processes at physical loads. In the subsequent years the Heart Rate Variability analysis begins widely to be used in USSR (Russia and Ukraine) in clinical and preventive medicine, and from 80-th years has applied in Western Europe and USA. Hundreds articles and reports about using of the heart rate variability analysis in clinical practice and applied physiology are at present annually published.

However, so far in earthly medicine the space technology of stress level valuation is not enough used. The important of this technology is determined by that the majority of diseases is results of overstrain and exhaustion of the mechanisms of physiological functions regulation and diagnostics of a regulatory systems state is the most effective on Heart Rate Variability parameters.

Therefore in a space medicine 10-balls scale of valuations of a stress level is developed, that permits to determine risk of diseases and to supervise results of fulfilment of the preventive recommendations.

The adaptation of large long-term experience of application Heat Rate Variability has allowed to create computer diagnostic systems **"CardioTensionTest™ 5.0"** and **"Varicard"**.

2 . Functionality's of systems

These systems allow:

- To quantitatively evaluate the emotional stress rate;
- To quantitatively evaluate the "regulation stability" under extreme conditions;
- To evaluate the regulatory systems tension level reflecting the activation rate of neuro-endocrine of "stress axes";
- To carry out medical control and prediction of an organism's functional possibilities, to diagnose the following states: a) satisfactory adaptation; b) functional tension; c) unsatisfactory adaptation; d) adaptation failure.
- To determine the functional state of a heart rhythm regulation system according to R.M. Bayevsky's classifier [1] pointing out five cardiac rhythm features: 1. Indication of summary effect of all regulatory influences; 2. Cardiac muscle automatism; 3. Regulatory influences on stability rate; 4. State and interaction of VNS parts (vegetative homeostasis); 5. Indication of subcortical nervous centres state.
- To evaluate arterial pressure regulation system activity (Ssw1);
- To evaluate thermal regulation system activity (Ssw2).
- "CardioTensionTest™ 5.0" and "Varicard" have substantial advantages over other available systems.

It is necessary to mark some important features of these systems, which increase reliability and reliability of results.

3. " CardioTensionTest™ 5.0 "

3.1. Detection of R-peaks and R-R intervals

Reliable automatic discrimination of R-peaks is of primary importance. In the available systems R-peaks are discriminated by means of an electronic amplitude filter, i.e. An R-peak is discriminated from other ECG peaks (P, T) by its higher amplitude. Such approach has low reliability because under emotional stress, in the periods of negative emotional state, in cases of hypoxia and myocardial ischemia of different etiology, a T-peak amplitude significantly increases.

Besides, hardware-based discrimination of R-peaks does not permit to account for the presence of artifacts (spikes, displacements and other ECG distortions) [2]. At the same time, discrimination of only one "false" R-peak (or omission of a real R-peak) causes a nonlinear distortion of the analysis results by 60-80 times [1].

The stage of detection consists of two steps - on a first step of the analysis the system uses methods of automatic detection.

3.2. Automatic detection

Automatic detection of R - peaks (waves) and R-R- intervals - not hardware, but computer detection of R-waves according to three specially designed independent criteria.

An original algorithm is used for this purpose that makes it possible to reliably detect R-waves not only for clinical purposes at rest, but also for investigations of under the conditions of operator's activity - operators, pilots, sports persons etc., as well as animals under the condition of free behaviour in chronic experiment.

On second step of recognition R- peaks in the system the quality control of detection, and then semiautomatic and hand-operated correction is carried out.

3.3. Visual checking of R peak detection

Makes it possible to check up visually on the monitor screen the detected R-waves with further manual correction (detection or elimination) of 'false' or omitted R-waves in a defect section.

3.4. Automatic editing

Detection or elimination of 'false' or omitted R-waves in a defect section basing on the original correction algorithm.

3.5. Manual correction

Manual correction (insertion or elimination) of 'false' or omitted R-waves in a defect section (especially important when investigating the subjects (operators) during their activity or functional tests.

4. Mathematical and statistical analysis

The reliability of R-peaks selection ensures at a stage of a mathematical and statistical analysis high reliability of results. The universal analysis is carried out which allows evaluating practically all levels of regulation.

Calculation of a set of well known from the literature mathematical and statistical values (31 value) reflecting the result of statistical, correlation and spectral analysis of the cardiac rhythm. Integral interference-proof from the point of view of computer processing index AI (anxiety index) and ART (anxiety reaction type index) are used;

4.1 Correlation analysis

Sequences of R-R (N-N) intervals, that makes it possible to estimate the degree of control centralisation, domination of one of the vegetative nervous system sections, quantitatively estimate the degree of emotional stress;

4.2. Spectral analysis

Sequence of R-R (N-N) intervals that makes it possible to estimate the degree of activation of subcortical nervous centres controlling the blood flow regulation apparatus, measure the degree of stress of the neuro-endocrine function regulation apparatus;

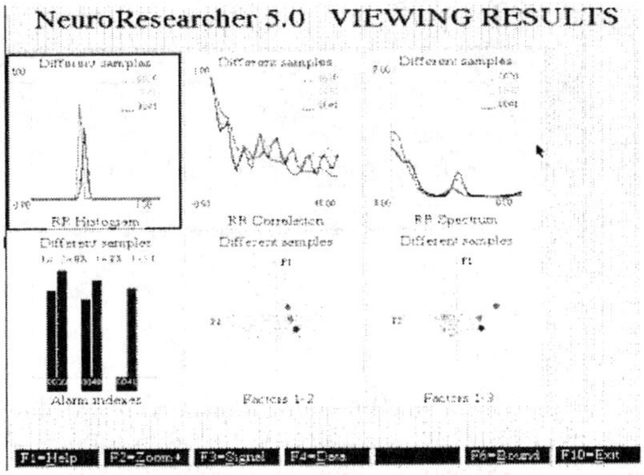

Fig.1. Visualization of result - in the form of charts of R-R- (N-N) interval distribution histograms, correlograms and spectra; results of factor analysis, possibility to present in one chart and compare several states simultaneously.

4.3. Multidimensional factor analysis

Makes it possible to compress information and reduce a large number of values to 2-3 factors [3]. This approach makes it possible to range (quantitatively estimate and compare) the subjects as to the level of stress of the regulation systems, 'regulation stability'; quantitative estimate the state of integrative function of hypothalamus. The ranging results are output to a 3D chart. There is a possibility to create factor models for various age groups and contingents of the subjects [3].

Large advantage "CardioTensionTest™ 5.0" is the possibility of inclusion it in the structure of the developed advanced system of the computer EEG "NeuroResearcher™ 5.0". It allows simultaneously to conduct a research of an EEG, and to compare results to data of a calculus of Heart Rate Variability.

5. " Varicard "

"Varicard" is specialised hardware-software complex for the Heart Rate Variability analysis is at present developed, in which are used as western standards of this technique, as created in a space medicine criterion of stress level estimation. Is allocated three zones (Fig. 2)(green, yellow and red) determining danger of development of diseases. In a complex structure there is base of knowledge, forming individual preventive and healthcare recommendation by results of valuation at stress level. The complex is tested in a number of clinical establishments, is used at mass preventive examinations of thousands people, as well as at investigation of the health in schools.

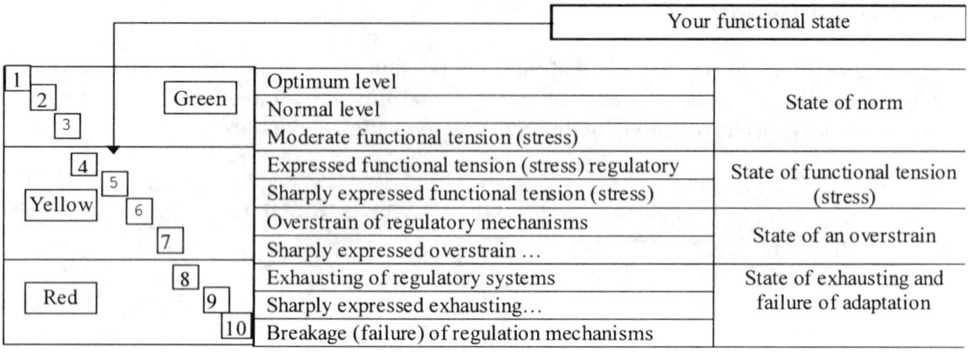

Fig.2. " A Ladder of states " and system of an evaluation of functional states of a type "Traffic Light".

6. Summary

The Heart Rate Variability analysis is modern technology of valuation of the health states in applied physiology, clinical practice, rehabilitation and preventive medicine. This technology was developed in space medicine as the method for stress level estimation. Widely application of this approach in different parts of human sciences is very important for understanding the unity and differences of the health and disease.

References

[1] R.M. Baevsky, O. I. Kirillov, S.M. Kleckin, Mathematical analysis of changes of cardiac rhythm under the stress,. Nauka, 1984, 221 p.

[2] O.Yu. Mayorov et al., Features of the vegetative status at adolescents with displastic cardiopathy. Ukrainian Journal of Cardiology. 1998, V.9, pp. 53 - 55.

[3] O.Yu. Mayorov, Some methodical and methodological approaches to mathematical analysis of cardiac rhythm under emotionally stressed activity and emotional stress. Proceedings of the Plenum of the Problem Commission of the USSR Academy of Medical Sciences "Mechanisms of system organisation of physiological functions", Kursk, 1990, pp. 81-88.

Medical Informatics Europe '99
P. Kokol et al. (Eds.)
IOS Press, 1999

An efficient algorithm for automatic decoding of ECG signals

Evgen A. PALAMARCHOUK
PALLAR Ltd, Porik str.-7, Vinnytsya-21, Ukraine

Abstract. Creating of computer ECG-conclusion, based on decodings of ECG-signals, as a rule includes three main stages - morphological analysis, comparison of obtained parameters and synthesis the conclusion. In a considered circuit the most critical point is the first stage. Here even the minor errors of automated, i.e. computer determination of elements, can provoke synthesis incorrect conclusions, in particular automated measurement of heart rate variability [1]. From this point of view it is extremely important to creat algorithms of decoding which are stable against parasites of electrical and biological origin, and also which are capable adequately to react to signal polymorphism [2]. Research in this direction have revealed the following.

1. Problems

So, the main problems of ECG-proccessing are:

- Correct delimitation of QRS-complexies. Just they are the base points for determination of amplitudes and width for all remaining of them of elements. The most frequently problems arise when their amplitudes are comparable or less then amplitududes of narrow and high P and T-waves. This phenomenon is characteristical for marked tachycardia.

- Correct distinguishing of Q and S-waves in complexes of a type SR (Sr), QR (Qr) or SR. A noise and the parasites essentially influence on the form of an initial phase theese waves. It allows easily to confuse them among themselves.

- The determination of P-waves is one of the most hard tasks. It is dealed with their low amplitudes and comparatively rather fuzzy form. The correct detection of P-waves sharply becomes complicated on a hum noise of parasites of a biological character (muscle tremor, phenomenon of RE-entry). The form and amplitude of such parasites is rather similar on P-waves and can cause errors. The detecting becomes complicated as well that there is no correspondence of the form and amplitude of P-waves to concrete ECG-leads. The similar problem concerns also with determination of T-waves.

- The migration of the rhythm driver (AV-blockade) causes not only transition of P-wave around QRS-complex, but also modification it of its form.

- Correct determinations of a site of isoelectric lines essentially influences on a delimitation (first of all on breadths) of P and T-waves P with low amplitudes. Additional problems gives the drift of global isoelectric line due to bad contacts of electrodes to the patient or breathing of the patient and also displacement of PQ and ST-segments.

- Confluence of P and T-waves on marked sinus tachycardia. This phenomenon influences on a delimitation of segments PQ and ST and also can infringe correct detecting of QRS-complex.

- Complexity of correct delimitation of sloping ascending or descending PQ or ST-segments.

2. Solutions

Problems mentioned above are worked out by using the complex approach to ECG-processing. In order to remove influence of QRS-polymorphism in various leads is productive to form a generalized power function of phased leads. The processing of it should be carried out by using methods of an adaptive filtration and iterative search is threshold of sensitivity with the purpose of approximate definition of QRS-complex position . On the second stage is necessary to define RR-intervals and breadths of QRS-complexes for localization possible extrasystoles. In this purpose in signals of each ECG-leads is necessary to search the separate ECG-elements (waves, intervals, segments ets.) and then to define their performances. It will give the information to further clarification of ECG-morphology. With the purpose of authentic definition of parameters of separate elements the ECG is expedient to use iterative procedures and methods of optimal filtration and correlation analysis with reference to each ECG-fragment. During processing for any element of the ECG there should be a certain measure of the probability which dependends on a condition of already detected parameters. In relation to it the probability evaluation of reliability of definition of parameters of an element is accumulated. Exceeding of the appointed threshold indicates that the element is detected and its caracteristics could be recorded to the register. Errors caused by the drift of "global" isoelectric line is expedient to reduce by definition of envelope of isoelectric line and then to detect local isoelectric lineы around of QRS-complexies. Such approach allows rather successfully suppress errors in definition of parameters of the displaced PQ and ST-segments and both boundaries of all waves and segments.

3. Outcomes

Indicated problems and solution methods were realized in a series of the versions of software for diagnostic complexies **CARDIO-5 - CARDIO-9** in which were used ECG-equipment with an amount of phaised channels from 3 up to 12. There were used 10-byte signals with an amount of readout from 100 up to 200 per second. The outcomes of their 5-year's operation have shown a regularity of selected methods of ECG-processing and their comparatively high reliability of decoding even in conditions of actual parasites. The worst results were marked while processing of ECG-signals with expressed violations of a rhythm. In this aspect using the combination of self-learning, reconstructive [3] algorithms and adaptive methods of ECG-processing is represented to be a very perspective.

References

[1] Heart rate variability. Standarts of measurment, physiological interpretation, and clinical use. European Heart Journal (1996) 17, 354-381.

[2] Bailey JJ, Berson AS, Garson A Jr et al. Recommendations for standardization and specifications in automated electrocardiography. Circulation 1990; 81: 730-9.

[3] Kennedy HN. Ambulatory (Holter) electrocardiography techology. Clin Cardiol 1992; 10: 341-56.

Medical Informatics Europe '99
P. Kokol et al. (Eds.)
IOS Press, 1999

Frequency Domain Methods For Measurement Of Heart Rate Variability

MARIANA BULICA[1], VICTOR DAN MOGA[2]
[1]*Computer Dept. Country Hosp. Timisoara*
[2]*Cardiology Clinic University of Medicine and Pharmacy Timisoara*

1. Introduction

Nowadays, surface electrocardiography is the basic noninvasive technique in the clinical study of the electrical signal from the heart. Heart rate is usually defined as the number of heart beats per unit of time. Heart rate variability (HRV) is the measure of variation from one cardiac cycle on the next, utilizing normal morphology. HRV should not be confused with the time averaged heart rate changes as seen in minimum and maximum heart rate or other heart rate measurements on ambulatory ECG recording.

The analysis of very rapid fluctuations in heart rate (expressed as heart rate variability) is hampered by the fact that the cardiac events are not regularly spaced in time. However, if we are interested in rapid fluctuations theoretically the unit of time mentioned above should be as small as possible. The analysis of fluctuation in heart rate has become increasingly important boths in physiological studies and in modeling of the neurocardiovascular system.

Furthermore, a number of diagnostic applications of this analysis is emanating, such as in the field of acute myocardial infarction, congestive heart failure, sudden cardiac death and diabetic neuropathy, neonatalogy and fetal monitoring. Very often the fluctuations are studied in the frequency domain.

During the past 13 years, the provocative hypothesis by Akselrod et al. that quantitative analysis of fluctuations in hemodynamic parameters is a powerful quantitative means of probing mechanism of short-term cardiovascular control, a new field of impetuous research.

We will therefore discriminate three ranges of the rate of the fluctuations (in terms of average duration of one cycle):

1). Slow variations: few minutes to hours.

The heart rate can be defined as twice the number of beats in a 30 seconds time bin.

2). Rapid fluctuations: some tens seconds to a few minutes.

3). Very fast fluctuations: few seconds (or less) to tens seconds

Detection of a cardiac event series from the ECG is necessary and attention has to be paid to both reliability and accuracy of the QRS detection. The usage of some HRV signal is discouraged and event series (spectral) analysis should be applied. In practice, very often the series is still assumed to be equidistant and spectral analysis is carried out by applying the Fast Fourier Transform to this series.

Electrocardiographic assessment of heart rate is necessary. The QRS complexes have to be detected and converted to short pulses.

Consequently, a heart rate variability (HRV) signal is to be derived, which can be subjected to spectral analysis. This is schematically shown in figure 1, where F.T. refers to Fourrier Transform.

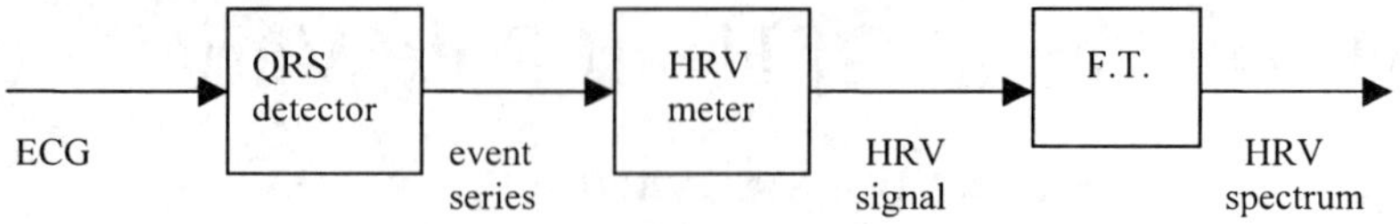

Figure 1. Spectral analysis of rapid fluctuations in heart rate

2. Method

To analyze cardiovascular variability signals, power spectrum analysis may be carried out either in nonparametric form (based upon the FFT algorithm) or in parametric form (based upon stochastic black-box modeling).

If heart rate were constant at 72 beats/minute it could easily be described at a frequency of 1.2 Hz. Since heart rate is not truly constant, multiple frequency components comprise its make-up.

The sinus node is highly innervated by the autonomic nervous system. Since the P wave is difficult to detect with precision, an assumption is made that the PR interval remains constant. Measurements are derived from the RR intervals. Successive heart beats are considered a series of events. Connecting the R to R intervals creates a rhythmatic pattern. Via spectral analysis, characteristic frequencies are extracted from the rhythm pattern, coupling them in order of range. In essence, spectral analysis measures the contribution of each of the many frequencies that exist in a given phenomenon (figure 2).

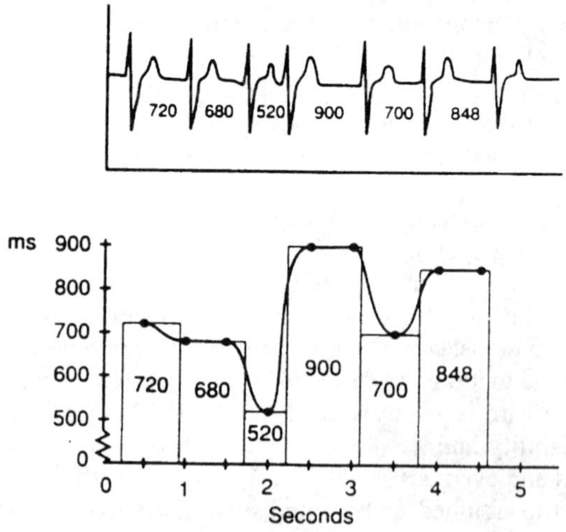

Figure 2. Measurements are derived from the R-R intervals.

Succesive heart beats are considered a series of events.

Connecting the R to R intervals creates a rhythmatic pattern.

Similar to the glass prism, spectral analysis uses a mathematical function called Fast Fourier Transform to separate the characteristic frequencies of the underlying rhythm (figure 3).

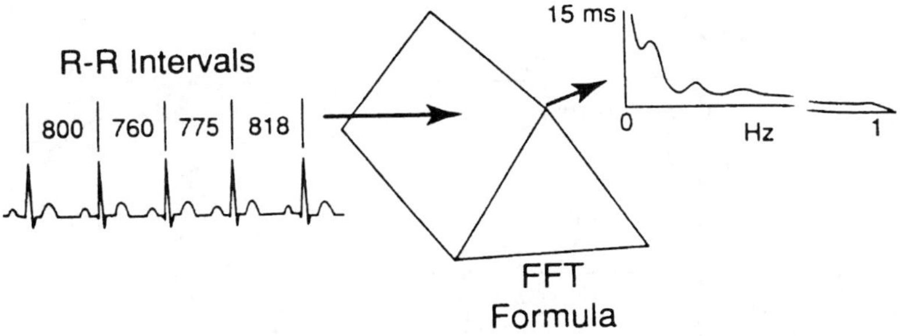

Figure 3. The Fast Fourier Transform (FFT) formula functions like a prism in analyzing heart rate variability.

Since respiration is a rhythmatic phenomenon, its measurement can be expressed in frequency.

Example:

10 breaths/minute = 1 breath/6 seconds;
breathing rate 1/6 seconds = 0.17 Hz.
OR
30 breaths/minute = 1 breath per 2 seconds;
breathing rate 1/2 seconds = 0.15 Hz.

Spectral analysis offers the clinician the proportional amount of variation at each component frequency. This may be illustrated by considering how a respiratory rate of 15 breaths/minute affects heart rate variability. The 15 breaths per minute translates to one breath every 4 seconds (1/4 of a respiratory cycle per second) equivalent to 0.25 Hz. (cycles/sec) on the frequency spectrum. A spectral peak would be seen at 0.25 Hz. The comparative height of this peak demonstrates its relative contribution to overall heart rate variability. This type of analysis becomes the basis for determining the pathophysiology of heart rate variability (figure 4).

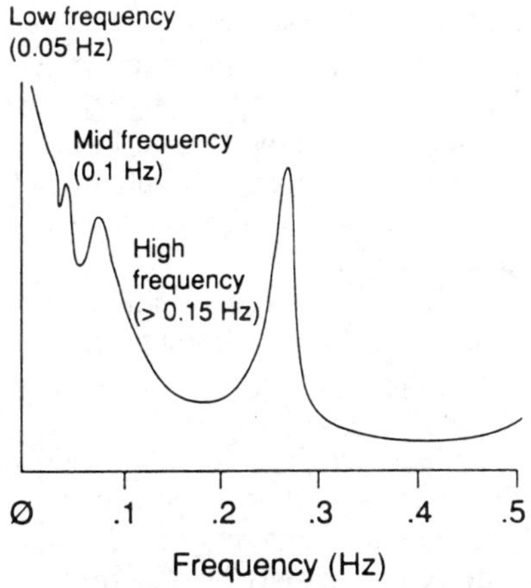

Figure 4. Power spectrum of instantaneous heart rate (HR) fluctuations featuring three main peaks: low-frequency peak (from 0.02 to 0.09 Hz), mid-frequency peak (from 0.09 to 0.15 Hz) and high-frequency peak (around respiratory frequency).

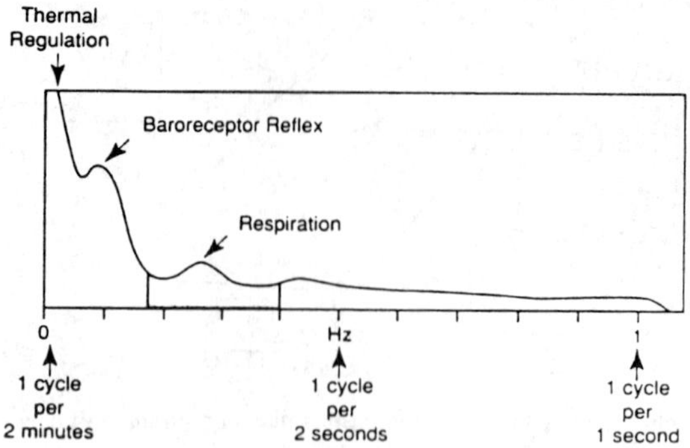

Figure 5. The cycling of various physiologic processes and their respective frequencies.

The spectral analysis of beat-by-beat RR interval shows two principal components:
1). Low frequency (LF), component generally centered around 0.05 to 0.15 Hz and whose change in power have been related to the sympathetic activity on the basis of pharmacological and clinical experiments;
2). High frequency (HF), component, in synchrony with the respiration rate (in the range between 0.15 and 0.5 Hz), which considered to be an expression of the respiration disturbances mediated by the vagal activity (parasympathetic) and are descreased by standing they are mediated solely by the parasympathetic system.

The power related to the LF and HF components is expressed in absolute values as well as in their ratio (LF/HF; so known autonomic index) and the related peak frequencies are useful parameters which help to quantify the sympatho-vagal balance activity.

The Fast Fourier Transform (FFT) accepts as input a time series of data samples (normal to normal coupling intervals) every half a second. The FFT returns a series of amplitudes for sine waves at many discrete frequencies.

The summation of those weighted sine waves would make a time signal that could be sampled to reproduce the original time series of samples, however the FFT output is not a continuos spectrum. The amplitude response from the FFT represents all the frequencies for each of the 128 output bins along the horizontal axis. These amplitudes are in milliseconds. To further explain this consider a time signal which is purely one frequency of variation within the entire sampling window. If the frequency was the center frequency of one of the bins in the FFT output spectrum, the output spectrum would contains zero values for every bin except one. That bin would contain zero-to-peak amplitude of the sinusoidal variation. The range is 0 to 15 ms.

More commonly seen in the literature than amplitude, power spectral density is drawn by squaring each component of the FFT output amplitude spectrum. The squaring function exaggerates the dynamic range, making the smaller amplitude components smaller and the bigger amplitude components bigger.

We have proposed to couple the analysis of HRV to the concept of sympatho-vagal balance. This assumes that the interplay between sympathetic and vagal modulations of sinus node pacemaker activity is organized in a reciprocal fashion, that increased activity in one system is accompanied by decreased activity by the other.

3. Results and disscussion

The study was performed in the Coronary Care Unit of the Cardiology Center Timisoara and data were analyzed in the Computer Department of the County Hospital Timisoara.

Acute myocardial infarction has been shown to result in autonomic imbalance that can be followed by power spectral analysis of the HRV. Power spectral analysis has the potential to quantify sympathetic and parasympathetic nervous system activity.

In our study, data were analyzed using first a ECG devices (PPG-HELLIGE EK 512 P CARDIOGNOST) with 12 leads, that use a “Arrhythmia” analyzer. Data were analyzed as heart rate (in digital form and also as a trend), trend of ventricular premature beats, trend of RR intervals (ms), and also as heart rate variability for short time intervals (10 –20 minutes) in time domain and frequency domain (figure 6).

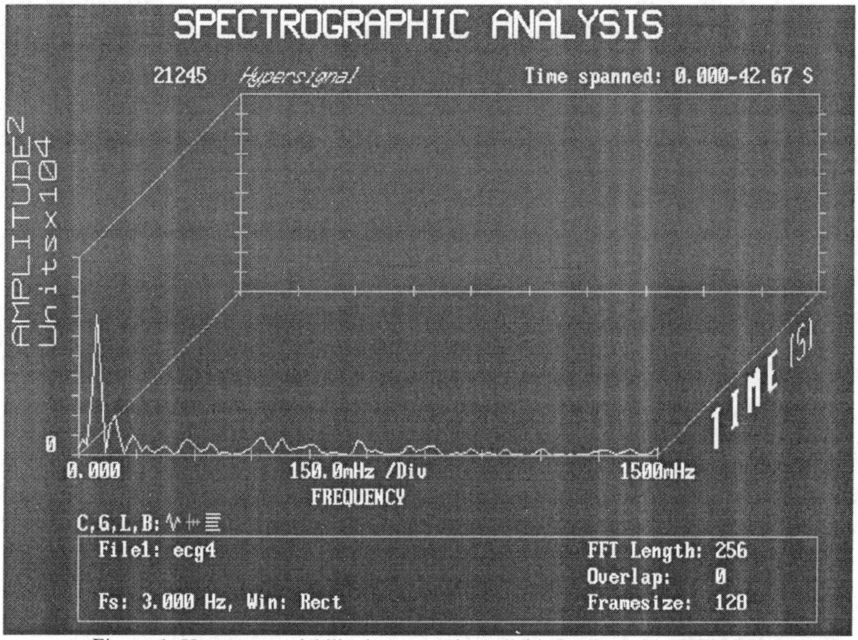

Figure 6. Heart rate variability in acute miocardial infarction with HSWORK program

Acute myocardial infarction is characterized by sympathetic activity and with loss of the high component of HRV, that means a higher risk for ventricular arrhythmias and arrhythmic death.

Data were analyzed off line. The software application was implemented a personal computer Pentium, 133 MHz. Since our software application is dealing with long-term recordings, one of the first problems encountered was the problem of "stationarity". The question was if spectral analysis performed in the entire 24-h period provide the same results as spectral results obtained from shorter segments (e.g. 5 min) averaged over the entire 24-h period.

Another problem is choosing the proper sampling rate. A low sampling rate may produce a jitter in the estimation of the R wave fiducial point which alters the spectrum considerably. The optimal range is 250 - 500 Mhz, while a lower sampling rate may behave satisfactorily only if an algorithm of interpolation is used.

We developed and implemented a software application for ECG processing. The application was written in Turbo Pascal and is running on MS-DOS operating system. The software application has a friendly interface and it is easy to use.

We implemented several signal processing techniques: fast Fourier transformation, different types of filters, autocorellation etc. The parameters required for running different processing techniques are established by the programme, but the user has the possibility to change them, function on type of the disease and type of the research performed.

We would like to develope a new version for our software application. This new version will work on Windows environment, which offers an easy to use man-machine interface and also supports network and multitasking functions. We will add new facilities for importing and exporting files using standard file formats (SCP, OEDIPE or CSE). Since acquired data occupies huge amount of disk space we will pay attention to compression techniques.

Medical Informatics Europe '99
P. Kokol et al. (Eds.)
IOS Press, 1999

A Signal Analysis Method for Impulse-like Eye Movements

Martti JUHOLA
Department of Computer Science, University of Tampere, P.O. Box 607, 33101 Tampere, Finland
Heikki AALTO and Timo HIRVONEN
Department of Otorhinolaryngology, Helsinki University Central Hospital, Finland

Abstract. Eye movement investigations are performed in several fields of medicine. We have developed signal analysis methods of eye movements studied in otoneurology for several years. Previously, we have designed methods for eye movement types of saccades, nystagmus, smooth pursuit, and vestibulo-ocular reflex. In this paper we extend and develop further our method to concern also impulse-like eye movements, i.e. a new type of eye movement tests for investigations of vertiginous patients. According to our preliminary results the use of our method is efficient to differentiate patients with inner ear diseases from normals.

1. Introduction

The eye movement signals were sampled in connection with otoneurological investigations, from patients suffering from inner ear diseases usually expressed by vertigo. Our earlier signal analysis methods [1-4] were primarily based on syntactic pattern recognition of eye movement waveforms from other phenomena in signals such as various noise and artifacts. With the syntactic recognition, common signal analysis techniques were applied. First, we designed a syntactic-based method for saccadic eye movements [1] which are step-like rapid eye movements from a target to another. Nystagmus [2] consists of bias reflexive "saw-tooth" movements that are repeated in changing form. Smooth pursuit or sinusoidal tracking eye movements [2,3] include sinusoidal waveforms that are stimulated when a subject follows stimulus movements like swinging pendulum. We advanced to vestibulo-ocular reflex eye movements [4] that resemble the former, but their sinusoidal waveforms contain greater frequencies. Their stimulus movements are not so regular as in the case of smooth pursuit, but are head movements of sinusoidal form which are approximately symmetrical to eye movements occurring at the same time.

Impulse-like eye movements include waveforms that appear suddenly according to the corresponding stimulus. In fact, they are physiologically vestibulo-ocular reflexive eye movements, but stimulated in a passive way concerning the subject, not actively by the subject. The stimulus is again a head movement rather symmetrically in the opposite direction (Fig. 1). This is not performed voluntarily by the patient himself as in the vestibulo-ocular test, but a stimulus movement is achieved by mechanically shaking the head of patient by using the helmet set firmly. The helmet is moved a little so that the head moves from the left to the right and then returns. This type of the eye movement test is recently introduced [5].

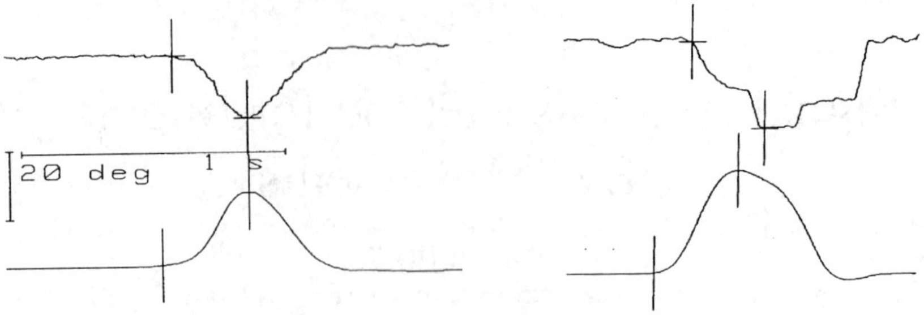

Fig. 1. The left signal pair consists of one impulse-type eye movement (upper curve) and the corresponding head movement (stimulus) performed by a normal. In the right pair there is a more "unsteady" form of the eye movement of a patient. The beginnings and maxima or minima of the waveforms recognised by the analysis program are indicated in the signals. Starting from those beginnings, values of eye movement parameters are computed.

2. Eye Movement Measurements

In an impulse-like eye movement test a subject is due to keep his gaze fixed to a predefined point during the whole measurement. His head is mechanically moved from the left to the right or in the opposite direction and then returned. The subject is seated in a clamped chair to keep the constant distance between the subject and the target point on the laboratory wall. The head movement has to be perfomed when the subject is relaxed not to resist the power moving his head. The head slightly rotates horizontally. When the gaze is fixed, the eyes make almost a symmetric movement compared to the head movement recorded at the same time (Fig. 1). These stimulus movements are performed after varying intervals that the subject is not able to guess the starting times.

Recording of eye and head movement signals was executed at a sampling frequency of 400 Hz that is sufficiently high. The amplitude resolution was 13 bits ($\pm$10 V). Eye movement signals were calibrated by making a separate saccade test where a constant angle was performed by the subject with his gaze from which a calibration value was computed. Skin electrodes were used with these electro-oculographic measurements [1-4]. We recorded about half a dozen signals per subject from two healthy normals and eight patients randomly selected from our laboratory. Thus, 16 normal signals and 44 patient signals were collected. The duration of each was 40 s. They were horizontal eye movements in the direction from the left (upwards in Fig. 1) to the right or vice versa.

3. Waveform Recognition

Waveforms of the signals were detected syntactically, i.e. after suitable preprocessing impulse-like waveforms were separated from the signals by using a parser in the recognition. First, a signal was digitally filtered in order to decrease noise. This low pass filtering can safely be run above an approximate cutoff frequency of 70 Hz [1-4]. This was made by employing a hybrid-median filter approriate to these signals [6]. The preprocessing includes the transformation of short (20 ms or 8 samples) consecutive signal segments into terminal symbols that are *a*, *b*, and *c*. A choice depends on the slope of each segment. If the slope is clearly rising, *a* is determined, if it is falling, *c* is taken, and otherwise *b*. A sequence of terminal symbols is obtained that corresponds to the signal.

The duration of each segment is short enough to ascertain that beginnings and maxima or minima of impulse-like eye movements are found. This syntactic strategy has well functioned in our earlier implementations [1-4,6]. Nonetheless, the syntactic recognition only searches for approximate locations of the beginnings and maxima or minima. Their exact locations are determined simply by looking for the fastest changes of the velocity curve (the first derivative of the positional signal) in the close neighbourhood of the detected approximate location of each beginning, maximum or minimum. A terminal symbol sequence is input to a parser generated for a formal language which specifies valid subsequences expressing impulse-like eye movement candidates, i.e. probable eye movements. These are checked and some of them are rejected as improbable impulse-like eye movements. The following formal grammar defines the formal language for accetable impulse-like eye movements. The start symbol is *S*. The other nonterminals are *A* and *B*.

$S \rightarrow baaA$ $A \rightarrow bc$ $S \rightarrow caaA$ $S \rightarrow bccB$ $B \rightarrow ba$ $S \rightarrow accB$
$A \rightarrow aA$ $A \rightarrow cb$ $A \rightarrow baA$ $B \rightarrow cB$ $B \rightarrow ab$ $B \rightarrow bcB$
$A \rightarrow bb$ $A \rightarrow cc$ $A \rightarrow caA$ $B \rightarrow bb$ $B \rightarrow aa$ $B \rightarrow acB$

The start symbol *S* commences a derivation of symbol sequence. Rules which have *A* on the lefthand side generate eye movements from the left to the right and those with *B* in the opposite direction. Occasional single symbols *b* in the middle of a sequence correspond to random short, approximately horizontal segments within an eye movement. Also single symbols *c* (conversely *a* within symbols *c*) inside a sequence of symbols *a* form rapid, very short segments caused by noise within eye movements. Clearly longer subsequences including several such successive "opposite" symbols are considered as very probable other parts than the rising or falling lefthand side (between the beginning and maximum or minimum; see Fig. 1) of an impulse-like eye movement. This lefthand side is namely the imperative part of the eye movement from which all results are computed as will be told later in the text. To exemplify a sequence of an impulse-like eye movement we present

baaabaacaabb

that is recognised, as a subsequence, by a suitable parser along with the preceding formal grammar from among a long terminal sequence of a whole signal. The first three symbols *baa* indicate a viable start of an eye movement. Terminals *a* then follow interrupted by single *b* and *c*. Two terminals *b* show an acceptable end of the subsequence that expresses the approximate location of the maximum of the impulse-like eye movement. To separate large artifacts or other disturbance, a checking module was constructed within the analysis program.

4. Computation of Eye Movement Parameters

After the exact determination of the above-mentioned beginnings in particular the parameter values are computed. Gain parameters are calculated in two ways. First, our program computes gain by amplitude as follows. The maximum of the angular velocity curve (the first derivative of the positional eye movement or head movement) is defined. Such a maximum is located within 100 ms [5] after the beginning of the impulse-like eye movement or corresponding head movement. The amplitude of the location of the maximum velocity is computed for both the eye movement and head movement signals concerning each detected and accepted impulse pair. The ratio of these two maximum velocity amplitudes is our gain by amplitude. Second, gain is computed from a ratio of slopes given by linear regression for the velocity curves during 100 ms of the eye movement and head movement signals [5]. Finally, latency is computed as a time difference of the beginning of the impulse-like eye movement and that of the corresponding head movement. The response eye movement usually follows a little after the stimulus head movement. Mean and standard deviations of all three parameter types are computed throughout all accepted impulses of the signals

5. Test Results

All test signals were run with our analysis program implemented with Pascal in a microcomputer. They were visually checked that no extraneous phenomena would have deteriorated even parts of them. Gain and latency parameters and their statistical results (Table 1) were computed for all normals and patients. Average gain computed by amplitude ratios was exactly the ideal gain value of 1 for the normals, but about one third (0.34) less for the patients. Similarly, average gain computed by linear regression was 0.32 less for the patients than for the normals. Average latency was almost double for the patients compared with the normals. The results were as may be excepted in the sense that healthy normals were able to perform more accurate gain values with less reaction times.

Table 1. Means and standard deviations of gain and latency parameters of the normals for 16 signals and those of the patients for 44 signals.

	normals		**patients**	
	mean	**standard deviation**	**mean**	**standard deviation**
gain by amplitude	1.00	0.22	0.66	0.20
gain by linear regression	0.82	0.21	0.50	0.21
latency [s]	0.022	0.014	0.042	0.031

6. Conclusion

Impulse-like eye movements seem to be a suitable means to investigate oculomotor performance of otoneurological patients. The syntactic recognition method developed was able to recognise and analyse these eye movements reliably and accurately.

References

[1] M. Juhola, A syntactic method for analysis of saccadic eye movements, *Pattern Recognition* **19** (1986) 353-359.

[2] M. Juhola, A syntactic method for analysis of nystagmus and smooth pursuit eye movements, *Computer Methods and Programs in Biomedicine* **26** (1988) 53-62.

[3] M. Juhola, A syntactic analysis method for sinusoidal tracking eye movements, *Computers in Biomedical Research* **24** (1991) 222-233.

[4] M. Juhola, A syntactic analysis method for eye movements of vestibulo-ocular reflex, *Computer Methods and Programs in Biomedicine* **46** (1995) 59-65.

[5] Tabak, H. Collewijn, L.J.J.M. Boumans and J. van der Steen, Gain and delay of human vestibulo-ocular reflexes to oscillation and steps of the head by a reactive torquet helmet. I. Normal subjects, *Acta Otololaryngologica* **117** (1997) 785-795.

[6] M. Juhola, I. Pyykkö, H. Aalto and T. Hirvonen. Effects of digital filtering on the parameters of vestibulo-ocular reflex signals, *Automedica* **16** (1998) 205-216.

Medical Informatics Europe '99
P. Kokol et al. (Eds.)
IOS Press, 1999

Lossless Compression of Eye Movement Signals

Timo TOSSAVAINEN, Martti JUHOLA
Department of Computer Science, University of Tampere, P.O. Box 607, 33101 Tampere, Finland
Antti KOSKI
Department of Computer Science, University of Turku, Turku, Finland

Abstract. Compression of digital signals is widely employed in several areas such as speech signals. Concerning biomedical signals almost merely ECG signals have so far been compressed, in fact, in very many applications. To our knowledge, this compression study is the first one presented in the case of eye movement signal which are investigated in several medical specialties. In this study eye movements are electro-oculographically recorded. Tests performed to signals of patients of an equilibrium laboratory gave compression ratios generated with essential lossless compression methods.

1. Introduction

Signal compression has been employed in several applications, also for biomedical signals. However, it seems to be that well-known, but practically the only biomedical signal type applied in compression is electrocardiography (ECG) [1,2]. Still the compression of other biomedical signal types is desirable. It diminishes storage space requirements and transmission time. These are crucial although computers become more efficient; at the same time more and more data are generated, too.

In lossy signal compression some information is allowed to be lost in hope that it is chiefly noise. Instead, in lossless compression it is required that no information is lost and thus a compressed signal can entirely be reversed to its original form. There is no guarantee that a lossy compression method would lose only noise. In applications physicians usually appreciate exact reconstruction of eye movement signals and prefer it to better compression ratios of lossy methods. Besides, biomedical signals are commonly filtered digitally before compression or any signal analysis operations to dampen noise. For these reasons, we were particularly interested in the lossless compression of eye movement signals.

We used eye movement signals measured at the equilibrium laboratory of Helsinki University Central Hospital, Finland. These signals are clinically used for otoneurological investigations, especially for patients suffering from inner ear diseases whose typical symptom is vertigo. Eye movements used particularly in otoneurology are saccades that are fast voluntary eye movements, nystagmus that is reflexive eye movement, sinusoidal tracking eye movements (smooth pursuit), and vestibulo-ocular reflex eye movements.

2. Eye Movement Recordings

Saccades (Fig. 1) are the fastest eye movements. A patient produces saccades when he watches a target of a light dot that is reflected on the opposite wall in the darkened test room. During all tests the patient is seated in a chair so that the distance from the patient's eyes is practically constant to the stimulation light dot. The laser light dot used in our tests jumps from a location to another on the wall. These jumps of the light dot that a patient is to follow with his gaze are controlled by a microcomputer to generate a fixed stimulation movement series which is random for the patient, since amplitudes of stimulation movements and times between movements vary in order to be unpredictable for a patient.

Sinusoidal tracking eye movements (Fig. 1) are yielded when a patient watches the light dot which horizontally moves on the wall. To generate stimulation movements the light dot glides fast or slowly depending on the phase of the sinusoidal angle. With two different frequencies and different amplitudes, the test is random from a patient's point of view.

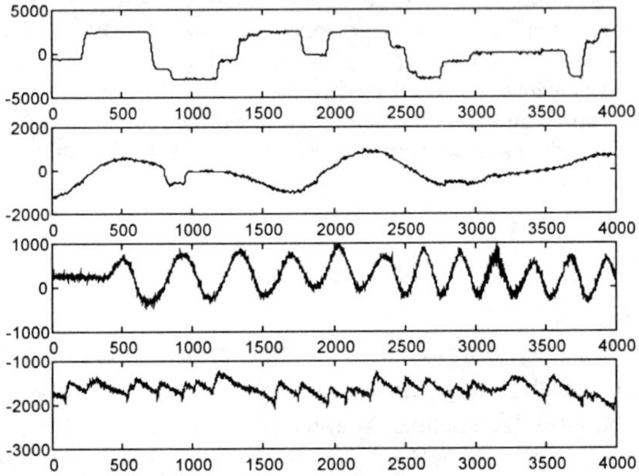

Fig. 1. The duration (horizontal axis) of these signal parts is 10 s. The vertical axis corresponds to amplitudes which vary between approximately 10° and 60°, but are here given, without the calibration, as original integers obtained from the analog-digital converter. The uppermost curve is from a saccadic eye movement signal. The second curve is from a sinusoidal tracking eye movement signal, the third segment is from a vestibulo-ocular reflex signal, and the lowermost segment from a nystagmus signal. They were horizontal eye movements in the direction from left (downwards in the figure) to right (upwards) or vice versa

In a vestibulo-ocular test a subject is due to move his head along with the stimulus of a beep sound, the frequency being increased from 0.5 Hz to 5.0 Hz. The subject moves his head repeatedly from left to right and back. His gaze has to be fixed to the same position. These (Fig. 1) resemble sinusoidal tracking movements, but with greater frequencies.

Involuntary nystagmus is irrigated by injecting warm or cool (37±7 °C) air or water into the auditory canal. The subject will normally have a rotating feeling that is seen as nystagmus, repeated saw-tooth type reflex of the eyes (Fig. 1) that soon fades out.

The recording was executed at 400 Hz, sufficently high to detect even the subtlest details from eye movement signals [3]. The amplitude resolution was 13 bits (±10 V). Eye movements were calibrated suitably. Skin electrodes were used with the measurements. The recording and signal analysis methods applied were described earlier [3]. Altogether, 69 signals were picked up from random otoneurological patients: 22 saccade, 18 sinusoidal tracking, 15 vestibulo-ocular and 14 nystagmus signals. The durations of the signal types were 20 s, 60 s or 80 s. Average signal to noise ratio was 32 dB.

3. Compression Methods Applied

Although the signals contained different numbers of samples, this does not affect the compression results, since all the compression ratios *CR* to be presented are expressed in the following form

$$CR = \frac{B_u}{B_c}$$

where B_u is the original number of bits in the uncompressed signal and B_c is that of the compressed signal (each original sample consists of 13 bits). The latter number of bits contains all additional "header" information possibly required by a compression method.

A basic technique to decrease the length of data is compression by differential pulse code modulation (DPCM). To estimate a sample, the error *e* between the sample and its estimate

$$e = x - \hat{x}$$

is computed and encoded with some compression method instead of the original sample. Since the error is considerably smaller than the original sample, less bits are needed to store the error. This simple technique attempts to reduce signal redundancy by taking intersample correlation into account. The decoding process computes in a reversed way by calculating the estimate and error and summing them up to produce the original sample. A suitable prediction model has to be applied to compute estimates for signal samples.

DPCM is applied as preprocessing and the error is then coded to a file. Another preprocessing is digital filtering that is used to eliminate noise outside the significant frequency band. For eye movements the sufficient cutoff frequency is 70 Hz [3]. Lowpass filtering increases signal redundancy by sweeping out signal variation. Compression ratios are then expected to increase. Both unfiltered and filtered signals were tested.

The simplest predictor for a sample estimate is

$$\hat{x}_i = x_{i-1}$$

where the next sample is estimated by using the preceding sample directly. This is the zero-order predictor. Correspondingly, the first-order predictor is

$$\hat{x}_i = x_{i-1} + (x_{i-1} - x_{i-2}) = 2x_{i-1} - x_{i-2}$$

where two preceding samples are employed to predict the following sample.

There are various techniques to encode the error of the actual sample and its estimate, e.g. Gamma code [4]. Golomb code is suitable for non-uniformly distributed integers. We applied its advanced variant, Exponential-Golomb [5], since this was very good [6]. Another type of universal code employed is Rice code [2], a special case of Golomb code.

Since traditional compression methods are frequently applied, we included Huffman coding, LZSS coding that is an advanced derivative from the famous LZ77 by Liv and Zempel [5] and LZW that is also a repaired version by Welch on the basis of LZ78. Another is also arithmetic coding [7].

DPCM uses a predictor to reduce the dynamic range of signals. In addition to the zero-order and first-order predictors, we used the Levinson-Durbin algorithm which generates an optimal linear predictor by utilising signal autocorrelation and previous samples [8]. We developed a variation where a buffer is filled, then the best parameter value is computed for the code and the buffer content is encoded with the Rice code [9]. We designed also another adaptive method, quite similar to the adaptive Rice method, but the encoding made with Exponential-Golomb. We executed the compression also by using directly the "raw material", i.e. signals themselves, without the prior DPCM. Results gained with these tests were considerably worse than with DPCM and so they are not reported.

4. Experimental Results

Means and standard deviations were computed over all the signals. The results gained are presented in Table 1 for the original unfiltered signals and for the same signals after filtering with a hybrid-median filter suitable for eye movement signals [3]. The results of FOP and LD (see Table 1) were not largely shown, since they were not superior; FOP was often inferior to the results regarding ZOP. In fact, LD ordinarily generated its first coefficient almost equal to 1. Consequently, it was quite like ZOP. This was also seen when a mean absolute error (MAE) and mean square error (MSE) were computed between the original signals and those predicted ones given by ZOP, FOP, and LD. On an average, the predictor performance was slightly better in the case of ZOP and LD.

Average results obtained by using the coding methods directly without the preprocessing of the DPCM technique were approximately only 1.04 – 1.27 even for the filtered signals.

Table 1 – Compression ratio results of the 69 eye movement signals.

	unfiltered		**filtered**	
	mean	**standard deviation**	**mean**	**standard deviation**
Gamma ZOP	1.79	0.50	2.31	0.82
Gamma FOP	1.58	0.52	1.95	0.64
Exponential-Golomb ZOP	2.08	0.54	2.45	0.54
Huffman ZOP	2.27	0.57	2.65	0.71
LZSS ZOP	1.02	0.13	1.14	0.23
LZW ZOP	1.87	0.57	2.26	0.74
LZW LD	1.82	0.54	2.16	0.66
Arithmetic ZOP	2.29	0.57	2.68	0.71
Adaptive Exp.-Golomb ZOP	2.23	0.53	2.64	0.65
variation with Rice ZOP	2.28	0.55	2.68	0.68

ZOP zero-order predictor, FOP first-order predictor, LD predictor with Levinson-Durbin algorithm (order 3)

It is worth noting that Huffman and arithmetic coding methods required relatively great numbers of storage for these rather short test signals. All compressed signals were finally decoded. These decoded signals were compared to the original input signals to ensure that the original and decoded signals were identical. We see that Huffman, arithmetic, our adaptive Exponential-Golomb coding, and our adaptive variation with Rice coding produced equally good compression ratios, about 2.3, for the unfiltered signals and 2.7 for the filtered signals. These are not high compared, for instance, to lossy ECG compression. On the other hand, no information was lost. Moreover, the practically lowest sampling frequency possible of 400 Hz was used. Doubtless DPCM method is always beneficial.

References

[1] S.M.S. Jalaleddine *et al.* ECG data compression techniques – a unified approach, *IEEE Transactions on Biomedical Engineering* **37** (1990) 329-343.
[2] C.P. Mammen and B. Ramamurthi, Vector quantization for compression of multichannel ECG, *IEEE Transactions on Biomedical Engineering* **37**(1990) 821-825.
[3] M. Juhola *et al.*, Effects of digital filtering on the parameters of vestibulo-ocular reflex signals, *Automedica*, **16** (1998) 205-216.
[4] P. Elias, Universal codeword sets and representations of the integers, *IEEE Transactions on Information Theory* **21** (1975) 194-203.
[5] J. Ziv and A. Lempel, A universal algorithm for sequential data compression, *IEEE Transactions on Information Theory* **23** (1977) 337-343.
[6] A. Koski, Lossless ECG encoding, *Computer Methods and Programs in Biomedicine*, **52** (1997) 23-33.
[7] I. Witten *et al.*, Arithmetic coding for data compression, *Communications of the ACM*, **30** (1987) 520-540.
[8] A. Cohen, Biomedical Signal Processing. CRS Press, Boca Raton, FL, USA, 1986.
[9] R.F. Rice, Some practical universal noiseless coding techniques. Jet Propulsion Laboratory, *JPL Publication* **79** (22), CA, Pasadena, CA, USA, 1979.

Medical Informatics Europe '99
P. Kokol et al. (Eds.)
IOS Press, 1999

Use of time-variant coherence as a general tool for analysis of interrelations between brain electrical processes

H. Witte*, M. Arnold*, W. Miltner**, T. Rosburg***, Ch. Schelenz****
**Institute of Medical Statistics, Computer Sciences and Documentation, **Institute of Psychology, ***Clinic of Psychiatry, ****Clinic of Anesthesiology and Intensive Care, Medical Faculty of the Friedrich Schiller University Jena, 07740 Jena, Germany*

1 Introduction

Functional or effective connectivity are operational measures which describe different aspects of interrelations of neuronal assemblies. The electrophysiological phenomena related to both kinds of connectivity reflect a 'temporal correlation between spatially remote neurophyiological events' [1]. Consequently, a method is needed which measures the temporal correlation between separate brain electrical processes. The coherence spectrum can be interpreted as the squared linear correlation coefficient between two signals for each frequency component. The time-variant coherence approach between two signals leads to a sequence of coherence spectra for each sampling point (coherence spectrogram). Therefore, by means of a defined location of EEG electrodes on the scalp, the spatial (topographic) information can be considered and the time variant coherence spectrum designates the temporal frequency-selective correlation.

The results of the first applications of such an analysis tool shed light on the cortical processing of ultra short-term cognitive processes [2, 3].

This study deals with aim to summarise results of three of our present applications [4, 5, 6] which can be seen as an extension of the concept of time-variant coherence analysing phenomena of connectivity between brain electrical processes:

1. The first application (<u>AP 1- conditioning</u>) supported observations that the development of correlation among cell assemblies of the brain is a basic element of associative learning or conditioning [4]. The 'subjects' task was to learn that a visual stimulus (red colour) was always terminated by a painful electrical stimulus (10-ms duration) applied to the left midfinger (condition A) whereas no such painful stimulus (condition B) was given at the end of another visual stimulus (green colour).
2. The second application (<u>AP 2- correction quality</u>) shows the utility of time-variant coherence for the evaluation of the correction quality after elimination of ocular artefacts in MEG data [5].
3. The third application (<u>AP 3- sedation depth</u>) demonstrates that the transient coupling of two brain electrical processes can be used as an indicator for the depth of sedation in intensive care patients [6].

All applications were based on adaptive autoregressive modelling of nonstationary time series by means of Kalman filtering [7]. This paper is focused on the different methodical concepts of signal processing on the basis of this fundamental algorithm.

2 Methods and Material

2.1 Definition of time-variant coherence (TVC)

The time-variant coherence analysis used in all applications of this study is based on the estimation of autoregressive (AR) coefficients updated at each sampling point by Kalman algorithm. The algorithm was described in detail by Arnold et al. [7]. Accordingly, the coherence

$$\gamma_n^2(f) = \frac{\left|S_{xy,n}(f)\right|^2}{S_{xx,n}(f) \cdot S_{yy,n}(f)}$$

can be computed from momentary estimations of autospectra ($S_{xx,n}$ and $S_{yy,n}$) of two time series $\{x_n\}$ and $\{y_n\}$ as well as from the momentary cross-spectrum ($S_{xy,n}$) as a function of frequency (f) and time (n). This procedure results in time sequence of coherence spectra. For example, the mean coherence within a frequency band can be extracted from this sequence and plotted as a time-variant parameter. Investigations regarding the AR model order were performed by means of Akaike's information criterion [8].

2.2 General concepts of signal processing

There are two different concepts in studying interrelations between electrical and/or magnetical sources by means of TVC:

1. The TVC between two EEG(MEG) channels can be computed. However, a pre-processing has been applied before. As a rule, the use of a reference-free EEG recording has been recommended [9]. Therefore, a high pass filtering of the genuine cortical signals of AP1 by a Laplacian was used. Furthermore, a rejection of ocular artefacts is necessary. AP2 deals with the aim to show, how the TVC can be used to control the rejection quality. The TVC between one EEG/MEG and one EOG channel was computed after artefact rejection.
2. The TVC between two time-variant parameters of one EEG/MEG channel can be used for the identification of interrelations of two unknown generator structures. This concept based on the assumption that different frequency ranges have been generated by different brain electrical processes. In general, the coupling or interrelations of frequency ranges can be described by bispectral analysis [10]. We used the envelope curves of EEG frequency components as one input signal of the TVC, the second input signal was a low-frequency component computed by means of filtering. This concept was used in AP 3.

2.3 Study design, subjects, data recording

AP 1 - Conditioning: The 'subjects' task was to learn that a visual stimulus (red colour) was always terminated by a painful electrical stimulus (10-ms duration) applied to the left midfinger (condition A) whereas no such painful stimulus (condition B) was given at the end of another visual stimulus (green colour). Duration of visual stimuli was 3000ms. Both visual stimuli were applied in random order for a total number of 120 trials with 60 stimuli representing each condition. The intertrial interval was 4 s. Sixteen healthy, right handed student volunteers (nine female) participated in the experiment. EEG data were recorded from 31 electrodes mounted on the subject's scalp according to the international 10-20-

system (with additional electrodes interspaced between standard electrodes. The electrode Cz was used as common reference, the sampling rate was 200 Hz.

AP 2 - Correction quality: For the magnetoencephalographic (MEG) investigations of the auditory evoked field (AEF) schizophrenic patients and controls were stimulated monaurally, using computer-generated tone-tips, delivered to the probands via a plastic tube. Auditory stimuli consisted of 1000Hz, 90dB tone pips with 50ms duration and 10ms rise- and fall-times, and a randomised interstimulus interval between 800 and 1800ms. Each session consisted of 270 trials and each trial had a length of 512 ms. The study group consisted of 17 medicated male schizophrenics and 17 age- and sex-matched healthy controls. Recordings were performed using a 31 channel first-order biomagnometer (Philips GmbH), positioned contralaterally to the stimulated ear over the temporal lobe. The EOG was recorded with a pair of electrodes, one positioned below the eye and the other one laterally above the eye ipsilateral to the MEG recording side. The sampling frequency of MEG and EOG was 1000 Hz. A down-sampling to lower rates was performed after digital low pass filtering.

AP 3 - sedation depth: The burst-suppression pattern of the EEG during sedation was used for investigations. A rising intracranial pressure, refractory to conventional therapy (ventricular drainage - if available, hyperventilation to a $PaCO_2$ below 4.6 kPa and infusion of Mannitol®), was the indication for increasing the basic sedation by adding i.v.-hypnotics. The investigations were carried out on a group of 12 patients with various neurosurgical diseases. All of them were given individual basic sedation to ensure controlled mechanical ventilation and safe nursing. The EEG was recorded from an eight channel analogous EEG (Neurofax 5610G, Nihon Kohden, Japan); the electrodes were placed in superior lengthwise positions according to the international 10-20 system with Cz as reference being the favoured recording modus in important clinical studies. The sampling frequency was 256 Hz. A down-sampling to a rate of 128 Hz was performed after digital low pass filtering with a upper cut-off frequency of 64 Hz.

3 Results

AP 1- Conditioning: Our methodical investigations led to an optimal computation scheme which can be summarised as follows. In a first step of pre-processing the correction of eye movement and blink interferences was performed by means of standard methods [11]. In a second step a current source density analysis was carried out in order to maximise the topographical distribution of sources and sinks to obtain reference-free measures for each electrode [12]. Pairs of electrodes (Fig. 1) between the two regions of interests I and II (electrodes covered the occipital lobe, the primary and secondary somatosensory projection areas of fingers on the homunculus of both hemispheres, and the midline of the brain) were considered for coherence analysis (electrode of region I versus electrode of region II) using all possible combinations. The mean coherence within the frequency range of 37-43 Hz (due to the theory of Singer [13]) was extracted as time-variant coherence parameter. The time-window for the detailed analysis covered the last 250 ms prior to the application of the painful stimulus (arrow in Fig. 1). In spite of using this time window the time-variant coherence was computed for each entire trial. The coherence measures extracted from the analysis window were transformed using Fisher's z-transformation and collapsed to averaged coherence measures for each subject, each pair of electrodes, and each condition of visual stimulation. The trial sequences were subdivided into five blocks of 12 trials (to trace the process of development of the coherence between different electrode sites throughout the course of acquisition. After testing the normal distribution, these mean coherences were submitted to an ANOVA analysis (repeated measurements) with the within factor blocks (five levels) and experimental condition.

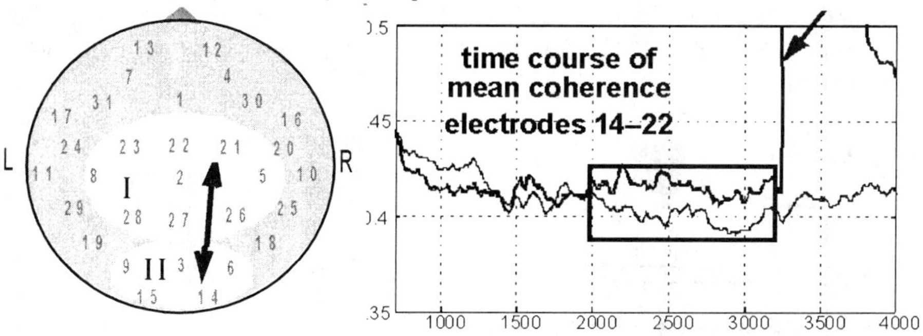

Fig. 1: Left: Electrode locations and regions of interests (I: occipital cortex; II fields of postcentral projection and of somatosensory association of left hand). Right: Result (grand mean) of time-variant coherence analysis between electrodes 14 and 22 (thick line: condition A; thin line: condition B).

The neurophysiological results gave evidence for the existence of a transient neural connectivity between occipital brain regions processing the visual stimulus and primary somatosensory brain regions processing the painful stimulus. Both regions seemed to communicate toward the end of the visual stimulus as a result of conditioning (learning). In detail, there is a clear evidence that condition A (visual stimulus followed by a painful stimulus) was associated with larger coherences then were seen for condition B (other visual stimulus which was not followed by a painful stimulus) between occipital electrode sites and electrode sites on the contralateral somatosensory projection area. One significant result (grand mean data about all subjects and trials) is represented in Fig. 1. The time-course of the mean coherence (37-43 Hz) is significantly different between condition A and B before the painful stimulus occurs. The difference are small but systematic across subjects and statistically significant ($p<0.05$ [4]).

AP 2- Correction quality : The computation scheme was given by Witte et al. [14] and modified for the use of time-variant coherence instead of FFT (fast Fourier transformation) based coherence estimation. Following methodical procedure can be suggested. After the correction [method, see [5]), the time-variant coherence was used to evaluate the correction quality. The corrected MEG interval and the corresponding EOG interval were used as input signals of TVC. It can be demonstrated that the time-course of TVC decreases significantly after correction for times when amplitudes of the EOG are large. In the extended (original) algorithm the ocular artefact can also be detected in evaluating the coherence spectrum. Accordingly, an extended version would be able to detect the artefact in a first run of the program and the correction quality could be determined in a second run.

AP 3 - Sedation depth : The processing scheme for this application is given in Fig 2 A. The EEG during burst-suppression patterns (BSP) was subdivided into a sequence of burst and suppression patterns using a modified version of our method for burst onset detection in neonatal EEG [15].

The following processing methods were started automatically by the segmentation algorithm (burst onset) and the results were averaged: (1) Estimation of the biamplitude; (2) Low-pass filtering 0-2.5Hz; (3) Calculation of the envelope curve of the frequency components within the frequency bands 3-7.5Hz and 8-12Hz. On the basis of visual inspection, burst-like EEG patterns were selected manually from the EEG during basic sedation. Such EEG patterns start with a high-amplitude (negative) wave ($\approx$1Hz). The EEG intervals separated were analysed given above. The envelope curve of EEG activity within the frequency bands 3-7.5Hz and 8-12Hz was computed by means of filtering [16]. The resulting continuous envelope curves (additionally filtered between 0.5-2.5Hz) and a low-frequency component of the EEG (0-2.5Hz) were used as input signals for an instantaneous coherence analysis.

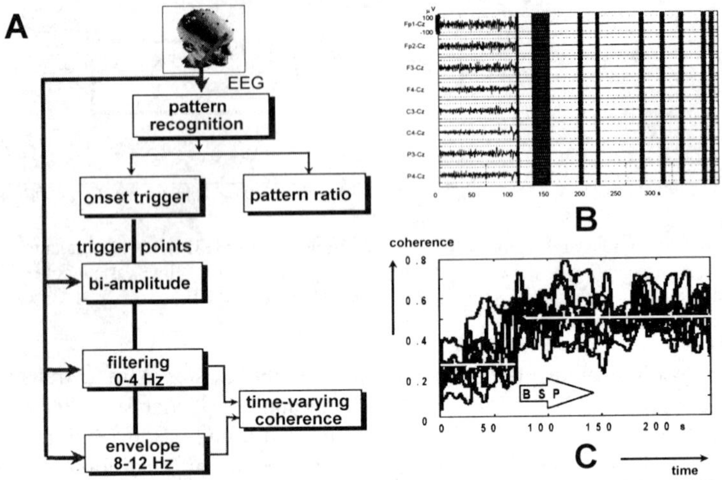

Fig. 2: (A) Processing scheme for EEG pattern analysis in sedated patients. (B) EEG recording entering BSP with segmentation in burst (grey background) and suppression patterns. (C) Superposition of all courses of the mean TVC within the frequency band 0.8 - 2.5Hz during EEG recording entering BSP (all patients N=12; Fp1-Cz).

In the biamplitude representations, two separable peaks with the co-ordinate range ≈4,5-5/2Hz and ≈9/0,5Hz can be recognised with the best expression at Fp1/2-Cz. These results can be derived from the grand mean data of the biamplitude (Fig. 2 C) as well as from the averaged biamplitude representations in each patient. These findings designate interrelations between the frequency ranges 0-2.5Hz⇔3-7.5Hz as well as 0-2.5Hz⇔8-12Hz.

An amplitude modulation seems to be the most probable reason for the appearance of the biamplitude peaks, i.e. a low-frequency component modulates the amplitude of faster EEG components. The degree of amplitude modulation can be quantified continuously by means of instantaneous coherence analysis between an envelope curve of the modulated component and the low-frequency component 0-2.5Hz (modulation component). The analysis was focused on the coherence between the low-pass filtered (0-2.5Hz) signal component and envelope (3-7.5Hz) as well as between the low-pass filtered (0-2.5Hz) signal component and envelope (8-12Hz), because corresponding peaks appeared in the biamplitude representation. The mean coherence values within the band 0.8-2.5Hz were derived from the resulting coherence spectrogram and plotted as time course. Fig. 2 C shows the superposition of all courses of the mean coherence within the frequency band 0.8-2.5Hz during EEG recording entering BSP (all patients N=12; Fp1-Cz). According to the design of our study, the different influences of the injuries, treatment regimes, drugs etc. on the interrelation effects cannot be separated, but a relation between the degree of interrelations and the depth of sedation can be postulated.

4 Discussion

It can be demonstrated that the time-variant coherence can be used as an efficient method in analysing interrelations between signals. Due to EEG/MEG analysis, this new approach leads to novel knowledge of transient interrelations between brain electrical processes. For the first time such ultra short-term effects could be demonstrated. The studies were performed on the basis of representative groups and the results have been evaluated statistically. The use of the Kalman filter algorithm for the estimation procedures has some advantage compared with other approaches. First, Kalman filters can be constructed for multivariate systems (i.e. partial and multiple coherences can be estimated in a time-variant manner) with stochastic variations of the parameters. The properties of the resulting estimates can be described theoretically. Furthermore, it is not necessary to search for a suitable set of base functions to model the temporal evolution of coefficients or to implement procedures for the detection of change points. Secondly, the Kalman filter is suitable for implementation on microcomputers. Because of its recursive structure, it allows on-line processing.

The study was supported by BMBF 01 ZZ 9602 and DFG Wi1166-2.

References

[1] Friston, K.J.: *Theoretical neurobiology and schizophrenia.* Br.Med.Bull. 52(1996), 644-655.

[2] Krause, W., Gibbons, H., Schack, B.: *Concept activation and coordination procedure require two different networks.* NeuroReport (1998), 1649-1653.

[3] Schack, B., Krause, W.: *Dynamic Power and Coherence Analysis of Ultra Short-Term Cognitive Processes - a methodical study.* Brain Topogr. 8 (1995) 127-136.

[4] Miltner, W.H.R. Braun, Ch., Arnold, M., Witte, H., Taub, E.: *Coherence of gamma-band activity as a basis of associative learning.* Nature (1999), accepted.

[5] Meier, T., Rosburg, M., Arnold, M., Sauer, H., Nowak, H., Witte, H.: *Quantification and rejection of ocular artifacts in auditive evoked fields in schizophrenics.* Electroenceph. Clin. Neurophysiol. 108(1998), 526-535.

[6] Witte, H., Schelenz, Ch., Specht, M., Jäger, H., Putsche, P., Arnold, M., Leistritz, L., Reinhart, K.: *Interrelations between EEG frequency components in sedated intensive care patients during burst-suppression period.* Neuroscience Letters 260(1999), in press.

[7] Arnold, M., Miltner, W., Witte, H., Bauer, R., Braun, Ch.: *Adaptive Measurement of Linear Dependence between Physiological Signals by means of Time-varying Multivariate AR-Modelling,* IEEE Transactions on Biomedical Engineering 45(1998), 553-562.

[8] Chen, H.H., Guo, L.: *Identification and stochastic adaptive control.* Boston, MA, Bikhäuser, 1991.

[9] Nunez, P.L., Srinivasan, R., Wijesinghe, R.S., et al.: *EEG coherence I. statistics, reference electrode, volume conduction, laplacians, cortical imaging, and interpretation at multiple scales.* Electroencephalopr. Clin. Neurophysiol. 103(1997), 499-515.

[10] Witte, H., Putsche, P., Eiselt, M., Hoffmann, K., Schack, B., Arnold, M., Jäger, H.: *Analysis of the interrelations between a low-frequency and a high-frequency signal component in human neonatal EEG during quiet sleep.* Neuroscience Letters 236(1997), 175-179.

[11] Gratton, G., Coles, M.G., Donchin, E.: *A new method for off-line removal of ocular artifact.* Electroencephalogr. Clin. Neurophysiol. 55(1983), 468-484.

[12] Nunez, P.L.: *Electrical fields of the brain.* New York, Oxford Uiversity Press, 1981.

[13] Gray, C.M., Konig, P., Engel, A.K., Singer, W.: *Oscillatory responses in cat visual cortex exhibit inter-columnar synchronization which reflects global stimulus properties.* Nature 338(1989), 334-337.

[14] Witte,H., Glaser,S., Rother,M.: *New spectral detection and elimination test algorithms of ECG and EOG artefacts in neonatal EEG recordings.* Med. & Biol. Eng. & Comput. 25 (1987), 127-130.

[15] Galicki,M., Witte,H., Dörschel,J., Eiselt,M., Grießbach,G.: *Common optimization of adaptive preprocessing units and a Neural Network during the learning period. Application in EEG pattern recognition.* Neural Networks 10(1997), 1153-1163.

[16] Arnold, M., Doering, A., Witte, H.,Eiselt, M., Grießbach, G.: *The use of adaptive Hilbert transformation in the analysis of the polygraphic data of neonates. A methodical investigation.* J. Clin. Monitoring 12(1996), 43-60.

Medical Informatics Europe '99
P. Kokol et al. (Eds.)
IOS Press, 1999

Computer EEG-monitoring of laserotherapy effects in patients with asteno-depressive syndrome

V.P. OMELCHENKO, I.S. BARANCHOOK, M.N. DMITRIEV
Rostov State Medical University, 29, Nahichevansky street, 344718, Rostov-on-Don, Russia

Abstract. Nowadays the low-intensive laserotherapy is shown to be an effective and non-hazardous method of asteno-depressive syndrome treatment. The differences of EEG-reactions to laser influences have been revealed in patients of different age groups. And the close negative correlation between the therapy effect, on the one hand, and the patient's age and the disease duration, on the other hand, has been shown. No significant changes of the patient's state or integrative EEG-indices have been evoked by a placebo application. The results showed the advantages of the low-intensive laserotherapy in asteno-depressive syndrome treatment and confirmed the significance of computer EEG-monitoring for prediction, control and correction of the state of the patient.

The considerable increase of mental disorders, associated with the asteno-depressive syndrome, has been noted in recent years (Klerman, Weisman, 1989; Alexandrovsky, 1993). It should be mentioned, that asteno-depressive syndrome is one of the main neuro-psychical disorders, found in persons, who took part in the liquidation of consequences of the Chernobil catastrophe (Golovenko, 1994). Taking into consideration the increasing occurence of such disorders and their acute social character, the problem of the brain functional state control and correction of its unfavourable shifts (which are necessary for early dyagnostics, choosing an adequate therapy and methods of patient's reabilitation) is of great interest.

The traditional therapy of such a pathology by antidepressants and benzodiasepines is complicated by some side effects and is characterised by considerably prolonged courses of therapy (Avrutsky, 1984, 1987). And as it was demonstrated in recent clinical and experimental studies, the low-intensity laserotherapy is an effective and non-hazardous method of asteno-depressive syndrome treatment (Kovalenko et al.,1993; Mrihin, 1995). That is why, not only the clinical testing of the method, but the elaboration of objective techniques for express-dyagnostics of initial state, the control of therapy effectiveness and, if necessary, its correction, are of great importance.

It should be noted that the improvement of the clinical state of the patients with asteno-depressive syndrome is usually accompanied by the "normalisation" of the whole EEG-pattern, its characteristics approaching to the indices of healthy subjects. Therefore the recording of biopotentials at certain time intervals for monitoring the CNS functional state dynamics during the course of the therapy was suggested (Omelchenko, 1990). This approach gives a chance of objective estimation in it EEG changes during the therapy and to relate them with clinical, biochemical, psychosomatic and other indices of the patient's state.

1. Subjects

42 patients (37 men and 5 women aged from 18 to 52; mean age 36±2,4), of the neurological department of the Rostov State Medical University took part in the experiments. All of them had asteno-depressive syndrome of different genesis and severity. Part of them - 26 men - were the Chernobil catastrophe liquidators.

30 patients (18 Chernobil liquidators (ChL) and 12 non-liquidators, composing a control group (CG)), underwent a complete the whole course of laserotherapy and the rest 12 subjects (8- ChL and 4 - CG) got a placebo. The control group was composed of 42 practically healthy subjects aged 17-54 without somatic pathology and mental disorders or pathological EEG manifestations.

2. Laserotherapy

Endonasal laserotherapy was carried out daily (morningly); the right and the left nasal cavity were alternated. The course of therapy consisted of 8-10 procedures. The influences were generated by the therapeutic laser devise "USOR" within an ifrared range. Technical characteristics were as follows: wavelenth - 0,891±0,002 mcm, impulse power -2,8±0,15 Wt, impulse generation frequency - 3000 Hz, exposure time - 256 s.

3. EEG Recording

EEG was recorded in an unipolar manner from bilateral placements over frontal, temporal, parietal and occipital sites, referenced to linked auricular electrodes. The EEG data were registered before, just after the 1st session (1-2 minutes later), and after the 3-4 and 8-10th laserotherapy sessions. For EEG recording and amplifying 8-channeled electroencephalographer "ORION" (Hungary) was used with a time constant 0,3 and 30 Hz bandwidth. EEG was registered on paper tape, divided into 8-seconds fragments. The latter were input into a computer (IBM PC). Preliminary input to a temporary file enabled the rapid artifacts rejections by a medical expert and saving in a database only the records contaning clinically significant data.

4. Data analysis

The parameters obtained by preliminary computer processing were the spectral power indices in the following common bands: delta (1-3 Hz), theta (4-7 Hz), alpha (8-13 Hz), beta (14-30 Hz), maximal and minimal amplitude of the rhythm, spectral power in each channel, computed as the sum of amplitude squares for the each reading, the rhythm index computed as the ratio of the rhythm time to the whole time of EEG registration (in %). On the basis of that data obtained, the separate descriptions of EEG for the right and left hemispheres conditioned by their patterns differences were given. To evaluate the interhemispheric asymmetry the frequency and amplitude characteristics of the collateral sites have been used.

The set of secondary EEG parameters, which were necessary for the estimation of EEG disorder severity have been estimated on the basis of the chosen sign. The characteristics included were as follows: the dominant activity, the amplitude of dominant activity, the dominant frequency in each band, the alpha-activity description, differences of alpha-activity in distinct sites, descriptions of beta- and slow-wave activity. Besides the regularity of dominant frequency and the character of modulation were determined for alpha-activity.

As a method for the evaluation of the therapy effect the integrative parameter ρ (x) (Omelchenko, 1990), characterizing the changes in the EEG under analysis from "the normal EEG" has been used:

$$\rho(x) = \sum_{i=1}^{N}\left(\frac{x_i - \bar{x}_i}{\sigma_i}\right)^2$$

where $\tilde{O}_i$ - the vector of the mean quantitative signs of EEG under analysis; $\overline{X}_i$ - the vector of the mean values of EEG signs for the group of healthy subjects, σ_i - the mean square deviation of Xi values for the group of healthy subjects; N - the signs quantity.

5. Results

According to the data obtaned all the patients had the common tendency of the EEG dynamics during laserotherapy. There was a marked non-linear dependence of laser radiation effect on EEG-indices. Both a significant decrements of "the distance to the normal level" and transition of main function values to those characteristics of healthy subjects and the opposite changes took place, correspondingly. There was a typical peak just ufter the 1st procedure and the opposite changes of indices to the initial value. Placebo therapy didn't evoke an improvement of the patient's state; integrative indices changed insignificantly in a random order with respect to the background level.

As it was marked, the absence of considerable changes of both indices after the 1st procedure could be the prognostic criterion of the absense of absolute remission after the therapy, though EEG-indices had a tendency to the normalization and a certain improvement of the clinical state took place.

Table 1 present the typical dynamics of both integrative indices of the brain bioelectrical activity during the lasero- and placebotherapy.

Table1: Changes of the monitoring indices during the laser and placebo therapy in patients with asteno-depressive syndrome

#	Patient	Metod	Background (before the therapy)	After the 1st session	After 4-5 sessions	After 8-10 sessions
			$\rho(x)$	$\rho(x)$	$\rho(x)$	$\rho(x)$
1.	D-ov	laser	654,66	142,87	200,35	80,44
2.	L-iy*	laser	1089,5	91,24	969,03	45,71
3.	Ch-ya	laser	247,13	31,09	252,69	59,21
4.	P-yan	laser	625,95	36,38	301,47	75,27
5.	M-ov*	laser	1236,81	991,92	1305,74	636,57
6.	S-in	laser	286,83	43,64	82,22	52,24
7.	K-va	laser	253,28	55,81	277,41	44,36
8.	A-uk*	laser	866,88	794,12	818,01	600,96
9.	K-b*	placebo	338,73	412,56	382,14	301,47
10.	I-a	placebo	226,62	217,48	270,09	210,87

* – Liquidator of the Chernobil catastrophe concequences

The results showed that the changes of integrative indices of the brain bioelectrical activity during the therapy correlated with a positive clinical dynamics with a certain forestall. The individual EEG reactions of the patients to laser radiation dependent on their age were revealed, as well as the dependence of positive dynamics of integral EEG-indices and, correspondingly, the therapy effectiveness from the duration of the pathology time. The treatment was more effective in younger patients with less pronounced pathological changes.

6. Discussion

In this work, the attempt to demonstrate the necessity and to justify the application of computer monitoring of the CNS functional state as high informative clinical method has been made. Moreover, the application of the method is practically unlimited and, besides the clinical practice (anesthesiology, cardiac surgery etc.) it could be used in scientific investigations, dealing with pharmocological preparations with a central effect as well as other methods of treatment, in particular, in laserotherapy of asteno-depressive syndrome considered in this work. We traced EEG indices dynamics in depressive patients in different phases of treatment. This enabled to predict the therapy effectiveness by the chosen integrative parameters. The elaborated metods are aimed at the standartization of such EEG researches in clinical and experimental medicine.

The maximum changes of the integrative parameters of the brain bioelectrical activity in patients with the complete consequent recovery occured after the 1st procedure, and the more explicit biostimulating effect being revealed on the background of the initially decreased level of cortical processes. These results can be used as a future prognostic criterion of the laserotherapy effectiveness. Further the EEG characteristics usially returned to the state, insignificantly differing from the initial one, followed by a gradual stabilization of investigated parameters, previous to the initial signs of the reduction of psychopathological symptoms.

During the analysis of the EEG integrative parameters an attention was paid to the fact that the therapy effectiveness depended directly on the severeness of the patient's initial state. It is obvious that the effective prognosis of the laserotherapy application could be given when the adaptational and compensatory possibilities of the organism aren't ehausted as a result of a continuous of pathological procass and the greater age of the patient.

So, in this work the important prognostic value of the bioelectrical activity of the brain for the objective estimation of the common functional stste of the CNS has been suggested. The data obtained demonstrate and justify the necessity of the EEG-investigations as well as abilities of the modern mathematical apparatus to achieve better results in the dyagnostics of the CNS functional state and monitoring of the therapy course using biopotentials recording.

7. Conclusions

On the basis of the data obtained we can speak about the effectiveness of astenodepressive patients treatment by the laserotherapy and the actuality of the method to the clinical practice.

The application of the integrative EEG-indices for the EEG-monitoring of the lasero- and placebotherapy effects in asteno-depressive patients gives the possibility to determine objectively the dynamics of the CNS functional state during the therapy, to evaluate the therapy effectiveness and to predict its consequences.

References

[1] Alexandrovsky U.A. (1993) *Pogranichnie psyhicheskie rasstroistva.* (Handbook). Moscow: Medicina. (In Russian).

[2] Golovenko S.V. (1994) Psychical and somatovegetative disorders durind the continuous exposition of the weak radiation doses. *Zhurnal nevropatologii i psihiatrii* , 94, 4, 63-65. (In Russian).

[3] Kovalenko V.M., Mrichin V.V., Kojin A.A. (1993) Non-medicamental correction of the psycho-vegetative status in liquidators of the Chernobil catastrophe concequences. In *Ecologicheski obuslovlennie zabolevanya.* Sbornic nauchnih trudov RODNMI. Rostov-on-Don. (In Russian).

[4] Mrihin V.V. (1995) *Experimental and clinical proof of the laserotherapy application in asteno-depressive syndrome treatment.* Thesis for the Ph.D. degree in medicine. Rostov-on-Don. (In Russian).

[5] Omelchenko V.P. (1990) *Computer analysis of the biopotentials of the brain as the basis for the evaluation and correction of the psychopathological states.* Thesis for the M.D. in biology. Kiev. (in Russian).

Medical Informatics Europe '99
P. Kokol et al. (Eds.)
IOS Press, 1999

Parametric Time-Varying Spectrum and its Application to SEMG Signals

Dean Korošec
Faculty of Electrical Engineering and Computer Science, University of Maribor,
it Smetanova 17, 2000 Maribor, Slovenia, dean.korosec@uni-mb.si

Abstract Frequency spectrum of surface electromyographic signals (SEMGs) exhibits a non-stationary nature even in case of constant level isometric muscle contractions. This changes are related to muscle fatigue processes and can be evaluated by methods for estimation of time-varying (TV) spectrum.

We describe a two estimation techniques: sliding window approach and decompostion of linear model coefficients trajectories. Drawback of the first is its large variance which causes unrealistic abrupt changes in the curve of overall dynamics, calculated either as the second derivative of the MF or as the ARMA distance between subsequent linear models forming the TV parametric spectrum. We demonstrate, that the second method is more appropriate for description of a slowly changing spectrum of surface EMG signals. Dynamics measures obtained from this estimation are proposed as an indication of the fatigue process character.

1 Introduction

Electromyographic signals

Electromyogram (EMG) is a signal obtained by a measurement of the electrical activity in a muscle [1]. Muscles consist of **muscle fibers** which are activated by **motoneurons**. Impulses coming from the spinal cord through a single motoneuron trigger a recruitment of several muscle fibers, these fibers form a group called **motor unit** (MU). Shape of the electrical response to the stimulation of motor unit is called **motor unit action potential** (MUAP) and contains a weighted (depending on the spatial distribution of fibers belonging to the MU) sum of electrical responses of each muscle fiber.

In frequency spectrum of SEMGs a phenomena called **spectral compression** can be observed, which is generally accepted to be in connection with muscle fatigue [3]. Different researchers have used mean (or median) frequency of the estimated power spectral density (PSD) or coefficients of the fitted autoregressive models to track and evaluate fatigue long before it is represented as a mechanical failure of the muscle - that is when the subject can not sustain the reference level of contraction any more. Especially AR models have been used for fatigue estimation or diagnostic classification, based on AR derived PSD.

Parametric frequency spectrum estimation: Linear modeling

Frequency spectrum of a signal can be obtained in several ways. Two main approaches are possible: (a) classical, **non-parametric** techniques, based on Fourier transform and (b) **parametric** or model based techniques, which try to describe the data as an output of a linear filter, where the input is random noise. Here we usually restrict our attention to the case, when the filter transfer function $H(z)$ can be expresed as a rational polynomial of $B(z)$ and $A(z)$ and call it a **linear model**. Power spectral density $S(\omega)$ (PSD) is then obtained as the square of the absolute value of the transfer function $H(z)$ evaluated on the unit circle:

$$|S(\omega)|^2 = |H(e^{j\omega})|^2 = \left|\frac{B(e^{j\omega})}{A(e^{j\omega})}\right|^2. \tag{1}$$

Regarding the order of A and B three types of linear models with typically different shape of the PSD can be obtained: AR or autoregressive , MA or moving average and ARMA or autoregressive moving average models.

2 Methods

Multichannel SEMG data acquisition

We used a 16-channel recording system, developed at the Centro di Biongegneria, Torino [4], to record surface electromyographic signals. System was used to record 15 single differential leads of SEMG out of 16 monopolar electrodes at 10 mm distance. Recordings were made on *biceps brachii* muscle of **normal subjects** with no neuro-muscular disorders under **isometric** conditions, guaranteed by the special gear providing a firm support for the subject's arm fixed at 90 degrees angle in the elbow. The 16th channel of the amplifier was used to acquire the torque data. Amplifier gain was set to 2000 and its range was -5 to +5 Volts. Digitalisation was done by using a 16-bit analogue/digital card with a sampling frequency of 1024 Hz. After a calibration to the **maximum voluntary contraction** (MVC) a subject was asked to sustain a desired contraction level (30 and 70% of MVC, controled visually on the torque monito) for 30 seconds.

Time-varying linear models

To extend the concept of ARMA (or AR) modeling to non-stationary we have to introduce time-varying model parameters $A(n)$ and $B(n)$. Let us denote a full set of a single ARMA model parameters by $\theta = [a_0\ a_1\ a_2\ \ldots\ a_P\ b_0\ b_1\ b_2 \ldots b_Q]'$. A complete set of parameters, describing the time-varying ARMA (TV ARMA) model over N time instances is then $\Theta = [\theta(0)\ \theta(1)\ \ldots\ \theta(N-1)]$ and its corresponding difference equation is

$$y(n) = \sum_{i=0}^{Q} b_i(n-i)w(n-i) - \sum_{i=1}^{P} a_i(n-i)y(n-i), \tag{2}$$

where $\theta(i)$ is a single ARMA model at time instance i, P and Q, are, respectively, AR and MA order and w is an uncorrelated white noise.

We used two approaches to the estimation of Θ. The simpler one is to assume, that the signal is slowly changing and therefore piece-wise stationary. In this case standard methods can be applied on windowed data segments and the obtained model is declared to be valid inside this window. Such approach is based on intuitively reasonable assumptions and is computationaly efficient. In the second solution of TV ARMA models parameters $b(n)$ and $a(n)$ are considered a linear combination of m basis functions [5]:

$$a_i(t) = \sum_{j=0}^{m} a_{ij} f_j(t). \tag{3}$$

As basis we used polynoms, altghough in general any functions can be used.By using the later approach, TV ARMA model is described by $m(P+1)(Q+1)$ parameters (let us denote them by ϑ), from which a full matrix Θ can be calculated. We used TV AR models only, since in this case estimation of φ can be obtained from a set of linear equations of the Yule-Walker type and AR models are appropriate for SEMG signals.

Distances between linear models and generalisation to time-varying case

For measurement and comparison of linear models a distance should be defined in a certain way [2]. While it is tempting to use **Euclidean distance** d_E between model coefficients θ it is not as efficient as other distances, based on comparison of spectra. Such measure is **log spectral deviation**, which is defined as the L_q norm of the difference between the logarithmic spectra. Most commonly the L_2 norm, **mean quadratic distance** d_{LS2} is used.

Any distance between stationary ARMA models θ_1 and θ_2 can be extended to TV ARMA models Θ_1 and Θ_2 by summation of partial distances over all time instances. Such generalisation is valid, since all metric properties (identity, symmetrie and triangular inequality) of d_{ARMA} are preserved also in d_{TVARMA}.

Degree of signal non-stationary over time can also be expressed by means of ARMA distances if signal is described by TV ARMA model Θ. Model dynamics over time (dyn_Θ) is then expressed as the measure of changes between the subsequent linear models:

$$dyn_\Theta(i) = d_{ARMA}\left(\theta(i), \theta(i+1)\right). \tag{4}$$

3 Results

Stationary SEMG spectrum

SEMG at higher level isometric contractions can be considered a random signal. Under the assumption of stationarity it can be modeled by stationary ARMA models. But there is an important question which needs to be answered before: the choice of the model order. For AR models criteria for order estimation exist, but they have not much practical value in case of non-true-autoregressive data. For SEMG signals different criteria also propose very different order, which may indicates that the choice of order is application dependent. And indeed: low order models (AR(2-8), ARMA(2,2) to ARMA(6,6)) are enough when one is interested only in the main frequency content (as in fatigue studies, for example), while estimation of the low frequency component (< 30 Hz), indicating the firing frequencies of the dominant MUs requires much higher order models (AR(30+), ARMA(10,10) and more).

Figure 1 shows spectrums of the two parts of the ninth lead of the 15-channel SEMG signal at 70% MVC. Both parts are 2 seconds long, the first is taken from the beginning of the recording and the second part starts after 25 seconds (25th to 27th second). For both signal parts their mean was removed before they were modeled by AR and ARMA models of different orders. Upper figure shows AR spectrums of models with 6, 20 and 50 coefficients, while lower figure depicts spectrums of ARMA(4,4), ARMA(10,10) and ARMA(30,30) models.

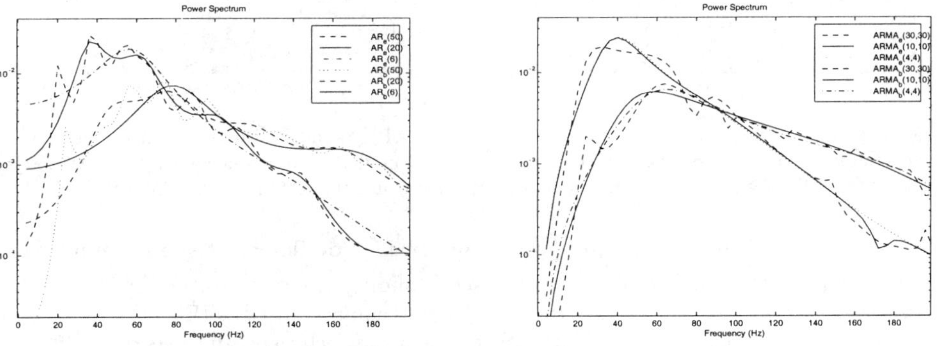

Figure 1: Left: Frequency spectrum of the TV AR models of orders 6, 20 and 50 for two segments of the SEMG signal (starting at 0 and 25 seconds, 2 seconds long). Right: Spectrums, corresponding to the same two signal segments, obtained from TV ARMA models of orders (4,4), (10,10) and (30,30).

Difference between spectrums of both segments is obvious. A strong shift toward lower frequencies is present in the signal after 25 seconds of contraction. Shift of the strongest frequency band is visible in both AR and ARMA models, obtained with any of the chosen number of parameters. On the other hand the low frequency component is visible only in models with relatively high number of parameters (more than 40). This component can be clearly seen in case of AR models, while ARMA spectrums exhibit it only in the first data segment and with 30 AR and 30 MA coefficients used.

Time-varying SEMG spectrum: sliding window approach

Fig. 2 shows an example of a sliding window estimation with AR(6) and ARMA(4,4), when we chose half a second windows (512 samples) with half overlap (window step: 256 samples). Evolution of the coefficients is smoother in case of AR model, but evolution of spectrum (Fig. 3) seem smoother for ARMA model. There is no difference between the two in estimation of the mean frequency (MF), which is indicated on both graphs of the figure 3 by dots.

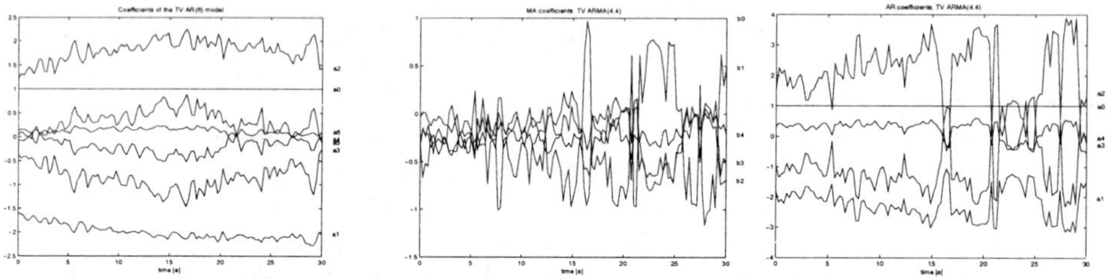

Figure 2: Left: Time-varying coefficients of the TV AR(6) model for the whole 30 second SEMG at 70% MVC. Center and right: MA and AR coefficients of the TV ARMA(4,4) model for the same signal. In both estimations sliding windows of lenght 0.5 second (512 samples) with half (256 samples) overlap were used.

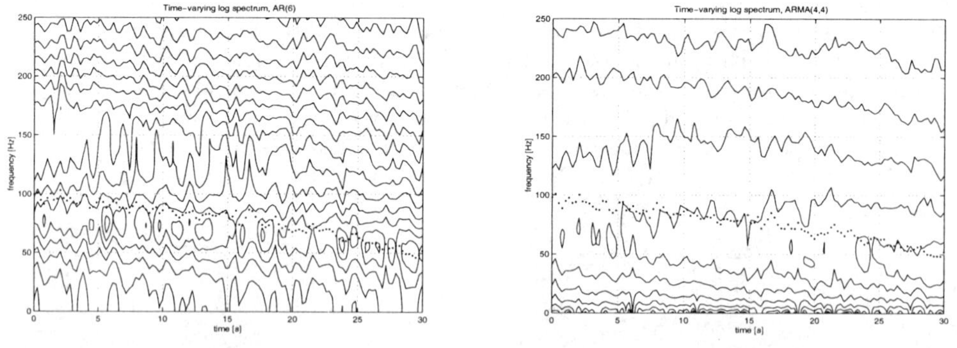

Figure 3: Left: Time-varying log spectrum of the TV AR(6) model with coefficients from Fig. 2. Right: Time-varying log spectrum of the TV ARMA(4,4) model. Only frequency range below 250 Hz is plotted and the mean frequency of the analytical spectrum is indicated by dots on both figures.

Time-varying SEMG spectrum: projection of TV coefficients to basis functions

Evolution of linear model coefficients observed in sliding window estimation indicates, that their trajectories could be well approximated by polynomial functions (Eq. 3). So we used polynoms up to the order 2 ($m = 3$) as basis function to which the coefficients of the TV AR model are projected. A very smooth time-varying spectrums were obtained, as shown on Fig. 4, where AR(6) and AR(40) models are presented. There is no significant difference of MF, but in AR(40) model a shift of the low frequency component, not seen in AR(6), can also be tracked as the lowest peak in the spectra at each time instant.

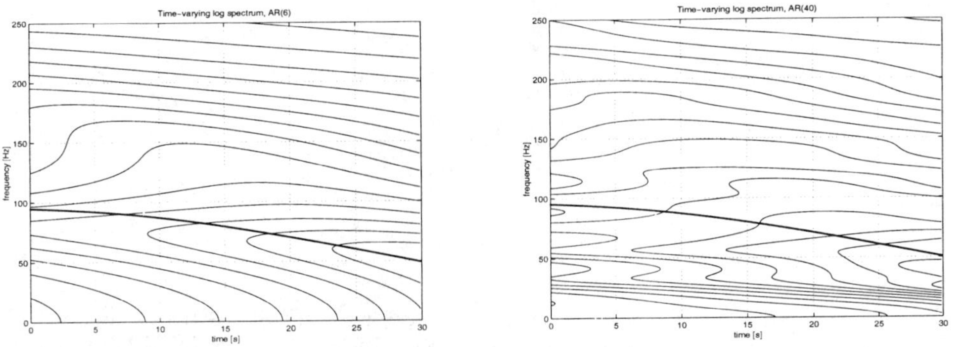

Figure 4: Time-varying logaritmic spectrum and evolution of its mean frequency, obtained by expanding model coefficients to the basis of polynomial function up to the second order. Left: AR(6), right: AR(40) model.

SEMG signal dynamics

Second derivative of the mean frequency should indicate at which periods its change was slower and when it was faster. But as the right graph in Fig. 5 shows, the second derivatives of MF obtained from 6 and 40 order AR models show very different behaviour although the estimated MF (Fig. 5, left) differ only slightly. A smooth trend of MF is needed to calculate derivatives, therefore a sliding window estimates can not be used.

Another view of when the changes in spectra are stronger can be provided by using ARMA distances and the dynamic measure, defined in Eq. 4. Fig. 6 (left) represents such measure using four different ARMA distances: cepstral, Euclidean, log spectral 1 and mean quadratic distance. They all indicate, that the spectrum is least changing in the middle of the recording (between $t = 10$ and $t = 20$ seconds) and do not differ much in case of different order models. But as integrals of those measures (Fig. 6, right) show, this only has a minor influence on cumulative change of the time-varying spectrum, which is constantly (almost linearly) growing. Mentioned measures of dynamic can not be applied to models obtained from sliding window estimation, since calculating gradient on noisy data has no particular meaning.

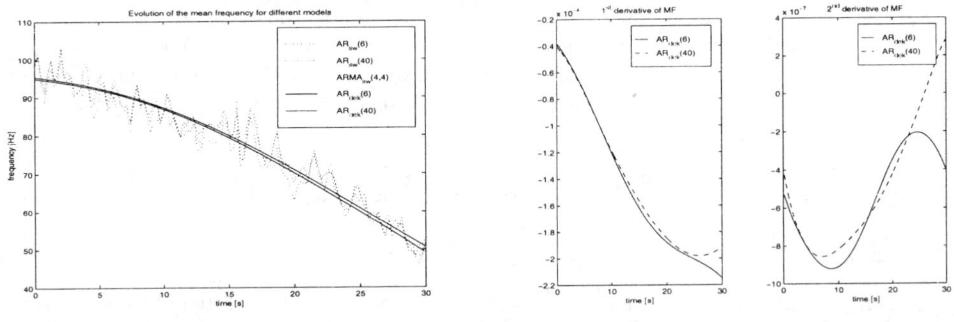

Figure 5: Left: Mean frequency trends for different order models. Dotted lines represent MF from models obtained by sliding window estimation (AR_{sw}), solid lines represent estimations by decomposition of coefficients (AR_{dek}). Center and right: first and second derivatives of the MF, obtained from AR_{dek} models of orders 6 and 40.

4 Conclusions

Linear modeling is a very appropriate tool for description of the frequency content of the SEMG signals. But since such signals are non-stationary, linear models have to be adapted to time-varying data. We presented two possible approaches: (a) sliding window approach, and (b) trajectory decomposition approach.

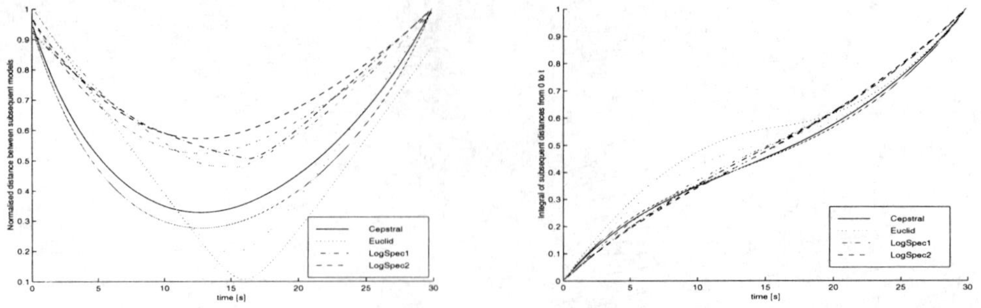

Figure 6: Left: Measures of changes in TV ARMA spectrum of the SEMG signal, measured by different ARMA distances betwen subsequent ARMA models. Right: Integrals of TV ARMA spectrum changes measures. In both graphs the same linestyle corresponds to the same distance. Dark lines are for $AR_{dek}(6)$ and bright lines are for $AR_{dek}(40)$ models.

We favourise AR models over ARMA, due to the following reasons: (a) estimation of AR models is relatively simple since they are governed by the set of linear equations; (b) AR models are superior in exhibitng the low frequency SEMG component; and (c) variance of the AR model estimation on shorter segments is lower than for ARMA models. On the other hand the spectrum of ARMA model is generally smoother and for low number of parameters (AR(6) vs. ARMA(4,4), for example) ARMA models provide more concentrated description of the main frequency band. MA models are not suitable for application on SEMG signals.

Estimation procedure where time-varying linear model coefficients are decomposed to the set of basis functions drastically decreases the number of parameters needed to describe the model. Coefficient trajectories are smooth and models give a smooth, continuous trends of the spectrum and MF changes. Such smooth trends are needed if we wish to observe the signal variation over time as the amount of spectrum or MF changes. If the question of signal dynamics is in which periods the changes in the frequency content of SEMG are more and when they are less evident we suggest to take into account the whole spectrum instead of its single variable (as mean frequency). Measures, based on TV ARMA distances (as proposed in Eq. and 4) are more reliable than observing the second derivative of MF, which is very sensitive to minor variations of the MF trend. In both cases a smooth estimation of time-varying spectrum as obtained from the coefficient decomposition method is advantageous to the sliding window estimation. This hold also if one is interested in SEMG low-frequency component. But for only obtaining the evolution of the mean frequency sliding window approach is sufficient.

References

[1] J. Basmajian and C. J. De Luca. *Muscles Alive, 5th ed.*, Williams and Wilkins, Baltimore, 1985.

[2] M. Basseville, “Distance measures for signal processing and pattern recognition”, *Signal Process.*, Vol. 18, 1989, pp. 349-369

[3] J. Duchęne, F. Goubel, "Surface Electromyogram during Voluntary Contraction: Processing Tools and Relation to Physiological Events", *Critical Reviews in Biomedical Engineering*, CRC Press, Volume 21, Issue 4, 1993, pp. 313-397

[4] R. Merletti, U. Dimanico, "Linear Electrode Array for Surface EMG", In *Proceedings of the 14th International Congress of EEG and Clinical Neurophysiology*, August 24-30, Florence, Italy.

[5] Y. Grenier, "Time-Dependent ARMA Modeling of Nonstationary Signals", *IEEE Transactions on Acoustics, Speech and Signal Processing*, Vol. ASSP-31, No. 4, August 1983

Medical Informatics Europe '99
P. Kokol et al. (Eds.)
IOS Press, 1999

Monte Carlo Simulation of the Radiographic Imaging Procedure for Electronically Designed Phantoms

D. Lazos, Z. Kolitsi and N. Pallikarakis
Medical Physics Department, School of Medicine, University of Patras, 265 00 Patras, Greece

Abstract. This paper presents a software simulation package of the entire X-ray projection radiography process including beam generation, absorber structure and composition, irradiation set up, radiation transport through the absorbing medium and image formation. This software tool is an augmented version of a previously presented system with expanded range of application by the implementation of Monte Carlo approach for the simulation of the radiation interaction at the absorber and the detector. Phantoms are created as composite objects from geometrical or voxelized primitives and can be subjected to simulated irradiation process. The acquired projection images represent the two dimensional spatial distribution of the energy absorbed in the detector and are formed at any geometry, taking into account energy spectrum, beam geometry and detector response.

1. Introduction

Computer simulation has proven a particularly useful and efficient research tool, in the study of image quality parameters in Diagnostic Radiology. Software phantoms, used in association with radiography simulation programs, allow the flexibility in defining and modifying their features in order to fit the specific requirements of each application.

The Monte Carlo method [1] is well established for the study of imaging systems in diagnostic radiology. It has been extensively used to study contrast, noise, absorbed dose and grid performance [2-4]. The method simulates the radiation-matter interaction by generating a large number of randomly selected particle paths, on the basis of the relevant theoretical framework.

This paper refers to the development and the implementation of a software application, that is used to create electronic phantoms and to subsequently subject them to a Monte Carlo simulated imaging procedure, in order to produce radiographic projection images. The software is an extension of our previous program [5], where the imaging procedure was analytically simulated for the primary component. The scatter component, on the other hand, can only be simulated by Monte Carlo methods, since none of the proposed analytical approaches can effectively calculate multiple scatter. Projection images represent the two dimensional intensity distribution of the radiation reaching or absorbed by the detector, and they are produced at selectable energy spectrum, irradiation geometry, parameters of antiscatter grid and detector response.

2. Description of the system

The program is comprised of two modules: the electronic phantom design and the radiographic image simulator module. The phantom modeling is based on constructed solid geometry [6]. Electronic phantoms are composed by geometrical or voxelized primitives, combined with the set operations union, intersection and difference, to build more complex objects. The geometrical primitives are user defined elementary geometrical objects, such as ellipsoids, cylinders, cuboids, pyramids, cones and wedges, with selectable composition, location and orientation [5]. Geometrical primitives of particular shape can be reconstructed by the contours of their sections with a sequence of parallel planes. The use of primitives of this type, however in Monte Carlo applications increases dramatically the computational times, since their surface representation by a large numbers of triangles results in large computational times in ray tracing calculations. In voxelized primitives, the volume of interest is divided into voxels and was represented by a three dimensional matrix carrying the information of the content of each voxel. The antiscatter grid is considered as a specific type of object and can be set to any position and orientation. It is modeled as a cuboid containing lead strips and interspace material, between two protective covers. Phantoms are displayed in three dimensions in the wire-frame form, with selectable viewing angle.

The geometric model, used, comprises the point-like X-ray source, the phantom, the antiscatter grid and the detector. Photon transport is simulated by tracing paths of photons emitted from the X-ray source, through the phantom, the grid and the detector.

The X-ray spectra are either calculated by a semiempirical model [7], for selectable values of the parameters of the X-ray generator, or taken from tabulated data [8]. The semi-empirical model computes spectra taking into account the selected tube voltages (kVp), target angle, inherent and added filtration. Both bremsstrahlung and characteristic x-rays are included. Off-axis spectra can also be calculated. The initial photon energy is calculated by inverse sampling of the source spectrum.

The program follows the histories of single photons emitted from the x-ray source as they pass through the phantom, the antiscatter grid and the detector. Photons are followed until they escape from the region of interest, or their energy drops below predefined cut-off energy. The distance between two successive interactions is sampled based on the relevant attenuation cross-sections, accounting for the different media, along the photon path. Three possible interactions are simulated, on the basis of Monte Carlo approach, according to their probabilities for the given material and energy: Photoelectric absorption, Compton scattering and Rayleigh (coherent) scattering. When photoelectric effect is chosen to occur, the photon history ends. Fluorescence photons are further traced for high atomic number materials, if the photon energy is higher than 10keV. In Compton scattering the binding effect of the electrons is taken into account. Modeling of Rayleigh scattering is based on measured values [9] of molecular form factors, instead of the ones calculated theoretically. The scattering angle in both scattering interactions, is selected by random sampling according to their differential cross-sections. Photon transport through antiscatter grids is also simulated by Monte Carlo method. Ray tracing is simplified since strips are spaced at equal intervals. Scattered or fluorescent photons of the grid are further traced. The detector is simulated either by a plate of selected dimensions and composition, that records the absorbed energy on a event by event basis, or by recording all radiation passing through a plane, positioned at the detector surface. Images are produced in 'row' format.

The Monte Carlo simulation program was developed in programming language "Borland C" and the interface in "Visual Basic". The application run on a Pentium II PC, with 64Mb RAM, working at 233MHz, under the Windows 98 platform. The program uses 100Kb of memory including code and explanatory comments. The library of photon interaction cross-sections and tabulated X-ray spectra requires 150Kb of disc space. The CPU-time per run depends strongly on the operating parameters and the required statistical precision. For a 3% fluctuation of the energy absorbed in the detector, and a 20cm thick phantom, a typical run time is 10 hours.

3. System Verification

A direct comparison of a Monte Carlo image, with the one obtained by a radiographic imaging system, cannot verify the entire accuracy of the program, since errors in a real image are significantly larger than typical errors in Monte Carlo method. For that reason the verification was attempted by comparisons with theoretical calculations (were the last are possible), separately for the primary and the scattered component of the image. The primary component calculations are verified by comparison between a Monte Carlo primary image of a test phantom and the corresponding one, produced by analytical calculations [5]. The test phantom, used for this purpose, is consisted of a cuboid of water containing two aluminum objects. A 50keV monoenergetic beam was simulated. Figures 1a shows the image of primary radiation obtained using the Monte Carlo method, while figure 1b shows the Monte Carlo and analytical gray scale profiles, of a vertical line of the image, passing through both objects. There is a good agreement between the profiles of the two images. The average difference between Monte Carlo and analytical values is of the order of 0.5%, for 120000 photons/pixel. For the verification of the scatter calculations, we compared the Monte Carlo derived scatter point-spread-functions (PSF) of a layer of water of various thicknesses, with the corresponding analytical ones. The comparison refers to the first order scatter. The analytical PSFs are derived by the model of Boone and Seibert [10], modified to include coherent scattering and binding effects in Compton scattering. Figure 2 shows both PSFs for a water layer, 10cm thick, at energy 50keV, with an air-gap 2cm.

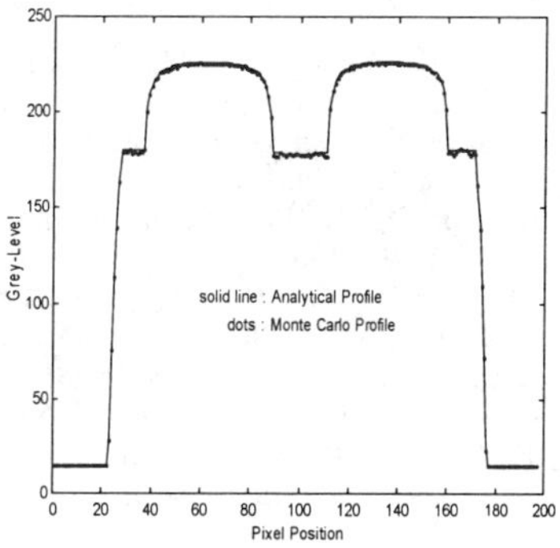

Figure 1. (a) Monte Carlo image of the primary radiation of the test phantom and (b) Monte Carlo and analytical profiles of a vertical line of the image.

4. Conclusions

This implementation has been successfully verified, as there is a good agreement between the Monte Carlo results and the theoretical expectations. As in all Monte Carlo implementations, the computation times are generally large, depending strongly on the operating parameters and the required statistical precision. A typical run time of this program is in the order of few tens of hours. A significant reduction of the computation

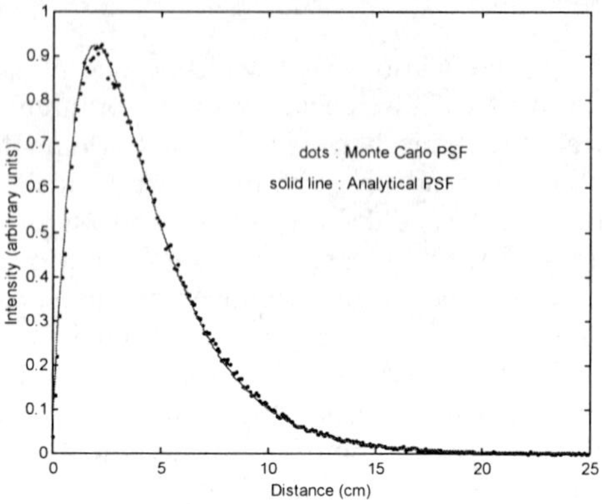

Figure 2. Monte Carlo and analytically derived PSFs.

time, to approximately one half, can be achieved by separately calculating the primary component of the image by fast and accurate analytical method [5].

References

[1] Andreo P, 1991, Monte Carlo techniques in medical radiation physics, *Phys. Med. Biol.* **36** 861-920.

[2] Sandborg M, Christoffersson J-O, Carlsson GA, Almen T and Dance DR, 1995, The physical performance of different x-ray contrast agents: calculations using a Monte Carlo code of the imaging chain, *Phys.Med.Biol.* **40**, 1209-1224

[3] Chan H P and Doi K, 1984, Radiation dose in diagnostic radiology: Monte Carlo simulation studies, *Med. Phys.* **11**, 480-490.

[4] Dance D R and Day G J 1983 The computation of scatter in mammography by Monte Carlo methods, *Phys. Med. Biol.* **29**, 237-247

[5] Lazos D, Kolitsi Z, Pallikarakis N, A software data generator for radiographic imaging investigations, *paper submitted to IEEE Trans. Biomed. Inform. Techn.*

[6] Wang H, Jaczszak RJ and Coleman RE, 1992, Solid geometry based object model for Monte Carlo simulated emission and transmission tomographic imaging systems, IEEE Trans, Med. Imaging **MI-11** 361-372.

[7] Tucker D M, Barnes G T, Chakraborty D P,1991, Semiempirical model for generating tungsten target x-ray spectra. *Med. Phys.* **18** 211-218

[8] Birch R, Marshall M and Ardran G M Catalog of spectral data for diagnostic X-rays. *The Hospital Physicists' Association, London.*

[9] Peplow E D and Verghese K, 1998, Measured molecular coherent scattering form factors of animal tissues, plastics and human breast tissue. *Phys. Med. Biol.* **43** 2431-2452.

[10] Boone J and Seibert A, 1988, An analytical model of scattered radiation distribution in diagnostic radiology *Med. Phys.* **15** 721-25.

Computed Tomography Image Analyzer: Segmentation Applying Active Contour Models - "Snakes"

Ružica MAKSIMOVIČ, Srdjan STANKOVIČ[1], Dragorad MILOVANOVIČ[1], Jelena MARINKOVIČ[2], Branislav GOLDNER, Miloš JANIČIJEVIČ, Petar M. SEFEROVIČ
Institute of Radiology, Koste Todorovica 8, Dept. II
[1]Faculty of Electrical Engineering, University of Belgrade,
[2]Institute of Social Medicine, Statistics and Health Research
Belgrade, Yugoslavia
E-mail: ruzica@EUnet.yu

Abstract. Many diagnostic and therapeutic procedures depend on medical images. In order to overcome imperfections of obtained images which are due to acquisition process and to obtain new information from available images, many techniques have been developed. In this study relatively new method of image segmentation, active contour model - "snakes" was applied in analyzing computed tomography (CT) images in patients with acute head trauma. Using this method, lesion to brain (LBR) and ventricle to brain ratio (VBR) were obtained accurately. Quantitative variable LBR, is significantly higher in patients with other pathologic CT findings and who do not survive during hospitalization. Thus, by applying segmentation "snakes" model it is possible to extract maximum information from available CT scans. These variables could be basis for medical decision making in patients with acute head trauma.

1. Introduction

Imaging techniques occupy a growing part of the practice of medicine and may intervene in the diagnostic, prognostic, or therapeutic decision making processes. Many procedures are based on image analysis in order to provide diagnosis and optimal therapy approach like in patients with acute head trauma. Patients with acute head trauma are seen in Emergency Department in epidemic dimension in developed countries. Despite introdusing new imaging techniqes in evaluation of patients with acute head trauma, computed tomography (CT) is the first diagnostic procedure in these patients [1]. Once images have been captured and corrected for distortions due to the acquisition process, various techniques for further image analysis could be applied [2]. One method that has been increasingly used for image segmentation is active contour models "snakes" [3]. Therefore, the aim of the study was to elucidate the significance of new quantitative parameters, obtained by active contour models "snakes" in clinical decision making in patients with acute head trauma.

2. Patients and methods

The study included patients with acute head trauma who were admitted to the Emergency Department in the six month period. In all patients 9 clinical variables, two variables from X-ray, and 18 characteristics from the first CT scans were recorded. Furthermore, two variables were obtained by analyzing CT images. In this study, digital - image analysis includes preprocessing phase which eliminates imperfections related to the image generation system and reduce noise in order to improve visibility of certain structures [3].

In the segmentation phase, elements of the image were separated. Using "snakes" model all elements of the image could be isolated but it is not possible to distinguish important information. This is the reason that physician set the control points which represent an initial estimation of the "snakes" model. It is followed by optimization techniques so as to improve the initial assessment.

"Snakes" could be considered as large scale interconnected dynamic systems whose equlibria correspond to the edges between the image areas with different characteristics. Advantages of active contour models over other techniques are that extraction and segmentation phase are in one process. The total energy amount of the contour is a sum of inner energy (E_{int}) that is determined by behavior of the contour (binding, stretching) and external energy (E_{ext}), that represents the influence of surrounding pixels on the contour:

$$E_{SNAKE}^{functional} = \int \{E_{\text{int}}(\mathbf{v}) + E_{ext}(\mathbf{v})\} ds = \sum_{i=1}^{N} \{E_i^{\text{int}} + E_i^{ext}\} \qquad [4]$$

In stationary state, if the overall procedure converges, i.e. if a system as a whole is stable, a contour represents the approximation of an edge, the border between two regions. Having in mind the properties of bio-medical images, this method represents a solution which is not possible to reach via classical methods of local edge detection, that do not have a property of continuity preservation and contour incompleteness. "Snakes" can be permanently mobile and can adjust to the contours of an object, that automatically enables us to observe its permanently functioning. When the best edge between two regions is achieved the motion of "snakes" model is completed. Existing of a "snake" at a given moment means unambiguously visualization of edges of an image, but also offers a possibility for calculating a quantitative indicators like volume, moving of center of mass etc. The simplest discrete active contour can be described as a string of rectilinear segments connected in a chain, whose location is defined by coordinates of N nodes (contact points of segments of mass m_i) [5]. The eigenproperties, the contour has to outperform are described by forces that act in nodes (compression force α_i, stretch resistance β_i and outer force f_i). Differential equation of a snake-model is:

$$m_i \ddot{x}_i + \gamma_i \dot{x}_i + \alpha_i + \beta_i = f_i \qquad [6]$$

The resulting force in the k-th node, determine location of a node in the next iteration. Iterative procedure is terminated when the resulting forces in all nodes became zero. The model is implemented in a software IMAGEX.C programmed in language MS Visual C++. This computer program is developed at the Faculty of Electrical Engineering, University of Belgrade [6]. For the purpose of digital image analysis, all CT films were scanned using drum scanner Hell DC320 in resolution 48 lines/centimeter as blue channel. This database was stored on CD-ROM as TIFF files (256 levels grey scale).

In CT images control points were set between ventricles and brain, lesion and brain (Figure 1a) and brain and endocranium (Figure 1b). This model was especially usefull in patienst with traumatic lesion with perifocal oedema without distinctive edge between two regions. Based on this model, two new variables were obtained. One is lesion to brain ratio which represents the volume of traumatic lesion in realtion to the volume of braine

(LBR) while the other represents the pressure of cerebral oedema to ventricles - ventricle to brain ratio (VBR).

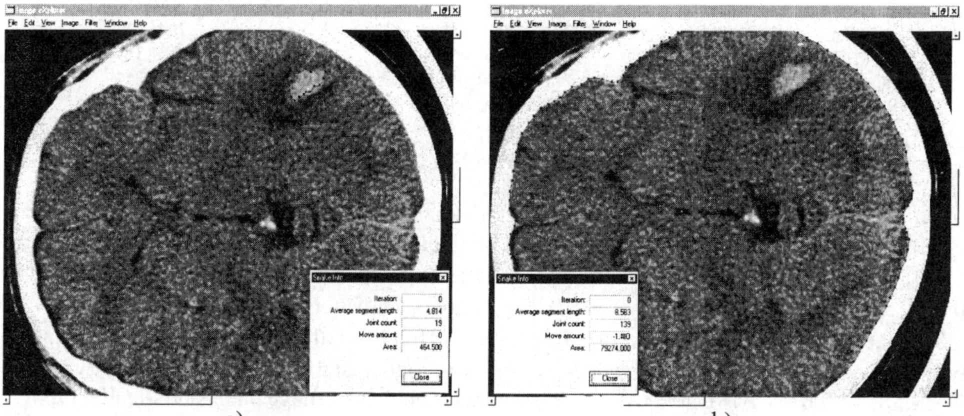

a) b)

Figure 1. Estimation of pixels number within the "snakes" model a) lesion b) endocranium on CT image for assessment LTB and VTB.

3. Results

Our study group consisted of 215 patients [mean age 42.4±23.5 years, 138/215 (64.2%) males]. On admission in each patient Glasgow Coma Score (GCS) was assessed for evaluation the level of consciousness as well as for the state of responsiveness. According to this score, most of the patients in this study had minor head injury [GCS >13, 117 (54.4%)], with moderate had injury GCS <8, was 27 (12.6%) pts, while the least number was patients with sever head injury [GCS<8, 71 (33.0%)]. During hospitalisation 72 (33.5%) died.

Table 1. Correlation clinical variables, VTB, and LTB

Clinical variable	VTB	LTB
Glasgow Coma Score	0.110	-0.457**
Intrahospital outcome	-0.062	0.515**

VTB - ventricle tobrain ratio, LTB - lesion to brain ratio, ** - p<0.01

VTB did not correlation with GCS and intrahospital outcome while LTB showed high statistical significant relationship, r=-0.457 and r=0.515, respectively (table 1). Patients with severe had injury had larger LTB (0.038±0.033) than patients with moderate (0.024±0.027) and mild head injury (0.003±0.009), F=53.12, p<0.01. Furthermore, patients who died during hospitalisation in Emergency Department had greater value of LTV (0.042 ±0.034) than those who survived (0.005±0.011), t=-11.38, p>0.01.

VTB was associated with cerebral edema, r=-0.273, table 2. Patients without cerebral edema had significantly higher value o VTB 0.027±0.011, then patients with local edema 0.025±0.016 or patients with diffuse cerebral edema 0.017±0.018, F=9.34, p<0.01.

Table 2. Correlation radiological variables, LTB, and VTB

Radiological variables	VTB	LTB
Fracture	-0.174	0.101
Pneumatocephalus	-0.124	0.071
Cerebral oedema	-0.273**	0.469**
Volume of basal cisterns	-0.026	0.383**
Subarachnoidal hemorrhage	-0.114	0.442**
Axonal lesion	-0.086	0.134*
VTB	-	-0.002

VTB - ventricle tobrain ratio, LTB - lesion to brain ratio, * - p<0.05, ** - p<0.01

With respect to LTB, there was statistical significant correlation with cerebral oedema, volume of basal cisterns, subarachnoidal hemorrhage, axonal lesion (r=0.469, r=0.383, r=0.442, r=0.134, respectively). In patients without oedema (0.001±0.005 0.021± 0.029 0.028±0.033 (F=31.91, p<0.01. In patients with normal basal cisterns LTB was 0.005±0.016, in those with collapsed it was 0.027±0.037 while in patients with obliterated basal cisterns LTB was 0.031±0.033, which was highly statistical significant difference, F=24.56, p<0.01. Also, patients with subarachnoid hemorrhage had statistically higher value of LTB 0.037±0.033 then those without hemorrhage, t=8,49, p<0.01. The same is true with patients with axonal lesion which had higher value of LTB 0.033±0.041 then patients without axonal lesion 0.016±0.025, t=-2.87, p<0.01.

4. Discussion

Most information we receive from images of object and processes they are involved in as well as by measuring their characteristics. Images could represent not only structure but also functional properties which are not accessible with other methods. In order to optimize object of interes parameters, numerous thechniques for acquisition and analyzing images have been developed in recent years [7].

Obtained images are imperfect due to acquisition process itself so that only certain characteristics could be seen, there is nonlinear distortion, limited spatial resolution and artifacts depending on the image acquisition process. Improvement of images could be achieved using different method of digital image analysis. Many different techniques for digital image processing and analysis are available, but the choice is to a large extent independent of the image formation process [8]. This process involves series of procedures in which the results of the proceeding step depends on the previous as well as on the operator□s knowledge and experience. In preprocessing phase using various techniques visibility of certain anatomical structures is improved. Next step in image analysis is identification region of interest or segmentation. Segmentation methods for medical images could be classified as regional and contour. Regional methods could be applied in analyzing images with significant level of noise. e.g. ultrasound images, while contour methods are more precise and they are used in analyzing images of high quality and resolution like CT [9]. Therefore, in this study active contour method - "snakes" model, was applied. Using this method precise, objective and quantitative assessment of volume of traumatic lesion and ventricles was performed.

Evaluation of CT images and other dynamic medical images arises many questions with no definite answers. Assessment of human expert will be always of utmost importance in process of medical decision making but with great help of contemporary method of digital image analysis. Using active contour models "snakes" it is possible to extract maximum information from CT images and which represent quantitative assessment of patients with acute head trauma. Variables obtained using this method were found to be significant predictors of intrahospital outcome and are therefore, important components in clinical decision making [10].

The future of digital image analysis is in developing system which will enable transfer images to homes end educational centres. In this way it would be possible to simulate and have an direct insight in process of interest which is especially important in interventional procedure, and to include in discussion collaborative groups from different sites [11]. Most of these activites is possible in the time being with introduction of personal computers which could be used for archieving, automatic analysis and storage of data base, and facilitate information management and informatin exhange between institutions.

5. Conclusion

Digital medical imaging analysis is ever increasing area in informatics which enable obtaining additional information on clinical status of patients. Digitizing medical images offer possibilities to construct an image from measurements, store and retrieve images, present images, improve image quality by image processing, and obtain new quantitative information. Using active contours models "snakes" two new image varibles were acquired, LTB and VTB which obtain quantitative and objective information on traumatic lesion and intracranial pressure respectively. LTB is a good indicator of clinical status in patients with acute head trauma and correlated with other pathologic CT findings. There was no statistical significant correlation with VTB (r=-0.002). Applying new method of image analysis, active contour model - "snakes" it is possible to assess intrahospital outcome in patients with acute head trauma. These information could have influence on optimizing consequente diagnostic and therapeutic procedure in these patients.

References

[1] C.B. Grossman, Cranial and intracranial injuries. In: C.B. Grossman (ed.), Magnetic resonance imaging and computed tomography of the head and spine. Williams and Wilkins, Baltimore, 1996, pp. 319-347.

[2] P. Degault, M. Fieschi, Medical imaging systems. In: J. K. Hannah, J.M. Ball (eds.), Introduction to clinical informatics, Springer Verlag, Berlin, 1997, pp. 139-153.

[3] S. Stankovic, D. Milovanovic, Contemporary methods in digital analysis of signals in medical diagnosis. *Informatics in medicine and farmacy* (1997) 31-36.

[4] L.D. Cohen, Note on active contour models and balloons. *CVGIP: Image understanding* **53**: (1991) 211-218.

[5] A. Vuckovic, D. Milovanovic, S. Stankovic, Nonlinear contrast enhancement of medical diagnostic images using Discrete Wavelet Transform. *ETRAN* (1997) 123-126.

[6] A. Vuckovic, S. Stankovic, D. Milovanovic, Wavelet neural networks. *TELFLOR* (1997), 424-427.

[7] R.K. Castleman, Images and digital processing. In: R.K. Castleman (ed.), Digital image processing. Prentice Hall, Englewood Cliffs, New Jersey 1979; pp. 1-13.

[8] N.R. Beck, Overview of imaging science, *Proc Natl Acad Sci* (1993) 974-979.

[9] M. Kass, A. Witkin, D. Terzopolous, Snakes: active contour models. *Int J Computer Vision* **1** (1988) 321-331.

[10] R. Maksimovic, D. Milovanovic, S. Stankovic, J. Marinkovic, B. Goldner, M. Janicijevic, Computed tomography image segmentation and artificial neural networks in clinical prognosis. *14th Biennial International Conference Biosignal 98; Proceedings* (1998) 45-47.

[11] D. Milovanovic, E. Jovanov, Z. Tomic, Image compression techniques for medical diagnostic imaging system. *YU INFO-TECH* (1995) 49-51.

Medical Informatics Europe '99
P. Kokol et al. (Eds.)
IOS Press, 1999

A new way for the analysis of the exocytosis

J.L. Sánchez, M.A. Brioso, F. Segura* and R. Borges*
*Depts. Física Fundamental y Experimental and * Medicina Física y Farmacología.*
Universidad de La Laguna. Tenerife. Spain

Abstract. Exocytosis is the most common way for cells to secrete substances. This is a wide distributed phenomenon that involves all cell types and all animal species from yeast to human. Catecholamine (CA) release from adrenal chromaffin cells occurs by the exocytosis of secretory vesicles also called chromaffin granules. Individual secretory events can be easily monitored by the use of carbon fibers encased in glass microelectrodes. Catecholamines oxidized at the electrode tip produce a transient electrical current wave called secretory spike. The typical secretory spike consists in a sharp elevation of current followed by a rapid exponential decrease to the basal level. A 35-50% of the spikes showed a pre-spike wave called "foot" which represents the CA release through the fusion pore. The time course of secretory spikes observed is altered by extracellular phenomena's like diffusion. It has been suggested that amperometric spikes can be described by the convolution of a Gaussian with a decreasing exponential. The exponential function is partially governed by the diffusion of the secreted substances towards the electrode. In this article a method to deconvolve both functions is proposed. This mathematical approach allows the observation of the original secretory profile -the Gaussian- without the distortion caused by the diffusional broadening of catecholamines.

1. Introduction

Many hormones and neurotransmitters are secreted by exocytosis. Catecholamines, like adrenaline, are stored in secretory vesicles until the moment of secretion to prevent their lysis by intracellular enzymes. In the chromaffin cell these vesicles are the most abundant organelle (15,000-25,000 vesicles/cell (1). Catecholamines together with other secretable substances are stored in very high concentrations within chromaffin granules. The concentration of soluble products has been estimated as high as 500-800 mM of CA, 130 mM of ATP and 80 mM of calcium. In addition, important concentrations of ascorbic acid, peptides or other nucleotides have been quantified (2). These enormous amounts largely exceed the osmotic equilibrium and reveal complex store mechanisms (3).

The use of amperometric techniques (4) allows the study of the exocytosis dynamics but they could also reveal direct information about how CA are stored and what the molecular mechanisms implicated in it storage are. Working with amperometric and voltametric techniques Wightman proposed that secretory spikes, observed upon the stimulation of chromaffin cells, can be mathematically simulated using a convolution of a Gaussian (with variance "σ") with a decreasing exponential (with time constant "τ") (5). These equations were obtained from the mathematical approach used in the sixties to fit gas chromatography peaks. The use of deconvolution not only allows the mathematical modeling of spikes but it could also reveal physiological processes masked by diffusional broadening. This method has been used to establish the role of the intragranular matrix in the store and release of adrenaline (5). In addition, this approach has been used to resolve complex spikes resulted from the coincidence of two or more secretory events.

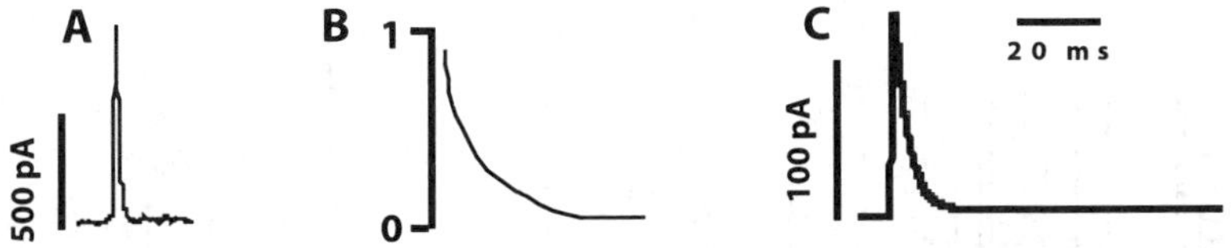

Figure 1: **Convolution of a Gaussian with a decreasing exponential.** Traces **A** and **B** show a computer-generated Gaussian and a decreasing exponential curves respectively. The convolved curve is shown on the trace **C**.

2. Materials and methods

Cell culture. Bovine adrenal medullar cells enriched in adrenaline using a single-step Urografin® gradient were prepared as previously described (6). Cells were planted in 12 mm-diameter glass coverslips placed in a 24 well plate at a density of 5 x 10^5 cells/well. Cells were incubated at 37°C in a 5% CO_2 environment at saturated humidity and were used within 1 and 4 days of culture. Experiments were carried out at room temperature (23° C).

Electrochemical detection of CA. Carbon fiber electrodes were prepared as described by Kawagoe et al (7) using 5-µm radius carbon fibers. Glass coverslips with adhering adrenal cells were bathed in Krebs-HEPES buffer solution (pH 7.35) and were placed in a perfusion chamber positioned on the stage of an inverted microscope. Amperometric measurements were performed with the carbon fiber microelectrode gently touching the cell membrane. Cells release was stimulated by pressure ejection of 5 mM Ba^{2+} for 5 s from a micropipette placed 25-30 µm away from the cell.

Data acquisition. Amperometric signals were low-pass filtered at 400 or 1000 Hz (Bessel filter), sampled at 4 kHz and recorded on the hard drive of a Power Macintosh G3 using a locally written program on LabVIEW (National Inst. Austin, TX, USA). Exocytotic events were digitally filtered, located and analyzed with locally written macros for IGOR (Wavemetrics Inc, Lake Oswego, OR, USA) and the areas of individual current spikes (Q), their amplitudes (I_{max}), and their widths at half-height ($t_{1/2}$) were determined as described previously (8). For evaluation of Q changes the quantity $Q^{1/3}$, which has a Gaussian distribution, was computed for each spike (5), (see below).

Materials. The culture medium, enzymes and drugs used were purchased from Sigma-Aldrich Co. (Madrid, Spain). Salts used were reagent-grade.

3. Results and discussion

Using amperometric techniques the exocytotic pathway can only be followed once CA start to diffuse towards the electrode surface. Although it is not clear what the physiological meaning of the functions resolved by deconvolution of secretory spikes it is known that diffusion of particles in a liquid media will follow an exponential decay. In this way a realistic assumption is to consider that the exponential term includes effects like diffusion or dispersion while the Gaussian could represent the CA flow on the pore before diffusion processes can take place. The whole system can hence be described as two systems in cascade.

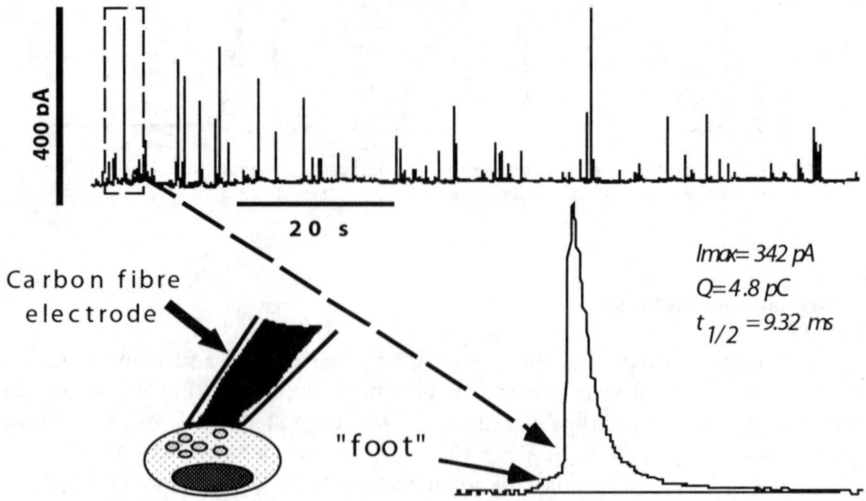

Figure 2. Amperometric recording of secretion from a single bovine chromaffin cell. Upper trace shows typical secretory spikes obtained upon stimulation with 5 mM $BaCl_2$. A detail of one spike is shown on the lower right trace. A glass encapsulating carbon fiber electrode is used as a sensor for CA, a scheme of the electrode size and position compared to the cell is shown.

Even when the electrode is touching the cell -there is a liquid limit layer- this layer is quantitatively large compared with granule diameter (≈ 100-300 nm). Products emitted must cross such limit layer before reaching the carbon fiber electrode. Hence, diffusion and dispersion are expected to occur. The figure 3 shows a cascade of two systems, where the first one produces the emission of CA and the second acts with a diminishing exponential function over it. It is not possible to predict the moment when a given granule exocytosis will occur, so no "input" for the first system can be modeled. Its output is the emission of CA through the fusion pore. Assuming that the liberated CA are the input of a system (whose impulse response is a diminishing exponential) then the output represents the actual measures (assuming the electrode has no effect over the measure). However, some difficulties can be found:

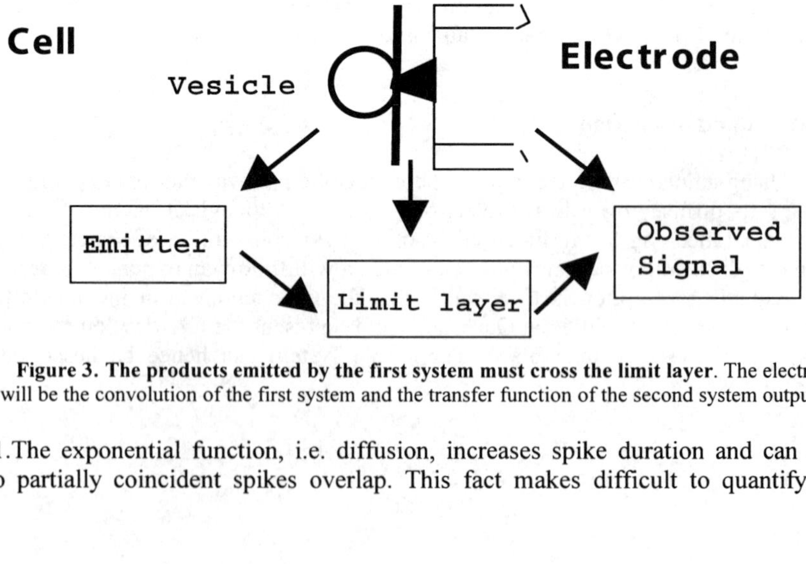

Figure 3. The products emitted by the first system must cross the limit layer. The electrode input will be the convolution of the first system and the transfer function of the second system outputs.

1.The exponential function, i.e. diffusion, increases spike duration and can cause that two partially coincident spikes overlap. This fact makes difficult to quantify each spike.

2. Due to the electronic noise, the beginning and end of small spikes are difficult to recognize. That can produce errors in the estimation of the spike area. In addition, subjective estimations of the beginning and the end can vary from one observer to another.

3.Although the electrode should not introduce artifacts in the measure, quantification of the real concentration of CA from the amperometric traces are under-estimated. However, the time-course and the dynamics of the secretory event are reliable.

Figure 2 shows a trace obtained after the stimulation of a chromaffin cell. Each secretory event can be temporary resolved as secretory spikes. This figure also shows the parameters directly obtained from spikes. Imax, indicates the concentration of CA at electrode tip and is expressed in pA; Q, is the area under the curve and indicates the amount of CA released expressed in pC. $t_{1/2}$, reflects the duration of the secretory event and is expressed in ms. As mentioned above, spike traces are disturbed by diffusion. Because diffusion can be modeled by a decreasing exponential, it is plausible that a wave resulting from the subtraction of the exponential component could reflect what is the real time-course of exocytosis at the cell membrane level. If this assumption were correct, the areas under curve (i.e. Q) of the original and the deconvolved spikes should be similar. Figure 4 shows an original and its deconvolved spike. As shown, the Imax obtained from the deconvolved spike is far larger than the original, whereas the opposite can be observed in $t_{1/2}$. These differences in the time courses can be explained because of the catecholamine concentration being larger at the fusion place and it should take place in a shorter time than that observed at the electrode surface. If the value of τ and the derivative of the output signal is estimated, the input value x(t) can be calculated. Such input represents the flow before being affected by the exponential process. The derivative from the observed wave is easy to obtain by numerical process. Due to the large variations in size and duration of a given population of spikes (Figure 2) it is not possible to calculate a fixed value of τ that can be extrapolated to the whole spike population. For this reason τ has to be estimated for each spike.

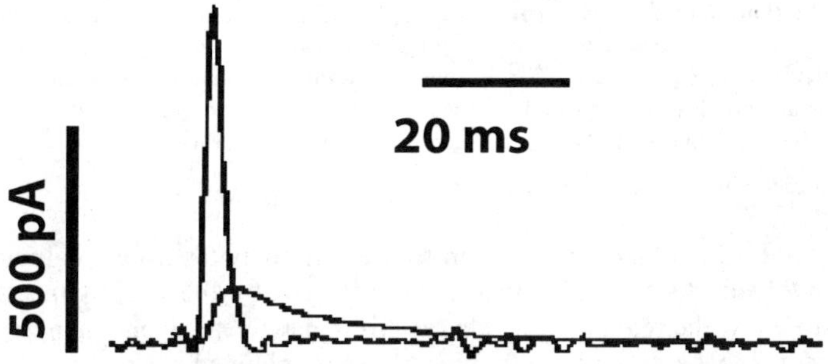

Figure 4. The effect of deconvolution on the spike shape. Traces show a secretory spike before deconvolution (lower and wider) and after deconvolution (higher and sharper). However, the areas calculated from both curves are not modified by the deconvolution process.

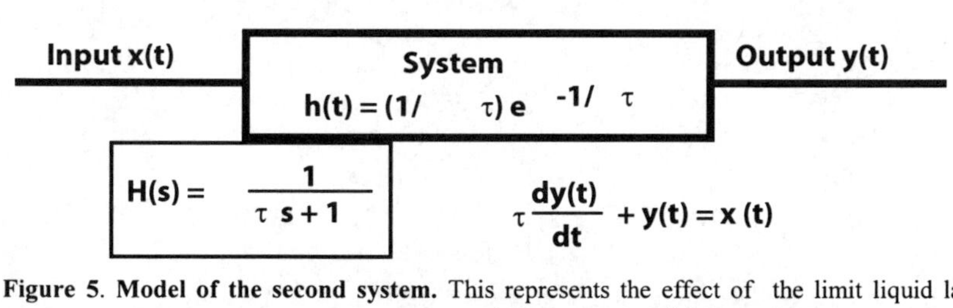

Figure 5. Model of the second system. This represents the effect of the limit liquid layer. The transfer function for a system which impulse response is defined as $1/t\ e^{-1/t}$ is given by:

Transfer function and differential equation of the exponential system.

In Control Theory, it is a well-known fact that the crossing of the initial slope of an decreasein exponential with the axis will give an estimation of the time constant. However, spike decay does not follow a pure exponential but it is mixed with a Gaussian. It can be shown that the if the line which fits the curve with maximum slope from the point τ= B is selected, the cross of this line with the axis will give an estimation of t+s, as can be observed in the next figure. An estimator of σ is the distance between the point at which the maximum of the peak occurs and the zero crossing of the 2nd derivative of y(t) to the right of the peak. So, the value of t can still be known. Moreover, the influence of the exponential can be eliminated in order to keep only with the term corresponding to the Gaussian as can be observed in the figure 6.

Behavior of the estimator over simulated peaks. To check the goodness of this method a number of simulated spikes has been introduced with pre-established σ and τ. In addition, the method has been applied to deconvolve both functions. In this example errors can be observed in the estimation are of the order of 5% and they are not bigger than 10% usually.

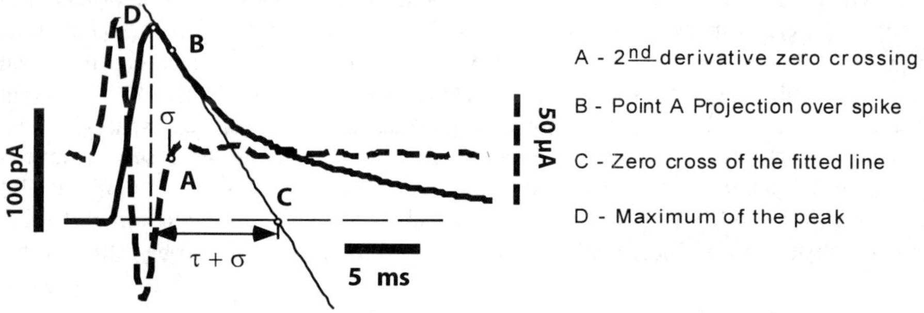

Figure 6. Method for estimating τ from the spike. The first step is to determine where the maximum of the peak is located (**D**). Then the crossing by zero of the second derivative to the right of this point is used to determine two parameters: i) σ is estimated as the distance between the abscissa of the maximum of the peak and point **A**. ii) $\tau+\sigma$ can be estimated as the distance between the maximum of the peak and the crossing of the fitted line with the axis **C** (horizontal dashed line). As we know σ, then τ can be obtained. σ^2 will represent the variance of the Gaussian.

Resolving a double peak. Traces from figure 7 show two partially coincident peaks after being deconvolved. As the peak area is not affected by the deconvolution process, now we are able to know the real area -i.e. charge- from each peak even when they overlaps in the original traces. Most authors have to reject those overlapped peaks.

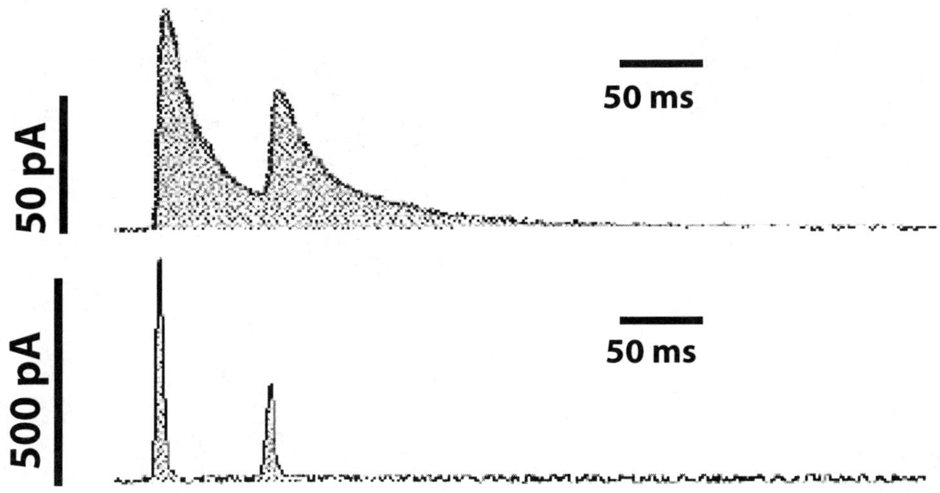

Figure 7. Deconvolution can resolve double peaks. Two partially coincident secretory events generate a double peak wave where individual areas cannot be calculate (upper trace). After deconvolution both secretory spikes can be completely separated and they do not overlap one onto the other.

4. Concluded remarks

The method presented here is intended for resolving a number of problems derived from the analysis of exocytotic phenomenon, using amperometric techniques. The use of this mathematical approach allows the partial removal of the disturbances due to the diffusion of secreted CA towards the working electrode. This procedure also permits a more objective way to establish the points where the spike starts and ends. In addition, it provides a good tool to resolve coincident secretory spikes.

Acknowledgments. Supported by a grant from DGICYT (No. PB97-1483). We are grateful to Dr. López de Vergara for his help in the preparation of this manuscript.

References

[1] H. Winkler Occurrence and mechanisms of exocytosis in adrenal medulla and sympathetic nerve. in Handbook of Experimental Pharmacology, 90/I. U. Trendelenburg and N. Weiner Eds. Springer-Verlag, Berlin. pp 44-118 (1988) .
[2] H. Winkler and EW. Westhead,The molecular organization of adrenal chromaffin granules. *Neuroscience.* **5** (1980) 1803-1823.
[3] R. Borges *et al.*,Effect of osmotic pressure on vesicular secretion from bovine adrenal chromaffin cells. *J. Biol. Chem.* **272** (1997) 8325-8331.
[4] DJ. Leszczyszyn *et al.*, Nicotinic-receptor mediated catecholamine secretion from individual chromaffin cell: chemical evidence of exocytosis. *J. Biol. Chem.* **265** (1990) 14736-14737.
[5] TJ. Schroeder *et al.*, Temporally resolved, independent stages of individual exocytotic secretion events. *Biophys. J.* **70** (1996) 1061-1068.
[6] MA. Moro *et al.*, Separation and culture of living adrenaline containing and noradrenaline-containing cells from bovine adrenal medullae. *Anal. Biochem.* 185, (1990) 243-248.
[7] KT. Kawagoe *et al.*, Principles of voltametry and microelectrode surface states. *J. Neurosci. Meth.* **48** (1993) 225-240.
[8] TJ. Schroeder *et al.*, Analysis of diffusional broadening of vesicular packets of catecholamines released from biological cells during exocytosis. *Anal. Chem.* **68** (1992) 3180-3186.
[9] A. Albillos *et al.*, The exocytotic event in chromaffin cells revealed by patch amperometry. *Nature Lond.* **389** (1997) 509-512.

Data Warehousing, Data Mining and Knowledge Discovery

Medical Informatics Europe '99
P. Kokol et al. (Eds.)
IOS Press, 1999

Knowledge Discovery for Advanced Clinical Data Management and Analysis

Ankica Babic[1,2]
1. Medical Informatics, Dept of Biomedical Engineering, Linkoping University, Sweden
2. Faculty of Electrical Engineering, University of Ljubljana, Slovenia

Abstract: Knowledge discovery is a broad research field in which methods are developed to support discovery of novel and potentially useful knowledge from clinical databases and registers in systems for patient care. However, the techniques available are not readily applicable in medical domains, due to, among other reasons, low user friendliness and lack of proper methodological background.
Data mining approaches to be explored and improved are predictive modelling, segmentation, dependency modelling, summarisation, and change and deviation detection/modelling (in data or knowledge).
Another and original contribution of the research is to build up efficient feedback loops. Human experts and available domain expert systems could provide suggestions as how to improve all major steps in the knowledge discovery process such as evaluation of knowledge, choice of data mining methods and data input.
A long tradition of collecting and maintaining clinical and administrative data could be found in fields of oncology, cardiology, coronary surgery, social and primary health care medicine All these areas, that gather data over long periods of time, could benefit from knowledge discovery.

1. Introduction to the field

Knowledge discovery is a process of identifying novel, valid and understandable patterns in data. This is done in order to explain existing data, make predictions or classifications about new data, and summarise the contents of large database to support decision making. Logical data visualisation, which is a part of the process, helps human experts in better understanding of data and in discovering deeper patterns. The approach requires less from the end user allowing him easier hypothesis building compared to conventional statistical methods.
Data mining, which is essential to the whole process, can handle large amounts of data and offer efficient techniques to discover new data patterns which can be visualised in a manner easily understandable by the users. In a multidimensional database, data mining typically begins when even the most advanced query approaches can no longer provide sought answers. It is used to extract general descriptive knowledge (generative models of data, symbolic descriptions of subsets, summarisation), as well as discriminative knowledge (to distinguish between K classes, for accurate classification, to separate spaces).
Practical realisation of the knowledge discovery process is dependent both on the area of the application and the choice of clinical and other tasks to be supported. Therefore, good results can be expected only for well-defined research problems. In all other cases, quality of data management and knowledge extraction will strongly depend on end user skills and support which might be given by knowledge engineers. The most important issues to be taken care of in implementing any knowledge discovery process are given in Table 1 [1].

Table 1. Practical tasks in knowledge discovery.

• automation,
• data transformation and dimensionality reduction,
• guarding against overfitting,
• modes of growth of data,
• interface to derive simplified forms of the extracted models for comprehensibility and visualisation,
• efficient and sufficient sampling schemes,
• in-memory vs. disk-based data processing,
• choice of optimal subset of techniques to span most tasks,
• interfaces to large data warehouses, and use of metadata to optimise access,
• client-server issues, where to perform the processing,
• exploiting parallelism, distributed computing over a network of computers.

The important direction concerns a selection of suitable methods from the data mining library. Depending on the nature of the knowledge discovery task, users preferences and other factors, the following considerations are to be taken into account:

- univariate vs. multivariate analysis,
- numerical data vs. categorical or mixed data,
- explanation requirements or comprehensibility,
- fuzzy vs. precise patterns,
- sample independence assumptions,
- availability of prior knowledge.

Practical motivation to build up an integrated environment for knowledge discovery has a foundation in the following facts:

- data volume is too large for classical analysis regimes,
- networking, increased opportunity for access by many end users,
- end users are also physicians and other non-statisticians.

2. Advanced methodological solutions

Machine learning techniques that have an ability to provide new knowledge have undergone intensive development [2,6]. Many of them provide solutions to complex questions usually offering flexible software implementation and valuable graphical presentation of the results. End users are not, however, generally aware of all the possible disadvantages of choosing a particular method. In addition, an attractive graphical presentation could mislead interpretation of the results. Both these aspects could become an obstacle for knowledge discovery. Therefore, we intend to study effects of learning from the clinical data. Table 2. presents quite detailed performance features to be considered in upgrading of the methods and minimisation of risks of inaccurate outcomes.

Table 2. Classification data methods as represented by their performance features.

	Advantages	Disadvantages
Decision Trees	• Can deal with high-dimensional data • Breaks data into symbolic partition (leaves, or rules) • Fast execution time with greedy search • Easy to implement	• Quick partitioning of data results in fast deterioration in attribute selection quality • Greedy search is too blind • Limited representation language • Search space is huge, even for limited node tests
Neural Networks	• If examples have attached class probabilities, and densities are smooth, then problem becomes a regression problem and neural nets have been shown to be effective at learning to predict actual probabilities accurately • Representational power • Implicit massive parallelism, though hard to implement in many architectures	• Training neural net to be consistent with training set is known to be NP-hard problem (for classification, NOT regression problems) • Network architecture choice (number of nodes, hidden layers, so forth) are by trial and error • Solution depends on initial weight settings • Learned function not easy to understand, virtually a black box classifier that offers no explanations to humans
Nearest Neighbour Method	• Deal with inexact matches of features • Explanation in terms of records used to reach a decision	• Computationally expensive: all records in the database being mined have to be ”touched”. Feature weight calculations are dynamic. The method, especially the first variant, is good for small databases, or sparse feature sets • Identifying k: Determining how many records to return can be tricky • Defining ”most appropriate”: The definition is problem dependent A computable similarity metric may be hard to define • No good method for deciding weights on attributes exists • Generalisation is hard
Bayesian Clustering	• Does not require distance measures • Gives probability of membership in each class rather than a single class assignment • Has natural measure of fit of models to data: probability if the provide data given the model assumptions • Forces user to make all assumptions explicit	• Requires selecting class models a priori. While this is difficult, it is actually better than making this assumption implicitly as any other program would do • Search model parameter space is very large • Have to worry about co-variances between variables

3. Evaluation insights and further development with respect to clinical demands

Common examples of knowledge discovery in oncology are navigation and searching in the databases, hypothesis testing, summarising experiment results, creating predictions and discrimination of the patient groups. Scientific data analyses puts even stronger demands on the whole process: basic processing, high-level science analysis and, finally, scientific discovery over large data sets.

In our research work we have developed and tested methods of several approaches to extract sought clinical knowledge [7]. Experiences of using multivariate statistics were enriched by implementing procedures of artificial intelligence [8,9,10]. In the field of asymptotic liver disease we have researched and strengthened a complete knowledge discovery cycle from the data to a standardised knowledge representation form [11]. In the field of oncology we have developed procedures for effective graphical representation that gave excellent insights into data clusters [12]. We have designed and implemented customised classification procedures when standard statistical techniques have not proven to be efficient enough [13].

The growing potential of knowledge discovery [1,15-18] enables development of a newer, advanced methods and efficient integration of already existing multivariate methods. *Cluster, discriminant and regression analyses* constitute a powerful analytical toolbox. Case based reasoning is another methodology that could provide significant support trough the integration into a knowledge base system.

4. Empowering knowledge discovering process

Expert validation and evaluation is a normal, required step in declaring any new facts and patterns as novel and relevant knowledge. Figure 1. suggests how this step of quality control could be implemented in an automated manner.

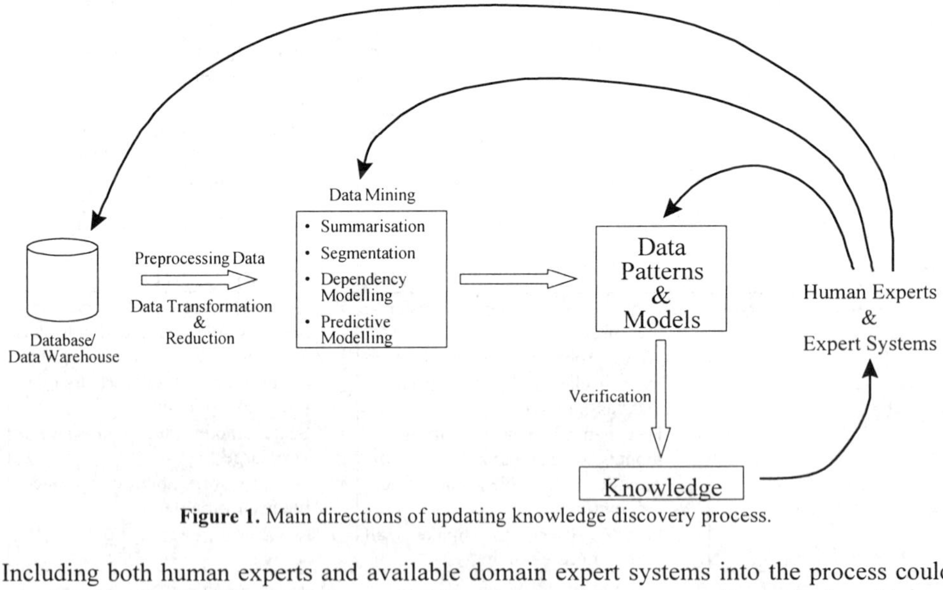

Figure 1. Main directions of updating knowledge discovery process.

Including both human experts and available domain expert systems into the process could provide a feedback information to practically all steps of the process. By analysing obtained data models, or even patterns, a user could come up with new explanations of the knowledge, or go back to either chose another method or select more suitable data. In this manner, and as described in [19], an evaluation of all suggested data analytical methods could be done.

Oncology is just one of the important research and application domains where awareness of potentials and usefulness of proposed research could be raised. Equally important is to propagate results of the research into other domains where data is collected and maintained, e.g. cardiology, coronary surgery [20,21], and many branches of social medicine [22].

References

[1] Fayyad U., Piatetsky-Shapiro G. and Smyth P.(1995), "From Knowledge Discovery to Data Mining: An overview. a chapter in Advances in Knowledge Discovery and Data Mining, U M Fayyad, G Piatetsky-Shapiro, P J Smyth and R Uthurusamy (Eds.) AAAI/MIT Press

[2] Wu X, Knowledge Acquisition from Data Bases, PhD Thesis 176, pp, Dept of Artificial Intelligence, University of Edinburgh, Edinburgh, Scotland, 1993.

[3] Wu X., K Eshell2: An Intelligent Learning Data Base System, Research and Development in Expert Systems IX, M A Bramer and R W Milne (Eds) Cambridge University Press, UK 1992.

[4] Wu X., Inductive Learning: Algorithms and Frontiers, Artificial Intelligence review, 7 (1993), 2:93-108.

[5] Wu X, Research Issues in Intelligent Learning Database Systems, Proceedings of the Seventh Annual Florida AI Research Symposium, Pensacola Beach, Florida, USA May 5-7, 1994.

[6] Wu X., Book: Knowledge Acquisition from databases, Ablex, USA, 1995.

[7] Babic Ankica. *Medical knowledge extraction, Application of data analysis methods to support clinical decisions*. PhD. dissertation. No. 322, Linköping University, 1993.

[8] Babic A, Aahlfeld H, Wigertz O, Bodemar G, Mathiesen U. Artificial neural networks in clustering and classification data on unspecified liver diseases. XIth Nordic Meeting on Medical and Biological Engineering, Lund, Sweden, p 136, 1993.

[9] Babic A, Krusinska E, Strömberg J.-E. Extraction of diagnostic rules using recursive partitioning systems. A Comparison of Approaches. Artificial Intelligence in Medicine, 4:373-387, Elsevier, 1992.

[10] Babic A. Case Studies in Machine Learning for Medical Knowledge Extraction. The SAIS94, Swedish artificial Intelligence workshop, Ronneby, Sweden, 1994

[11] Babic A, Bodemar G, Mathiesen U, Aahlfeldt H, Franzen L, Wigertz O. Machine Learning to Support Diagnostics in the Domain of Asymptomatic Liver Disease. In R.A. Greeneset al. (Eds) MEDINFO'95 Proceedings, IMIA, 8th Wrold Congress on Medical Informatics, Vancouver, Canada, pp 809-813, 1995

[12] Zganec M, Babic A., M Us-Krasovec, B Palcic. 3D Presentation of the nuclear cell features in quantitative cytometry. In Proc AMIA Annual Fall Symposium, Washington DC, James J Cimino, ed. Hanley & Belfus, 1996, pp 679-683.

[13] Siska A, Babic A., Pavesic N., Studies of responsiveness in the R-EGFR and Rcerb-B2 oncogenes spaces: a customized application for thyroid lesions. In Proc MIE'97, Technology and Informatics 43, C Pappas, N Maglaveras, J-R Scherrer eds, Greece. IOS Press, Netherlands, 1997, pp 634-637.

[14] Matheus C, Chan P, G Piatetsky-Shapiro, Systems for Knowledge Discovery in Databases, Special Issue on Learning and Discovery in Databases, IEEE Transactions on Knowledge and Data Engineering, Dec. 1993

[15] Parsaye K. and Chignell M., 1993. Intelligent Database Tools & Applications, John Wiley.

[16] N Cerone and M Tsuchiya, guest editors, Special Issue on Learning and Discovery in Databases, IEEE Transactions on Knowledge and Data Engineering, 5(6) Dec 1993.

[17] G Piatetsky-Shapiro, guest editor, Special issue on Knowledge Discovery in Databases and Knowledge Bases, International Journal of Intelligent Systems, Vol 7, no 7, Sep 1992,

[18] G Piatetsky-Sharpio, guest editor , Special issue on Knowledge Discovery in Databases, Journal of Intelligent Information Systems, 3(4), Dec 1994,.

[19] Harrell Jr FE, Lee KL, Mark DB. Multivariable prognostic models: issues in developing models, evaluating assumptions and adequacy, and measuring and reducing errors. *Stat Med* 1996;**15**:361-87.

[20] Higgins TL, Estafanous FG, Loop FD, Beck GJ, Blum JM, Paranandi L. Stratification of morbidity and mortality outcome by preoperative risk factors in coronary artery bypass patients. A clinical severity score [published erratum appears in jama 1992 oct 14;268(14):1860] [see comments]. *JAMA* 1992;**267**:2344-8.

[21] O'Connor G.T., Plume S.K., Olmstead E.M., Morton J.R., Maloney C.T., Nugent W.C., Hernandez F., Clough R., Leavitt, B.J., Coffin L.H., Marrin C.A.S., Wennberg J.E., Birkmeyer J.D., Charlesworth D.C., Malenka D.J., Quinton H.B., Kasper J.F., A Regional Intervention to Improve the Hospital Mortality Associated With Coronary Artery Bypass Graft Surgery, *JAMA* 1996, 275: 841-6.

[22] Iezzoni LI, Ash AS, Shwartz M, Daley J, Hughes JS, Mackiernan YD. Predicting who dies depends on how severity is measured: implications for evaluating patient outcomes [see comments]. *Ann Intern Med* 1995;123:763-70.

Medical Informatics Europe '99
P. Kokol et al. (Eds.)
IOS Press, 1999

Application of the medical data warehousing architecture Epidware to epidemiological follow-up : data extraction and transformation

Elmostafa Kerkri[a], Catherine Quantin[a], Kokou Yetongnon[b], FA Allaert[a,c] and Liliane Dusserre[a]
[a] *Dijon University Hospital, medical informatics Department, Dijon, France BP 1542- 21034 Dijon Cedex- France- emkerkri@u-bourgogne.fr*
[b] *University of Burgundy, Electronic and Informatic Engineering Laboratory, Dijon, France*
[c] *W2 "data security" European Federation of Medical Informatics*

Abstract. In this paper, we present an application of EPIDWARE, medical data warehousing architecture, to our epidemiological follow-up project. The aim of this project is to extract and regroup information from various information systems for epidemiological studies. We give a description of the requirements of the epidemiological follow-up project such as anonymity of medical data information and data file linkage procedure. We introduce the concept of Data Warehousing Architecture. The particularities of data extraction and transformation are presented and discussed.

Key words. data warehousing; epidemiological follow-up; data extraction and transformation; medical information systems; data anonymity and linkage

1 Introduction

Computer science has been used in medical applications since the 1970's. Health care systems in industrialised nations have undergone hospital output evaluation based on a classification of hospital stays called Diagnosis Related Groups (DRGs) aimed at curbing hospital expenditure. In 1985, the implementation of the application of the information system program (Programme de Médicalisation des systèmes d'information - PMSI) began in France. In 1996, the PMSI was enlarged to private medical sector and the Health ministry initiated the national medical network project Réseau Santé Social. The aim of this project is to propose an Intranet to enable medical professionals either to send information to sickness benefits organisms, or to exchange medical information between themselves.

This evolution in the application of computer science to healthcare followed the evolution in informatics, characterised by the transition towards microcomputers, towards networks and the Internet, and towards relational or object oriented databases.

Since 1992, Data warehouse technologies are used as components of decision support environment aimed at collecting and organising relevant information to aid decision-makers. Data warehouse technology can also be used in medical management. Besides this economic aim, we suggest using this technology to link recorded medical information concerning a given pathology in a given region in view of epidemiological studies. These studies would also allow the optimisation of health expenses by limiting redundancies in examinations and procedures for the same patient while improving patient care. However, in order to respect the European legislation concerning personal data processing, and so to guarantee confidentiality, integrity and availability of data, this regrouping of information should be composed of different steps such as anonymity of the data, secured file transfer and linkage [3].

In the first part of this paper we present the "Epidemiological Follow-up" project and the necessary stages for its implementation. The second part is devoted to the data warehousing EPIDWARE architecture.

2 Development of the architecture EPIDWARE for epidemiological follow-up

2.1 The epidemiological follow-up project

To carry out epidemiological follow-up of diseases such as cardiovascular diseases or cancers, for example, it is necessary to link information recorded by different health structures participating in the care of a given patient. Diagnoses made by the Anatomo-pathology laboratory, type of the surgical operation and of chemotherapy treatments, the localisation and the duration of the different hospitalisations, and if possible the date of death.

To respect the European legislation concerning medical file linkage, we have developed an anonymous record linkage procedure [7,8,9], which is composed of two steps: an anonymity procedure and the record linkage of rendered anonymous files. The question now is to integrate the different files coming from different sources into a decisional database (data warehouse) while ensuring the regrouping of the information concerning a given patient.

2.2 Data warehousing concept

In the databases technology area, Data warehouse is defined as a collection of decision support functionalities / environment to allow decision-makers to take more rapid and relevant decisions. The Data warehouse has to insure the coherence of information of the enterprise and to facilitate its access. These objectives imply the integration of request tools and other tools for information analysis and presentation. Data have to be carefully gathered from different information sources, then cleaned and filtered and to be distributed only after validation of their quality. Thus, information provided by data warehouse is not a crude data but an information that assist and helps the decision-makers. It is subject oriented, aggregated, easily accessible, reliable, relevant, non-volatile and possesses a specific temporal context [1,2,4,5].

The principle of data warehousing is to extract useful information, to combine and to consolidate them into a coherent data repository to provide a single image of activity reality. This improves data quality and allows users to retrieve necessary data by themselves [6]. The coherence of data is measured globally, based on the viewpoint of the manager who seeks for example if data is complete and without contradiction [5].

2.3 EPIDWARE architecture

The implementation process of a data warehouse is generally progressive. Often, it begins with the implementation of a data mart (a data warehouse relative to a given department/activity). Then, two types of development are possible according to the organisational choice of the administrative staff of enterprise: progressive centralisation of strategic data or implementation of as much data marts as specific services.

The modelling of the target data structure (a data mart or a data warehouse) constitutes the initial stage of data warehousing. Builders establish, with the direction of the enterprise, a dictionary of data description (metadata). They also specify extraction, translation and integration tools. Once implemented, the data warehouse has to be updated to ensure that the format of data corresponds to the user's need, which may change later on. More, changes in sources of information have to be propagated on the data warehouse.

Once extracted, data are aggregated and filtered so as to harmonise their formats and to eliminate redundancies. The attribution of coherent values to non initialised variables (, completes the stages which precede the information loading in the Data warehouse.

Information sources: Information sources (Figure1), can be multiple [1]: database systems, files systems, document HTML or knowledge bases. In medical context, information sources are in public or private hospitals, biomedical analysis laboratories, radiology departments. And data are related either to patient identity or to medical information.

Wrapper: Is mainly composed by a three elements: the Translator, the Monitor and the Anonymity tool. **Translator**'s role is to translate data from the format and the model of the information sources to the format and the model of the data warehouse. The translation consists in making the underlying information source appearing as subscribing to the data model used by the warehousing system. For example, if the information source has a data file structure but the warehouse uses a relational data model, then the wrapper/monitor has to have an interface presenting data of the information source as if they were relational[1].

The detection of data changes concerning the data warehouse and their propagation to the integrator is the main role of the **Monitor**. Then, the changes occurring on data have to be translated by the wrapper, from the format and the model of the information source, to the format and model of the data warehouse, just as for data themselves. Another approach consists in ignoring the functionality of change detection and transmitting periodically whole data copies from the information source to the data warehouse. The Integrator can

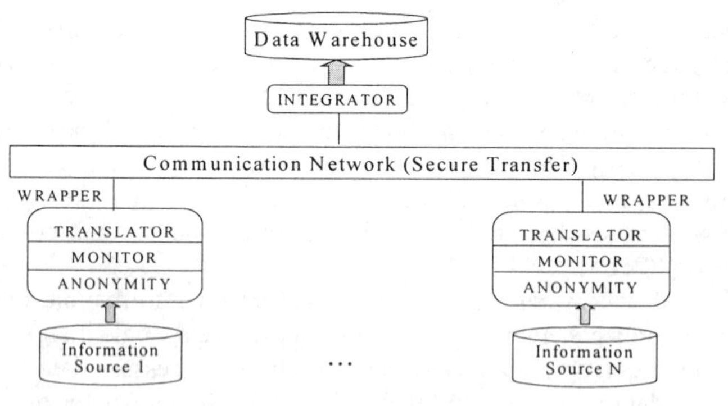

Figure 1. EPIDWARE Architecture

[1] Most of the commercial Data Warehousing systems suppose that the information sources and the Data Warehouse are relational.

then combine these data with those of the data warehouse coming from other sources, or ask all sources for other information to complete data of the warehouse. However, if the continuous access of updated information is required, it is preferable to adopt the principle of change detection and their propagation to data of the warehouse. The first stage of **Anonymity** procedure is included in the Wrapper functionalities.

Integrator: To load information in the data warehouse, the integrator must filter, refine, integrate and combine information coming from the local sources. It provides decision-maker with a clear, relevant and non-redundant view of patient medical information. To achieve the above, the integrator include some additional functionalities. First, it receives change notifications from the wrapper and updates the data warehouse. Second, it applies the second stage of anonymity to the received files. Finally, it links received medical files to regroup medical information of each patient.

2.4 Data extraction

The particularity of our project is that most administrative and medical information sources are outside our hospital. Usually, we do not meet any difficulty with the database systems bought from computer companies specialised in medical fields. But some hospitals use software without any technical documentation and it is thus difficult to locate, for example, the database tables of discharge abstracts containing associate diagnoses and the corresponding acts. Moreover, sometimes information needed for epidemiological studies is missing, for example the term of the pregnancy for perinatology studies, which then require a completion of the data set manually.

Another problem is to eliminate duplicated data, due to a lack of quality of administrative information. In some cases we have data redundancy characterised by as many records, for each hospital stay of the patient, as numbers of therapeutic procedures and associate diagnoses coded for this stay. In order to solve the problem of regrouping all these records in a single one, we have implemented a solution, consisting of three steps. The first step is to eliminate redundancy by therapeutic procedure, the second step consists of doing the same thing with the associate diagnoses, and the third, of joining the two files resulting from the two first steps. This solution was implemented with Visual Basic and SQL for Microsoft Query.

In a particular application of neonatalogy follow-up, the problem of the connection between the record of a baby and his mother was posed. If the mother and her babe do not have the same name, we need to use our linkage procedure [8,9] to know the medical information about the mother. In practice, giving successive identification numbers to the baby and his mother enables to link the babe and his mother records. This seemed to solve the problem, but not completely because we have to pay attention to the case of twins for example. We proposed a general solution by creating a new variable, namely the identification number of the mother, in the baby's record.

2.5 Data transformation

Data are translated according to the metadata specifications. For example, date of birth must be coded as DDMMYYYY, so we have to translate it from any other format to this one. In other way, date of birth is indirectly nominative, thus the second translation is to compute the age of the patient from his date of birth. The zip code, which is also indirectly nominative, must be replaced by a geographical code.

The most important transformation concerns nominative variables such as the name, the first name and the maiden name. The first stage consists in spelling treatment [9] that contains rules and facts. This step is necessary because of typing errors, in particular for homonyms. Obviously, the knowledge base of the spelling treatment must be adapted to the language used. The second stage consists in an irreversible transformation of all nominative variables.

3 Discussion and conclusion

The advantage of EPIDWARE information system is to combine data warehouse techniques with an anonymity procedure to design an epidemiological follow-up system. It is very useful, from an epidemiological point of view to be able to integrate and to consolidate inconsistent medical data from various legacy systems into one coherent data set and to improve data quality by extracting relevant and pertinent information. We cannot ignore the difficulties of obtaining information, which may even imply manual copying from existing databases. Indeed, the data-processing solutions proposed depend on the concerned information sources' specificity. Though, these solutions will progressively constitute a data extraction toolkit well adapted to most information sources so that manual intervention would be exceptional. In the same idea, the set of transformation roles will be completed in order to take into account new information sources particularities.

Epidemiologists can benefit also from direct access to the information needed without requiring the help of computer scientists, using requests on databases already implemented. Of course, this necessitates a certain sense of anticipation. At last, this architecture relieves epidemiologists from concerns about the respect of legal security aspects as it guarantees data confidentiality and secures information processing.

Acknowledgements. This work was supported by the Burgundy Regional Council, France Telecom and the French "Ligue Bourguignonne" against cancer.

References

[1]]Widom J, Research problems in Data Warehousing, Proc. Of 4th Int'l CKIM, Nov. 1995.

[2] Franco JM & EDS- Institut prometétéus, Le Data Warehousing, ed Eyrolles, Paris, janvier 1997

[3] Quantin C., Kerkri E. Allaert FA, Bouzelat H, Dusserre L. Security aspects of medicale file regrouping for the epidemiological follow-up. In Cesnim B, McCray A, Scherrer JR (eds), Proceeding Medinfo'98, pp. 1135-1137

[4] Inmon WH & Hackthorn RD. Using the data warehouse, Wiley-QED Publication, 1994

[5] Kimball R. The Data Warehouse Toolkit.(French version by Raimond C.) Paris: International Thomson Publishing France, 1997.

[6] Sakaguchi T. and Frolik Mark N. A Review of the Data Warehousing Literature. Web: http://www.people.memphis.edu/~tsakagch/dw-web.htm. Jan. 31, 1996.

[7] Bouzelat H, Quantin C, Duserre L. Extraction and Anonymity. Protocol of Medical file. JAMIA 1996 Symposium Supplement:323-7.

[8] Quantin C., Bouzelat H, Allaert FA, Benhamiche AM, Faivre J, Dusserre L. How to ensure data security of an epidemiological follow-up: quality assessment of an anonymous record linkage procedure. Int J of Medical Informatics, 49 (1998) 117-122.

[9] Quantin C., Bouzelat H, Allaert FA, Benhamiche AM, Faivre J, Dusserre Development of an automatic record hash coding and linkage procedure to warrant epidemiological follow-up data confidentiality. Methods of Information in Medicine. 1998; 37:271-277.

Medical Informatics Europe '99
P. Kokol et al. (Eds.)
IOS Press, 1999

Statistical approaches for evaluation of genetic risk factor of peripheral arterial occlusive disease

Svatoš J. [1], Orendáč M. [2], Mušková B. [2], Hyánek J. [3], Kožich V. [2], Zvárová J. [1]
[1] *European Center for Medical Informatics, Statistics and Epidemiology of Charles University and Academy of Sciences, Prague, Czech Republic*
[2] *Institute of Inherited Metabolic Diseases, 1st Faculty of Medicine, Charles University, Prague, Czech Republic*
[3] *Dept. of Clinical Biochemistry, Na Homolce Hospital, Prague, Czech Republic*

Abstract: In the paper we show results of medical study from statistical point of view. The medical study was aimed to study genetic risk factors of peripheral arterial occlusive diseases in Czech population. Two genes, CBS and MTHFR were examined, as various genotypes of these genes are thought to have impact on amino thiols, who participate in variety of reactions in vasculature. Statistical part of the study was responsible for analysis and interpretation of collected data.

1. Introduction

In recent time, statistical methods gain greater importance for genetic risk factors analysis, which can be observed in various types of statistical studies, either population or family studies. We will demonstrate approaches for of genetic risk factors analysis in population studies. Application of statistical methods for risk factor identification will be our concern.

Influence of heterozygozity in the cystathionine-β-synthase (CBS) on premature atherosclerosis was studied in works during late 80's to mid 90's (Boers et al. 1985 ,1989, Clarke et al.1991 [1], Kožich et al.1995, Kluitmans et al. 1996 [2]). First three of them suggest that heterozygosity in CBS, associated with mild hyperhomocysteinemia is a cause of premature atherosclerosis, while two recent do not find more prevalent CBS mutations among vascular diseased patients. As in 1995 an insertion of 68bps in the CBS exon 8, 844ins68 was described (Sebastio et al. 1995, [3]), new possibility of association between CBS gene and premature atherosclerosis arised and was consequently studied by Sperandeo et al., 1996 [4], Tsai et al., 1996 [5], Kluitmans et al., 1997 [6], de Franchis et al.(1997).

2. Study of risk factors of PAOD

2.1 Design of study

Total number of cases in this study was 162, from that 124 men ,38 women. One patient was removed from the study because of extremely high homocysteine level (tHcy plasma level 78 μmol/l). Cases were recruited from about 600 individuals who underwent treatment at the Na Homolce Hospital in Prague, Czech Rep. in the period between April 1996 and September 1997. These patients suffered from at least 75% stenosis of femoral artery (about 2/3 of the cases), carotid artery (about 1/4 of the cases) or other peripheral artery. Exlusive criteria involved for selection of cases were: age over 65 years, diabetes, heavy smoking (over 40 cigarettes per day), renal insufficiency and/or plasma creatinine level over 120 mmol/l, hypercholesterolemia (either total cholesterol plasma level over 6.5 mmol/l or intake of hypolipidemic drugs in currently normocholesterolemic individuals) and hyper-triglyceridemia (plasma level over 2.2 mmol/l). For the men was age range 37 to 65 years with mean 54.8 years. For the women was age range 41 to 65 yearswith mean 52.8 years).

Total Hcy and Cys plasma levels under fasting conditions were examined in all cases. One patient was excluded from the group of cases due to extreme tHcy plasma level (78mmol/l).

The control group of healthy individuals was unmatched and recruited randomly from two sources within Prague area: 250 children undergoing a routine pediatric examination, aged under 16, and 150 blood donors with age range 21 to 87 years, mean age 36.2 years.

2.2 Medical hypotheses

As amino thiols such as homocysteine (Hcy), cysteine (Cys) and glutathione (Gl) actively participate in a variety of reactions in vasculature, it is reasonable to suppose, that mechanisms involving amino thiols levels can be associated with atheroslerosis. While Gl is recognized as an antioxidative agent, Hcy is considered a prooxidative factor in atherogenesis. Association between highly elevated plasma Hcy levels and atherosclerosis was first proposed by McCully in [7]. Subsequent studies suggested that even mild elevation of total Hcy (tHcy) levels may be associated with occlusive vascular diseases. Mild hyperhomocysteinemia (mHHC), defined differently in various studies, is now accepted as an independent risk factor for atherosclerosis [8].There are two pathways of concern, the remethylation pathway and the transsulfuration pathway. Disturbances in Hcy metabolism are currently assessed by measuring either concentrations of fasting tHcy which presumably detect impairment in the remethylation pathway, or by methionine loading test which may reveal disorders in the transsulfuration pathway. Disturbed Hcy metabolism is caused by factors of both exo-genous (deficiency of folates, B6 and B12 vitamines, excessive coffee consumption) and endogenous origin. Some of the non-genetic endogenous factors are renal insufficiency and lower cortisol and estradiol plasma levels. Genetic causes of mHHC may include various defects in any enzymatic step of the two metabolic pathways of Hcy.

Moreover, familial occurrence of mHHC strongly suggests that inheritance plays an important role in the development of this trait. Majority of studies that examined genetic causes of mHHC had analyzed disturbances in the methylenetetrahydrofolate reductase (MTHFR) and cystathionine-β-synthase (CBS) genes. Various researchers studied influence of MTHFR gene as possible risk factor for coronary artery disease and influence of homozygosity in 677C→T polymorphism was further studied.

To ascertain whether heterozygosity for 844ins68 in the CBS gene and/or homozygosity for the 677C→T in the MTHFR locus are risk factors for PAOD, we performed a case-control study. We also analyzed relation between individual MTHFR/CBS genotypes, and fasting levels of sulfur amino acids Hcy and Cys. Our aim was to assess the contribution of above genetic abnormalities to etiology and pathogenesis of PAOD in Czech population.

2.3 Statistical methods and their description

The medical hypotheses described above were transformed into statistical hypotheses and tested using variety of methods. Chi-square tests were performed to test Hardy-Weinberg equilibrium, if the conditions for using of chi-square were not met (at least one expected frequency low under HWE), a permutation test was used. The conditions can be broken when there is either small number of observations or large number of alleles, because the asymptotic considerations do not work under such conditions and resulting distribution of test statistic does not follow chi-square distribution with appropriate number of degrees of freedom. Only first of these two possibilities threatened in analyzed study, as only two alleles were thought for CBS and for MTHFR. A note to low expected frequencies: There are different criteria to define "low frequency", but reasonable one is, that all expected frequencies should be at least one, stronger criterion defines the smallest expected number to be five. Contingency tables of prevalences in controls and cases were examined using chi-square test or, if conditions were not met, Fischer's exact test. Main principle of exact tests lies in counting exact probability of each contingency table with given marginals, supposing that the null hypothesis (independence) holds. Confidence intervals for allelic and genotype frequencies were constructed by means of normal approximation, because of sufficient number of observations (161 patients, 400 controls). When influence of MTHFR and CBS genotypes on metabolite levels was examined, ANOVA test was used, or, if the conditions for ANOVA were violated, a median test was performed. The violation was caused by skewed distribution of metabolite levels, variances did not differ significantly.

We used statistical software STATISTICA for ANOVA, median test and chi-square tests and StatXact for exact tests. EpiInfo was used for establishing confidence intervals.

3. Results of statistical evaluation

Allele and genotype frequencies were computed and HWE was tested for both MTHFR and CBS. Throughout following tables, T means the MTHFR polymorphism (mutant allele), C wild type MTHFR allele (677C), I the CBS 844ins68-bearing allele, N the CBS wild type allele (without 844ins68). Codes CC, CT, TT, NN, NI describe genotypes.

Table 1 MTHFR and CBS allele frequencies in cases and controls

MTHFR					CBS				
	Cases		Controls			Cases		Controls	
Allele	n	%	n	%	Allele	n	%	n	%
C	214	66.5	530	66.2	N	295	91.6	756	94.5
T	108	33.5	270	33.8	I	27	8.4	44	5.5
Total	322	100	800	100	Total	322	100	800	100

Table 2 MHFTR and CBS genotype frequencies in cases and controls

	MTHFR				CBS				
	Cases		Controls			Cases		Controls	
Genotype	n	%	n	%	Genotype	n	%	n	%
CC	72	44.7	171	42.8	NN	134	83.2	356	89.0
CT	70	43.5	188	47.0	NI	27	16.8	44	11.0
TT	19	11.8	41	10.2	II	0	0.0	0	0.0
Total	**161**	**100**	**400**	**100**	**Total**	**161**	**100**	**400**	**100**

Odds ratio (OR, given as ad/bc ratio in 2-by-2 table) for NI genotype statistically significantly differs from 1, when tested against one-sided alternative by exact Fischer's test, p=0,045. Use of one-tailed test is reasonable here, because the medical hypothesis, based on study of metabolite pathways and their connection to risk of vascular disease expects that possible difference should be in only one direction (NI heterozygotes may have problems more frequently than NN homozygotes). HWE was tested using chi-square test for MTHFR data, exact test for CBS data (as there was small expected frequency for BB genotype). Table 3 covers the results.

Table 3 Test of HWE

	Cases			Controls		
Gene	Chi-sqr	df	p	Chi-sqr	df	p
MTHFR	0.099	1	0.753	0.128	1	0.721
CBS	---	---	0.614	---	---	1.000

Prevalences of MTHFR T allele and TT genotype frequencies were determined for both cases and controls. The 95% CI was computed for the prevalences. The same was done for CBS I allele frequency and NI genotype frequency. The results are given in Table 4.

Table 4 Prevalence of individual genotypes

	Allele/genotype	Cases	Controls
MTHFR	T freq. and 95%CI	0.34 (0.28-0.39)	0.34(0.30-0.37)
	TT freq. and 95%CI	0.118 (0.067-0.169)	0.102 (0.072-0.133)
CBS	I freq. and 95%CI	0.084 (0.053-0.115)	0.055 (0.039-0.071)
	NI freq. and 95%CI	0.168 (0.101-0.227)	0.110 (0.078-0.141)

OR for MTHFR was clearly non-significant (p=0.67), but difference between cases and controls in CBS was significant (p=0.045) when tested against one-sided alternative using

Fischer's test.To test independence of CBS and MTHFR genotypes, another table was constructed, containing counts of each combination of MTHFR and CBS genotypes.

Table 5 Prevalence of combinations

	CC / NN	CT / NN	TT / NN	CC / NI	CT / NI	TT / NI	Total
Cases	63	53	18	9	17	1	161
row %	39.1	32.9	11.2	5.6	10.6	0.6	100.0
Controls	157	168	31	14	20	10	400
row %	39.3	42.0	7.7	3.5	5.0	2.5	100.0

Permutation test p value=0.1545 does not indicate difference between populations of controls and cases. For studying of possible correlation between genotypes and metabolite levels, ANOVA was performed, one-way for MTHFR and one-way for CBS. Results of ANOVA (MTHFR) are shown in Table 6, results for CBS were clearly nonsignificant.

Table 6 ANOVA of metabolite levels on MTHFR genotypes

	CC			CT			TT			ANOVA	
Metabolites	n	Mean	SD	n	Mean	SD	n	Mean	SD	Test	p
tHcy (mmol/l)	71	12.2	3.5	70	12.9	4.9	19	14.1	5.6	M-test	0.076
Cys (mmol/l)	66	227.1	44.4	68	229.4	49.9	19	219.7	37.5	F-test	0.720
Cys/tHcy ratio	66	19.7	5.4	68	19.5	5.8	19	18.1	8.0	M-test	0.088

No statistically significant differences were found between metabolite levels in different MTHFR genotypes, although the p-value for tHcy 0.076 approaches statistical significance.

4. Conclusion

Frequencies obtained from sample give insight to MTHFR and CBS distribution in Czech population. HWE was not rejected for both groups and both genes. Moreover, difference between cases and controls in CBS allele frequencies was significant, supporting medical hypothesis and slightly elevated in tHcy levels in MTHFR T homozygotes supports hypothesis about genetic influence in mHHC, yet not statistically significantly (p=0.076).

Acknowledgement

Study was supported by The Grant Agency of Ministry of Health of the Czech Republic (M/26-3).

References

[1] Clarke et al: Hyperhomocysteinemia: An independent risk factor for vascular disease, NEJM 1991, 324, No.17, pp.1149-1155
[2] Kluijtmans et al: Molecular genetic analysis in mild hyperhomocysteinemia: A common mutation in the MTHFR gene is a genetic risk factor for cardiovascular disease, Am J Hum Genet (1996), 58:35-41
[3] Sebastio et al: The molecular basis of homocystinuria due to cystathionine β-synthase deficiency in Italian families, and report of four novel mutations. Am J Hum Genet 56: 1324-1333, 1995
[4] M.P.Sperandeo et al.: A 68bp Insertion Found in a Homocystinuric Patient Is a Common Variant and Is skipped by Alternative Splicing of the Cystathionine β-synthase mRNA. Am J Hum Genet 59:1391-1393, 1996
[5] High prevalence of a mutation in the CBS gene, Tsai et al. Am J Hum Genet, 59:1262-1267, 1996
[6] Kluijtmans et al: Thermolabile methylenetetrahydrofolate reductase in coronary artery disease, Circulation Vol.96, No.8, pp.2573-2577 (1997)
[7] Vascular pathology of homocysteinaemia: implications for the pathogenesis of atherosclerosis. Mc Cully Am J Patol 1969, 56:111-128
[8] A quantitative assessment of plasma homocysteine as a risk factor for vascular disease, Boushey CJ JAMA 1995, 274:1049-1057

Medical Informatics Europe '99
P. Kokol et al. (Eds.)
IOS Press, 1999

Data warehousing as a basis for web-based documentation of data mining and analysis

Johan Karlsson[1], Patrik Eklund[1], Carl-Gunnar Hallgren[2], Jan-Gunnar Sjödin[3]
[1] *Umeå University, Department of Computing Science, SE-901 87 Umeå, Sweden*
[2] *Ersboda Health Centre, SE-906 25 Umeå, Sweden*
[3] *Umeå University, Department of Urology and Andrology, SE-901 85 Umeå, Sweden*

Abstract. In this paper we present a case study for data warehousing intended to support data mining and analysis. We also describe a prototype for data retrieval. Further we discuss some technical issues related to a particular choice of a patient record environment.

1. Introduction

In this paper we discuss the establishing of a data warehouse for the purpose of enabling high quality and fast documentation of data analysis. We will discuss the end-user perspective in a particular clinical environment. These developments demonstrate the benefits of retrieval tools in conjunction with support for generated web-based documentation.

Developments are done related to a regional record system used in clinics and health centres within the County Council of Västerbotten in Northern Sweden. This work is part of data warehousing and data mining developments for these record systems. Generation of documentation, involving aspects of guideline development, is discussed in [6].

Work on data warehousing as described in this paper has been inspired also by successful warehousing for patient administrative information in Västerbotten [15]. This system includes regular downloading of information and uses standard software for statistics and reporting. A comparable system was reported in [19] for the provision of various service statistics. A retrieval system oriented towards elaborated user-interface design together with selections from vocabularies can be found in [12].

Developments in this paper are partly based on a previous approach to data warehousing as described in [5], where a data retrieval system for MUMPS based record systems was developed for use within a laboratory environment. Search criteria given by users were converted to querying code, and resulting data files delivered to the end-user, thus minimising retrieval time from the end-user point of view. A similar approach was reported in [2], which describes graphical query generation based on object-oriented user views.

Note the distinction between our presentation of documentation and other approaches related to medical reporting which are based on concept representation, see e.g. [13, 7, 11]. Our approach is, however, in a natural and obvious way related to terminology as the record system includes parts of terminology. Concerning software and technological issues of terminologies, our influence comes from developments within Spriterm [14]. These approaches obviously are in no conflict, as the latter represents more of a top-down approach, and the warehousing bottom-up approach needs to be grounded to technological issues with terminologies in the forefront. In the bottom-up approach we always need to deal with technological platforms, and even more so, always have to anticipate involvement of neighbouring technologies, e.g. the inclusion of information residing in PACS/RIS systems.

A prototype including image retrieval in PACS installations is found in [17], and possibilities of using meta-patient-record approaches is described more generally in [18]. In the warehousing approach we also need to build upon standards, thus being dependent on record system middleware components as developed in [8, 16].

2. Case study: Lower urinary tract symptoms

The initial target group for the data warehouse is male patients with LUTS (Lower Urinary Tract Symptoms). These patients have symptoms such as a weak or interrupted flow of urine, difficulty urinating, frequent urination, pain or a burning sensation during urination, blood in the urine, urinary leakage etc. The symptoms are often vague and can have many causes. Patients may have conditions such as prostate cancer, enlarged prostate (Benign Prostatic Hyperplasia, BPH) or combinations of the two, neurological diseases and diabetes. Treatment of LUTS depends on the diagnosis and degree of symptoms. Thus from watchful waiting to major surgery.

The data that will be included in the data warehouse will be acquired from databases at the urology department of the University Hospital in Umeå. The patients that had an enlarged prostate and were operated upon, were more extensively tested and the data were subsequently more complete. For that reason, the initial data warehouse will only contain data on such patients. Discussions with the physicians at the department have resulted in a set of laboratory tests that was considered important for diagnosing these patients; PSA (Prostate Specific Anti-gen), IPSS (International Prostate Symptom Scoring) given by the patient before and after the operation, flow voided volume (urine flow, ml/s), remaining urine (amount of urine that remains in the bladder after urination, ml), blood in urine (yes/no) and IPSS difference (as measured after the operation).

3. Web-based documentation

In general, the process of producing web-based documentation contains modules for respectively retrieval of data, acquisition and representation of knowledge, and creation of the final web-based system. Knowledge acquisition in form of decision structure identification, as provided by the process of mining, enrichment and refinement of data into decision support, obviously invites to a vision of a automated documentation within which evidence-based documentation including corresponding executable DSSs are produced by end-users for end-users. Initial suggestions for a system architecture was suggested in [9].

Decision support usually means text-based guidelines. But since the documents that the proposed system will produce are web-based, executable elements can be added. We believe this will result in more dynamic guidelines that will give additional support to the end-users. Historically, expert systems have been developed during close co-operation between a domain expert and a computer engineer. It is our contention that various computational models, either of feedforward or inference type, can serve as underlying mechanisms in the expert systems. These models would of course only be applicable to certain diseases. They would be based on data acquired from a data mining module. Since the documentation is web-based, important aspects such as availability and easy maintenance are met.

4. Technical aspects

Data mining involves a wide range of technicalities, which in an integrated environment must be considered in relation to existing systems. For data warehousing, and in particular for the retrieval systems, development platforms must be carefully selected so as to provide an efficient environment for development and maintenance of systems, and at the same time not to disable integration capabilities.

In order to maintain platform independence, we use Java technology [1]. The Java platform was first announced in 1994, where one of its main advantages was the "write once, run everywhere" philosophy that allowed developers to construct programs that would run on any platform with a Java virtual machine (JVM) without recompilation. The aspect of platform independence has recently been made topical when the County Council of Västerbotten decided to change operating system to Windows NT. The task of updating existing medical applications to this new platform will demand considerable time and resources. Applications developed in Java would, if written correctly, be immediately available for use under the new operating system.

We also need a flexible way to access the data warehouse. JDBC (Java Database Connectivity) is an API that provides database access from Java applications or applets. It abstracts the necessary functions, thus allowing platform independent access to databases. If additional technology, such as JNDI (Java Naming and Directory Interface), is used, applications can retrieve information about the database, e.g., its name. This makes the applications even more dynamic.

Additional work will be necessary if the structure of the database is changed, i.e., if tables or fields are added or changed. The use of a repository, as suggested in [10], is a typical suggestion in order to minimise the work required in such cases.

The urology clinic at the University Hospital, Umeå, uses BMS Cross from IBM for managing their patient records. This system is based upon the DB/2 database engine. As most vendors, also IBM supports JDBC.

Some data in the records is written as free text, and thus some problems will arise when such data is extracted for inclusion in the data warehouse. However, the hospital is currently introducing new routines for journal entry. The content will be tagged to make the data more accessible and exchangeable. The record system complies to using terminologies, even if the user is not fully enforced to include structured data only.

5. A prototype system for data retrieval

The data warehouse must include efficient, flexible and user-friendly retrieval tools. Retrieval can be broken down in steps shown in Figure 1.

A description of a disease is acquired from a medical expert. This description will typically consist of the selected disease together with the laboratory tests that are important when diagnosing the disease. This information is translated to a SQL-statement by the code generator. A retrieval program is transferred over to the information pool (data warehouse) and a raw data set is returned.

Since physical input in itself does not always indicate all the dynamics of the measurements, it is necessary to organise and combine the data. One example where this is important is when symptom values vary over time.

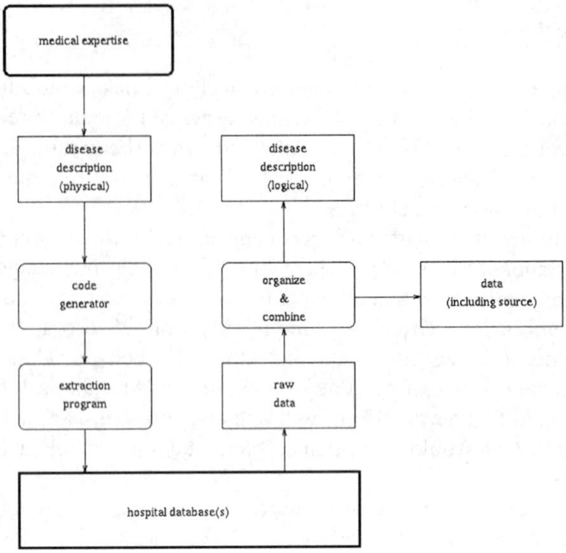

Figure 1

A prototype retrieval program is shown in the Figure 2.

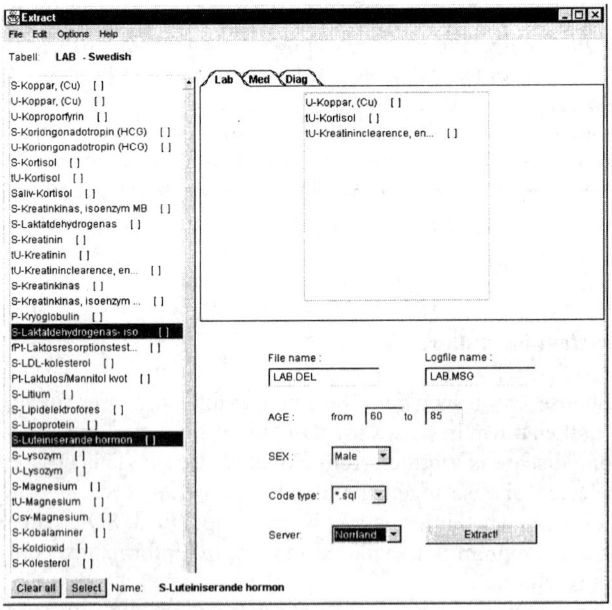

Figure 2

This system enables a user to browse and select various laboratory results, medicines and diagnoses. The application produces an SQL request that is exported to the data warehouse.

The prototype, written in Java, was developed earlier to fit another patient record environment, and JDBC capability is now being added.

Acknowledgements

This work is funded by the Foundation for Knowledge and Competence Development (KK-foundation, Sweden, http://www.kks.se) and is part of IT in health and health care within the area of IT-R&D. Research and development is related to work within the Centre for Medical Informatics and Telematics in Norrland, CMIT (http://www.cs.umu.se/~medinfo/cmit), covering health care IT needs in northern Sweden.

References

[1] Arnold, K., Gosling, J.: The Java™ Programming Language, Addison Wesley (1998)
[2] Banhart, F., Klaeren, H.: A Graphical Query Generator for Clinical Research Databases. Methods Inf Med, 34 (1995) 328-339
[3] van Bemmel, J., Musen, M.A. (eds.): Medical Informatics. Springer-Verlag, Berlin Heidelberg New York (1997)
[4] Ceusters, W., Spyns, P., De Moor, G., Martin, W. (eds.): Syntactic-Semantic Tagging of Medical Texts: The Multi-TALE Project. IOS Press, Amsterdam Berlin Oxford Tokyo Washington, DC (1998)
[5] Eklund, P., Forsström, J., Holm, A., Nyström, M., Selén, G.: Rule Generation as an Alternative to Knowledge Acquisition. Fuzzy Sets and Systems, 66 (1994) 195-205
[6] Eklund, P., Karlsson, J.: Data mining and structuring of executable data analysis reports: Guideline development and implementation in a narrow sense. Submitted.
[7] GALEN project. Home page URL: http://www.cs.man.ac.uk/mig/galen. (1997)
[8] HANSA project. Home page URL: http://www2.echo.lu/telematics/health/hansa.html. (1998)
[9] Karlsson, J.: A Generic System for Developing Medical Decision Support. Graduation thesis for MSc degree, UMNAD 232.98, Umeå University, Department of Computing Science (1998)
[10] Niinimäki, J., Selén, G., Kailajärvi, M., Grönroos, P., Irjala, K., Forsström, J.J.: Medical Data Warehouse, an Investment for Better Medical Care. In: Brender, J., et al. (eds.): Medical Informatics Europe '96. IOS Press (1996) 766-770
[11] Moorman, P.: Towards Formal Medical Reporting. Thesis. Erasmus Universiteit Rotterdam, (1995)
[12] Poon, A.D., Fagan, L.M., Shortliffe, E.H.: The PEN-Ivory Proj-ect: Exploring User-interface Design for the Selection of Items from Large Controlled Vocabularies of Medicine. JAMIA, 3 (1996) 168-183
[13] Rector, A.L (ed.): Terminology and Concept Representation (Theme Issue). Artif Intell Med, 15 no 1 (1999)
[14] Spriterm 2.01. The Swedish Institute for Health Service Devel-opment (December 1998)
[15] Strukturanalys 2000 (projekt). Västerbottens läns landsting. (1998)
[16] SYNAPSES project. Home page URL: http://www.cs.tcd.ie/synapses/public/index.html. (1997)
[17] Taira, R.K., Johnson, D.B., Bhushan, V., Rivera, M., Wong, C., Huang, L., Aberle, D.R., Greaves, M., Goldin, J.G.: A Concept-based Retrieval System for Thoracic Radiology. J Digit Imaging, 9 (1996) 25-36
[18] Weser, A.J., Kleinholz, L., Söderström, P.O., Eklund, P., De Moor, G., Williams, H., Venters, G., Mahr, B.: In: Brender, J., et al. (eds.): Co-operative Health Information Networks "CHIN". Medical Informatics Europe '96. IOS Press (1996) 1068-1072
[19] Woelk, G.B., Moyo, I.M.: Development of a Computerized In-formation System in the Harare City Health Department. Methods Inf Med, 34 (1995) 297-301

Medical Informatics Europe '99
P. Kokol et al. (Eds.)
IOS Press, 1999

Treatment of Missing Values with Imputation for the Analysis of Otologic Data

Jorma LAURIKKALA[a], Erna KENTALA[b], Martti JUHOLA[a], Ilmari PYYKKÖ[c]
[a] *Department of Computer Science, University of Tampere, P.O.Box 607, 33101 Tampere, Finland. E-mail: jpl@cs.uta.fi*
[b] *Department of Otorhinolaryngology, Helsinki University Hospital, Helsinki, Finland*
[c] *Department of Otorhinolaryngology, Karolinska Hospital, Stockholm, Sweden*

Abstract. Usefulness of imputation in the treatment of missing values in an otologic database was studied. Missing values were filled in with means (ME), regression (LR) and Expectation-Maximization (EM) imputation methods. A random imputation method (RA) provided baseline results. ME, LR and EM methods agreed on 41-42% of the imputed missing values. The level of agreement between these and RA method was 20-22%. Despite the moderate agreement, discriminant functions were similar and accurate (prediction accuracy 83-99%) for each diagnosis. A lot of data were missing in otoneurotologic tests which have less weight in the diagnosis of vertiginous patients. Consequently, the disagreement of the methods did not affect discriminant analysis. Imputation seems to be a useful method to treat missing data in this database, but future research requires more complete data and advanced imputation methods.
Keywords: Imputation; Missing data; Discriminant analysis; Otoneurology

1. Introduction

Missing data values are common in the medical data. One obvious source of incomplete information is the everyday diagnostic work, where some patients may be quickly diagnosed on the basis of symptoms, while in the hard cases, all available tests and measurements are needed to reach the diagnosis. A part of the data is not recorded sometimes, because it is considered unimportant. Data may also be lost because of haste or by omission. Incomplete data rarely hinders the diagnostic work-up, but when statistical analysis is considered, missing data values are often a major problem, because the standard multivariate analyses usually assume complete data.

Complete-case analysis [1] is a feasible solution when there are few missing values, but otherwise excluding incomplete cases may lead to a considerable loss of information and biased estimates. Available-case analysis [1] uses all cases where a variable is present, but analysis is difficult, since the number of available cases changes from variable to variable. Imputation [1,2] is a method where complete data is created by filling in the missing data values. The analysis of imputed data and the presentation of the results are easier in comparison to available-case analysis. The most serious drawback is the possible distortion of the associations between variables.

This study reports the initial work to treat missing values in otologic data with imputation methods. The usefulness of imputation was evaluated on the basis of the agreement level of the imputed values and the characteristics of the discriminant functions that were generated from the imputed data. The data were retrieved from the patient database of the otoneurologic expert system ONE [3] which is designed to help physicians in the diagnosis of diseases involving vertigo.

2. Materials and Methods

The database [3,4] was collected in the vestibular unit of the Helsinki University Hospital. We focused on the six largest patient groups with vertigo (*N*=564), these being vestibular schwannoma (*N*=128), benign positional vertigo (*N*=59), Meniere's disease (*N*=243), sudden deafness (*N*=21), traumatic vertigo (*N*=53) and vestibular neuritis (*N*=60) [5]. The 38 most important variables [6,7] were used in this study (see Table 1).

Table 1. Missing value frequencies of the 38 variables.

Variable	N	%	Variable	N	%
Age at first symptoms	11	2.0	Ear operation	134	23.8
Vertigo			Occurrence of head injury	21	3.7
- Duration of vertigo symptoms	7	1.2	- Head trauma	29	5.1
- Frequency of vertigo attacks	45	8.0	- Ear trauma	50	8.9
- Intensity of a vertigo attack	16	2.8	- Noise trauma	50	8.9
- Duration of a vertigo attack	49	8.7	Spontanic nystagmus test	136	24.1
- Score for rotational vertigo	32	5.7	Electronystagmography		
- Score for floating sensation	32	5.7	- Spontanic nystagmus	77	13.7
- Score for position induced vertigo	14	2.5	- Caloric asymmetry	48	8.5
- Unsteadiness	71	12.6	- Response with 44°C right	113	20.0
- Sudden falls	3	0.5	- Response with 44°C left	118	20.9
Hearing loss			Posturography		
- Duration of hearing loss	26	4.6	- Eyes open	105	18.6
- Type of hearing loss	428	75.9	- Eyes closed	105	18.6
- Hearing loss of right ear	38	6.7	Pursuit eye movements		
- Hearing loss of left ear	35	6.2	- Gain amplitude	86	15.2
- Fluctuation in hearing	203	36.0	- Gain latency	117	20.7
Tinnitus			Tone burst audiometry		
- Severity of tinnitus	14	2.5	- 500 Hz right	14	2.5
- Duration of tinnitus	31	5.5	- 500 Hz left	17	3.0
Severity of nausea	7	1.2	- 2000 Hz right	14	2.5
Lightheadedness	0	0	- 2000 Hz left	15	2.7
Ear illness	34	6.0			

The total of 11% of the data was missing. Type of hearing loss (75.9%), fluctuation in hearing (36.0%), spontanic nystagmus (24.1%) and ear operation (23.8%) variables had the most missing data. Also, otoneurotologic tests (electronystagmography, posturography and pursuit eye movements) had high missing value rates especially in vestibular schwannoma and Meniere's disease groups. These tests had 33% of all the missing values. Complete-case analysis was not clearly an option, because only 50 of all the 564 cases were complete. Data were missing due to unanswered questions, tests done only when diagnostic aid was expected and retrospective data collection (spontanic nystagmus test).

The data were repaired by the patient groups using means (ME), regression (LR) and Expectation-Maximization (EM) imputation methods. ME imputation [1,2] is a simple method where the missing values of a variable are replaced with the mean of available variable values. LR imputation [1,2] is a more sophisticated method which computes a linear regression equation of a given variable on the remaining variables and then uses the equation to impute the missing values. ME and LR imputation produce unbiased results only when the data are missing completely at random (MCAR) [1], i.e. the pattern of missing values does not depend on the data values. EM imputation [1,2] is a model-based iterative procedure which utilizes the principle of maximum likelihood to impute without bias when data are missing at random (MAR) [1]. MAR assumption holds if the pattern of missing data is related to the observed data only. Although we assume MAR, ME and LR imputation were applied, because these methods are still commonly used. In addition, the amount of missing data was moderate.

To provide baseline results, missing data values were filled in randomly (RA) with values selected with uniform probability from the value domain of the variable. Stepwise discriminant analysis was conducted with a data set containing 70% of the repaired data (N=388). The remaining data (N=176) formed a testing set which was used to evaluate the prediction accuracy of discriminant functions. The prediction accuracy ((correctly classified cases / all cases in the testing set)·100%) of the functions was calculated in the testing set using the discriminant function coefficients and the cut-off value obtained from analysis.

3. Results

ME, LR and EM methods agreed on 41-42% of imputed values and these methods produced the same values as RA method for 20-22% of missing values. Examination of the imputed values by the variables showed that the level of agreement decreased as the value range of a variable increased. The imputed values of the nominal variables, all of which were binary, had the highest level of agreement, the ordinal variables had a moderate level of agreement, and the mainly quantitative measurement, i.e. otoneurotologic tests and audiometry, related variables had the lowest level of agreement.

The prediction accuracies, true-positive (TP) and true-negative (TN) rates of the discriminant functions are shown in Table 2. TP rate = (TP cases / positive cases in the testing set)·100%. Similarly, TN rate = (TN cases / negative cases in the testing set)·100%. For each diagnosis, nearly all coefficients present in all the three discriminant functions, generated from the ME, LR and EM imputed data, had the same direction (i.e. sign). The only coefficient triplet that had contradictory directions was that of unsteadiness in the sudden deafness group. All coefficient pairs, i.e. coefficients present in two of the three functions, had the same direction.

Table 2. Prediction accuracies (A) in percents of the discriminant functions for the six otologic diseases. P=true-positive rate, N=true-negative rate, VS=vestibular schwannoma, BPV=benign positional vertigo, MEN=Meniere's disease, SUD=sudden deafness, TRV=traumatic vertigo, VN=vestibular neuritis.

Diagnosis	RA method			ME method			LR method			EM method		
	A	P	N	A	P	N	A	P	N	A	P	N
VS	94	91	95	98	98	98	96	93	97	95	95	95
BPV	92	94	91	94	100	94	94	100	93	95	100	94
MEN	90	87	92	98	99	97	92	92	91	92	96	90
SUD	88	56	89	85	33	87	88	56	90	83	33	86
TRV	97	100	97	99	100	99	99	100	99	99	100	99
VN	96	89	96	99	94	100	99	100	99	97	94	98
Mean	93	86	93	96	87	96	95	90	95	94	86	94

4. Discussion

The agreement among the ME, LR and EM imputation was only moderate (41-42%). Reason is most likely the differences in the imputation methods. ME and LR imputation assume that the data is MCAR, while EM imputation generates unbiased data under the less restrictive MAR assumption. When the value domain of an attribute was small, the methods had high agreement. As the number of possible values increased, it was more likely that the imputed values differed. Expectedly, the baseline method RA had a low level of agreement (20-22%) with the actual imputation methods. The functions generated from ME, LR and EM imputed data were highly accurate (92-99%) for all diagnoses, except sudden deafness (83-85%). The true-positive rate for sudden deafness diagnosis was especially low (33-56%). Discriminant analysis failed with this diagnosis probably due to the small number of cases. Traumatic vertigo was easiest to classify.

It may be reasonable to consider the results based on the EM imputed data as the most reliable, because EM method assumed that the data is MAR. The highest predictive accuracy of the functions obtained from the ME imputed data was as expected, because the multivariate analyses are known to often produce excessively accurate result with this type of data. However, the mean prediction accuracies were very close to one another, being 96%, 95% and 94% for ME, LR and EM imputed data, respectively. In addition, true-positive and true-negative rates differed clearly only for the sudden deafness diagnosis. This suggests that the functions obtained from the EM imputed data were quite similar to functions created from the ME and LR imputed data, even if the agreement between the imputed values was moderate. In addition, all but one coefficient triplet and all coefficient pairs had the same direction and a considerable number of the coefficients in the functions belonged to the triplets.

Contrary to expectations, the functions obtained from the RA imputed data were quite accurate having mean accuracy as high as 93% (88-97%). Also, Wilk's lambdas were significant ($p<0.01$) indicating that these functions were good. Furthermore, Kruskal-Wallis test revealed no significant ($p<0.01$) difference between the four prediction accuracy groups defined by the imputation methods. These results and the similarity of the discriminant functions suggest that at least part of the variables with the highest missing value rates were not crucial in the diagnostic work-up. Differences in the imputed data did not affect much the discriminant analysis, because less important diagnostic data were missing.

It is likely that the otoneurotologic tests were these less important data. A lot of test data (33%) were missing, and the imputed values of the measurement data had the lowest level of agreement. Also, few neurotologic tests related variables were present in the discriminant functions. These results are in accord with the earlier research suggesting that neurotologic and audiometric information is of minor importance in the diagnosis of six otologic diseases involving vertigo [5].

There are limitations to this study. Firstly, more reliable results could have been obtained, if we had had enough complete cases to create, at least, a complete testing data set. Secondly, application of several advanced imputation methods assuming MAR might have given better means to evaluate the usefulness of the ME and LR imputation methods. Thirdly, all methods imputed data having both qualitative and quantitative variables. In conclusion, imputation seems to be a useful method to deal with missing data in our otologic database, but future work should focus on the limitations discussed.

References

[1] R.J.A. Little and D.B. Rubin, Statistical Analysis with Missing Data. John Wiley & Sons, 1987.
[2] M.A. Hill, SPSS Missing Value Analysis 7.5. SPSS Inc., Chicago, 1997.
[3] E . Kentala, I. Pyykkö, Y. Auramo and M. Juhola, Otoneurological expert system, *Ann Otol Rhinol Laryngol* **105** (1996) 654-658.
[4] E. Kentala, I. Pyykkö, Y. Auramo and M. Juhola, Database for vertigo, *Otolaryngol Head Neck Surg* **112** (1995) 383-390.
[5] E. Kentala, Characteristics of six otologic diseases involving vertigo, *Am J Otol* (1996) 882-892.
[6] E. Kentala, J. Laurikkala, I. Pyykkö and M. Juhola, Discovering diagnostic rules from a neurotologic database with genetic algorithms, *Ann Otol Rhinol Laryngol.* (in press)
[7] E. Kentala, K. Viikki, I. Pyykkö and M. Juhola, Production of diagnostic rules from a neurotologic database with decision trees, *Ann Otol Rhinol Laryngol.* (accepted)

Medical Informatics Europe '99
P. Kokol et al. (Eds.)
IOS Press, 1999

Data Warehousing as a Tool for Quality Management in Oncology

S. Hölzer, A.G. Tafazzoli, U. Altmann, W. Wächter, J. Dudeck
Institute of Medical Informatics, Justus-Liebig-University Gießen,
Heinrich-Buff-Ring 44, D-35392 Gießen, Germany

Abstract: At present, physicians are constrained by their limited skills to integrate and understand the growing amount of electronic medical information. To handle, extract, integrate, analyse and take advantage of the gathered information regarding the quality of patient care, the concept of a data warehouse seems to be especially interesting in medicine. Medical data warehousing allows the physicians to take advantage of all the operational data they have been collecting over the years. Our purpose is to build a data warehouse in order to use all available information about cancer patients. We think that with the sensible use of this tool, there are economic benefits for the Society and an improvement of quality of medical care for patients.

Keywords: Data Warehouse, Analytical Processing, Quality Management, Oncology, Tumour Documentation, Medical Informatics

1. Introduction

The intelligent management of information is essential to the efficient operation of any large enterprise or institution. Particularly in the health care domain with its dynamically changing environment this management has become important to provide up-to-date patient care. The increasing use of computers by the medical profession as well as in the administrative area has led to large amounts of structured and unstructured, clinical and non-clinical data. To co-ordinate the flow of information and to distribute it adequately hospital information systems have been developed. On the other hand, the health professional has to perform more and better clinical work with stagnant resources. Our purpose is to build a data warehouse in order to use all available information about cancer patients. This tool seems to be especially beneficial to evaluate actual patient care and optimise the provided quality of care.

2. Material and Methods

In this context we intend to outline the general concept of a data warehouse, demonstrate its possible application in health care and medical research, and point out current problems. Subsequently, we explain the idea and give practical examples dealing with typical data of oncological patients as a very specialised category of medical data.
Medical knowledge is increasing very fast. Large amounts of clinical and non-clinical (e.g. administrative) data are routinely collected into computer systems and are available for analysis under certain conditions. This growing infrastructure can improve the

management of health care and the understanding of disease if adequate tools to extract relevant information are developed. At present, physicians are constrained by their limited skills to integrate and understand growing amount of electronic medical information. They lack an essential enzyme to digest this material. The volume of data is irrelevant if it isn't organised so that it adds value. Value to an organisation means turning data into actionable information. Value to a medical institution means turning data into information which can improve quality of patient care, understanding of disease, and economic use of resources. Data warehouses, a term of the business and financial world, manage large amounts of historical and reference data for decision making and reporting [1,2]. They consist of three major components. Tools to extract, transform and load operational and external data sources; a database to store and manage the data; and end-user tools to reference and analyse the data.

Information about patients, their medical history and disease specific items are collected at different levels, e.g. hospitals, general practitioners, clinical registries, epidemiological registries, pharmacies, health insurance companies, public health centres and so on. To gather this spread information is a big challenge. Only data available in a structured form can be useful for central analytical processing. Gaining access to previously unavailable information sources, building documentation facilities and infrastructure (e.g. hospital information systems, distributed electronic medical records) are first steps in creating a data warehouse. This means that the success of a data warehouse depends to a great extend on the quality of the underlying databases [3]. This informational system (data warehouse) is different from the operational systems such as e.g. hospital information systems. Our intention is to optimise the collection of data of oncological patients from various sources (operational systems) into our data warehouse. The management of tumour patients almost always includes a multicentric and interdisciplinary approach. This way, information from these patients is collected in the hospital by physicians of surgery, radiology, radiotherapy, pathology and by the administration (Admission, Discharge, Transfer). Other, external information comes from the above mentioned institutions. Tumour centres gather these information sources and transfer them to our central database. But the integration of medical data is still a big problem. There is no application consistency in encoding, key structure and naming convention. Some data exist in many places with different names; some data are labelled the same in different places but are still the same and some data are in the same places with the same name but reflect a different measurement of data ....

As data pass from the operational environment to the data warehouse environment, they are integrated.

3. Results and Discussion

Whereas at the institutional level (hospital) communication standards such as HL 7 or EDIFACT are well established, a data exchange format called BDT (abbreviation for the German word: Behandlungsdatenträger) exists at the level of ambulatory care in Germany. In order to facilitate in part this process of integration, an extension of this special data exchange format for oncological data was designed. A basic data set for cancer patients is also available in Germany (Basisdokumentation für Tumorkranke). On the basis of this Domain Information Model the above mentioned extension of the data exchange format was defined [4].

Thus we are able to easily collect the information deriving from operational databases of hospital departments, tumour registries and so on by using the standardised data exchange format. But the integration of other sources rests problematic. In a pilot project we are collecting data for patients with a special tumour (thyroid carcinoma) in cooperation with the Commission on Cancer of the American College of Surgeons in the United States: Information from both National Cancer Databases (NCDB in the US and Germany) plus data from cancer centres involved in this project are gathered. This way, we are combining information of cross-sectional studies and specially designed prospective studies. A data warehouse is time variant because it is associated with specific time periods [5]. The time horizon of our data is about 8 years. Data warehouse data is snapshots taken as of some moment in time. We load data in different cycles (monthly or annually). In medicine there is a strong need to have the relevant information topical and up-to-date. As more applications will come on-line in the future more frequent refresh cycles are possible. Following that, the concept of the data warehouse offers different ideas and techniques to manage and analyse data that make it especially useful for physicians.

As mentioned above, data warehouses are separated logically and physically from operational systems and optimised for the retrieval of information. It has the advantage to being accessible by health professionals on their own terms, regardless of their understanding of underlying data structures. The benefit consists of viewing the integrated data, of running large queries without impacting operational systems and of analysing "what if" scenarios. The analysis of time trends based on historical information is essential in medical research. For example, a gynecologist can recognise trends in breast cancer staging or shifts in the use of different treatments (surgery, radiotherapy, adjuvant chemotherapy ...). One can get clinical, epidemiological, social or even economic data of a geographic region, a period, a tumour stage selected for patients with certain risk factors or other conditions. This process is known as drilling down. Drill downs can continue until the user gets hold of the necessary information.

Data can also be sliced into user-defined views. This makes it possible to view and to work with it in multiple dimensions. This multidimensional database usually contains a star model which represents data as an array where each perspective is a subject around which analysis is performed. The data warehouse is oriented to the major subject areas that are in our case the patient or the quality of care for the patient. Getting the answer to typical questions from raw data of an oncological patient often requires such viewing from various perspectives. For example, a physician of nuclear medicine, treating patients with thyroid carcinoma, wants to know which groups of his patients (depending on histological type, stage, age, sex) get a real benefit (survival time, time of remission, post-treatment side effects and complications ...) of a selected therapy (applied radio-iodine activity, number of cycles ...). To overcome the constraints of small numbers of patients in the generated subgroups even for rare neoplasms, information sources of long term follow-up are combined with data of regional and time limited cross-sectional studies.

Additional options of a data warehouse include ranking, sorting, exception filtering and visualisation. At the information access layer we are using standard applications such as Microsoft Excel and SPSS statistical packages for analysing and visualisation. One has to take into account that the medical knowledge of associations between the parameters is complex and different sorts of bias increase the probability of misinterpretations. Open Database Connectivity (ODBC) and Standard Query Language (ORACLE and Microsoft ACCESS databases) are important components of the data access layer. But the technical details are not contents of this paper.

In the future we intend to organise our central tumour database to become a data warehouse with more and more up-to-date (online) and clinical relevant information. The development of features that will provide analysis, query, and reporting for the health professional to access useful information quickly and easily seems to be the most difficult and sophisticated step. Integrating more and more data of better quality from distributed sources will improve the validity of such a tool. Thus, data warehousing could become essential for the quality management in medicine [6-8].

4. Conclusion

Medical data warehousing allows the physicians to take advantage of all the operational data they have been collecting over the years. These data are a valuable corporate asset, yet seem seldom to be used strategically. The great value of analysing large quantity of medical information is to illuminate hidden problems and to point to their solutions. The interesting feature of data warehousing is its ability to provide the answers to questions not yet asked, by finding trends, patterns or anomalies in data. This feature could become very valuable in handling a growing amount of medical data. With its sensible use there are economic benefits for the Society and an improvement of quality of medical care for patients.

Acknowledgements

This project is supported by the German Federal Ministry of Health.

References

[1] Neil R. Technology Tutorial 1 - Data warehouse. *Information Week* 1996; No. 571
[2] Neil R. Technology Tutorial 2 - Data warehouse. *Information Week* 1996; No. 572
[3] Holthuis J, Muksch H, Reiser M. Das Data Warehouse Konzept - ein Überblick. *Wirtschaftsinformatik* 1996; 38: 421-433.
[4] Altmann, U, Wächter, W, Müller, A, Funken, O, Sembritzki, J, Lichtner, F, Gehlen, E, Dudeck, J. Datenaustausch in der Onkologie mittels BDT. *Medizinische Informatik, Biometrie und Epidemiologie.* Greiser,E, Wischnewsky, M (Editors) 1998, 83: 247-250.
[5] Mundy J. From the ground up: Building a data warehouse. *Sybase Server Magazine* Fall 1995
[6] Hölzer S, Dudeck J. Patient Care Evaluation Studies: Applying this concept of quality management in oncology. *Medical Informatics Europe* 1997; 834-838.
[7] Hölzer S, Dudeck J. Patient Care Evaluation Studien als Werkzeug der Qualitätssicherung in der Onkologie - Ist eine Übertragung auf Deutsche Verhältnisse möglich? *Biomedical Journal* 1998; 51:8-11.
[8] Hölzer, S, Dudeck, J., and Clive, R. Realising a Co-ordinated Approach to Quality Management in Oncology. Cesnik, B., McCray, A. T., and Scherrer, J. R. *MedInfo ,Proceedings of the Ninth World Congress on Medical Informatics* 1998, 890-890.

Medical Informatics Europe '99
P. Kokol et al. (Eds.)
IOS Press, 1999

Naive Bayesian-Based Nomogram for Prediction of Prostate Cancer Recurrence

Janez Demšar[1], Blaž Zupan[1,2], Michael W. Kattan[3], J. Robert Beck[4] and Ivan Bratko[1]

[1] Faculty of Computer Science, University of Ljubljana, Slovenia
[2] J. Stefan Institute, Ljubljana, Slovenia
[4] Memorial Sloan Kettering Cancer Center, New York, U.S.A.
[3] Baylor College of Medicine, Houston, U.S.A.

Abstract

This paper introduces a schema with naive-Bayesian classifier and patient weighting technique to develop a prostate cancer recurrence prediction model from patient data. We propose the graphical presentation of naive-Bayesian classifier with a nomogram, which can be used both for prediction or can provide means to data analysis. The resulting model was experimentally evaluated; the results were favorable both in terms of interpretability and predictive accuracy.

1 Introduction

In medicine, it is often required to use purposely collected data in order to construct models that either serve for prediction and support in medical decision making, or are used solely for data analysis. Machine learning offers various methods for efficient construction of descriptive models from data. At its best, the modern modeling technique should offer both: accuracy of the developed model and transparency so that the decision maker knows *why* and *how* the model derives the decision. Machine learning methods may support both perspectives, and are as such increasingly used in developing fields of Intelligent Medical Data Analysis [4] and Medical Data Mining [8].

When modeling is used for the survival analysis, specific mechanisms for proper treatment and modeling of the data are required. Namely, the survival data normally include the *censor* variable that indicates whether some outcome under observation (like death or recurrence of a disease) has occurred within some patient specific *follow-up time*. Therefore, the modeling technique has then to consider that for some patients the follow-up may end before the event occurs. This paper offers a solution to this problem by introducing a weighting technique that lowers the importance of patients with short follow-up time and for whom the event does not occur, i.e., the patients for which one know the event did not occur (yet) but does not know whether it will occur in the future.

The paper considers the survival analysis problem for prostate cancer recurrence after prostatectomy. For this problem, the physician is mainly interested if after the operation the cancer will recur, so that the survival analysis problem actually translates to the pure classification problem. This is in a sense different from classical survival analysis, which essentially estimates the probability of recurrence given the follow-up time, but as a consequence, this approach allows the use of broader range of classification-based machine learning techniques.

We propose the schema that uses naive Bayesian classifier to construct the model for prostate cancer recurrence prediction. Naive Bayes is one of the simplest but, surprisingly, one of the often most accurate machine learning predictors, especially for medical domains [3]. In order to appropriately use it for derivation of prognostic models for prostate cancer recurrence, we couple it with the above mentioned patient data weighting technique. We present the naive Bayesian predictor as a nomogram, and show how this can be used for prediction as well as for data analysis. To evaluate the quality of naive Bayes, we compare its performance with Cox proportional hazards model, a standard statistical method for survival analysis.

2 Methods

The approach presented in this paper incorporates three techniques. Example weighting is used to appropriately consider survival data when building classification models. We use naive Bayesian technique to induce the model from data, and represent the derived model graphically using the nomogram. Besides the physician's interpretation and validation of the model, three different statistics are used to assess the model's performance.

2.1 Example weighting

Survival analysis normally estimates the hazard for an event to occur or the expected time before the event occurs ("survival time" of an individual). From machine learning point of view, this is more a kind of regression problem, which we can turn into a classification problem by discretizing the class value: setting a limit T_f divides the examples into two classes – to those *surviving* the period T_f and those *failing* before that time.

The main difficulty with this approach is handling the *censoring* which is specific for survival data. There can be examples which are known to be "alive" at time $T_0 < T_f$, after which the trace of them was lost or they have failed for an unrelated reason. Statistical methods for survival analysis are time-aware and can take such examples into account till T_0 and ignore them afterwards. Machine learning methods cannot handle "disappearing examples". Skipping them completely could, on the other hand, significantly change the statistical properties of example set and influence the results [2, 6].

To cope with this, we weight the examples with the weights depending on the follow-up time and the class of the example. Failing examples and examples which are not censored before the time T_f are confident and have a weight of 1. Examples with follow-up times shorter that T_f ("disappearing examples") are assigned a follow-up time dependent weight $W(T)$, which monotonically increases from $W(0) = 0$ to $W(T_f) = 1$. We use the null Martingale residual (NMR) [7, 2], which is computed from the example set itself and is proportional to the risk of deceasing given only the follow-up time (and not the values of attributes). Intuitively, the lower the risk of recurrence, the more likely it is that the patient that is non-recurrent is also a good example for the patients that never recur. Thus, we weighted the non-recurrent patients with weights that were proportional to $1 - \text{NMR}$. We also assumed that the non-recurrent patients with follow-up time of more than 5 years never recur. The weights were linearly scaled so that a patient with hypothetical follow-up time of 0 would have a weight equal to 0, and a patient with a follow-up time of 5 years or more would have a weight equal to 1.

2.2 Naive Bayesian nomograms

The naive Bayesian classifier estimates the probabilities of classes for the given example by using the formula

$$P(r_k|V) = P(r_k) \prod_{i=1}^{n} \frac{P(r_k|v_i)}{P(r_k)}$$

where $P(r_k)$ is the priori probability of class r_k and $P(r_k|v_i)$ is the conditional probability of class r_k if i-th attribute has the value v_i; both are estimated from the training set of examples. Since the formula (naively) assumes the independence of attributes, the computed probabilities can be larger than 1 and do not necessarily sum to 1. If the naive Bayesian classifier is to be used as a class probability predictor, the probabilities must be normalized.

To get an explainable form of the classifier, we turn the product into a sum, by computing $\ln P(r_k|V)$ instead of $P(r_k|V)$.

$$\begin{aligned} \ln P(r_k|V) = \ln P(r_k) \quad &+ \quad \textstyle\sum_{i=1}^{n} \ln \frac{P(r_k|v_i)}{P(r_k)} \\ = B(r_k) \quad &+ \quad \textstyle\sum_{i=1}^{n} w_{k,i,v_i} \end{aligned}$$

In this form, each class r_k has its base probability, abbreviated by $B(r_k)$, which can be increased or decreased by different attributes, abbreviated by w_{k,i,v_i}. The value of w_{k,i,v_i} is positive if the probability of r_k after knowing that i-th attribute's values is v_i is greater than priori probability of r_k, and negative if it is smaller. Therefore each term of the sum can be interpreted as the weighted vote of the i-th predictor for or against the class r_k.

Values of w_{k,i,v_i} can be plotted in a *nomogram*. Nomogram consists of vertical bars, one bar for each attribute-class combination. Values w_{k,i,v_i} for all possible triples (k, i, v_i) are computed and plotted, with class k and attribute i selecting the bar, w_{k,i,v_i} is used as coordinate and v_i is printed as a label. If there are only two possible classes, the nomogram can be further simplified by using the two sides of the same bar for both classes, therefore having only one bar for each attribute.

Nomograms can also be used for predicting class or the probabilities of classes for a given example. The values of w_{k,i,v_i} for the chosen class and example's values of attributes must be summed, added to the base probability and, if probabilities and not just the most probable class are needed, exponentialized and normalized. Except for the summing and normalizing, the calculation can be done graphically, using a lookup graph tabulating the function $f_{r_k}(x) = e^{B(r_k)+x}$ for each r_k. An example of a nomogram is shown in Figure 1. Note that nomograms can be used to present the naive Bayesian classifier in general and not only when used in survival analysis.

2.3 Measuring the quality of models

To compare predictive accuracy of Cox proportional hazards model and naive Bayes, we used a standard technique of stratified 10-fold cross validation [5], which averages over 10 experiments, each time deriving and testing the model on different datasets. Given the patient's data, both models derived the probability of recurrence, where for Cox model the probability was estimated for the patients to recur within 5 years after the prostatectomy.

Three different quality measures are used. *Classification accuracy* (CA) is expressed in percent of patients in the test set that were classified correctly. A probability higher than 0.5 was considered as a prediction for a patient to recur. The examples are weighted, so that, if a surviving example with a short follow-up time is misclassified the error is smaller than in the case of misclassifying a surviving example with a long follow time.

Average probability assigned to the correct class (AP) averages the probability of recurrence assigned to the recurrent patients and probability of non-recurrence for non-recurrent patients in the test dataset. As for CA, the probabilities are weighted.

Another measure, *concordance index (CI)* [1], estimates the probability that, given two randomly drawn examples, the example which fails first is predicted a higher probability of failing. CI is computed from the testing data as the proportion of consistent example pairs over the set of usable example pairs. A pair is usable if the example with a shorter follow-up time fails (while the other example may fail later or not at all), and consistent if the example with a shorter follow-up time is assigned the higher probability of failing.

3 Experiments on prostate cancer recurrence data

The above ideas were tested on the prostate cancer recurrence data. We used the naive Bayes algorithm from the ML* package, which can handle weighted examples and supports adding new statistics, such as concordance index which has not been included in ML* before.

3.1 Patients data

We have used the data from 967 patients admitted to The Methodist Hospital (Houston, TX) with the intent to operate on their clinically localized prostate cancer between June 1983 and December 1996. The dataset used consists of the following routinely measured clinical variables as predictors of recurrence: pretreatment serum PSA levels (`prepsa`), primary (`bxgg1`) and secondary Gleason grade (`bxgg2`) in the biopsy specimen, and clinical stage assigned using the TNM system (`uicc`). Treatment failure was defined as either clinical evidence of cancer recurrence or an abnormal postoperative PSA (0.4 ng/ml and rising) on at least one additional evaluation. Of 967 patients, 189 (19.5%) recurred.

3.2 Nomogram

The nomogram in Figure 1, derived from naive Bayesian classifier, shows the impact of individual attributes on probability of recurrence (upper labels) and non-recurrence (lower labels). The values right of zero favor (non)recurrence and the values on the left speak against it. For example observe `bxgg2` and non-recurrence: values of 5 and 4 vote *against*, and values 3, 2, 1 vote *for* non-recurrence. The lookup graph below helps converting the sums of impacts of attributes to probabilities, again using the upper values for computing the recurrence and lower for non-recurrence.

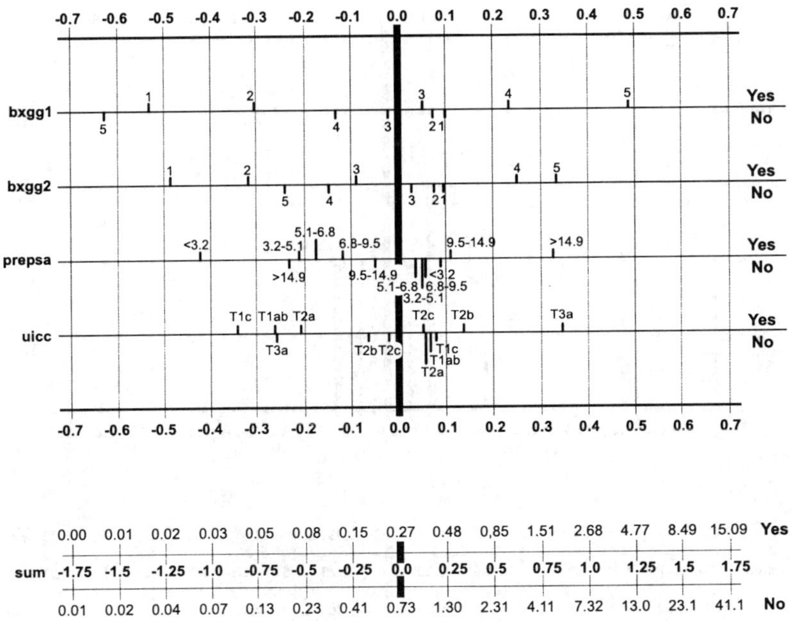

Figure 1: Nomogram showing the impacts of different values of attributes, derived from the probability estimates by naive Bayes

Figure 2 shows the use of the nomogram on a patient `(bxgg1=1, bxgg2=3, prepsa=11, uicc=T2a)`. The solid lines show the calculation for recurrence and the dotted for non-recurrence. Summing the values of impacts gives -0.54-0.09+0.11-0.21=-0.71 for recurrence and 0.1+0.03-0.05+0.05=0.13 against, from which we can already predict that the patient will not recur. Approximation by the lookup table gives "probabilities" of 0.06 for recurrence and 1 against, predicting the patient will not recur. Obtained probabilities should be normalized by multiplying by $(0.06+1)^{-1}$, which gives probabilities 0.057 for and 0.943 against recurrence.

3.3 Evaluation of the model

The performance of naive Bayesian classifier was compared with performance of the standard Cox model of proportional hazards. Results for different evaluation statistics are shown in Table 1. Overall, the performance of both modeling techniques is similar, with exception of weighted average probability assigned to the correct class, where Cox performance is significantly lower.

Table 1: Results of performance evaluation

modeling technique	weighted classification accuracy	weighted avg. prob. assigned to correct class	concordance index
naive Bayes	75.5	0.706	0.759
Cox	75.8	0.625	0.756
default	73.1	0.606	0.5

The "default" line shows the performance of a classifier which always predicts the majority class with its priori probability (in our case, it predicts non-recurrence with probability 0.731). An interesting point to be mentioned here is the fact that, judging only by classification accuracy, both methods seem to be useless since they do not predict much better than the default classifier. The other two criteria, especially

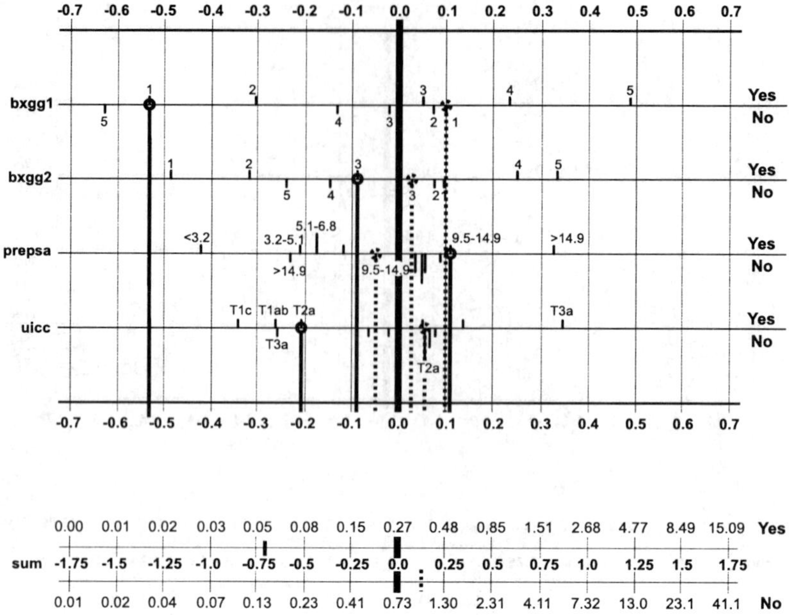

Figure 2: An example of computing probabilities of recurrence and non-recurrence from the nomogram. (Certain labels have been erased to increase the clarity of the figure.)

the concordance index, reveal a much better picture: although most of the patients are still classified as non-recurrent, both methods can successfully identify the patients with higher possibility of recurrence.

Another criteria for evaluation of a modeling technique is interpretability of the derived models and their concordance to the general knowledge. In case of naive Bayesian classifier nomogram reveals that the two Gleason scores are the most important factors for the decision as their values are most dispersed through the score line. In general, the impacts of attributes are as expected. The only anomaly occurs in `uicc`: `T1ab` would be expected to appear before `T1c` for recurrence and after `T1c` for non-recurrence. We believe that, while this anomalist is due to specific set of patients that were considered (sampling problem), it requires additional investigation on (preferably) different data set.

4 Conclusion

We have proposed the method to construct naive Bayesian-based nomogram from preoperative patient data for predicting the prostate cancer recurrence after prostatectomy. The experimental evaluation which used a patient data from The Methodist Hospital (Houston, TX) showed that the nomogram can be used both for data analysis and recurrence prediction. For the later, naive Bayes was favorably compared to Cox proportional hazards model.

The implications of this work may be two fold. First, the proposed schema can be used for general survival analysis problems when only the prediction of event, and not its time-dependent probability, is in question. Note that, besides naive Bayes, any classifier induction tool may be used that supports the inclusion of example weights. Second, the nomogram as a graphical device for presentation and utility can be used beyond survival analysis for any classification setup where naive Bayes is applicable.

Acknowledgment

Support for this work was provided by the Ministry of Science and Technology of Slovenia as a USA-Slovenia Cooperation in Science and Technology Grant, and by Developmental Support from Information Technology Program at Baylor College of Medicine.

References

[1] F. E. Harrell, R. M. Califf, D. B. Pryor, K. L. Lee, and R. A. Rosati. Evaluating the yield of medical tests. *Journal of American Medical Association*, 247(18):2543–2546, 1982.

[2] M. W. Kattan, H. Ishida, P. T. Scardino, and J. R. Beck. Applying a neural network to prostate cancer survival data. In N. Lavrač, E. Keravnou, and B. Zupan, editors, *Intelligent data analysis in medicine and pharmacology*, pages 295–306. Kluwer, Boston, 1997.

[3] I. Kononenko, I. Bratko, and M. Kukar. Application of machine learning to medical diagnosis. In *Machine Learning and Data Mining: Methods and Applications*, pages 389–408. John Wiley & Sons, Chichester, 1998.

[4] N. Lavrač, E. Keravnou, and B. Zupan, editors. *Intelligent data analysis in medicine and pharmacology*, Boston, 1997. Kluwer.

[5] D. Michie, D. J. Spiegelhalter, and C. C. Taylor, editors. *Machine learning, neural and statistical classification*. Ellis Horwood, 1994.

[6] B. D. Ripley and R. M. Ripley. Neural networks as statistical methods in survival analysis. In R. Dybowski and V. Gant, editors, *Artificial Neural Networks: Prospects for Medicine*. Landes Biosciences Publishers, 1998.

[7] T. M. Therneau, P. M. Grambsch, and T. R. Fleming. Martingale-based residuals for survival models. *Biometrika*, 77(1):147–160, 1990.

[8] B. Zupan, N. Lavrač, and E. Keravnou. Data mining techniques and applications in medicine (editorial). *Artificial Intelligence in Medicine*, 15, 1999 (in press).

Medical Informatics Europe '99
P. Kokol et al. (Eds.)
IOS Press, 1999

Increasing the Diversity of Medical Data Mining through Distributed Object Technology

Martin Holeňa[1], Anna Sochorová[1], Jana Zvárová[2]
Institute of Computer Science, Academy of Sciences, Prague (1),
Euromise, Charles University and Academy of Sciences, Prague (2)

Abstract. Data mining has been recently experiencing a boom of interest from researchers and software producers. In medicine, however, its applications are still rather rare. In this paper, we argue that this is primarily due to the requirements of reproducibility of results and diversity of available data mining tools, both of which are crucially important for medical research. We propose to tackle the diversity requirement by means of distributed object technologies. The results presented here rely on our experience with medical data mining using the method GUHA and with further developing that method.

1. Introduction

Some 15 years ago, the term *data mining* was used rather derogatorily, to denote a search for the best fitting model or the most significant hypothesis by trying a large number of models or hypotheses on the same body of data, not worrying about the requirement of reproducibility of the obtained results [6], [22]. In this paper, we argue that it is this requirement, together with the required diversity of data mining tools, that cause the still low acceptance of medical data mining, compared with the boom of interest data mining experiences in some other application domains such as marketing and finance [14], [23]. To deal with data mining in the context of those requirements is the objective of our paper. In the following two sections, the role of data mining in medicine is discussed, and our experience with medical data mining using the method GUHA is sketched. The last two sections then analyse the diversity requirement and its existing solutions, outlining the possible impact of that analysis on our prospective data mining strategy.

2. Role of data mining in medicine

Data mining is usually defined somehow like a *nontrivial search for interesting relationships and patterns hidden in data* with the aim of *knowledge discovery* from those data [4], [9], [10], [29]. In the context of medicine, it is important to note that the concept of *knowledge* is understood differently in data mining and in medical research:

- Medical research is mostly concerned with law-like, objectively valid knowledge. In some respect, the objective of each medical research study is to extend, detail or correct the existing medical knowledge, typically through confirming or refuting either some in advance postulated conjecture, or some already available piece of knowledge. To achieve an objective validity of the knowledge, all steps through which it can be established, including the performed data analysis, are required to be exactly *reproducible*.
- Data mining, in contrast, is concerned with knowledge about the data in a particular database or dataset. Though that knowledge is usually also established through

evaluating some hypotheses, with the purpose of confirming or rejecting them, these hypotheses are typically not postulated by humans, but are automatically generated during a search in a predefined hypotheses space [3], [14], [29], [34]. Due to the limitation to particular databases and datasets, data mining is not concerned about the reproducibility of results.

This comparison clearly shows that data mining is not able to substitute rigorous data analysis with respect to the cognitive task of medical research. On the other hand, it can be very well employed for the often tedious exploratory pre-processing of the data, which is needed especially in situations when the data have not been collected with any particular conjecture in mind, but simply as a result of an improved computer support of the health care process. It is this kind of data the amount of which has been growing most rapidly since hospital information systems came into use [7], [23]. In the context of exploratory data analysis, data mining can play a twofold role. First, some of its results can serve as conjectures for further research. Due to the exhaustive search that data mining methods perform, they can sometimes suggest interesting conjectures that would not be considered otherwise [21], [23]. Second, the high degree of automation inherent to data mining makes the initial exploratory analysis of the available data less time consuming, thus freeing the data analyst to focus on the ultimate confirmatory analysis [2], [14].

In addition, the importance of data mining for the management of hospitals and healthcare centres should be mentioned. It concerns mining data about costs and revenues, personal and material resources, quantity and quality of the provided care, bed occupancy etc. In this respect, data mining plays its more traditional role – to replace the overwhelming amount of data through a manageable number of association rules, classifications, fitted models and the like [4], [9], [18], [32].

3. Our own experience – the method GUHA

So far, we have tackled our medical data mining tasks using a sophisticated method called *General Unary Hypotheses Automaton (GUHA)*. It is one of the earliest methods for automated discovery of knowledge from data, theoretically elaborated and first implemented in the seventies [13]. However, it is only in the last years that, as the result of an increased performance of the ubiquitous personal computers, GUHA has found a broad acceptance, witnessed by more than a dozen new applications published since 1995.

Basically, GUHA relies on interconnecting logic and statistics. Such a connection, encountered also in the more recent data mining systems Explora and 49er [21], [34], allows to combine the strengths of both approaches:

- logic helps to reduce the complexity of the search for valid hypotheses;
- statistics helps to filter patterns inherent to the data from random influences or noise.

The interested readers are referred to the book [13] for the original GUHA method, and to [12], [15], [16], [27], [28] for its most important later extensions, developed under the participation of the present authors.

The hypotheses generated by GUHA are sentences of a *observational calculus*, for which *dichotomous data matrices* are used as *models*, which in turn are viewed as realizations of *random samples*. By means of common dichotomization transformations of nominal or ordinal features, GUHA can handle those kinds of features as well. *A monadic observational predicate calculus* (MOPC) is a collection of a finite number of *unary predicates*, and of an at most countable number of *generalized quantifiers*. From predicates, *open formulae* can be built by means of the usual connectives ¬, & and ∨, whereas generalized quantifiers yield *closed formulae* when applied to open formulae.

As an example, the following two sentences were among those output by GUHA in a research study of epilepsy, reported in [33]:

SEX = MALE & DISEASE DURATION > 10 YEARS & ONLY GRAND MAL SEIZURES $\sim^F$ MEMORY QUOTIENT > 90,

DISEASE DURATION > 10 YEARS & ONLY GRAND MAL SEIZURES & DISEASE COURSE = GOOD $\sim^F$ MEMORY QUOTIENT > 90.

Both sentences are closed formulae of a MOPC containing the unary predicates SEX = MALE, DISEASE DURATION > 10 YEARS, ONLY GRAND MAL SEIZURES, DISEASE COURSE = GOOD, and MEMORY QUOTIENT > 90. The first four of them are used to build the open formulae on the left side of the symbol $\sim^F$, denoting the *Fisher quantifier*. This generalized quantifier captures performing, on the considered data matrix, the one-sided Fisher exact test of independence in contingency tables. Its truth function is defined

$$\mathrm{Tr}_{\sim_F}(M) = \begin{cases} 1 & \text{if} \quad a_M \geq n_M s \;\&\; a_M d_M \geq b_M c_M \;\&\; \displaystyle\sum_{i=a_M}^{\min(r_M,k_M)} \frac{\binom{k_M}{i}\binom{l_M}{r_M - i}}{\binom{n_M}{r_M}} \leq \alpha \\ 0 & \text{else,} \end{cases}$$

where M is a two-column model, viewed as a realization of a random sample, a_M, b_M, c_M, d_M are cardinalities of occurrences of the vectors (1,1), (1,0), (0,1), (0,0), respectively, among the rows of M (i.e., $a_M + b_M + c_M + d_M = n_M$, where n_M is the sample size), $s \in (0,1]$ is a prescribed minimal support for a sentence to be generated, and $\alpha \in (0,½]$ is a given constant capturing the significance level of the test.

As a typical data mining method, GUHA tests each hypothesis separately. However, it can be combined with multiple hypotheses testing methods (e.g., Bonferroni, Hochberg, Holm, Shaffer, Simes) to arrive to sets of sentences valid at global or multiple significance levels.

Among the recent applications of GUHA, there were four belonging to the area of medical data mining:

- In the *biochemistry of cancer cells*, hypotheses generated by GUHA helped to elucidate some of the mechanisms driving the rise of metastases of a primary tumour [20].
- In a *clinical research of epilepsy*, GUHA was applied to search possible relationships of 13 clinical variables commonly used to characterize the disease to the occurrence of memory disturbances in epileptic patients [33].
- In a *preventive care screening study*, GUHA helped to find dependencies between the life style, the family history, and the state of health of first-year medical students [26].
- In the *psychotherapeutic medicine*, the GUHA method has been used to investigate the patterns of conflict episodes of clinically inconspicuous persons [25], which should serve as a control-group information for clinical research studies of various psychic diseases.

4. The diversity requirement and distributed object technologies

In the application domains in which data mining has been most successful so far, it typically has been used for some specific repeatedly performed task, such as analysing consumer behaviour, or proposing bank clients likely to take high credits [8], [24]. In medicine, the situation is completely different. Different research studies may lead to different data mining tasks (e.g., classification, clustering, association rules mining, sequence mining). Moreover, even in the case of a particular task, different methods may be appropriate (e.g., Bayesian classification, decision trees, or artificial neural networks in the case of classification).

Even large data mining suites (such as Decision Support Suite, Enterprise Miner, Intelligent Miner, or MineSet), besides being usually too expensive for the healthcare sector, do not implement every existing or newly emerging method. Therefore, successful application of data mining in medical research requires diverse data mining tools to be simultaneously accessible, or to be easily added if necessary.

A general solution to the diversity requirement provide distributed object technologies (DOTs), i.e. middleware technologies allowing clients to pass requests to objects implementing diverse data mining functionality in a distributed environment. Such a situation is schematically depicted in Figure 1.

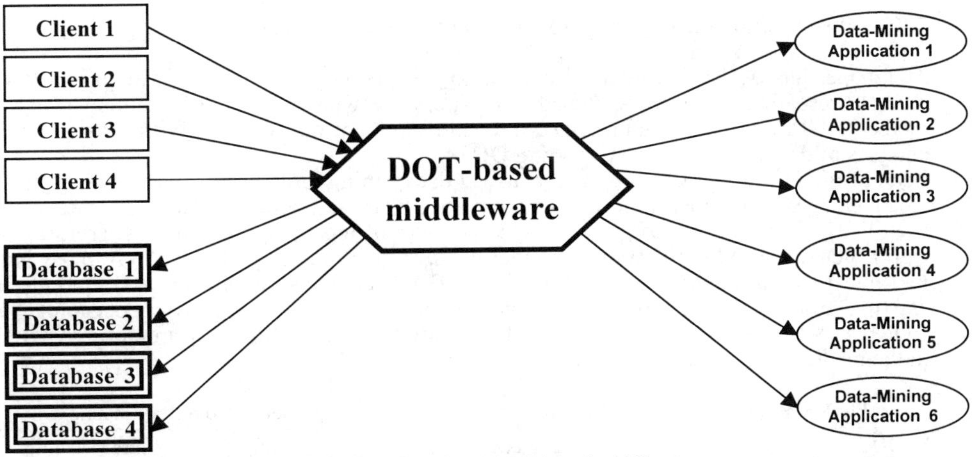

Figure 1: Data mining using a DOT-based middleware

Developers of data mining tools increasingly often realize the need for an underlying DOT, and they start providing their products with corresponding interfaces. Recently, we have performed a market analysis of available data mining tools supporting some DOT. The main results of that analysis are summarized in Table 1.

Table 1: Important data mining tools supporting distributed object technologies. Based on [1], [5], [11], [19], [30], [31] and the web pages of the producers.

data-mining tool	producer	supported DOT	basic feature(s)
ActiveSuite	Sheridan	ActiveX	concentrates on hierarchical data; mainly OLAP
Daisy (Data Analysis Interactively)	Daisy Analysis	ActiveX	conceived as an ActiveX component for interactive, mainly graphical, data analysis
Darwin / Spectrum	Thinking Machines / Cabletron	CORBA	the Darwin tool above the Spectrum data warehouse
Decision Centre	Imperial College / Fujitsu	CORBA, JavaBeans	both DOTs used to invoke data mining applications; databases accessed via JDBC
Decision Support Suite	Pilot Software	ActiveX	local / remote (in web) mining; mainly OLAP capabilities
DynamiCube	Hallogram	ActiveX	an ActiveX component; mainly OLAP capabilities
Expression / Sequence Explorer	Millenium Pharmaceuticals	CORBA	specialized for RNA expression + DNA sequence mining
Infosleuth	MCC	CORBA, JavaBeans	data mining agent – one of many agents, which are invoked either via RMI, or via CORBA
JWAVE	Visual Numerics	JavaBeans	PV-WAVE applications for data mining and visualisation
KnowledgeStudio	Angoss	ActiveX	8 own methods + bi-directional interface to SAS
OASIS	UCLA Data Mining Laboratory	CORBA	for mining scientific data; Java GUI above CORBA
ONISA	Frauenhofer Computer Graphics Institute	CORBA	CORBA-based metaserver routes data mining requests to database servers
SuperNova	Meditech	ActiveX	only simple data mining, but specialized for medicine
VisualAge	IBM	JavaBeans	for data mining against DB2 Universal Databases
XpertRule	Attar Software	ActiveX	association rules and decision trees; SQL client-server

5. Conclusion and consequences for our data mining strategy

This paper has dealt with medical data mining in the context of specific requirements of medical research. We have sketched our experience with medical data mining using the method GUHA and have summarized the main results of our recent comprehensive market analysis of data mining tools supporting DOTs.
Each of the DOTs supported by the analysed data mining tools has its own advantages and disadvantages. The most important of them are juxtaposed below in Table 2. Observe that each DOT allows access to quite a large spectrum of legacy applications. Therefore, they can be actually used with a much broader class of data mining tools than only those listed in Table 1. In particular, we want to use CORBA to enable simultaneous access to GUHA and two tools based on artificial neural networks and fuzzy logic. Our decision to use CORBA as the underlying DOT is due to our previous engagement in promoting CORBA in the medical domain [17].

Table 2: Main pros and contras of the distributed object technologies supported by data mining tools.

DOT	advantages	disadvantages
ActiveX	easy to use, access to all applications supporting OLE (often encountered in the medical domain)	not fully object-oriented, proprietary
CORBA	fully object-oriented, medical standardization (CORBAmed) access to applications in IDL-mapped languages (C, C++, Java...),	complex, little support by important software producers
JavaBeans	fully object-oriented, access to all Java applications + to CORBA applications via the Java-IDL mapping	dependent on the Java language, complex

References

[1] A. Al-Attar. Data mining – beyond algorithms. Technical report, Attar Software, 1998.
[2] C. Chatfield. Model uncertainty, data mining and statistical inference. Journal of the Royal Statistical Society. Series A, 158:419–466, 1995.
[3] P. Cheeseman and J. Stutz. Bayesian classification (autoclass): Theory and results. In [8], pages 153–180.
[4] M.S. Chen, J. Han, and P.S. Yu. Data mining: An overview from a database perspective. IEEE Transactions on Knowledge and Data Engineering, 8:866–883, 1996.
[5] T. Clark. Response to CORBAmed life sciences research request for information. Technical report, Millenium Pharmaceuticals, Inc., 1997.
[6] F.T. Denton. Data mining as an industry. The Review of Economics and Statistics, 67:124–127, 1985.
[7] J. Dudeck, B. Blobel, W. Lordieck, and T. Bürkle, editors. New Technologies in Hospital Information Systems. IOS Press, Amsterdam, 1997.
[8] U.M. Fayyad, G. Piatetsky-Shapiro, P. Smyth, and R. Uthurusamy, editors. Advances in Knowledge Discovery and Data Mining. AAAI Press, Menlo Park, 1996.
[9] U.M. Fayyad, G. Piatetsky-Shapiro, and P. Smyth. From data mining to knowledge discovery: An overview. In [8], pages 1–36.
[10] W.J. Frawley, G. Piatetsky-Shapiro, and C.J. Matheus. Knowledge discovery in databases: An overview. In G. Piatetsky-Shapiro and W. Frawley, editors, Knowledge Discovery in Databases, pages 1–27. AAAI Press, Menlo Park, 1991.
[11] Y. Guo, D. Yang, and S. Hedvall. Software architecture for DecisionCentre: A web-based distributed data mining system. Technical report, Imperial College London, 1998.
[12] P. Hájek. The new version of the GUHA procedure ASSOC (generating hypotheses on associations) – mathematical foundations. In COMPSTAT 1984 – Proceedings in Computational Statistics, pages 360–365, 1984.
[13] P. Hájek and T. Havránek. Mechanizing Hypothesis Formation. Springer-Verlag, Berlin, 1978.
[14] D. Harmancová, M. Holeňa, and A. Sochorová. Overview of the GUHA method for automating knowledge discovery in statistical data sets. In [24], pages 39–52.
[15] M. Holeňa. Exploratory data processing using a fuzzy generalization of the GUHA approach. In J.F. Baldwin, editor, Fuzzy Logic, pages 213–229. John Wiley and Sons, New York, 1996.
[16] M. Holeňa. Fuzzy hypotheses for GUHA implications. Fuzzy Sets and Systems, 98:101–125, 1998.

[17] M. Holeňa and B. Blobel. Healthcare information system approaches based on middleware concepts. In [7], pages 178–185.
[18] M. Holsheimer and A. Siebes. Data mining. The search for knowledge in databases. Technical report, CWI, Amsterdam, 1994.
[19] M. Jern. Information drill-down using web tools. Technical report, Advanced Visual Systems, 1998.
[20] J. Kaušitz, P. Kulliffay, B. Puterová, and L. Pecen. Prognostic meaning of cystolic concentrations of ER, PS2, Cath-D, TPS, TK and cAMP in primary breast carcinomas for patient risk estimation and therapy selection. To appear in International Journal of Human Tumor Markers.
[21] W. Klösgen. Explora: A multipattern and multistrategy discovery assistant. In [8], pages 249–272.
[22] M.C. Lovell. Data mining. The Review of Economics and Statistics, 65:1–12, 1983.
[23] N. Lavrac, E.T. Keravnou, and B. Zupan. Intelligent data analysis in medicine and pharmacology. Proceedings of the First International Workshop. Kluwer Academic Publishers, Dordrecht, 1996.
[24] M. Noirhomme-Fraiture, editor. Proceedings of KESDA'98 – International Conference on Knowledge Extraction from Statistical Data, 1998.
[25] D. Pokorný and A. Sochorová. Do we use stereotypes in our relationship to the others? Technical report, Dept. of Psychotherapy, University of Ulm, 1996.
[26] H. Provazníková, N. Štullerová, and J. Štullcr. Health and options in preventive care for first year students at the 3rd medical faculty of Charles University in Prague. To appear in Journal of American College Health.
[27] J. Rauch. Logical problems of statistical data analysis in data bases. In Proceedings of the Eleventh International Seminar on Data Base Management Systems, pages 53–63, 1988.
[28] J. Rauch. Logical calculi for knowledge discovery in databases. In J. Komorowski and J. Żytkov, editors, Principles of Data Mining and Knowledge Discovery, pages 47–57. Springer-Verlag, Berlin, 1997.
[29] A. Siebes. KESO: data mining and statistics. In [24], pages 1–13.
[30] M.A. Sokolewicz. ONISA: The open networked information system architecture. Technical report, Frauenhofer Computer Graphics Institute, 1998.
[31] Visual Numerics, Inc. JWAVE System Introduction, 1998.
[32] M.J. Zaki, S. Parathasarathy, M. Ogihara, and W. Li. New parallel algorithms for fast discovery of association rules. Data Mining and Knowledge Discovery, 1:343–373, 1997.
[33] J. Zvárová, J. Preiss, and A. Sochorová. Analysis of data about epileptic patients using GUHA method. International Journal of Medical Informatics, 45:59–64, 1997.
[34] J.M. Żytkov and R. Zembowicz. Contingency tables as the foundation for concepts, concept hierarchies and rules: The 49er system approach. Fundamenta Informaticae, 30:383–399, 1997.

Medical Informatics Europe '99
P. Kokol et al. (Eds.)
IOS Press, 1999

Outpatient Health Care Statistics Data warehouse - logical design

Srečko Natek
Vizija d.o.o., Ljubljanska 42, Celje, Slovenia

Abstract. Outpatient Health Care Statistics on a state level is a central point where all relevant statistic data are collected from various sources from all over the country. Various and complex requirements for processing and reporting data makes Outpatient Health Care Statistics on a state level a perfect example for efficient implementing of Data warehouse technology. The research investigates logical design of data warehouse with a special attention on a different data modeling technique in various phases of a logical data warehouse design. The research shows that a requirement for processing statistical data determines the design decision and thus the scope and semantic value of final data warehouse.

Keywords
Data Warehousing, Health Care Statistics, Health Care Information System

1 Introduction

Outpatient Health Care Statistics on a state level depends on the data that come from all health care centers, physicians and other institutions on a primary health care level in Slovenia. To ensure statistic data integrity, coming from a different health care software applications, several requirements were defined by Institute of Public Health of the Republic of Slovenia, including data structure for reporting about Disease and Conditions for Outpatient Health Care. To ensure cost effective solution for Outpatient Health Care Statistics on a state level, the following technology was employed: floppy disks for data transfer, Paradox for data store and Delphi application is used to merge data from different providers and for basic statistical and reporting purposes. The project which developed and implemented the solution for Outpatient Health Care Statistics offered some excellent results. **But is it possible to make it perfect?** This questions was the major challenge of our research. Is it possible to employ the latest data warehouse and OLAP technology and the very latest data warehouse design techniques, to create a better solution?

Knowing the existing solution very well, due to being involved in designing and implementing it, having in mind the existing market of data warehouse technology and the latest design technique, we made the following initial hypotheses:

1. It is possible to make a better OLAP solution without changing data transfer structure; changing data transfer structure to the lowest level of details could further more improve the solutions, but on a higher cost level.
2. Microsoft SQL Server 7.0 with included data warehouse OLAP technology is the suitable technology for our solution.

The research was divided into two parts. The first part investigates the differences in designing data models for logical, data transfer and data warehouse purposes. The differences, designing decisions, possible results are discussed and the first hypothesis was confirmed. The second part covers the implementation phases of designed data warehouse with special attention on data transformations and physical design. The second hypothesis was also confirmed. The second part of research was described by Dejan Zilli: Outpatient Health Care Statistics Data warehouse – implementation.

2 Logical data model for Outpatient Health Care Statistics for Diseases and Conditions

Logical data model for Outpatient Health Care Statistics for Diseases and Conditions reflects the real world medicine entities on a primary level. Picture 1 shows the most complex logical data model without technology limitations. The model simply explains that Outpatient Health Care Statistics for Diseases and Conditions need data (instances of diseases and conditions) assigned to the reporting period (twice a year: the first half of the year and then the whole year), community of the provider (territory dimension), reporting unit (from national data base), basic activity (e.g. general medicine etc.), specialty / field (pediatric specialty), type of diagnosis (draft diagnosis and final diagnosis), diagnosis classification (ICD–10 code, also for injuries at work), external cause (also ICD-10 code), age (group and category), sex, insurance category (e.g. workers etc.) and duration of pregnancy (valid only for some ICD-10 groups).

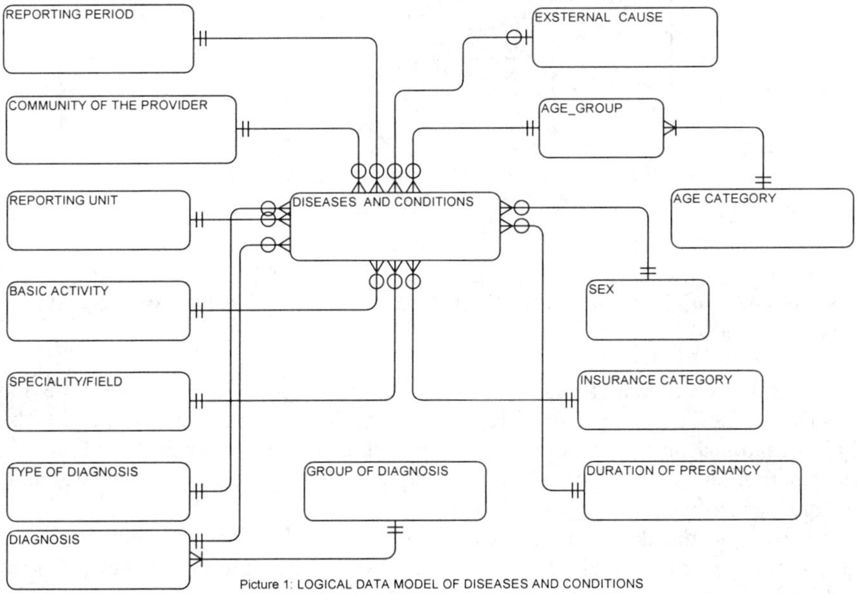

Picture 1: LOGICAL DATA MODEL OF DISEASES AND CONDITIONS

3 Data transfer model for Outpatient Health Care Statistics for Diseases and Conditions

Data transfer data model, presented in Picture 2, documents the existing standard data structure. The designer of the model made some important decisions, which were necessary in order to achieve cost effective solutions without employing data warehouse technology. Unfortunately the designers did not follow any international data standard like HL-7. Data structure follows technical limitations of floppy disk data transfer and tries to minimize the volume of data in data transfer and later data store phases. In any way the electronic data transfer should replace the existing floppy data transfer. The most important differences in compare with the most complex logical model in Picture 1 are:

- the primary key is not assigned to all referential entities of the logical model, thus the level of details is higher than in the logical model; the designer decided that the age / sex, insurance category, injuries at work and pregnancy duration do not interact in such extend that the lowest level of detail is necessary for statistical purposes;
- the age group in conjunction with sex, insurance category, injuries at work and pregnancy duration instances became attributes, dependent on reporting period, community, reporting unit, basic activity, specialty / field, type of diagnosis, diagnosis and external cause;
- the group of diagnosis is implemented as an redundant attribute.

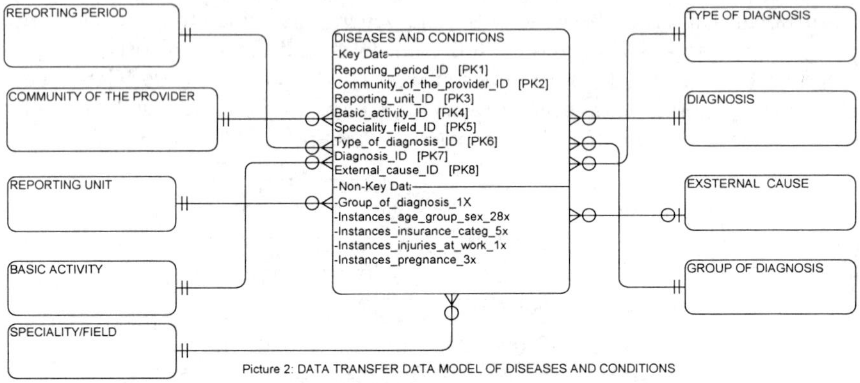

Picture 2: DATA TRANSFER DATA MODEL OF DISEASES AND CONDITIONS

4 Data warehouse models for Outpatient Health Care Statistics for diseases and conditions

Logical data warehouse design follows several design principles [4]. The most important design criteria is the usage of data warehouse. This is a semantic principle which is mainly concentrated on the question of **how detailed the data warehouse should be?** The answer determine the amount of data we expect and the amount of data warehouse development effort, as well as operational costs.

In our example the designer decided that the lowest level of possible details (see picture 1) is not needed. Therefore data transfer data model employs some previously mentioned limitations and thus produces higher granularity. Without described limitations a designer should accept the logical data model on the lowest detailed level as the data warehouse model. In this case all current answers and of course all detailed ones impossible with the current solution, would be possible from such data warehouse. A different data transfer model from the existing one should be accordingly designed. Another data transfer and data warehouse technology should be employed on a bigger amount of data and, of course, on a higher cost level. This research tries to overcome some of the problems, caused by the disintegration of data warehouse to four schemes and later four OLAP cubes, by designing and implementing a OLAP virtual cube, which is described in detail in the second part of the research.

On the assumption that no improvement in the final requirements are needed and that the existing data transfer model is the optimum solution, the following data warehouse and OLAP design should be appropriate for our solution. Because of special design principles of data warehouse where star and snowflake structure [4] are the optimum data models, four snowflake data models were designed:

- Four models are needed for optimum OLAP possibilities [2,6,7]. Common data warehouse can not be defined from existing data transfer model, because the lovest detailed level was lost by purpose.
- All four models have similar fact tables, where primary key is compound from several standard dimensions: the reporting period, community of the provider, reporting unit, basic activity, specialty / field, type of diagnosis, diagnosis code, group of diagnosis and the external cause (mandatory only in the picture 6: injuries at work, in all other cases external cause is present only for a certain diagnosis code which represents injuries at work).
- All fact tables consists of numeric attributes, continuously valued and additive across time [4].
- Some shared dimensions have further level of hierarchy: the reporting period (calendar hierarchy: half of the year/ year), reporting unit (organizational hierarchy) and diagnosis (group of diagnosis).
- All four models are basically star schema, except the group of diagnoses connected with the diagnosis and the age group connected with the age category – snowflake schema.
- All four models have only one attribute – "instances" according to the primary key.
- All four models share common dimensions.
- Beside common – shared dimensions 3 models employ special dimensions: in picture 3 the age_group and sex, in picture 4 the insurance category and in picture 5 the duration_of_pregnancy.
- Nearly all of the described dimensions are basically slowly changing dimensions [4] which means that they are slowly changing over the time. The research incorporates the simplest method of solving the problems, namely overwriting the old values with losing the ability to track the history. If the decision maker requests a more precise solution, the data warehouse model can be promoted to such capabilities, following the well known techniques [4].

Picture 3 describes a 1. data warehouse model in which instances are dependent on common – shared dimensions together with age groups and sex dimensions. Age dimensions have a further level of hierarchy – the age category.

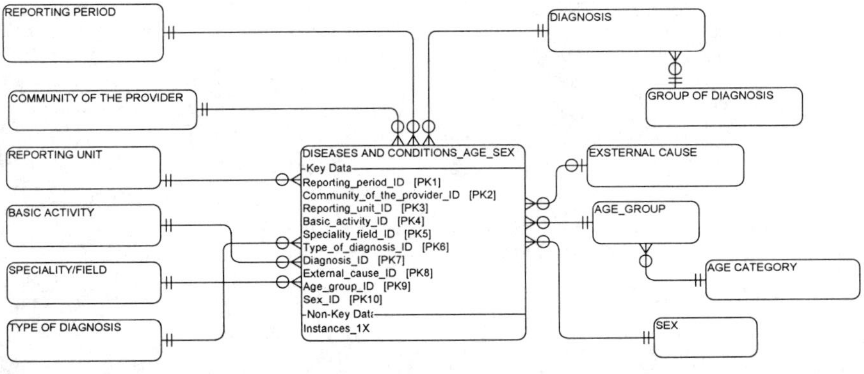

Picture3: DATA WAREHOUSE MODEL OF DISEASES AND CONDITIONS BY AGE AND SEX

The 2. data warehouse model is similar to the one from picture 3, but instances depend on common – shared dimensions, together with the insurance category.

The 3. data warehouse model is similar to one from picture 3, but instances depend on common – shared dimensions together with the duration of pregnancy. Of course there is a semantic question if an external cause is really connected with a diagnosis or not.

The 4. data warehouse data model is similar to one from picture 3, but instances depend only on common – shared dimensions, but the diagnosis covers only injuries at work.

After the data warehouse and OLAP cubes were built, using SQL 7.0 technology, the Excel 2000 was used as client for statistical and data retrieval analysis. The capability of the system easily support all existing statistical analysis and far more. So the end user should benefit from OLAP solution.

5 Conclusion

The results of the research clearly confirm both hypotheses. Better solutions can be designed and implemented to fulfill all of the goals of a data warehouse [4]: provide access to statistical data on national level, ensure consistent data and combine all the data in such a warehouse. In addition the Microsoft data warehouse technology SQL 7.0 with its OLAP capabilities are confirmed. So data are stored for all statistical purposes to effectively support the Ministry of Health in managing the Health care national policy.

References

[1] Anahory S., Murray D.: Data warehouse in the real world, Addison Wesley, 1997
[2] Inmon W.H., Welch J.D., Glassey K.L.: Managing the Data Warehouse, John Wiley & Sons, Inc., 1979
[3] Inmon W.H.: Building the Data Warehouse, 2.ed. Wiley, 1996
[4] Kimball Ralph: The Data Warehouse Toolkit, John Wiley & Sons, Inc. 1996
[5] Microsoft Corporation, The Microsoft Data Warehousing Strategy: A platform for improved decision-making through easier data access and analysis, USA, 1998
[6] Microsoft Corporation, Microsoft SQL 7.0 Decision Support Services: Lowering the Cost of Business Intelligence, USA, 1998
[7] Microsoft Corporation: http://www.microsoft.com/sql/beta : Microsoft SQL Server 7.0
[8] Silverston L., Inmon W.H., Graziano K.: The Data Model Resource Book, Wiley, 1997
[9] Zilli D.: Outpatient Health Care Statistics Data warehouse – implementation, MIE 99
[10] Willcocks L.P., Feeny D.F., Islei G.: Managing IT as a Strategic Resource, The McGraw-Hill, 1997
[11] Berndt D.J.: A data warehouse to support comprehensive assessment for tracking community health, Proc Amia Symp. 1998, 250-4

Medical Informatics Europe '99
P. Kokol et al. (Eds.)
IOS Press, 1999

Applying Data Mining in Healthcare: An Info-Structure for Delivering 'Data-Driven' Strategic Services

Syed Sibte Raza ABIDI
Health Informatics Research Group, School of Computer Sciences, Universiti Sains Malaysia, 11800 Penang, Malaysia

Abstract. Presently, there is a growing demand from the healthcare community to leverage upon and transform the vast quantities of healthcare data into value-added, 'decision-quality' knowledge, vis-à-vis, *strategic knowledge services* oriented towards healthcare management and planning. To meet this end, we present a *Strategic Knowledge Services Info-structure* that leverages on existing healthcare knowledge/data bases to derive decision-quality knowledge—knowledge that is extracted from healthcare data through services akin to *knowledge discovery in databases and data mining*.

1. Introduction

Prime facie, the healthcare enterprise—say hospitals, clinics community centres, etc.—is 'data rich' but 'knowledge poor'. The prevailing scenario is that IT based healthcare systems are consistently churning out volumes of healthcare data; the data may be superficially or partially introspected and exploited by humans for limited and visible intents and purposes; and finally the data is stored in data warehouses either for record keeping or in anticipation of any future use. What is apparent here is that there is a lack of judgement amongst healthcare practitioners with regards to the 'hidden' potential of healthcare data. Thus, there is a strong case for operationalising the seemingly placid healthcare data in to 'health enterprise knowledge', which can then be used for strategic decision making, for instance to abet the planning of healthcare delivery.

The above proposal is not alien to the healthcare industry; one such process that the healthcare industry is well aware of is 'Outcomes Measurement'—a means of searching, or more appropriately 'mining', for previously unknown, actionable information/knowledge from large health databases. By understanding what worked—or did not work—healthcare providers are then able to identify areas for improvement or capitalise on successful methods [1].

In this paper we propose a *Strategic Knowledge Services (SKS) Info-structure* that leverages on existing healthcare data bases to derive decision-quality knowledge—knowledge that is extracted from healthcare data through services akin to *knowledge discovery in databases and data mining* [2] [3]. Here, we will discuss the architectural blueprint of the proposed *SKS Info-structure.* We conclude that the proposed SKS info-structure can add value to routinely collected patient level data and can therefore serve as a management resource to healthcare administrators and policy makers.

2. Introducing Strategic Knowledge Services

Strategic Knowledge Services (SKS) can best be defined as a suite of data-driven strategic services—based on knowledge discovery and data mining techniques—to facilitate the derivation (or extraction) of 'decision-quality' information/knowledge from (a) nation-wide healthcare databases and (b) the health enterprise's knowledge bases, thereby leading to the delivery of value-added, focused and pro-active healthcare services.

Typical SKS may include: data mining for helping health-care providers cut costs and improve care is by showing which treatments statistically have been most effective; benchmarking for knowing how various physicians and hospitals compare with their peers; outcomes measurement to identify people statistically at risk for certain ailments so that they can be treated before the condition escalates into something expensive and potentially fatal; trend analysis of diseases/epidemics [4] [5], treatment patterns, hospital admissions, drug patterns and so on; what-if scenario analysis; comparing medical practices (of a segment of practitioners) with medical business rules; market research; point-of-need generation of statistics; publication of regulatory and best-practices reports; feedback routing to R&D institutions (e.g. drug effectiveness on outcomes of treatment); analysis for healthcare financing; data analysis for formulating health policies and planning; data analysis for epidemiological or health surveillance; examining resource allocations and so on [6].

3. Architecture of the SKS Info-Structure

Our proposed SKS info-structure manifests a suite of 'modules' that facilitate the transformation of data to knowledge to wisdom. Conceptually, the SKS info-structure has a multi-tier architecture that effectuates a confluence of knowledge management and data mining techniques. Figure 1 gives an overview of the 4-tier architecture of the proposed SKS info-structure.

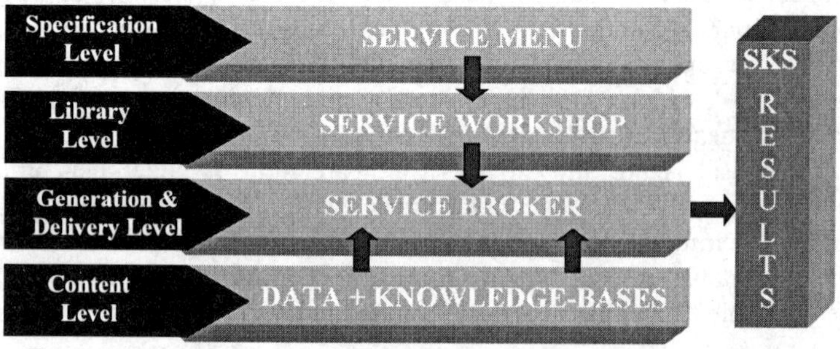

Figure 1: An overview of the multi-tier architecture of the SKS info-structure

In procedural terms, the scheme for the provision SKS is quite simple: (1) specification of the user's desired strategic service(s); (2) procurement of the necessary knowledge and methods (in terms of SKS modules) relevant to the SKS's specification; (3) generating the specified strategic service by the systematic manipulation of the SKS modules in concert with data and knowledge from the data and knowledge repositories; and finally (4) the delivery of the SKS results to users [7].

The SKS info-structure can be visualised as having four distinct levels, characterised by the roles/aspects pertaining to the overall processes underlying the generation and delivery of SKS. The top level—the *Specification Level*—is responsible for the specification of a particular SKS by users. The second level—the *Library Level*—stores knowledge pertinent to the provision of a variety of SKS; each designated SKS is stored as a specific *SKS module* (encapsulating the processing methods and knowledge). Next, the third level—the *Generation & Delivery Level*—is the main workplace (i.e. the info-structure's engine) where the strategic services are generated by the execution of the SKS modules (as per their processing script) in tandem with pertinent data and knowledge drawn from a variety of databases and knowledge-bases. The results/findings/conclusions/ recommendations of the concluded SKS are then delivered to the users. Finally, the *Content Layer* houses the enterprise-wide data and knowledge stored in one or more databases and knowledge-bases. Figure 2 gives the architecture of the SKS info-structure.

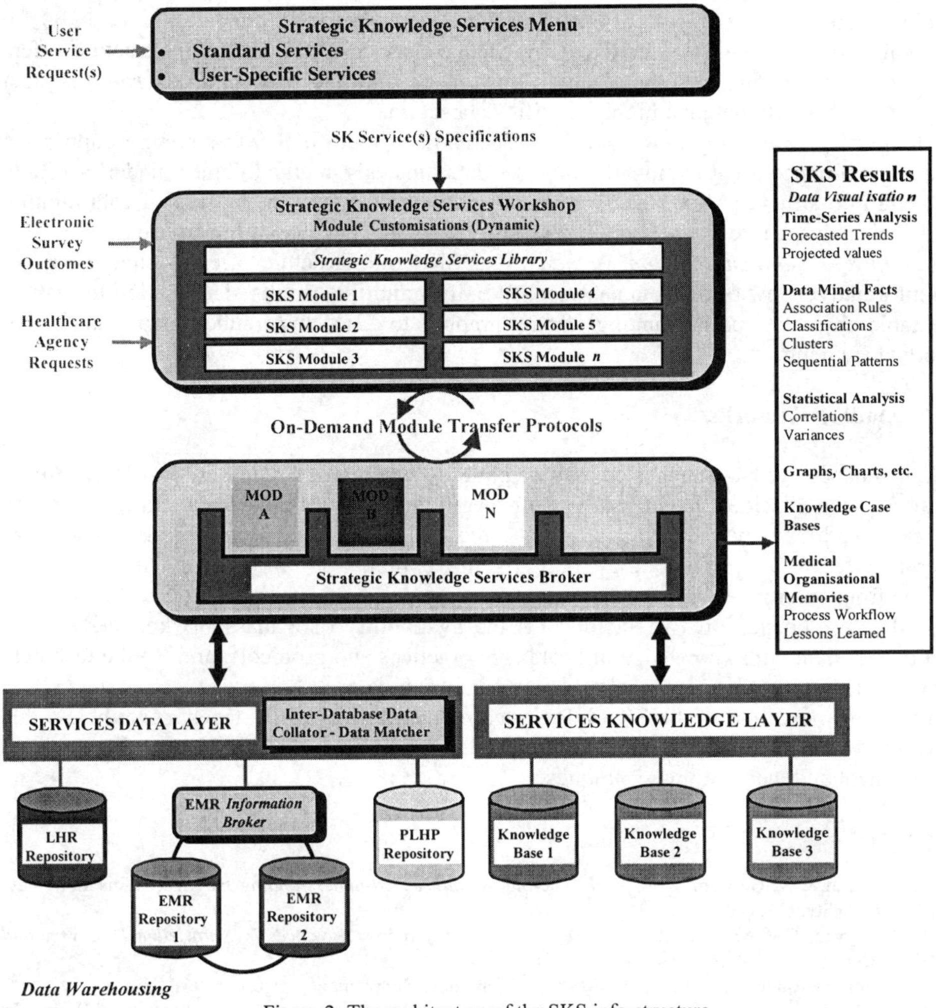

Figure 2: The architecture of the SKS info-structure

4. Features of the SKS Info-Structure

Functionally, the proposed SKS info-structure supports a number of innovative features, such as:

Data Collation: Comprehensive data analysis by collating data from multiple data repositories—where each data repository may contain logically different health-related information—to form a virtual, seamless and continuous data source.

Suite of Strategic Knowledge Services: A wide range of SKS that address the demands of multiple clients—healthcare agencies, insurance and the pharmaceutical industry. The SKS are categorised into four prominent classes (whereas within each class we have numerous sub-SKS): (1) Treatment Management; (2) Pharmaceutical Requirements; (3) Healthcare Planning and Services and (4) Best Practices Benchmarking.

User-Specific Strategic Knowledge Service Requests: To incorporate usage and temporal constraints, we allow users to dynamically choose both (a) data items of interest and (b) the data analysis techniques.

Addition of New Strategic Knowledge Services: Our SKS info-structure caters for the limitless increase in the breadth of knowledge that can be derived from data.

Combination of Multiple Strategic Knowledge Services: Our SKS info-structure offers the possibility for an 'intelligent' amalgamation of multiple *data analysis routines* in a principled manner to obtain a highly specific data service.

Multiple Data & Knowledge Analysis Techniques: Our SKS info-structure supports a unique confluence of functionally diverse data analysis methodologies under a single umbrella info-structure. For instance, we will provide data analysis by way of data mining, statistical analysis, rule extraction, time-series forecasting, benchmarking and so on.

Multiple Result Visualisation Methods: Our SKS info-structure offers a comprehensive and informative view of the data analysed. We offer multiple results visualisation formats—selectable by the user—ranging from graphs to 3D hypercube maps to active reports/documents.

5. Concluding Remarks

In this paper, we have suggested that the possible synergy of *Healthcare* and *Data Mining* techniques can provide a paradigm for the generation of knowledge-driven strategic services that can go a long way in addressing some of the challenges faced by any modern healthcare enterprise [8]. Our methodology purports the exploitation of experiential knowledge, derived from enterprise-wide databases, for strategic decision-making. The feasibility of our methodology depends on two factors: (a) the availability of a mass of 'knowledge-rich' (healthcare) data with knowledge of healthcare practices and protocols, and (b) the technical capability to extract 'decision-quality' knowledge from data.

The implementation of the SKS info-structure is still in its early stages, nevertheless this project provides us an opportunity to experiment with and analyse the efficacy of knowledge management and data mining techniques.

References

[1] A. Weigend & N. Gershenfeld (eds), *Predicting the future and understanding the past*, Addison Wesley, Redwood City, CA, (1993).

[2] U.M. Fayyad, G.P. Shapiro, P. Smyth & R. Uthurusamy (eds.), *Advances in Knowledge Discovery and Data Mining*, AAAI Press, California, (1996).

[3] B. Moxon, Defining Data Mining, DBMS Data Warehouse Supplement, August (1996).

[4] S.S.R. Abidi & A. Goh, Applying Knowledge Discovery to Predict Infectious Disease Epidemics. In *Lecture Notes in Artificial Intelligence 1531- PRICAI'98: Topics in Artificial Intelligence*, H. Lee & H. Motoda (eds.). Berlin:Springer Verlag (1998).

[5] S.S.R. Abidi & A. Goh, Neural Network Based Forecasting of Bacteria-Antibiotic Interactions for Infectious Disease Control". *9th World Congress on Medical Informatics (MedInfo'98)*, Seoul, (1998).

[6] S.S.R. Abidi & Z. Yusoff, Data Driven Healthcare Management: From a Philosophy to an IT Info-Structure. *International Conference on Multimedia & Information Technology*, Kuala Lumpur, (1998).

[7] M.S. Turtle, Bringing knowledge to the point of care. *Proceeding of Healthcare Information Management Systems (HIMSS) Society Annual Meeting*, Texas (1995).

[8] J. Flower, The Future of Healthcare, Encyclopaedia of the Future, Macmillan & Co., (1995).

Medical Informatics Europe '99
P. Kokol et al. (Eds.)
IOS Press, 1999

Quantitative Data Analysis for Exploring Outcomes in Cardiac Surgery

Albert Kircher[1,3], Johan Antonsson[1], Ankica Babic Ph.D.[1,4], Henrik Casimir-Ahn, MD, Ph.D.[2]
1 Medical Informatics, Department of Biomed. Engineering, Linköping University, Sweden
2 Linköping Hearth Center, Linköping University Hospital, Sweden
3 Institute of Electrical and Biomedical Technology, Technical University Graz, Austria
4 Faculty of Electrical Engineering, University of Ljubljana, Slovenia

Abstract: The article focuses on possibilities of statistical knowledge exploration to predict outcomes of surgical treatments. The outcomes were defined in relation to the measured peri- and intraoperative data, as well as follow-up patient questionnaire. Clinical consequences are expected in terms of a smaller data set with a better ability to predict the surgery outcomes and a better cost performance. The important questions that could discriminate quality of life (QoL) were:
Relief from surgery?, Has cardiac surgery effected earlier symptoms? Work capacity? Consultations after the surgery?
The performed data analysis proved to be efficient in the complex data set that was collected. Pain relief was identified to be significant, while relations between measured blood laboratory profile and later QoL were weak.

1. Introduction

We intended to analyze possibilities of extracting medical knowledge from data in order to carry out an outcomes analysis. We aimed at characterizing/differentiating patient subgroups against QoL and physiological well-being defined in terms of pain relief, risk of repeated infarction and angina pectoris. Second goal was to evaluate a questionnaire developed by Prof. Henrik Casimir-Ahn of the Linköping Heart Center in Sweden, who used his own clinical experience to formulate a simple, short quality of life questionnaire which relates patients' physical well-being to the patient experienced QoL (Table 2).

Other studies have successfully used discriminant and regression analysis to learn from medical data. As pointed out by Epstein, it was initially hoped that outcome analysis would begin to compare medical treatments not only on the basis of saving lives, but also in terms of making those lives better [1]. Duits et al. [2] have summarized and compared a huge number of existing QoL instruments. The effects of CABG on QoL and return to work were studied in [3] using a set of standardized questionnaires. Another study of postoperative six month recovery after CABG showed no big difference in physiological status, but the emotional side of QoL was improved [4].

2. Material and Methods

The study sample consisted of 102 Swedish patients (35 women, 77 men, 60±7.7 years, each 46 variables, see Table 1), who had CABG surgery. Clustering, multivariate regression and discriminant analysis were used. Dimensions, flow and occlusions of the grafts were measured to obtain an objective picture of the surgery success. Such a technical approach is not common due to high costs of the invasive examination.

Table 1. Categories of input data and number of collected variables aside the follow-up questionnaire.

Laboratory tests	Alanine (ALT) and Aspartate (AST) aminotransferase, Creatine kinase (CKMB)	9
Surgery variables	Duration, crossclamp time, ECC (extra corporal circulation) time, ECC termination, aorta quality, infarctions,	6
Grafts	Type, dimension, flow, number and information about the occlusion	18

Successful surgery outcome relates to good perception of one's life, pain relief, no symptoms of angina pectoris or postoperative infarctions.

Different approaches to define the quality of life have been reported [5]; we analyzed patients' reported QoL against their biochemical, hemodynamic and follow-up findings. Patients were interviewed using the questionnaire showed in Table 2.

Table 2. Patient follow-up questionnaire.

Item	Question	Type
Regret	Do you regret the surgery?	Yes/No
QoL	How do you look at your own quality of life?	1-5
Symptom	How is your physical ability without getting pain?	1-5
AP	Have you still got angina pectoris after the surgery?	Yes/No
Medication	Do you still need medication?	Yes/No
Hospitalization	Have you needed to stay in a hospital?	Yes/No
Smoking	Do you (still) smoke?	Yes/No
Change in symptoms	How do you think the cardiac surgery has effected your earlier symptoms?	1-5
Consultations	Have you needed consultations after the surgery?	Yes/No
Infarction	Have you had another infarction after surgery?	Yes/No
Breath	Do you have shortness of breath?	Yes/No
Relief	Did you get a relief from the surgery?	Yes/No
Working capacity	How is your own view of your working capacity?	1-5

3. Results and Discussion

Data reduction was performed, together with other methods, by deleting the variables with the lowest variance. This process has to be done cautiously, because some of the events, though being rare, may contain significant information (ex. mortality) [6]. Cluster analysis, performed in all four data groups (see Table 1), allowed the finding of patients classified as outliers. The blood profile showed 2 main clusters, 76 patients with normal aminotransferase values (AST, ALT) formed the dominant cluster, while 4 patients formed a cluster of extremely high values.

To analyze the improvements in QoL, discriminant analysis was utilized to search for any data that could differentiate between the subgroups. Discrimination around grouping variable QoL two and three was relevant, since it contained most of the patient cases. Flow and dimensions of left anterior descendent, marginal branches, diagonal branch, right coronary artery and jump grafts were measured.

Table 3. Mean values for AST and ALT before the surgery and of the flow in LAD and in MARG with respect to QoL.

QoL	AST before surgery	ALT before surgery	LAD flow	MARG flow
	[μkat/liter]	[μkat/liter]	[l/min]	[l/min]
2 (good)	0.528	0.515	1.70±0.42 (n=23)	1.56±0.55 (n=17)
3 (moderate)	0.436	0.442	1.77±0.39 (n=67)	1.55±0.40 (n=57)

74 % of cases correctly classified

The laboratory data shows that there was a difference in values of ALT and AST before the surgery with accuracy of 74%. Table 3 shows no significant difference in the flow measurements in patient groups who reported good to moderate quality of life. Their well-being is most probably connected to other factors such as previous experiences and coping abilities.

The intention was to provide a detailed dynamic profile which is not commonly done in standardized patient management. This can provide answers to the question of whether implanted grafts were functional. A minimal number of occluded grafts is considered as one of the main factors of the surgery success.

Discrimination between the patients that felt pain relief, and those who did not, relates to the values of ALT during and after the surgery with 90% obtained accuracy. Patients who felt relieved had fewer occluded grafts in comparison to the others who still suffered from the pain with a classification accuracy of 90%.

Table 4. Mean values of ALT, number of occluded grafts and flow with respect to pain relief.

Relief through surgery	ALT during surgery	ALT after the surgery	Occluded grafts	LAD flow	MARG flow
	[μkat/liter]	[μkat/liter]	Number	[l/min]	[l/min]
YES	0.482	0.488	0.24	1.76±0.38 (n=85)	1.59±0.40 (n=71)
NO	0.999	0.851	0.64	1.70±0.48 (n=10)	1.22±0.61 (n=9)

90 % of cases correctly classified

Measurements of the flow in LAD and MARG grafts could not significantly separate the patient groups with different reports on pain relief. This means that more than physiological factors has to be taken into account to explain such an outcome. Discrepancy could be caused by unbalanced data subsets (85 vs. 10 and 71 vs. 9 patients with pain relief yes/no).

To analyze QoL we applied discrimination between two or three QoL values at the same time, because of the unbalanced distribution of QoL. The first variables investigated were the QoL values 2 and 3, which contained the majority of patient cases. Then we analyzed a small group containing QoL values 1, 4 and 5, which represents the extremes. Finally the neighboring values of QoL were analyzed, that means values of 1 and 2 as well as 3, 4 and 5 together. In this way we gained a detailed and complete picture of the all five QoL values.

Table 5. Discriminant accuracy in investigated patient groups for postoperative follow-up variables.

QoL values	Significant variables	Correct class.	Nr of patients
1,2	Working capacity	89.3%	25
2,3	Change in symptoms, infarction, breath, relief	82.8%	89
1,4,5	Change in symptoms	83.3%	6
3,4,5	Change in symptoms, working capacity, consultations, relief	100%	70

Table 5 shows that the correct classification was 100% (with a significance level < 0.08) in the group with QoL values 3, 4 and 5. This result should not be taken as completely reliable, but as highly sensitive to the patient group with lowest life quality.

68 patients of QoL = 3 were compared to one patient with QoL = 4 and one patient with QoL = 5. This motivates a new investigation with a larger group containing patients with similar QoL experience. A need to explore more data of patients sharing the same quality of life is once again obvious.

An Internet based questionnaire could be a comfortable way for a patient to avoid expressing too personal or complex issues making the questionnaire less biased. However, more psychological items could be added to the questionnaire.

Patients should be able to reflect over physiological questions in an easy way, by answering simple and direct questions.

The course of data examination led from eliminating data of poor quality, identifying risk factors and finally, formulating a set of predictive models. In terms of data analysis this corresponds to applications of variance, cluster, multivariate discriminant and regression analyses. The variable CKMB, from which important informations concerning the postsurgical status of the cardiac muscle were expected, turned out not to be relevant for the surgery outcomes. ALT and AST transamenases are considered informative, but far from being sufficient to create any predictive outcome model.

The introductory overview has pointed out psychological concerns to be principal dimensions in QoL instruments. In this study we have taken care of hemodynamic parameters, which are rarely reported in the literature.

4. Conclusions

Advanced statistical analyses were performed in an elaborate way, but without a resulting prognostic model that could relate the most significant clinical observation to the better outcome of cardiac artery bypass surgery. Cost effectiveness of the study was not satisfying given the limited usefulness of its results for clinical practice.

More promising were results relating to the QoL questionnaire. Psychological concerns were taken into account which has ensured a more reliable instrument for assessing patient well-being. Insights into patient self-perception of life quality could be used to improve patient care.

There are several ways to evaluate this questionnaire. To test responsiveness, the simplest would be to interview patients before and after the surgical treatment. If an obvious change can be seen, it could be concluded that the surgery provided some comfort and thus improved certain aspects of life quality. We investigated the content validity, while the construct validity is to be tested against some other established QoL measurements.

The study has shown several difficulties of extracting knowledge from data collected in a regular clinical setting. It was not possible to compensate for lack of data quality, such as the occurrence of missing data, but a detailed study could be carried out showing the multidimensional and complex nature of the outcome analysis.

This research has been supported by the Swedish Research Council for Engineering Sciences (TFR).

References

[1] Epstein RS, Measuring Quality of Life, How does care affect a patient's quality of life? One physician explores the scientific foundations for quality-of-life studies and the factors needed to produce valid results, Healthplan, November/December 1997, Vol. 38, No. 6.

[2] Duits AA, Boeke S, Taams MA, et al, Prediction of Quality of Life After Coronary Artery Bypass Graft Surgery: A Review and Evaluation of Multiple, Recent Studies, Psychosom Medicine 59:257-268 (1997).

[3] Speziale G, Bilotta F, Ruvolo G, et al, Return to work and quality of life measurement in coronary artery bypass grafting, Eur J Cardio-thorac Surg (1996) 10:852-858.

[4] Guadagnoli E, Ayanian JZ, Cleary PD, Comparison of Patient-Reported Outcomes After Elective Coronary Artery Bypass Grafting in Patients Aged >= and < 65 Years, Am J Cardiol 1992;70:60-64.

[5] Antonsson J, Babic A, Quality of Life Using Physiological Profile in Artery Bypass Surgery Patients, AMIA ´99 Annual Symposium, 1999, submitted

[6] Marshall G, Hendersson WG, Moritz Tem et al., Statistical Methods and Strategies for Working with Large Databases, Medical Care, 1995, Vol. 33, Number 10, pp OS35 . OS42.

Training and Education

Medical Informatics Europe '99
P. Kokol et al. (Eds.)
IOS Press, 1999

Post-Doc: Satisfying the Information Needs of General Practitioners in Continuing Medical Education and Daily Practice

Dickmann C. (1), Baaren J. van der (2), Spitzer K. (1)
(1) Institut für Medizinische Informatik der RWTH Aachen, Germany
(2) Vakgroep Medische Informatica, Universiteit Maastricht, The Netherlands

Abstract. The learning needs of General Practitioners (GPs) are not optimally covered by traditional ways of Continuing Medical Education (CME). The European-funded Post-Doc project sets up a model for a European internet-based infrastructure and learning environment to support GPs' individual CME activities, focusing on problems of daily work. It integrates education, information and communication for both daily work and learning at home. Based upon a user requirements analysis, the service includes multimedia training applications, selections of relevant information sources, a calendar of events, and communication facilities. The service is intended to fit in existing health care structures and accreditation systems. Because of different languages and user requirements in Post-Doc's regions each region builds an own website. The regional prototypes are built and evaluated in cooperation with small core user groups. This regional approach proved feasible and also influenced the network structure with regional demonstrator websites and one master website including central functionality.

1. Introduction and Objectives of the Post-Doc project

GPs, seeing patients with diseases from nearly all medical fields [1], must be lifelong learners and keep up with the exploding medical knowledge [2]. Their role as regionally acting "gate-keepers" in many health care systems requires profound medical knowledge and information on regional structures and events. Therefore, it is highly important for them to find relevant information for daily work and needs of CME by an acceptable effort.

Traditional CME can be time-consuming, inefficient or expensive (e.g. library searches, congresses) [2]. Computer-based CME can significantly support the acquisition of desired pieces of knowledge [2]. Most GPs in Post-Doc's countries have access to a modern computer at home or in practice [1]. WWW-based education by multimedia, interactive and collaborative training is technologically mature to be used, with barriers mainly from psycho-social, economic and political factors [3, 4]. Thus, important aspects of learning in medicine like interaction or group processes [4, 5] can be realized by internet-based training.

Post-Doc, taking place in the Euroregion Maastricht-Liège-Hasselt-Aachen, investigates structural and content requirements and the feasibility of an internet-based CME service for GPs for a European level. The service is intended to suit the GP's informational and CME needs at home and at practice. Problems are cultural differences in medicine, the expensive construction of multimedia applications and the co-operation between designers, medical experts, GPs and GP organizations. Four training applications are developed whose online accreditation is prepared. Guidelines for a European internet-based CME environment will be formulated. This paper presents first results of the Post-Doc project on the construction of an infrastructure and prototypes for an integrated learning environment.

2. Methods

Regional core user groups of 5-10 GPs were formed that follow the whole project. Their requirements, elicited by group discussions, brainstorming, questionnaires and hands-on workshops [6], are the basis for the construction of the prototype.

In collaboration with telecommunication providers a network infrastructure assuring sufficient performance for multimedia data transfer was established. High bandwidth components link the universities hosting the WWW servers (ATM, TEN-34). GPs are connected to the network by cable TV, ADSL, and ISDN [7].

A video server for real-time streaming video is built [7] and will be integrated in an interactive multimedia database developed in the European project ELECTRA.

Regional websites as demonstrators of the learning environment were built in close collaboration of users and designers, partly by prototyping. One master website integrates and coordinates common functionality. The web-based Post-Doc environment is built using standard techniques of HTML, Javascript, Java and database access. GPs, clinical experts and computer scientists collaborate in the development of the training applications.

These components will be integrated into one coherent environment in summer 1999, followed by an evaluation period with extended regional user groups of 30-50 GPs each.

3. Results

The GPs' requirements were: use of native language, orientation towards practice, feedback and discussion with the authors of training modules, self-tests instead of external evaluation of one's training performance, a clear quality control, access to the service from the practice and the home, short download times, a clear screen layout, and an easy-to-use functionality [6]. GPs judged multimedia presentations to be of high and communication of low importance [6]. Requirements for accreditation differed in the three countries [6]. GPs will accept an efficient new means of CME if it meets regional and national needs.

According to those needs, four regional websites in native languages were set up with a first common prototype. Similar types of information were grouped together:

- "About Post-Doc": Help desk and general information on the project and website.
- "CME": A collection of online CME courses, programs, and events.
- "Training": Post-Doc training modules, other internet-based learning tools and courses.
- "Library": Relevant medical information sources like Medline, databases, video servers.
- "News": Relevant news from the entire health care sector.
- "Events": An agenda of any CME activities and related information (e.g. proceedings).
- "Colleagues": An address book of registered GPs and their medical profiles.
- "Discussion": Email, discussion fora, contact to medical experts, mailing lists and chat.
- "Organizations": Links to organizations of GPs, patients and the health care system.

Websites are open to the public, except the communication area and some training applications. The requirements of fast information access and a clear and easy-to-use graphical user interface were met by a coherent design, good contrasts of colours and large buttons to be clicked without superfluous graphics. This design was uniquely accepted by the GPs.

The evaluation of this first prototype showed that the classification of functions by types of information did not fully capture the GPs' way of thinking. They think in categories of actions (e.g. "looking up facts") and organ systems or medical topics (e.g. "information of hyperthyreoidism belongs to endocrine disorders or internal medicine"). While Dutch doctors desired to index medical information by the International Classification of Primary

Care (ICPC) which is well known to them, German doctors prefer a combination of medical fields (e.g. cardiology) and organ systems. Most GPs had problems with the distinctions of information types in the user interface (e.g.: Why is a real-life course not placed in "Training" but only in "CME"?). Their way of interpreting the user interface is highly individual and cannot be strictly categorized. Therefore, different points of view on the same piece of information must be presented. Again, GPs stressed the need to quickly find information by keyword search, well-organized content structure, and to get the news presented on the starting page. Repeatedly, the communication functionality was rated by the doctors to be of minor importance. According to the -again regionally different- requirements, each prototype was modified, especially concerning indexes and cross-references. Main functional categories were redefined as: "About Post-Doc", "Training online", "Lookup" (existing WWW resources), "Medical Fields" (medical index for all information presented), "News", "Events" (CME agenda), and "Contact" (addresses, communication).

Three user's roles were defined to give an individual GP direct control over his level of participation in the service and the environment's contents, avoiding bureaucratic efforts or organizational impediments: 1. Unregistered visitors merely obtain public information and may send requests and suggestions to the Post-Doc service team via email. 2. Registered users have a password that lets them access the whole functionality and professional information. 3. Editors have a special password that also permits them to enter data directly into databases behind central information like CME events or news. However, GPs do not agree to a mainly self-maintained content provision, ranging from willingness to participate in one region (Liège) to predominant refusal in another (Aachen). Thus, the organizational aspects of the CME service do not seem to be trivial and have to be further clarified.

The regional project structure adequately supported the collaboration of clinical experts, GPs and designers by allowing more frequent meetings because of short distances.

4. Discussion

The difficulties of medical professionals to efficiently obtain individually needed information for CME activities and for daily practice are well known [1, 2]. This was corroborated by the GPs participating in the Post-Doc project by judging well-structured and -indexed information more important for the learning environment than communication facilities. The large amount of medical information on the web, being "scattered" over numerous providers and being of varying quality [6] does not seem sufficient to match these information needs. Highly usable applications for medical professionals should be specifically built according to their own needs [2], contrasting to many existing medical websites targeted at both doctors and medical students. Post-Doc, integrating multimedia training applications in a rich information environment, offers this specifity of service because it was constructed based on GPs' requirements, also respecting their organizational conditions.

A literature survey performed by one of the authors on the search term "medicine and multimedia" (INSPEC literature database) with the purpose of identifying recent publications describing a user-centred integrated multimedia education revealed the following: Of articles published in 1997 and 1998, less then 20% describe the perspective or work on the integration of educational services into a more general information environment. In about 25% of these abstracts it was noted that the mentioned service was suitable for educating health care professionals either in actual or future times, in contrary to most abstracts describing projects for educating students. One important difference between students and the GPs questioned in the Post-Doc project is that the former like quizzes and being tested externally while the latter have a stable self-image and reject external judgement [6] which leads to different concepts for training applications. This orientating survey leaves the impression that the integration of more or less isolated medical education or information systems into one environment being specifically configured for the needs of a professional target group is still seldomly done, showing that the Post-Doc environment is filling this gap. A university-centred integrative approach towards professional cooperative networks exists in Rennes, France [8]. A highly informative WWW catalogue of international resources on Primary Care is found in [9] but it lacks the regional or national orientation and the collaborative aspect. The participatory design of the Post-Doc service ensures a selection of information, knowledge and skill training being relevant for GPs. In contrast to broadly orientated websites or even medical search engines, Post-Doc's GPs themselves create a filter that ensures relevance and quality of the service's contents. The collaboration of universitarian specialists and GPs can bridge the gap between theoretically and practically orientated medicine that should not be regarded as a binary opposition [5]. It can be concluded that Post-Doc is superior to many existing approaches to WWW-based education services for medical professionals by offering a framework for the integration of GPs' different educational and informational needs, respecting regional or national conditions and preferences.

Educating students in medical informatics is going to shape new generations of doctors that will be familiar with techniques [2] posing problems to many adult GPs nowadays. Nevertheless, the stepwise introduction of services like Post-Doc may gradually increase the efficiency and quality of GPs' work even in the near future.

It can be seen as a shortcoming of the project that no generic tools are created for supporting a quick adaptation of the system or individually resp. adaptive interfaces. But this remains a problem to solve for most existing information systems nowadays [10].

Future work will consist of refinement of the services, a thorough evaluation and the setting up of management and quality-assuring structures. Especially the service's management by providers and the degree of the GPs' participation must be settled in a mutually satisfactory manner because this constitutes the most important success factor for the continuation of the service after the end of the Post-Doc project. Concepts on the integration of links to computer-based patient records, of secure communications or of patient-GP or GP-hospital collaboration should be addressed in the more remote future [10].

Acknowledgements. The authors wish to express their gratefulness to the participating GPs and the project partners as well as the EU funding this work.

References

[1] A.M. van Ginneken *et al.*, The Patient Record. In: Bemmel J.H. van, Musen M.A. (eds.), Handbook of Medical Informatics. ISBN: 3 540 63351 0. Springer-Verlag, Heidelberg, 1997, pp. 105-115

[2] A. Hasman, Education and health informatics. *International Journal of Medical Informatics* **52** (1998) 209-216

[3] P. Cravener, Education on the Web: A Rejoinder. *IEEE Computer*, September (1998) 107-108

[4] U. Giani, P. Martone, Distance learning, problem based learning and dynamic knowledge networks, *International Journal of Medical Informatics* **50** (1998) 273-278

[5] W.J. Clancey, The Learning Process in the Epistemology of Medical Information, *Methods of Information in Medicine* **43** (1995) 122-130

[6] J.J. van Lochem *et al.*, Post-Doc deliverable D02.01: User Requirements Analysis, July 1998

[7] B. Daems *et al.*, Post-Doc deliverable D04.01: Functional specifications (of the DIVSA and the BIMN), June 1998

[8] P. Denier *et al.*, A network of Web multimedia medical information servers for a medical school and university hospital, *International Journal of Medical Informatics* **46** (1997) 41-51

[9] University of Bergen, Department of Public Health and Primary Health Care: http://www.uib.no/isf/guide/family.htm, January 1999

[10] J.R. Moehr, Informatics in the Service of Health, a Look to the Future, *Methods of Information in Medicine* **37** (1998) 165-170

Medical Informatics Europe '99
P. Kokol et al. (Eds.)
IOS Press, 1999

The interactive use of networking multimedia - innovative education resource for professionals and patients

H. K. MATTHIES [1], G. F. WALTER [2], A. BRANDIS [2], A. C. STAN [2], A. AMMANN [3], U. von JAN [1], A. J. PORTH [1]

[1] *Medical Computing Center, Hannover Medical School, D-30623 Hannover, Germany*
[2] *Institute of Neuropathology, Hannover Medical School, D-30623 Hannover, Germany*
[3] *Quintessence Publishing Co. ltd., Ifenpfad 2-4, D-12107 Berlin, Germany*

Abstract. The combination of new and rapidly developing interactive multimedia computers and applications with electronic networks will require a restructuring of our traditional approach to strategic planning and organizational structure. World-wide telecommunication networks (using satellites, cable) are now facilitating the global pooling of healthcare information and medical knowledge independent of location. The development of multimedia information and communication systems demands cooperative working teams of authors, who are able to master several areas of medical knowledge as well as the presentation of these in different multimedia forms. The assemblage of telematics and services offers a base for multimedia applications, for example teleteaching, telelearning, telepublishing, teleconsulting, teleconferencing, telemedicine etc. The expansion of the internet will also lead to the formation of interdisciplinary "Global Education Networks". The theory and practice of education are undergoing dramatic changes. Lifelong learning and adaptation of medical practice to new knowledge and new techniques will be even more important in the future.

1. Using Multimedia Technologies for Education

The internet technology is rapidly emerging as the most powerful medium of mass communication. Its WWW (World Wide Web) service has become a very important media for providing medical knowledge. Printed publications are more and more supplemented by electronical methods of publishing. Unfortunately the kinds of knowledge presentation in electronical media are often very similar to the traditional "patterns" that are used in printed books and scientific journals and are often only supplemented by hyperlinks and multimedia elements. The development of multimedia information and communication systems therefore demands cooperative working teams of authors, who are able to master several areas of medical knowledge as well as the presentation of these in different multimedia forms (text, graphics, images, audio, video). This way has opened up new possibilities and qualities for the training of medical students in universities and for further education of hospital physicians as well as for practicing professionals. The user's interaction with the information is made possible by visualization and simulation. Of significant importance are the possibilities of simulating diagnostic and therapeutic methods close to reality so that patients later can be treated more precisely by a perfectly prepared team. The learners can vary the parameters of experimental series of tests independently. In addition to internet services, the medical information is offered on

CD/DVD-ROM and can be used in multimedia PCs. Such offline-media does not cause a pressure of time by the user and allows repetitions whenever necessary.

Often electronic publishing groups offer medical information systems online as Web based multimedia communication systems (for instance the Health Online Service multimedica [5], Physicians Online [6], Virtual Hospital at the University of Iowa [7]). Such systems contain knowledge from renowned experts. Special support for diagnostic and therapeutic strategies are available. These Web applications are useful for distance education and training of practicing physicians, specialists of all fields in practice and clinical environments, students as well as providing health news for patients and consumers.

2. The G8 Global Healthcare Applications Project (GHAP)

The G8 is an informal forum of the seven major industrialized democracies plus Russia. Ministers met in Brussels in 1995 and identified 11 pilot project areas for international co-operation, one is the GHAP. The G8 GHAP aims at improving quality and cost efficiency of healthcare delivery through telematics tools. It has ten sub-projects [8]. Because this paper is only about education support possibilities we will only present the last two sub-projects

- Medical Image Reference Center (MEDIREC)
- IOA – International Online Academy (Special interactive TV and multimedia programs for professionals and public in dentistry and oral medicine).

3. The G8 GHAP sub-project MEDIREC

The objectives of this sub-project are to support clinical activities, contribute to medical education and training, and facilitate medical research. The proposed reference centers would include clinical and pathological images (still and moving) and typical, rare and difficult to diagnose cases. The G8 sub-project MEDIREC is co-ordinated by Japan [9]. English language Medical Image Reference Centers are developed at the

- National Cancer Center Research Institute in Tokyo
  MEDIREC / Images of Cancer
- National Cardiovascular Center in Osaka
  MEDIREC / Images of Cardiovascular Diseases
- University of Regensburg
  MEDIREC / Images of Dermatology
- Hannover Medical School
  MEDIREC / Images of Neurological and Neuromuscular Diseases

Accessing such image databases via internet is possible. Data collection mechanisms, online publishing, and organization (including regional co-ordination centers), for example, have been proposed. A technical group will ensure interoperability with other image databases and will develop an information security management for file and image transfer.

In co-operation with the research centers specified above, a multilingual "MEDIREC / Images of Neurological and Neuromuscular Diseases" is being developed at the Hannover Medical School [10]. Efficient Web based database access to the MEDIREC at the Hannover Medical School is made possible via an Oracle Application Server that uses Java-based programs to answer requests, i.e. all authorized internet users may access the data using a standard web browser (e.g. Netscape, Microsoft Internet Explorer). An editorial board is responsible for the quality assurance of contents. The case examples for the MEDIREC in Hannover were prepared by the Institute of Neuropathology as well as the Medical Computing Center. The search masks and appropriate search results (fig. 1) can be displayed in several languages (WHO recommendation).

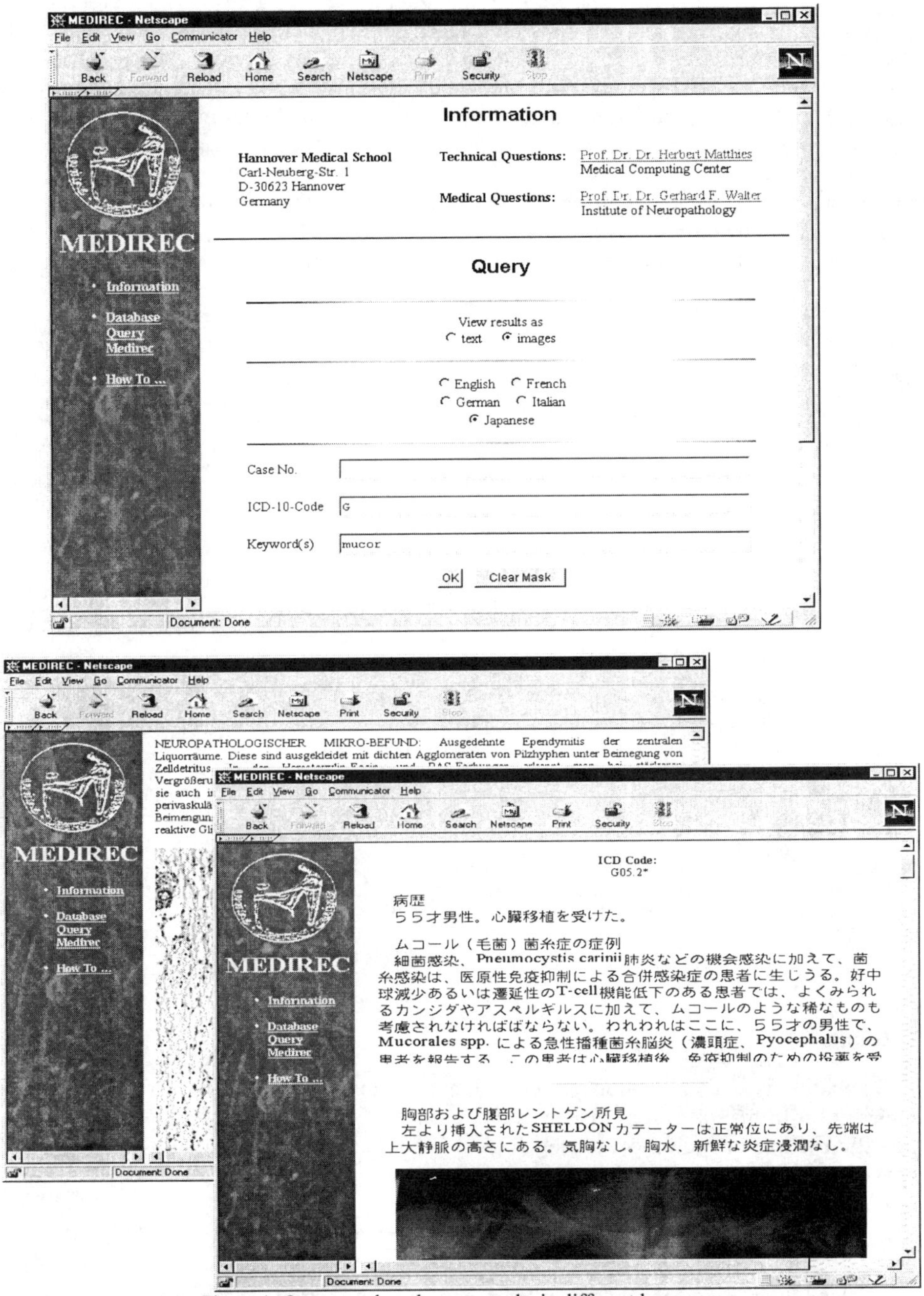

Figure 1: Query mask and query results in different languages

4. The G8 GHAP sub-project IOA

The expansion of the Internet will also lead to the formation of interdisciplinary "Global Education Networks". Such an exemplary network (fig. 2) will be realized in the G8 GHAP sub-project "MEDlive/IOA". The aim of the interactive "MEDlive" is to promote the international knowledge and information exchange in dentistry and oral medicine with telecommunication services, e.g. digital broadcast and internet services. The "International Online Academy of Dentistry and Oral Medicine" (IOA) is part of "MEDlive" and provides means for high quality, structured and certified education and continuing education. One day each week, video on-demand is available as a test program via satellite television receivers (ASTRA) or television-based Web browsers. Project coordinator is the international Quintessence Publishing Group [11] in Berlin. The aim of this engagement is to strengthen innovation, to assure the quality of content and to support the qualification and competence of the professionals on the road to the information society.

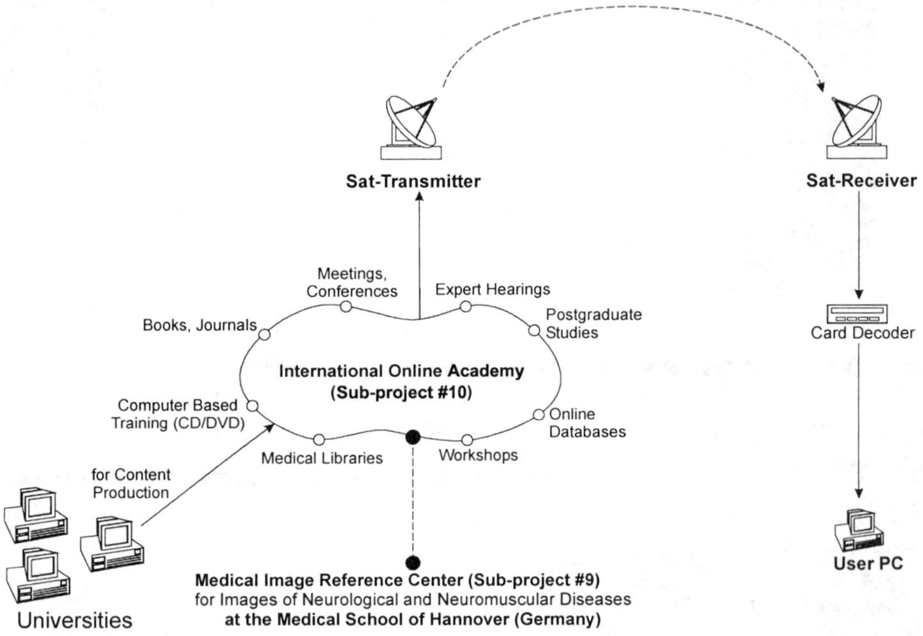

Figure 2: Link between MEDIREC and the G8 GHAP sub-project IOA

5. Results

Telematics is a combination of telecommunications and informatics resulting in the transfer of information across distances. High rates of data transmission are necessary for the efficient use of multimedia technologies. Modern telematics infrastructures allow for instance

- flexible possibilities for distance learning
- world wide access to certified knowledge bases and digital image archives
- as well as simulations of and training for surgical procedures
- flexible training for the support of diagnosis and therapy by using visualization and simulation

- decision support for diagnostics and therapy
- creation of digital video libraries of clinical treatments.

The new information and communication systems open up new forms of learning and make it possible to combine classroom instruction/lecture and multimedia applications. New educational technologies and course contents will be required.

First experiences have shown that in addition to medical lectures, specific offers for further education are required in dealing with electronical information sources. Learners' motivation will be improved by the access to multimedially supported teaching materials and contents. Problem-oriented learning will thus be possible and the quality of education will increase in general.

Multimedia technologies simplify the access to information from databases and electronical libraries. Renowned experts can give online support for healthcare professionals and patients. Knowledge and research results can nowadays be published and offered much quicker by the available telematics infrastructures. In contrast to printed books or video tapes, multimedia applications can permanently and easily be activated.

The theory and practice of education are undergoing dramatic changes. An innovative education resource for professionals and patients is the interactive use of multimedia applications in telecommunication networks. Video on-demand via satellite television receivers or television-based Web browsers will play an important role as effective user interfaces for access to broad range of knowledge and information resources. Learning is independent of time and location. The expansion of the internet will also lead to the formation of interdisciplinary "Global Education Networks" that focus on learning, not teaching. The challenge is not only for academic staff to change their work habits, but also for students to accept a changing concept of university education. Lifelong learning and adaptation of medical practice to new knowledge and new techniques will be even more important in the future.

References

[1] J.H. van Bemmel, Medical Informatics, Art or Science? In: *Int. J. Med. Inform.* **35**, 1996, pp. 157-172.

[2] H.K. Matthies, H. Poliwoda, K. Bob, H. Link, A.J. Porth, Multimedia Applications for Healthcare Professionals and Education. In: R. Haux et al. (Eds.), Health and Medical Informatics Education. Abstract Vol., Newcastle (Australia) 1997, pp. 96-97.

[3] L. Alpay, P. Murray, Challenges for delivering healthcare education through telematics. In: *Int. J. Med. Inform.* **50**, 1998, pp. 273-278.

[4] B. Richards, A.W. Colman, R.A. Hollingsworth, The current and future role of the internet in patient education. In: *Int. J. Med. Inform.* **50**, 1998, pp. 279-285.

[5] http://www.multimedica.de/

[6] http://www.po.com/

[7] http://www.vh.org/

[8] http://www.gip.int/g8

[9] http://www.medirec.ncc.go.jp/

[10] H.K. Matthies, G.F. Walter, A.C. Stan, A. Ammann, U. von Jan, A.J. Porth, The G7 GHAP sub-project "Medical Image Reference Center" at the Hannover Medical School. In: H.U. Lemke et al. (Eds.), Computer Assisted Radiology and Surgery. Elsevier Science B.V., Amsterdam 1999, i.p.

[11] http://quinline.globaldent.com/

[12] H.K. Matthies, A. Ammann, G.F. Walter, U. von Jan, A.J. Porth, Innovative Multimedia-Anwendungen für Global Education Networks. In: E. Baron (Ed.), Elektronische Medien in der wissenschaftlichen Weiterbildung, TU Braunschweig, 1999, pp. 193-203.

Medical Informatics Europe '99
P. Kokol et al. (Eds.)
IOS Press, 1999

WWW as a Teaching Resource for Introductory Medical Informatics in Primary Care

IR Young , PJ McCullagh and WG Kernohan*
*School of Information & Software Engineering and *School of Health Sciences*
University of Ulster, Northern Ireland, UK.

Abstract. This pro and contra report assesses the current state of the WWW as a teaching aid for Medical Informatics, using the experience gained from the delivery of a module to a heterogeneous group of health workers enrolled in an MSc/PgDip in Primary Care. The students were expected to act as both information consumers in a directed bibliographic retrieval task and information providers for Primary Care. The students' perceptions as to the usefulness and local relevance of current resources on the world wide web (WWW) are discussed.

1. Introduction

Medical Informatics has become an established discipline for advanced education, training and continuing professional development achieving European [1,2] and International recognition [3]. As the area is closely linked to the rapidly changing discipline of Informatics, curricula and guidelines for courses continue to evolve [4]. This report uses the experience gained from the delivery of a module in Medical Informatics to a heterogeneous group of workers in the field of Primary Care[1]. The group studying the module comprised 20 professionals in full-time employment. Six were general practitioners, 7 had a managerial role in Primary Care, 4 were nurse practitioners, two were health visitors and one was a podiatrist. The module comprised a weekly 3 hour class located in a computer laboratory with Internet access. The syllabus comprised the following main themes: Information Retrieval, Data Management, Classification, Telecommunication and Telemedicine, Diagnostic Methods, Decision Support. Although some aspects of the course could be classified as IT use, the objective was to provide an introduction to Health and Medical Informatics (HMI) specialisation in Primary Care [5].

The module was 100% assessed by coursework. Four of the participants had prior information skills, but the rest could be classified as Informatics novices. All were enthusiastic and motivated to complete the programme and deliver three set assignments as follows.

- Bibliographic information retrieval.
- Development of a small (work-related) medical database application (Microsoft Access).

[1] The module at M2 level comprised 150 student effort hours with 36 contact hours. It was delivered by Informatics lecturers with prior expertise in biomedical engineering and database technology. Clinical support was provided by health practitioners working at School of Health Sciences. The module was a prerequisite for a follow up course on Evidence Based Practice.

- Authoring and publishing a tutorial on a relevant medical informatics topic on WWW.

The WWW is a rich source of information, but it is important for the novice to have a good starting point and backup materials that do not rely on a computer and Internet access. Van Bemmel and Musen[6] have provided an appropriate text, with an associated web site and this was adopted as the core resource.

Pro

- Comprehensive up-to date treatment of Medical Informatics from authenticated source.
- Indexed for appropriate sub-disciplines, Medicine, Health Sciences, Health Care, Medical Informatics and level of expertise.
- WWW site provides excellent links to other key sites.

Contra

- Too much material for a single introductory module without sufficient emphasis on Primary Care.
- Textbook intended as general purpose Medical Informatics source and hence not targeted specifically towards Primary care.
- WWW support material not fully developed, particularly with regard to tutorial material (at time of delivery).
- Limited number of UK-specific and NHS heath links relevant to these students (e.g. GP-UK: http://www.schin.ncl.ac.uk/gpuk/gpuk_home.htm).
- Textbook intended to cover European medical informatics and not specifically UK oriented.

The outcome of this was that a course specific website was developed to provide links to supplementary material (http://www.infj.ulst.ac.uk/~cbnk23/medinfo.htm).

2. Bibliographic information retrieval

The participants were set a directed information retrieval task, in the area of *Meningococcal Meningitis and Public Health.* This task was chosen as it was relevant to most of the sub-disciplines within the group, and was also appropriate to the university environment, as a student awareness promotion had been initiated, due to previous recent isolated outbreaks. It is also an area of high public concern with incidence at a 15 year high in UK. The assignment was based on a similar Medline search proposed by Jenders [7] with a topic *Aspirin and kidney failure.*

To enable the class to complete the assignment, a number of supervised Internet searches of NLM's PUBMED database (http://www.ncbi.nlm.nih.gov/PubMed/) were provided. Students were required to compile statistics on the volume and year of publishing of articles found, to summarise the five most appropriate abstracts and comment on their relevance to Primary Care in Northern Ireland.

Once connected to PUBMED, the participants had little difficulty in obtaining information. However the participants agreed that planned searching and fully utilising the facilities available was extremely important in using time productively. It was important to:

- Use logical operators (AND, OR, NOT) and strings (e.g. "Meningococcal Meningitis") to refine searches more precisely.
- Use the MeSH browser available in PUBMED.

Documents are assigned to specific Medical Subject Headings (MeSH) by a team of medical experts. By assignment of *major topic* status the classifier determines that the term is representative of the document and this categorisation can be used to efficiently search the database. Meningitis, Meningococcal is a MeSH term found within the *Bacterial infections and mycoses* and *Nervous System Diseases* portions of *Diseases*.
- Restrict the date over which the search was made.

In all 47 "relevant papers" were retrieved, with a number of key papers identified, see Table 1.

Table 1 - Sample of Papers retrieved with more than two citations

Primary Author	Area	Local Relevance	Citations
Hastings	UK University	High	11
Imrey	UK University	High	3
Riorden	UK	Medium	10
Stuart	UK school	High	7
Tikhomirov	WHO \ Africa	Low	7

Hastings et al [8] indicate that the relative risk was increased in the 30 day period following an outbreak, although the absolute risk was still low. Prescribing chemoprophylaxis to household members may prevent 50% cases of further infection. Raised awareness is also crucial in reducing fatality among household members who developed the disease. Riordan et al [9] advocate raising awareness in primary care staff. This is achieved by education and research and results in children presenting at A&E department with a petechial rash receiving antibiotic treatment within 60 minutes.

Stuart et al [10] emphasise the importance of microbiological confirmation. Intervention is recommended for groups with two or more confirmed or probable cases in a school group within a 4 week period. Tikhomirov et al [11] working for the World Health Organisation examine meningococcal meningitis on a global scale. In sub-Sahara Africa occurrence rates of 500/100,000 are ten times the number for Europe. Factors which influence infectivity include immunity, diet and living conditions. In Europe most cases are caused by type B or C whereas in Africa type A is more prevalent. Imrey et al [12] indicate that the carriage of bacteria was higher in campus bar staff than a control group by a factor of 3.8. Carriage was also higher in students who used the bar and had taken alcohol the previous week. This is an interesting finding, given the nature of the assignment, but was only cited by three of the participants.

Pro
- Many students had little or no experience of computer usage and thus acquiring basic file handling skills, Web navigation and document retrieval skills is of great benefit.
- These generic skills are relatively easy to learn using on-line tutorials such as Netskills (http://www.netskills.ac.uk).
- Provides a useful basis for an evidence based medicine approach to problem solving.
- Quick access to appropriate abstracts, with possibility for author search, efficient indexing by MESH term and date restrictions.

Contra

- Initially there was a degree of user resistance due to unfamiliarity with computer technology.
- The majority of students did not have access to the WWW in their workplaces but this situation is gradually changing.
- Applicability of material to Primary Care in Northern Ireland. In particular some strains of the disease are not prevalent in Europe.
- Full articles not available via WWW. Full papers must be retrieved using standard library procedures, with the residual delay.
- Not all papers have documented abstracts. Hence it is possible for a search to identify a potentially important document, only to discover that the abstract is not available.

Participants' opinion on the applicability to Primary Care of the information retrieved in this "snapshot" study was divided. Overall nine were positive as to the benefits of the general evidence based approach contributing to local health care, with another nine expressing both positive and negative views and two having more negative opinions. Of the two students who were negative, one had expressed negative opinions about computing from the outset of the course.

3. Publishing a tutorial on a relevant medical informatics topic on WWW

The students, having gained expertise in WWW browsing, were required to produce a tutorial summarising health care and technical issues in a medical informatics topic of relevance to Primary Care and publish this on WWW, as an information provider. Sample topics included Year2000 problem, NHSNet, Telemedicine, Security of Medical Information and Decision Support Systems.

Pro

- Use of specific medical search engines (e.g. MedHunt http://www.hon.ch/cgi-bin/find).
- Useful Information provision (e.g. COCO Project http://www.teb.upm.es/coco/coco.html).
- Tutorial accessible to other students for peer tutoring.
- Students could address an area of particular relevance.

Contra

- Sites need to be authenticated to assure the quality and independence of information provided.
- Irrelevant and outdated links may waste time and cause some confusion.
- Performance of Internet may be unacceptably slow, particularly for image and multimedia sites sourced in US domains accessed at peak times after 1 pm. (E.g. Visible Human Site http://www.nlm.nih.gov/research/visible/visible_human.html).
- Resources for some topics were less available (e.g. Decision Support in Primary Healthcare).

4. Conclusion

The are many advantages of the WWW for the delivery of a course on Medical Informatics. Problems regarding authentication, applicability and the performance are offset by the amount of useful material and the ease of information retrieval when using appropriate search tools. In our experience, the relevance of the information retrieved is directly related to the information skills of the user. An introductory Medical Informatics course can prime the student so that they can avail themselves of the opportunity and demands of the evidence based approach to Primary Care. These skills are particularly important as more training materials resulting from Concerted Action IT EDUCTRA (http://www.fundesco.es/it-eductra/download.htm) have become available and initiatives such as NHSNet become central to UK health care. As the amount of medically related information expands in the highly deregulated Internet, busy professionals also need help to evaluate the quality [13] and independence of information and there is an obvious need for trusted and possibly kite-marked sites.

Although the students were studying for an MSc\PgDip in Primary Care, the heterogeneous backgrounds of the group caused some difficulties with prior IT skills and the perceived relevance of the material. In subsequent delivery of the course it is proposed to either run a preliminary IT skills course or require exemption using criteria such as European Computer Driving Licence (http://speke.ukc.ac.uk/ess/IT/ECDL/index.htm) for exemption. In the latter, the WWW is a distinct advantage as students having gained appropriate basic skills can focus on relevant topics. The information provision assignment was used to address this problem with students encouraged to pick a topic of particular relevance to their discipline.

Whilst local lectures and laboratory sessions cannot be completely eliminated, the WWW also offers potential for the use of more distance learning, permitting structured delivery and interactive assessment with software such as Topclass (http://www.wbtsystems.com/). This can also facilitate student centred learning.

The experience of Primary Care workers on our MSc. in Primary Care in completing tutorials on both bibliographic retrieval and medical informatics tutorial demonstrates both the feasibility and applicability of using the WWW to support medical informatics education.

In summary the WWW provided some relevant material, and with appropriate guidance, a student can quickly learn sufficient skills to use the WWW as part of evidence based approach to Primary Care. The need for filtering and authentication of sites is apparent, and it important to skill potential users as this happens.

References

[1] A. Hasman, A. Albert, P. Wainwright,, R. Klar, and M. Sosa, Education and Training in Health Informatics in Europe: Health, Technology and Informatics 25, IOS Press, Amsterdam, 1995.

[2] J. Zvarova, R. Engelbrecht and J. van Bemmel, Education and training in medical informatics, statistics and epidemiology in EuroMISE, Int Journal of Medical Informatics 45 (1997) 3-8.

[3] R. Haux, J. Frank and P. Knaup, The IMIA WG1 Database on Health and Medical Informatics Programs and Courses: A Call for Participation. Yearbook of Medical Informatics 98 ed JH van Bemmell and AT McCray, Schattauer, Stuttgart 1998

[4] R. Haux, W. Swinkels, M. Ball, P. Knaup, K. Lun, Special Issue Transformation of Health Care through Innovative Use of Information Technology for the 21st Century. International Journal of Medical Informatics, **50** (1998)1-300.

[5] IMIA Recommendation on Education in Health and Medical Informatics. Draft version March 99, http://www.rzuser.uni-heidelberg.de/~d16/rec.htm

[6] J.H. Van Bemmel and M.A. Musen, Handbook of Medical Informatics, Springer, Heidelberg, 1997 159-170. http://www.mieur.nl/mihandbook/r_3_3/handbook/home.htm
[7] R. Jenders, R. Sideli, and G. Hripcsak, MDIF G4001 Introduction to Medical Informatics Online Lecture Notes http://www.cpmc.columbia.edu/edu/textbook
[8] L. Hastings,J. Stuart, J. Andrews and N. Begg, A retrospective survey of clusters of meningococcal disease
in England and Wales, 1993 to 1995: estimated risks of further cases in household and educational settings. Commun Dis Rep CDR Rev **12;7(13)** (1997) 195-200.
[9] F. Riordan, A. Thompson, J. Sills and C. Hart, Prospective study of "door to needle time" in meningococcal
disease. J Accid Emerg Med **Jul;15(4)** (1998) 249-51.
[10] J. Stuart, P. Monk, D. Lewis, et al. Management of clusters of meningococcal disease. PHIS Meningococcus Working Group and Public Health Medicine Environmental Group. Commun Dis Rep CDR
Rev **10;7(1)** (1997) 3-5.
[11] E. Tikhomirov, M. Santamaria and K. Esteves, Meningococcal disease: public health burden and control.
World Health Stat Q. **50(3-4)** (1997) 170-7.
[12] P. Imrey, L. Jackson, P. Ludwinski, et al. Meningococcal carriage, alcohol consumption and campus bar patronage in a serogroup C meningococcal disease outbreak. Am J Epidemiol., **143(6)** (1996) 624-30
[13] J. Wyatt Commentary: Measuring quality and impact of the world wide web. In: Yearbook of Medical Informatics 98, Schattauer, Stuttgart, 1998, pp. 180-182.

Medical Informatics Europe '99
P. Kokol et al. (Eds.)
IOS Press, 1999

The Electronic Learning Zone in health informatics

John Bryant and Thomas Olsson
European Institute of Health and Medical Sciences
University of Surrey
Stirling House, Surrey Research Park,
Guildford GU2 5RF, United Kingdom
e-mail: j.bryant@surrey.ac.uk

Abstract. This paper outlines developments in health informatics education arising from the rapid development of the Internet and the growing importance of lifelong learning. The drivers for change in educational delivery are examined and examples of related uses of the Internet are given. The development of the Electronic Learning Zone at the University of Surrey is described and the paper concludes with the probable future extensions to support lifelong learning.

Keywords: health informatics, education, Internet

1. Introduction

It is sometimes thought that health informatics is a new field. This is true in that it lacks the prerequisite of the classical definition of a scientific discipline, namely an independent methodology. However, it has long been recognised that health informatics is fundamental to medicine, and has been since the origins of the latter [1]. The need to provide education in health informatics is also well recognised [2] and the challenge of gaining widespread acceptance and incorporation of informatics in clinical practice has been expounded frequently [3]. Consider the developments in the field of health informatics education. What might be considered the milestones across time? It is known that prehistoric man practised rudimentary medicine as long ago as 10,000 BC [4]. Indeed the first anatomical model may have been the Venus of Willendorf. However, the landmark contributions throughout history were probably the invention of paper in China around 105 AD, the printing press in the fifteenth century, and the stored program computer in 1948. Many people now recognise the Internet as the twentieth century's landmark contribution. Indeed, some futurologists suggest that health and education are the two main lifelong pursuits that future informatics will affect in many ways [5]. This paper describes an attempt to harness the Internet in the cause of health informatics education.

2. Drivers for change

There are four main drivers for change which have influenced the developments described in this paper. They are the growth of the Internet, the growth in availability of tools to access and use the Internet, the drive for lifelong learning, and the introduction of Europe-wide postgraduate courses. These drivers are discussed further in the following sections.

Since the introduction of the Internet in the late 1960's, the amount of users has risen to well over 100 million. The largest addition was brought about by the introduction of the World Wide Web in the late 1980's. Current growth is approximately 20 million pages per month, and there are now at least 275 million distinct pages on the Web [6]. This growth is also demonstrated by the increase in the number of web sites and hosts (Table 1).

Table 1: Growth of the Internet. Figures from Internet Valley [7].

Date	Hosts	Web Sites
1998	36,739,000	4,270,000
1997	19,540,000	1,200,000
1996	12,881,000	300,000
1995	6,642,000	25,000
1994	3,212,000	3,000
1993	1,776,000	150
1992	992,000	50
↕		
1989	130,000	
↕		
1981	210	
↕		
1969	4	

This expansion has been reflected in the health field. A simple Internet search for health related information, using a standard search engine and the search terms 'health AND medicine', was undertaken by Sosa-Iudicissa and Bernard [8] in late 1995. This resulted in around 2,000 hits and when repeated in early 1997 the number had risen to over 1.5 million. To confirm the growth, the authors of this paper performed a similar search in early 1999. The number of hits had again risen – to approximately 24 million!

A contributing factor to, or possibly a consequence of, the growth in use of the Internet in recent years is the wide availability of Internet and intranet technologies. To access information sources stored on these networks, the user has a wide choice of free tools, mainly browsers. The most popular browsers are Microsoft Internet Explorer and Netscape Navigator. These either come bundled from the Internet service provider, or can be obtained from magazine cover disks, or can be freely obtained from the Internet. Various software to facilitate the display of video clips and playing of audio clips are also freely available. Additionally, the cost of gaining access to the Internet has fallen dramatically in recent times. As a result, the user base has shifted from hardcore researchers to more or less everyone with a computer.

A further driver is the concept of lifelong learning, which educationalists and governments across Europe and the rest of the world have been promoting for a number of years. It has frequently been acknowledged [9] that employee competence is a crucial element of competitiveness. In many rapidly developing sectors the present competence, particularly technical competence, becomes obsolete in two to three years' time. Hence, employees working in such fields need continuous updating and upgrading. In the United Kingdom this has been implemented for some time in the nursing field and for general medical practitioners. These ideas are even more important in the field of health informatics, based as it is on probably the fastest changing technologies and sciences of today.

The final driver for the development of the ELZ has been the introduction of a European postgraduate degree in health informatics, based on a curriculum model developed by Aarts et al [10]. The programme has been developed, and is delivered, jointly by the Universities of Surrey and Manchester in the United Kingdom and Fontys University in the Netherlands. Students are recruited from across Europe and undertake periodic taught modules at each of the three universities. Effective communication among the universities and the students is therefore a vital ingredient for a successful learning experience. The availability and reliability of electronic communication using e-mail and/or the Web has therefore been essential to the successful delivery of the course.

3. The ELZ at the University of Surrey

There is already considerable precedent for successfully supporting health informatics communities using the Internet. The International Medical Informatics Association (IMIA) has been carrying out all its business using the Internet for some time [11]. Fully refereed professional journals, for example Sociological Research Online [12], conduct their business exclusively via the Internet, as do a number of international conferences, for example MEDNET 98 [13].

The response to the drivers for change, described previously, has been to begin the development of an Electronic Learning Zone (ELZ) within the European Institute of Health and Medical Sciences (the Institute) at the University of Surrey. A preliminary analysis has shown that there are three main stakeholders in the ELZ, namely the students, the academic staff, and the course administrators. Later in this paper, a fourth important stakeholder is identified. Each of these stakeholders has different requirements, the responses to which are described in the following sections.

3.1 Supporting the administration

Although the ELZ is primarily an educational resource, it needs also to support the routine administration of the educational courses. This starts with marketing to attract new students. An ever increasing number of students learn about courses from Internet access to academic web sites. A recent survey showed that almost fifty percent of new informatics students either learnt about, or made first contact with, the Institute via the Internet. Although conventional advertising in professional journals is still used, this is decreasing in favour of reliance on an enhanced Web site and the use of e-mail via appropriate discussion groups. Prospective students can register interest directly via an online registration form. Most, but not yet all, of the routine administration of registration for a course can be handled electronically. Indeed for the postgraduate health informatics students, Internet access and e-mail facilities are already a pre-requisite for registration. Once registered, students require an ongoing source of information about the academic staff, the course timetables, the physical location of taught modules, accommodation availability, maps and directions etc. All this information is provided within the ELZ, which also facilitates examination processing and results publication.

3.2 Supporting the students

More important than providing administrative support is the provision of learning resources to support the students in their studies. There are numerous, and often obvious, elements to this area of the ELZ. Obvious elements include mailing lists and discussion groups. There are a number of the latter that are used to discuss both general topics and the content of specific modules within the course. A searchable bibliographic database is being built up, based initially on the suggested reading lists for the course and extended by new material as this becomes known. From this, students can also identify the required reading for their area of study. Current research within the Institute into the construction of a bibliographic database covering the grey literature will subsequently be merged with the master database, thus providing a substantial resource for both the students and the academic staff.

Much of the lecture material is developed using presentation software, for example Microsoft PowerPoint. Following delivery of a lecture, the presentation and various supporting material is made available, and directly re-playable, in the ELZ. Such presentations are also 'imported' from alternative co-operating courses and seminars. It has already been demonstrated that a typical PowerPoint presentation can be implemented in this way in a matter of minutes. Work will shortly be under way to automate this process.

3.3 Supporting the academic staff

The academic staff at the various sites gain very similar benefits from the ELZ to those gained by the students. Some additional benefit can be gained from the provision of similar closed-access facilities only accessible by the academic staff. For example closed discussion groups allow the academics to collaborate on and debate the development of new material. Equally, closed presentations provide an ideal means to quality assure new material and to ensure appropriate integration and consistency of input across the syllabus. Finally and perhaps obviously, student-tutor contact is maintained primarily using e-mail. This does not preclude telephone conversation nor personal contact whilst the students are on campus - rather it supports and enhances the relationship.

3.4 The technology

The development of the ELZ, whilst not necessarily easy, has been relatively cheap by comparison with conventional software development. This is because much of the software needed for construction is freely available. The basis for the ELZ is plain HTML (the mark-up language used on the Web). As both staff and students are likely to use the ELZ at home and at work, the probability of access via dial-up connection is high. In addition, a survey indicated that finding a common software platform would be very difficult. The decision was hence taken that higher-end techniques such as Java, streaming audio and animations would be kept to a minimum. However, the requirement to work at a low common denominator may not prevail in the future. The ELZ is therefore designed in such a way that it should be possible to take advantage of appropriate future technologies. Initially, during the evaluation of need, cost was a major issue. The Institute already operated its own Internet server and no additional cost was incurred in this area. As mentioned previously, software such as Microsoft Office is used within the Institute and this automates much of the creation of material. The remaining software needed has been obtained in the public domain, including software for establishing and managing the discussion groups, designing and implementing the Web site, and establishing and maintaining searchable databases.

4. The ELZ in the future

There are currently two major developments planned to take the ELZ into the twenty-first century. These concern the development of a new health informatics knowledgebase and the establishment of a lifelong learning club. These proposals are described in the following sections.

Postgraduate health informatics students are required to undertake a series of assignments based on developments and activities in their own working environment. These activities are centred on the application of the ideas discussed during the taught elements of postgraduate study. However, the students are all in full time employment in relatively senior positions and the assignments are based around real-life problems rather than artificially generated ones. The reports resulting from these assignments, once formally assessed, will therefore form the core of a knowledgebase of real experiences. Submission to the knowledgebase will be automated so that it becomes the final sub-process in the marking process. Each report will be key-worded to ensure that the resultant knowledgebase is fully searchable. At present, thirty such reports are being piloted to ensure the development of an appropriate index of keywords. This will initially be based on the National Library of Medicine's subject headings (MeSH) but will subsequently be upgraded to incorporate new ideas, for example extensions to MESH [14] and labelling techniques such as med-PICS [15]. It is expected that more than one hundred new entries will be available annually. Access to the knowledgebase will be via membership of the ELZ although discussions are currently underway to make the knowledgebase more openly accessible and possibly to include suitably assessed entries from other collaborating academic centres.

Earlier in the paper reference was made to a fourth stakeholder in the ELZ. Further examination of the concept of lifelong learning suggests that learning will increasingly be embedded in work, and training will be conducted at the workplace. It is essential, therefore, that the employer be part of a partnership with academia to provide appropriate lifelong learning which supports current and future work. To achieve this, Otala [9] suggests a tripartite framework based on the employee, the employer and the university. If one accepts that the employer is the fourth stakeholder, then the ELZ must support such a framework including both the employers and the concept of lifelong learning. The Otala model can be extended to illustrate this (Figure 1).

Today, most existing academic institutes already support alumni societies. In an ideal world these societies would form the backbone for lifelong learning. Currently, however, most rely on periodic meetings and newsletters. In today's busy world this approach is thought unsatisfactory. Within the Institute, it is proposed that the ELZ should be the framework within which lifelong learning is achieved. By providing access to both the employers and the alumni, the foundations will be laid down for a lifelong learning club, linking the workplace with the academic centre and with students, both past and present. The alumni will not only have access to their own learning resources, but also to those in current use. They will be able to practise continual professional self-development by participating in discussion groups, joining on-line tutorials, searching and retrieving material from the knowledgebase, and contributing to periodic online workshops. The employer also will have direct access to the extensive resources developed within the ELZ.

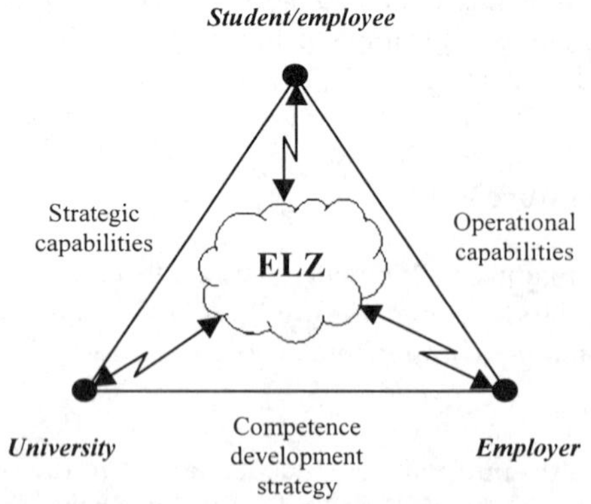

Figure 1. Lifelong learning and the Electronic Learning Zone

In conclusion, it is believed that the ELZ should be self-evolving, that is, it must adapt to the needs of the people using it and the environment within which it is used. Hence it is not locked into a specific format, nor is the content fixed. Today's important knowledge may become less relevant in the future. By having an evolving ELZ, closely related to the needs of its users, the latter have a reliable, relevant, one-stop shop for information in the health informatics field. The ELZ therefore attempts to address Olsson and Wright's 'general versus specific' problem [16] of accessing information on the Internet. The problem is that today's search engines tend to fall into two categories wherein they are either very general in their approach or else they are designed to address very specific tasks. Hence there is a tendency for people to rely on sources of information which they know and trust, and can restrict their ability to locate new and valid sources. The alumni can help to alleviate this problem by developing and promoting new links to other valuable sources. The other stakeholders can also assist with the future development of this and other areas of the ELZ. Some notable visionaries have foreseen the need for increased use of information and communication technologies within education. Bill Gates, for example, predicts that this 'will lead to downstream benefits in every area of society' [17]. The authors believe that the ELZ is an appropriate contribution to this vision.

References

[1] F. Wingert, Medical Informatics. Springer-Verlag, 1979.

[2] R. Haux, A. Hasman, F.J. Leven, D.J. Protti and M.A. Musen, Education and training in Medical Informatics. In: J.H. van Bemmel and M.A. Musen (eds.), Handbook of Medical Informatics. Springer, 1997, pp. 537-547.

[3] A. Hasman and M. Sosa , Education and training of health informatics in Europe. In: A. Hasman, A. Albert, P. Wainwright, R. Klar and M. Sosa (eds.), Education and Training in Health Informatics in Europe. IOS Press, 1995, pp. 13-24.

[4] R. Porter, The Cambridge Illustrated History of Medicine. Cambridge University Press, 1996.

[5] M. Dertouzos, What will be. How the new world of information will change our lives. Piatkus, 1998.

[6] DIGITAL, Systems Research Centre. http://www.research.digital.com/SRC/whatsnew/sem.html [Accessed 11 January 1999].

[7] Internet Valley. http://www.internetvalley.com/intvalstat.html [Accessed 14 December 1998].

[8] M. Sosa-Iudicissa and P.G. Bernard, Navigating the Internet in Search of Medical and Health Information. In: M. Sosa-Iudicissa, N. Oliveri, C.A. Gamboa and J. Roberts (eds.), Internet, Telematics and Health. IOS Press, 1997, pp. 423-432.

[9] L. Otala, Industry-University Partnership: Implementing Lifelong Learning. *Journal of European Industrial Training* **18:8** (1994) 13-18.

[10] J.E.C.M. Aarts, V.J. Peel and G. Wright, Human and organisational issues in health care informatics. In: J. Mantas (ed.), Health telematics education. IOS Press, 1997, pp. 241-248.

[11] T. Kleinoeder and O. Rienhoff, A Global Intranet for an International Scientific Society. In: B. Cesnik, A.T. McCray and J-R. Scherrer (eds.), MEDINFO 98. IOS Press, 1998, pp. 197-201.

[12] *Sociological Research Online*. http://www.socresonline.org.uk

[13] MEDNET 98 - The Third Annual World Congress on the Internet in Medicine. http://mednet.qut.edu.au/mednet98.htm

[14] M.C. Sievert, D.E Moxley, N.J. Ogg and T.B. Patrick, Thesaurus of Health Informatics. IOS Press, 1998.

[15] G. Eysenbach and T.L. Diepgen, Towards quality management of medical information on the internet: evaluation, labelling, and filtering of information. *British Medical Journal* **317** (1998) 1496-1500.

[16] D.T. Olsson and G. Wright, General or Specific – the Internet Pandemonium. 3rd European Conference on Health Telematics Education. Athens, Greece 18-20 June 1998.

[17] W. Gates, The Road Ahead. Viking, 1995.

Medical Informatics Europe '99
P. Kokol et al. (Eds.)
IOS Press, 1999

Medical Informatics in the Medical Curriculum - When?

Josipa Kern
Andrija Štampar School of Public Health, Medical School, University of Zagreb
Rockefellerova 4, 10000 Zagreb, Croatia, e-mail: jkern@snz.hr

Abstract. Undergraduate teaching of medical informatics (MI) at the Medical School University of Zagreb has been changing its position in the medical curriculum. Nowadays, this subject is positioned in the second year of the medical curriculum. The aim of this paper is to find out what the students of the second year (S2Y) and of the sixth year (S6Y) think about the position of MI in the medical curriculum. The results of students' opinions have shown that MI should be positioned: in the last two years (63% of S2Y, 36% of S6Y), in the middle (11% of S2Y, 21% of S6Y), and at the beginning of the medical curriculum (26% of S2Y, 43% of S6Y) . However, analysing this question according to previous experience of the students of both groups, it can be concluded that: the *S6Y* with *more previous experience* shift the subject towards the *end* of the medical curriculum, and the *S2Y* with *more previous experience* shift the subject towards the *beginning* of the medical curriculum. According to our long-term experience and students' opinion, the most relevant MI subjects, any kind of medical application, should necessarily come at the end of the medical curriculum.

1. Introduction

Medical informatics (MI) can be considered as development, evaluation and application of information technology in medicine and health care [1]. Medical informatics has to contribute to research, education and to the practice of health care in order to improve diagnostics, therapy and health care organisation [2]. Therefore, teaching of medical informatics is important for students of medicine and health care, realising that they will be the health professionals of the future (3). Medical informatics practice cannot be imagined without medical knowledge, without physicians, medical professionals, without people taking part in medicine and health care. Consequently, medical curriculum should contain the medical informatics subject. It is important to find its best position in the medical curriculum.

1.1. History of medical informatics teaching in Croatia

Teaching of medical informatics subjects for postgraduate students in Croatia started at the Medical School, University of Zagreb, in 1966 but more elaborated proposal for education of health personnel appeared in 1969 [4,5]. According to this proposal the most efficient education would be achieved in collaboration with universities, and teaching should be planned at different levels (undergraduate, postgraduate and refreshment levels). As a result of this proposal, in 1970 compulsory appreciation courses in medical informatics were introduced at the undergraduate and postgraduate levels for all medical students at the Medical School in Zagreb. A very strong impetus to the development of medical informatics on both teaching and research was given by setting up the University Computing Centre in Zagreb in 1972 operating a multiprocessing timesharing system (UNIVAC 1110) with terminals installed at the Medical School.

Our beginnings coincided with a period in which serious attempts were made to design the first information systems in the medical field. One should not be astonished that the need of such systems for computer educated and trained staff was one of the leading points in defining the goals of informatics education of health personnel. That fact was recognised in our consideration from the very beginnings since the computer technology in the country was scarce at that time and was predominantly used for general data processing in other fields with very few applications in diagnostics, therapy and other medical tasks.

1.2. Medical Informatics at the Medical School University of Zagreb

Undergraduate teaching of medical informatics at the Medical School University of Zagreb has been changing its position in the medical curriculum: it started in the third year, was shifted to the first year, then to the end of the curriculum, and now it is placed at the second year in the curriculum. The elements of the teaching program comprised definition of medical informatics and its importance in medicine and health care, terminology, structure and organisation of health data, elements of hardware, software and computer networking in health care applications, health information systems and a review and analysis of medical informatics applications in particular medical fields including telemedicine and the internet in medicine generally. Practical work is provided both in medical database design and handling and usage of application software, both general (word processing, database design, spreadsheet, statistical software) and medically oriented (register of drugs, computer assisted learning, medical decision making, electronic journals reading, searching for medical information through the internet, etc.).

1.3. The aim of the study

The aim of this paper is to discuss the question, when to start with medical informatics (MI) education - at the beginning, in the middle, or at the end of medical curriculum, or what the best time for teaching of medical informatics is, and when medical students are ready to handle these subjects.

2. Material and methods

Searching for an appropriate position of MI subjects in the medical curriculum, thanks to the fact that two generations of undergraduate students were taught at the same time, two groups of medical students were examined: the students (n=222) of the second year (S2Y) and the students (n=159) of the sixth year (S6Y). Both groups were asked several questions, immediately after the last lecture: (1) previous experience of the student, (2) is MI subject interesting – student's opinion, (3) is MI useful for physician – student's opinion, (4) which subjects the student considers as interesting, (5) is the student able to evaluate MI application, (6) appropriate position of MI in the medical curriculum – student's opinion, (7) willingness to learn more of MI, and (8) which topics to add and/or change in the course of MI.

The previous experience includes experience in word processing, spreadsheet and database design, in surfing on the Internet and using e-mail, in programming, playing games and using special medical application software. The second and the third question, on interests and usefulness, reflect a general impression. An interesting MI subject is expected to be chosen from the list of practical issues the student meets during the MI course. 'Capability for evaluation' means that the student feels to be able to say that a particular medical application (especially information it provides, e.g. information about drugs in registry of drugs) is appropriate or not for implementation in medicine and health care. The question about the appropriate position offers three possibilities (beginning, middle and the end of the medical curriculum). 'Learn more of MI' means postgraduate education in MI (which exists at the Medical School University of Zagreb since 1984). The last question is open for a free answer.

3. Results

The results are showen in Figures 1-3. The previous experience, especially programming, is supposed to come from previous education, high school or other. Experience in games reflects the absence of a 'fear of information technology'. Experience in medical applications reflects the highest level of student's interest in MI. The results (Fig.1) have shown that the S2Y have much more computer experience than the S6Y. The frequency of non-experienced students is 30% in the S6Y and 14% in the S2Y. The Office (word processing, spreadsheet and database design), especially word processing, is the software most students used to practice.

The question 'What is interesting?' (Fig.2) shows quite a different pattern. Medical applications (registry of drugs, computer assisted learning, making diagnosis) and Office (word processing, spreadsheet and database system), especially database design and use, are the most interesting features for the S6Y. The S2Y prefer surfing through the Internet. Medical applications have a rank number two. Data preparing cannot be recognised at all as a feature of interest for the students of medicine of the second year.

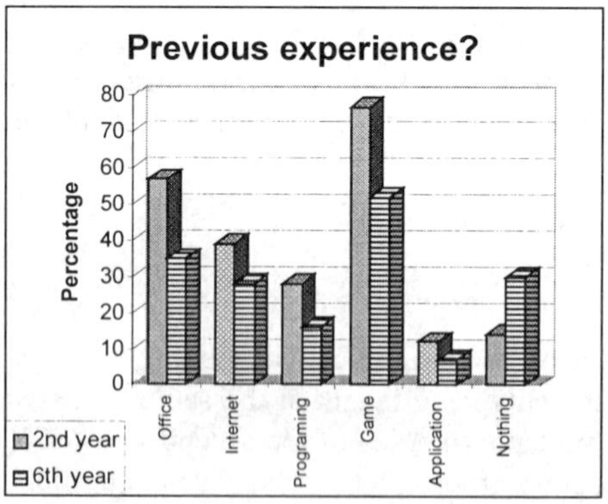

Fig.1. Previous experience of the Croatian medical students

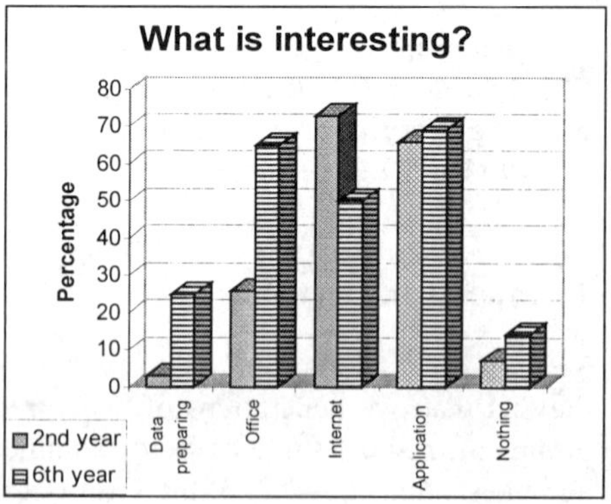

Fig.2 Most interesting features

General attitudes of students towards MI are not negative, especially of the S6Y. They feel that MI is interesting for them (78%) and useful for medical doctors (89%). The S2Y feel ambiguous towards the statement 'MI is interesting' (42% 'Yes', about 36% 'Yes and No', about 22% 'No'). However they vote for the statement 'MI is useful' (77%).

At the end of MI education, 29% of the S6Y feel able to say which medical applications are appropriate for a medical doctor. Some of them (39%) say 'No, I can't evaluate MI application from the medical doctor's point of view'. Some of them (32%) are not sure whether they are able or not to make the evaluation. Most of the S2Y are sure they are not able to evaluate MI applications. Both groups want to learn more about MI, about 60% of the S6Y and 45% of the S2Y.

The opinion (Fig.3) of the majority of the S2Y (63%) is that MI should be positioned in the last two years, 26% vote for the first two years, and 11% for the middle of the medical curriculum. The S6Y vote for the beginning (43%), for the middle (21%) and for the end of medical curriculum (36%). However, analysing this question according to the previous experience of students of both groups it can be concluded that:

- the *sixth* year students with more previous experience shift the subject towards the *end* of the medical curriculum, and
- the *second* year students with more previous experience shift the subject towards the *beginning* of the medical curriculum.

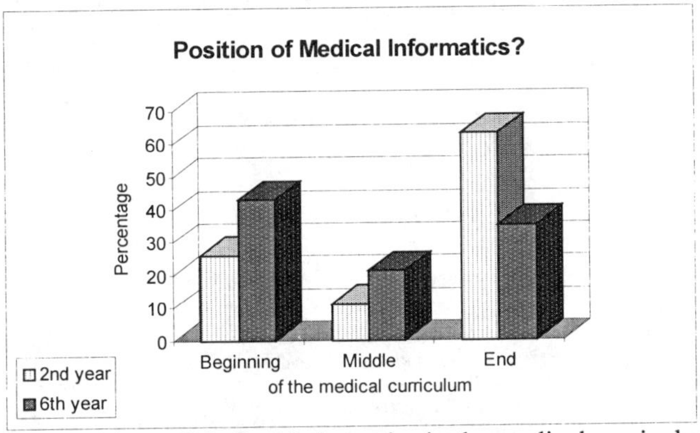

Fig.3. Position of Medical Informatics in the medical curriculum

4. Conclusion

An overview of results is indicative. It can be expected that the new generations of medical students would come with much more experience in general informatics (programming, word processing, spreadsheet and database software, as well as the Internet) to medical schools. It can be supposed that the S6Y, insisting on shifting MI subject towards the beginning of the curriculum, do that because they do not have enough skills in using IT. They want to learn much more about using the computer as soon as possible. On the contrary, the majority of the S2Y think that MI should be positioned at the end of the curriculum, because they have some experience in general informatics. Students of both groups insist on more practical work (question: Which topics to add and/or change in the course of MI?') in spite of the fact that about 70% of all teachings is practice in computer laboratory. They also insist on more hours for MI. Some of them propose to learn about MI all the six years through. At the same time many of them want to learn more about MI during the postgraduate education.

According to our long-term experience and students' opinion on the most relevant MI subjects, any kind of medical application should necessarily come at the end of the medical curriculum. Then, when the students have sufficient medical knowledge, they become able to understand medical contents of the application, and it can be expected that they are able to understand and evaluate these applications from the medical doctor's point of view.

References

[1] E. Coiera, Medical Informatics, *BMJ* **310** (1995) 1381-1386.

[2] R. Haux, Medical Informatics - A Key to the Future of Medicine and Health Care. *Methods of Information in Medicine* **34** (1995) 454-457.

[3] J.H. Vanbemmel and J.S. Duisterhout, Education and Training of Medical Informatics in the Medical Curriculum. *International Journal of Medical Informatics* **50** (1998) 49-58.

[4] Gj. Deželić, Medical Informatics Teaching at Medical Schools: Problems and Prospects. In: Adlassing KP, Dorda W, Grabner G (Eds.) Medizinische Informatik, R. Oldenbourg Verlag, Vienna-Munich, 1981, pp.82-89.

[5] Gj. Deželić and J. Kern, Education in Medical Informatics: Croatian Experience. *Medicinska Informatika* **2** (1995) 105-109.

Medical Informatics Europe '99
P. Kokol et al. (Eds.)
IOS Press, 1999

Communication between the Higher Education and Industry

*Rodica Dimitriu, **Mariana Bazavan, ***Radu Sima, ****Diana Lungeanu,****Gh. Mihalas
**Romanian Society of Automation and Technical Informatics,*
***Romanian National Center for Health Statistics, *** Sintec Ltd. Baia-Mare,*
*****University of Medicine and Pharmacy Timisoara*

Abstract The paper presents the starting premise and the general frame of the Tempus Project CME-02555-96, entitled "Know How Transfer form University to Industry". It is intended to be a study for establishing a frame and methods for communication between academic, scientific and research bodies and industry. This project continues the efforts made in the RENEHEMA Tempus project aiming to support the improvement of communication between higher education and industry. Following the conclusions of the RENEHEMA conference the strategy adopted by the management board focused on the Internet technology and free market mechanisms to fulfill the project objectives.

1. General Background

The partners in this project have a thorough background regarding their cooperation. Most of the representatives of the institutions in this consortium took the advantage of the PHARE Tempus courses from the EuroMISE Center in Prague. On this occasion they established excellent contacts with Prof. Bernard Richards, UMIST Department of Medical Informatics, who was a remarkable adviser for Medical Informatics development in Romania, along all these three years of cooperation. University of Medicine & Pharmacy Timisoara, National Center for Health Statistics, Bucharest, Romanian Society of Control and Technical Informatics, Bucharest, were part or participated in the Tempus CME "Regional Network for Healthcare Management" that laid the basis of the present project. Sintec Ltd., Baia-Mare and Health Information Consulting, Faversham, Kent were also deeply involved in medical informatics development in Romania and due to their cooperation with the team that launched the Tempus project were asked to bring their support given their experience in free market mechanisms and healthcare management systems respectively.

2. Previous Work

The national survey on communication needs showed that there is a critical issue for hospitals, district health authorities, sanitary police departments and drug stores. The medical research units showed a lower interest probably due to the difficulties crossed by the research all over Romania after the transition process started in 1990 that induced frustration and lack of confidence. On the opposite the research centres are interested being connected to a communication network (100%) while the healthcare units are of lower enthusiasm. This result was biased by the confusion of many subjects that considered the network a technical infrastructure rather than an organisational frame for communication. The majority of the subjects are oriented mainly to the training opportunities and the offer of the market. The low interest in commercial offers shows clearly that the demand/supply mechanisms are not working properly yet. [1]

The debates in RENEHEMA conference based on the national survey results and on the presentations on healthcare reform IT infrastructure development in Romania led to the conclusion that: [2]

- Romania is currently subject to a transition process from a centralized to a free market economy. The decentralizing process destroyed the traditional links between different kind of bodies and now these links must be rebuilt according to the structural changes occurred as a result of the transition. For a good management a high quality information is necessary and also a good cooperation between institutions supporting health care process.
- The information need is controlled by the physician need, which determines the activity in management, education, research, and industry. Import needs should be avoided.
- Improving communication and delivering the information where, when, and how it is needed might help graduate and postgraduate multidisciplinary education.
- Information must be produced, validated on the market an offered to different type of clients. This process creates a new culture and the people should be educated to accept the change.
- At present, the communication infrastructures in Romania are too weak and there is a great need for improving infrastructure at the national level
- A national strategy/plan with legislation and legal framework is needed as a top priority

3. Objectives of the Project

The project proposed by University of Medicine and Pharmacy Timisoara represents a study to establish a frame and methods for communication between academic, scientific and research bodies and industry. This frame must be able to support (i) the development of interdisciplinary fields in Romania, (ii) the improvement of communication between the higher education and industry, (iii) development of applied informatics colleges in Romania.

This project aims to support the process of university reform at management level developing tools for enabling education orienting, training quality assessment, strategy development and cooperation with other bodies.

4. Project Development

To reach the project goals it was necessary to collect and deliver information concerning the hot priorities of the health care. At present the feed back of the healthcare market to the higher education is quite low and it is very difficult for the universities to asses and plan their development at a structural level and to adjust the curriculum. On the other hand, industry is not able to absorb the qualified manpower prepared by universities, leading to a dramatic waste of resources. Only functional information facilities with wide access may lay the basis for creation a frame able to synthesize appropriate methods to stimulate and control the development process of adjusting prepared manpower and harmonize research activity according to the industry demand.

The real conditions in Romania consistently changed since the project application had been submitted to the EU. The health care reform produced migration of the manpower in other fields of activity and the Healthcare Management Information System project lounched by the Ministry of Health is raising new priorities regarding the manpower. The initial form of the project envisaged debates on three main topics: (i) measuring feedback of the manpower in medical informatics (ii) medical informatics map in Romania (iii) and the part to be acted by research in medical informatics.

The current priorities of health care in the country determined the management board of the project to adjust the debate topics to: (i) demand/supply of training in medical informatics versus the needs for training in the field (ii) medical informatics products national register (iii) and dissemination of research results in the health care system.

In order to increase the impact, we decided that the results of the project would be disseminated by means of WEB pages concentrating all the information collected and processed in the project. A WEB site can be an information facility able to support an efficient awareness campaign and, at the same time, it can be a useful and easy to access mean to access the needed information.

This decision laid both on the conclusions issued by the RENEHEMA project and on the analysis of the current developments of Internet usage. During the short stays of the Romanian specialists in UK it was agreed that the experience of our EU partners must be valued in consulting activities.

Considering that information must be produced, validated on the market and sold to different type of clients and that process creates a new culture we decided that data collection must be performed by the national Center for Health Statistics and Romanian Society of Automation and Technical Informatics. This way, we could tackle the problem both from the state and professionals point of view.

Improving communication and delivering information where, when, and how it is needed may help graduate and postgraduate multidisciplinary education. This was the reason the University of Medicine and Pharmacy is in charge with structuring the information for the WEB site.

To avoid producing information on a volunteer basis, as well as wasting efforts to develop local IT infrastructures with scarce resources we involved our partner Sintec Ltd., which is an Internet service provider, to host and maintain the WEB site.

5. Future Development

The dynamic of the labour market has a significant impact on the private sector. It is already observed that there is a decline in the state sector and increase in the private one and much more there is a constantly decrease in employment rate leading to a reduction of the activity rate. [3]

Rate of activity

	1990	1991	1992	1993	1994	1995
Labour force	10840	11123	11387	11227	11235	10491
Working age population	15324.4	15377.3	15153.6	15212.8	15271.5	15315.9
Rate of activity(%)	70.7	72.3	75.1	73.8	73.6	68.5

Source: National Comission for Statistics and CRIMM foundation Calculations.

The Annual Report 1997 shows that the wages dynamic of the occupied population is not the same in different industrial branches.

Relative Wages

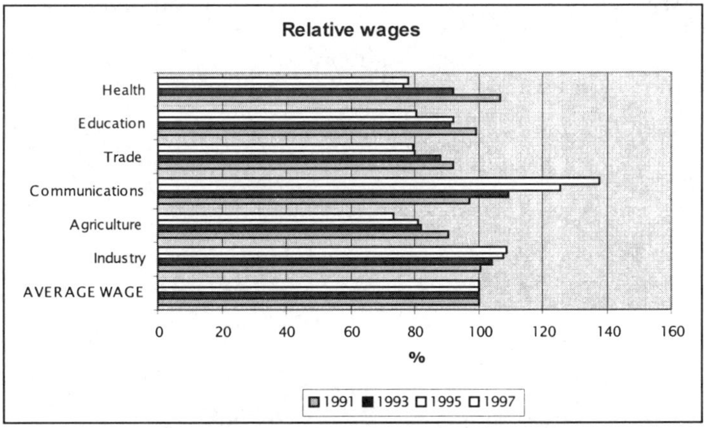

Source: National Comission for Statistics and CRIMM foundation Calculations.

The figures presented above emphasize the difficult environment of the WEB site development. We expect low rate of response from all the bodies acting in or connected to the health care field. Despite the discouraging aspect of the socio-economic environment, we think that developing an information facility is a must. The RENEHEMA project findings: (i) the information should be made available only to those with a need to know and who are authorized to use it and (ii) the information must be sold on the market was considered in another way. The funding strategy of the new information is based on the free market mechanism. The Tempus Phare funds were used to establish the development frame, structure and functioning rules of the site and to create the initial information core. The site is intended to become self sustainable by building and hosting commercial objects to drag funds. After the end of the project allowing only scientific and technical information to be posted on the WEB will preserve the Tempus spirit. The funds for the development are expected from companies who want to use the site for promoting new and valuable solutions.

6. Conclusions

The seminars organised as debate forums analyzed the methods and means to develop a new information facility for health care supported by Internet technology. Participants, who represented all the parts involved in the project and invited guests contributed with their creative opinions to the deliverables of the meeting.

The Internet site INFOSAN was designed to collect the feedback of the market in order the ring of higher education, research and industry to have a frame for more efficient closing.

A three months advertising campaign in the main health and computing publications doubled the number of the visitors (the site has 1000 hits) but the feedback of the market is still low. Only the private and nongovernmental healthcare units and small enterprises sent questions and information to be posted.

Starting with the fall semester 1999 the University of Medicine and Pharmacy Timisoara will be involved in the development of the INFOSAN site.

References

[1] I Jipescu, F. Filip, R. Dimitriu, National Survey on Communication Needs for Healthcare, Tempus/PHARE Conference, Sinaia, 1996.

[2] F Filip, G Mihalas, R Dimitriu, I Jipescu, D Lungeanu, A Popescu, M Bazavan, An Approach to Establishing a Health Information Market, in MIE97 Proceedings, ISBN 90 5199 343 9. IOS Press, , Amsterdam 1997, pp. 869-873.

[3] Annual Report 1997 on The Private Sector of Small and Medium-Sized Enterprises in Romania published by the Romanian Government, 1998

Medical Informatics Europe '99
P. Kokol et al. (Eds.)
IOS Press, 1999

CISMeF: Cataloque and Index of French speaking health resources

SJ. Darmoni (a), JP. Leroy (a), F. Baudic (b), M. Douyère (a), J. Piot (b), B. Thirion (b)
(a) Computer and Networks Department, (b) Medical Library,
Rouen University Hospital, 1 rue de Germont 76031 Rouen Cedex

Abstract. In 1999, the Internet has become a major source of health information. The objective of CISMeF is to catalogue and index the main French-speaking sites and documents concerning health. Currently, the number of resources already totalled over 6,100 with a mean of 75 new sites each week. CISMeF contains a thematic index, including medical specialities and an alphabetic index. CISMeF uses two standard tools for organising information: the MeSH (Medical Subject Heading) thesaurus from the Medline bibliographic database (National Library of Medicine) and the Dublin Core metadata format. A brief description of the site is systematically added. CISMeF respects the Net Scoring, criteria to assess the quality of health information on the Internet. The CISMeF project fulfils a valuable tool for the French-speaking health community: 2,500 machines visit the Web site each working day.

MeSH key-words: Abstracting and indexing; Cataloging; Internet; Vocabulary controlled

1. Introduction

In 1999, the Internet can be considered as a major source of scientific and health information. For the health professional, to find the accurate information on the Internet is not so easy; therefore, there is a profusion of directories such as Yahoo and search engines such as Altavista. In a previous study [1], we demonstrated that manually catalogues vs. search engines were less sensitive but far more specific.

The objective of CISMeF is to assist health professional during his/her search of electronic information and knowledge available on the Internet. CISMeF is a project initiated by the Rouen University Hospital (RUH). Its Universal Resource Locator (URL) is http://www.chu-rouen.fr/cismef. CISMeF began in February 1995 with the creation of the RUH's Web site. The scope of CISMeF covers healthcare disciplines and medical sciences.

2. Material and methods

– *Hardware and software.* CISMeF was implemented in February 1995 on a Sun running Sun Unix. CISMeF is a Web Site using the NCSA freeware http server. The Gestats and Webtrends programs evaluate the use of the Web page after excluding requests by our Hospital Information System computers and image files.

– *Standards.* CISMeF is entirely based on static HTML. CISMeF uses two standard tools for organising information: the MeSH (Medical Subject Heading) thesaurus from the Medline bibliographic database (US National Library of Medicine) and the Dublin Core metadata format [2].

- Methodology and realisation of the catalogue:

Since its creation, CISMeF has only catalogued and indexed French-speaking health resources, independently of its origin. The CISMeF method entails a five-fold process: resource collection, filtering, description, classification, and index.

Resource collection: A deputy medical librarian (J.P.) performs the resource collection on French-speaking health resources on a daily basis. She checks French-speaking directories and search engines, especially their "what's new" pages. A total of 420 health webmasters (7% of the sites included in CISMeF) have sent us an Email or a specific form to be indexed in CISMeF. Indexing priority is given to Internet sites of institutions and scientific societies. Resources include sites and high quality documents, issued especially from evidence-based medicine, practice guidelines, consensus development conference, teaching material, and technical report.

CISMeF respects the Net Scoring [3], which consists of 48 criteria to assess the quality of health information on the Internet. These criteria are grouped in eight categories: credibility, content, links, design, interactivity, quantitative aspects, ethics, and accessibility. Some of the criteria are inspired by a US white paper [4]. The description of a site should permit the evaluation of the quality of its content. Some sites and documents are not introduced in CISMeF, because they do not respect basic particularly ethical criteria.

Catalogue and index: Cataloguing a site is necessary because it helps to estimate, in advance, the type of information, which saves time for the end-user, and to evaluate its content. Resources included in CISMeF are described by the following elements from the Dublin core project [http://purl.org/DC/about/element_set.htm]: title, author or creator, subject and keywords, description, publisher, date, resource type, format, identifier, and language. We also include the following elements from the Dublin core metadata format in the metadata of CISMeF's HTML documents: language, and keywords and their synonyms in English and in French. We have organised our catalogue with the MeSH thesaurus, which is precise, rigorous and annually updated. We also use the French translation of this thesaurus, performed by the French Medlars Center, the National Institute for Health and Medical Research (INSERM).

In CISMeF, each keyword is "de facto" a MeSH Major Topic. MeSH subheading permits a focus on a sub-field of a MeSH term, e.g. chloride/toxicity. We also use a French translation of the MeSH subheadings, which is less systematically used in CISMeF compared to Medline. CISMeF resource type is a generalisation of the publication type of Medline. We have added types which are specific of the resources available on the Internet, such as association, patient information, community networks (see http://www.chu-rouen.fr/documed/typeressource.html). Resource type describes the nature of the resource and MeSH describes the subject of the resource.

Example of a description of a document indexed in CISMeF:

> Adolescent pregnancy [http://www.cps.ca/english/statements/AM/am94-02.htm]. Adolescent Medicine Committee, Canadian Paediatric Society (CPS). In : Canadian Journal of Paediatrics 1994; 1(2): 58-60 [prevention, diagnosis, management, counselling, bibliography]. -Ca
> *keywords : adolescence ; pregnancy in adolescence*
> *resource type : clinical practice guideline*

Structure of the CISMeF catalogue: CISMeF contains a thematic index, including medical specialities and an alphabetic index. A brief description of any site indexed in CISMeF is systematically added. To index the health resources CISMeF uses five levels of hierarchy: (1) CISMeF “meta-term” (2) MeSH category (3) MeSH keyword (4) MeSH subheading (5) CISMeF resource type. The levels 1 and 5 are specific of CISMeF. The levels 2, 3 and 4 are using the Medline database structure.

The CISMeF “meta-term” is generally a medical speciality or a biological science, e.g., cardiology or bacteriology. For example on the cardiology page, the sites of general interest about this speciality are indexed and described, followed by a list of starting points of related categories and others associated MeSH terms. In CISMeF, each MeSH term (level 3 of the CISMeF structure) corresponds to a HTML document, which is organised first with MeSH subheading (level 4), then for each subheading, the resource types (level 5). The alphabetic index uses the MeSH terms in English and their French translation, which permits bilingual search. Alphabetic and thematic indices are available, and also a general index for permuted utilisation. Currently, CISMeF contains indexed 6,118 resources with 1,444 MeSH terms. A mean of 75 sites and documents are indexed each week and approximately 32 new MeSH terms are added in the same time.

3. Results

CISMeF is efficient an end-user-friendly solution to find French-speaking worldwide health resources on the Internet. Two-thirds of these sites and documents are located in France, 20% are from Canada, in particular the Quebec Province, 5% from Switzerland, 4% from Africa and 3% from Belgium. This Web site is principally and initially oriented for the health professional, although the general public may also have access to it. Many sites are devoted to both. There are no HTML documents with restricted access in the CISMeF Web site. Thus our traditional "end-users" are now not only healthcare practitioners but also patients, their families and health consumers. One deputy medical librarian (J.P.) performs the resource collection and the information watch. Two deputy medical librarians (F.B. and M.D.) describe and index resources. The chief medical librarian (B.T.) is a 'super-indexer' in charge of checking the indexing. There is a 30-minute meeting daily with the medical informaticians (S.J.D. and/or J-P.L.) for double-checking. Since February 1995, some new features have been added to optimise the navigability and the access to the information for the end-user: (a) use of an internal search engine (full-text search), (b) a general index, and (c) a "what's new" page to easily display the newly indexed sites on a weekly basis. Since January 1997 it also includes an archive of the what's new pages. Two guides to use CISMeF are also on line, one for basic search and one for advanced search. CISMeF is accessible by the lowest common denominator of current browser technology. Since December 1996, CISMeF has an Editorial Board, following the policy of the hospital managers to control its development, its quality, its validity, its reliability, its consistency and its coherence. The editorial board peer reviews each document and site included in CISMeF. If necessary, we use external peer reviewing.

Use patterns of the Web site: Analysis of a representative period, the month of March 1999, showed that every working day approximately 2,500 machines visited our site (excluding ours). During the entire month, users from 68,601 computers made 280,195 requests for HTML documents originating from 114 different countries (33.58% from France, 23.48% from USA, and 8.03% from Canada). These statistics underestimate the real figures due to the practice of file cacheing. The CISMeF "Web impact factor" [5] (number of sites, which have at least one hyperlink to our site) was over 550. Over 110 press articles released information about our Web site. In March 1998, CISMeF has obtained the label "Experimentation of public interest" by an inter-ministry committee (procedure " Information Highways").

4. Discussion

The Internet facilitates the communication among the health professionals and with the general public, and also improves the information access. We distinguish several tools in the retrieval of health information on the Internet: - *level 1*: search engine, generalist or more specialised ones, such as MedHunt; - *level 2*: catalogue and index without thesaurus, such as and Medical Matrix, US; - *level 3*: catalogue and index with thesaurus, such as the UMLS (Unified Medical Language System) metathesaurus and MeSH thesaurus. The latter thesaurus is used in the following health catalogues, MedWebPlus, CliniWeb [6], Oregon Health Sciences

University-US, and DDRT (Diseases, Disorders and Related Topics, Medical Library and Medical Information Center, Karolinska Institute, Stockholm, Sweden) ; - *level 4*: catalogue and index with thesaurus, metadata, and description of sites. CISMeF and two other catalogues have now reached this level: OMNI (Organising Medical Networked Information - UK) [7] and HON (Health on the Net - Switzerland) [8]. OMNI and MedWebPlus, Us are also using the UMLS metathesaurus to provide a conceptual network to the subject headings. OMNI, HON, and CliniWeb have also developed a structured database (dynamic HTML) which permits better searches. This improvement will be developed for CISMeF in 1999. OMNI and CISMeF are using the Dublin Core metadata format, which is expected to become the dominant metadata format for Internet resource description.

One main objective of CISMeF is to promote best medical practice and teaching. Therefore, we index high-quality documents available on the Internet on a priority basis. Further challenges that CISMeF needs to address in the next months are to expand sites and high-quality documents, especially patient information, and to collaborate more closely with similar services, particularly in Europe (DDRT, HON and OMNI).

Acknowledgements

CISMeF was supported in part by the grant n° 1998 06 016 from the Agence Universitaire de la Francophonie in the program "French-speaking Virtual University". The authors thank Richard Medeiros for his advice in the editing of this manuscript.

References

[1] SJ Darmoni, B. Thirion,. Indexing the Web ? A comparative study of three medical Web servers on the Internet: Cliniweb ,"Diseases, Disorders and Related Topics", *Omni. Mednet 96, European Congress of the Internet in Medicine* (1996) 5-6.
Available from Internet: <http://www.mednet.org.uk/mednet/dl4.htm>.
[2] S Weibel, H. Juha, DC-5: The Helsinki Metadata Workshop; A Report on the Workshop and Subsequent Developments. *D-Lib Magazine* February (1998)
Available from Internet: <http://www.dlib.org/dlib/february98/02weibel.html>.
[3] Centrale Sante. Net Scoring : criteres de qualite de l'information de sante sur l'Internet; 20 Apr 1998 [Web document, accessed 27 Apr 1999].
Available from Internet: <http://www.chu-rouen.fr/dsii/publi/critqualv2.html>.
[4] J. Ambre, R. Guard, FM Perveiler, J. Renner, H. Rippen, Health Information Technology Institute. Working Draft White Paper: Criteria for Assessing the Quality of Health Information; 20 Apr 1998 [Web document, accessed 27 Apr 1999].
Available from Internet: <http://www.mitretek.org/hiti/showcase/documents/criteria.html>.
[5] P. Ingwersen, The calculation of WEB impact factor, *Journal of Documentation* **54** **(2)** (1998) 236-243.
[6] WR. Hersh, KE. Brown, LC. Donohoe, EM Campbell, AE Horacek, CliniWeb: managing clinical information on the World Wide Web, *Journal of the American Medical Informatics Association* **3(4):** (1996) 273-280.
[7] F.Norman, Organising Medical Networks' information (OMNI). *Med. Inf.* **23** (1998) 43-51.
[8] C. Boyer, O. Baujard, V. Baujard, S. Aurel, M. Selby, RD. Appel, Health On the Net automated database of health and medical information, *International Journal of Medical Informatics* **47(1-2)** (1997) 27-29.

Medical Informatics Europe '99
P. Kokol et al. (Eds.)
IOS Press, 1999

Medical Informatics Educational Tasks Seen from Practical Perspective

Diana LUNGEANU[1], Rodica DIMITRIU[2], Mariana BAZAVAN[3], Radu SIMA[4], Bernard RICHARDS[5], Roderick NEAME[6], Jeanette MURPHY[7], George MIHALAS[1]
Tempus-Phare Project CME-02555-96
(1) Medical Informatics Department, University of Medicine and Pharmacy Timisoara, P-ta E.Murgu 2, 1900-Timisoara, Romania; (2) Romanian Society of Control and Technical Informatics; (3) Computing Centre for Health Statistics, Romania; (4) Sintec Ltd. Baia-Mare, Romania; (5) UMIST, Manchester, UK; (6) Health Information Consulting Ltd., UK; (7) University College London Medical School, UK

Abstract. This paper tries to synthesize the discussions of a seminar on medical informatics educational tasks held in May 1998 in Sinaia, Romania, within the frame of the Tempus-Phare Project CME-02555-96 entitled "Know How Transfer from University to Industry" and coordinated by the University of Medicine and Pharmacy Timisoara, Romania. Special emphasis was paid to particular features of medical education requirements in East European countries, with particular reference to Romania.

1. Introduction

The Tempus-Phare Project CME-02555-96 entitled "Know How (Technology) Transfer from University to Industry" aimed to create a common platform for communication between education and practice and to support the development of interdisciplinary fields in Romania, focusing mainly on medical informatics. The project was intended to support the process of university reform, as well as the healthcare system reform, enabling cooperation between the academic, scientific, research, and practice fields in establishing needs and developing new strategies.

Three seminars were organized as debate forums, each of them dedicated to one of the three main fields: education, research, and production. They were followed by a plenary session for conclusions' presentation and synthesis. Some outstanding scientific personalities and high level governmental representatives attended the seminars.

2. Education and Training. Target Groups for Medical Informatics Education

We considered that an important distinction has to be made between two different phases of instruction:

- **education** – the preparation phase for long term knowledge and skill development, which provides the theoretical foundation;
- **training** – the practical activity phase, concerning knowledge and skills for near future mainly focused on using some specific products.

Moreover, in order to have a thorough understanding and a complete overview of the large palette of activities covered by "healthcare delivery", we thought a scheme of medical information flow would be useful – figure 1.

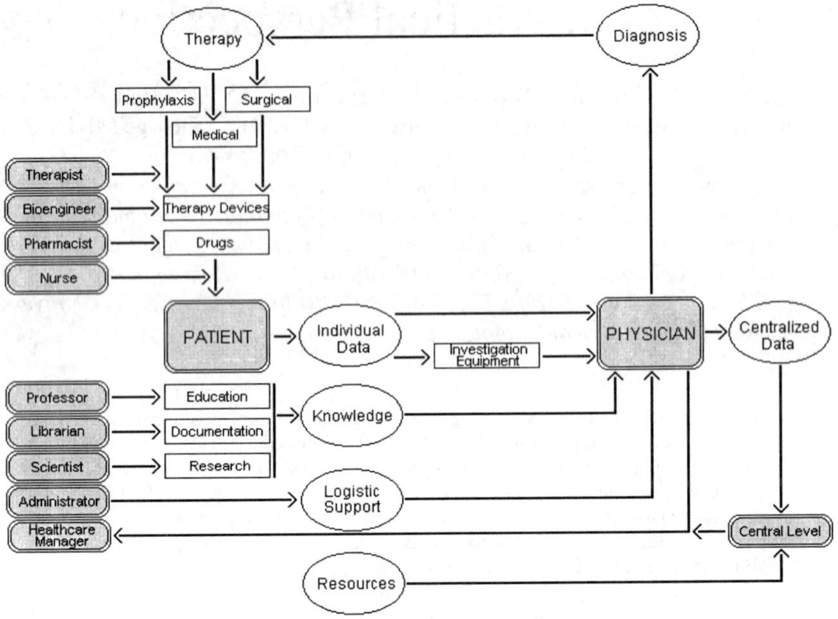

Figure 1 – Scheme of medical information flow

As the scheme emphasizes, it is important to be aware that **education** should involve not only the future doctors' education, but also the education of other categories of personnel: nurses, pharmacists, therapists, bioengineers, technicians, healthcare managers, documentarists, software producers, researchers, etc. Moreover, the patient's education should be considered and we have to be aware that the educational objectives are specific for each category.

At the beginning of the new age of communication we enter in, an increasing attention is oriented toward the industrial challenge for a better communication [1]. In addition to this, the more demanding is the work market, the more willing are the healthcare professionals to improve their education and training [2], with all the implied economic benefits. Therefore, the education system has to adapt itself to the market demands. Moreover, new facilities are offered: Internet and the Web sites are already widely seen as ideal platforms for interdisciplinary communication, as well as tools for healthcare professionals' education [3].

The participants in the seminar on education took all the aspects presented above into consideration. The discussion emphasized the importance of building strong connections between education, research, industry, and healthcare. An aspect that was stressed was the value of a Web site built as a virtual dialogue centre.

3. Present State of Medical Informatics Education in Romania

The participants in the seminar agreed that for medical students (including dentists and pharmacists) the present education met the basic requirements in most schools [4]. Furthermore, some nursing schools have just started educational programs on medical informatics and this is expected to be generalized in the next years.

However, some improvements have to be made: even if graduate studies in medical informatics and bioengineering have also started, the links with the healthcare communities are still poor, most of the specialists are misused or underused. The common feeling of some participants was that there was a general confusion at high governmental levels, lack of legal basis, as well as some lack of interest for these interdisciplinary aspects.

Another important issue discussed was the healthcare management, where there is still no possibility to specialize.

The doctoral level studies in medical informatics are also an important unsolved problem in Romania: there is a lack of legal frame concerning the relation between the titles awarded and the institutions able to do this. Therefore, in Romania, only the medical doctors may receive the Ph.D. title in medical informatics.

4. Conclusions

A successful strategy for the healthcare reform should be based on a realistic estimation of the present state and a thorough analysis of the available resources. As the role of education is to provide future human resources, a long-term strategy should start with a good educational program.

The Recommendation No. R (20) 21 of the Council of Europe, Committee of Ministers [5] was presented and considered to be a good introduction to the proposals to the governmental authorities, concerning the improvement of the present state. Moreover, several proposals for each category of personnel were made and sent to the appropriate institution.

We do hope that the Web site (***http://www.infosan.ro***) we built as an interdisciplinary dialogue platform will be a valuable help for a better communication between universities and practice.

References

[1] De Benedetti C. The industrial challenge. In: Laires M.F. et al. (Eds), *Health in the Communication Age*. Amsterdam: IOS Press, 1995, p. 21-22.

[2] Vimarlund V. et al. The economic implications of users willingness to increase knowledge capital in health informatics. In: Cesnik B. et al. (Eds.), *MEDINFO 98*. Amsterdam: IOS Press, 1998, p. 711-715.

[3] Murphy J. et al. Designing, implementing and evaluating a Web site for health informatics. In: Richards B. (Ed.), *Healthcare computing 1998*. BJHC Ltd. 1998, p. 189-199.

[4] Mihalas G.I., Lungeanu D. Strategy for medical informatics education at the University of Medicine and Pharmacy in Timisoara. In: van Bemmel J.H., McCray A.T. (Eds), *Yearbook of Medical Informatics 1997*. Stuttgart: Shattauer 1997, p. 113-119.

[5] Council of Europe. Committee of Ministers. Recommendation No. R (90) 21. In Hasman A. et al (Eds.), *Education and training in health informatics in Europe*. Amsterdam: IOS Press, 1995, p.3-6.

Medical Informatics Europe '99
P. Kokol et al. (Eds.)
IOS Press, 1999

An Orthopaedic Discussion Group, linking and teaching the Orthopaedic Community

Ian Callanan[1]
Ursula Gormalley[2]
Tim O'Brien[2]
1.*Mater Hospital, Dublin, Ireland*
2.*Cappagh Hospital, Dublin, Ireland*

Abstract. Since its inception, the Internet has created many new opportunities for the dissemination of knowledge between individuals. One of the areas most affected by these changes has been healthcare, both in terms of service provision and in the arena of medical education. Other healthcare professionals have described the educational resources available on the Net but few have illustrated the advantages of educational and conversant interaction between members of a surgical speciality or the maturing process that takes place within that group. We describe how the initiation and continued development of an Internet-based discussion group has benefited the orthopaedic profession in Ireland. We identify problems detected to date and possible difficulties in the future of the discussion group.

1. History of the group

The Orthopaedic Discussion Group was set up by the Professor Tim O'Brien, of the Department of Orthopaedic Surgery of the Royal College of Surgeons in Ireland in 1996 at Cappagh Hospital. This is an elective orthopaedic institution which acts as the centre of postgraduate orthopaedic education for the Republic of Ireland.

The primary aim of the discussion group has been to facilitate the discussion of difficult, interesting or unusual cases. Initially the group consisted of a small number of consultants and senior registrars who worked in the hospital and who had a strong interest in new technology. A steady expansion of members has taken place since then. Since the group's existence has never been publicly announced, new members have been added, at their own request, after word of mouth contact and recommendation.

There are 59 consultants and 72 registrars / senior registrars in Ireland. Of these, 21 consultants and 47 registrars / senior registrars are on the discussion group. In total there are 93 members of the discussion group.

2. Workings of the group

The initial message from a subscriber consists of a brief history and description of an orthopaedic problem accompanied by the relevant x-rays or clinical pictures. Respondents have the opportunity to reply to the submission with suggestions, opinions, researched treatises or further questions. To allow for categorisation, threading and subsequent filing, cases are usually named after the institution from which they have been sent. As the group has expanded and the numbers of contributions has grown, submissions previously numbered in sequence from each hospital are further indexed by appending one of several descriptive terms to the title, namely spot, current, archival. This also serves to alert group members to the nature of the case and in particular the sensitivity of commenting on and discussion about cases under active treatment. However, within the group, case taxonomy has not always been adhered to. Cases proven to be of specific interest are subsequently summarised for publication in the Irish Journal of Trauma and Orthopaedic Surgery.

3. Discussion

More than 100 cases have been discussed on the group to date. These range from cases where the submission related to a spot diagnosis with one or two comments to those more complex and contentious submissions where between 10 and 14 replies were received. Replies vary from single sentence comments to pages of comment and research on the topic under discussion. Submission of cases is always by consent of the principal surgeon, even though he may not be a member of the group. Precautions are taken to ensure the confidentiality of all cases submitted to the group. All patient identifiers are removed from images, x-rays and reports prior to submission; cases under active treatment are specifically highlighted as such.

Since most orthopaedic cases centre on interpretation of radiological findings, scanning of x-rays is a necessary adjunct to case presentation on the group. In the early life of the group, access to flatbed scanners with transparency adapters was limited, submissions were limited to those from members with access to the professorial unit. However it is now commonplace for many of the orthopaedic trainees to have purchased their own scanner or have ready access to one in their hospital's orthopaedic department. Many trainees have also purchased digital cameras directly due to participation in the discussion group.

Concurrently, an Internet instruction course was set up under the auspices of the professorial unit for the training of orthopaedic staff in basic and intermediate usage of Net facilities. Though admission to the course was open to all, early promotion was confined to those in close contact with the hospital, in order to create a cohort of trained Internet users within the speciality. Subsequent courses have included participants from all areas of medical and paramedical disciplines. Five of these courses have been held over the past 18 months and there is a waiting list for future courses.

Though the discussion group is semi-moderated (all messages can be posted directly to the group but Professor O'Brien can request that further correspondence should not be entered into on that subject) it's development has been almost completely self-driven. It has taken a direction without the imposition of rules, dictats or formal plans. This might be due to the "immediacy" of discussions that take place on the group, allowing the members to espouse a communal intent of future direction almost simultaneously.

As membership of the discussion group has increased, the number and variety of the submissions has enlarged. A number of aspects of this increased throughput should be considered.

1. The use of and participation in the discussion group has now become a significant element in the continuing orthopaedic education of trainees.
2. The group has facilitated the distance learning programme for those trainees working in regional centres around the country, with members highlighting topics discussed in lectures and conferences both in Dublin and internationally.
3. To have submitted case material or responses to the discussion group is acknowledged as a career enhancing move
4. The quality of response has progressed from that of personal opinion, conjecture and unsupported ideas to researched and illustrated answers to both specific orthopaedic questions and general surgical topics. This trend towards evidence based medicine is an

important side effect of group participation and facilitates training for subsequent completion of the inter-collegiate examinations. The elevation of standard of response has been driven from within, where individual contributors feel that their reply needs to be equivalent to or better than their perceived peers are. Even though these peers might be more or less experienced, interaction through the Internet seems to create a levelling effect between trainees of different experience, reducing the hierarchical distinctions associated with face to face contact.

The identifiable difficulties associated with the inception of the group are;

I. The large number of "lurkers" or "voyeurs", who though members, feel reluctant or unwilling for whatever reason to contribute to the group. Opinion on these individuals is divided, with some more active participants resenting their presence on the group and others patiently waiting for them to summon up the interest, courage or ability to interact with their net colleagues.

II. Timing of logging on and contributing to the group. Since most group members access the group from home rather than the workplace, there is a danger of eventual fatigue or frustration with this concept of Internet based learning unless net interaction is regarded as a more integral part of the working day.

III. There exists the danger of disinterest developing from information overload. This might arise principally from two distinct aspects of group participation. Firstly, the number of cases has grown steadily since the group's inception; with between 4 and 10 messages being broadcast each night. Those that do not log on each and every night might find the volume and diversity of information downloaded too large, diverse and intensive to consider responding to the cases submitted. Also, what was previously heralded as a relaxed and unconstrained medium for information sharing has been turned into an exercise in competitive answering by those individuals who put so much time and effort into their replies. There is a danger that individuals might find the opportunity of responding to a problem too daunting to consider, resulting in an increase rather than a decrease in the proportion of "lurkers" in the group.

4. Conclusion

The use of an internet-based discussion group in orthopaedics has significantly expanded the educational and communication opportunities for the Irish orthopaedic profession both nationally and internationally. It has become an important adjunct to training as well as improving the web skills of members while providing a forum for correspondence between participants. The group has survived the initial honeymoon period, where enthusiasm and eagerness propagate an internet culture within the speciality and has maintained a momentum which will serve to safeguard its continued existence.

Table 1. Composition of the orthopaedic mailing list.

Consultants	Dublin	12
	Outside Dublin	9
	Abroad	6
Senior Registrars	Dublin	11
	Outside Dublin	2
	Abroad (Visiting Fellows)	8
Registrars	Dublin	20
	Outside Dublin	14
	Abroad	4
Hospitals		7

Medical Informatics Europe '99
P. Kokol et al. (Eds.)
IOS Press, 1999

Education and training possibilities in Europe for chaining ambulatory and hospital inpatients care

F.H. ROGER FRANCE*
Centre for Medical Informatics , Université Catholique de Louvain
10, av. Hippocrate, B-1200 Brussels

Abstract. Although there is a trend to the development of the electronic patient record, the need for uniform classification systems to document diagnoses and procedures is still there. In the European Union, some research projects or concerted actions promote the concept of episodes of care, meaning that the clinical status of a patient might be followed by different health professionals in various health care settings (ambulatory care, emergency, inpatient, long term care) through medical record summaries. An inventory of teaching and training tools related to information systems that classify diagnoses in various health care settings has been made during the year 1998. Its results show that casemix tools are mainly used for hospital inpatients, much less for outpatients and almost never yet to link episodes of care. Computerised training tools exist in several countries for coding as well as for grouping patients but this area appears still too knew in the field of education because of a lack of European health policy to use uniform data sets in order to measure the degree of efficiency as well as the quality of health care delivery systems in the European union country members.

1. Introduction

Health care delivery systems are a national matter jealously guarded by each European country. This is due to social and cultural factors that have contributed to the history of the financing system as well as to organisation of health care in each nation. Diagnoses, procedures, and other patients characteristics can be described in a similar way. A European uniform minimum basic data set has been proposed already in 1991 for the European Union and applied nearly uniformly in many European countries for acute care[1]. More variations exist for ambulatory and long term care. The possibility to compare medical practices in various countries using different financing and organisation systems might provide a living laboratory of successful and less successful measures that could be recommended in order to improve either efficiency or quality of care.

The episode of care concept[2] has been developed in order to make a link between different practices based on diagnoses or a set of interrelated risks that could explain the request for care. This concept should could allow to estimate its cost more globally than in a divided approach. It has been promoted by a proposal of concerted action, the "Chaine

* This paper has been supported by the European Union Health Telematics programme in the CHAINE concerted action (N° 4820). Views expressed in this paper are those of the author and do not represent these of the Commission of the European Communities

project", that existed only in 1998 and allowed to proceed to a first survey of educational and training tools available in Europe in this area.

2. Purposes of the survey

An inventory was proposed in order to identify institutions that could provide education and training in case mix grouping methods using diagnoses related group (DRGs) or other patient classification systems (All Patients DRGs, All Patients Refined DRGs, HRG (health related groups), GHM (groupes homogènes de malades), APGs "Ambulatory Patients Groups", ACGs "Ambulatory Care Groups", DCGs "Diagnostic Cost Groups", DS "Disease Staging", PMC "Patient Management Categories", ...). Another objective was to determine if computer aided tools existed in this area, developed in Europe.

Finally, external factors contributing to the development of such education and training were investigated as the situation could differ very much between countries.

3. Method

38 questionnaires were sent to current members of EFMI Working Group 1 as well as to members of PCS Europe during the month of October 1998. Among the European Union made of 15 countries, answers were received only from 7 countries. They were Belgium, Denmark, France, Italy, Portugal, Sweden and United Kingdom. No answer was received from Austria, Finland, Germany, Greece, Ireland, Luxembourg, Netherlands and Spain.

Among non-member countries of the European Union, answers were received from Czekia and Switzerland. A repetitive sending of the questionnaire was not followed by more answers by the end of December 1998.

This study could not be continued because of the premature ending of the "Chaine Concerted Action".

4. Results

The low number of answers to the questionnaire might simply reflect the lack of application of the episode of care concept in most European countries.

Only two countries have not yet implemented the Minimum Basic Data Set in Europe since 1991 : Greece and Luxembourg. In all others, medical record summaries are mainly used for acute care inpatients. Although plans exist for health care financing in the next future in Austria as well as in Switzerland, the case mix approach is less popular in the Netherlands as well as in Finland and Germany or Ireland. Portugal has conducted data collection for ambulatory care, but has not linked these data to inpatient DRGs. Spain did not apply the episode of care concept either.

The following trends were observed through the EuroChaine Inventory :

4.1. Lack of incentives for education and training in this area

In the European Union, objectives of the Minimum Basic Data Set differ by country. Those that answered to the questionnaire had some education programmes because case mix is used there for financial purpose as well as for quality of care. These applications exist in Belgium, France, Sweden and Czechia and expected by the year 2000 in Denmark.

Other purposes can be stimulating, mainly population based statistics : United Kingdom as well as Switzerland have such an objective. When used, case mix tools are utilised mainly for hospital inpatient and much less for outpatient data.

In ambulatory care there are only experiments. The most used grouper in Europe is APG (Ambulatory Patient Group), a 3M method that distinguishes three kinds of outpatients : those having had a surgical operation as day cases, those having had a technical procedure requiring time, personnel and a specific room and finally visits that did'nt imply any technology. These outpatients visits could vary in time as well as in ordering ancillary tests and treatments.

APG experiments in Europe were described as being mostly experimental and local. A main difficulty is that APGs are based on CPT4 classification developed in the USA for procedures, updated by the American Medical Association (AMA) every sixth month[3].

APG are tested currently in Belgium, France, Italy, Sweden and United Kingdom. Other incentives are still lacking. Although quality of care indicators are developed in many European countries as a new trend, they are not yet generalised and not necessarily based on Minimum Basic Data Sets. They are described as present in Belgium, France, Italy, Israel and United Kingdom.

Another important factor that requires education is missing : there is not enough professional recognition in the area of health informatics except for coders in some countries (Belgium, Israel, Switzerland, United Kingdom). Graduates in health informatics, coordinators of quality of care and health economists have a variable professional status by country, symptomatic for a lack of official recognition.

4.2. *Lack of standards in education and training programmes*

The survey considered several levels in education and training programmes :

- at the University level, more and more programmes exist[4] to teach health informaticians, health economists and coordinators for the development of quality of care. They were mentioned in answers from Belgium, Denmark, France, Sweden, Switzerland, United Kingdom and the USA. However, specific courses on case mix and on the episode of care concept are not mandatory for physicians, pharmacists, nurses, health administrators, biomedical statisticians, except for some Schools of Public Health in Belgium and France. Programme content is highly variable by institution, without any prototype promoted yet. HTLM based CD-ROM and Internet projects are developed in various countries (Belgium, France, Sweden, Switzerland, UK and the USA).
- Non university training is assured in several European countries to train data entry coders (diagnostic and procedures encoding), mainly by government supported educational programmes or by hospital associations (in Belgium, Denmark, France, Israel, Sweden, Switzerland, UK).
- Some industrial companies, such as 3M, provide a market training for case-mix uses. In countries where new health care financing systems are based on diagnosis grouping, some small and medium enterprises provide also training methods.

4.3. *Inventory of computerized training tools in 1998*

The following computer-aided training tools have been mentioned by the respondents to the Eurochaine Survey in 1998 :

COUNTRY	***COMPUTERIZED TRAINING TOOL***
Belgium	• coding standards (Min. Public Health and 7 Universities) • Case Mix uses and feed backs (CD-ROMs) (CIES, CIM, Univ. Cath. Louvain) • Encoding tools ACODAM (CIM-Univ. Cath. Louvain) 3M groupers, code finder
Czechia	• DRG view programme
France	• Coding lessons (AUNIS, ENSP)
Sweden	• ICD-10 training tools
Switzerland	• Knowledge finder (NLM, KSF) • DIDAC (Geneva Univ.) • Bâle Website for medical education
United Kingdom	• ICD-10 Training : TENDON (OPCS) • Case Mix Training : National Case-Mix Office, Package version 1

4.4. *Discussion*

Results of the present survey are still preliminary but they already show that training and education follow the development of new areas of knowledge.

As far as financial systems are not taking more into account diagnosis grouping, the urgent need for an appropriate educational system is not perceived.

Even health informatics, quality of care development and health economics are not mandatory courses in medical schools. The professional status of personel in charge of these new developments is not well recognised.

In the near future, one might expect important changes in this area, as health cost containment as well as the development of quality of care become priority areas in most European countries. The concept of episode of care will most likely be applied more widely and a request for well trained personnel might become widely necessary.

In order to face such challenge, it appears important to prepare education and training programmes in each European country. Two elements might have a great influence for the future :

- Interuniversity credits system is developed progressively. There are two components : the accreditation of an education and training programme (types of courses and exercises) and credits by hours of work of students (and not of teachers, as now). Each student could get a credit for formal courses and for computer aided training.

- The development of new education and training tools is needed in order to enable the diffusion of knowledge needed for health care management. As soon as case-mix and episode of care concepts will be applied, the need for training will be so large that current education methods won't be sufficient for the demand. Computer aided training solutions might offer adequate solutions for a rapid coverage of the various health professions that should be aware of new financing and quality of care evaluation methods. Distance learning through internet can provide education and training programmes that are only in a development stage nowadays.

References

[1] F.H. Roger France, Hospital Information Systems in Europe : Trends towards uniformity in patient record summaries. In "Diagnosis Related Groups in Europe : Uses and perspectives", (M. Casas and M. Wiley, Eds). Springer Verlag, Berlin Heidelberg, 1993, pp. 3-16.

[2] P. Iggulden and I. Herbert, Developing the Episode of Care Model. in Proceedings of 14th PCS/E Conference, Manchester, 1998, p. 21-27

[3] American Medical Association, Physician's Current Procedural Terminology (CPT4) Fourth Edition, 1988, Chicago

[4] A. Hasman, A. Albert, P.K Wainwright, R. Klar and M. Sosa, Education and Training in Health Informatics in Europe, State of the Art - Guidelines – Applications, Volume 25 in Studies in Health Technology and Informatics 1995, 286 pp.

Medical Informatics Europe '99
P. Kokol et al. (Eds.)
IOS Press, 1999

Globalisation and the Cultural Impact on Distance Education

Wendy McPhee[1] and Christian Nøhr[2]
[1]*Center of Medical Informatics, Monash University, Australia*
[2]*Virtual Center of Medical Informatics, Department of Development and Planning, Aalborg University, Denmark*

1. Introduction

The role of a distance educator in today's quest for the delivery of knowledge to a global community must begin with the question - "What do I need to consider about my own culture before I embark on the delivery of education to a culture that predicably will be different to my own?"

With the delivery of distance (or flexible) learning in today's society the changing roles of both the teacher and the learner need to be seriously considered. This is particularly relevant with the use of new technologies to deliver courses in locations with entirely different cultural and academic traditions. International education of this kind currently faces challenges in facilitating cross-cultural learning. Some of the challenges we face could be due to persistent problems of limited communications technologies, lack of teacher training, inadequate competence at university administration and general cultural differences such as acceptable level of student support. Global changes call for the development of new pedagogues with new communication technologies in ways which are sensitive to issues of cultural diversity.

Education by distance faces many challenges as we are all aware, these are all well documented [1]. We all know that the feelings of isolation, time management, compatibility of technology are some of the issues that need to be carefully thought about. When one contemplates the extra hurdles of dealing with a country that has a different language and a different culture then the considerations of delivering education needs to be viewed with a more in depth perspective. Are we as educators able to consider these differences whilst sitting inside our own culture?

Aalborg University felt that it was time to step outside of their very successful national program [2] and test what barriers and success it encountered with their program on an international level.

This paper, in a summative fashion, reflects on the cultural impact of 'tried and true' successful distance education teaching modalities used at Aalborg University in their distance education program, in an Australian setting.

2. Method

The modalities that are used by an Australian Masters of Information Technology - Health Informatics program that are compared with a cultural view are:

- Computer medicated communication (CMC)

- Residential gatherings
- The provision of coursework materials
- Verbal communication

Within each modality a number of key intents are identified and the main outcomes are assessed from the distance student's point of view.

3. Results

The result of the assessment is shown in the table below.

CULTURAL IMPACT ASSESSMENT		
Modality	**Intent (Denmark)**	**Outcome (Australia)**
CMC	Conference system as a backbone for communication between students and teachers	Technically the product chosen worked well, it was easy to install and quite user friendly
	Successful group discussion and supervisor communication to minimise the feeling of isolation and to enable collaboration between students and supervisors	Due to the lack of a common language, an in depth communication about professional issues was almost impossible. Spontaneous communication difficult This caused the feeling of isolation.
Residential gatherings	Face to face contact – student to student and student to supervisor	Language proved to be quite a barrier for real participation on behalf of the students, however the supervisors were most helpful
	Delivery of lectures as an introduction to subjects	The lecturers were uncomfortable with the delivery of their lecture material in English.
	Research project discussion with the forming of groups of students for project work	The students were not sufficiently prepared for professional discussions in another language. The feeling of distance and, the difference between the countries healthcare made the challenge of working together on a research project unmanageable.
Coursework	The necessary provision of reference material and text books for the course	A number of books were in Danish, therefore a comparable English text needed to be found. Often reference material that is easy to obtain in one country is difficult to find in another Some textbooks when translated to English had a loss of meaning and flow. Examples of Healthcare need to move outside a National example and have more of a global application.
Verbal communication	Synchronous communication Reduce isolation Personal contact Interaction and guidance when needed.	Heightened isolation - time zones are awkward. Different calendars - eg: summer/winter when one hemisphere is on summer vacation the other is in winter and working!!

4. Discussion

A program in health informatics can be very successful within one nation, and achieve good results within neighboring countries. But when the program is diffused to more distant countries unforeseen problems may occur. The situation is very similar to the transfer of IT systems, where one very well functioning system can prove to be of limited or no value to organizations in even near by countries.

In the Babel project [3] cultural preferences in development and implementation of health informatics systems have been investigated and a model for handling cultural diversity has been developed [4]. Given the definition of culture as used in the Babel project and defined *as the acquired preference in problem solving,* then problem solving could be understood in a very broad sense, which includes learning situations. As culture is defined as something which is acquired, it could magnify the implications in a learning situation and hence be very complex to deal with in educational programs. However just to be aware of the implications would be an important factor in the implementation of distance learning programs.

The traditional difference between the teacher and the student should be re examined in the light of cross cultural exchange, modalities should be examined to make sure that they are applicable, manageable or learnable in a different cultural environment.

5. Conclusion

Tested and successful modalities within a national environment that have very positive outcomes for distance education revealed the potential to have a less of a positive effect when delivered to an international student.

Cultural exchange is difficult for both the teacher and the student. The teachers/supervisors need to carefully consider as many issues as possible. A visit to the participating country could make this task easier for both the student and the teacher, or could, on the other hand, exacerbate the problems encountered.

Supervisors need to be responsible for facilitation between the cultures, and the administration and the management within the organisation need to support the faculty in acquiring the competence in international and cross cultural teaching.

Students need to understand the possibilities of cultural impact and consider what ramifications this could lead to before they make a commitment to the program. They should also understand that undertaking international distance education programs where there is likely to be a cultural difference, requires a high level of dedication. The student should have the opportunity to make an informed decision when participating in cross cultural distance education.

Many questions need to be asked - Is it possible for distance educations and students to address these issues when their own culture could bias the decision? Do cultural differences make a real impact on learning outcomes? How could cultural differences enhance the learning experience? It is useful to consider the above questions and many others when addressing the delivery of distance education across differing cultural platforms.

References

[1] http://seamonkey.ed.asu.edu/~mcisaac/disted/final98/finalam.html

[2] Christian Nøhr, Ann Bygholm, Ole Hejlesen: "Strategic Planning of the Master Programme in Health Informatics at Aalborg University: Targeting and updating the Programme to Meet Explicit Customer Needs", International Journal of Medical Informatics, vol. 50, no. 1-3, 207-213, 1998.

[3] http://www2.echo.lu/telematics/teleng/babel.html

[4] Michel Demeester: "Cultural Aspects of Information Technology Implementation". International Journal of Medical Informatics. (In print)

Internet/Intranet

Medical Informatics Europe '99
P. Kokol et al. (Eds.)
IOS Press, 1999

The Case-based Internet Textbook ODITEB for Multi-modal Diagnosis of Tumors – Development, Features and First Experiences

Alexander Horsch[1], Thomas Balbach[1], Markus Hogg[2], Fabian Sturm[1], Christo Minov[1]
[1]*Institut für Medizinische Statistik und Epidemiologie (IMSE)*
[2]*Institut für Röntgendiagnostik*
Klinikum rechts der Isar der Technischen Universität München
Ismaninger Str. 22, 81675 München
http://www.imse.med.tu-muenchen.de/mi/

Abstract. Internet technologies offer the chance to build high-quality learning media for the education in medicine. In particular, the teaching of diagnostics with medical imaging can be supported by the excellent visualization and interaction capabilities. In cooperation with three radiological departments at German universities in Munich, Erlangen and Würzburg the distributed case-based Internet textbook ODITEB[1] for tumor diagnosis of the GI-tract, liver, pancreas and thorax has been developed. It offers a growing collection of didactically prepared cases located on servers at the provider sites Munich, Erlangen and Würzburg, functionality similar to a real CT console, original DICOM data, X-rays and endoscopic and endosonographic videos, and expert-guided tours through the cases. In a first evaluation in summer 1998, 32 medical students graded the application with 1.9 ('good') on a scale from 1 ('very good') to 5 ('very bad').

1. Introduction

Diagnostic imaging is a rapidly developing area in medicine. To raise the teaching level gets more and more important [1]. Most of the nowadays learning material is paper-based. But printed media have proven to be inadequate for teaching the difficult diagnostics with modern medical imaging. Their major disadvantages are the restriction to comparably few "typical" images and the lack of image manipulation capabilities. The possibility of working interactively with the images is of high value for effective learning, since one can achieve retention rates of up to 90% by this kind of active learners participation [2].

An increasing number of publications on computer-based education show that Internet technologies with the World Wide Web as user interface will play a major role in distributed education settings of the future [2-5].

With the distributed radiological Internet-based textbook ODITEB (Open Distributed TExt Book) [6-7] for the diagnosis of tumors of the GI-tract, liver, pancreas and thorax, a learning medium has been developed that goes far beyond the potential of a printed book by fully utilizing available Internet technologies. Emphasis was laid on a comprehensive and growing collection of cases stored at different provider sites (Technische Universität München, Universität Erlangen, Universität Würzburg). The cases are didactically prepared by means of expert-guided diagnostic tours stored together with the image data.

[1] Funded by the DFN-Verein and the German Ministry of Research and Education

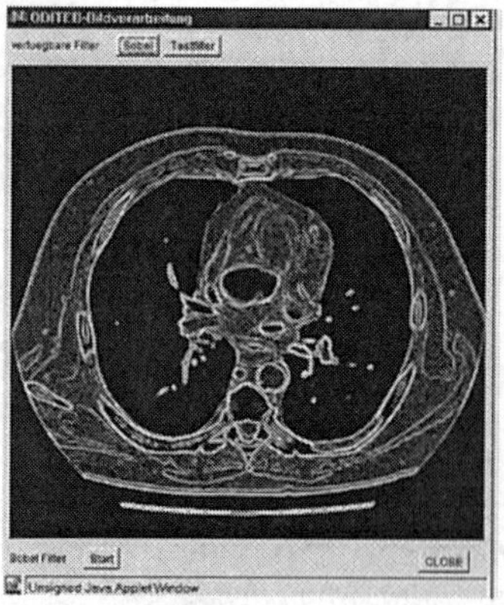

Figure 1: Image processing with ODITEB

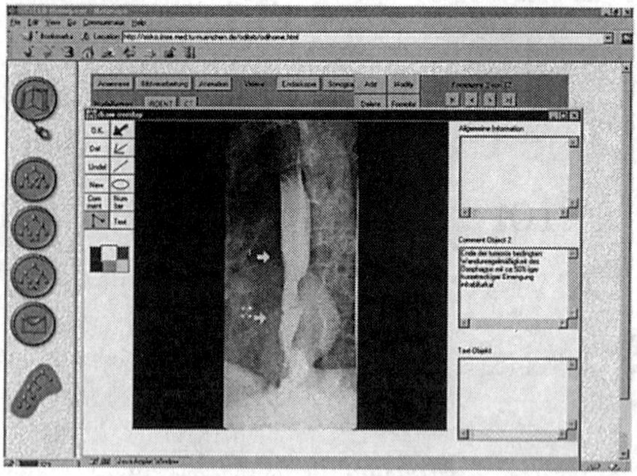

Figure 2: Authoring with the ODITEB viewer

2. Development

2.1. Basic Design Approach

When ODITEB was designed the basic approach was to join and preserve, as far as possible, the advantages of existing learning media and educational setting, and to avoid, if possible, their disadvantages. High availability of the learning medium, individual usage, comprehensiveness (depending on the authors), two-sense learning (audio/video), demonstration of difficult cases, interactive image manipulation and, to a certain extent, interaction with the expert are the advantages that can be achieved with a case-based Internet textbook [6].

In order to implement this approach three major concepts were used: (1) three-layer architecture (dynamic case layer, intermediate query layer, static instruction layer) (2) case pool distribution (3) active learners experience (interactive exploration of original image data). [6]

2.2. Hardware and Software

For the development of the ODITEB Java Applet a SGI-Indy running IRIX 5.3 and a PC running Windows NT 4.0 were used. The applet is based on the Java Development Kit 1.0 for reasons of compatibility to older browser versions. All ODITEB case servers are PCs with Linux as operating system, an Apache web server version 1.3 and WAIS as case indexing system. CGI scripts are written in Perl.

3. Features

3.1. Text Content

The textbook addresses two target groups, students of medicine and students of medical informatics. For the first group, a hypertext structure following medical terminology is provided. Starting with the selection of the tumor location, the student gets a short overview of the state of the art of diagnostics for that location. This overview includes information about clinical symptoms, diagnostic steps, normal anatomy, TNM classification and differential diagnosis. From hyperlinks within the texts the student gets lists of example cases depending on the textual context. Each list is the result of a query over all cases stored in the distributed case collection via WAIS. Each list entry is a hyperlink to the case. When a case is selected, the case viewer is started (see 3.2) and the case can be worked on. For the second group of students the hypertext part follows the terminology of image processing which comprises topics like image transformation or segmentation. It is structured similar to the medical part.

3.2. *The Case Viewer*

This Java applet provides a platform-independent mean for the visualization and exploration of original (anonymized) DICOM 3.0 data from CT and MRI as well as X-Ray images and endoscopy and endoscopic ultrasound (EUS) videos. It provides user-interactive image visualization functions like graylevel windowing according to Houndsfield or image processing (see figure 1) and allows to work up the guided diagnostic tours through the cases with comments from the expert (generated by the expert during case authoring, see 3.3). The viewer gives nearly the same functionality as a real CT or MRI console, extended by the handling of the further modalities and the guided diagnostic tours.

3.3. *Authoring*

Authoring comprises the didactical preparation of the image material collected for a case. Result of this authoring is a guided diagnostic tour through the image material following the clinical diagnostic schema. The expert virtually walks along the usual workflow and selects the most relevant images from the material that would be available at the respective point of time within the diagnostic process. To perform this task, the author uses the normal ODITEB viewer and enters the authoring tool. This tool is shown as a separate popup window overlaying the regular ODITEB image area (see figure 2). While walking through the case material, the author selects graphical elements from a palette, places them on the image and types in his comments. An author can add, modify and delete a case. In a form he types in the anamnesis of the patient, additional medical information, the type of tumor, the medical indexing like tumor location, histology and tumor staging.

4. First Experiences

4.1. *Design and performance of a small usability issue*

The evaluation of the project ODITEB was designed as a usability issue, which took place at the Technische Universität München in the half-year term of summer 1998. Out of 75 students of the sixth term class in radiology, 32 students (17 female and 15 male) participated voluntarily. Most of them had already computer experience. In a prospective and a retrospective survey the students filled out anonymously a questionnaire.

The aim of the evaluation of ODITEB was the assessment of the following criterions: (1) user interface and navigation elements; (2) efficiency as learning media compared with conventional printed media; (3) acceptance by medical students; (4) suggestions for improvement.

There was a prospective survey initiated at the beginning of the sixth term to learn about the students' expectations and requests to the ODITEB textbook. Later on, at the end of the sixth term, a second retrospective survey was performed on the students' collected experiences. All 64 questionnaires were analyzed for statistical statements afterwards.

4.2. *Results*

All questions with scalable answering possibilities were based on a scale ranging from 1 for 'very good' to 5 for 'very bad'. Overall the statistical analysis resulted in a positive grading. The assessment of the general impression of ODITEB resulted in the arithmetical mean value 1.93. This is nearly the same as the result of the question about the navigation concept of ODITEB, which was regarded as self-explaining by 75% of the students, justifying the efforts made for design and structure of the navigation buttons. The graphical user interface was judged particularly good with an arithmetical mean value of 2.03.

The students also were asked whether they had been able to acquire new knowledge using ODITEB and whether learning was more efficient than with other learning media. Indeed, 18 of the 32 participating students could acquire new knowledge in contrast to 14 who did not. Compared to that it is surprising, that only 10 students confirmed that learning with ODITEB is more efficient than learning with conventional textbook. This has to be seen on the background of a test the students have to pass at the end of the term. This test was based only on knowledge supplied in the radiological lectures and not on particular knowledge provided by ODITEB.

As major advantages of ODITEB the students mentioned: (1) easy user interface; (2) good visual presentation; (3) very good image quality of the original image data; (4) high motivation to learn with ODITEB because of interactivity. On the other hand they stated the following disadvantages: (1) long lasting download times due to the huge amount of the original image data; (2) instability regarding to some hardware equipment. The students suggested to (1) extend the case pool itself; (2) increase the number of commented cases; (3) create a possibility to use ODITEB at home with the bandwidth restrictions of a modem connection.

5. Discussion and conclusions

The consequent utilization of the multimedia capabilities of the Internet by the ODITEB textbook led to an application with high acceptance by the students. Although multimedia technologies like ODITEB will not completely replace the conventional printed media, for most of the students the interactive manipulation of image data is an important added-value in their learning setting. In near future broader bandwith capacities will simplify using extensive multimedia applications like ODITEB at home. The implementation of the technology and the provision of the contents was cost-intensive (about 4 manyear equivalents). Further extensions and the transfer to other medical domains shall be initiated in cooperation with commercial partners.

Acknowledgement

We wish to thank our sponsors, the DFN-Verein, Berlin, and the German Ministry of Research and Education. Special thanks for providing the content we owe to our colleagues in the radiology departments, Carl Ganter, Thomas Treumann, Paul Hellerhoff and their director Paul Gerhardt (Munich), Alexander Tschammler and his chief Dietbert Hahn (Würzburg), Alexander Cavallaro, Ekkehard Fiedler and their chief Werner Bautz (Erlangen), to the collegues in the department of surgery, Lukas Prantl and his chief H.-J. Dittler (endoscopy).

References

[1] Wu E, Lian Z. Raise the teaching and research level to fit development of diagnostic imageology. Chin Med J Engl 1996: 109 (1): 62-4

[2] Dounavis P, Karistinou E, Diomidus Marianna, Mantas J. Using World Wide Web technology for educating Students in the Health Care Sector. In: Pappas C, Maglavera N, Scherrer J-R (eds): Medical Informatics Europe '97,. Amsterdam et al.: IOS Press, 1997, 686-690

[3] Downie AC. Teaching radiology on the Internet. Clin Radiol 1997: 52 (1):4-7

[4] Bernard E. S, Frantescu A, Bernard S, Vernic C: WEB-MO – A Computer Aided Learning on WWW. In: Cesnik B, McCray A.T, Scherrer J.-R (eds): Medinfo '98. Amsterdam et al: IOS Press, 1998, 745-747

[5] Scalzetti EM. Radiology teaching-file cases on the World-Wide Web: a second-generation viewer. Am J Roentgenol 1997: 168 (3):615-7

[6] Horsch A, Hellerhoff P, Hogg M, Ahlbrink H, Balbach T, Liß T, Minov K, Gerhardt P: Concepts of a Web-based Open Distributed Textbook for the Multimodal Diagnostics of Gastrointestinal Tumours with MRI, CT and Video-endoscopy Addressing Students of Medicine and Students of Medical Informatics as two Different Target Groups. In: Cesnik B, McCray A.T, Scherrer J.-R (eds): Medinfo '98. Amsterdam et al: IOS Press, 1998, 793-797

[7] Balbach T, Liß T, Horsch A: Visualisierung und Kommentierung von DICOM-Daten - Ein Java-Applet. In: Lehmann T, Metzler V, Spitzer K, Tolxdorff T (Hrsg.): Bildverarbeitung für die Medizin 1998. Algorithmen - Systeme - Anwendungen. Berlin, Heidelberg, New York et al.: Springer, 1998, 338-342

Medical Informatics Europe '99
P. Kokol et al. (Eds.)
IOS Press, 1999

From Bridges to Super-Highways: Transmitting Meaning Within and Between Professions, and Across Time and Space - Beginning the Process

*Ann J Sheridan, **Michael J Rigby, ***Ronald J Draper
**Principal Nurse Tutor, St. John of God Hospital, Dublin, Ireland.*
***Lecturer, Centre for Health Planning and Management, Keele University, UK.*
****Consultant Psychiatrist, Hospitaller Order of St. John of God, Dublin, Ireland.*

Abstract. As development of health informatics, including electronic patient records, proceeds apace there is an innate tendency to focus on acute and primary care, and upon bio-pathological data sets. This is where virtually all research and investment is being directed. However, the core purpose of health care (and mental health care in particular) is to improve and maintain the individual's functioning and sense of well-being, not simply to eliminate adverse pathology. It is therefore vital for health care records to contain subjective, descriptive, and self-expressed components if the record is to have true health meaning. This in turn raises challenges about meaning and context, terms and language. Most informatic systems run the risk of being Islands of Automation, linked at best by bridges conveying data sets rather than knowledge. If health informatics is really to serve people and their health, attention needs to be given to developing the recording, communication, and understanding of perception through shared meaning. Only then will informatics systems be full supporters of the people's health, and record system linkages become Super-Highways of Knowledge between patients and their supporting professionals.

1. Introduction - the Communication of Health Perceptions

Mental health services (which comprise 10% of all healthcare need and expenditure) are by their nature diverse, with care being provided by numerous professional groups in a variety of settings. Moreover, mental health care is dependant upon patients' subjective descriptions of their feeling states which are then interpreted according to the perspective of the individuals who record these occurrences. Therefore, the patient record has a pivotal role as a means of communication and co-ordination of care.

Somatic (acute physical care) services may feel that their recording and communication requirements are more objective, empirical and straightforward, but this denies the essential human focus of healthcare - the enabling of persons to optimise their health, wellbeing, and functioning in society. Whilst mental health services are fundamentally based on patient perception and wellbeing, other services are enriched if they too adopt functioning and belief components, and avoid the trap of developing a solely biological data warehouse model of electronic records matching a repair shop model of health care.

However, the recordings made by individual clinicians and the meaning attributed to these, which form the basis of clinical decision making in mental health and should inform clinical care in all sectors, have a high linguistic and interpretative vulnerability. The reliance on patients' subjective accounts, and subsequent interpretation of this data by various professional disciplines, presents a number of challenges when attempting to progress towards a truly holistic and integrated approach to patient care. The major challenge is that of sharing the meaning of the data in a way which reflects the patients' reality and coherently informs clinical intervention.

2. Meaning and Language

Attempting to define meaning has occupied the minds of linguists and philosophers for centuries and as yet has not been satisfactorily resolved [1]. While there is no generally accepted definition of meaning, this does not absolve health care professionals from exploring and grappling with such issues. Semiology and anthropology emphasise the structural nature of meaning. Within these perspectives meaning is determined by symbols, which are associated with social life and determine thought and perception. Thus meaning is socially constructed and language has a critical role in shaping the social construction of reality.

In the health care setting the meaning-making process is a social one, and being able to make sense of what is going on as a health care professional requires making sense of this sociability [1]. Making sense of sociability, however, requires more than simply attaching a personal meaning to the experiences of others. Sharing meaning in social relationships involves the deep processes of understanding someone else's ways of thinking about their experiences in the world [2].

Language is the medium by which meaning is conveyed between persons. However, this is more than a vocabulary comprising words with attached definitions - semantic rules are necessary to provide the context, which creates significant meaning. Moreover, the meanings of words also change with culture and geography, and this is particularly significant with vernacular language, which is often a key element of patient self-expression and description of their health problems and perceptions. Given the intensely personal and dialogue-based nature of mental health care and its related assessment and recording, recognition of the context-specificity of words, and of formal terms, is essential in the long-identified challenge of developing a common language of care [3].

Within the health care domain there exists among professionals a variety of conceptual systems that inform the construction of meaning. Navigating through such complex systems increases the risk of misunderstanding within and between professional disciplines. Moreover, and inappropriately, they have the effect of alienating the patient [4].

How then do we begin the process of attempting to reconcile our differences? How do we build bridges within and between disciplines and with patients in an attempt to make health care meaningful and effective?

3. Meeting the Challenge

Within mental health care the patient record is the primary means through which meaning is transmitted, and in this recognition of the value of the integrated record mental health has been ahead of other domains [5]. The significance of the record is further enhanced given the likelihood of such a document supporting the patient for a considerable portion of their life span. Added to the complexity of transmitting meaning for a particular episode of care between professionals and patients is the challenge of transmitting it across a time span complicated by changes in knowledge, understanding and fashions in approaches to treatment and care.

The value of the electronic record in mental health as a means of building bridges between care providers for an individual patient has been identified [6]. However, without a means of conveying meaning across those bridges they remain merely expensive architectural impositions on the landscape. In attempting to meet these challenges the Hospitaller Order of St. John of God is proceeding towards developing an holistic, integrated electronic patient record which represents the patient rather than a multiplicity of differently formulated views of the patient [7]. In so doing it is drawing on earlier lessons and analyses [8-10] and in particular the importance of accommodating human values as the core element [11].

However, simply structuring the record to collate and present facts is not enough - such structures of themselves merely act as navigation tools around Islands of Automation [12]. The patient record, rather than being a static account of discreet episodes of care, must become a dynamic tool, which is an active means of transmitting meaning between individuals. Included in the dynamic record must be components, which represent patient circumstances and preferences, and future plans of action mapped against purpose and intended outcome [13,14]. The dynamic element of the record must include automatic indication of when health or care delivery deviate from the expected or the intended [15,16], and all these factors must be capable of meaningful anonymised aggregation to provide service level information.

4. The Hospitaller Order of St. John of God Project

The Hospitaller Order of St. John of God, County Dublin, a mental health service provider, is working towards a comprehensive, clinically driven patient-based record, available on multiple sites, in real time, which would capture, store, retrieve and process a longitudinal and holistic representation of the patient's health status in order to support multidisciplinary care and treatment [7,17]. The system is modular, comprising Active X components. It was initially developed as a series of simulations using Borland's Delphi. Following extensive end user feedback [18] it has been rebuilt using a Visual Basic front end running on Windows NT and an SQL Server, and after prototyping is in process of phased roll out. Input is stored both as textual reports and coded for statistical output. A Viewer displays a list of all stored data items within an individual patient record as active keys to the data with options to view the stored report or through construct views which display selected data for specific purposes. As the data are stored according to contacts and episodes a longitudinal view of the patient's care and treatment over many years and multiple episodes can be obtained with easy access to historical data.

Point and click data entry, utilising recognised clinical frameworks such as the Mental State Examination and Orem's model of nursing [19], result in meaning being captured in a clear context and from an unambiguous professional viewpoint, including labelling as mild, mocerate, or severe; where drop-down sub-menus still do not enable sufficient detail or specificity the opportunity to add text is given. To complement this structured and context-specific record core, text fields give opportunity for richness of message, but with the drawbacks of possible degradation of meaning through ambiguity of language, and limitations on searches.

5. Deeper Personalised Meaning - The Tall Order

However, having built these bridges linking professionals and services, what deeper meaning will travel over them? In so far as bio-pathologic data are concerned, and completed structured assessments, there is no major problem. But that is only part of the optimal mental health record. It is the building in of the attitudinal and evaluative information, in structured unambiguous terminological format [4], which is the challenge. Given the lack of corporate progress internationally in these areas of terminology, it is a tall order for a single health care provider to achieve alone. The Order has therefore been actively seeking solutions to what are important issues in developing clinical communication and record-keeping, linked to modern information technology opportunities, and endeavouring to find others interesting in pushing for progress.

6. A Catalogue of Frustration

International terminology systems such as ICD10 and DSMIII are diagnostic, and do not accommodate the topics of interventions or intentions. Likewise, nursing taxonomies have adopted this diagnostic approach which presupposes the existence of a curative intervention. Such systems tend to ignore or at least shy away from dealing with the less concrete and more complex situations which are the everyday reality of patients' lives and professional practice in mental health [4]. Proposals have been put to the European Health Informatics Standards Body CEN TC251 by one of the co-authors to develop a meta-taxonomy for mental health interventions, and secondly to define a generic framework for care plans. Both proposals have been accepted onto the group's 'long list', but neither has reached the top of the list to obtain resources in the face of competing bids from apparently more attractive domains. More specifically in mental health, a group convened informally by the World Health Organisation identified the issues which needed addressing [20], and a visioning paper took the debate into the American setting [21], but again only moral support but no finite action resulted. A European collaboration paper in the policy context [22] met a similar fate. There are no specifically mental health initiatives within the European Telematics Application programme (TAP), nor in earlier EU research phases, whilst the generic programmes give little support to mental health, and approaches have not been fruitful. This lack of input also applied when the project addressed the hitherto unanswered aspects of data protection and ethics for persons not mentally competent at particular moments of time [23].

In the setting of health informatics bodies, the frustration is similar. A proposal to develop a working group of the International Medical Informatics Association (IMIA) to consider issues specific to mental health (but which would, like the mental competence issue, be likely to illuminate the wider health informatics field), which was encouraged by one outgoing IMIA President, did not produce any formal response when considered by the IMIA Board. Fortunately, the World Psychiatric Association is more progressive, with the recent establishment of an Informatics and Telecommunications section, and has resulted in special workshop strands at the biennially alternating global and European meetings. Unfortunately, important though this is, it is perforce primarily a uni-disciplinary and reporting occasion.

7. Conclusion - Under-Used Bridges

Practitioners in mental health should find the process of transmitting meaning, and not just bio-pathologic facts and schedules of physical interventions, an essential core of their work. Therefore, as health informatics techniques are harnessed in mental health to further improve care delivery, information systems should be capable of holding and transmitting such patient-based subjective meaning. It should also transcend different professional models of care when applying to one individual [24].

However, mental health professionals should not be alone in the health community in this respect. If health is truly to be considered in the terms enshrined in the World Health Organisation's founding charter as being "a state of complete physical, mental, and social well-being, and not merely the absence of disease or infirmity" [25], and with the increasing recognition that health should now be defined in relation to the individual and his or her expectations, and to his or her optimum level of functioning in everyday living [26], then all health practitioners have a need to be able to communicate this richer meaning.

The Hospitaller Order of St. John of God, in its desire to run a modern, quality-based service, has sought to build informatics bridges. That has been challenging, but not impossible. However, in terms of transmitting across those bridges meaningful and relevant information and knowledge, as opposed to bio-pathological data and images, it feels at a very early pioneering stage. More worrying, it finds itself very much alone in caring about this problem.

Possibly, and hopefully, a scientific conference in the setting of a newly emergent democracy which is building on strong cultural values but reviewing its methodology afresh will provide an appropriate and fruitful setting to enable rediscovery of healthcare meaning. This kind of proven fresh thinking and return to core human values is needed in the quest for the optimisation of health information and thus health informatics - namely to develop an effective focus on recording the perceived and expressed personal health status and functioning of the individual person, thereby turning informatics bridges into super-highways of knowledge.

References

[1] Crawford P, Browne B, Nolan P: Communicating Caring - The Language of Nursing, Stanley Thornes, Cheltenham, 1998.

[2] Duck S: Meaningful Relationships, Sage, London, 1994.

[3] Swayne J: A Common language of Care?; *Journal of Interprofessional Care*, **7**, 1, 29-35, 1993.

[4] Sheridan A, Draper R, Rigby M: The Importance of a Holistic, Patient Based and Multi-Disciplinary Approach to Terms and Coding for Success in EPR Systems - A Case Study from Mental Health; in Moorman PW, van der Lei J, Musen MA: Preceedings of IMIA Working Group 17, Rotterdam, 8-10 October 1998 – EPRiMP: The International Working Conference on Electronic Patients Records in Medical Practice; Erasmus University, Rotterdam, 1998, Annexe 1-4.

[5] Williams JG, R. Roberts R, Rigby MJ: Integrated Patient Records - Another Move Towards Quality for Patients? (editorial); *Quality in Health* Care **2**,2, 73-74, 1993.

[6] Rigby MJ: An Electronic Patient Information System in Mental Health - An Integrated Solution for Better Care and Management, in Adlassnig K-P, Grabner G, Bergtsson S, Hansen R (eds.): Medical Informatics Europe 1991, Proceedings Vienna, Austria, 1991; Springer-Verlag, Berlin, 1991.

[7] Draper R, Hamilton I, Rigby M: Developing an Electronic Patient Record for Mental Health; in Proceedings 2nd. Annual Conference and Scientific Symposium, 13th. November 1997, Grand Hotel, Malahide, Co. Dublin; Health Informatics Society of Ireland, Dublin, 1998, 1-10.

[8] Rigby MJ, Robins SC: A Networked Patient-Based Integrated Care System as a Basis for the Achievement of Quality in Practice; in Roger-France F, Noothoven van Goor J, Staehr-Johansen K: Case-Based Telematic Systems Towards Equity in Health Care (Studies in Health Technology and Informatics Vol. 14); IOS Press, Amsterdam, 1994.

[9] Rigby M, Robins S: Practical Success of an Electronic Patient Record System in Community Care: A Manifestation of the Vision and Discussion of the Issues; in Runnenberg J (ed.): The Future of Patient Records - Care for Records for Care (Proceedings of the 8th European Health Records Conference, 21-24 May 1995, Maastricht); Dutch Association for Medical Records Administration, Hoorn, 1995, 403-410.

[10] Rigby MJ, Roberts R, Williams JG: Objectives and Prerequisites to Success for Integrated Patient Records; *Computer Methods and Programs in Biomedicine*, **48**, 121-125, 1995.

[11] Rigby MJ, Robins SC: Human Values as the Core Focus of Community Health Computing; in Barahona P, Veloso M, Bryant J (eds.): Proceedings of the Twelfth International Congress of the European Federation of Medical Informatics, Lisbon, Portugal, 22-26 May 1994; Portuguese Association for Medical Informatics, Lisbon, 1994.

[12] Song L, Ho J, Ho S: The Integrated Patient Information System; *Computers in Nursing*; **15**, 2, S14-S22, 1997.

[13] Rigby M: Reviewing and Developing Architectural and Technological Concepts to Meet the Needs of Long-Term Holistic Health Services; in Moorman PW, van der Lei J, Musen MA (eds.): Preceedings of IMIA Working Group 17, Rotterdam, 8-10 October 1998 – EPRiMP: The International Working Conference on Electronic Patients Records in Medical Practice; Department of Medical Records, Erasmus University, Rotterdam, 1998, 338-343.

[14] Rigby M: Realising the Fundamental Role of Information in Health Care Delivery and Management (Reducing the Zone of Confusion); Nuffield Trust, London, 1999.

[15] Rigby M, Robins S: Practical Success of an Electronic Patient Record System in Community Care - A Manifestation of the Vision and Discussion of the Issues; *International Journal of Bio-Medical Computing*, **42**, 117-122, 1996.

[16] Mooney M, Barry S, Draper R: The Electronic Patient Record as a Guarantor of Personalised Mental Health Care; in Cesnik B, McCray AT, Scherrer J-R (eds.): Medinfo 98 9th World Congress in Medical Informatics, Proceedings; IOS Press, Amsterdam, 1998, 14-17.

[17] Draper RJ, Rigby MJ, Hamilton I: The End User as Key to Successful Implementation of Electronic Patient Records for Mental Health; in Moorman PW, van der Lei J, Musen MA (eds.): Preceedings of IMIA Working Group 17, Rotterdam, 8-10 October 1998 – EPRiMP: The International Working Conference on Electronic Patients Records in Medical Practice; Erasmus University, Rotterdam, 1998, 232-236.

[18] Draper RJ Sheridan AJ Rigby MJ: A Mental Health EHCR – Buying or Building. Proceedings of EUROREC '99 Third European Conference on Electronic Health Care Records, Seville, 6-7 May 1999.

[19] Orem D: Nursing Concepts of Practice (Third edition); McGraw-Hill, New York, 1985.

[20] Rigby M: The Vision of WHO's Mental Health Informatics Standards Working Group - Forging a Development Path for Mental Health Informatics; *MIM News - Belgische Vereniging voor Medische Informatica VZW/Societé Belge d'Informatique Medicale ASBL*; **October 1995**, 3-8.

[21] Rigby M: A Global View of Behavioral Health Informatics Initiatives - The Vision for Tomorrow must start Today; *Behavioral Healthcare Tomorrow*, **5**, 6, 25-29, 1996.

[22] Rigby M, Lindmark J, Furlan PM: The Importance of Developing an Informatics Framework for Mental Health; *Health Policy*, **45**, 57-67, 1998.

[23] Rigby M, Hamilton R, Draper R: Towards an Ethical Protocol in Mental Health Informatics; in Cesnik B, McCray AT, Scherrer J-R (eds.): Medinfo 98 9th World Congress in Medical Informatics, Proceedings; IOS Press, Amsterdam, 1998, 1223-1227.

[24] Roberts R, Rigby MJ, Williams JG: Compatibilities and Incompatibilities Between Different Professional Terminology for Patient Healthcare Needs, and Comparative Benefits for Patient Classifications; in Hofdijk J (ed.): Proceedings of the 12th International PCS/E Event and 8th Australian Casemix Conference, 16th-21st September 1996, Sydney, Australia; University of New South Wales, Sydney, 1996.

[25] World Health Organisation: Handbook of Resolutions and Decisions, Vol. II, 1973-1984; World Health Organisation, Geneva, 1985.

[26] World Health Organisation Regional Office for Europe: Targets for Health for All; World Health Organisation, Geneva, 1985.

Medical Informatics Europe '99
P. Kokol et al. (Eds.)
IOS Press, 1999

Are healthcare professionals really prepared to deal with information-empowered citizens?

Jean Roberts
First Consulting Group, Macclesfield
Chair, **medinfo2001** *Organising Committee*
jmroberts@fcg.com

1. Introduction

Traditionally, healthcare practitioners have had a constructive dialogue amongst themselves about patient diagnosis, therapy & treatment. Up until recently, that dialogue was substantially intra-professional. As the model of care delivery has become more team-oriented, the professions have to communicate across professional divides to achieve successful care outcomes, & are also put in the position of having to enter into an enhanced interactive debate about health issues with informed members of the public. This paper explores the challenges which are about to present across the world; albeit they will emerge in different countries at different time points. Also explored are the drivers & inhibitors faced by healthcare practitioners in meeting the issues raised by more 'informed' patients & clients.

2. Current status

Professionals in healthcare are increasingly working together, but there are still some cultural reservations & organisational barriers to be addressed. The electronic revolution is driving such harmonisation forward, through introducing the unavoidable capability to interact with remote personnel, reference & knowledge bases & service delivery mechanisms. The work in G8 sub-groups [1] is looking at many of the issues implicit in rationalising & harmonising technological aspects in order to widen the effectiveness of international interaction. Some of the prime issues are outlined below, because their resolution has an effect on how 'well' citizens' demands can be satisfied.

One of the catalysts to professional team working is the enabling by informatics technology of the shared patient record. The content of a 'good' electronic patient record contains input & assessment from medical staffs, nursing professionals & other direct care professionals such as physiotherapists. That record exists for the duration of an episode of care, & usually is 'closed' but not deleted after the patient has left the care facility, for example - is discharged from an inpatient hospital stay.

In a similar manner, a general practitioner (family physician) keeps their own record of non-hospital interventions - which can be anything from a septic cut or common cold to the stable maintenance of a long term chronic clinical condition. Rarely, before informatics played such a supportive part, did anything but the barest of patient history outlines go with the patient as they crossed the clinical boundaries between the community & hospitals.

From the citizen's perspective – the client / patient side, a substantive decision is usually made to seek healthcare or advice. This proactive initiative may be a visit to the local trauma unit in what is perceived as an emergency; an appointment made with a local primary care physician or, in some countries, a self-referral for a probable specific condition for a specialist consultation. In some healthcare delivery environments, this process may result in a considerable 'lag' between the individual's determination that they feel they need a clinical assessment, & the time at which that assessment actually occurs. In addition, individuals rarely inform the healthcare delivery agencies when their demographic or personal circumstances change or give a 'good' summary account of their previous clinical history when meeting a new delivery agency or professional. In the light of the likelihood of intermittent & infrequent interactions, the data held to represent the 'situation' of an individual in the various locations where previous care interventions have taken place, will at best be inconsistent between such care delivery agencies.

Even when a situation arises, perhaps through an accident when there is no forethought about such a clinical condition occurring, the citizen may well employ the various information sources to enhance their knowledge after the fact, & still make informed demands on healthcare professionals in a follow-up context.

The typical traditional situation is fragmented records, across delivery agency boundaries or divisively between professions. A number of national, international & global initiatives (such as GEHR[2], Clinical Coding Consortia[3], GALEN[4], IMIA WG16[5], CEN/TC251[6], ISHTAR[7], G8-ENABLE[8] are looking to address the professional issues, including :

- Record content harmonisation & record structures rationalisation
- Coding of clinical terms for international consistency, comparability, analysis & opportunities for effective dialogue
- Robust message passing, satisfying both technical performance & privacy concerns
- Inter-professional collective requirements to achieve holistic clinical interpretation & care delivery

The points made above address professional & organisational issues. Increasingly the individual member of the public is demanding to take a more proactive part in not only their own care, but also the determination & design of that care. They wish to explore options & be included in the consideration & incorporation of lifestyle changes that may result in care avoidance rather than treatment interventions.

3. Transition situation

Inter-professional initiatives are moving towards being able to provide integrated care – the holistic picture of what is being done, why & with what outcome – for individual case management & for strategic planning & monitoring of the demands & effectiveness of health-related resource use in general.

Agencies like the NHS in the UK, federal bodies in the USA, other governmental groups in Australasia, Europe & beyond, are investing in infrastructure projects which can facilitate inter-professional & inter-agency working; initiatives like :

- Unique patient identification (to enable record linkage between organisations to produce a (partial) holistic picture of an individual clinical history)

- Networking backbone, which presents the opportunity for sharing of clinical data between authorised professionals for individual patient/client & research use
- Development of clinically-acceptable datasets; by the professions for the professions
- Consideration of tele-solutions, involving third parties, for effective healthcare

However, to date, little activity has realised widespread support for the emerging role of the citizen in their own health management, or has addressed the future interaction between public & professional. Research projects such as Healthpoint (Scotland) [9] have not, to date, achieved a critical operational mass as the value of individual involvement in care has not been fully capitalised upon. It is suggested that 'bottom up' pressure from the citizens themselves, in a number of ways, will increase & therefore healthcare professionals must consider their ability to respond to this – in both clinical & technological terms.

4. Citizen's emerging electronic interactions

It is expected that the informed citizen achieves that 'informed' status in a number of ways & for a number of reasons, typically :

- The technology & propensity of the general media to report 'heath-related' issues, especially with heroic human-interest or possible mis-management dimensions
- The increasing global perspective on health issues; even where, for example in rural South America, there is little technological healthcare support [10], there are television channels where the local population can see projected scenarios (documentaries & stylised edu-tainment series) to frame their own expectations
- The availability, to anyone with the inclination to enquire, of previously ring-fenced academic & other reference sources on health topics
- Some personal situation or circumstance prompts the individual into collecting data on a particular health-related topic from any available source; for example –the illness of a child may prompt a parent to seek knowledge from general & specific / qualified & unqualified sources such as lifestyle & text books, friends, other professionals, & increasingly electronic sources
- The increasing mobility of population exposes individuals to experience of a greater range of options than traditional 'living at home' will present

5. Potential pitfalls to citizens empowerment about health

There is an adage in the UK that 'a little knowledge is a dangerous thing'. It is possible that a piece of raw data, available to a citizen, will not become useful information, or useable knowledge without further preparatory steps being taken. If we take, for the purposes of this paper, the view that nothing is useful without effort, then there are actions that may be taken to avoid potential distortion of clinical situations / practice as seen by citizens currently :

- The media reporting of health-related issues should take account of the capacity of the planned (& unexpected) audiences to understand the clinical concepts presented & frame their communication accordingly.
- Any communication relating to authoritative clinical material should describe its origins, credentials & veracity in understandable terms for its potential audiences.
- Professionals should seriously & proactively consider how 'best' to involve the general citizen in their own health management, rather than await the demand

- Citizens too should be kept informed of progress, pitfalls & potential towards the open society; their expectations of 'full informed status' today should be more realistically grounded in a reasoned understanding of issues.

Communication may take a number of forms, such as : individual (access to personal clinical records & assistance with their meaning); local (facilities definition & performance criteria relating to local healthcare delivery & local factors); and international (specifications of standards of care in general, description of progress in epidemic conditions, disaster management capabilities, research progress).

The Internet & its widespread accessibility have broken down barriers between professionals & public further. They present an ongoing challenge to healthcare practitioners. Citizens are now able to investigate what they perceive to be their 'clinical condition'. Armed with material from Internet public domain repositories, 'Joe Public' (a typical citizen) presents at the healthcare practitioner's clinic, surgery or private rooms, with a pre-researched perception of their own condition, covering :

- what they are suffering from, how it should be treated
- what drugs or therapy they expect to receive, how they recognised the condition

6. Potential pitfalls for the professional

Even presenting a *professional* with raw data has its problems, some previously encountered & resolved with printed & other traditional communications & reference sources. There are a number of real challenges to a healthcare professional from this type of electronic environmental situation :

- setting into a local context, information which may be from another country, health system or even be misleading or inappropriate to the specific person's overall condition
- rapidly, in a typically short consultation, entering into natural dialogue about prior documentation, & its interpretation, that may have been in complex clinical jargon
- explaining to a patient with certain expectations that there are inappropriate criteria within what they have found / or believe, relative to their particular condition & the way current 'clinical best practice' can deal with it in their country

In addition, as the general public starts to communicate via electronic mail, over their own home computer systems, the questioning & demands made on healthcare delivery systems may increasingly not occur in a face-to-face manner. Question to pose to all healthcare practitioners include :

- 'How will you cope with general mail when the bulk of it no longer comes in an envelope & requires a typed response, but comes over e-mail with an expectation of a much faster immediate reply'?
- 'How will you deal when the previous phone calls (perhaps filtered by your reception staff) for advice are sitting in the In-tray of your email service provider every morning, & arrive thereafter with invasive sound-alerts throughout the day'?

Where the patient / client increasingly interacts with the professional, armed with data gleaned from readily generally accessible sources, this will raise the spectrum of professional reluctance to relinquish the perceived 'elitist' state of being the professional who knows. That antagonism must be faced up to & minimised as the overall electronic environment will not go away.

7. What can be done

Certain countries are introducing advice call centre capabilities [11] staffed by generally informed professionals. This is generating a need for more investment in guidance & protocols that express, incontrovertibly & audibly, what clinical interventions could & should be recommended in certain clinical circumstances. This type of decision support takes a considerable amount of investment in comprehensive design, risk management evaluation & risk avoidance procedures, & in customisation to ensure advice can be appropriately refined, is understandable to the requestor & clinical & organisational liability is minimised. In addition to 'good' (whatever that is clinically deemed to be) advice leading to satisfactory individual outcomes, these types of service need to be evaluated organisationally against factors such as : efficiency of service (cost & quality aspects); effectiveness of use of professional resources & stimulation of professional motivation; and necessary investment in cultural changes, to enable acceptability of such service types by the ultimate end-users (the citizens). Citizens & professionals have to feel comfortable with the electronic interventions that are emerging into the dialogue of health. There is a need for much further work on impact assessment, ongoing information about evaluating progress & discussion about concerns, preservation of clinical confidence & professional trust, & actual contribution to better health.

8. Summary

The new Global Information Society increasingly incorporates electronic tools in every walk of life. The e-communication revolution should not be welcomed just because it exists, but rather taken as a possible catalyst to better performance, however that is perceived. Healthcare practitioners must harness the good will & motivation of citizens to play proactive parts in the health & lifestyle management for themselves, their families & their communities. Citizens must recognise that they do not become 'experts' overnight & must work with professional practitioners to the benefit of health status per se. There are still a number of substantial challenges to be faced & a need for considerable parallel & collective development if we (professionals & public) are to contribute effectively together in healthcare in the future.

References

[1] Barriers to a Global Information Society - Recommendations for International Action, Rogers, R Reardon, J (IOS Press, 1999)
[2] www.ehto.be/aim/volume2/gehr.html
[3] www.coding.nhsia.nhs.uk
[4] www2.echo.lu/telematics/health/galen.html
[5] www.ehto.be/imiawg16 or www.imia.org
[6] www.cen.org
[7] www2.echo.lu/telematics/health/ishtar.html
[8] www.ehto.be/sp5
[9] Jones, R. McLachlan, K. HEALTHPOINT : a public access health information system. Health Computing 90 (pp 65-69)
[10] Jones, R. Information for Citizens, health promotion & patient education IT EDUCTRA Product 4.10 www/fundesco.es/~it-eductra
[11] Sosa, M et al (eds.) Internet, Telematics & Health (IOS Press, 1998)
[12] Wired For Sound, Health Service Journal (29th January 1998)

Medical Informatics Europe '99
P. Kokol et al. (Eds.)
IOS Press, 1999

An Internet Implementation of an International Clinical Study

R. A. Hollingsworth[+], C. Hay[+], B.Richards*
[+] *Central Manchester Healthcare Trust*
* *Medical Informatics Department, UMIST, Manchester, England, M60 1QD*

Abstract. This paper describes a clinical study that is being conducted in 15 countries world-wide via the internet. The study concerns the removal of Factor VIII inhibitors in haemophilic children. The suitability of the Internet for this type of study is explored together with the technology (Active Server Pages, Secure Sockets Layer) that is involved in the creation of such a system.

1. Introduction

Here at the UMIST Department of Medical Informatics we have been involved in the development of numerous clinical information systems over the past two decades and as such we keep in touch with the latest technological developments. Some of the most recent developments are the Internet related technologies, Active Server Pages and dynamic HTML.

The writer is currently in charge of the I.T. side of a project that concerns a multi-national clinical study. The study is being conducted in 15 countries with 40 participating Centres. The study aims to discover the best treatment regime for the removal of factor VIII inhibitors from haemophilic children. Due to the rarity of this disorder it was necessary to involve many countries in order to recruit the required number of patients. The large geographical dispersion of Centres makes the Internet[1] the ideal medium for this study.

2. Internet Technology

Using the Internet technologies brings tremendous benefits[2] to a project of this type:-

- Elimination of the complexities involved with geographical dispersion
- The provision of dynamic content from databases with real-time interactive capabilities
- Implementation and development cost savings
- Platform independence
- High specification computers are not required to run these systems

Two main advances in Internet technology made its use for this study possible. Firstly the ability to include executable code within web pages, and secondly the ability to retrieve and store information using databases. Examples of these types of technology are Active Server Pages (ASP) and Active Data Objects (ADO). Active Server Pages allow the inclusion of code within web pages, and Active Data Objects enable information retrieval from databases using the Microsoft ODBC database connectivity standard.

3. The User Interface

The new generation of web browsers and the coding and formatting facilities they provide allow for the production of user-friendly systems within the Internet environment. These types of systems were previously only possible with packages such as Microsoft ACCESS, and Visual Basic[3].

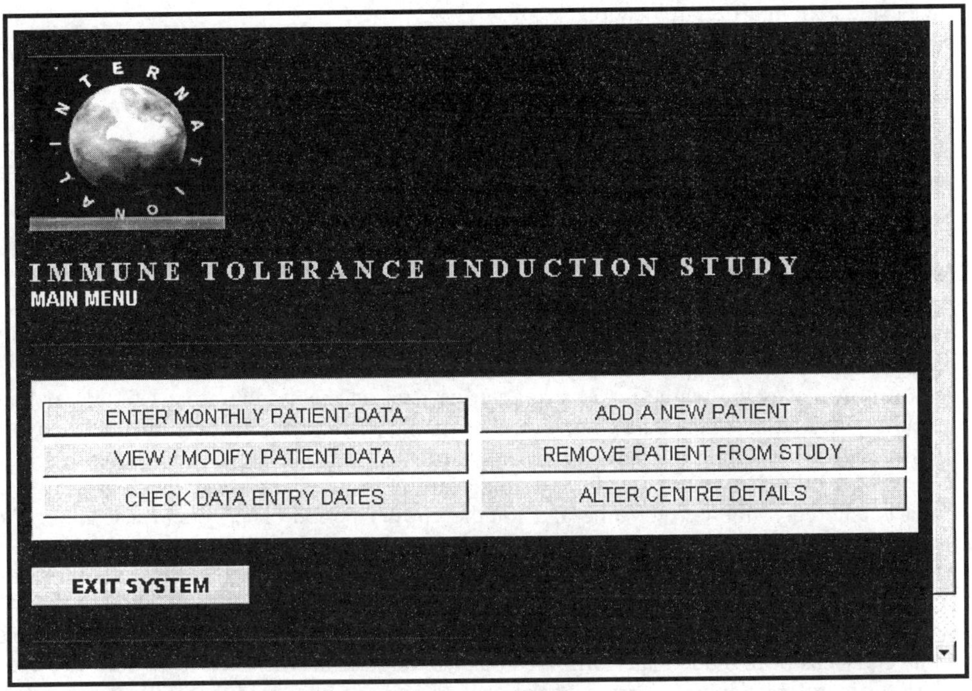

Figure 1. User Interface

For this system a user interface has been developed in which the aim was to give the system an appearance of an application rather than a web page. To do this the web browser menus have been removed giving no visual references to the use of a browser. Navigating around the system is achieved by selecting options from the 'MAIN MENU' shown in Figure 1.

4. Security

The first area of concern with a system of this type is that of security. The Internet is an open medium designed for access to one and all. For this reason it is important that proper security safeguards are in place to prevent unauthorised system access.

There are three main areas for consideration: Interception of transmitted data, unauthorised access to the system, and physical attack or environmental damage to server.

To stop people intercepting information as it passes from the client to the server the system uses a technology known as Secure Sockets Layer (SSL). This technology allows the transmitted data to be encrypted using a key. This makes it almost impossible for someone to make sense of any intercepted data.

In order to prevent unauthorised access to the system, users accessing the system must log onto a web user account set up on the server. Once they have logged onto the server they must then enter their password and username details for the system if they have already registered. If not already registered for the system the Centre must go through an on-line registration process.

To protect the system from any physical damage the server is located in a secure area of the hospital with card key access. In the event of fire, flood, etc. regular back up copies are made and kept in different locations.

5. System Facilities

The system provides centres with a number of facilities. Firstly the ability for a centre to register their centre and patients (see Figure 2) on-line without the need for any manual input from administrative personnel. The centres can also enter patient data, view and modify patient data, check data entry times for their patients, remove patients from the study and also alter their own centre details.

These features have been implemented in such a way as to guide a user through use of the system. As a registered patient progresses to the different stages of the study the system automatically adjusts itself to match the patient's current position in the study. In this way it makes the whole process of entering data on the system almost foolproof thus ensuring the quality of the data entered. One example of these automatic adjustments is that at the end of each month's data entry the system sets the date for the next month's data entry. This is varied automatically depending on the stage of the study thus ensuring that data is entered at the correct time and for the correct period. The system also alters the questions in the monthly data entry questionnaire and the forms displayed at each month's data entry time (see Figure 3), this ensures the correct information is collected. Automatic validation of the data that is entered is also provided to further ensure quality of data.

During data entry, study protocol information is displayed to the user, for example if an entry has been made which will mean that different data will need to be collected then the user is automatically informed of the change and the new data that will be requested. This gives the user further guidance in successfully following the study protocol and therefore does not rely on the user to both know and follow the protocol.

An automated email facility is contained within the system, this is designed to cut down on the amount of administrative input necessary for the running of the study. The system automatically emails centres to remind them when their patients are due for data entry. Should a centre be overdue on a patient's data entry then an email is automatically sent to the study co-ordinator informing them. Emails are also sent to the study co-ordinator when a new centre registers or a new patient is registered.

For security purposes two Audit Logs are created by the system and stored in the study database. The first Audit Log stores information about data changes and contains the following, the field altered, the old value, the new value, the patient, the time of alteration, and the person making the change. The second Audit Log keeps track of the pages visited by a user from the moment that they log onto the system.

An Information Management System has also been constructed for use by the study administrators to monitor the progress of the study and to extract information in the form of reports, for example audit log reports, newly registered centres etc.

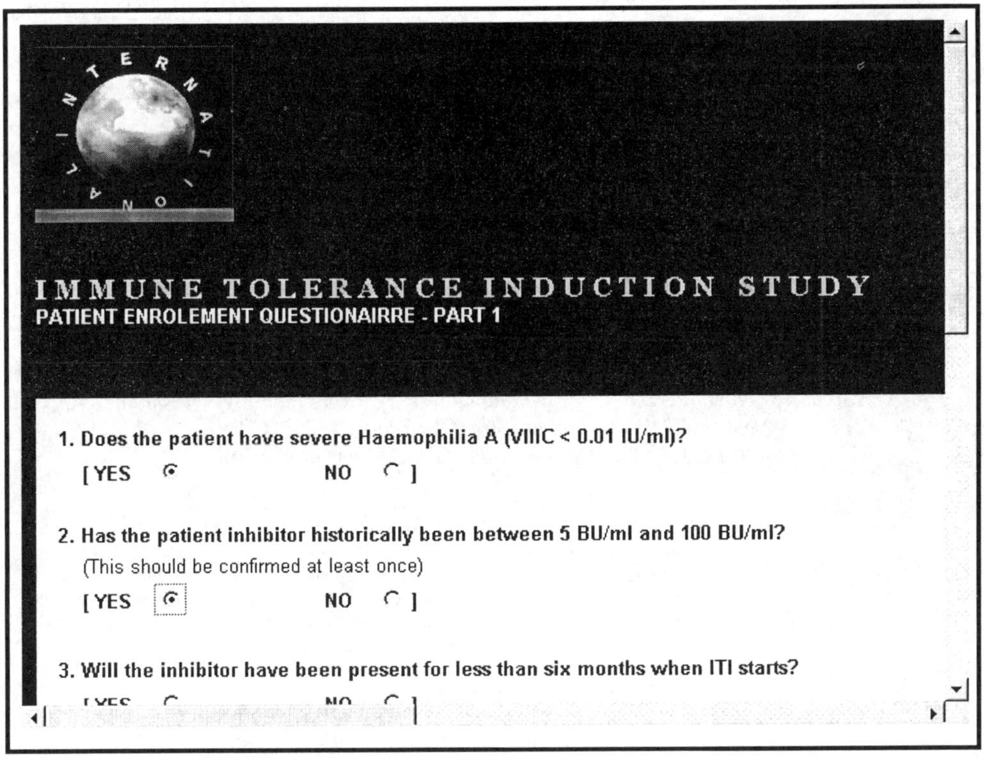

Figure 2. Patient Enrolment

6. Conclusion

The use of the Internet for this system will both improve the quality of data and reduce the amount of administration that would have otherwise been necessary using a solely paper-based approach. The Internet approach is most certainly the way forward for not just this type of project but also for projects such as patient appointment systems, and laboratory results services etc[4].

References

[1] Kelly MA, Oldham J. The Internet and randomised controlled trials. Int J Med Inf 1997 Nov;47(1-2):91-9.

[2] Menduno M. Prognosis: wired. Why Internet technology is the next medical breakthrough. Hosp Health Netw. 1998 Nov 5;72(21):28-30, 32-5, 3.

[3] Hollingsworth R., B.Richards, A Multi-Media Hospital Equipment Database. MEDINFO 95 Proceedings, Eds. R.A.Greenes et al. North-Holland Publishing Company, p624-25.

[4] Nakamura A, Baba M, Matsuto. Communications between hospital laboratory personnel and physicians. *Rinsho Byori* 1998 Nov;46(11):1103-10.

Medical Informatics Europe '99
P. Kokol et al. (Eds.)
IOS Press, 1999

Accessing a WWW Reference Library of 3D Models of Pathological Organs to Support Medical Education

Michele CRUDELE[1], Gordon J. CLAPWORTHY[2], Feng DONG[2,3],
Meleagros A. KROKOS[2], Nikos VASILONIKOLIDAKIS[4] and Giuliano SALCITO[5]
[1] *"Campus Bio-Medico", University of Rome, Via Longoni 83, Rome 00155, Italy*
[2] *Computer & Information Sciences, De Montfort University, Milton Keynes MK7 6HP, UK*
[3] *State Key Lab of CAD & CG, Zhejiang University, Hangzhou, P. R. of China*
[4] *Neurosoft Ltd., 24 Kofidou Street, Nea Ionia 14231, Greece*
[5] *CITEC Ltd., Via Alessandro Farnese 3, Rome 00192, Italy*

Abstract. A major aspiration of the medical community is to use multimedia databases to disseminate important research or clinical information and for education. We describe a WWW reference library of 3D models of human organs containing pathological and normal organs organised in cases, together with a variety of educational and supporting tools. Although the emphasis is chiefly on the teaching of medical students and the continuing education of physicians, the library is also a potentially-valuable resource for diagnostic investigation. This paper describes the environment, methodologies and tools for supporting 3D models in medical education. The prototype of the system is currently being completed; the full system is scheduled for public access in the year 2000 through multimedia publishers.

1. Introduction

The medical community is keen to support the creation of distributed multimedia databases on the WWW for disseminating important research and/or clinical information and for education [1]. Radiological information usually comes in the form of 2D images. Radiologists' experience and long training provides them with an ability to envisage the spatial relationships associated with anatomical structures appearing in a succession of 2D scans. However, non-radiologists find it rather difficult, and the availability of 3D models can be extremely helpful in providing insights into the medical conditions displayed.

The pilot project IAEVA [2] developed an integrated methodology for constructing organised WWW databases of 3D models of pathological human organs and providing relevant retrieval and manipulation mechanisms. Other databases of 3D models usually focus on the NIH-Visible Human project, i.e. scans of a male and a female cadaver that contain no particular pathological structures [3].

The results of IAEVA are now being exploited by the development of a WWW-based medical visualisation system - primarily intended for student or continuing education - under the DGXIII EC-funded IAEVA-II project. Algorithms for accelerating transmission and manipulation of 3D models over the Internet have been developed, and advanced educational tools are now provided. The system can operate on standard configurations: PC, mouse and keyboard interaction, no dedicated graphics accelerator and no sophisticated communication connections. The distributed database allows medical providers to insert/update 3D models of human pathological organs easily through their WWW servers. However, users are unaware of this: they are simply provided with a single entry point into the database [4].

2. Construction of the 3D Models

Creating the database of 3D models requires the extraction of meaningful information, by use of interactive techniques, from sequences of 2D radiological images. Currently those captured from Computed Tomography (CT) and Magnetic Resonance Imaging (MRI) are used, but other technologies could be incorporated without difficulty.

3D surface models are employed due to their fast rendering and transmission times. Demand for *3D volumetric models* is increasing rapidly, but for Internet-based work, the sizes of the models currently prohibit general use. As soon as lines with sufficiently high-bandwidth become more widespread, volumetric models will be incorporated into the system. One available solution is the adoption of Internet via satellite at downstream speeds between 300Kbps and 2 Mbit/s. The upstream can be any PSTN or ISDN connection. If the models are stored in the main network of the satellite provider, bottlenecks are generally avoided and the highest speeds can be maintained. One of the authors is experimenting in Italy with this technology which can be very useful in locations where good lines are unavailable[5].

The processing algorithms associated with volumetric models are more demanding than those associated with surface models and, until now, their use has called for specialised hardware and large computer memory. The rapidly-decreasing cost of computer hardware and the evolution of relatively cheap, highly-specified graphics cards are making it feasible to consider using PCs for these tasks. However, within the scope of IAEVA-II – a WWW-based medical education system for standard PC configurations and Internet connections – 3D surface models are currently of higher priority than volumetric models.

The surface models are formed of polygons and are displayed using the marching cubes algorithm, which is perhaps the most widely-used method for such models [6]. Depending upon the shape complexity of the anatomical structure under consideration, hundreds of thousands (or perhaps millions) of polygons are produced.

Simplification algorithms can address polygon-count reduction [7], but adequate models may still contain an excessive number of polygons; commonly, a trade-off is made between display speed, accuracy and storage requirements.

Optimisation of rendering and Internet-transmission times for 3D models containing large numbers of polygons is achieved through *multi-resolution algorithms* [8]. For a particular 3D model, a continuous range of Levels of Detail (LoDs) is captured. For rendering, different LoDs are displayed – these depend upon the user's viewpoint and the particular interaction. For transmission, a coarse LoD is transmitted initially followed by a sequence of finer LoDs, so the quality of the model is upgraded incrementally.

One of the toughest points in constructing surface models is segmentation, that is the identification of specific structures. A completely automatic process cannot be achieved in all cases, and problems arise while dealing with MRI. The IAEVA-II project is therefore providing the physicians in charge of building the models with a set of semi-automatic tools.

3. The Database

The database could be any ODBC SQL-compliant RDBMS. In IAEVA, Microsoft SQL was used; IAEVA-II uses Microsoft Access for ease of management. As soon as the size increases, upgrading the database to a more reliable RDBMS is a straightforward task. The Internet connection is performed through ASP pages. The structure is relational, with tables for keywords (classification systems), for 2D images (raw images and thumbnails) and for 3D models, which may be stored in any other server over the Internet. Textual data about a case is stored along with author, source and reference.

To speed the navigation through the coding systems, instead of providing a dynamic access to the classification codes and their huge description tables, a full set of web pages has been generated with all the levels of the tree structure of ACR codes and MeSH terms. This generation needs to be recompiled every time a coding system releases a new version: this happens at most every year. Tests have proved that the speed advantage in using static pages overcomes the annoying process of pages regeneration, which lasts only a couple of hours every year.

At least three categories of users are allowed to search the database: final users, authorised users, medical providers. Each category has its path through a password-based mechanism, in order to allow different functionalities.

4. User Interaction

The library resides on the platforms of the two largest European medical Internet publishers and is accessible through their Web servers. Users can access it via an ordinary Internet service provider and an appropriate plug-in for their WWW browser.

Automatic presentation of the library contents is an option for inexperienced users; a searching tool on various attributes of organs and their pathologies is provided for more experienced users. Searches are conducted through keywords according to internationally-accepted medical terminology standards (Section 5).

3D models are transmitted over the Internet incrementally – crude information to which users can respond is received rapidly by transmitting the coarsest LoD for the model as shown in Figure 1. Afterwards, while users remain inactive, refinement occurs progressively; information for finer and finer LoDs is transmitted and these LoDs are displayed. This operating scenario allows, if necessary, the termination of downloading at an early stage and furthermore ensures that the final 3D model is the one desired, displayed in full detail. Results so far indicate that expected delays in response times are between 30 seconds and 1 minute.

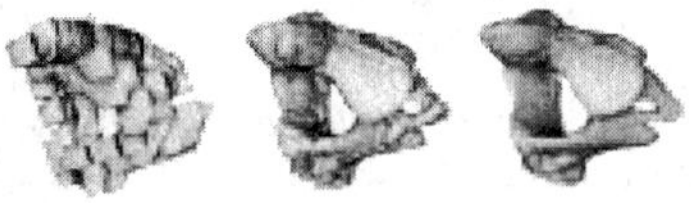

Figure 1

Upon downloading the model required, users can perform a number of operations, view, manipulate (rotate, translate, zoom, etc.), change colour/brightness/ opacity, dissect, employ embedded hyperlinks to gain extra information, or participate in discussion groups on the particular organ pathology. To allow for real-time interactivity, 3D models are rendered by coarser LoDs during rotation, translation or zooming and once the manipulation operation is completed, the fully-detailed LoD model is again displayed almost instantly.

5. Classification and Coding Procedures

A central issue in collecting medical images for databases is classification and coding. Any efficient searching mechanism relies on the indexing system. Every image or case has a code which represents its content in a short but meaningful, unambiguous string.

There is no unique coding system available in medicine, and efforts range from simply defining some codes for statistical purposes, up to automatic extraction from natural language descriptions [9]. The problem has been addressed since the very beginning of the IAEVA project. Accepting that the most advanced automatic coding systems are still in very preliminary versions, and allowing for the multilingual scenario of the university hospitals involved in this project, we have decided to partially solve the problem by using the most common classification and terminology among the members of the consortium.

Therefore, ACR has been chosen to code every image and MeSH terms are added by the medical content providers to increase the level of detail in explaining the content. ACR is widely used by radiologists and is very simple to use for both coding and retrieval. MeSH [10], while not being a proper pathology coding system, is the standard in indexing medical literature, because it is used by the U.S. National Library of Medicine for the MEDLINE database. Through the mapping tables built by the UMLS project, MeSH terms can be cross-referenced into other classification systems. The process require manual intervention for solving ambiguities. So far UMLS has not yet implemented the latest version of ACR, but there are plans to add it in a future annual release. To facilitate the coding phase, an assisted Web-based tool has been developed which allows physicians to navigate through the tree-structured ACR and MeSH terms, which are stored using both the code and the description.

6. Interactive Questionnaires

Self-evaluation questionnaires related to 2D images, 3D models, or cases are provided to give users the opportunity of assessing their knowledge of the field. The medical providers produce the questionnaires. The general structure of a questionnaire is a multiple-response choice, with a minimum of three choices. One, more than one, or none, of the proposed choices is the correct answer. The questions number between five and thirty.

The questionnaire is generated over the Internet without any specific client software, soon after 2D images or 3D models have been provided. The questionnaire has a reference to the unique identifier of the 3D model. Other models can be associated with the same questionnaire, or other questionnaires linked to the model. The links are stored in the main database of the IAEVA-II server. The questionnaire itself is a URL and is generated using ASP technology.

The option to build a questionnaire is also given to some users (mainly teachers) for use in conjunction with the Bulletin Board System. The teacher can select a model or group of models (e.g. a case) and build a questionnaire linked to it. This relies on the structure of the BBS; it is not stored into the database. The questionnaires are not designed to act as a formal evaluating system as this would require a complex system for student identification.

7. Bulletin Board System

Any authorised user (e.g. a teacher) can start a discussion about a case, protecting the "electronic forum" with a password, sent via e-mail to his/her students. They can then study the case using the material provided by their professor, and post their comments and answers into the Bulletin Board (BBS). At the end of the pre-arranged period, the teacher can verify the students' answers, replying to individual or general questions.

The BBS is a simplified version of a typical Internet "digital forum". It is not a permanent and general source of information, but a one-time facility for a specific educational purpose. This approach relies on the importance of quality control. As IAEVA-II will be a public service, all information must be verified and controlled by a board of reviewers. The so called "public" discussion about a case will therefore not be open for writing to everybody: it will contain only the reviewers' annotations.

The teacher can also build interactive multiple-choice questionnaires for self-assessment. The results are stored in a database which can be browsed by the teacher. As it has been seen previously, there is no system available for ensuring the identity of the student, beside the name for logging in (which can be a pseudonym): therefore the whole system has a limited validity for knowledge evaluation.

8. Supporting Education

A major enhancement of IAEVA-II, as compared to IAEVA, is the provision of video-recorded short lessons by leading physicians. Some of the cases or 3D models are linked to video clips, which give the user audio explanations while showing the professor talking. We make use of streaming video technology, now capable of delivering very good audio quality and fairly acceptable motion images, while using standard Internet connections down to 20 Kbps. Microsoft Windows Media technology [11] was chosen for this purpose because it provides a complete set of free of charge tools under the Windows NT environment used for the IAEVA-II server.

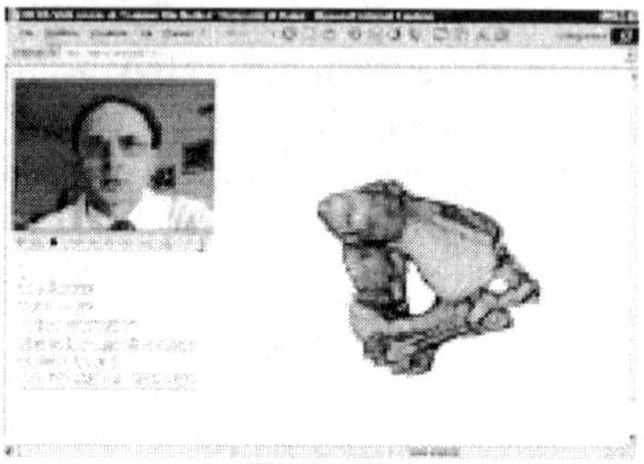

Figure 2

By adapting a methodology developed by one of the authors [12], shown in Figure 2, the images can be displayed alongside the teacher while he is discussing them. Therefore, it is possible to explain characteristics of the images as if they were being shown in a classroom.

The effort demanded of the medical providers in producing the video clip is kept to the minimum. It requires a consumer-quality video camera and a good microphone. Most of the work is done while digitally-encoding the videotape, in order to set the triggers that point to the model or the images. Tests have proved that the running video of the speaking teacher is more accepted by students than voice only.

Streaming video will also be used for a lower resolution preview of some animations generated by 3D reconstructing tools, such as a fly-through in a trachea or the rotation of the view point of a tumour in the lungs. Downgrading an uncompressed 78 Mbytes Quicktime 24 seconds movie to a RealVideo [13] 116 Kbytes file, capable of real time streaming over a normal 34 Kbps line, produced a result which was considered exceptionally good by major radiologists and physicians. Further tests with the latest compression algorithms can widen the use of such formats allowing a much wider audience.

9. Conclusions

The prototype IAEVA-II server is being completed [14] and the partners are testing all procedures. The public service will become operational in 2000 and will be run by medical Internet publishers, Euromultimedia [15] and Health Online Service [16], for their subscribers.

Acknowledgements

This project has been supported by the European Commission DGXIII, Telematics Application Project IAEVA-II (HC4009) and by Hewlett-Packard, project MEDICALIZE. We thank Stefano Dessena and Roberto Diana for the help in building the educational tools.

References

[1] G. Clapworthy and M. Krokos, The Graphical Demands on Medical Visualisation Systems Using the WWW: A Case Study, Proc Information Visualisation '97, IEEE Press, pp 296-305, 1997
[2] M. Krokos *et al.*, Organisation, Transmission, and Manipulation of Pathological Human Organs on the WWW, Proc MIE '97, IOS Press, pp. 99-103, 1997
[3] http://WWW.nlm.nih.gov/research/visible.
[4] M. Crudele *et al.*, A Distributed Database of 3D Models of Human Organs, 10th IEEE Symposium on Computer-Based Medical Systems, Maribor, Slovenia, 11-13 June, 1997
[5] http://hermes.unicampus.it
[6] W. Lorensen and H. Cline, Marching Cubes: A High-Resolution 3D Surface-Construction Algorithm, Computer Graphics, Vol 21, No 4, pp 38-44, 1987
[7] W. Schroeder et al., Decimation of Triangle Meshes, Computer Graphics, Vol 26, No 2, pp 65-69, 1992
[8] W. Schroeder, A Topology Modifying Progressive Decimation Algorithm, Visualisation '97, IEEE Computer Society Press, pp 205-212.
[9] C. Lovis, Trends and Pitfalls with Nomenclatures and Classifications in Medicine, International Journal of Medical Informatics, Vol 52, 1998, pp.141-148.
[10] http://www.nlm.nih.gov/mesh/meshhome.html
[11] http://www.microsoft.com/windows/windowsmedia/
[12] M. Crudele: Delivering Video Teaching Courses through the Internet: Technical Issues, Congresso Aica '98, Naples, 18-20 November, 1998. See also http://projects.elis.org/mpp.
[13] http://www.real.com
[14] http://iaeva.unicampus.it
[15] http://medic-online.net/
[16] http://www.multimedica.de/

Medical Informatics Europe '99
P. Kokol et al. (Eds.)
IOS Press, 1999

Sharing Electronic Medical Record on the WWW using InterCare architecture and smart cards

Mikko Rotonen (1), Pekka Ruotsalainen (2) Atte Kaskihalme (3) Matti Aarnio (4)
1 Development Manager, Uusimaa Hospital District, Finland
2 Head of Unit, National Research and Development Centre for Welfare and Health, Finland
3 Unit Manager, Siemens Business Services, Finland
4 It-manager, Jorvi Hospital/Uusimaa Hospital District, Finland

Abstract. Southern-Finland is a partner of the European Commission funded telematics project, InterCare, which is developing and demonstrating the www – based regional architecture and application integrated with smart cards. The InterCare project will combine the results from the most important EC funded healthcare telematics projects in their respective areas – Cardlink 2, Hector, Star, Synapses and TrustHealth. The primary objective is to achieve a convergence of results and to demonstrate & promote the synergy between projects from different areas of the healthcare telematics programme.

Keywords. WWW, Intranet, Internet, smart cards, security, regional telematics services, service chain, old legacy system face lift by browser interface, integration

1. Introduction

InterCare project in Finland will cover administratively ¼ of the population of Finland. The project is located in the Capital City area and the following organisation are involved in the project: The Helsinki City Health Department provides primary healthcare services and, via Helsinki Hospital District, specialised care to the citizens of Helsinki. Geographically, Helsinki is divided into seven districts. Each district has primary healthcare centres which is responsible for the provision of health services in its district. Uusimaa Hospital District (UHD) is Finland's biggest hospital District and it operates in 9 hospitals for the population of Uusimaa region. In Uusimaa region there are 24 primary healthcare centres, but they are operated by the municipalities. The primary healthcare centres use the services of the Uusimaa Hospital District by referring their patients to the hospitals of the Uusimaa Hospital District. The Helsinki University Central Hospital (HUCH) serves as a referral hospital for the Helsinki Hospital District and the Uusimaa Hospital District with the total population of 1.3 million. HUCH occupies a special position in Finnish health care as it serves the whole country in the treatment of certain diseases that are very rare or require specialist knowledge or costly equipment. Patients referred to HUCH from primary healthcare centres or by private doctors are either hospitalised or seen in outpatient clinics. HUCH is owned by the municipalities of the Province of Uusimaa. The hospital is divided into a number of responsibility centres, either clinical departments or internal service units.

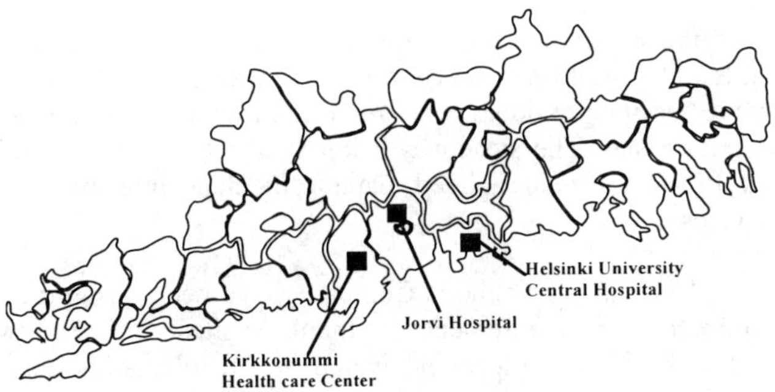

Figure 3: InterCare Region (Uusimaa Province) in Finland

2. Objectives

All the above mentioned organisations are strengthening their co-operation in order to provide seamless care for their patients. They are also currently making a division of labour to improve efficiency. This can only be done if the information needed to organise and provide care can be delivered seamlessly to the organisation treating the patient.

3. Methods

From the architectural point of view there are three basic types of services in the regional server:

1. Information services (yellow pages) available for anyone
2. Information services available only for the registered users
3. Social and healthcare related interactive services (regional social and healthcare services)

Information services include both yellow pages services (preventive information, self care guidelines, etc.) as well as guidance on how to access and use different regional services. Also a service to assist on writing applications for regional social and healthcare services and email are included in the information services. These services are open for anyone to use.

Certain more personal services can be offered to registered users. These services can be based on the additional user information (for example user home address, responsible social and primary healthcare centre) available to the authentication procedures required.

- Service chain follow up: the most important patient service items and their status information can be retrieved from the regional server. The service status here includes the information if the service has been booked, currently being executed or already provided to the customer. Some of the technical aspects of the regional architecture and an overview of the implementation plan and the required interfaces, are depicted in the following diagram:
- The data security of the service chain will be defined and demonstrated. The definitions will include functional and technical requirements for security system (based on TrustHealth results). The functional and technical integration of star applications to smart card systems will to be defined based on Cardlink 2 results. The value of smart cards carrying electronic identity and critical medical data will be demonstrated.

- The citizens of the Kirkkonummi community have a maximum of 2,800 multi-technology cards to be used for authorisation/authentication for the access of telematic. All the healthcare service providers will use these cards to access the telematic services in the demonstration site. The system will interconnect to the emergency system and other services to obtain value added patient medical information to the mobile emergency services.

The project group and Helsinki Telephone Company have been designing the architecture and defining the infrastructure requirements for the three sites. The study will provide the design guidelines for the base platform on which health telematics applications can be developed. Moreover, this study will identify the configuration for the local hardware and software for connecting the sites to the regional Intranet. On this basis InterCare will deliver the specialised integrated applications and services that the project will produce.

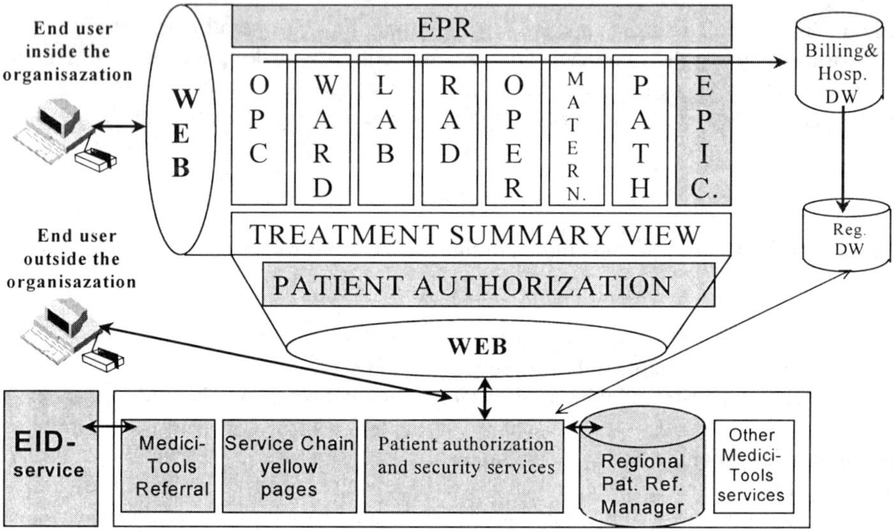

Regional Architecture

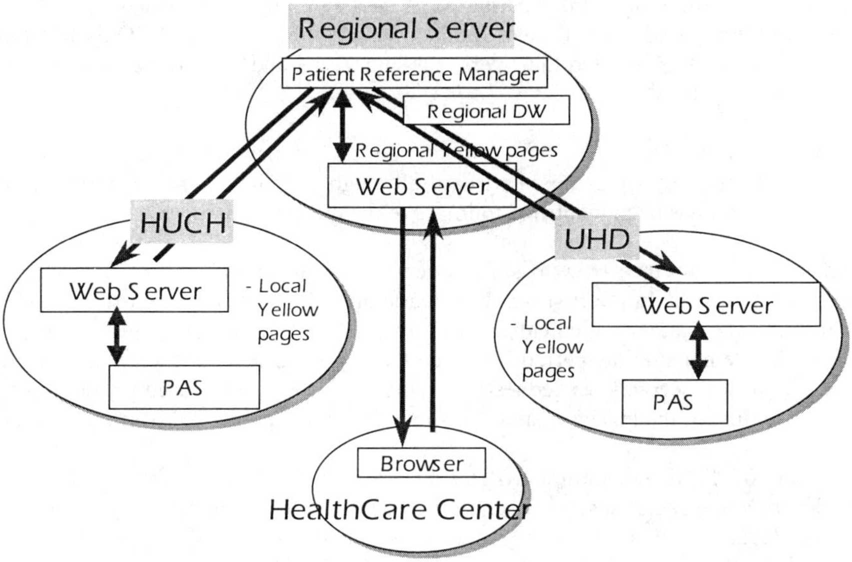

The smart cards have two different roles; a key card (security) and personal medical data delivery tool. The smart card has capacity of 16 kilos and the 32-bit workstation software is running in Microsoft NT developed and programmed by Siemens Business Services Oy Finland. The developed system is very modern and flexible.

HealthCard - Compliance with PC/SC Standards

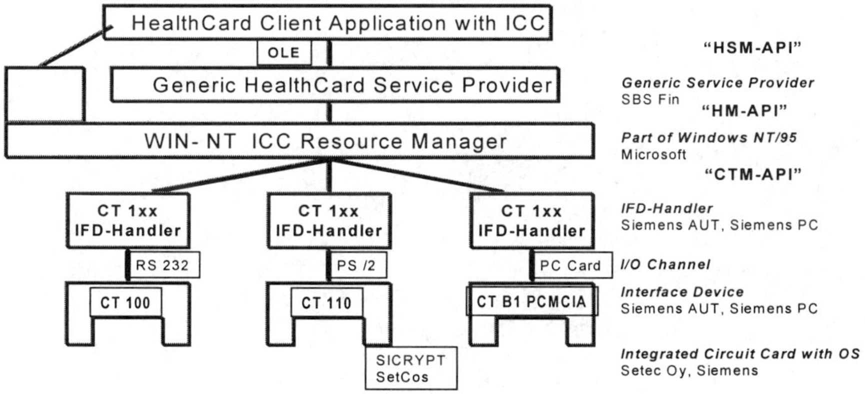

4. Conclusions

The demonstration of the smart cards has started in the beginning of the January 1999. The citizens were very interested in the project and has accepted the smart cards. Only less than 2 % of the chosen citizens rejected their personal smart card and most of the very elderly citizens living in the elderly home.

The physicians and nursing staff have already developed new ways to communicate between different units by using the smart card although they have email system. Even small signals (ccu etc) has been identified to improve the quality of care.

The demonstrations of the www-based patient medical record browsing will be demonstrated in two parts. In the first part the smart card of the citizen as a key card is the only way to enter the patient's medical records. In the alfa-testing period just before the beginning of the demonstration period showed, that systems response time in the real environment is under 2 seconds per request. It seems that using www-based techniques the average response time of the legacy systems in shorter than using terminal based technique.

The second part of the demonstration will be based on the regional reference database, which will improve the security services and other services. It will be the only connecting method to the legacy systems in the regional level and in the use of the service chain. Before entering to the second part, the security aspects have defined and the needed new application have been developed. The objectives of this part is to demonstrate the rights of the citizen based the new legislation of the data protection and the rights of the patient.

Medical Informatics Europe '99
P. Kokol et al. (Eds.)
IOS Press, 1999

The Need for Evaluation when Managing the IMIA.ORG Web-site

Thomas KLEINOEDER, Udo JAHN *, Otto RIENHOFF *
Dept. of Nephrology & Rheumatology, University Hospital Goettingen,
Robert Koch Str. 40, D-37075 Goettingen, Germany
** Dept. of Medical Informatics, University Hospital Goettingen,*
Robert Koch Str. 40, D-37075 Goettingen, Germany

Abstract. The International Medical Informatics Association (IMIA) has built up a web-site to support international scientific exchange and facilitate organizational tasks. Regular monitoring is required to get information on whether the site is actually used and by whom. Main aspects of the evaluation are function, structure and contents. As main evaluation methods the logfile analysis and user questionnaires are used. The number of visits to IMIA´s web-site has constantly increased in the last year. In January 1998 the site had 418 visits, in December 1998 there were 6002 visits. The user questionnaire showed that the web-site offers an adequate platform for the members. It is concluded that the members as the main target group are reached by the services and in addition that the growing number of non-members require further development of the public part of the site.

1. Background Information

The International Medical Informatics Association (IMIA) is a world-wide organization of Medical Informatics societies. More than 40 national societies, and a similar number of institutional and corresponding members are linked together within IMIA. About 100 international experts are key figures representing more than 20.000 members of the national Medical Informatics societies.

In Summer 1996, IMIA started to build up its electronic services. The first application after a gopher-server was the electronic distribution of the Newsletter via WWW. In 1997, the content of the public web-site has been constantly extended. A password protected area with member lists and a document archive was created in the same year. Since 1998, a member-database is available as well as web-based email-services. The goal of IMIA´s electronic services is to support international scientific exchange and facilitate organizational tasks [1].

2. Methods and Description of Application

Regular monitoring of a web-site is required to get information on whether a web-site is actually used, and by whom. The evaluation is a constant process to recognize the changing needs of the users. In the past a lot of criteria for the evaluation of medical web-sites have been published [2][3][4]. Many authors criticize the lack of reliable methods for evaluating the impact of a web-site [5][6]. Therefore measures of process and structure are proposed to be used as indirect indicators of quality [5]. Function, structure and content are the main aspects of the evaluation [7].

In general monitoring of a web-site is done by analyzing the web-server log-files. These records have to be interpreted very carefully. In the log file the IP-addresses of the visitors and the requested html-pages are stored. To analyze the data, clear goals have to be defined. One task is to find out whether the site is visited by the intended audience. It is very difficult to exclude "accidental visitors" who are following a link from a search engine and who are not continuing their visit to the site. Another evaluation method is a user questionnaire. This method often fails as a result of low feedback [8]. In the case of IMIA user questionnaires are used at the General Assembly with a feedback rate of 90 percent.

For IMIA it is essential to find out whether its members are using the site. When analyzing the log-file, it is not possible to identify members who are visiting the public area of the site. The requests of the index page of the password-protected part of the site represent the visits of members to this area. Non-members cannot request this page as a result of the password protection. To get more information on the user behavior and requirements a questionnaire on technical and content issues is distributed to the attendants at the yearly general-assembly.

IMIA´s electronic services are used for the preparation of the General Assembly and the Board Meetings. Daily communication is mainly based on email. Documents are distributed via email as ASCII text or attached pdf-file (portable document format). All documents are put into the password-protected area of the web-site in the archive. To evaluate the preparation of meetings in each of the last two years a user-questionnaire was distributed at the General Assembly. Most of the national representatives, working group chairs and board members are present.

Table 1

Evaluation of IMIA´s Web-Site

Criteria		Method
Function	Accessibility / Availability	Logfiles + User Questionnaire
	Use of site	Logfiles + User Questionnaire
	Profile of users	Logfiles + User Questionnaire
	Links to IMIA	Link Analysis
	Navigation	User Questionnaire
Structure	Performance	User Questionnaire
	Technical requirements	User Questionnaire
	Ease of use	User Questionnaire
	References	Publication Guidelines
	Currency / Updates	Publication Guidelines
	Quality of links to other sites	Regular manual check
Content	Quality of content and services	User Questionnaire
	Reliability	User Questionnaire

To evaluate IMIA´s electronic services three evaluation methods are regularly used:

1. IMIA´s web-server is running under Windows NT, as web-server the MS Internet Information Server is installed. The log-files of the server are analyzed using the shareware version of Marketwave Hitlist. Weekly and monthly reports are generated automatically. Visits to the site and requests of selected key-pages are counted. In addition the visitor countries and the kind of entries from search engines are extracted. A visit is a collection of requests for all pages and graphics seen by a particular visitor at one time. The requests by the office staff at the Department of Medical Informatics in Goettingen where the site is managed are not counted in the statistics.

2. For each General Assembly, a user-questionnaire is prepared. Technical questions regarding soft- and hardware are included as well as questions on web-access and performance. In addition, the users are asked about their experiences with the services.
3. To complete the monitoring a regular link analysis is done using the Altavista Search engine. This task has the intention to find links to IMIA´s Homepage and put them in relation to the number of visits.

In addition a basic set of publication guidelines for the publication on IMIA´s web-server including information for style, references, currency and updates are used. The links from the web-site are regularly checked by the office staff. Table 1 summarizes the evaluation criteria of IMIA´s web-site and the applied evaluation methods.

3. Results

The number of visits to IMIA´s web-site has constantly increased in the last year. In January 1998 the site had 413 visits, in December 1998 there were already 6.002 visits. In total 42.554 visits were counted. About 85 percent of the users started their visit at the homepage before requesting other pages. The most popular page at the public site was the coming-events list beside the links-page to the national member societies and other Medical Informatics resources. Most of the visitors came from the United States (17.392). Less frequent were visits from Germany (1.795), the Netherlands (1.235), and the United Kingdom (1.162). About 10 percent of the visitors are accessing the site by using search engines. In 60 percent Altavista is used, in 21 percent Yahoo followed by Lycos (9 percent) and Hotbot (8 percent). The number of visits to the index-page of the password protected area for board members and national representatives increased in the year of 1998. About 200 request where counted in December 98 in contrast to 42 visits in January 1998. The number of possible users is about 50 people.

Additional information was obtained by the analysis of the questionnaire. In 1997 and 1998, about 90 percent of the attendants at the IMIA General Assembly visited IMIA´s web-site. At the public area the coming-events list and the links-page were most attractive for the members. The emails sent out before the General Assembly reached all members, except one. In this case email-problems were known. The pdf-format for the documentation was well accepted by 90 percent of the members. The analysis of the technical equipment used by the members yield an important result for the technical development. The Windows 95 Operating System is used by 70 percent, 30 percent are using DOS, Windows 3.11, Windows NT, Unix or MacOS.

Most of the members have Internet access via the high-speed university/company network. S-VGA is the most common screen-resolution. As web-browser about half of the members uses Netscape Communicator 4 the others Internet Explorer 4. Regarding the email clients there is a very heterogeneous environment to be found with at least 8 different software products.

4. Conclusions

Constant monitoring of the site gave us the possibility to analyze the user behavior and draw conclusions for the further development of the services. The promotion and development of the services in 1997 and 1998 focused on IMIA´s members. Regarding the number of visits of the password protected area from different locations in relation to the number of possible users of the service one can conclude that the site was accepted by IMIA´s members. This conclusion is confirmed by the comments given by the members in the user questionnaire.

Surprisingly, the number of visits at the public area of the web-site increased tenfold without further promotion in 1998. In mid 1997, the site had only few links from Medical Informatics sites which were related to IMIA. In January 1999, there were more than 200 links to IMIA´s homepage. This might be one reason for the increasing traffic at the site. The analysis of the user-questionnaire showed that the members were satisfied with the system performance. The increasing number of visitors of the public area did not cause performance problems. This can be attributed to the fact that the server is running on a fast machine, and that the web-site is not graphic intensive. Taking into account the evaluation results of the public area and the sufficient performance for the member services it can be concluded that the public area should be extended. Since 1998 IMIA´s electronic services have received enough recognition to base the further development of IMIA on the functions of these services.

References

[1] Kleinoeder T, Rienhoff O: A Global Intranet for an International Scientific Society. MedInfo 98, Seoul, Proceedings, 1998, 197-201, IOS Press, Amsterdam.

[2] Silberg M, Lundberg GD, Musacchio RA: Assessing, controlling, and assuring the quality of medical information on the internet. Caveat lector et viewor – let the reader and viewer beware. JAMA 1997; 277; 1244-5

[3] Kim P, Eng TR, Deering MJ, Maxfield A: Published criteria for evaluating health related web sites: Review. BMJ 1999; 318; 647-9

[4] Jadad AR, Gagliardi A: Rating Health Information on the Internet. JAMA 1998; 279; 611-4

[5] Eysenbach G, Diepgen TL: Towards quality management of medical information on the internet: evaluation, labeling, and filtering of information. BMJ 1998; 317; 1496-500

[6] van Bemmel JH, Musen MA: Handbook of Medical Informatics. 1997; Springer; Heidelberg

[7] Bonati M, Impicciatore P, Pandolfini C: Quality on the Internet. BMJ 1998; 317; 1501

[8] Wyatt JC: Commentary: Measuring quality and impact of the world wide web. BMJ 1997; 314: 1879.

Medical Informatics Europe '99
P. Kokol et al. (Eds.)
IOS Press, 1999

WWW search engine for Slovenian and English medical documents

Jure Dimec[*], Sašo Džeroski[**], Ljupčo Todorovski[*], Dimitar Hristovski[*]
[*]*Institute of Biomedical Informatics, Faculty of Medicine, Vrazov trg 2, 1105 Ljubljana, Slovenia*
{jure.dimec | ljupco.todorovski | dimitar.hristovski}@mf.uni-lj.si
[**]*Institute Jožef Stefan, Jamova 39, 1111 Ljubljana, Slovenia*
saso.dzeroski@ijs.si

Abstract. The information tool for the organization and searching of Slovenian and English medical documents is presented. The tool, partly still in development phases, performs automatic subject description of documents, searching with natural language queries and ranking of search hits according to their relevance. The search engine allows the searcher to use relevance feedback in order to perform incremental improvement of search results.
The machine learning system TILDE for learning user profiles was also applied. Documents marked by the user as relevant or non-relevant are used to find characteristics that distinguish relevant documents from non-relevant ones.

1. Introduction

World Wide Web (WWW) is increasingly useful as a source of information in research and development. In the flood of documents aimed at different user populations the idea of digital library is steadily gaining importance. Digital library *sensu stricto* could be described as a collection of electronic documents accessible on network on which some sort of quality control was performed and as a suite of information tools for discovery and presentation of these documents. Among information tools, search engines are the most important.

Digital libraries in their present-day rudimentary forms only partially solve the problems rooted in the abundance of untrustworthy documents on Internet. Good information tool designed for the demanding user should enable him or her to search through information sources organised in local digital library(es) and, at the same time, offer an individualised discovery and access to the wealth of potentially useful documents elsewhere on WWW.

In this paper we would like to report on our work on both tasks. We are (a) developing the database of automatically built subject descriptions of unstructured and structured documents archived in our digital library, (b) developing a search engine for searching this database with natural language queries, and (c) building the user profiles with descriptions of users' information needs. User profiles built with the machine learning methodology will automate the discovery of relevant documents on WWW. With respect to documents published, medicine in Slovenia is predominantly bilingual, Slovenian and English languages being almost equally important, therefore all language-dependent procedures are dealing with these languages.

The paper begins with the description of automatic indexing. The third and fourth sections are devoted to the search engine and to the arguments for developing it from the scratch. The fifth section presents preliminary experiments in building user profiles with machine learning system TILDE.

2. Database with subject descriptions of Slovenian and English medical documents

Dynamic nature and number of information sources on Internet make indexing with keywords or subject headings attributed by human experts virtually impossible. The task is realisable only with automatic indexing – the approach used for the construction of databases of famous search services like AltaVista, Excite, Infoseek, and others. With some simplification, the automatic indexing could be described as a three-step procedure:

1. using of stop-words list to eliminate the words with minimal informational value;
2. stemming to normalise the different forms of the same word to the same stem; and
3. weighting of the remaining stems to reflect their informational value.

We use all three steps for documents in both languages but only processing of Slovenian documents is described here. For automatic indexing of English documents we use methods often described in literature [e.g. 1].

At the time of reporting the pilot database installation consists of documents from electronic versions of two medical journals: Slovenian edition of JAMA (Journal of the American Medical Association, http://www.mf.uni-lj.si/jama/jama-slo-e.html) and ISIS (Journal of Slovenian Chamber of Medicine, http://www.mf.uni-lj.si/isis/isis.html) and bibliographic records with abstracts from national database Biomedicina Slovenica (http://www.mf.uni-lj.si/cgi-bin/wow/bs_frm?lang=ENG).

2.1. *Stop-words and stemming*

Each word from document to some extent represents the document's subject and is a candidate for being an index term. Words called stop-words are exceptions. Stop-words are words that are evenly distributed in document base and as a consequence bear the least amount of information in documents. They mainly belong to several word groups like propositions, adverbs, pronouns, etc. Slovenian stop-words list presently contains near 1600 words and word forms, which is much compared to typical English lists with 250 – 400 words. Words found in list are excluded from further processing.

The quality of stemming, which is also language-dependent procedure, is a critical factor and the quality of both automatic indexing and searching depends on it to the great extent. With stemming we try to determine the string of characters that represents all forms of the word and discriminates them from other words. Often, but not always, the stem corresponds to the word root. While reports exist on little or medium importance of stemming of English documents it is very important in languages with rich morphology. Of such languages the Slovenian is a good example.

We are aware of two previous successful attempts to develop statistical algorithms for stemming of Slovenian texts and used for construction of document databases [2, 3]. Both were based on longest match principle and used extensive lists of word endings, 1205 and 5276 endings, respectively. In longest match algorithms the list of endings is searched for the longest ending that could be mapped to the terminal part of the word and ending is cut off the word. These algorithms often exhibit overstemming producing too short stems and they are less adequate for medical sublanguage due to abundance of words of Greek or Latin origin. In our project we developed new algorithm, which works as a combination of stemming rules and a set of valid stem examples.

We use three groups of the stemming rules firing consecutively: rules for endings that divide the word at the consonant-vowel pair, rules for the remaining consonant-consonant pairs, and recoding rules. The cursor marking the potential division point between stem and ending is gradually moving from right to left, one character at the time. At each character the full stemming is performed (if possible) and if it succeeds and the resulting stem is found in the list of legal stems, the procedure is finished. In the case when the stem is never found in the list of legal stems it enters the temporary list, that have to be occasionally inspected, corrected, and merged with the legal list. This new stemmer, which could be attributed as the shortest match algorithm, is evolutive, self-learning, and is found to be better adapted to the medical sublanguage.

2.2. Weighting of stems

Weight of the stem denotes the share of information that this particular stem contributes to the whole information load of the document. It depends mainly on the stem's frequencies in the document (intradocument frequency) and in the database (interdocument frequency). Basically, the higher intradocument stem frequency means more important aspect of the content the stem is about; and lower interdocument stem frequency results in higher ability of stem to discriminate documents that contain it from others in database. Both measures are combined in stem weight in particular document.

Unavoidable characteristic of Internet is its dynamic state, which prevents the computation of the final stem weights during automatic indexing. Parameters derived from interdocument frequencies could be taken into account only during searching thus reflecting the database state at that moment. Documents in digital library are marked with HTML (Hypertext Markup Language) therefore it is possible to augment stem weights with additional (ad hoc) values of HTML tags. We can expect the word from text body to be less important than the word which is emphasised and this one again less important than the title word.

3. Searching

A good search engine is expected to process queries as natural language sentences and rank resulting pointers to documents according to the computed relevance. Relevance is defined as a measure of similarity between a query and a document. In general it is computed as a sum of stem weights common to the query and the document. In our work we used Croft's probabilistic method [5] supplemented with the value of HTML tags.

All big search engines on WWW use ranking of search hits. Analyses show that the majority of queries are short, two or three words long, causing the quality of ranking that is suboptimal. The searcher is forced to browse through a good part of ranked list (which is often very long) or to change the query and repeat the searching. To avoid this shortcoming we implemented the searching method called relevance feedback, known from the classical document retrieval as one of the methods that give the best search results [4, 5]. The method is based on the interactive dialog with the searcher who provides identifications of relevant documents. Big WWW search services don't use the method because it needs unique identity of searcher or uninterrupted (statefull) search session that is difficult to accomplish with usual CGI programs and HTTP protocol. The course of relevance feedback searching is three-step:

1. the searcher performs first, normal search;
2. receives search hits, inspects several top-ranked documents and mark those that he finds relevant;
3. system automatically reformulates query and performs new search.

The core of the procedure is query reformulation. The system recalculates weights of all stems from the query using the probabilities of their occurrence in relevant and non-relevant documents. Searching with the reformulated query includes new documents to the hit list and changes the positions of previously found documents so those relevant ones climb the list upwards. After receiving each hit list the searcher repeats the inspection of top ranked and previously uninspected documents and mark the relevant. Steps 2 and 3 are repeated as long as there are new relevant documents near the top of the list or the searcher gives up.

4. Why another search engine?

Public search services like AltaVista, Excite, and some others index the predominant part of WWW (according to their authoring institutions), including pages on Slovenian servers. Then, why are we developing new search engine for which it is clear that it can not substitute the big ones?

Automatic indexing is highly language-dependent procedure determining the success of searching. The *lingua franca* of WWW pages is English and indexing is adapted for that language, although some search engines are able to process queries in limited number of other languages. While using them the documents in Slovenian mainly remain hidden. For the time being we are not aware of any working search engine for Slovenian documents that doesn't avoid language-dependent functions by requiring manual truncation of query words although we are aware of two very promising lines of work. We believe that our system at least partly fills this empty space.

We conceive the database of subject descriptions and pointers to documents, search engine, and modules for personalised document discovery as a tool for the advanced use of digital library of medical documents. We are indexing only documents that undergone some sort of quality control and that are useful for students or in professional and research work in Slovenian medicine. One of the consequences of this commitment is relatively small database.

The amount of stored data and relatively limited size of users' population gives us the possibility to implement functions that big search services still can not afford themselves. It is our firm opinion that good search engine should borrow from the behaviour of each of the two existing information retrieval words – local, possibly client/server systems used with bibliographic databases, and big public search services on WWW. We believe that good and exhaustive search could not be performed in one pass therefore user should be able to evolutively improve search results.

The server, search engine and client were written in Java. The search engine is implemented with TxtIndex4, search engine kernel in Java, provided by Novi Forum [10].

5. Learning relevance of documents

In the context of user interests' profiles, documents marked by the user of the search engine as relevant or non-relevant are used to find characteristics that distinguish relevant documents from non-relevant ones. Given the examples of relevant and non-relevant documents, machine learning methods are used to build a model that can be used to predict the relevance of new documents.

Machine learning methods have been already used for predicting the relevance of documents on the WWW within the WebWatcher project [7] and also for modeling individual user's information interests as profiles within the Personal WebWatcher project [8]. However, none of this methods deals with documents in the Slovenian language.

We used machine learning methods for predicting the relevance of English and Slovenian documents from examples. We used the collection of 770 short documents (abstracts from some leading Slovenian medical journals) – half of them in Slovenian and the other half their English translations. Three human experts marked the documents as relevant or non-relevant with respect to 50 different queries, which we assume correspond to 50 topics of interest. We consider each of them as a learning problem, where the relevant documents are positive and the non-relevant ones are negative examples. Therefore, each learning problem has 770 examples. Two series of experiments were performed. The documents were represented as sets of words in the first, and as sets of stems in the second series.

TILDE [9] machine learning system was used to generate logical decision trees that distinguish relevant documents from non-relevant ones. The trees can in most cases be transformed into decision lists of keywords that indicate relevant documents. The motivation for using TILDE was the fact that it can also use background knowledge, such as MeSH or UMLS, in the learning process. Although we did not use such knowledge in the experiments presented here, we plan to do so in the future.

Consider query number 10: "Nastanek, diagnostika in zdravljenje ulkusa, še posebej razjede želodca in dvanajstnika" (in Slovenian) or "The origin, diagnosis and treatment of ulcer, especially duodenal and gastric ulcerations" (in English). From the examples for the query (in the set of 770 documents, only 8 are marked as relevant), TILDE generates the following decision tree:

```
ulcer ?
+--yes: rel_10
+--no: ulkusa ?
   +--yes: rel_10
   +--no: not_rel_10
```

The tree can be interpreted as follows: "If the document includes the word *ulcer*, then it is relevant. The document is also relevant, if it does not include the word *ulcer*, but it include the word *ulkusa* (Slovenian for 'of the ulcer'). Otherwise the document is non-relevant."

In the case of query number 14 ("Kirurško (operativno) zdravljenje zlomov kosti" or "Surgical (operative) treatment of bone fractures") TILDE generated a tree which can be interpreted as follows: "The document is relevant, if it includes one of the words: *fracture*, *zlome*, *calcaneal*, *zlomih* or *zlomov*." The tree misclassifies one of the relevant documents as non-relevant. Note here that Slovene is a highly inflected language: *zlome*, *zlomih* and *zlomov* are all plural forms of the word *zlom* (fracture).

Finally, consider query number 31: "Uporaba ultrazvoka v diagnostiki" or "Use of ultrasound in diagnosis". There was 22 relevant documents for this query out of all 770 documents in the collection. The tree generated by TILDE can be interpreted as follows. A document is relevant, if it includes one of the words *ultrazvočni*, *sonography*, *ultrazvokom*, *ultrasound*, *echocardiographic*, *ehokardiografija*, *hoechst*, *laser* or *ultrazvočno*. Otherwise it is non-relevant. The tree misclassifies three relevant documents as non-relevant and two non-relevant documents as relevant.

In the decision tree for query number 14 the words *zlome*, *zlomih* and *zlomov* appeared. All of them have the same stem *zlom*. Also, in the tree for the query number 31 three words with the stem *ultrazv* appeared (*ultrazvočni*, *ultrazvokom*, *ultrazvočno*). This motivated us to use stemmed versions of the documents, which would probably produce more concise trees/decision lists distinguishing between relevant and non-relevant documents.

When using a set of stems instead of words the decision tree for the query number 14 is: "A document is relevant, if it includes the stem *zlom* or the stem *calcaneu*. Otherwise, the relevance depends on the stem *fractur*: if the stem *fractur* appears and stems *bas* and *manag* do not appear, the document is relevant, else the document is relevant, if it icludes stems *spin* and *oper*, else it is non-relevant. The tree based on stems misclassifies one non-relevant document as relevant.

For the query number 31 TILDE generated the following tree. A document is relevant, if it includes at least one of the stems *ultrazvoč*, *digit*, *ultrasound*, *echocardiograph*, *sonograph*, *ehokardiograf* or *lh*. If the document includes stem *cist*, then it is relevant in case when it does not include stem *premer*. The tree misclassifies two non-relevant documents as relevant.

As we expected, the decision trees based on stems distinguish relevant documents from non-relevant ones better. In the two example queries described above, the misclassification error is smaller when using stems instead of words. Furthermore, none of the relevant documents was misclassified as non-relevant which was not the case with the trees based on words. This is very important, because there are few relevant documents for each query.

Finally, we used some of the learned profiles to generate queries for WWW search engines (e.g. AltaVista). The profiles generated from the set of words abstract representation were used here. The keywords appearing in the profile (identified by the machine learning approach) are used to form a query. The generated queries were submitted to the search engine and the search results inspected manually. Reasonable search results were obtained, especially for profiles on topics with larger numbers of relevant documents.

6. Further work

Having all the necessary elements in place, we will incorporate the above methodology into a search mechanism that will be made available to medical researchers. In addition to the use of machine learning methods for generating user profiles as described in the paper, the system will also include automatically generating queries for different WWW search engines from these profiles. We also plan to incorporate a clustering approach to present the search results of queries generated from profiles. The user will also be able to browse this clustered and ranked list of hits and add more relevant documents to his/her profile.

Acknowledgement

The work presented in this paper was partly supported by the subproject "Intelligent Information Storage and Retrieval of Slovenian and English Medical Documents on Internet" of the INCO COPERNICUS project CRII Cooperative Research in Information Infrastructure, and partly by the project "Digital Library of Slovenian Medical Documents" funded by Slovenian Ministry of Science and Technology.

References

[1] Porter MF. An algorithm for suffix stripping. Program. 14. 1980:130-7.
[2] Dimec J. Computer analysis of Slovenian information language in biomedicine (in Slovenian). M. Sc. thesis. Ljubljana: Medicinska fakulteta, 1989; 77.
[3] Popovič M, Willett P. Processing of documents and queries in a Slovene language free text retrieval system. Literary and Linguistic Computing. 5. 1990:183-90.
[4] Harman D. Relevance feedback and other query modification techniques. In: Frakes WB, Baeza-Yates, editors. Information Retrieval. Data Structures & Algorithms, Englewood Cliffs: Prentice hall, 1992; 241-63
[5] Croft WB. Experiments with representation in a document retrieval system. Research and Development in Information Technology, 1983; 2(1)1-21.
[6] Dimec J. Analysis of information content in different types of Slovenian medical texts and their searching with non-Boolean methods (in Slovenian). Ph. D. thesis. Ljubljana: Medicinska fakulteta, 1995; 108.
[7] Joachims T, Freitag D, Mitchell TM. Web Watcher: A tour guide for the WWW. Proc. IJCAI-97, 15th Intl. Joint Conference on Artificial Intelligence, 1997.
[8] Mladenič D. Personal WebWatcher: Implementation and design. Work report IJS-DP 7472, 1996. Ljubljana, Institute Jožef Stefan.
[9] Blockeel H, De Raedt L. Experiments with Top-down Induction of Logical Decision Trees. Artificial Intelligence, 1998 (in print).
[10] Novi Forum d.o.o. URL: http://www.noviforum.si/

Medical Informatics Europe '99
P. Kokol et al. (Eds.)
IOS Press, 1999

Analysis of free MEDLINE on the WWW

Eva Klemenčič, Ljupčo Todorovski
Institute for Biomedical Informatics, Medical Faculty, Vrazov trg 2, Ljubljana, Slovenia
Email: Eva.Klemencic@mf.uni-lj.si

Abstract. In the paper, a survey of free MEDLINE access on the WWW is given. We compared five different vendors that provide free unlimited access to MEDLINE. The comparison of different search parameters was made: number of search statements, number of search fields, ability to combine search statements, number of search limits. The possibilities of using MESH thesaurus during the search are also explored. At last, we compared and evaluated the results of two search queries, obtained with searching MEDLINE, provided by five vendors mentioned above.

1. Introduction

The aim of this survey was to overview MEDLINE vendors on the WWW. Among them, we were especially interested in vendors providing free unlimited access to MEDLINE. For these providers, we explored the search possibilities including the use of controlled terms and Medical Subject Headings vocabulary hierarchy.

MEDLINE [1] is a bibliographic database, which covers the field of biomedicine and is created and regularly updated by the National Library of Medicine in USA. It contains articles from 3,800 international medical journals. MEDLINE is weekly updated and 31,000 records are added each month. MEDLINE consists of three parts: OLDMEDLINE contains data from 1960 to 1965 and includes 770,000 records; MEDLINE contains data from 1966 to the present and at the present time (January 1999) includes above 9 millions records; and PREMEDLINE (MEDLINE in process) includes 25,000 to 100,000 records. The records are hold in PREMEDLINE only so long, that the indexing process is finished: after that, they are moved to MEDLINE.

The rest of the paper is oganized as follows. The survey of MEDLINE vendors on the WWW is given is Section 2. Next section gives the results of comparing the search possibilities of five free MEDLINE vendors. The results of two search queries are evaluated and compared in Section 4. Finaly, the comparison of different free MEDLINE is summarized in Section 5.

2. MEDLINE vendors on the WWW

We made a systematically survey of MEDLINE vendors that can be found on the WWW. First, we classify them in three categories: commercial vendors (paid access), vendors that require (usally on-line) registration and vendors that provide free unlimited access to MEDLINE. The example vendor in the first category is OVID [2]. They charge the users for every search query. The vendors in the second category require (usually on-line) registration and/or subscription to obtain username and password, which are necessary for MEDLINE access. There are number of vendors in this category, some of them are listed in Table 1. Finally, vendors providing free unlimited access to MEDLINE including the corresponding URL address are listed in Table 2. All the URL addresses in Tables 1 and 2 were accessed in the beginning of January 1999.

Table 1: MEDLINE vendors that require registration

MEDLINE vendor name	URL address
Avicenna	http://www.avicenna.com
BioMedNet	http://www.biomednet.com
Community of science	http://medline.cos.com
Health communcation network	http://www.hcn.net.au
MEDSCAPE	http://www.medscape.com
PaperChase	http://fleming.bidmc.harvard.edu/MEDLINE/start.htm

Note here, that Table 2 includes only free vendors that contain all MEDLINE records and not subsets of them. Namely, there are also subsets of MEDLINE available on the WWW, which are specialised for particular medical field: ophthalmology (`http://www.ophthoguide.com/ophtho`), neurosurgery, dentistry, cardiology and orthopaedics.

Table 2: Free MEDLINE vendors

MEDLINE vendor name	URL address
DIMDI	http://gripsdb.dimdi.de/engl/guieng.html
HealthGate	http://www.healthgate.com/HealthGate/MEDLINE/search.shtml
HealthWorld	http://www.healthy.net/library/search/medline.htm
Infotrieve Online	http://www.infotrieve.com/freemedline
Internet Greateful MED	http://igm.nlm.nih.gov
MEDLINE Fool!	http://www.medportal.com
PubMED	http://www.ncbi.nlm.nih.gov/PubMed

3. Comparison of the search possibilities

After we collected links to different MEDLINE vendors on the WWW, we started the comparison of the free searchable ones. The examination of their home pages shows that there are only five really different search engines for accessing MEDLINE. Furthermore, for these five MEDLINE search engines, we evaluated the following parameters: maximal number of search sessions, possibility of combining the results of different search sessions, number of fields available for searching, posibility of limiting the search results and possibility of researching only in one appointed year. The results of the evaluation are resumed in Table 3.

Table 3: Free MEDLINE analysis

MEDLINE vendor	Num. of sessions	Num. of fields	Period
DIMDI	4	9	1998
HealthGate	5	4	last 2 years
HealthWorld	4	8	1993-1997
Infotrieve	4	8	1995-1998
Internet Grateful MED	3	3	1998
MEDLINE Fool!	1	12	1997-1998
PubMed	1	3	last 12 months

From now on, our analysis is concentrated on the five MEDLINE vendors providing different search possibilities: DIMDI, HealthGate, HealthWorld, Infotrieve and NLM (Internet Grateful MED, PubMed). The next step of our survey was the determination of possible number of limits used for narrowing the search scope and diminishing the large number of retrieved records. This is reviewed in Table 4. In the same table we also showed the possibilities of searching with subject headings.

Because of only some possibilities of limiting the search scope are offered the set of hits can not be narrowed to some reasonable size for purpose of displaying and/or printing. Therefore, unlimited searching can serve only for a purpose of getting quick and orientating results and not for getting answers to complex search queries.

Table 4: Number of limits and use of subject headings in different free MEDLINE vendors

MEDLINE vendor	Num. of limits	Subject heading
DIMDI	2	explode MeSH term
HealthGate	3	keyword
Internet grateful MED	7	subject
Infotrieve	5	MeSH term
PubMed	1	keyword

3.1. Searching with subject headings

The most important feature in searching MEDLINE is the use of subject headings and tree hierarchy. NLM creates the hierarchically organized vocabulary called Medical Subject Headings (MeSH) [1], which include about 18,000 controlled terms, named subject headings or MeSH terms. The location of a single MeSH term in the MeSH hierarchy is given in MeSH tree structures. Single subject heading can be broad or more specific. Exploring of MeSH hierarchy during the search can spare a lot of time. For searching specific aspect of MeSH terms we can add subheadings, also called qualifiers. However, none of the free MEDLINE vendors can make use of the subheadings during the defining of the search query. The DIMDI GRIPS-WEB Search engine allows user the use of the "explode" command to include all more specific MeSH terms from the MeSH hierarchy.

Some of the free MEDLINE vendors allow user to browse the MeSH hierarchy. Two different browsers are available: using the one we can see only alphabetic list of MeSH terms, and the other gives better insight into the tree location of the given subject heading through all categories.

4. Two example queries

At last we compare the search results, obtained with serarching MEDLINE from five vendors, on two example queries. Each example query consists of combination of two terms. Where available, we used MeSH term field for searching. Also, where possible, we limited the set of search results to the results from year 1998.The results of the queries are surveyed in Tables 5 and 6.

Table 5: Number of citations retrieved in different free MEDLINE for the query: ticks and lyme disease

MEDLINE vendor	ticks	lyme disease	Both	Period
DIMDI	289	279	63	1998
HealthGate	553	624	152	2 years
Infotrieve	1208	206672	592	1995-1998
Internet Greatful MED	374	119	100	1998
PubMed	456	424	120	1 year

The example queries could not be formulated equally for all MEDLINE vendors. Namely, the search results can not be limited to one-year period in some of the search engines, used by free MEDLINE vendors.

Table 6: Number of citations retrieved in different free MEDLINE for the query: mercury and environmental exposure

MEDLINE vendor	mercury	environmental exposure	Both	Period
DIMDI	222	2275	68	1998
HealthGate	826	3773	95	2 years
Infotrieve	1122	14559	314	1995-1998
Internet Grateful MED	489	2529	97	1998
PubMed	617	3127	111	1 year

5. Discussion

It is very hard to compare the number of search results obtained from different MEDLINE vendors. First, only two search engines allow the user to limit the results to the ones from the year 1998 (see Table 3).

The main differencies between MEDLINE providers can be noticed when the quality of the searching is being explored. Only DIMDI offers the use of the exploded MeSH terms. Internet Grateful Med enables searching by subject only. The subject comprises MeSH terms and keywords at the same time. Infotrieve enables searching by MeSH terms without using the MeSH hierarchy. Other two MEDLINE vendors (HealthGate and Pub Med) offer only keyword searching.

We are not aware of any other studies concerned with comparison of different free MEDLINE vendors. Surveys that consider the use of Internet Grateful Med [3], or measure the response times from different geographic locations (for Internet Grateful Med again) [4], can be found. Some of them describe only the possibilities of searching NLM databases on WWW [5, 6].

After the evaluation of different free MEDLINE vendors, we can conclude that free MEDLINE is appropriate to use for getting quick answers to simple search queries. The quality of search improves with the possibility of using the hierarchy of MeSH terms, and is even better, if the user is able to browse trough the MeSH tree hierarchy. The free MEDLINE vendors on the WWW make MEDLINE available to the great number of end-users and improve the accessibility of bibliographic information, but the quality of the search results is usually not very good. From all search possibilitites provided with the MEDLINE organizational structure, only a small part of them are freely available to the users.

References

[1] U.S. National Library of Medicine (NLM) [WWW page], 1999. http://www.nlm.nih.gov [Accessed: January, 1999].

[2] Ovid Technologies, Inc. Homepage [WWW page], 1999. http://www.ovid.com [Accessed: January, 1999].

[3] F.B. Wood et al., Transitioning to the Internet: Results of a National Library of Medicine User Survey, Bulletin of the Medical Library Association 85(1997)331-340.

[4] F.B. Wood et al., Evaluation Internet End-to end Performance: Overview of Test Methodology and Results, Journal of the American Medical Informatics Association 5(1998)528-545.

[5] R. Sikorski et al., Medical Literature Made Easy: Querying Databases on the Internet, Journal of the American Medical Association 26(1997)959-960.

[6] R. Kisley, Medical Databases on the Internet: part 1, Journal of the Royal Society of Medicine 90(1997)610-611.

Medical Informatics Europe '99
P. Kokol et al. (Eds.)
IOS Press, 1999

Organization and dissemination of multimedia medical databases on the WWW

Ljupčo Todorovski[1], Samo Ribarič[2], Jure Dimec[1], Emil Hudomalj[1], Tomaž Lunder[3]
[1]*Institute for Biomedical Informatics, Medical Faculty, Vrazov trg 2, Ljubljana, Slovenia*
Email: {Ljupco.Todorovski,Jure.Dimec,Emil.Hudomalj}@mf.uni-lj.si
[2]*Institute of Pathophysiology, Medical Faculty, Zaloška 4, Ljubljana, Slovenia*
Email: ribaric@ibmi.mf.uni-lj.si
[3]*Department and Chair of Dermatovenerology, University Medical Centre, Zaloška 2, Ljubljana, Slovenia*

Abstract. In the paper, we focus on the problem of building and disseminating multimedia medical databases on the World Wide Web (WWW). The current results of the ongoing project of building a prototype dermatology images database and its WWW presentation are presented. The dermatology database is part of an ambitious plan concerning an organization of a network of medical institutions building distributed and federated multimedia databases of a much wider scale.

1. Introduction

The amount of knowledge in the field of medicine is vast and increasing daily. Conventional methods of storage and dissemination of knowledge (i.e. books and journals) are not sufficient because they cannot offer updated information on a daily basis, are not always available, and are handicapped with high printing costs. In addition, practising physicians have a very limited amount of time to search books and journals for specific information essential for their work.

Therefore, from the physician's and medical student's viewpoint, the ideal medical database has to (1) be accessible to everyone, anytime, anywhere, (2) be updated on a daily basis, (3) combine text, images and video clips, (4) pool medical data, knowledge and experience on an international scale and (5) be flexible enough to be used in medical practice, for training, and teaching purposes. At present, the only practical solution that meets these requirements is the organization of multimedia medical databases on the World Wide Web (WWW) [3]. Traditionally, the first step in the preparation of multimedia medical databases is the transfer of text, images and video clips into digital form [1]. The necessary technology (hardware and software) is developing rapidly, is widely available and affordable.

We believe that at least three prerequisites should exist to successfully build a multimedia database. First of all, the appropriate amount of quality data should be available. Second, their owners should be aware of the benefits of storing medical data on the WWW. And third, a fair computer and network infrastructure should be available.

In Slovenia, the central medical institution is the University Medical Centre and the central education institution for medicine is the Medical Faculty at the University of Ljubljana. Their departments have archives of tens of thousands slides, images and video clips that can be used for teaching purposes. Some of the owners use computer networks since the late eighties and many others since 1993 when computer network at Medical

Faculty was established and connected to Internet. They have knowledge and enthusiasm to actively participate in building multimedia databases. In 1998, University Medical Centre connected their communication infrastructure to Internet as well.

2. Pilot Project

Some of the key problems that could appear when building a multimedia medical database for physicians and medical students are (1) selection and preparation of data, (2) developing a versatile information system for storage and retrieval of data, and (3) presentation of the data in an information system on the WWW. These problems require the organization of interdisciplinary teams of computer experts and physicians.

These problems are addressed in the ongoing pilot project at the Institute for Biomedical Informatics at Medical Faculty in Ljubljana. The Institute is collaborating with several departments of the University Medical Centre in Ljubljana to design multimedia medical databases on the WWW. A prototype of a bilingual (Slovenian and English), multimedia medical database, for the field of dermatology, is running on the Medical Faculty's WWW server (`http://www.mf.uni-lj.si/mmd/derma/`).

The dermatology database is an example for the presentation of a multi-purpose medical database. The first step was the development of a simple versatile relational medical image database structure. Versatility of the database structure allows its use for storing images and video clips from different areas of medicine other than dermatology. The record for every image (or video clip) in the database, beside the image itself, contains the international diagnosis code of the depicted disease, text description of the image and diagnosis, localization, and type of the disease. The last two attributes can take values from the predefined hierarchies.

The Chair and Department of Dermatovenerology, at the Medical Faculty and University Medical Centre in Ljubljana selected and digitized the images and also prepared and entered the data about the images in the database. Furthermore, the tools for transforming the medical image database into WWW presentation consisting of HyperText Markup Language (HTML) pages were developed at the Institute for Biomedical Informatics. For WWW server performance reasons, static HTML pages are used wherever possible, rather then building pages dynamically using database queries. However, static HTML pages should be re-created after database updates. The WWW presentation provides the user with four different ways of using the dermatology images database.

1. Browsing. The simplest way of browsing the database is using the index of all images sorted alphabetically by diagnosis. Other two indexes allow browsing through the hierarchies of the localization and the type of the disease. Each of them allows the user to move up and down the hierarchy tree and get thumbnails of all the images in the current category. The thumbnails are linked to the HTML pages presenting the corresponding image.

2. Searching. Query form allows users to combine two search criteria: localization and type of disease. The results of the search are HTML pages generated dynamically using database queries. Each HTML page contains up to 15 thumbnails linked with the corresponding HTML presentations of the images.

3. Self-testing. To allow the use of the database as a teaching tool for medical students a feature of self-testing is also added to the WWW presentation. The questions are built dynamically on the basis of a randomly chosen image and four randomly chosen wrong answers in addition to the right one. At the end of the test the user is provided with the score as well as the corrections to wrong answers (see Figure 1).

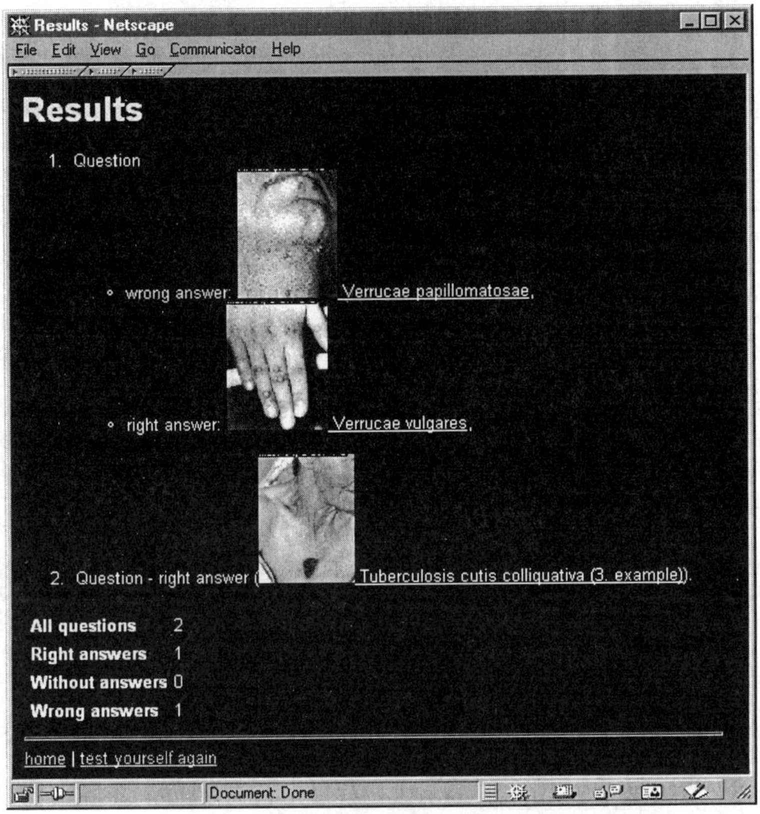

Figure 1: The HTML page displaying the score of the test.

4. Comparison with images from different sources. Finally, the WWW presentation of the database also allows its use as a reference database for physicians, providing the possibility to compare their own images, stored on their personal computers or somewhere on the WWW, with the images from the database.

The pilot project does not include only the development of dermatological images database on the WWW. Multimedia databases for the fields of plastic surgery, opthalmology, cardiology and neurology (including video clips) are in preparation and will be available on the WWW by the end of 1999.

3. Future work

Future work on the multimedia medical databases has several objectives: (1) to increase the number and quality of medical images and video clips in each medical database as well as the number of collaborating departments from the University Medical Centre, (2) to develop new tools for the presentation and integration of video clips, images and text on the WWW, and (3) to exchange and pool medical data among medical institutions on an international level and organize an international network of servers that provide prompt and world-wide access to multi-lingual, multimedia medical databases.

Preliminary steps along the first objective on the national level are already done. Beside the five departments, which are currently developing their databases, contacts are made with ten other departments of the University Medical Centre in Ljubljana. Five of them already agreed to build databases of images and video clips, and disseminate them on the WWW in the next three years.

We see multimedia medical databases as a basis for the development of future information and educational tools. To reach this goal, mechanisms should be developed to enrich the multimedia content with additional knowledge of arbitrary types. For the time being, we are enhancing the database structure to include links to some other resources available on the WWW. These links will provide the physicians an overview of a great amount of information about their topics of interest. For instance, this additional information can take a form of references to the articles published in journals and proceedings. For this purpose we will include links to the bibliographic databases, such as Biomedicina Slovenica (Slovene national biomedical bibliography) [4] and Medline [6] to the HTML pages. Links to the WWW version of medical textbooks and manuals (for example, we are negotiating to include links to the Merck Manual [5]) providing additional information on specific diseases could be also included in the database.

It was already shown (see e.g. [2]) that the usability of the digital library as a daily reference tool is in close connection with its size and coverage of the topic it is specialized for. The amount of work necessary for building a digital library with sufficient coverage exceeds the capacity of a single institution. Therefore, the co-operative work of different medical institutions on an international level is necessary. The Internet technology allows and stimulates such co-operative work. The co-operation of the institutions should be flexible, so that the institutions with different interests and different levels of informatics infrastructure development would be stimulated to collaborate in the project.

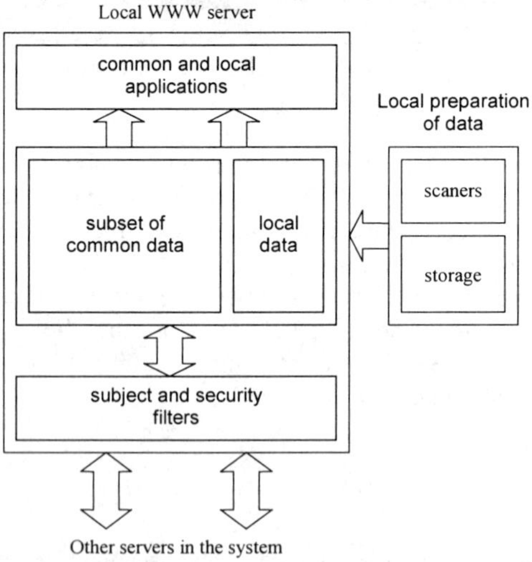

Figure 2: The structrure of the server node of the international distributed multimedia medical database

The organization scheme of each of the database servers is shown in Figure 2. The mediator of the network of servers will (1) install and maintain the hardware necessary for the storage and accessibility of the database, (2) mediate the co-operative work, (3) define the protocols for database updates, and (4) build and maintain the user interface for accessing the database. Software at each network server should perform several tasks concerning the availability of the data. It should (1) forward data to the topologically neighboring servers, (2) copy data which are important for local use and cashing, (3) issue data provided by the owner of the server, and (4) respect rules agreed on a network level, like routing tables, security etc.

The preparation and input of the images and video clips into the database should be organized locally at each co-operating institution. Preparation of the data includes image/video digitalization, providing relevant textual information (keywords, diagnosis, treatment, etc.), and links to related resources available on the WWW. Each collaborating institution can choose from several possible ways of organizing its local environment. At the most basic level, some of the institutions could decide to mirror the database and quicken their data access. Also, the most advanced collaborating institutions may wish to build their local databases, gathering local medical data, probably in their national language.

4. Conclusions

A prototype of a bilingual (Slovenian and English), multimedia medical database, for the field of dermatology, running on the Medical Faculty's WWW server is presented. This dermatology database is an example for the presentation of a multi-purpose medical database on the WWW.

The prototype dermatology database should be enhanced in different ways. First, we will increase the number and quality of images and also build similar databases for different fields of medicine. Also new tools for integrating links to different multimedia medical resources on the WWW should be developed. Finally, we propose the organization of an international, multilingual, multimedia, medical database based on a co-operative work of different medical institutions. The pooling of medical data, knowledge and experience on an international scale will have two advantages. It will increase the amount of medical information available on the WWW and improve its organization at the same time. The latter will simplify the search and retrieval of the medical information on the WWW.

Acknowledgements

The workstation for preparation of the dermatology library was sponsored by MSD IDEA INC. (A subsidiary of Merck & CO., INC., Whitehouse Station, N.J., USA.) The library content reflects the opinions of its authors, and not necessarily those of the sponsor, and is presented as a service to the medical profession. The work is also supported by the Slovenian Ministry for science and technology within the research project "Digital library of Slovenian medical documents".

References

[1] Bittorf, N.C. Krejci-Papa, T.L. Diepgen. Development of a Dermatologic Image Atlas with World Wide Access for the Continuous Education of Physicians. *J. telemedicine and Telecare*, 1995; 1: 45-53.

[2] M. Borghuis, H. Brinckman, A. Fischer, K. Hunter, E. van der Loo, R. ter Mors, P. Mostert, J. Zijlstra. TULIP project final report. `http://www.elsevier.nl/homepage/about/resproj/trmenu.htm`.

[3] DermIS - Dermatology Internet Service (WWW page). `http://www.derma.med.uni-erlangen.de/index_e.htm`. Accessed: January, 1999.

[4] D. Hristovski, A. Rožić-Hristovski. Organizing Slovene medical bibliography on the World Wide Web. *Journal of American Medical Informatics Association* 1997; (Suppl): 862.

[5] Merck Publications (WWW page). `http://www.merck.com/pubs/`. Accessed: January, 1999.

[6] U.S. National Library of Medicine (NLM) (WWW page). `http://www.nlm.nih.gov/`. Accessed: January, 1999.

Medical Informatics Europe '99
P. Kokol et al. (Eds.)
IOS Press, 1999

GIN AUSTRIA
Assuring quality and relevance on Internet-Health-Informations for patients

Georg Göbel, Karl Peter Pfeiffer
Institute of Biostatistics und Documentation, University of Innsbruck, Schöpfstraße 41/1, A-6020 Innsbruck, Austria

Abstract. GIN AUSTRIA (Gesundheitsinformationsnetz AUSTRIA) offers patients and consumers reliable medical knowledge about diseases, wellness and disease management in an understandable way and enables them to quick and incessant access to informations about the Austrian health system and Austrian health organizations. To improve the quality of the database and to achieve full customer (patients, citizens) satisfaction a systematic approach for implementing total quality management is also applied. Focusing the attention on understanding and responding to customer needs, systematic and continous improving of the IS and total involvement of all participants are the three core TQM principles at this project. The second focus of the project is the development and the implementation (prototype) of a medical dictionary or rather medical thesaurus as interface for patients, who are not used to scientific terms and expressions. This interface is based on the controlled vocabulary of the MeSH-Thesaurus (german version).

1 Introduction

In 1995 the GIN project has been started at the Institute of Biostatistics and Documentation at the Medical Faculty of the University of Innsbruck. The project was designed to provide consumer-oriented health and wellness information for patients and citizens of Austria and to enable Austrian residents to quick and incessant access to informations about the Austrian health system and Austrian health organizations. Main medical topics are disease information, wellness information, alternative therapies information, physician referral and insurance/health planning information. Links to important websites and addresses of potential contact persons/institutions complete informations of the system.
The main goal of the project is the development of an Austrian Health Information System, which provides customers reliable medical knowledge and referrals about the most important medical subjects and comprehensive informations about the Austrian Health-System.

2 Status report

2.1 Hardware and Software Platforms

GIN runs as database backed Website on a standard-PC (Pentium II, 266 MHz, 128 MB RAM, Windows NT, MS-IIS3). The main part (95%) of data is being stored in a RDBMS (MS Access97). Customer Information-enquiries are handled by a Middleware script-language-program (Cold Fusion 3.0). Cold Fusion makes it very simple to pass data to the data source and to receive and format data for dynamic display.
The University of Innsbruck maintains an Internet segment featuring a 100-Mbps (FDDI) backbone (INNET), with 10-Mbps Ethernet links within the buildings. The GIN-Server is connected to this backbone. The INNET connects to the internet via the Austrian Acadamic Network ACONET (ATM technology - 8Mbps). Customers may visit GIN directly over the Internet (HTTP protocol). HTML3-Browsers (Netscape3, MS Internet-Explorer3) are recommended as minimal software configuration for clients. To improve the performance GIN will be transferred to higher platforms till the end of 1999 (Pentium 450, 320 MB RAM, Oracle 8i). Data input and data maintance are presently done by members of the GIN staff over a Web interface (HTML-Form).

2.2 Target groups

The primary target groups of GIN are "healthy" citizens and patients seeking for advice. Understandable informations, which are based on responsible and competent information sources, should enable these groups to make timely decisions about their health maintenance. GIN is provided to "Health-Professionals" (physicians, therapists) as information-platform for their own contributes or publications and as IS for their patients.

2.3 Contents

GIN customers have access to informations via two ways: On one hand the contact-data (name, address, telephone number, email-address) of about 8500 Austrian healthcare institutions are stored in the database, on the other hand informations about different medical topics are available. Table 1 gives an overview of the structure of available information of GIN.
Starting from the indicated target groups in table 1 (content-matrix [1, p.20]) the more detailled database contents will be systematically planned and gathered via further information-matrices (drill-down-analysis). The information-matrix patient/disease for example includes the detailled items: definition, factors, symptoms, diagnosis, consequences, therapies, prophylaxis-prevention-precaution. This means that every kind of disease being stored within the database has to be structured similarly.

Tab. 1 "Main Matrix"

Institutions	Medical topics	
	Patients, Citizens	Health Professionals
Contact - data adress, phone, email	Informations about diseases, wellness, health maintenance. "basics"	Informations about diseases, professional health literature *(in development process)*
Enhanced informations about physicians, organizations (e.g. specializations)	Alternative therapies, result of investigations	Links to Evidence-based-medicine Sites *(in development process)*
Additional and Background informations (Patients rights, Health System in Austria)	Referrals and practical experiences of patients, physicians, therapists,...	
Links to other important sites		Links to Professional IS (Medline,...)

At the moment customers can work with the system either via a hierarchical navigation system or via fulltext-search aid. As a result of a query the user obtains a list of available database-contents which are arranged according to the type of information but not ranked. Used terms of the query and their frequencies are being stored.

2.4 Quality Assurance/Quality Control (QA/QC)

Many evaluations and reports (not unique to medicine) show us the absence of QA/QC - programs as one of the key problems of internet information [2;3]. According to different suggestions [e.g. 4] and main principles of QA/QC [5] a systematic approach for implementing total quality management (TQM) is applied.

In order to give a comprehensive, easy understandable description of the purpose of the project, all members of the GIN-staff designed in a first step a "Mission Statement" and - in a second step - goals [5], which cover the organization's broad intent, by defining what is to be attained through sustained effort over the long time (Tab. 2):

Tab.2 Mission statement und GIN-Goals

Mission - statement "GIN AUSTRIA provides quick and incessant access to reliable and up-to-date informations referring to diseases, wellness, disease management and Austrian health-care institutions. We facilitate and support the process of communication between Austrian health-care institutions and citizens by means of advanced information technologies." The GIN Goals are: • To provide comprehensive informations about Austrian health-care institutions on the Internet. • To support customer's health and wellness maintenance by providing informations about health promotion and health education • To improve exchange of informations between Austrian health-care institutions and citizens by means of advanced information technologies • To provide citizens, patients and employees of health-care institutions permanent and widespread access to health-related multimedia informations • To develop an Austrian and further international Health-Information-Net, which contents consider a high quality level (Ring of Excellence) • To focus on applied research in the field of information systems and services for citizens

3 Current Development

Beside systematic enhancement of contents two action lines are being focused: the further development of the QA/QC-program and research on a MeSH-based search aid for patients.

3.1 QA/QC-program

Obtaining quality criterias for all parts of GIN (hardware, software, user-interactions, logistics of information, user-support, data security, documentation, evaluation) is the objective in this field of the GIN project. This has seemed most urgent in the field logistics of information [2]: Selecting information sources, information gathering, interpretation, representation, integration and maintenance of data [8].
GIN content is selected in the same sense that scientific journals select from available materials. Materials proposed for inclusion in GIN are reviewed by at least two members of the GIN-staff, partially papers are referred to outside experts if necessary.
For instance, guidelines for authors who want to compose GIN-articles are adopted from [4]:

- All Contents are presented correctly and comprehensively.
- The content is adapted to the specified target group .
- Personal opinions are explicitly marked.
- Authors, editors, release dates and version numbers are documented.
- Quotations and reference sources are marked as such, attributed and documented.
- Medical contents are linked to existing coding schemes and professional nomenclatures.

These guidelines serve as a starting point for the concept of a comprehensive checklist for the presentation of new articles within GIN. Other criterias in the field information-logistic/data-maintenance concern the following items: updating, date of the last update, information about the changes, Off-site-link checking.

3.2 MeSH-based Thesaurus (GIN-Search):

The reason for this main focus is the fact that the access to useful data and informations that provide high quality and reliability is still very tricky and difficult, especially for customers - patients or their relatives for example - who do not know basic clinical terms or expressions.
With this project an efficient search aid for health-information-systems is being developed. Thereby the customer will be able to obtain relevant information even if he doesn't know any clinical terms in the range of his question. This also means that already existing datasources (even external ones) can be contained by using metadata or offered to the customer as information sources respectively. In this context "to contain existing datasources" means to provide access to stored informations by metadata, whereby these metadata can be simple URLs. The use of the MeSH-Thesaurus [7] should ease the connection to other datasources and the use by "non-physicians". Furthermore an extension of the (German) MeSH-Version with "non-medical-expert-expressions" can be necessary.
Another aim is the most possible independence from HW/SW-platforms. Therefore the concept suggests a three-layer client/server-architecture.

Example: A customer is looking for informations about the topic "vaccination/vaccinate" *(german: "Impfung/impfen")*. There are two ways: He/she can search these expressions directly or he/she will first try to find a better search term (e.g. synonyms or related term) via the Thesaurus and adopt the new term into his/her query. Furthermore the customer has the opportunity to filter and rank the information by several criterias (e.g. medical topics, institutions, regions, target groups). As a result the customer obtains a hitlist which matches to his/her search term (e.g. ranked by the chosen criterias in alphabetical order), whereby (similar to MEDLINE) accordant metadata will be indicated.

The first approach was a specification of the essential structure and functionalities. Thereby it was assumed that external datasources will be contained but the development of the prototype will be based on GIN data only.

The design-objectives of GIN-Search are:

- GIN - Search is put on existing WWW-IS as modular part.
- Different kinds of datasources are integrated by an interface (e.g. "normal" HTML-Sites, RDBMS, OODBS).
- GIN - Search integrates heterogenous datasources to one homogenous "information-pool".
- GIN - Search bases on a 3-layer Client/Server concept, where GIN - Search acts as a broker between the presentation-layer and the datasource-layer.
- Access of clients is possible by Internet (HTML, XML, Java). As far as possible all components of GIN - Search should run on most platforms (Windows NT, UNIX).
- The controlled vocabulary of MeSH-Thesaurus (german version) is used as search aid for users and for indexing datasources. The MeSH-Thesaurus has to be extended by "non-physician-expressions" if necessary.

According to [10] Table 3 shows the structure and the program-parts of GIN - Search.

Tab.3 GIN - Search scheme

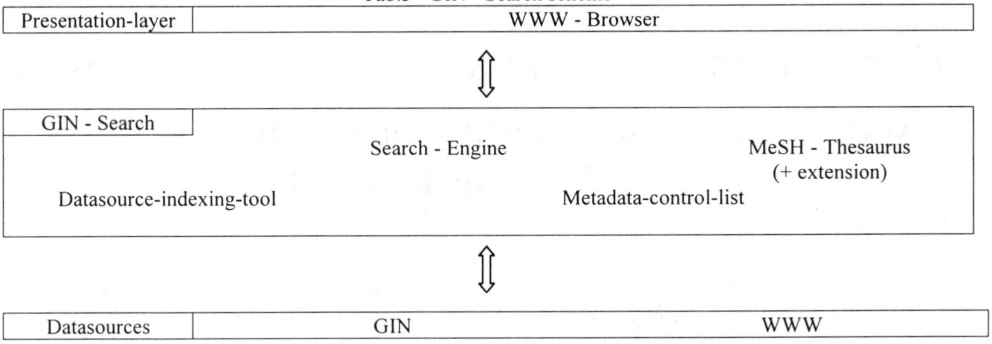

Some SW-components are required to satisfy the features of a powerful medical search-engine for patients: MeSH-Thesaurus, which is available on Internet, search-engine, Metadata-control-list, Datasource-indexing-Tool.

In a first step, an Access-Tool to the MeSH-Thesaurus (german version) was build in Java programming language. Users may use the Thesaurus directly via Internet and are able to look at the MeSH Tree, to examine specific terms and to find out associated terms by usual features of the MeSH-Thesaurus (DIN 1463) [9].
For addition of any extensions to the MeSH-Thesaurus used terms of the query and their frequencies are being stored, similarly to the fulltext-search-engine.

4 Next steps

At the QA/QC-program both designed quality-standards have to be implemented completely and advancement of comprehensive quality-criterias are planned. Regarding to the search-function the next steps will be the field test of the MeSH-Thesaurus, an evaluation and systematization of the search terms so far used by customers and the development of the missing components of GIN-Search. (**URL:** http://gin.uibk.ac.at)

References

[1] **Grabowski** H./**Rude** S (Hrsg.). *Informationslogistik.* B.G. Teubner. Stuttgart 1999

[2] Eysenbach G./Diepgen T. *Towards quality management of medical information on the internet.* BMJ Vol 317, p1496. Nov. 28, 1998.

[3] **Sherter** Alain L. *Disease Management on the Web.* Health Data Management 1998 Vol.6/Num 10; p34.

[4] **Schulz** S. a.o. *Qualitätskriterienkatalog für elektronische Publikationen in der Medizin.* http://www.imbi.uni-freiburg.de/medinf/mi_home.htm

[5] **Tenner**, Arthur R. *Total Quality Management.* Addison-Wesley Publishing. New York 1992

[6] **Lawrence** S./**Giles** C.L. *Searching the WWW.* Science 1998 April 3; 280 (5360):98.

[7] **König** J./**Dorda** W./**Erhart** G. *Erfolgreiche Suche in medizinischen Datenbanken.* Springer Medizin Verlag. Wien 1996.

[8] **Petkoff** B. *Wissensmanagement.* Addison-Wesley Publishing. Bonn 1998

[9] **Ferber** R. Data Mining und Information Retrieval. Vorlesungsskript, GMD-IPSI http://www.darmstadt.gmd.de/~ferber/dm-ir/PDF-neu/vb.pdf

[10] **Boles** D./**Dreger** M./**Großjohann** K.*Konzeption eines Informationsvermittlungssystems für heterogene, verteilte Informationsquellen im Internet.* http://www-is.informatik.uni-oldenburg.de/~dibo/paper/emisa/index.html

Medical Informatics Europe '99
P. Kokol et al. (Eds.)
IOS Press, 1999

Generalisation and extension of a web-based data collection system for clinical studies using Java and CORBA

H.P. Eich, C. Ohmann
Theoretical Surgery Unit, Dept. of General and Trauma Surgery, Heinrich-Heine – University Düsseldorf, Germany, {eich, ohmannch}@uni-duesseldorf.de

Abstract. Inadequate informatical support of multi-centre clinical trials lead to pure quality. In order to support a multi-centre clinical trial a data collection via WWW and Internet based on Java has been developed. In this study a generalisation and extension of this prototype has been performed. The prototype has been applied to another clinical trial and a knowledge server based on C++ has been integrated via CORBA. The investigation and implementation of security aspects of web-based data collection is now under evaluation.

1. Introduction

Multi-centre clinical trials bear the risk of errors in patient recruitment, protocol failures and documentation errors. These difficulties can lead to poor quality of multi-centre trials [1]. Major reasons are: information deficiency, no informatical support of the performance of the study and inadequate tools for documentation.

The internet is an ideal platform to support clinical trials. Any participant is able to send data to the collecting centre at any time. First approaches to collect data via the World Wide Web (WWW) have been made [2]. In this approach data had to be integrated in another step in the database by members of the collecting centre. With the WWW many of the problems described above can be solved. Applications are platform independent, access is inexpensive and makes an distribution of up-to-date information possible 24 hours a day [3]. Special tools can be provided by the study centre to ensure the quality of the data collection (e.g. automatic evaluation of inclusion/exclusion criteria, randomisation, electronic forms with plausibility checks). A prototype for a multi-centre data collection in an world-wide survey of the World Organisation of Gastroenterology (OMGE) on Appendicitis and HIV/AIDS[1] has been set-up. The system is developed entirely in Java and is currently under evaluation [4,5].

It was the aim of the investigation to improve the prototype with respect to two aspects: First, how this prototype can be generalised to be used for other clinical fields with only little effort and second, how additional study software (e.g. knowledge server for scores) can be integrated via a CORBA approach.

[1] http://www.tc.uni-duesseldorf.de/partners/OMGE/projects/HIV/

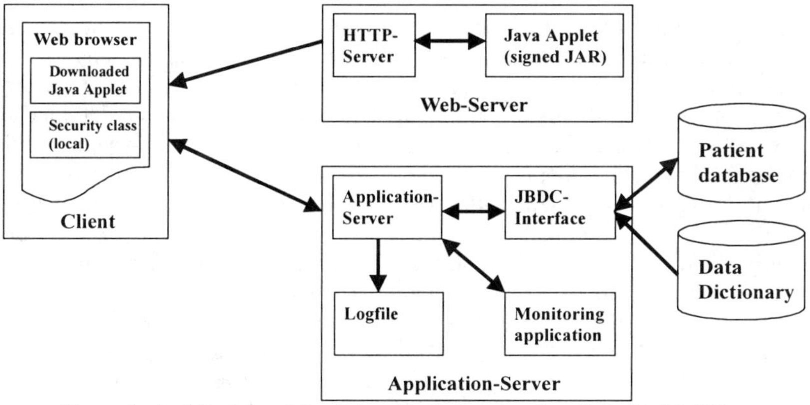

Figure 1: Architecture of the data collection system for clinical trials [5]

2. Methods

The architecture of the web-based data collection prototype for clinical trials is presented in figure 1. It is a so-called 3-tier model, because the database cannot be directly accessed by the client. The database is controlled by the application server. A client with a Java capable web browser logs into the web server and downloads the documentation program, which then connects to the application server. If the client cannot prove his identity, the connection is refused. The application server checks the presence of a unique Java class file containing a key which has to be installed on the client machine. The system was developed on a Pentium PC under Windows 95 with the Integrated Development Environment (IDE) Visual J++ by Microsoft. The server platform consists of a Pentium PC with Windows NT4 and the Information Server 3 of Microsoft. The underlying Relational Database Management System (RDBMS) is Microsoft Access together with the JDBC-ODBC-bridge of Sun Microsystems.

A main design feature is the integration of a central data dictionary to handle all terminological aspects. First of all, it supports an effective database structure of the patient database, since only term identifiers are stored without any additional terminological information. The terminology with semantic links is capable to build-up a complex hierarchy of terms. This supports a semi-automatic development of electronic forms for documentation [4]. Additional information of the parameters to be documented, like valid ranges and units can be can be checked on-line during documentation process to ensure the quality of the collected data. The terminology can be used for other tasks in the same clinical field like decision-support (guidelines, scores, etc.) or retrieval of information (e.g. Medline). With the terminology separated in a data dictionary it should be easy to use the same program for a different clinical field.

To show how flexible the documentation tool with the data dictionary approach is, the system should be applied in an international survey on Behcet's disease[2]. Gastrointestinal involvement in Behcet's disease appears to range between rare and 50 % in different parts of the world. This may be the result of true differences or variations in ascertainment. In practice there are practically no large series of patients with gastrointestinal involvement of Behcet's disease (GIBD) in the literature. The only feasible way to study this disease is to build up a world-wide survey to get a database with an adequate sample size.

[2] http://www.tc.uni-duesseldorf.de/partners/OMGE/projects/Behcet/behcet.htm

The documentation tool for clinical trials should be extended with other independent program modules. Motivated is this task by the necessity to integrate small decision-aids for clinical trials, such as scores, algorithms, guidelines, protocols, etc. In a prototype a scoring system for appendicitis should be applicable directly to study data and the result should be stored as clinical data in the patient record. The scoring system should not be integrated directly into the documentation tool not to harm its ability of generalisation. An existing knowledge-based system with integrated scoring systems and sets of rules for the clinical field of acute abdominal pain should be reused for this task [6]. This program is written in Borland C++ on IBM-compatible PCs as a stand-alone system. It was developed with object-oriented methods and has a modular design that separates the graphical user interface (GUI), from the problem and the underlying database. The system should be reused as a knowledge server to be consulted by other systems via the internet, such as our web based data collection system. A link between the Java-based documentation tool and the knowledge based system written in C++ should be established via a CORBA middleware approach [7]. The system was developed with a data dictionary to separate the structure of the knowledge modules from terminology.

For a prototypical integration of a scoring system implemented in a knowledge server with a web-based data collection module different approaches can be taken into consideration. In principle there are two approaches possible to link the application server of the knowledge server: Java Native Interface (JNI) and a CORBA interface. With JNI it is possible to execute C++ methods directly with the great disadvantage of loosing the platform independence. The decision was made to link the application server to the knowledge server via CORBA (figure 2). The interface for data exchange was defined with the Interface Definition Language (IDL) and was then translated to Java and C++. The version 3.0 of ORBacus[3] was used, which is free for non-commercial applications and can be used under UNIX and Microsoft 95 / NT. The knowledge server is implemented on an IBM-compatible PC but can be helt remote from the study data collection server. Since both systems are linked to the same data dictionary a terminological link is easily established. The trigger event to execute a score on actual data is when the user saves the patient data. In this moment the client checks if all necessary data is present and the application server can therefore apply the score to them. Missing data would be prompted by the client.

3. Results

For development of the data dictionary for Behcet's disease about 200 clinical terms including links, parameters, values, units were stored in a data dictionary. Three electronic forms (diagnosis, treatment, outcome) were developed semi-automatically for data collection in a period of less than one week (see figure 3). There was no need to change one line of code, all information was assembled in databases.
In a prototype the German appendicitis score implemented in the C++ knowledge server has been linked to a web-based data collection module (figure 4).

[3] http://www.ooc.com/ob

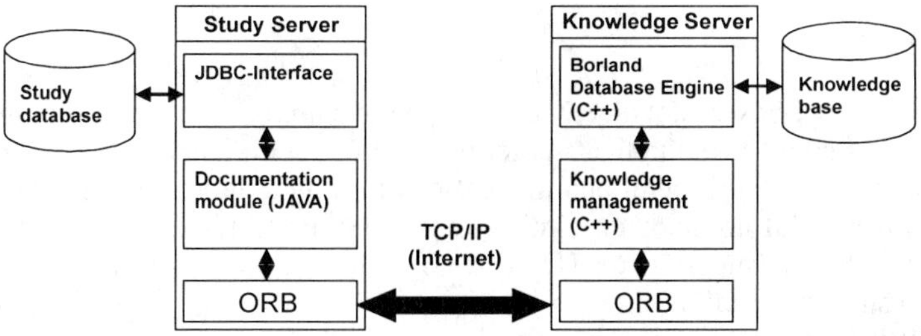

Figure 2: Conception of a Internet-based Documentation module for clinical trials and a knowledge server

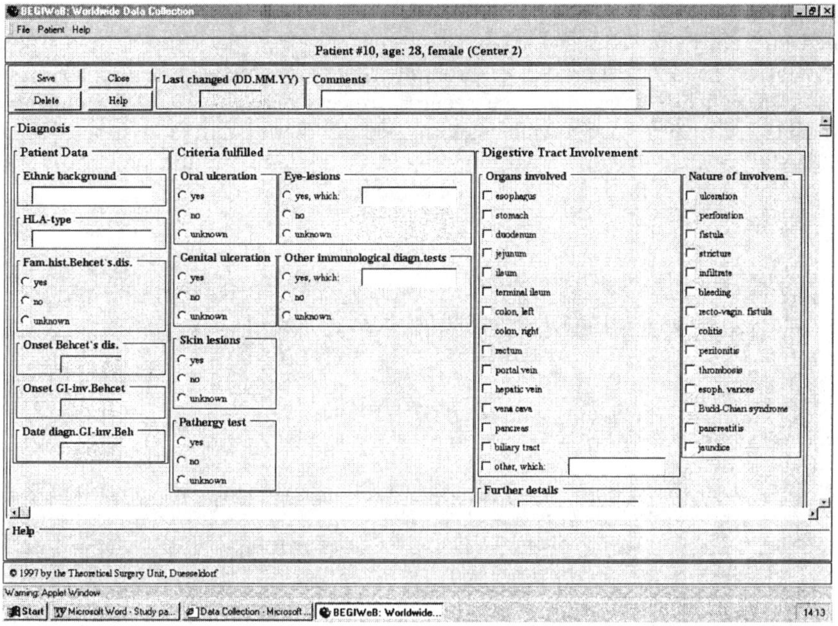

Figure 3: Screen shot of the form-based data entry for the diagnosis of Behcet's disease

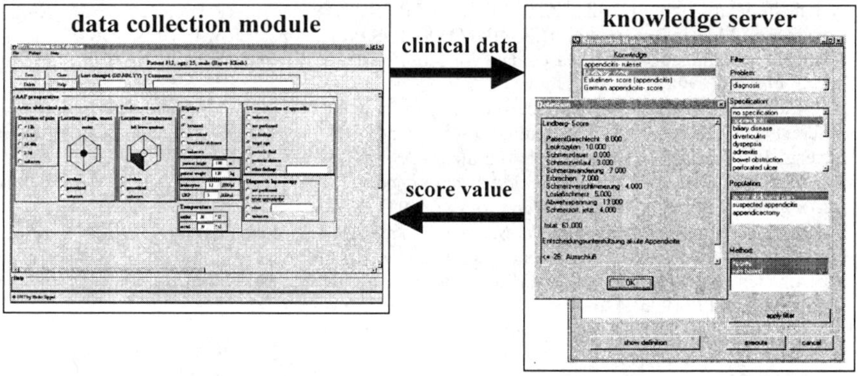

Figure 4: Information exchange between the study data collection tool and the knowledge server

4. Discussion

Concerning the Java-based documentation tool for clinical trials the combination of Java/JDBC makes sophisticated client/server applications with database access possible. A complex GUI can be created semi-automatically with a data dictionary approach. Support of a new clinical trial in another clinical field can be achieved in short time. The architecture is clearly superior to HTML/CGI combinations for data collection [8]. Moreover, transmitting data via Internet bares great security risks. The underlying network protocol TCP/IP contains no adequate security layer. Sun Microsystems has included tools for data encryption into its JDK. However, legal problems forbid higher level encryption technology in some countries and the export of such a technology is prohibited by law. Therefore, only anonymous data are collected at the moment. A link to personal data is kept only in the participating centre. On the server side all connections to the database are monitored and any connection to a non-registered user will be refused. A new project funded by the German Research Association (Deutsche Forschungsgemeinschaft) has been set-up to systematically investigate the security aspects of web-based data collection in clinical trials. A major issue is the performance of the system and user acceptance. Evaluation studies have to show the availability of the system, the time and effort to use it and the satisfaction with the interface and the content of the prototypes.

Acknowledgement

The work was supported by grant of the German Research Association (Deutsche Forschungsgemeinschaft, Oh 39/3-2).

References

[1] M. Evans, A.V. Pullock, The inadequacy of published random control trials of antibacterial prophylaxis in colorectal surgery. *Dis Colon Rectum* **30** (1987) 743-746.

[2] L.B. Afrin, V. Kuppuswamy, B. Slater, R.K. Stuart RK, Electronic clinical trial distribution via World Wide Web: A prototype for reducing costs and errors, improving accrual, and saving trees. *Journal of the American Informatics Association* **4** (1997) 25.

[3] H.J. Lowe, E.C. Lomax, S.E. Polonky, The World Wide Web: a review of an emerging Internet-based technology for the distribution of biomedical information. *Journal of the American Medical Informatics Association* **3** (1996) 1-14.

[4] H. Sippel, H.P. Eich, C. Ohmann, Data collection in multi-centre clinical trials via Internet – A generic system in Java. In: B. Cesnik, A.T. McCray, J.R. Scherrer (eds.), Proceedings of the Ninth World Congress on Medical Informatics (MEDINFO'98). IOS Press, Amsterdam **1** (1998) 93 - 97.

[5] H. Sippel, C. Ohmann, A web-based data collection system for clinical trial studies using Java. *Medical Informatics* **23** (1998) 223-229.

[6] H.P. Eich, C. Ohmann, K. Lang, Decision support in acute abdominal pain using an expert system for different knowledge bases. Proceedings of the tenth IEEE symposium on computer-based medical systems. IEEE computer society, Los Alamitos, CA (1997) 2-7.

[7] B. Blobel, M. Holena, Comparing middleware concepts for advanced healthcare system architectures. *International Journal of Medical Informatics* **46** (1997) 69-85.

[8] T. Kiuchi, Y. Ohashi, M. Konishi, Y. Mandai, T. Kosgue, T. Kakizoe. A World Wide Web-based user interface for a data management system for use in multi-institutional clinical trials. Development and experimental operation of an automated patient registration and random allocation system. *Controlled Clinical Trials* **17** (1995) 476-493.

Medical Informatics Europe '99
P. Kokol et al. (Eds.)
IOS Press, 1999

Evaluation of medical knowledge using electronic textbooks and ExaMe program on Internet

Jana ZVÁROVÁ, Karel ZVÁRA Jr., Petr HANZLÍČEK, Jan NEUSTADT, Pavel ROŠICKÝ, Karel BURIÁNEK, Růžena AUGUSTINOVÁ, Jakub PROX
European Center for Medical Informatics, Statistics and Epidemiology of Charles University and Academy of Sciences
Pod vodarenskou vezi 2, 182 07 Prague 8, The Czech Republic

Abstract. In the paper we describe the function of the ExaMe program that serves for evaluation of students' knowledge using Internet. Evaluation is based on the knowledge base of a given course. Two types of evaluation tests are described. The fixed test is appropriate for examination of students by the teacher in computer classroom connected to Internet. By this test the evaluation is done in the limited time period and all students are tested with the same evaluation test. The automatic test is appropriate for self-evaluation and self-study by students on remote places. The student can ask the ExaMe program for the test of different difficulty levels and state the number of questions required. Finally the first experience with the ExaMe program in practice is given. The application of the ExaMe program is shown in connection with IT EDUCTRA electronic products and electronic textbook on biomedical statistics.

1. Introduction

Education is the basis for research and development in all areas of business and also in health care. However, health care professionals can benefit from new information and communication technologies. Quick access to many information sources using Internet has been opened. The rapid development of information society technologies and applications is also opening new ways of education and training. There are broad international efforts to speed this process by medical informatics education of students, nurses, physicians, health managers and other health care professionals and by changing a learning environment using new information and communication technologies. The International Medical Informatics Association (IMIA) has recognized the importance of medical informatics education and training a long time ago. Working Group 1 (WG1) on Education held the IMIA conferences in Lyon, France 1974 [1], Chamonix, France, 1983 [2], Victoria, Canada, 1989 [3], Prague, Czech Republic 1990 [4], Heidelberg/Heibron, Germany, 1992 [5] and Sydney, Australia 1997 [6]. The 6th International Conference on Health and Medical Informatics Education in Sydney [6] focused not only on great needs for medical informatics education but also on increasing requirements to produce, deliver and distribute information and education services without constraints of time and distance. Then the use of new information and communication technologies in the learning environment is inevitable.

European countries have been very supported to promote new ways and tools of education by European Commission programmes. The overview of results of several European projects can be found in [7]. One of the European projects EuroMISE (European

Education in Medical Informatics, Statistics and Epidemiology) was running in the period of three years 1993 - 1995 under the scheme of the TEMPUS-PHARE programme, giving assistance to central and eastern European countries [8], [9]. The results of the project has influenced teaching activities provided by the European Center of Medical Informatics, Statistics and Epidemiology of Charles University and Academy of Sciences (EuroMISE Center) in pre-graduate and post-graduate education of students and long-life education of health professionals. Medical informatics courses in English were developed in broad European co-operation focusing on teaching of teachers and health professionals from central and eastern European countries. These courses have been running each year in European co-operation since 1994. The medical informatics courses held in the years 1997 and 1998 could benefit also from the use of educational materials developed in the IT EDUCTRA (Information Technologies EDUcation and TRAining) project running under the Fourth Framework Programme of European Commission. Within the IT EDUCTRA project new educational materials in English have been developed covering the interdisciplinary field of medicine, health care, informatics and telematics. The EuroMISE Center is one of the dissemination centers of IT EDUCTRA educational materials and other products. IT EDUCTRA products can improve existing course curricula and act as a catalyst for self-learning [10]. Selected IT EDUCTRA educational materials and tools were translated to other languages. For local educational needs in the Czech Republic, the EuroMISE center provided translations in Czech. Further, the electronic textbook on Biomedical Statistics for teaching of interdisciplinary courses in this field was developed.

The important part of the educational processes is the evaluation of students' knowledge. For this purpose the program ExaMe as an Internet application was developed. First applications of the ExaMe program concerned with evaluation of students' knowledge attained from IT EDUCTRA educational materials and other medical informatics and medical statistics courses held at the EuroMISE Center.

2. ExaMe program

The ExaMe program for evaluation of students' knowledge has been developed to enhance the possibilities for independent and distance learning and to ease the self-study of individuals. The ExaMe program is an Internet application. The only interface between ExaMe program and its user is a Web browser. The main purpose of the ExaMe program is to evaluate quickly students' knowledge gathered in the learning phase from a given course. The course consists of all teaching materials and tools that can be used by students to acquire the knowledge. Now we describe in more details the main parts of the ExaMe program.

2.1. Knowledge base of the ExaMe program

The knowledge base used by the ExaMe program is created by knowledge bases of courses. For each course *knowledge base* contains the source database of questions with scores and answers with weights and comments. For each question scores define its importance and difficulty. For each answer points define its weight and comments explain, why the answer is wrong or correct in details.

For a given course teacher or a group of teachers formulate *questions with multiple answers*. The numbers of questions and answers are not a priori limited. Some answers are wrong and some are correct. For each question at least one answer must be correct, but more correct answers are possible. Each question is connected with scores reflecting its *difficulty* and *importance.* One selected category among five categories (very easy, easy, average, difficult, very difficult) defines the difficulty of a question. Similarly, one category selected among five categories (not important, little important, moderately important, important, very important) defines the importance of a question. Teachers define categories when creating the knowledge base of the course. *Scores of categories* are integers with the values from 1 to 5. For the difficulty, the score 1 means " very easy" and the score 5 "very difficult" question. Similarly, for the importance the score 1 means "not important" and the score 5 "very important" question.

Each *answer* is weighted with *points.* Points for correct answers are positive and points for wrong answers are negative. For the ExaME program the range of points from -5 (very bad answer) to +5 (very good answer) are recommended. Teachers give points when creating the knowledge base of the course. Therefore the knowledge base of a given course can grow according to the needs of teachers, it means new questions with scores and answers with points can be added any time.

2.2 Fixed and automatic evaluation tests

There are two user groups of the ExaMe program: *teachers* and *students*. Their role can be seen from two types of evaluation tests provided by the ExaMe program.

The first type of the evaluation of students' knowledge can be done by a *fixed test*. A teacher creates the fixed test using the knowledge base of the course. The teacher sets up the test by specifying from the knowledge base which questions to use and which answers to offer (Figure 1). Then all students are examined by the same test. The most appropriate application of a fixed test is for examination of students in computer classroom connected to Internet. The teacher can follow the examination procedure, stop the examination after the a priori stated period of time and give the final results of the examination to students immediately.

The second type is called the *automatic test*. The ExaME program generates different test for each student using the knowledge base of a selected course (questions, answers, scores and points) that were developed by teachers. Automatic test for a given course is used only if the number of questions in the source database is higher then 150 and at least 30 questions for each level of difficulty is created. Then students can choose the number of questions in the test (maximally 30 questions) and select one level among five different levels (very easy, easy, medium, difficult, very difficult) of overall difficulty of the test. In this case the ExaMe program randomly generates the test required. The application of automatic tests is appropriate for distance learning, self-study and self-evaluation using Internet. In this case students can evaluate their knowledge using the ExaMe program from remote places. Simultaneously, the results of evaluation are connected with explanation given by comments in the knowledge base, why the answers are wrong or correct. It has a stimulating effect in the process of self-study and makes the learning process more effective.

2.3. Standardization and adjustation of the ExaMe tests

Evaluation of students' knowledge by the ExaMe program is based on the following standardization and adjustation procedures of fixed and automatic tests.

Adjustation of the question q

Let us denote

x_q the total number of points reached by a student for the question q,

$x_q^{(MAX)}$ the maximal number of points for the question q,

$x_q^{(MIN)}$ the minimal number of points for the question q

I_q the importance for the question q.

If $x_q^{(MAX)} \neq x_q^{(MIN)}$, then we find a constant $k_q > 0$ such that $| x_q^{(MIN)} | = k_q \, x_q^{(MAX)}$.

The adjustation procedure is given by multiplying of all points for correct answers by the constant k_q. After the adjustation procedure we recalculate the maximal and minimal number of points for the question q. Adjusted maximal number of points for the question q equals to the absolute value of the minimal number of points for the question q. Further we assume that all questions in the test are already adjusted, it means

$| x_q^{(MIN)} | = x_q^{(MAX)}$.

Standardization of the question q

For adjusted questions we calculate

$x_q^{(+)} = x_q - x_q^{(MAX)}$ and $x_q^{(-)} = x_q - x_q^{(MIN)}$.

Then we standardize the value of the question q into the interval [-1; +1] as follows

$u_q = (x_q^{(-)} + x_q^{(+)}) / (x_q^{(MAX)} - x_q^{(MIN)})$.

Using the importance I_q for each question q we calculate the *total score* reached by a student as $y = \Sigma\, I_q \, u_q$.

Let us denote $y^{(MAX)} = \Sigma\, I_q$, $y^{(MIN)} = - \Sigma\, I_q$, $y^{(-)} = y - y^{(MIN)}$ and $y^{(+)} = y - y^{(MAX)}$.

Then the results of the total standardized score reached by a student in the test is calculated as

$z = (y^{(-)} + y^{(+)}) / (y^{(MAX)} - y^{(MIN)})$.

The *total standardized score* lies between the values -1 and +1. This value is displayed in both fixed and automatic tests as the final result. Students should not pass the test if the total standardized score is less or equal zero. The value of zero is also reached in two following cases. First, when a student marked all answers in the test and second, when a student marked no answer in the test. In case of positive total standardized score the categorization of its values into classes (in accordance with the used classification scale for the educational system and the course objectives) is possible. Evaluation of student´s knowledge by fixed or automatic test is concluded with the calculation of the total standardized score. Moreover, for each answer students can see an explanation why their answers were or correct. The explanation why the answers were wrong has a strong influence on the quality and efficiency of the learning processes.

3. Experience with the ExaMe program applications

The European Medical Informatics courses have been given each year since 1994. More then 100 participants from CEE and EU countries successfully completed the Course and received the certificate. Each year the Course covers selected medical informatics topics and is based on collective knowledge and teaching materials developed in the last five years in two European projects, namely EuroMISE (TEMPUS-PHARE programme) and IT EDUCTRA (4th framework programme). The ExaMe program was firstly applied in the European Medical Informatics Course held at the EuroMISE Center in Prague, September 1998. Both the EFMI WG6 and the IMIA WG1 on health and medical informatics education endorsed the Course. The Course was running in English for two weeks for 20 participants. It consisted of lectures, demonstrations, practical exercises and hand-on experience. The networked laboratory of workstations at the EuroMISE Center, with Internet access, served for the Course purposes.

The Course provided the opportunity to receive overview of medical informatics field. The knowledge base of the Course was developed by the teachers from the co-operating universities [9]. The fixed test created from this knowledge base was used in the final evaluation. Since 1998 the ExaMe program has been used in medical informatics and medical statistics pre-graduate courses at Charles University. The first electronic textbook on Biomedical Statistics for interdisciplinary courses was finished and its printed version published [12]. The knowledge base for the ExaME program was derived from the electronic textbook. Now it has been used for ExaME evaluation by both fixed and automatic tests.

4. Conclusions

The ExaMe program opens new possibilities for evaluation of students'knowledge using Internet. Its development was motivated by co-operation in IT EDUCTRA project. It should enhance the possibilities for independent and distance learning and to ease the self-study and self-evaluation

The ExaMe program provides two types of evaluation tests. The most appropriate application of a fixed test is for examination of students in computer classroom connected to Internet. The application of automatic tests is appropriate for distance learning, self-study and self-evaluation using Internet. In this case students can from remote places evaluate their knowledge using the ExaMe program.

The program is available for all IT EDUCTRA partners, to use developed sources of questions, answers and weights based on IT EDUCTRA products. The use of the program by other users for development of knowledge base of course and running the fixed tests in remote classrooms or automatic tests in remote places using Internet is possible after fulfilling the conditions of registration given at the Internet address http://www.euromise.cz.

Acknowledgement

Research was partially supported with the EC project IT EDUCTRA no. HC 1108

References

[1] Anderson J, Gremy F, Pages JC (Eds.), Education in Informatics of Health Personnel. Amsterdam:North Holland, 1974

[2] Pages JC, Levy AH, Gremy F, Anderson J (Eds.), Meeting the Challenge: Informatics and Medical Education. Amsterdam:Noth Holland 1983

[3] Salamon R, Moehr JR, Protti DJ (Eds.) Medical Informatics &Education. Victoria:University of Victoria Press, 1989

[4] Bemmel van JH, Zvárová J (Eds.), Knowledge, Information and Medical Education. Amsterdam: North Holland, 1991

[5] Haux R, Leven FJ, Moehr JR, Protti DJ, eds. Health and Medical Informatics Education. Special issue of Meth. Inform Med 33, 3, 1994

[6] Haux R, Swinkels W, Ball MJ, Knaup P, Lun KC. (Eds), Transformation of Healthcae\re through innovative use of Information Technology for 21st Century. Special issue of Int J. Med Inform 50, 1-3, 1998

[7] Hasman A., Albert A, Wainwright, Klar R. and Sosa M. (Eds.), Education and Training in Health Informatics in Europe, IOS Press 1995

[8] Zvárová J.: Education in the methodology field of health care - EuroMISE, Methods of information in medicine 3, 33, 1994, 315 - 317

[9] Zvárová J., Engelbrecht R., van Bemmel J.H.: Education in medical informatics, statistics and epidemiology, Int J Med Inform 45, 1/2, 1997, 3 - 8

[10] Hasman A.: Education and training in health informatics: the IT EDUCTRA project. Int J Med Inform 50, 1998, 179 - 185

[11] van Bemmel JH, Musen J, eds. Handbook of Medical Informatics. Springer, Heidelberg 1997

[12] Zvárová J.: Biomedical Statistics I., Carolinum Printing House, Prague 1999

Medical Informatics Europe '99
P. Kokol et al. (Eds.)
IOS Press, 1999

A JAVA Implementation of a Medical Knowledge Base for Decision Support

Vivian Ambrosiadou*, Dimitris Goulis**, Venky Shankararaman* and George Shamtani*
**Department of Computer Science, University of Hertfordshire, AL10 9AB, UK*
***Imperial College School of Medicine, University of London, W2 1NY, UK*

Abstract. Distributed decision support is a challenging issue requiring the implementation of advanced computer science techniques together with tools of development which offer ease of communication and efficiency of searching and control performance. This paper presents a JAVA implementation of a knowledge base model called ARISTOTELES which may be used in order to support the development of the medical knowledge base by clinicians in diverse specialised areas of interest. The advantages that are evident by the application of such a cognitive model are ease of knowledge acquisition, modular construction of the knowledge base and greater acceptance from clinicians.

1. Introduction

A number of different approaches support decision making in medicine. These may be divided into five main approaches as follows [1, 2]: the **Decision Tree Model**, the **Statistical Model**, the **Production Rule System Model**, the **Pathophysiological Model** and the **Cognitive Model**.

In terms of ease of knowledge acquisition and effective decision support, the cognitive model approach which attempts to replicate the human thinking process offers great promise since medical experts can better relate to systems developed using this approach. Additionally, by providing a suitable knowledge editor, the medical expert can develop the underlying knowledge map in the domain of interest. This alleviates the need for knowledge engineers thus partly overcoming the "knowledge acquisition bottleneck". A further advantage of the cognitive model approach is the modular construction of the associative knowledge map. Initially, the system may have limited application for a particular set of diseases, but as more nodes (or frames) are added, the scope of the system widens. Some examples of systems based on the cognitive model include INTERNIST [3] and NEUROLOGIST [4].

The present research is based on the cognitive model approach. The overall objective is to develop a distributed decision support system which can be accessed over the Internet using an underlying medical knowledge base developed as a associative network of nodes and arrows. In this paper we restrict the discussion to the implementation of the knowledge model - ARISTOTELES and the prototype editor that allows clinicians to build the knowledge model without the need for programming.

2. ARISTOTELES Medical Knowledge Base

The ARISTOTELES knowledge model represents medical knowledge as a set of nodes and arrows, akin to the structured semantic network representation. The underlying knowledge map has eight types of nodes, which are linked by forty-one type of arrows. Two nodes correspond to the disease-diagnosis and the treatment respectively. The remaining six node types correspond to the three main components of any medical consultation : history, examination and laboratory tests. Three of the node types are dedicated to "questions", that is medical questioning, performance of physical examination and ordering of laboratory tests, and three to "answers", that is symptoms (problems admitted by the patient), signs (abnormalities discovered by the doctor) and results of investigation. Knowledge in a node is represented as attribute-value pairs. The model currently supports nineteen different types of node attributes which covers all the eight primary node types. The basic unit of ARISTOTELES is the **knowledge item**. Each one is composed by two nodes connected by one arrow which establishes a 1:1 relationship between the nodes. The connection between the nodes establishes the underlying medical knowledge. In contrast to traditional semantic networks [5], the ARISTOTELES model supports attribute-value pairs for arrows. For example, the arrow type *Treatment* that connects a *Disease Node* (*Graves' disease*) to a *Treatment Node* (*carbimazole*) may be represented by attribute-value pairs such as Attribute: Severity Value: Very severe.

The arrows in the model serve two purposes. First, they support navigation between the nodes and second they support decision making by enabling the inference of new knowledge based on given evidence.

3. Implementation of the Knowledge Editor

A prototype of the knowledge editor, AIMKE (ARISTOTELES Medical Knowledge Editor) has been implemented which supports the acquisition of medical knowledge based on the ARISTOTELES model. The editor provides the necessary tools to allow non-programmers (clinical experts) to develop the knowledge consisting of the nodes, arrows and their attributes and values. The knowledge editor has been designed and implemented using object oriented technology in Java. Java language was chosen since it allows the editor to be portable and machine independent, distributed over a heterogeneous network and accessed through a web browser.

3.1. System Architecture

In order to ensure an object-oriented architecture, the AIMKE system has been designed using the model-view-controller (MVC) paradigm. In the present implementation, the **model** refers to the underlying ARISTOTELES medical knowledge, the **view** is

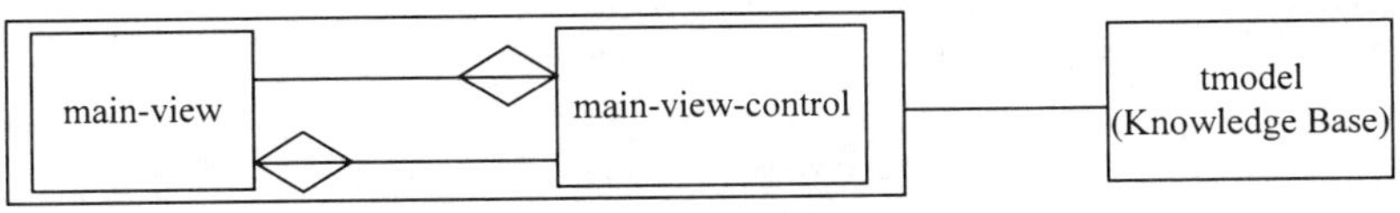

Figure 1 Architecture of the AIMKE

responsible for presenting this knowledge to the user, and the **controller** handles the user input. Accordingly, the view, which represents the editor interface, is separated from the underlying medical knowledge. This approach allows both structures to be easily extended. The architecture of the knowledge editor is as shown in Figure 1. The *main-view* and the *main-view-control* are the view and the controller classes respectively. As seen from the figure, in the current implementation, the controller is embedded in the view class. The *tmodel* class refers to the underlying ARISTOTELES medical model.

3.2. Knowledge Base

The knowledge base is structured around the ARISTOTELES model. In contrast to other approaches using a Database Management System (DBMS), to represent frame based information [6], AIMKE uses objects to store the medical knowledge represented as nodes and arrows. The use of objects is seen to provide better support for a platform independent distributed knowledge architecture.

Nodes are arranged in an inheritance hierarchy with an abstract class called *node* at the top of the hierarchy. The disease node (*dis_node*) and the treatment node (*tre_node*) directly inherit from this abstract class. In order to define the medical feature and values nodes, two abstract classes namely, *feature_node* and *value_node* are also defined which are sub classes of the abstract class *node*. Accordinly, history, examination and laboratory tests and values inherit from these abstract classes. As in the case of nodes, arrows which establish relationship between nodes are also arranged in an inheritance hierarchy with the an abstract class called *arrow* at the top of the hierarchy.

Once the ARISTOTELES model is populated with a specific medical knowledge domain such as "Respiratory Diseases", a clinician may interact with it in two ways. Firstly, as a knowledge map where the clinician may browse through the network of nodes and arrows. Secondly, as a decision support tool, where an inference engine will guide the clinician in making decisions regarding treatment of the disease based on the given symptoms and other patient related information.

When being used as a decision support tool, the system would start by asking the user a set of pre-defined questions to elicit information about the patient. An inference engine will use this information to match nodes to the symptoms. The system creates a set of symptom nodes from the questions. Where the set matches or is a subset of a rule the inference engine creates a list of hypotheses that it will use to search for a solution. The inference engine may have a hypothesis that symptoms A+B+C equal disease E and the inference engine is matching a set of symptoms A+B. The inference engine starting from node E would travel to value node C to its associated test node N through the has value/has test arrow. The system creates a set of test nodes that it would use to eliminate the test and hypothesis from the search. If the test does not match, the system asks whether the test has been performed and if the answer is 'yes' it extends the set of symptom nodes. The system then retries the set of symptoms against the hypotheses. The cycle is repeated until there is a complete match. If partial match is made, where a test result is missing, the system will suggest a test after it has checked the complete list of hypotheses.

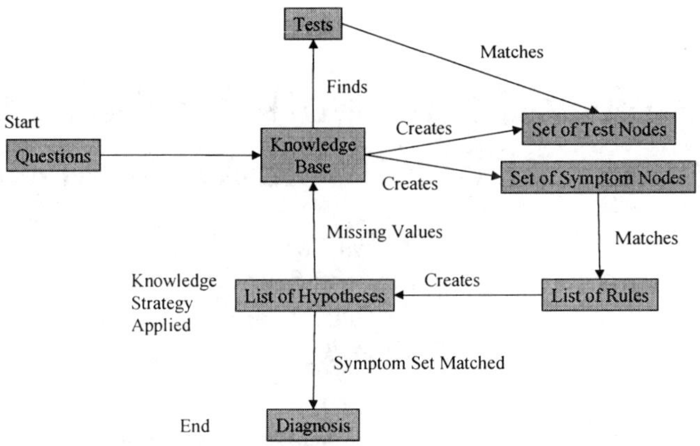

Figure 2 Use of the System as a Decision Support Tool

The view class creates a frame for the application that displays information about the knowledge base, such as its status and the nodes and arrows currently available. The user can select a node to edit, and can select a pair of nodes to link with an arrow.

The AIMKE was developed in an object oriented manner. The OMT methodology was used to specify the knowledge editor. The editor was written in Java, with a Java class being defined for each different type of node and arrow.

4. Conclusions

The implementation of a suitable interface and the mechanism for holding the medical knowledge as classes has been completed. Future work will be directed towards implementing the diagnosis module in LISP programming language and integrating it with the knowledge editor developed in Java.

References

[1] Anbar M. *Your Humble Consultant - Computer-Assisted Medical Decisions*. In: Computers in Medicine. Edited by M Anbar, Computer Science Press. 1987, pp227-260.

[2] Bradley G W. *Disease, Diagnosis and Decisions*. 1993. John Wiley and Sons.

[3] Miller R A, Pople H E and Myers J D. *INTERNIST I. An Experimental Computer Based Diagnostic Consultant for General Internal Medicine*. New England Journal of Medicie. 1982, 307, pp468-476.

[4] Catanzarite V and Greenburg A. *Neurologist - A Computer Programme for Diagnoses in Neurology*. In: Proceedings of the Third Symposium of Computer Applications in Medical Care. IEEE. 1979 pp 64-72.

[5] Luger G F and Stubblefield W A. *Artificial Intelligence: Structures and Strategies for Complex Problem Solving*. 1998. Addison Wesley Longman, Inc.

[6] Abernethy N F and Altman R B. SOPHIA: Providing Basic Knowledge Services with a Common DBMS. In: Proceedings of the 5th KRDB Workshop, Seatlle, WA, 31-May 1998.

Medical Informatics Europe '99
P. Kokol et al. (Eds.)
IOS Press, 1999

Java-based Framework for the Secure Distribution of Electronic Medical Records

Alwyn Goh
USM Computer Sciences
11800 Penang, Malaysia
Email: alwyn@cs.usm.my

Abstract: In this paper, we present a Java-based framework for the processing, storage and delivery of Electronic Medical Records (EMR). The choice of Java as a developmental and operational environment ensures operability over a wide-range of client-side platforms, with our on-going work emphasising migration towards Extensible Markup Language (XML) capable Web browser clients. Telemedicine in support of womb-to-tomb healthcare as articulated by the Multimedia Supercorridor (MSC) Telemedicine initiative—which motivated this project—will require high-volume data exchange over an insecure public-access Wide Area Network (WAN), thereby requiring a hybrid cryptosystem with both symmetric and asymmetric components. Our prototype framework features a pre-transaction authentication and key negotiation sequence which can be readily modified for client-side environments ranging from Web browsers without local storage capability to workstations with serial connectivity to a tamper-proof device, and also for point-to-multipoint transaction processes.

Keywords: Electronic Medical Record, Transaction Processing, Java Client-Server, Authentication, Secure Transactions

1 Introduction

MSC-based Telemedicine conceptualises various *information-enriched* products and services [1] for the healthcare community and general population. A wide cross-section of public healthcare facilities—major hospitals down to local clinics—will be eventually provided with WAN connectivity, through which the application-layer services will be delivered. MSC-based Telemedicine has the declared intention of initiating a paradigm shift in healthcare, in which systems and services currently designed to deliver a *curative* response would would henceforth be focussed on generating and implementing a *preventive* Lifetime Health Plan (LHP) based on exhaustive Lifetime Health Record (LHR) documentation. It bears pointing out that healthcare is one of the most basic social services rendered to the general population, hence an effective system would have the potential of contributing directly to an improvement in the quality of life.

The specific healthcare products and services articulated in the Concept Request for Proposal (CRFP) [2] documents have in common the requirement for a *standard* cross-system transaction-enabling framework. In this paper we describe an object-based transaction system designed to enable the automatic exchange of messages constructed and interpreted in compliance with a well-established and internationally recognised standard. When work on this project started in 1997, our choice for the messaging format was the United Nations (UN) sanctioned Electronic Data Interchange for Administration,

Commerce and Transportation (EDIFACT) standard. The usage of EDIFACT for healthcare messaging has been widely explored [3, 4, 5, 6]; but can be considered to be somewhat out-of-place in the context of Personal Computers (PC), thin-clients and the World Wide Web (WWW). The combination of EDI-like documents represented using Extensible Markup Language (XML) [7] looks to be particularly promising as a developmental basis, this will be also discussed in the following section.

2 Document Representation and Manipulation

The EDIFACT standard actually specifies both syntax and semantics [8], the former of which is designed to facilitate representation of arbitrarily complex relationships between various data elements organised in terms of the following hierarchy:-

- *Interchanges*: composed of Messages
- *Messages*: composed of Segment Groups and Segments
- *Segment Groups*: composed Segment Groups and Segments
- *Segments*: composed of Composite Data Elements and Data Elements
- *Composite Data Elements*: composed of Data Elements

with individual objects being either conditional or mandatory. Multiple instances of a particular object are also allowed subject to specified repetition factors. An EDIFACT interchange can be visualised as a progressively nested sequence of linked-lists, as shown in Figure 1 below:-

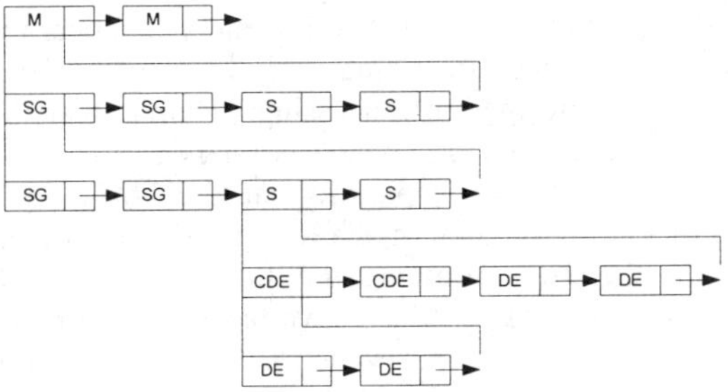

Fig 1: Typical EDIFACT Object

which can be mapped into textual form through usage of simple construction rules. EDIFACT semantics are encapsulated at the message level, with each message type intended for usage within a certain application-layer context. The UN maintains a periodically updated message directory [8], with almost 200 message types representing a broad range of administrative and commercial transactions.

The coding/decoding of EDIFACT documents, their storage within a Relational DBMS (RDMS) and their interactive representation to an enduser is discussed in [5] and [6]. The representation issue is particularly complex, and required the application of GUI design principles strongly reflecting the hierarchical linked-list structure of the transaction object. EDIFACT objects can be intuitively manipulated using nested panels and scroll-panels, with positional layout dictated by type-specific structuring features. For example, the two adjacent scroll-panels in Figure 2.1 represent segment groups GR1 and GR2 within a MEDPID message. GR2— which contains nested segment groups GR3, GR4 and GR5—is the more complex of the two, hence the inclusion of nested panels as shown in Figure 2.2. Transaction objects can be created, viewed or edited; with legitimate operations (ie adding a new segment) controlled using object-specific parameters. Most GUI elements are intuitive, ie the usage of button-set {*Previous*, *Next*, *New*, *Delete*} to navigate segments within a segment group and pull-down menus for enumerated responses. Java applications for any EDIFACT message-type can be therefore be straightforwardly assembled from a relatively small set of generic GUI object modules.

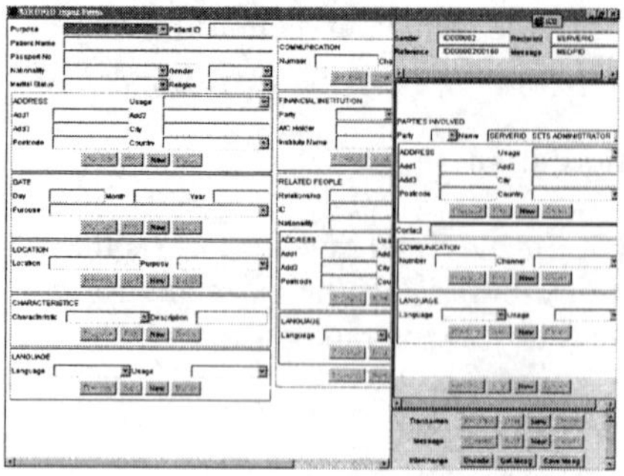

Fig 2.1: Object-based GUI Layout

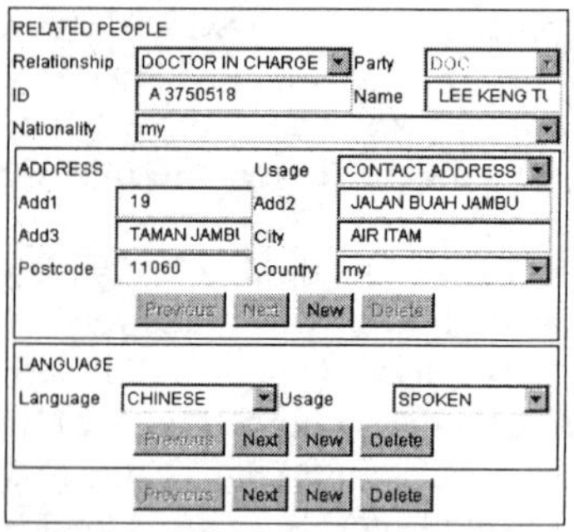

Fig 2.2: GUI Linking and Nesting

The size and complexity of the resulting GUI applications precludes implementation as a Web-downloaded applet functioning within a browser-client. An alternative approach would be to re-use the object construction syntax for presentation, this is in fact the main motivation in our ongoing investigation into XML-based encoding. On the most basic level, XML [7] is a generalisation of HTML in that user-defined tags are allowed. In the XML-model, documents are parsed for *validity* with respect some semantically meaningful document-type template, which is an extension of the syntactical *well-formedness* allowed in HTML. Document parse trees can subsequently be manipulated as objects for database storage, re-transmission or information processing. Human-readability is handled via the Extensible Stylesheet Language (XSL), which is intended to allow the mapping of well-formed documents into some *native* display format ie HTML. HTML-based presentation also allows for the embedding of multimedia and programmed elements (ie Java applets) into *rich* data models, thereby combining the structural capabilities of XML with the transparent object-integrability of HTML. Java-based functionality would be especially important for browser-based *thin* clients, which is a de facto architectural requirement to ensure the widespread accessibility critical for the success of MSC Telemedicine. The overall configuration of such a system would resemble Figure 3 below.

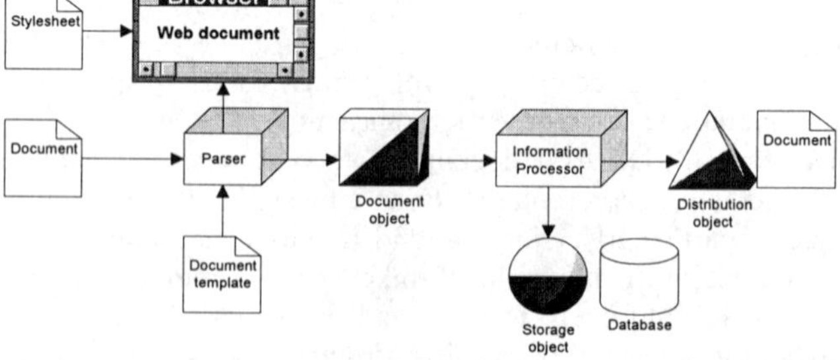

Fig 3: Transactional Architecture Based on Document-Object Modelling

3 Node Authentication and Inter-Node Security

Traditional EDI assumes the existence of a secure network environment over which transactions occur, with easy enforceability due to the strictly controlled number of network-connected terminals. Such assumptions would clearly not apply to any system designed to facilitate message distribution over a public-access WAN ie the Internet. The necessity for incorporating security and authentication components adds considerably to the operational overhead, nevertheless this is unavoidable given the legal and ethical sensitivities [10] pertaining to EMR-related information.

The transaction documents discussed in the previous section would be fairly large (even after compression) for practical EDI applications; hence the necessity for bulk encryption using some symmetric cipher, preferably one more secure than Data Encryption Standard (DES) and faster than Triple-DES (T-DES). Our system features the International Data Encryption Algorithm (IDEA) block cipher in Cipher Block Chaining (CBC) mode, thereby ensuring only one plaintext-ciphertext pair per message per session-key. This was deemed a sensible precaution given that a single session would typically be used for the exchange of multiple EDI messages, each of which contribute a large number of 64-bit ciphertext blocks. Such a scheme would, however, require session-key negotiation prior to the commencement of message exchange.

In most transactions, the roles of service provider and consumer are highly context-sensitive and frequently interchangeable within a particular session; hence the basic unacceptability of key-management protocols in which a single transaction participant selects the session-key. Alternatives—ie Needham-Schroeder (Kerberos), Neumann-Stubblebine or Woo-Lam—in which a trusted third party determines the session-key are unattractive due to the transactional overhead placed on a limited number of nodes within the transactional community. In addition, operational support of point-to-multipoint transactional modes would also require that the key-management protocol be extensible to accomodate multi-party computation and reducible for client-side platforms without local storage. All these requirements can be satisfied extending the Secure Remote Password (SRP) protocol [11] to enable bidirectional node-to-node (as opposed unidirectional client-to-server) authentication and mutual key-negotiation. The resultant protocol sequence enhances *standard* Diffie-Hellman (DH) by incorporating:-

- *Permanent and session-specific key-pairs*: the former enabling formulation of an elegantly combining authentication and key-negotiation sequence
- *Challenge-response sequence*: to enable detection of man-in-the-middle attacks, which is a well-known vulnerability associated with standard DH
- *Zero-knowledge proofs*: to verify correct conclusion of the key-negotiation sequence without potentially damaging information exposure

thereby providing security equivalent to the station-to-station [12] and other DH variants supported by the Secure Socket Layer (SSL) framework without the necessity for explicit signature verification during key-negotiation.

All transactions within the trading community can be conceptualised as occurring between a pair of nodes (initiator A and respondant B), with the involvement of a trusted Certificate Authority (CA) to distribute signed discrete logarithm public-keys, with our implementation featuring Digital Signature Algorithm (DSA) in particular. Successful authentication and key-negotiation as described in Table 1 below assumes prior downloading of public-keys associated with all other transaction nodes. Nodes A and B respectively own key-pair (α, A = $g^{\alpha} \bmod p$) and (β, B = $g^{\beta} \bmod p$), with each node possessing the public-key associated with the other. All private-keys are assumed to be securely stored, ideally on a smartcard capable of performing computations without key exposure. Note the community-wide usage of modular basis p and exponent g, which results in more economical cryptosystem management compared with authentication mechanisms based on Rivest-Shamir-Adleman (RSA) algorithm. The pre-transaction handshaking then proceeds as follows:-

Table 1: Authentication and Key-Negotiation Sequence

Step	*Party*	*Computation*	
1	Node A	Generate u, λ w = $g^{u} \bmod p$ Transmit (w, λ)	(u, w) = A session key-pair λ = A-to-B challenge parameter
2	Node B	Generate x, μ y = $g^{x} \bmod p$ χ = $(wA^{\mu})^{(x+\lambda\beta)} \bmod p$ k = H(χ) M_1 = H(w, y, k) Transmit (y, μ, M_1)	(x, y) = B session key-pair μ = B-to-A challenge parameter Note χ = $g^{(u+\alpha\mu)(x+\lambda\beta)} \bmod p$ k = symmetric session-key
3	Node A	χ = $(yB^{\lambda})^{(u+\mu\alpha)} \bmod p$ k = H(χ) Verify M_1 M_2 = H(w, y, k, M_1) Transmit M_2	Note χ = $g^{(x+\beta\lambda)(u+\mu\alpha)} \bmod p$
4	Node B	Verify M_2	

with Secure Hash Algorithm (SHA) used as the one-way hash function. Successful key-negotiation allows resultant message traffic M to be secured as E_K(M, sign(M)), with sign(M) being the DSA signature and k the unique session-key. The above-described mechanism allows for fine-tuned access control regulation—with each server maintaining a tabulation of permitted transactions associated with any given client—thereby allowing for protocol termination after step (1) in the event of an insufficiently privileged client (A) or an overloaded server (B).

4 Concluding Remarks

It is probably not an exaggeration to claim that MSC Telemedicine constitutes one the boldest policy initiatives with regards the widespread application of advanced technology in healthcare. An operational system implemented along the lines discussed in this paper would enjoy significant advantages over both *traditional* EDI-like and ad hoc Web-based transaction processing. The generic nature of open-standard object documents also makes it conceptually straightforward to incorporate commercial and governmental transactions, the only requirement being the definition of appropriate messaging specifications and the setting-up of additional transaction servers. Progressive evolution towards browser-client architectures would enable service delivery via public-access Internet terminals and home

PCs, thereby opening up MSC Telemedicine—and related commercial services ie sale of pharmaceuticals—to much larger population segments.

The initial implementation of MSC Telemedicine will, due to financial constraints, be scaled-down compared to the original CRFP conceptualisation Nevertheless even a *skeleton* solution—designed with sufficient allowances for future *plug-in* components—would have a dramatic impact on both administrative and clinical practices. The type of system proposed in this paper are in fact extremely amenable to such a roll-out strategy, with browser-clients completely eliminating the need for previously installed components and administratively-expensive version control.

One should also note that none of the systems and services envisaged in this paper are inherently bandwidth-intensive or latency-sensitive. It is therefore not unreasonable to anticipate the development and deployment of *lightweight* client-server systems intended to deliver healthcare and commercial services over generic public-access WANs, as opposed dedicated high-bandwidth environments. Such systems would, in fact, be ideal in that large-scale deployment could commence without significant investments in endpoint hardware and network infrastructure.

References

[1] Govt of Malaysia. *CRFP Telemedicine Flagship Applications: Personalised Health Information (PHI), Continuing Medical Education (CME), Teleconsultation and Lifetime Health Plan.* (1997)

[2] SSR Abidi, A Goh & Y Zaharin. *Telemedicine and Medical Informatics in the Multimedia Super Corridor: The Malaysian Vision.* Proc World Congress on Medical Informatics: Seoul, Korea. (1997)

[3] K Pramataris, G Doukidis, G Giaglis & J Raptakis. *The EUROMIDES EDI Prototype System.* Information Exchange for Medical Devices (Eds N Pallikarakis, N Anselmann & A Pernice): IOS Press. (1996)

[4] JL Monteagudo. *Data Exchange in the European Pharmacovigilance.* Information Exchange for Medical Devices (Eds N Pallikarakis, N Anselmann & A Pernice): IOS Press. (1996)

[5] DCL Ngo. *A Generic EDI Application Software.* Proc Conf on Research and Development in Computer Science (REDECS): Penang, Malaysia. (1997)

[6] A Goh, SW Leong & LC Tai. *Secure Transaction Processing Framework for Medical Informatics and Electronic Commerce in the Multimedia Super-Corridor.* Congress of Scientific and Technical Organisations in Malaysia (COSTAM): Penang, Malaysia. (1998)

[7] M Hogan. *XML and the Internet: Driving the Future of EDI.* http://www.poet.com/edi.html (1998)

[8] UN Economic Commision for Europe. *UN Rules and Directories for EDIFACT.* http://www.unece.org/trade/untdid/welcom1.htm (1998)

[9] World Wide Web Consortium (W3C). *XML Version 1.0.* http://www.w3.org/TR/PR-xml.html (1997)

[10] N Gaunt & F Roger-France. *Security of the Electronic Healthcare Record: Professional and Ethical Implications.* Towards Security in Medical Telematics (Eds B Barber, A Treacher & K Louwerse): IOS Press. (1994)

[11] Thomas Wu. *The Secure Remote Password Protocol.* http://srp.stanford.edu/srp/ (1998)

[12] W Diffie, PC van Oorschot and MJ Wiener. *Authentication and Authenticated Key Exchanges.* Design, Codes and Cryptography. (1992)

Resource Management

Medical Informatics Europe '99
P. Kokol et al. (Eds.)
IOS Press, 1999

NISPLAN – projecting hospital beds and hospital stays

Stein Østerlund Petersen
SINTEF Unimed, N-7465 Trondheim, Norway

Abstract. The paper describes a computer model for projections of hospital stays and hospital beds, developed by NIS Health Services Research in Norway. The model takes into account demographic changes, changes in medical technology, needs for hospital services, morbidity and hospital structure and population preferences as to choice of hospital. It has been used in several projects in Norway, both by central and local authorities.

1. Introduction

At NIS Health Services Research (NIS) at SINTEF Unimed a computer program has been developed to project hospital stays and hospital beds. The projection model is based on expected demographic changes, expected changes in morbidity, medical technology, population based needs for hospital services and the hospital structure within a defined geographic area. The model estimates the annual number of hospital stays and hospital beds for specified patient groups for future years, as for example the year 2005 or 2010. The model has been used in cooperation with several Norwegian hospitals and counties as well as the Norwegian Ministry of Health and Social Affairs.

The model aggregates the patients at a certain hospital or within a certain geographic area into suitable groups and performs separate projections for each group. In this context the DRG system has proved very useful. Hence the model is mainly based on groups defined according to DRG. It operates independently on each group, and estimates the number of hospital stays and hospital beds according to registered annual data from one or more previous years. It takes into account expected changes in demography (sex- and age composition of the actual population), medical technology, the need for hospital services, preferences by the population in choice of hospital and expected changes in length of stay. Except the demographic variables, the user is free to set the rate of change for the other parameters and to experiment with different scenarios. As for the demographic variables, these are based on the national population projections from Statistics Norway.

2. Parameters involved

Demographic changes and variations are important when deciding the volume and the contents of future health services. For example is the total population of Norway expected to increase by 6,4 pct. from 1996 to 2010, while the increase for the group of persons 80 years and more will be close to 25 pct. On the other hand there will be a major decrease in the population 20-39 years of age and for those below the age of 5. Knowing that the morbidity and the morbidity pattern are closely related to age and sex, these demographic changes will most certain have a dramatic effect for Norwegian hospitals, both regarding the number of patients to be treated and the patient mix within the hospitals.

The NISPLAN model used registered population figures by sex and 5-year age groups when forecasting hospital use within a geographic area. This area could be the predefined catchment area for a hospital, a county, a health region or the country as a whole. Furthermore medical and administrative hospital data have to be available. In Norway, the Norwegian Patient Register (NPR) handles patient information data. This organization war established in 1997 by the Ministry of Health and Social Affairs, and is administered by the company SINTEF Unimed. NIS and NPR work closely together, making it easy to obtain necessary for projection purposes.

The morbidity pattern of the population is an important variable in the model. Even though the morbidity seldom shows rapid changes, when we look 15-20 years into the future, a trend that seem unimportant today, may have caused great changes both in hospitalization rates and the causes for hospitalization.

The most complicated variable to is of course the evolution of medical technology. This is by far the most important variable and the hardest to project. NISPLAN approaches the topic from two different angles. One is to look at the population-based rates for hospital stays and how they may be influenced by technology improvements; another is based on changes in the length of stay for different patient groups. The first will affect the number of hospital stays, while the other will affect the number of bed days and hence the need for hospital beds.

At a certain hospital or within a certain geographical area it is not always so that all hospital services are equally covered. Better or other kinds of service may be found elsewhere. It is then necessary to identify patient groups where there is a mismatch between the supply and the demand for hospital services and to build some corrections into the model parameters. Waiting lists and comparisons with other hospitals and counties may be a fruitful way to deal with these aspects of hospital projections. In the model various assumptions are described as changes in the population based hospitalization rates.

Within a certain geographical area a patient may quite often choose between several hospitals. There may be various levels of specialization between the hospitals, from the smaller local hospitals to the larger regional or university hospitals. Not only will the distribution of patients in the future depend on factors as demography, needs, morbidity and technology, but to a large extent what kind of services that will be established at the various hospitals. In countries and regions where there are a free choice of hospital this is a crucial part of the planning process. This will most probably be introduced throughout the whole of Norway from next year on. In NISPLAN this is handled by describing the patient flow from one area to the hospitals in question, and by describing the patient flow from other areas than the catchment area to a certain hospital.

There is a direct mathematical link from changes in the length of stay for a certain patient group and to the number of beds needed. For example, there was an increase of more than 50 000 hospital stays in Norway from 1992 to 1997. In the same period the number of hospital beds increased with only 100 – that is one new bed per 500 extra admissions. The reason this could happen was a decrease in the average length of stay at Norwegian hospitals of about 0,5 days, while the occupancy rate was more or less constant on 85 per cent It is therefore obvious that model has to take changes in the average length of stay into account, and that the estimates here will be crucial for the success or failure of the model estimates. In the model, the distribution of bed days is aggregated in 5 groups, from 0-4 days as the lower group to 30 days and more as the highest. This gives a more precise and detailed picture of the question of length of stay than just one figure – the overall length of stay for each group will do.

3. Model output

The following figures are calculated through the model:

- Number of hospital stays at a specific hospital or from a specific geographic area, for each patient group and for each year.
- Average length of stay for each patient group and year.
- Number of bed for each patient group and year.
- The same figures for the total number of patients.

NISPLAN is a useful tool when it is necessary to combine a multiple set of factors simultaneously. The model handles the mathematical operations involved and shows how different assumptions influences the number of hospital stays and hospital beds. The crucial point is of course to decide how the various factors will develop over time. This decision is not done by the computer program, but is the essential input from the hospital planners. The DRG system has proved useful, both for the sake of overview and clarity, and as a means for bringing planners and medical experts together within a common language.

4. Concluding remarks

The projects where the model has been used in Norway have shown that

- It is easy to detect the effect of various assumptions for future trends.
- It is a common tool for planners and medical experts.
- It sorts out the important factors from those of minor importance.
- It makes it easy to compare different alternatives – for example high and low alternatives for the reduction of average length of stay.

The model will stimulate fruitful discussions, and change focus from the estimated figures themselves, to the assumptions leading to these estimates. This is of course a valuable effect in itself.

At the moment, plans for a new and updated version of the model are discussed. This involves outpatient services, economic and financial figures, personnel and space for buildings and medical services. An idea discussed is also to let the users access the model through the Internet. Then there are some problems with data security that has to be sorted out.

Medical Informatics Europe '99
P. Kokol et al. (Eds.)
IOS Press, 1999

Automated computer-assisted evaluation of diagnosis-and-procedure-reports in Austrian hospitals

Hagenbichler*, E.; Klingler** , D., Neuner** , L., Pfeiffer, K.-P.***
* *Jörgerstr. 3/35, A-1170 Wien.;* ** *AKH Linz, A-4020 Linz;*
*** *Inst. f. Biostatistik, Univ.-Klinik Innsbruck, A-6020 Innsbruck*

Abstract. Austria's 320 hospitals with 73.000 beds have to transmit a minimum basic data set for each hospital stay with diagnosis and procedures as well as scores for use in intensive care units (last only in performance-oriented financed hospitals). Based on these data, 160 hospitals or 53.000 beds are financed through performance oriented flat rates per case (LDFs - Leistungsorientierte Diagnosen-Fallpauschalen). Those LDFs are in some principles similar to DRG's (diagnosis related groups), but have been developed by the Federal Ministry of Labor, Health and Social Affairs (BMAGS). 1.94 million data sets of hospital stays, which were reported for financing in the year 1997 had to be analyzed for their correctness and plausibility. For this aim the "Scoringprogramm" of the BMAGS is in use. We describe in detail how many diagnoses and procedures are automatically checked with diagnosis, sex, age, length of stay etc. 1.6% warnings resulted from this checking, and no errors have been reported. The checking routines have to be further developed. At present data seem to be used only with caution for epidemiology or for analyzing medical quality. For financing purposes it might be reliable, especially if data quality commissions are enlarged and if evaluation of data with medical records is improved.

1. Background

Austrian hospitals are obliged to transmit an anonymous Minimum Basic Data Set (MBDS) for each hospital stay to the provincial funds, which is then forwarded to the Federal Ministry of Labor, Health and Social Affairs (BMAGS) [1]. It is a must that one main diagnosis and up to 9 additional diagnoses are being documented among other information like age, sex, ward, admission and discharge dates and administrative data. Since 1999 there is the possibility to gather the diagnosis voluntarily on the basis of ICD-10 (International Statistical Classification of Diseases and related health problems, 10th Revision, WHO – World Health Organization) [2]. This diagnosis will then be automatically encoded into the (mandatory) Austrian version of ICD-9-code numbers for the reason of hospital financing [3]. For this purpose an unequivocal translation table has been provided by the BMAGS [4].

Furthermore hospitals are obliged to document up to 9 medical procedures including their quantities. The documentation of medical procedures is based on an Austrian-specific catalog of medical procedures. In 1999 this catalog comes with 925 medical procedures and with 8 scores for therapeutic-intervention and severity-of-illness, whereas the 8 scores are used for the documentation of the performance in intensive care units (ICUs) only in performance-oriented financed hospitals.

Since 1998, these 8 scores have to be documented since 1998 using a different data set [5,6]. At admission one of the following scores has to be documented – depending on the patient's age: either SAPS II (Simplified Acute Physiology Score) [6,7], TRISS (a combination of Trauma Score and Injury Severity Score) [6,8], CRIB (Clinical Risk Index for Babies) [6,9], SNAP (Score for Neonatal Acute Physiology) [6,10] or PRISMIII (Pediatric Risk of Mortality Score) [6,11]. For daily documentation the following are in use: TISS-28 (Therapeutic Intervention Scoring System) [6,12], NTISS (Neonatal TISS) [6,13] or PedTISS (pediatric TISS) [6,14].

The correct use and hints for the software implementation and for plausibility checks of these classifications, catalogs and scores are described in a handbook and in additional publications of the BMAGS [3,6,15,16,17,18,19]. In the year 1997 there were earlier versions of the Austrian version of the ICD-9 and of the catalog of procedures in use [20,21].

Based upon this documentation and through performance-oriented flat rates per case (LDFs - Leistungsorientierte Diagnosen-Fallpauschalen) - that in some principles are similar to diagnosis related groups (DRG) - (but which we have especially developed in Austria), the scores (which represent the costs) have been calculated for the hospitals all over Austria in the same way since 1997. Days on ICUs are paid in addition. The paid cost for one day on a specific ICU is mainly determined through the average of TISS-points per day of the year before.

Some private hospitals and trauma surgery hospitals are exceptions of this financing system. For instance, in 1997 about 20.000 beds (roughly 160 smaller hospitals) were excepted and 53.000 beds (about 160 hospitals) were included in this financing system [22]. Before 1997 and in the private and trauma surgery hospitals nowadays a daily flat-rate was or respectively is paid.

1.94 million data sets of hospital stays (one for each stay), which were reported for financing in the year 1997 had to be put to the proof for their completeness and plausibility.

In the following we present the software tool for the year 1997 and for 1999, which we have developed for the routine check and the plausibility, and which is available free of charge on the internet in its actual version (http://www.bmags.gv.at, Scoringprogramm Version 3.1) [23]. We will also describe how these goals have been reached and which further checking routines will have to be developed.

As the new Austrian performance-oriented hospital financing system (LKF – Leistungsorientierte Krankenanstaltenfinanzierung) [24] is based upon these data, the correctness of these data is not only of big importance from an epidemiological point of view, but also from an economic one!

2. Results

We investigated the checking routines for the plausibility as defined by the BMAGS, which are mandatory in use and which are represented as software tools, namely "Scoringprogramm Version1.2" for the year 1997 [25] and "Version 3.1" for the year 1999 [23]; "Intensivscoringprogramm Version 2.1" [26] is used for the collection of data in ICUs for the year 1999.

The scoring program serves for calculating the points for financing the hospital stay of the patient, for checking the plausibility of data, and, if necessary, also for encoding the diagnosis and procedures in the hospital.

The scoring program is implemented under Windows 3.1. A C-source-code is available. Free disk space less than 6 MB is needed for the program itself (3 MB of the 6 MB are needed for documentation files). With the program the BMAGS - as the overall responsible organization for data quality - checks the plausibility of the data, which takes approximately one working day when using a standard PC for checking ca. 2 million data sets of one year [22].

The program of 1999 for the data of ICUs (under Windows 3.1; 4 MB disk space needed) checks completeness, the lab results in relation to medical minimum/maximum human limits and also for the combination of various parameters of the scores, e.g. "treatment of metabolic alkalosis or acidosis" with the respective "pH-value".

On the one hand the scoring program of 1997 evaluates formal criteria of completeness. On the other hand there are different other criteria. First diagnoses are checked in relation to age. 516 diagnoses out of 6.151 diagnoses are checked with age restrictions, e.g. "ICD-9 - 647.8 – toxoplasmosis during pregnancy" with age limits from 5 to 60 years, or "ICD-9 - 769 – IRDS (infants respiratory distress syndrome)" is checked with age limits from 0 to 4, or "ICD-9 - 797 – senility" with limits from 65 to 150. In 1999 there are 520 out of 6774 diagnoses with age restrictions.

For 1997 there are 628 diagnoses related to sex. Examples are "ICD-9 - 174 - malignant neoplasm of the mamma" with sex female, or "ICD-9 – 600 - hyperplasia of the prostate" with sex male. In 1999 there are 661 sex restrictions.

Rare and / or notifiable forms of disease are also checked in 71 cases in 1997 (in 1999: 64 cases), e.g. "ICD-9 - 050 – smallpox", or "ICD-9 – 001 - cholera".

A large part of all medical procedures (as of 1997: out of a catalog with 812 medical procedures [20], in 1999 with a total of 925 medical procedures [19]) is evaluated in connection to diagnosis (1997: 14.216 relations, 1999: 18.568 relations). The diagnosis is cross-checked only with the first three digits of the ICD-9-code. Thus in 1997, 767 diagnoses out of 937 three digits codes were checked as being plausible with 598 procedures out of the above mentioned 812. The median of one diagnosis is checking with 11 procedures (minimum 1, maximum 298), whereas the median checking of one procedure is with 13 diagnoses (minimum 1, maximum 146). In 1999 there are 858 diagnoses out of 937 three digits codes checked as plausible with 697 procedures out of the above mentioned 925. The median of one diagnosis is checking with 12 procedures (minimum 1, maximum 351), whereas the median checking of one procedure is with 16 diagnoses (minimum 1, maximum 232).

Furthermore checking is being done in respect to the number of performed medical procedures (all procedures with an upper high and very high limit). For example a coding of a "laparascopic appendectomy" or a "cholecystectomy" more often than one time during one hospital stay will cause a warning (upper high limit), but if it is coded more than four times it is doubtlessly an error (very high limit). In these cases, one can discuss if it makes sense to increase the very high limit to more than 4, and indeed a reduction of this limit has been done to 3 and probably will be done to 1 in the future.

In 1997 the checking of procedures in connection with male/female sex of patients had 69 relations, in 1999 78 relations. Examples are "hysterectomy" with female or "operation of a phimosis" with male patients.

In 1997 the checking of procedures with age occurred 17 times, in 1999 20 times, e.g. "Caesarian operation" only for patients aging between 5 and 60; or some age-pre-defined operations like "operation of the diaphragm in children under the age of 1 month".

Since 1999, 126 diagnoses are checked also if they are the only plausible cause for hospitalization. Maybe these patients should be rather treated as out-patients in the clinic than as in-patients in the ward, and the same may be true with superficial wounds, and some other specific symptoms.

823 diagnoses are checked if they are approved of as a cause for a "0-day-hospital-stay" (i.e. admission and normal discharge within the same day). Here the diagnosis seems to be too serious for being treated as 0-day-hospital-stay, e.g. "coma" or "sepsis".

Since 1999 medical procedures are also checked for their plausibility if performed within a "0-day-hospital-stay" and normal discharge (538 procedures, e.g. "heart transplantation" and other major operations, "therapy within a stroke unit", etc.) or if they could be rather handled as out-patients, such as with "transesophageal echocardiography" or maybe also with "chronic hemodialysis" (19 relations).

"Post-mortem examination" is cross-checked if it fits to the type of discharge (dead).

The generated warning and error hints usually necessitate to check the data with the medical records.

If the check for age, sex and the higher limit of the number of medical procedures produces an "error" result, this hospital stay of the respective patient will not be financed until the error is corrected. The other checking routines produce a "warning" result, so that a control with the medical record is necessary.

Very commonly occurring warnings concerned the combination of diagnosis with the procedure, e.g. "removal of osteosynthesis material" with the previous diagnosis of the acute bone fracture instead of the correct diagnosis, the delayed consequence of this fracture. Other warnings resulted from a misunderstanding of the definition of a procedure as for example in "continuous measurement of the intracranial pressure", where many physicians counted this "per day" instead of "per the whole time while continuously measuring" [22].

After an introduction phase we realized, however, that in some cases, the restrictions were too rigorous, so the checking routines needed adaptation. We also realized that there were many procedures which were not clearly defined, so we had to define a new and more precise description and counting of procedures.

Indeed in some cases also the choice of the correct diagnosis as main diagnosis was changed, there had been some misunderstandings with the coding hospital physician as well as with the administrative hospital employees. Also combinations of medical procedures have been coded, which were an implicit part of the main procedure, e.g. a therapeutic arthroscopy where also a diagnostic arthroscopy during the same procedure has been coded (because one has to look into the patient). Another example is the coding of two tonsillectomies during one operation because of the argument that both tonsils had been removed.

In 1997 there were approximately 1.6 % automatically produced warnings (ca. 32.000 of approx. 1,940.000 transmitted data sets) [22]. No errors have been reported [22].

The results of the evaluation are reported to the provincial funds (so-called "Landesfonds"), and they usually give feedback to the hospitals, although the hospitals are obliged to make this evaluation by themselves.

The provincial funds have established groups or commissions for checking the data plausibility ("data quality groups/commissions"). At the current state, these groups are working more or less intensively. Before the introduction of the LKF-system the various health insurance organizations took a bigger influence in the evaluation of the medical treatment, especially concerning the length of stay and allowance for treatment as in-patient.

3. Further developments

Future evaluation criteria should relate the diagnosis with the type of medical department, and therefore evaluate the correct choice of the main diagnosis. Further criteria could be a linking of all hospital stays of a patient in the same hospital to check the type of admission.

Further checking routines could be extended to the principle of severity-of-illness of diagnoses (including their combination). Also the severity-of-illness of one or more medical procedures and their relation with length of stay, type of department, type of admission and discharge (e.g. death) could be further developed. The analysis of combination of procedures should be of great importance, and therefore it would be necessary to know the date of the procedure (which we do not know at present).

Last but not least, an analysis of statistical relations in collectives of patients can be made regarding to type of hospital (e.g. in relation to the points that represent costs). A tool for producing statistically valid samples could be useful. A relation to other official reports should be made (e.g. carcinoma register or mortality statistics), allowing further evaluation of data.

In the future one should put more attention to the evaluation and interpretation of diagnosis-and-procedure-reports as tools for planning and information provision in the public health sector. Therefore methods which are now in use in the field of artificial intelligence (e.g. knowledge-based expert systems, data-mining and neural networks) should be further developed and implemented for this purpose.

4. Conclusion

The software, currently available free of charge, covers a lot of questions for automatic evaluation of data and their plausibility to choose suspicious data sets. After checking the medical records, these data sets have to be corrected if necessary.

However, the current quality and quantity of data is not sufficient to give detailed information on questions of medical quality and of epidemiology. But the data can be quite helpful for financing purposes and if one accepts a relatively broad range of acuity for spreading the financial means.

But even for this purpose the evaluation of data has to be increased through the work of the data quality groups or commissions.

The random sampling of patients data sets and checking them with the medical records will always be necessary.

References

[1] http://www.ris.bka.gv.at Dokumentation im Gesundheitswesen. BGBl Nr. 745/1996 and 783/1996.
[2] http://www.bmags.gv.at ICD-10 BMAGS 1999
[3] http://www.bmags.gv.at ICD-9 BMAGS 1998
[4] http://www.bmags.gv.at Überleitungstabelle ICD-10 nach ICD-9
[5] http://www.ris.bka.gv.at Dokumentation im Gesundheitswesen. BGBl II Nr. 63/1998 and 473/1998
[6] http://www.bmags.gv.at Medizinisches Dokumentationshandbuch (inkl. 2 Anhänge)
[7] SAPS-II: Le Gall JR, Lemeshow St, Saulnier F. A new Simplified Acute Physiology Score (SAPS II) based on a European/North American Multicenter Study. JAMA 1993; 270(24): 2957-2963.
[8] TRISS: Boyd CR, Tolson MA, Copes WS. Evaluating Trauma Care: The TRISS Method. The Journal of Trauma. April 1987.
[9] CRIB: The International Neonatal Network. The CRIB (clinical risk index for babies) score: a tool for assessing initial neonatal risk and comparing performance of neonatal intensive care units. Lancet 1993; 342: 193-198.
[10] SNAP: Richardson, Douglas K., et al. Score for Neonatal Acute Physiology: A Physiologic Severity Index for Neonatal Intensive Care. Pediatrics. 1993;91:617-623
[11] PRISMIII: Pollack, Murray M, et al. PRISM III: An updated Pediatric Risk of Mortality score. Crit Care Med. 1996;24: 743-752.
[12] TISS-28: Miranda DR, De Rijk A, Schaufeli W. Simplified Therapeutic Interventions Scoring System: The TISS-28 items - Results from a multicenter study. Crit-Care-Med 1996; 24(1): 64-73.
[13] NTISS: Gray, James E., et al. Neonatal Therapeutic Intervention Scoring System: A Therapy-Based Severity-of-Illness Index. Pediatrics. 1992;90: 561-567.
[14] PedTISS: Pollack, Murray M, Capron, Carolanne. The Pediatric Risk of Mortality and the Therapeutic Intervention Scoring System. In: Essentials of Pediatric Intensive Care. Levin, Daniel L., Quality Medical Pub. 1990; 31-37
[15] http://www.bmags.gv.at Satzartenbeschreibung + Corrigenda
[16] http://www.bmags.gv.at 1. LKF-Intensiv-Rundschreiben
[17] http://www.bmags.gv.at 2. LKF-Intensiv-Rundschreiben
[18] http://www.bmags.gv.at 7. LKF-Rundschreiben
[19] http://www.bmags.gv.at MEL-Katalog BMAGS 1999.
[20] ICD-9-BMGK 1997. BMAGS Gruppe VII/A, Stubenring 1, A-1010 Vienna.
[21] MEL-Katalog BMGK1997. Katalog medizinischer Einzelleistungen.
[22] Information by BMAGS, Gruppe VII/A, Stubenring 1, A-1010 Vienna.
[23] http://www.bmags.gv.at Scoringprogramm V.3.1
[24] http://www.ris.bka.gv.at Vereinbarung gemäß Art. 15a B-VG über die Reform im Gesundheitswesen und der Krankenanstalten. BGBl I Nr. 111/1997
[25] Scoringprogramm V.1.2. für 1997. BMAGS, Gruppe VII/A, Stubenring 1, A-1010 Vienna.
[26] Intensiv-Scoringprogramm V.2.1. für 1999. BMAGS, Gruppe VII/A, Stubenring 1, A-1010 Vienna.

Medical Informatics Europe '99
P. Kokol et al. (Eds.)
IOS Press, 1999

Healthcare Users and Computerised Resources

Gaye Stephens[1], Peter Gaffney[2], Jane Grimson[1]
1 Dept. of Computer Science, Trinity College Dublin, Ireland
2 Clinical Chemistry Laboratory, Tallaght Hospital, Dublin,Ireland

Abstract: This paper concerns users' views on computerised resources. The focus concerns a software tool that could be used to allow safety conscious user manipulation of the combination of these computerised resources. It is of concern to the authors that computerised resources used in healthcare should reflect users' working practices rather than working practices being changed to reflect computerised resources.

1. Introduction

Two areas of work being pursued in the medical informatics domain concern

1. Integration of computerised services(CORBAmed[4],OpenLabs[5])
2. Federation of patient information(Synapses[6][7], HISA[9]).

As a by product of technologies deployed in these areas users may achieve more control over the specification of the systems they use. Computer systems should reflect user's work and users should not have to modify their work to suit the computer systems. This reflection of user's work should change its scale and focus as the scale and focus of the user's work changes. In order for users to capitalise on this focus they need two things

1. A view on the computerised services and information available in their domain.
2. The ability to specify their requirements of this view.

Using a software tool called User Resources Integration Environment(URIE) users are provided with a view on available resources and the ability to specify their requirements of this view. Any specification of requirements must fit in with healthcare procedures and practices currently operational in their domain and site.

This work is not about finding technical solutions to integration problems. As much technical detail as possible should be removed to allow users focus on the healthcare specific resources at hand.

2. Work currently being pursued

As stated above there are two areas of work that could be looked at with a view to seeing how they can help users gain more control over their computerised resources. There is a considerable amount of research and development being undertaken at the moment in these areas[1,4,5,6,9,10]. Some other work carried out with a view to integrating computer resources includes $Meteor_2$ work flow management system[2] which uses an immunisation tracking system as an example application and a remittance processing system from the commercial world[3]. Both of these applications take a workflow management view of integrating computerised resources. The research used to develop these applications could be used in URIE but it is important to point out that the work presented here concentrates on two things

1. a mechanism or tool by which a user could combine services offered by computerised resources
2. dynamically specifying the mapping between information produced by these services and the presentation of this information.

For example purposes, users from the clinical chemistry and ICU domains are considered and in this paper the OpenLabs[5] and Synapses[6,7] EU funded projects are referred to. The OpenLabs project designed, implemented and integrated clinical laboratory computerised services and Synapses demonstrates the federation of patient information into a flexible, medically safe Electronic HealthCare Records (EHCR).

2.1 Integration of Computerised services

OpenLabs components which facilitate healthcare workers in all tasks from initial ordering of laboratory investigations to reporting of results were defined, implemented and integrated. These components can be distributed across a hospital's network and integrated as required using the Client/Server paradigm. The OpenLabs system provided many advantages to the computerisation of the laboratories including

- definition of components
- plug and play components
- integration technology independence,
- scaleability of laboratory computerisation.

If the OpenLabs project is looked at from a users perspective it can be further improved. At present the user aspects of the OpenLabs components are designed to suit an individual set of situations that exists in the laboratory at the time of design. Users from the clinical laboratory in St. James' Hospital Dublin were heavily involved in the design of some of the OpenLabs components and as a result their components reflect their work practices very well. However if the work practices change a re-write of the user aspects of the client applications would be necessary. The components cannot easily change their scale or focus as the user's work practices and content changes.

The main advantage that the OpenLabs project lends here is that components exist independently from each other and from their integration technology.

2.2 Federation of patient information

The Synapses project embarked on the difficult task of defining a model which could federate patient information from various sources and represent it as an EHCR. All legal and medical requirements of this type of data and its transfer from place to place had to be considered.

The final Synapses model, the SynOM, is a flexible one which could be used to represent information other than EHCR information. This SynOM is supported by a dynamically modifiable dictionary which in the case of an EHCR details the specific healthcare record objects which can be included in specific types of healthcare records. This dictionary is called the SynOD. It is our intention to use the idea of the SynOM and SynOD in the definition of computerised components and the transfer of information from one component to another.

2.3 The user's perspective

In summary, from the user's perspective we want

1. A view on the computerised services and information available in their domain. To address this requirement we use the OpenLabs idea of representing computerised services and resources as components which can be integrated. The intention is to define laboratory components and register them in a library which is made available to URIE. An important feature of the definition of these components is that independence exists between the data presentation and the data processing thus allowing for dynamic change of focus and scale of a user's work.
2. The ability to specify their requirements of this view. Once the components are defined and registered a mechanism is required to combine them. The concepts of SynOM and SynOD contribute to component exchange mechanism.

3. User Resource Integration Environment (URIE)

URIE is a software tool that graphically allows a user to combine their site specific computerised resources within the constraints of work practices and safeguards resulting in an end-user application.

3.1 Scope of URIE

The work being carried out here concerns the design and implementation of URIE. The design work will follow the client/server paradigm and will be independent of technology and domains. The following constraints apply to the implementation of URIE: The clinical laboratory and ICU are the domains of concern, Use of the client/server paradigm, Use of CORBA[10]- Orbix implementation- for communication handling.

3.2 Requirements

URIE requires a set of registered components. We have divided the set of components in two. The first division includes the computerised services components and the patient information components. We call these components working components. In any set of working components there can be multitask components which represent many tasks and there can be single task components. The granularity of the components depends on the domain and the computerised resources available. In theory the entire set of computerised resources of a site could be represented as one working component. Remember as stated earlier that these working components are independent of the presentation aspects of their information. The second division comprises what we call facilitator components. At present we have identified two key facilitator components: the User interface component and the Procedures component.

3.2.1 User interface component (UIC)

The UIC is a component which accesses a set of user interfaces. There must be entries in this component to represent the presentation of information provided by working components. Mapping user interfaces to information provided by the working components is complex. The following scenarios exist

- A working component produces one set of information. This set can be related to one or more than one user interface in the UIC.
- A working component may produce more than one set of information. These sets can be combined and related to one or more than one user interface in the UIC.
- A working component may produce more than one set of information which can be individually related to more than one user interface in the UIC.

3.2.2 Procedure component

The procedure component enforces work practices and safeguards. The component will have access to a set of electronic rules that say which components can and cannot be connected. For example it would not make sense for a component representing a laboratory analyser to be directly connected with a post-analytical component without some type of authorisation procedure being applied. This component will be active throughout the time that the user is specifying their requirements.
In summary URIE requires four things

- a set of components
- a registration of Components including the UIC and the Procedure component
- a UIC component with access to User Interfaces and
- a Procedure component with access to electronic work practice rules.

3.3 Using URIE

1. URIE accesses the component library and connects to the registered components.
2. There is a tool bar with buttons representing the individual, available components. The buttons are enabled as URIE establishes connection with the components.
3. The user opens a work-sheet places the components of interest on it.
4. Using the mouse they then connect the components together. This entire operation is overseen by the Procedure component. The users will specify which aspects of the components they are interested in. Each component has a set of editable properties including tasks offered, Data requirements, Data produced, Performance times, Communication Protocols supported
5. Next the UIC must be considered. Each line which connects one component to another represents an information flow. The user must select a user interface from the UIC to associate with these flows. Lines can be grouped together if groups of information are to be displayed on the same user interface. The information represented by a single line could be split up if required or it could be deemed medically unsafe to split this data up. In either case the Procedure component should look after what the user is allowed to do.
6. Finally the worksheet is saved. The clients system has been specified.

In order to run the specified system an application shell is required. This shell can read in the specified worksheet, establish connections to the relevant components and call on the relevant user interfaces. As the user-interfaces are loaded they call on their associated components to provide them with information which they display.

4. Further work

The work for the immediate future concerns detailed design of URIE and a shell to run applications produced. These will be used to build some elements of an OpenLabs environment. Much of the work will focus on making URIE as user accessible as possible and looking at the issues around selection of user interfaces. Some of the tasks to be addressed are as follows.

1. Three OpenLabs components are being considered, the Advanced Instrument Interface (AII)[5], the Advanced Instrument Workstation (AIW)[5] and Patient Result Validation (PRV)[5]. These components whether multitask or singletask will be described by domain experts and registered in the component registration library.
2. The UIC needs to be built. Some design work has been carried out on this component and the technical issues are being compared and considered.
3. The rules governing component combination must be determined and represented in computer format.
4. The URIE tool and the application shell needs to be further refined.

The development environment includes Orbix, Visual C++ and Visual Basic. It has yet to be seen if a tool such as URIE can be built and operated in a cost effective and efficient manner. At all times during design and implementation performance, reliability, maintainability and security issues will be considered.

5. Conclusions

By taking a user's view on current medical informatics work it is possible to give users more control over available resources. This control can be delivered in a safety conscious way. A system such as URIE will contribute to the solution of scaleability problems encountered in the client aspects of systems.

However this is not a solution which can be immediately used in a hospital, it needs backup and support of system administration and development personnel. A common protocol for defining components is required. The most difficult aspect of the work centres around selection and operation of the user interfaces to match the information flows.

This proposal is not solely applicable to the healthcare domain but is valid for any domain that has a number of computerised resources to combine and is trying approach a scaleability problem.

References

[1] Synapses- Synapses in the context of Healthcare Information Systems, Pier-Angelo Sottile p. 30-39 of New Technologies in Hospital Information Systems, edited by J. Dudeck, B. Blobel, W. Lordieck, T. Bürkle, The IOS press 1997.

[2] WebWork- WebWork: Meteor$_2$'s Web-Based Workflow Management System, J.Miller, D. Palaniswami, A. Sheth, K. Kochut, H. Singh, Journal of intelligent systems, Volume 10 No. 2 March/April 1998.

[3] Complex User Modifiable Workflow, Jesse T. Quatse, IA Corporation, Workflow handbook 1997, edited by Peter Lawrence, published in association with the Workflow Management Co-alition, 1997.
[4] http://www.omg.org/homepages/corbamed/
[5] OpenLabs -Computer Methods and Programs in Biomedicine, Special issue, edited by R. O'Moore, T. Groth, W. Grimson, G. Boran, Volume 50 N0. 2, Elsevier Science Ireland, July 1996.
[6] Synapses Public Web site: http://www.cs.tcd.ie/synapses/public.
[7] 'A CORBA-Based Integration of Distributed Electronic Healthcare Records Using the Synapses Approach', J. Grimson, W. Grimson, D. Berry, G. Stephens, E. Felton, D. Kalra, P. Toussaint, and O.W. Weier., IEEE Transactions on Information Technology in Biomedicine, Volume 2, Number 3, September 1998, pp. 124-138.
[8] User control of Healthcare Information, G. Stephens, P. Gaffney, J. Grimson, B. Grimson, HISI 98 Conference Dublin.
[9] http://csis.pace.edu/~rada/research/papers/edustand/Organstand.htm- Tutorial on the Healthcare Information System Architecture HISA standard.
[10] CORBAmed: Promoting a Homogeneous IT Environment in Hospitals, D. Berry, W. Grimson, HISI 98 Conference Dublin.

Medical Informatics Europe '99
P. Kokol et al. (Eds.)
IOS Press, 1999

Bed Utilization Performances Of Slovenian And Croatian Acute Hospitals Systems

Marjan Premik[1] Vladimir Mayer[2] Marina Kuzman[2] Miroslav Mayer[2]
[1] *University of Ljubljana, Faculty of Medicine Institute of Social Medicine*
[2] *Croatian National Institute of Public Health*

Abstract. With Barber-Johnson-Yates scattergrams (BJYS), the performances of Slovenian and Croatian acute hospital system were explored by taking turnover interval as a predictor variable, length of stay as a dependent variable, and by looking at the variables of bed throughput and percentage of bed emptiness on installed network.
The growing influences on the Slovenian hospital system of a cost-containment policy and of the past war on the Croatian hospital system are the best illustrations of the informatics potential inherent in BJYS presentations for the exploratory data analysis (EDA) used to identify systematic relations between variables in a setting of not complete *a priori* expectations of these relations.
Key words: acute hospital system performance, Slovenia, Croatia.

The Barber-Johnson's method of pictorial representation of hospital bed use was developed in 1973 [1]. In 1982 came a suggestion that the Yates' variant be widely used for hospital bed utilization analyses in the United Kingdom [2]. Despite being based on data collection during routine follow-ups of hospital activity [3], it still does not play its proper role in international comparisons of acute hospital systems [4].

1. Materials and methods

In calculating these four hospital bed performance indicators

- <u>length of stay</u>: 365 * bed occupancy/discharges + deaths
- <u>throughput</u>: discharges + deaths/available beds
- <u>turnover interval</u>: (available beds - occupied beds) * 365/discharges + deaths
- <u>% bed emptiness</u>: (available beds - occupied beds)/available beds * 100

the basic data on hospital activity (bed availability, bed occupancy, patient discharges and deaths) from the annuals authored by the Institute of Public Health of the Republic of Slovenia and by the Croatian National Institute of Public Health were used [5,6].

As recommended by Yates [3], the BJY diagram matrix was completed using the Statistica for Windows software release 5.1 (98 edition) linear regression modules [7]. Under the same module, all scattergrams were designed taking the turnover interval as a predictor and length of stay as a dependent variable. The acute hospital systems of the two countries marked with ellipses (confidence bands 0.95) were standardized manually on a scale equal to that of the matrix, and linked with the "merge graph" command. Other exploratory data analyses were performed by using cluster analyses, classification trees and discriminant analysis modules.

2. Results

The intensity of bed use in Slovenian and Croatian acute hospital systems in the 1986-96 period depended on their respective developmental stages and the socioeconomic settings in which they were operating.

Consolidated in the early 1980s [8,9], the Slovenian hospital system only exerted an obvious cost-containment pressure on hospital bed utilization from 1990 to 1991 (Fig. 1).

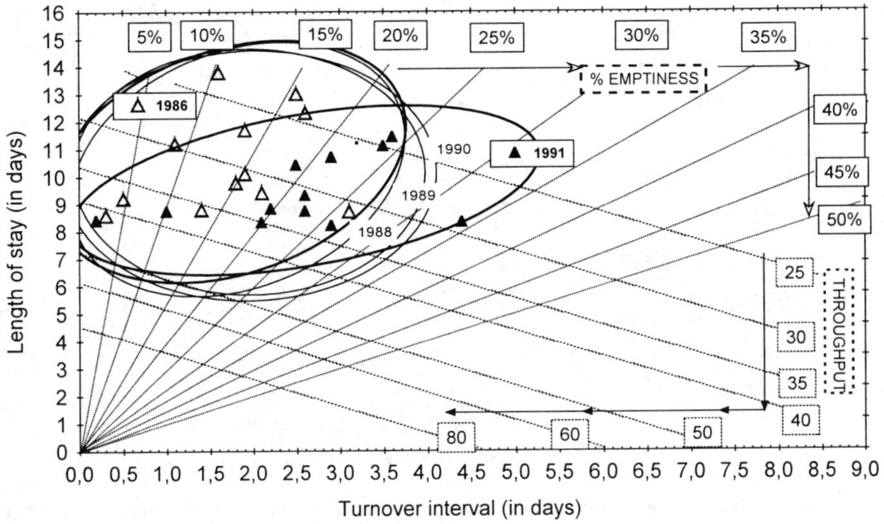

Fig. 1 The Barber-Johnson-Yates diagram of Slovenian acute hospital system performances 1986-91

The war in Croatia left some hospital facilities destroyed and others practicing a restrictive chronic patient admission policies as well as curtailing the length of stay. These policies were intended to free hospital facilities for a possible massive admission of war victims [10] (Fig. 2).

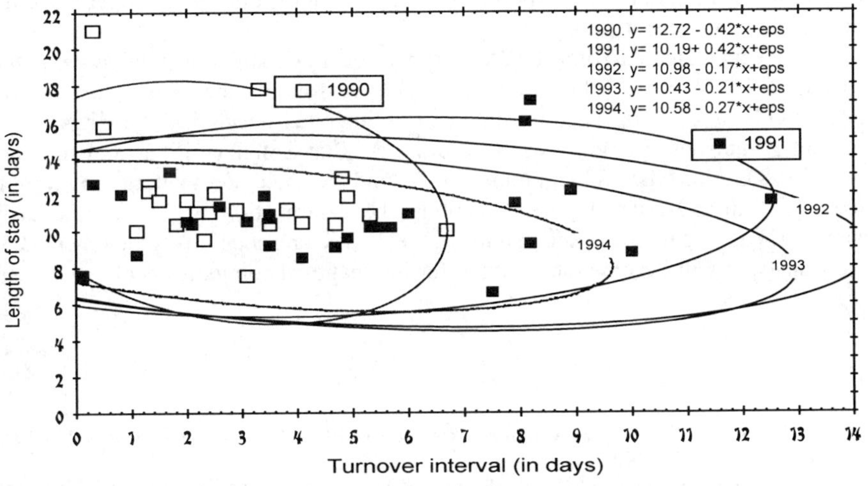

Fig. 2 Croatian acute hospital system performances 1990-94

In subsequent years in both systems, the average values of the four basic hospital performance indicators exhibited the trends of reduced length of stay, extended turnover interval accompanied by an increase in empty facilities, and a relative stagnation in the average number of patients treated per hospital bed. This trend was stronger in the Slovenian acute hospital system (Fig. 3). For 1996, discriminant function analysis of both systems showed that the main factor discriminating the two systems is the average percentage of empty beds (partial lambda 0.81; p<0.003)and turnover interval (partial lambda 0.89; p<0.026).

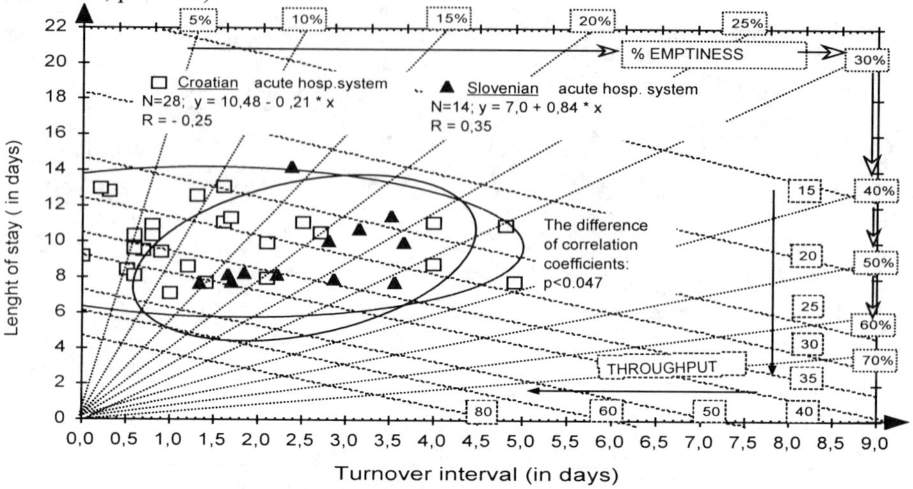

Fig. 3 The Barber-Johnson-Yates diagram of Slovenian and Croatian acute hospital system performances 1996

3. Discussion

Although it was conceived in 1973 [1], and further developed in 1982 [2,3] with the suggestion of the Yates' variant for wide application in hospital bed management, the Barber-Johnson scattergram information technology has not yet taken its proper place in the area of international comparisons [4].

In our experience based on BJYS presentations in Croatian hospital system studies over the period 1986-91 [10,11], the most likely reason for the limited use of BJYS presentations elsewhere is the need for time-consuming precise technical drawings.

Under Statistics for Windows release 4.5 A (Stat Soft Inc. 1993) and the current version 5.1 (98 edition), BJYS diagram matrices can be created and scattergrams combined dynamically. An EDA development enabling the examination of 35 hospital activity indicators [12] is a pointer to the future where BJYS presentations supplemented with statistical analyses will become the standard for international comparisons of acute hospital systems.

References

[1] Barber B, Johnson D. The Presentation of Acute Hospital In-patient Statistics. Hospital and Health Services Review 1973, 69: 11-4.

[2] Godber G. Foreword. In: Yates J. ed. Hospital Beds: A Problem for Diagnosis and Management? Heinemann Medical Books Ltd, London 1982, IV.

[3] Yates J. Hospital Beds; A Problem for Diagnosis and Management? Heinemann Medical Books Ltd, London 1982, 1-116.

[4] Mayer V, Premik M, Kovacic L, Kuzman M. Slovenian and Croatian acute hospital system performances in 1990, 1991 and 1995: A Barber-Johnson-Yates presentation. Med inform 1997, 3:57-60.

[5] Croatian National Institute of Public Health. Croatian Health Service Yearbook 1996. Zagreb 1997, 197-216.

[6] Institute of Public Health of the Republic of Slovenia. Health Statistical Annual Slovenia 1996. Zdrav Var 1997 (Suppl- 5):277-391.

[7] Multiple regression. In Stat Soft. Inc (1998) STATISTICA for Windows (Computer program manual) Tulusa 28000 East 14th Street USA.

[8] Ravnikar B, Erzen N, Paucic M. Kastelic I. Bolnisnicno gravitacisko podrocje v SR Sloveniji leta 1984 in primerjava z letom 1982. Zdrav var 1986; 1:5-74.

[9] Premik M. Javnozdravstveni informacijski sistemi. In: Premik M, editor. Zbornik prispevkov s kongresa Drustva za medicinsko informatiko Slovenije, 1996 sep 22-25; Bled. Ljubljana: Drustvo za medicinsko informatiko Slovenije, 1996:7-14.

[10] Mayer V, Trnski D., Vidakovic Z, Kuzman M., Tomic B. Barber-Johnson's bed utilization analyses in the system of hospital-type health care in Croatia in peace - and war-time conditions: 1986-91, Lijec vjesn 1994;116:65-69.

[11] Ministry of Science and Technology of Croatia: Project 3-01-124 data base Svibor 2. Zagreb 1995:1-17.

[12] Davidge J. IACC demonstration performance indicator: computer package. Data base IACC Birmingham 1995.

Medical Informatics Europe '99
P. Kokol et al. (Eds.)
IOS Press, 1999

The optimization of turnaround time for blood samples in an emergency clinical laboratory

Vesna Prijatelj[1], Andrej Vučkovič[2], Darko Černe[3]
[1]*Information Centre, University Medical Centre, Zaloška 2, 1000 Ljubljana, Slovenia*
[2]*Andrej Vučkovič, Kobis l.t.d ,Kidričeva 11, 1236 Trzin, Slovenia*
[3]*Institute of Clinical Chemistry and Biochemistry, University Medical Centre, Zaloška 7, 1000 Ljubljana, Slovenia*

Abstract. The University Medical Centre Ljubljana is a 3200-bed general hospital. A laboratory information system, developed to improve the reliability and usefulness of test results, was installed in the emergency laboratory in November 1994. At that time, all test requests received by the laboratory were treated as equally urgent, but in December 1994, a reorganisation took place, which involved the introduction of a priority system. We conducted a study in the period from November 1994 to September 1995. The turnaround time for blood analyses was evaluated by the method of case study. The influence of information technology and organisational changes on individual components of the turnaround time was assessed.

This study has shown a positive effect of the recently introduced information technology and organisational changes on the turnaround time. The median turnaround time improved for all phases of the laboratory process. The greatest improvement occurred in validity check time.

Keywords: turnaround time, clinical laboratory, information system, optimisation, priority system

1. Introduction

Laboratory testing provides essential information that aids in both diagnosis and treatment of critically ill patients[8]. For a laboratory test to be useful, it must be available in a timely manner. On occasion, the outcome of a life-threatening event may depend on how accurately and rapidly a laboratory test is performed and results reported back to the clinician [3]. Improving the turnaround time for urgent laboratory examinations is a principal problem in laboratory services.

Turnaround time is a complex process that begins with the physician's initiation of a laboratory order, continues with the acquisition of the appropriate specimen, proceeds with the actual analysis time, and concludes with the transmission of the results to the physician. Improving laboratory turnaround time requires a complete systems review of all of these factors from inception of the order through a completed result that is available to whomever needs the information [4]. Today, many laboratories can electronically follow specimens from receipt in the laboratory to the time analysis is completed and released to the clinic. Some advanced hospital laboratory computer systems can track specimens from the time of order entry on the patient's hospital floor. Laboratory computerisation now allows us to look closely at laboratory performance based on the time it takes to process, analyse, and report a test result [2].

The purpose of this report is to assess the influence of the information technology and organisational changes on the turnaround time in our laboratory. Our initial experience with the use of a laboratory information system (LIS) is presented.

2. Materials and Methods

The University Medical Centre Ljubljana is a 3200 - bed general hospital and the largest medical institution in Slovenia. It has a central emergency laboratory, which performs 50% of all tests requested for in-patients and 20 % of all tests for patients visiting the out-patient clinics.

A laboratory information system (LIS), designed to improve the reliability and usefulness of test results, was installed in the emergency laboratory in November 1994. The aims pursued in designing the system were to reduce the likelihood of data entry error and improve the efficiency of the personnel. The LIS has also been used to identify processes delayed and specimens lost.

At the time when the LIS was installed, all test requests arriving in the laboratory were treated as equally urgent, but in December 1994, a reorganisation took place, which involved the introduction of a priority system. Four priority levels were defined and the expected turnaround times were determined for each priority level as follows:

1st - tests requested by emergency department (1-20 min)
2nd - tests requested by ICUs (21-40 min)
3rd - tests requested by ICUs (41-90 min)
4th - tests requested by other departments (>90 min).

We have adjusted and improved the LIS to comply with the new organisation of work. Every five minutes, the software checks the registered times for all tests that are in progress, compares them with the expected times for the corresponding priority level, and prints out any results that have not been validated by the expected time. The laboratory personnel must identify the cause for each missing result. Possible causes include a delay in sample analysis or validation of the result, analysing instrument error or wrong priority.

A study was conducted in the emergency laboratory in the period from November 1994 to September 1995. Turnaround times for sodium determinations, blood cell counts and blood gas analysis were measured, and the data were analysed.

The total laboratory turnaround time was defined as the time from specimen arrival in the laboratory until release of the validated result into the LIS. Two components of the turnaround time were identified: analysis time and validity check time. Analysis time is the time from specimen arrival in the laboratory until receipt of the result by the PC. Validity check time is the time from receipt of the result by the PC until release of the validated result into the LIS [6].

The turnaround times for blood tests were analysed by the method of case study. The tests were grouped according to priority, and the mean monthly values were calculated for each test. The statistical tools used included Qpro and Dbase IV.

3. Results

The mean monthly values of the total laboratory turnaround time, analysis time and validity check time for blood tests for the months of November 1994 (completed LIS installation), December 1994 (introduction the priority list), January 1995 (process stabilisation) and September 1995 (end of study) are shown in table 1.

Table 1: The mean monthly values of the total laboratory turnaround time, analysis time and validity check time for blood tests: blood cell count, sodium determination and blood gas analysis

date	total turnaround time (min)			analysis time (min)			validity check time (min)		
	blood cell count	sodium determ.	blood gas analysis	blood cell count	sodium determ.	blood gas analysis	blood cell count	sodium determ.	blood gas analysis
Nov'94	80.4	78.9	54.7	31.9	48.3	28.4	48.5	30.6	26.3
Dec'94	60.2	69.2	39.6	25.0	46.2	19.9	35.2	23.0	19.7
Jan'95	32.8	62.7	21.2	24.3	52.9	18.4	8.5	9.8	2.8
Sep'95	25.3	44.1	17.2	19.8	36.1	15.7	5.6	8.0	1.5

The median turnaround time improved for all phases of the laboratory process. The greatest improvement occurred in validity check time for blood test results. From November'94 to September '95 the validity check time for blood cell counts improved by 88.5%, for blood gas analyses by 94.3%, and for sodium determinations by 73.9%.

The median validity check time for all tests improved by 25% after installation of the LIS. The greatest improvement occurred after the organisational change in December 1994.

This improvements resulted in a shorter total laboratory turnaround time for each test. From November '94 to September '95 the total laboratory turnaround time for blood gas analyses improved by 68.6%, for blood cell counts by 68.5%, and for sodium determinations by 44.1%.

4. Discussion

During our initial evaluation, we observed that laboratory test turnaround time varied depending on the specific test. However, on analysing the process, we realised that all laboratory tests could be broken down into two phases: analysis and validation. By studying each of the processes involved in laboratory area, we identified and instituted changes that would make the process more efficient. Those changes included implementing a LIS and using a priority system. With these measures we managed to reduce the turnaround time in our laboratory to an acceptable level.

By statistically analysing the turnaround components, we were able to focus our attention on the cause of delays rather than deal with only the analytic processes. In analysing the data, we found that the greatest delay was caused by the results not being validated by the expected time.

5. Conclusion

For a clinical laboratory test to be useful to the clinician, results should be available in a timely fashion. Few studies have examined turnaround times [1,7]. Slow turnaround and sluggish response by the clinical laboratory in the emergency department is unacceptable. Responsibility for delays needs to be clarified, and because they adversely affect the quality of service, the laboratory must ensure that appropriate action is taken [5]. Each of the processes taking place within the laboratory must be analysed in order to identify the causes of delays and plan changes that will contribute to better laboratory performance.

We examined turnaround time as an indicator of quality laboratory performance and efficiency. The results of our study confirm that improvements in organisation, management and information technology may provide effective ways to speed up turnaround time and achieve quality laboratory service.

References

[1] EI. Bluth, DJ. Lambert, TP. Lohman, Improvement in 'turnaround time' laboratory turnaround time, *Archives of Internal Medicine*, 1992,152:837-840

[2] LH. Hilborne, RK. Oye, McArdle, Use specimen turnaround time as a component of laboratory quality, A Comparison of Clinical Expectations with Laboratory Performance, *American Journal of Clinical Pathology,* 1989, 92(5):613-618

[3] DR. Misiano, ME. Meyerhoff, ME. Collison, Current and Future Directions in the Technology Relating to Bedside Testing of Critically Ill Patients, *Chest*, 1990, 97:204S-212S

[4] JS. Nosanchuk, R. Keefner, Cost analysis of point-of-care laboratory testing in a community hospital, *American Journal of Clinical Pathology,* 1995, 103(2):240-243

[5] M. Peters, PM. Broughton, PG. Nightingale, Use of information technology for auditing effective use of laboratory services, *Journal of Clinical Pathology*, 1991, 44(7):539-42

[6] V. Prijatelj, The optimization of turnaround time for blood samples in an emergency clinical laboratory of the University Medical Centre Ljubljana, M.Sc. thesis. University of Maribor, Faculty of organizational sciences, Kranj, 1986

[7] S. Saxena, ET. Wong, Does the Emergency Department Need a Dedicated turnaround time Laboratory? Continuous Quality Improvement as a Management Tool for the Clinical Laboratory, *American Journal of Clinical Pathology,* 1993, 100:606-610

[8] GP. Zaloga, Evaluation of beside testing options for the critical care unit, *Chest,* 1990, 97:185S-190S

Intelligent Medical Systems

Medical Informatics Europe '99
P. Kokol et al. (Eds.)
IOS Press, 1999

MOBISIM - Package for Simulation in Molecular Biology

George I MIHALAS[1], Gratian MACOVIEVICI[2], Zeno SIMON[3], Georgeta MIHALAS[1], Gabriel BALEA[1], Diana LUNGEANU[1]

[1] *University of Medicine and Pharmacy, P-ta Eftimie Murgu 2, 1900 Timisoara, Romania,* [2] *University "Politehnica" Timisoara,* [3] *West University Timisoara*

Abstract. A computer program for simulation of protein synthesis regulatory processes is described. A short theoretical background reveals the requirements of a simulation program. Our program, MOBISIM, offers several facilities and a user-friendly interface for molecular biologists. An example illustrates the graphical representation both as time evolution of the system or as phase diagram.

1. Introduction

An important role in gene activity control is played by specific activator and repressor transcription factors which bind to specific regulator DNA sequences Interactions between genes coding such transcription factors should explain the different stable or oscillatory gene activities characteristic for various tissues. A set of models has been built for several systems with interconnected genes. We have published our first model in 1985 [1], which has not been extended due to the scarce experimental support [3]. Meanwhile several new findings [4, 5] made us reconsider and develop the model [6, 7]. An important role in model refinement was brought by a set of computer programs developed in our laboratory [1, 8, 9].

2. Theoretical background

A typical sequences of gene control of protein synthesis comprises three steps (fig.1):
- *transcription:* mRNA structure is copied from the synthesis gene SG of the nuclear DNA, with a rate dependent on the activation degree of the regulatory gene R located uphill
- *translation:* protein P is synthesised with a rate proportional to mRNA concentration
- *regulation:* the regulatory gene R might either promote/enhance or inhibit/repress SG.

The regulatory gene activity might be controlled either by its own protein (selfregulation), or by other proteins, produced by other genes, named interconnected genes (inter-reulation).

Both mRNA and protein have a natural decay.

Using the notations of fig. 1, we can build the general model for a typical "unit of protein synthesis":

$$\begin{cases} \dfrac{dy}{dt} = \varphi \cdot F(x, x', t) - \eta y \\ \dfrac{dx}{dt} = \psi \cdot y - \lambda x \end{cases} \tag{1}$$

The general form cannot be integrated, so the easiest way to analyse such models is to study their simulations.

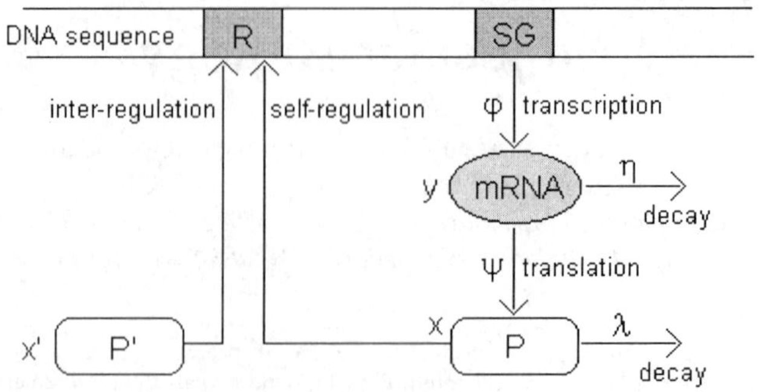

Fig. 1. Scheme of regulatory processes

The particular form of the activation function F is the determinant factor of most peculiarities found in different cases:

a) *self regulated gene* [1, 2]:

$$F(x) = \frac{Ax^n}{K_1 + x^n} + \frac{Bx^n}{K_2 + x^n} \qquad (2)$$

Three steady states might be obtained with this model; there is an experimental support for such case [3].

b) *threshold activation of interconnected genes:*

$$F_1(x_1, x_2) = \begin{cases} 0 \text{ for } x_1 < x_A \\ 1 \text{ for } x_1 \geq x_A \end{cases} \qquad (3)$$

These discontinuous (stepwise) activation functions with two or three intervals correspond to threshold phenomena. In particular instances the system of differential equations type (1) can be integrated on intervals

c) *delayed activation*:

The real phenomena comprise a delay between the moment of a certain concentration change and the moment of its effect; we have added all the delays of one cycle as a single delay, τ, and attributed it to the longest lasting event, i.e. activation:

$$F(t) = F(x(t - \tau)) \qquad (4)$$

which means that we compute the activation function at moment t from the concentration value of the regulatory protein at an earlier moment, $t - \tau$.

This short presentation of the basic theoretical background reveals the main features, which have to be covered by a simulation software dedicated to these phenomena [6, 7].

3. Requirements for a simulation program in molecular biology

a) Variables. The most common output of a simulation program modelling a process, is a graphical plot representing the evolution of one or more variables.

b) Iteration refinement. Classical methods (Runge-Kutta) are used for differential equation systems. The iteration step (dt) should be extremely small, especially for fast variations. The program should accept its adjustment.

c) Scaling: an automatic choice of the appropriate scale for each variable is advisable. However, one may prefer changing the scales for a better comparison.

d) Parameters. A set of default values for all the parameters is customary used but an important feature of a simulation program is to offer simple facilities for changing their values. These values should always be displayed aside the graph.

e) Parameter influence on graphical representation. A common procedure in simulation studies is to estimate the influence of (some of) the parameters on the evolution of a certain variable. In this case one would rather prefer to have a set of curves representing the evolution of only one variable for the set of different values of that parameter.

f) Phase diagram. The behaviour of systems comprising several regulatory mechanisms require a graphical plot having any (chosen) pair of variables on the axes, called phase diagram. One can better see the trends of the system towards steady states (attractors), or towards oscillations.

g) Operation facilities like adding a text for the graph, saving the parameters used for a graphical representation, reading parameters from a file, changing colours etc. - should also be available.

4. Description of MOBISIM

Our program is a Pascal application fulfilling the requirements. It has three modules:

- the **main module** comprising the variables and constants sections. The set of differential equations type (1) and the set of analytical equations type (2) or (3) or (4). The description of these equations is not automated, they have to be introduced as Pascal lines, specifying the parameters used. Actually all manual operations are included in this module. The core procedure computes the elements of the matrix corresponding to time evolution of the variables (and activation functions), calling the Runge-Kutta procedure for each iteration. After these computations, the graphical representation module is called.
- the **Runge-Kutta module,** (fourth order) in a general form (for any number of differential equations type (1)); this procedure is called in each iterative step.
- the **graphical representation module,** carries the tasks of scaling and representing the evolution of the desired variables or the phase diagram. One can change the variables to be represented, the limits of scales or the graph type (evolution or phase diagram).

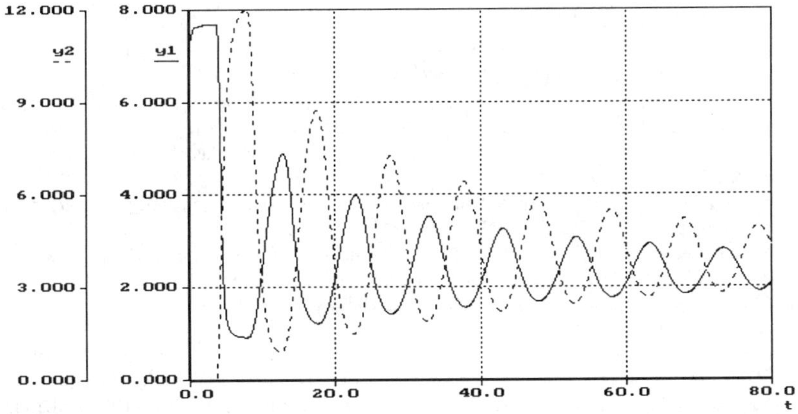

Fig.2. Time evolution of a system of two interrelated genes for a model with delay

5. Results and conclusions

An application of MOBISIM on a biosystem of two interrelated genes, p53 and mdm2, [4, 5] is presented below. Depending on the values of the parameters, the biosystem can evoluate either towards a steady state showing damped oscillations (fig. 2), or towards permanent oscillations. The corresponding phase diagram is presented in fig. 3.

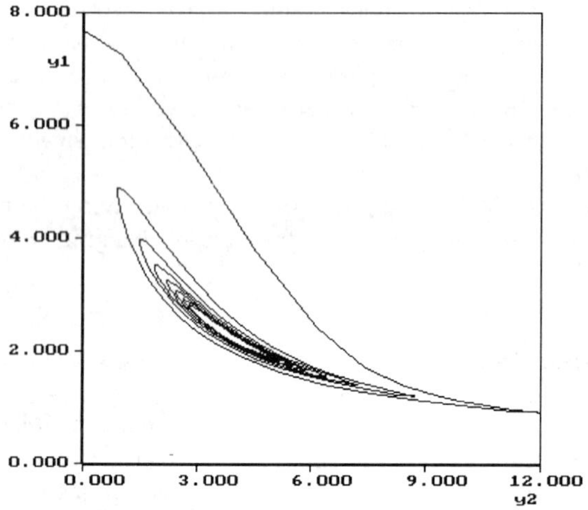

Fig. 3. The phase diagram for a system of interrelated genes with damped oscillations

Even the program was designed for molecular biology, it is quite general and it has also been applied to immunology [8] and physiology [9].

Acknowledgements

This work was partially supported by grants no 470 & 919/1996 of the Romanian Ministry of Research and Technology.

References

[1] Mihalas G I, Niculescu-Duvaz I, Simon Z: Trigger with positive control for gene activity regulation. Computer simulation. *Stud. Biophys (Berlin)* **107** (1985) 223-229.

[2] Ptashne M P, Buchman K, Humarajan M A, Jeffrey A, Maurer R, Mayer B, Sauer R T: Autoregulation and function of a repressor in the lambda bacteriophague. *Science* **194** (1976) 156-159.

[3] Bishop J O, Morton J G, Rosbach M, Richardson M: Tree abundance classes in Wela cell messenger RNA. *Nature* **250** (1974) 149-155.

[4] Picksley S M, Lane D P: The p53-mdm2 autoregulatory feedback-loop - a paradigm for the regulation of growth control by p53? *Bioessays* **15** (1993) 689-690.

[5] Haupt Y, Maya R et al: mdm2 promotes the rapid degradation of p53. *Nature* **387** (1997) 296-299.

[6] Simon Z, Voiculetz N: Trigger models for gene activity regulation in carcinogenesis. In *Modeling of Cancer Genesis and Prevention*, eds: Voiculetz N, Balaban A T, Niculescu-Duvaz I, Simon Z, (CRC Press, Boca Raton, Fla 1993) 13-68.

[7] Mihalas G I: Modeling and simulation in medicine and life sciences. *Med. Informatics* **23** (1998) 93-96.

[8] Mihalas G I, Simon Z, Macovievici G: Modeling and Computer Simulation of the Humoral Immune Response Based on the Immune Network Theory. *XVII-th Intel. Biometrics Conf.*, 1994, vol.**2**, 43.

[9] Mihalas G I, Mihalas Georgeta: Simularea proceselor adaptive de neurobiofizica. *Fiziologia* **8** (1998) 19

Medical Informatics Europe '99
P. Kokol et al. (Eds.)
IOS Press, 1999

Automatization of Physicians' Phone-in Hours

Jari TURUNEN*, Pekka LOULA* & Heikki SOININEN**
**Tampere University of Technology, Pori*
P.O. Box 30, FIN-28601 Pori, Finland. Email: turunenj@pori.tut.fi
***Kokemaki Health Center FIN-32800, Kokemaki, Finland*

Abstract. In this paper we present a computer-based system that is designed to reduce the number of patient calls in physicians' phone-in hours. Simultaneously it will offer a parallel alternative channel for the patients to listen to their laboratory results. The system requirements were reliability, security and the low costs. The results showed after a two-month test period that the tailored system proved extremely successful. The average time that the physician saved by using this system was over 4 minutes and doctors can leave the messages to the server also outside the phone-in hours.

1. Introduction

Traditionally the use of telephone in the health centers has been restricted to patient and health-care personnel communication. In Finland the patients can ask their test results directly from the physician who can also make conclusions from the results or in some cases from the nurse who can only tell the test results. The patients can call the physician during the physician's phone-in hour to hear their test results and conclusions.

The basic idea for the system was that the doctor can record an individual message to the computer and the patient can call the computer and listen to the message whenever he/she wants to. Computer-telephony interaction experiments have been done in the other countries. The telephone-linked care system to chronic patients for information providing and support has been successfully tested in [1]. Basically the use of computer-telephony interaction has been restricted to the interactive expert systems [2] [3] where the patient get the advice after answering the computer-made questions using the numeric keypad. In [4], the computer-telephony system was used as a decision making support tool for nurses when evaluating the patients. The test results of these papers were promising and showed the importance of the automated telephone systems. Our goal was to find a mechanism that can reduce the work of the personnel and serve the patients' information needs better than earlier. The demands for the system were: low cost, easy-to-use, scalability, data-security, time-saving and reliability.

Kokemaki health center was chosen to be the test place for our system and the system was tested during a two-month period. There are 9000 inhabitants in Kokemaki district and about 20 % of the people are over 65 years old. The small industry is the biggest employee in the area. The average number of telephone queries is 84 calls per 1000 inhabitants and 167 calls per 1000 patients.This project is a part of "Health Care Informatics Center of Excellence in Satakunta (HC-ICE)" launched C-MEDI2 project. The initiative to this project came from the field where the physicians' phone-in hours sometimes can be best described as a "chaos". However the need for ordinary phone-in hours cannot be denied but the automatic "answering" system that will work parallel with the old system started to seem appropriate. In this paper we present the results of our study that were collected within the two-month test period.

2. Technical Properties of the system

The cheapest way to produce a new system is to find a similar system or as similar as possible that is easily configured to the new direction. Our solution was to build software to the generally accepted system that is in world-wide use in, for example, different remote-ordering systems.

The stand-alone server that is connected to the local telephone network proved to be cost-effective. The system was built on 90 MHz Pentium PC-computer, with Dialogic Corporation's D/80 and LSI/81 telephone cards. The LSI/81 card is telephone interface card according to the CCITT POTS and Recommendation E standards. The D/80 voice card plays the messages and listens to the users' response. The operating system was IBM OS/2 WARP version 4. The information is stored on the local hard disk in Microsoft WAV-format.

The security is handled by keeping the server in a locked room. There is no other access to the server than authorised personnel only. Via telephone lines it is not possible to listen to or leave the messages without knowing the patients' or physicians' ID-code. The use of this system needs only a telephone that can produce DTMF (Dynamic Time Modulation Frequency) tones including for example wireless GSM phones. The model of the system is in figure 1. This system is capable of handling 8 telephone lines and in the experiment 2 lines were reserved for the patients, one for the doctors and one for the redirected calls for the reception assistant. This system is expandable with 8 lines by obtaining a new card pair.

3. Functionality of the system

The doctor calls the server and gives his own ID-code to the server via the telephone keypad. If the code is accepted then she or he can leave a message to the patient. The doctor can also record a standard message that can be used later with other patients. This system was designed so that every doctor could record his or her individual standard messages. The doctor can also make combinations with spoken and standard messages, for example, "Good day, this is doctor N.N. Your test results were normal" and continue with a formerly recorded standard message "There is no need for further checking ".

When the doctor is leaving the message for the patient, she/he keys in an individual patient ID-code number and leaves a message to the patient in question. These recorded messages are stored in the server's hard disk and the ID-code based database is updated.

The patient can call the phone server whenever she/he wants. After keying in the ID-code number the server will ask from the patient is ID-code is correct. "You gave the numbers 1,2,3... was it right?" This prevents unauthorised testing and hacking for other ID-code number combinations. After verifying the ID-code the computer will search the message associated with the ID-code in question. If there is, the computer prompts "There is a message for a person M.M. Are you sure that you want to hear it?" and plays the recorded message after a positive answer from the patient.

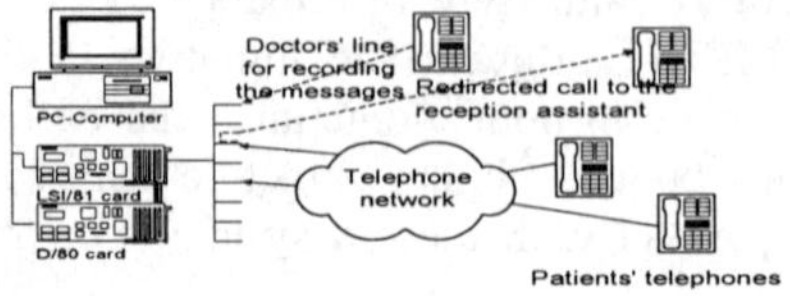

Figure 1: The structure of the system.

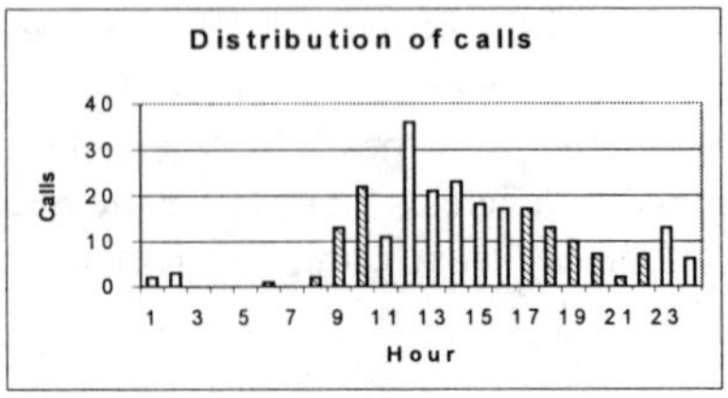

Figure 2: The distribution of calls.

If the patient message has not yet been recorded to the server the computer gives a default message to the patient "Your results are not yet available, the results are updated daily, please try again later". After listening to the message, there is a possibility to link the call to the reception assistant to make a new appointment with the physician.

4. Results

Reference base-line material

5 doctors recorded the reference base-line material without the automated phone-in server consisting of 227 patient calls within 30 phone-in hours before the pilot study period. The baseline material (the results and conclusions) consisted of all types of phone-in material. The average time that a doctor spends with a patient was 7 minutes 54 seconds.

Two-month study period

Within the two month automated study period (Oct-Dec 1998) doctors recorded 94 messages. The average time for recording one message was 3 minutes 27 seconds. It should be noted that during this study the very private and sensitive messages (for example results that may indicate "bad news" such as cancer and HIV and which require human contact) were excluded by the doctors and left to the ordinary phone-in hours. 456 ordinary phone-in calls were made within the period so this means that 17 % of the calls were transferred to the server. The patients mostly used line 1 (87,7 % of patient calls) although both telephone line numbers had been given by the doctors. This indicates that the patients do not need to call anymore within certain phone-in hours and the second line is only "experimental", so it is not needed for sharing the rush-hour call traffic.

Within the two-month study period (Oct-Dec 1998) patients made 244 calls to the server. The patient calls can be classified as follows in table 1:

Table 1: The distribution of calls and the average times

Calls	Number of calls	% of calls	Average time/call
Succeeded calls	159	65.2 %	0:01:52
- Answer	[67]	[27.5 %]	0:02:20
- No answer	[92]	[37.7 %]	0:01:31
--Redirected calls to the reception assistant	[[7]]	[[2.9 %]]	0:03:15
Failed calls	85	34.8 %	0:02:16

The *succeeded calls* mean that the patient was able to interact with the server. The *answer* means that the doctor's comments and the test results were successfully recorded and listened to. The *no answer* means that the results were not recorded to the server before the patient called or the patient was too eager to listen to them. *Redirected calls* were mostly asking confirmation from the reception assistant: "Why are my results not in the server?" The conclusion *Failed calls* was made in the situations where there was no interaction between the patient and the server. This number includes patients who do not have enough courage to start the interaction the first time. It may also include the small number of potential efforts by hackers. The average time for listening to the recorded message was 2 minutes 20 seconds. The server is available 24 hours per day so the patient can get her/his results whenever she/he wants to. The patients' calls are shown in figure 2. This diagram includes all the patients' calls made within the two month period to the server. The results show that the calls culminate in the afternoon. There is one peak that indicates patients want to hear the results after lunch break.

5. Discussion

The new approach for telephone services has been presented. It has proved its reliability and cost effectiveness. Time saving was remarkable and it should be noted that the doctors did the recordings beside their normal work. There is no need for specific time to leave the messages. The average time saving for doctor per patient is 4 minutes 27 seconds. The study was restricted only for the doctors' use but other personnel hoped that the system should be expanded to the informational use (such as opening and closing times, nursing care information and in some cases simple test results that do not need doctoral consultation) in the future. The robustness and easiness have created the overall acceptability of the system.

However there are certain things that should be taken into account. It is usually in Finland that the patient's permission should always be asked in order to put the patient-specific information to the hard disk and the doctor should evaluate the patient's ability to use the telephone before asking the patient to join the system.

The patients have been pleased with the system and its usability; comments like "There is no need for queueing" or "The ordinary phone-in hours are terrible" are common.

After the patient has listened to the results, the system will back-up the patient information to another hard disk and destroy them from the first one to free up its hard-disk space and for the data security. The system also clears the database entry considering the specific ID-code. In continuous use the data should be backed up with media that suits better for archiving, for example writable CD-ROM.

The number of lines was overestimated. Within the two-month period the averaged peak hour traffic per line was about 2 % of the maximum number of calls, so this system can serve a considerably bigger population than 9000 inhabitants.

Some parts of the system are useless. In practice, there are no needs for standard messages. The messages to be recorded are so different and individual that it is faster to speak the whole message than join some standard message to the basic message. The direct call to the reception assistant is also useless, only 3 % of calls were redirected. The patients need some thinking time in cases when the message is like "You should make a new appointment with the doctor as soon as possible".

The pilot patients managed well with this experiment. 65.2 % had enough courage and ability to interact with the new service in the Kokemaki district. It seems that the system reached the easy-to-use demand that was set on it. The data security was also accomplished.

A further development project has been launched based on this experiment where the Clinic of pediatrics of the Satakunta central hospital and the company Votek Oy which is specialized in computer telephony (CTI) products, are together developing the system. Votek Oy concentrates in this project to integrate the system to the turn-key solution.

References

[1] Friedman RH, Stollerman JE, Mahoney DM, Rozenblyum L. The virtual visit: using telecommunications technology to take care of patients. *Journal of American Med Inform Assoc* 1997 Nov-Dec;4(6):413-25 Evans Memorial Department of Clinical Research, Boston Medical Center, Boston University School of Medicine, MA 02118, USA.

[2] Meneghini LF, Albisser AM, Goldberg RB, Mintz DH. *An electronic case manager for diabetes control.* Diabetes Care *1998 Apr;21(4):591-6* Diabetes Research Institute, Eleanor and Joseph Kosow Diagnostic and Treatment Center, University of Miami School of Medicine, FL 33101, USA.

[3] Baer L, Greist JH. An interactive computer-administered self-assessment and self-help program for behavior therapy. *Journal of Clinical Psychiatry* 1997;58 Suppl 12:23-8 Department of Psychiatry, Harvard Medical School, Boston, Mass., USA.

[4] Dale J, Crouch R, Lloyd D. Primary care: nurse-led telephone triage and advice out-of-hours. *Nurs. Stand* 1998 Aug 12-18;12(47):41-5 Post Graduate Medical School, University of Warwick, Coventry.

Medical Informatics Europe '99
P. Kokol et al. (Eds.)
IOS Press, 1999

AIDMAN - Advanced Informatics Distributed Medical Access Network

M Clarke, R W Jones, N Kanellopoulos*, D Lioupis*, A Nassiopoulos+
Brunel University, Uxbridge, UK
* *Patras University, & Computer Technology Institute, Greece*
+ *TEI of Athens, Greece*

Abstract. We describe AIDMAN, a pilot project in which health clinics in remote areas of Greece are connected with mainland hospitals, to provide routine clinical service for both chronic health care and accident and emergency. Clinical practice is supported through the use of the Virtual Consultation Workstation that is being developed and evaluated specifically for the project and which is based on readily available commercial products and international standards. The communication infrastructure remains a major obstacle to any telemedicine project, and for this reason, satellite communication is used in the AIDMAN project to overcome the current lack of digital links and bandwidth. The proposed system will provide real time video, high definition image, shared applications and data over a link running at 128 kbps. In this paper we discuss the design of the AIDMAN system, the Virtual Consultation Workstation and the communication channel.

1. Introduction

Provision of health care to remote areas will always remain problematic and the normal solutions demand that either the patient travels to the specialist, or vice versa. This is time consuming and inefficient of human resource, not to mention the low quality service. Telemedicine provides an alternative solution, where patient and specialist remain in their own location but are brought together through an electronic medium. The solution is attractive in regions of low population unable to support medical specialities, which tend to be concentrated in the regions of dense population. The goal is to develop a system that can provide as effective a service as the face to face consultation. Many projects have proven the concept in a number of medical specialities, but these have each remained isolated within their speciality. However, the health centres provide a general medical service, and therefore the challenge is to identify a number of specialities that can be supported concurrently by telemedicine and combine them into an integrated service that is shared. Certain specialities may require add-on equipment, but in general the system should be capable of supporting outpatient clinic activity for any discipline. This will make the system significantly more cost effective, especially where yield in any one speciality is small.

Dermatology has been shown to adapt well to telemedicine, with rates of correct diagnosis and equivalent treatment plans consistently comparing well with face to face consultation [1, 2, 3, 4]. It can be successful even using low cost video conferencing equipment and modest data rates [5] and is well accepted by both patients and the doctors [6, 7, 8]. Its ability to remove the need for face to face follow up or referral is particularly noteworthy [9, 10]. Some have used electronic reports incorporating digital images, using a store and forward techniques, e.g. e-mail or file based transfer, but this has rarely proved adequate alone, with successful diagnosis being significantly lower than video based techniques [11, 12]. At best it may be seen as a method of triage.

Telepsychiatry has been much studied, particularly in under-populated areas. There have been trials in several branches of psychiatry, each reporting success [13, 14, 15].

Teleradiology is well developed and has included projects such as ultrasound for obstetrics [16], oncology [17] and other radiology referral [18], but such projects would appear more suited to inter-hospital services as they have tended to use very high bandwidth links.

Emerging standards such as DICOM [19, 20] for storing and transmitting images, and multimedia enabled applications and e-mail protocols, make telemedicine possible using readily available packages. The continuing development of WWW protocols and browsers can provide a standard graphical user interface for many applications [21].

Telecardiology does not appear as well developed as other telemedicine areas, particularly for chronic care, with its application to date being limited mainly to emergency cases [22] or interpretation of a resting ecg [23, 24, 25]. However, no telecardiology project has reported the use of ambulatory monitoring reporting systems based in the health clinic, with the report being transmitted to the clinician for interpretation, nor is there any report of exercise electrocardiography being undertaken in the remote site. Only one study describes the coupling of telecardiology with video conferencing for a consultation between clinician and patient [26].

There have been a few projects where support has been provided for accident and emergency service in remote areas. The purpose is to determine those patients that must be transferred to the main hospital to receive specialist treatment for their injuries that may not be available in the remote centres and those that can be managed in the remote centre given specialist support. This clearly will have significant cost benefits, with one study showing that up to 60% of patients are transferred unnecessarily [27].

Very few telemedicine projects use satellite links, and those that exist have been developed to support emergency situations where trained medical staff are not on hand. Generally these have been based on store and forward techniques [28].

2. The AIDMAN Project

The AIDMAN project investigates the provision of high speed, high quality digital telemedical links to remote areas, employing satellite technology and, consequently, the impact on the range of technologies that can be provided for delivery of medical care. Four Hellenic hospitals have been chosen in order to implement the AIDMAN project, namely between the K.A.T. hospital in Athens and three primary care health centres in Greece, Corfu, Myconos and Mytilini, which, currently, have access to analogue telephone lines using modems operating at a typical maximum possible speed of about 9600 baud due to the poor quality and noise on the lines. Routine clinical service for chronic health care, and accident and emergency care and its follow up are going to be supported.

The clinical system will be based on the concept of the virtual consultation, where the workstation will attempt to bring the patient and consultant as close together as possible through the use of video-conferencing, high definition images, shared access to data and applications and any other peripherals or medical systems necessary to present clinical data to both ends.

2.1. The Virtual Consultation

The face to face consultation will often involve all five physical senses, and frequently the sixth, intuition. The virtual consultation must be able to provide a communication channel for each of these if the same success as the face to face consultation is to be achieved. We have used low cost video conferencing to give sight and sound, and augment this, by using still digital pictures, to provide high definition views. Video is interactive, and affords the opportunity to question the patient and elicit vital information that may help lead to a correct diagnosis; a significant advantage over any store and forward technique. During the consultation the patient is accompanied by a medically trained person, who can be the hands and nose of the consultant and can also operate the camera to achieve an optimum view or angle to aid diagnosis. The medically trained person can have another significantly more important role, that of an advocate for the patient during the consultation. The effects on the AIDMAN system in this aspect is to be closely investigated.

2.2. Clinical Applications

The major goal is to involve as many specialities as possible in the project in order that the system is used to its maximum and thus be cost effective. The system is designed to be a general purpose tool, and not the property of any one speciality, though clearly some specialities will require specific extra equipment in order to be properly supported. In the initial phase we will support dermatology, orthopaedics, cardiology, and vascular surgery.

2.3. Applications

The initial design for the virtual workstation is based on a Pentium II machine and includes desktop video conferencing (Proshare System 500), a digital video camera for simultaneous analogue video and high resolution digital still image, flat bed scanner, sound card and hands free speaker phone. The workstation will be connected digitally to any local x-ray machines or CT-scanners, so that images may be viewed and made available to the remote site. Where a link to such equipment is not possible, then images will be scanned into the system instead. This is sufficient to support the majority of the clinical application areas.

In order to support telecardiology, Holter ecg and blood pressure recorders and analysers will be installed in the health centres, so that reports and example waveforms can be forwarded to the cardiologist for review. We are also investigating the use of a PC based exercise ecg system, with reports being forwarded to the cardiologist, but this will require training of the doctor in the techniques of supervising exercise ecgs.

2.4. Communication Infrastructure

The communication infrastructure in significant parts of Greece still relies on analogue lines, which are incapable of providing the service proposed. This is unlikely to change in the foreseeable future. For this reason, a satellite link with a bandwidth of 128 kbps or more is used to carry real time video and data between the island sites and a main hub in Athens. A simple point to point link has been used before with success, using bandwidth as low as 64 kbps [27]. However, in our project, we share the link between several sites, which keeps the costs down and makes more effective use of an expensive resource. In addition, the link is only capable of carrying a single video transmission at a time, and to ensure high quality, data should not be carried over the link at the same time. In practice this means that the link has to be booked for a clinic session and is not available to others for data transfer. The bandwidth is available 24 hours a day for emergency use and could be taken over from a clinic at short notice if necessary. The system is planned to go into pilot operation on a reduced daytime only basis in the second quarter of 1999 for testing and to provide a service for training. The full system is planned to go live in the first quarter of 2000. We will present details of preliminary performance at the meeting.

The satellite link provides a clear channel, capable of carrying any protocol. The problem lies in controlling access and reserving bandwidth for each application. Video-conferencing must have access to a minimum reserved bandwidth if performance is to be guaranteed.

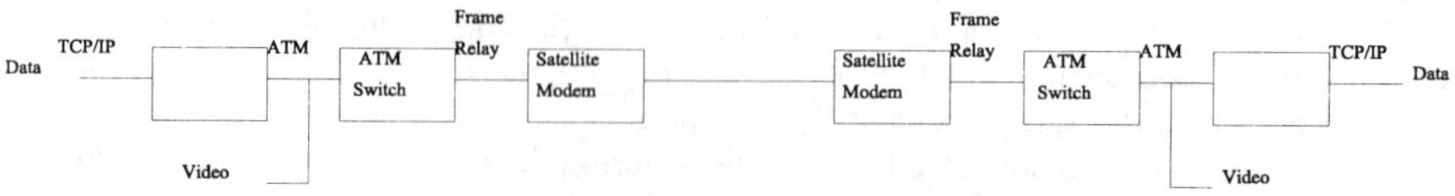

Figure 1. An ATM Network

An ATM network, such as figure 1, would provide the desired functionality, but at the moment there are few applications that are written for an ATM network and thus able to take advantage of this quality of service. Network equipment is also expensive.

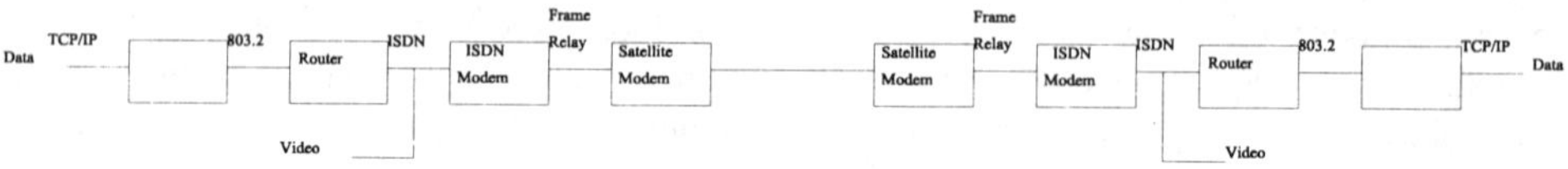

Figure 2. An ISDN Network

Alternatively, the link could be set up as a circuit switched channel, figure 2, with the whole of the channel bandwidth being taken by a single application, in this case data or video. For our purpose, the ISDN service is emulated over frame relay and is used separately for the video conferencing and the bridge-router. The solution provides a channel with ideal properties for the video conferencing, but the ISDN modem adds cost.

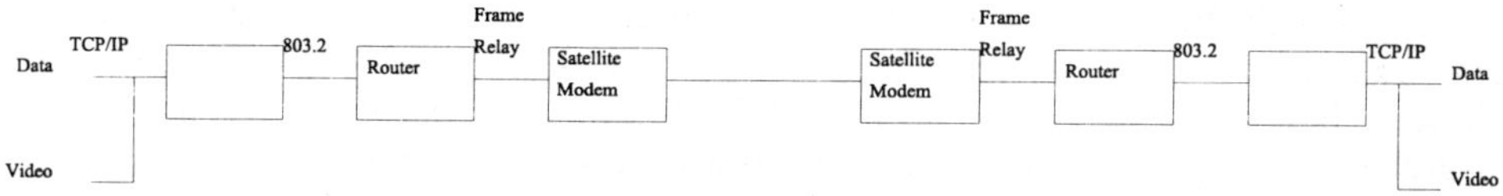

Figure 3. A TCP/IP Network

A third option is to run all the applications over TCP/IP, as in figure 3, and apply rigorous control of the applications that are running in the environment. Control of the link is done in an ad hoc fashion. Although not ideal, it is expedient at this stage of proving the concept, as it allows a common protocol such as TCP/IP, and for which many applications have been written, to be employed. This will allow easy integration of applications and sites using the network. As network protocols develop, we would anticipate TCP/IP V6 to be used, and thus provide guaranteed quality of service.

We will model each of the above three options during the project and compare them in terms of end to end performance, flexibility and cost. The best alternative will be chosen and implemented.

3. Discussion

The AIDMAN project is designed to capitalise on a number of important developments: the rapid fall in cost of technology; a growing level of expertise of IT in the medical profession; a greater awareness and acceptance of technology. The rapidly falling costs for video-conferencing, together with a maturing of this technology, now puts systems on the desk for a cost of only a few hundred Euros. This will only get better and thus the cost of the equipment is no longer a prohibiting factor. In addition, the increase in use of the satellite links is bound to lower significantly the currently high operational cost. Acceptance of technology by the medical profession has often been a hurdle, but the increased awareness of e-mail and WWW means that they are not only accepting, but are now demanding new applications. Studies have proven that the technology is equally accepted by the patient, particularly when significant benefit is seen [29] and this gives us confidence.

One important assessment that must be made by the AIDMAN project must be its socio-economic advantages. It is not enough to deploy technology merely because it is possible. However, the economic advantages are not easily measured [30], as many do not appear as direct costs to the health service, and assumptions regarding their levels must be made. Clearly the choice will govern one's conclusions [31]. Telemedicine is more expensive compared to the current arrangements as the patient currently bears the cost of travel to the mainland and the loss of earnings and productivity. There is also the likelihood of finding more disease that needs treating. However, any cost benefit analysis must include the indirect costs, together with a price for convenience and timely diagnosis. What price a life? There will be tangible economic benefits, such as a reduction in the number of patients being referred or evacuated unnecessarily, and by being able to manage the investigation and treatment of patients in a more economic way.

An obvious and important side effect of such projects is the educational benefits. It is common for relatively inexperienced doctors to be posted in the health centres in remote regions. When these doctors are involved in the consultation, they learn from the expert of the central hospital.

4. Conclusion

We are at an early stage in the AIDMAN project, and success will best be measured by the uptake following the pilot phase. Success of telemedicine projects has repeatedly been shown to be dependent on the perceived need of the service and on the motivation of those involved. Projects undertaken in isolation and under contrived circumstances have almost always failed at the end of their funding. The AIDMAN project attempts to address real needs, and is designed to provide tangible benefits such that those involved will be motivated to make the project succeed.

Acknowledgements

The AIDMAN Project is funded by the Commission of the European Communities Directorate General XIII – Contract TEN 45593 (FS).

References

[1] Gilmour E, et al, Comparison of teleconsultations and face-to-face consultations: preliminary results of a United Kingdom multicentre teledermatology study. *British Journal of Dermatology,* **139** (1):81-7, 1998 Jul.

[2] Loane MA, et al, Diagnostic accuracy and clinical management by realtime teledermatology. Results from the Northern Ireland arms of the UK Multicentre Teledermatology Trial. *Journal of Telemedicine & Telecare*, **4** (2):95-100, 1998.

[3] Lowitt MH, et al, Teledermatology and in-person examinations: a comparison of patient and physician perceptions and diagnostic agreement, *Archives of Dermatology*, **134** (4):471-6, 1998 Apr.

[4] Lesher JL Jr, et al, Telemedicine evaluation of cutaneous diseases: a blinded comparative study, *Journal of the American Academy of Dermatology*, **38** (1):27-31, 1998 Jan.

[5] Tsuchiya H, Telemedicine using a desktop conference system (Phoenix) in Kyushu, Japan, *Telemedicine Journal*, **4** (1):43-8, 1998 Spring.

[6] Freeman K, Groves-Phillips S, Lewis L, Telemedicine and Education, *World Congress on Telemedicine*, **Nov 1995** pp188.

[7] Freeman K, Wynn-Jones J, Groves-Phillips S, Lewis L, Teleconsulting - a practical account of pitfalls, problems and promise, experience from the TEAM project group, *Journal of Telemedicine & Telecare*, **2** Suppl 1:11-13, 1996.

[8] Low S J, Lewis L, Goldberg B, Transforming the Patient Experience Through Telemedicine, **HC '96** Harrogate.

[9] Oakley AM. Duffill MB. Reeve P, Practising dermatology via telemedicine, *New Zealand Medical Journal*, **111** (1071):296-9, 1998 Aug 14.

[10] Jones DH, et al, Teledermatology in the Highlands of Scotland, *Journal of Telemedicine & Telecare*, **2** Suppl 1:7-9, 1996.

[11] Zelickson BD, Homan L, Teledermatology in the nursing home, *Archives of Dermatology*, **133** (2):171-4, 1997 Feb.

[12] Kvedar JC, et al, The substitution of digital images for dermatologic physical examination, *Archives of Dermatology*, **133** (2):161-7, 1997 Feb.

[13] Mannion L, et al, Telepsychiatry: an island pilot project, *Journal of Telemedicine & Telecare*, **4** Suppl 1:62-3, 1998.

[14] Brown FW, Rural telepsychiatry, *Psychiatric Services*, **49** (7):963-4, 1998 Jul.

[15] Blackmon LA, Kaak HO, Ranseen J, Consumer satisfaction with telemedicine child psychiatry consultation in rural Kentucky, *Psychiatric Services*, **48** (11):1464-6, 1997 Nov.

[16] Fisk NM, et al, Fetal telemedicine: interactive transfer of realtime ultrasound and video via ISDN for remote consultation, *Journal of Telemedicine & Telecare*, **1** (1):38-44, 1995.

[17] Doolittle GC, et al, A cost measurement study for a tele-oncology practice, *Journal of Telemedicine & Telecare*, **4** (2):84-8, 1998.

[18] Eichelberg M, Hewett AJ, Jensch P, RETAIN - an ATM pilot project for applications in health care, *Journal of Telemedicine & Telecare*, **2** Suppl 1:13-6, 1996.

[19] http://www.rsna.org/REG/practiceres/dicom/index.html

[20] Ratib O, Hoehn H, Girard C, Parisot C, PAPYRUS 3.0: DICOM-compatible file format, *Medical Informatics*, **19** (2):171-8, 1994 Apr-Jun.

[21] Forslund DW, Phillips RL, Kilman DG, Cook JL, Experiences with a distributed virtual patient record system, *Proceedings/AMIA Annual Fall Symposium*, 483-7, 1996

[22] Bertazzoni G, Genuini I, Aguglia F, Telecar: an Italian telecardiology project, *Journal of Telemedicine & Telecare*, **2** (3):132-5, 1996.

[23] Mavrogeni S, et al, Telecardiology services in the Aegean islands, *Journal of Telemedicine & Telecare*, **2** Suppl 1:74-6, 1996.

[24] Economakos G, et al, ECG handling on a telemedicine platform, *Journal of Telemedicine & Telecare*, **2** Suppl 1:71-4, 1996.

[25] Tsagaris MJ, et al, The contribution of telemedicine to cardiology, *Journal of Telemedicine & Telecare*, **3** Suppl 1:63-4, 1997.

[26] Shanit D, Greenbaum RA, Towards a comprehensive telecardiology monitoring centre for community-based services, *Journal of Telemedicine & Telecare*, **3** Suppl 1:60-2, 1997.

[27] Armstrong IJ, Haston WS, Medical decision support for remote general practitioners using telemedicine, *Journal of Telemedicine & Telecare*, **3** (1):27-34, 1997.

[28] Anogianakis G, et al, Medical emergency aid through telematics (MERMAID), *Telemed 95, London, UK:135*, 1995, Nov.

[29] Harrison R, Clayton W, Wallace P, Can telemedicine be used to improve communication between primary and secondary care?, *BMJ*, **313** (7069):1377-80; discussion 1380-1, 1996 Nov 30.

[30] McIntosh E, Cairns J, A framework for the economic evaluation of telemedicine, *Journal of Telemedicine & Telecare*, **3** (3):132-9, 1997.

[31] Halvorsen PA, Kristiansen IS, Radiology services for remote communities: cost minimisation study of telemedicine, *BMJ*, **312** (7042):1333-6, 1996 May 25.

Medical Informatics Europe '99
P. Kokol et al. (Eds.)
IOS Press, 1999

Multimedia Stimulation for Psychophysiological Investigation

P.J. McCullagh, G.P. Gent, H.G. McAllister
School of Information & Software Engineering, University of Ulster, Northern Ireland, UK

Abstract. This paper describes a multimedia approach to sensory stimulation in psychophysiological studies. High resolution colour images are presented to a subject by a Delphi stimulus program, controlled by a data acquisition system which concurrently records cognitive Event Related Potentials from the subject. The acquisition PC is linked to the stimulus PC using serial communications and requests slide material using a character based protocol. The sound card in the data acquisition system can present concurrent complex auditory stimuli for multimedia experiments.

1. Introduction

Event-related potentials (ERPs) are electrical signals reflecting the neurochemical processes within the brain, which may be recorded non-invasively from the human scalp using electrodes, amplifiers and data acquisition system [1]. ERPs occur in response to auditory and visual stimuli but due to poor signal to noise ratio, are measured by presenting repeated stimuli and averaging acquired epochs of the electroencephalogram. This process decreases the background noise in proportion to the square root of the number of stimuli. The main use of ERPs has been in psychophysiological studies as a means of investigating cognitive processes.

Due to hardware advances multimedia PCs are capable of storing, processing and displaying high resolution images in photographic quality colour. This technology has been utilised in the generation and display of visual stimuli for presentation in psychophysiological studies. When linked to a data acquisition system, visual evoked potentials (VEPs) [2] and event related potentials (ERPs) [3] may be elicited and used to study sensory and cognitive processes in the brain, with high temporal resolution. To this end, a program (ViStim) was designed to present visual stimuli on a PC and to communicate with data acquisition software executing concurrently on an acquisition system. Although similar systems have been developed (E.g. Neuroscan, http:\\www.neuroscan.com) the approach produces flexible and more configurable paradigms, appropriate to a research environment.

Traditionally auditory stimuli have been used in the assessment of hearing and have comprised tones of various amplitudes and frequencies and white noise, presented using an audiometer, a precisely calibrated instrument. However for ERP studies there is a requirement for the synthesis of diverse yet controllable complex stimuli, without the requirement for calibration. The addition of sound to the multimedia PC provides a flexible alternative to the audiometer. This paper describes a software unit which facilitates the programming of a family of sound cards (Sound Blaster, Creative Labs Inc.) to generate complex stimuli for ERP experiments. It updates and augments software which facilitated the generation of simple tones and noise [4].

2. Hardware and Software

A stimulus PC is linked to a data acquisition system via a serial port. The data acquisition system comprises electrodes attached to a subject's scalp, physiological amplifiers, 16 channel A/D converter (Amplicon PC30AT), and appropriate software. The stimulus PC replaces dual slide projectors with shutter control and relay hardware [5]. Auditory stimuli may be concurrently presented using a sound card located in the data acquisition machine [6].

ViStim is a Microsoft Windows based program, written in Delphi (Borland), an object oriented, event driven language. Delphi was selected as it utilises visual component programming techniques for interface and program design, permitting rapid prototype development, and produces fast executable code. The program comprises image presentation and serial communications modules.

Serial communications driver

The presentation software is controlled by the acquisition system. A serial link (9600 baud) is established and the stimulus PC reads a message string from the communications port which after decoding, permits selection of the appropriate slide. Current design permits up to three categories of visual stimuli, with each category comprising up to 40 different slides, see Table 1. The number of conditions can easily be increased, subject to memory limitations in the presentation PC. The data acquisition system previously triggered slide projector instrumentation via an I/O port (PC30AT) and modifications to the software are required to send a suitable message string to the serial port for transmission to the stimulus PC. E.g. *"Show Slide 5, Condition 2"* is indicated by transmitting Chr(102), Chr(45).

Table 1 Character Based Communication Protocol

Character	**Function**
Chr(32)	Open Communications Link
Chr(101)	Set Condition to 1, E.g. Neutral slides
Chr(102)	Set Condition to 2, E.g. Phobic slides
Chr(103)	Set Condition to 3, E.g. Control slides
Chr(41)..Chr(80)	Slide number - 40, E.g. Chr(45) = Slide 5
Chr(33)	Close Communications Link

Purpose written slide displayer

This was developed to permit direct display of images from files. ViStim supports Bitmaps (BMP files) which may be presented efficiently as they are stored without compression. However conversion from other common formats such as GIF (Graphics Interchange Format) and JPEG (Joint Photographic Experts Group) is achieved using graphic utilities which are readily available on the Internet (E.g. Paint Shop Pro, http://www.jasc.com/psp5.html). The files once created and stored can be loaded at start-up from a set of defaults, stored in an initialisation file, or loaded manually once the program is running.

Delphi permits images to be loaded from file and stored as pictures on forms. The background is stored as a blank slide `Form[0,1]` and condition slides are loaded from file to new forms which are created, as required (`Form[condition 1..3, slide 1..40]`) at initialisation. The presentation requires the decoding of the communication protocol and the translation to a show/hide sequence, see Table 2.

Table 2 Slide display and auditory presentation example, as deduced from communications protocol

Commands	Function
Form[0,1].show, Form[0,1].hide	Show blank slide for prestimulus duration, sweep 1
Form[1,7].show, Form[1,7].hide Start condition 1 auditory stimulus, Stop condition 1 auditory stimulus	E.g. Show condition 1, slide 7 for stimulus duration and /or present auditory stimulus: 1kHz tone for stimulus duration
Form[0,1].show, Form[0,1].hide	Show blank slide for remainder of sweep 1
Form[0,1].show, Form[0,1].hide	Show blank slide for prestimulus duration, sweep 2
Form[2,3].show, Form[2,3].hide Start condition 2 auditory stimulus Stop condition 2 auditory stimulus	E.g. Show condition 2, slide 3 for stimulus duration and /or present auditory stimulus: 2kHz tone for stimulus duration
Form[0,1].show, Form[0,1].hide	Show blank slide for remainder of sweep 2

3. Discussion

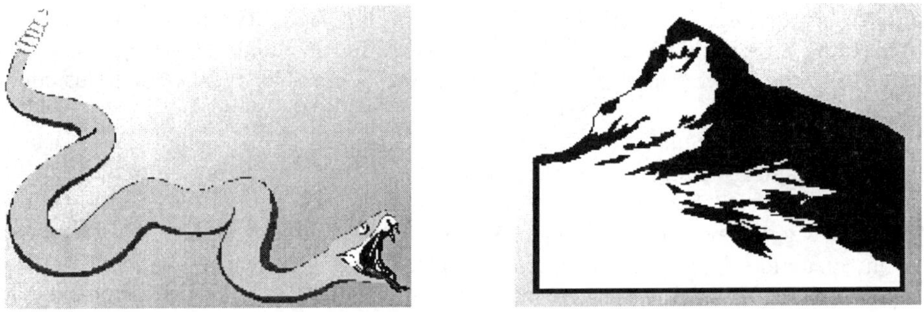

Figure 1 Sample visual stimuli, comprising phobic and neutral psychological stimuli. (The images appear in colour in psychophysiological experiments)

The system described provides a flexible solution for experiments which require a combination of visual and auditory stimulation, using standard hardware and is widely applicable to many studies in psychophysiology. The visual presentation may be used in the recording of a number of ERPs, including visual P300 and the contingent negative variation (CNV). Both paradigms comprise two conditions or categories of stimuli. A typical phobic study would comprise target stimuli such as images of spiders or rodents and neutral stimuli such as landscapes, see Figure 1. In the P300 paradigm, a rare image (15% probability of occurrence) will produce a positive component at approximately 300 msec after the stimulus for improbable average (condition 2), see Figure 2.

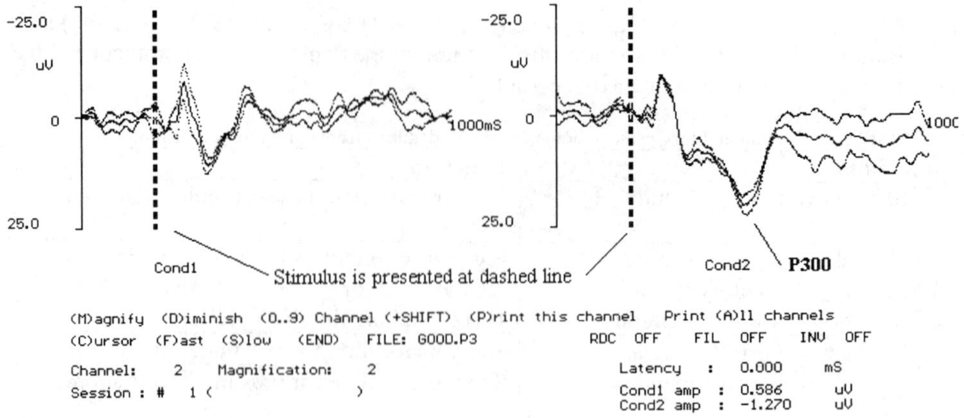

Figure 2 P300 component of the ERP. Condition 2 comprises 1 second averaged EEG to stimuli which occur at a probability of 15%. Each waveform comprises two subaverages of 16 sweeps and the overall average.

The CNV paradigm requires a warning stimulus, an imperative stimulus and an aversive stimulus. The imperative stimulus requires the user to perform an action such as pressing a button to avoid the aversive stimulus. The stimuli can be auditory, visual or a combination. For example a typical CNV can be elicited by presenting an auditory warning tone followed by a visual imperative stimulus which requires a response. The aversive stimulus could be an unpleasant noise.

Simple auditory stimuli such as tones may be generated by the Sound Blaster hardware using FM synthesis and more complex sounds or samples may be pre-processed and stored as VOC files (Creative Labs format) using a utility such as Goldwave (http://www.goldwave.com), see Figure 3. In this example the sound has been processed for use in an auditory hallucination experiment. This sound is currently presented by the data acquisition machine, synchronised to visual presentation. Auditory presentation by the stimulus machine is desirable and could be implemented by updates to the stimulus program and a more complex communications protocol. Control of the features of the sound card is possible with multimedia Delphi components (http://www.swiftsoft.de/mmtools.html).

The speed of slide update on the screen is critical in perceptual studies. The stimulus PC must be of a Pentium II (>133MHz) specification. Use of a lower specification PC can necessitate the reduction in the size and/or colour depth of images to reduce file size, as slides are cached from disc. In conclusion, ViStim provides a versatile display of any type of bit mapped visual stimulus in a Windows environment. Synchronisation with a data acquisition system incorporating flexible auditory stimulus generation provides a powerful tool for electrophysiological studies.

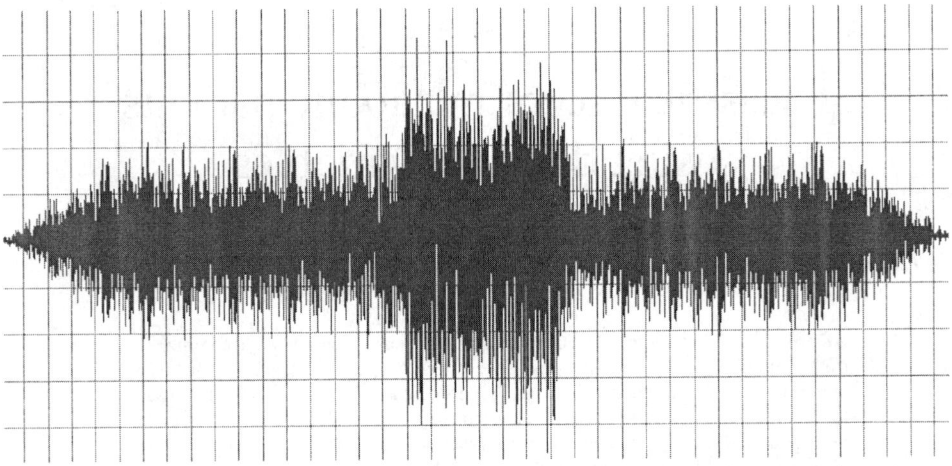

Figure 3 Speech epoch ("Who") recorded and mixed with background noise using Goldwave software. The software permits manipulation of background noise level and the temporal reverse of the speech segment in a target / acoustically matched non-target experiment.

References

[1] P.J. McCullagh, H.G. McAllister, M.F. Regan. "Multi channel data acquisition and analysis of EEG and Event Related Potentials". Innovation et Technologie en Biologie et Medecine, Vol 13, No. 6, (1992), 693-703.

[2] K.H. Chiappa, "Evoked Potientals in Clinical Medicine". Raven Press, New York, 1985.

[3] T.W. Picton, S.A. Hillyard. Endogenous event-related potentials. in: T.W. PICTON, (ed), "Handbook of Electroencephalography and Clinical Neurophysiology Vol 3: Human Event-Related Potentials", Amsterdam:Elservier, (1988), 361-426.

[4] McCullagh P J, McAllister H G, Armstrong G A and Regan M F. PC software library for the production of auditory stimuli in cognitive event-related potential experiments. Computer Methods and Programs in Biomedicine 45 (1994) 283-289.

[5] P.J. McCullagh, R.J. McClelland and M.F. Regan. "Computerised Paradigms for Eliciting the Contingent Negative Variation Event Related Potential". Proceedings of the 14th annual international conference of the IEEE Engineering in Medicine and Biology Society, (1992), 2481-2483.

[6] P.J. McCullagh. "Application of Multimedia Technology to the recording of Cognitive Event Related Potentials". Proceedings of the 16th annual international conference of the IEEE Engineering in Medicine and Biology Society, (1994), 241-242.

Medical Informatics Europe '99
P. Kokol et al. (Eds.)
IOS Press, 1999

Classification of metabolic patients using dynamic variables

Stepan SVACINA, Tomas HAAS, Martin MATOULEK, Klara NEDELNIKOVA
Charles University, 1st Medical Faculty, Katerinska 32, 121 08 Prague 2, Czech Republic

Abstract. The severity of metabolic syndrome is usually determined according to static variables (blood glucose, insulin level, body mass index etc.) The most important classification is dynamic and prognostic classification which can be used to determine the ability to decrease elevated metabolite and hormone levels or to lose weight. Different mathematical approaches were used to determine these phenomena : 1. Mathematical modelling e.g. (Bergman minimal model or glycation model). 2. Predictive calculations using multiple regression (using static and dynamic parameters to determine weight loss in obesity treatment). 3. One day starvation test (finding very variable hormone and metabolic changes in obese patients). We can conclude There are 3 types of metabolic parameters: A. Static (basic) description, B. Functional (actual) description, C. Dynamic- stability describing variables. Mathematical modelling is a complicated method needing many blood samples. It is very invasive for patients and it is difficult to be repeated. Predictive importance can have also repeated measured metabolic data which are able to classify the stability (fixation) of metabolic state. Some basic parameters and simple dynamic tests like one day starvation test can be used in prognostic classification of patients who are able to change their fixed metabolic state.

1. Introduction

The metabolic X syndrome is a very important and common human disease defined by Reaven [1]. It is a combination of common diseases (type 2 diabetes, hypertension, obesity, hypertriglyceridemia, hyperuricemia and some hormonal, coagulation and fibrinolytic changes). It is one of most important factors leading to atherosclerosis. The leading and perhaps primary pathogenetic feature is insulin resistance and hyperinsulinaemia. Many features of these diseases can be described mathematically. Since 10 years some of these problems are discussed in the conferences Computers in Diabetes which take part every two years in Europe. The most important approach describing quantitatively insulin resistance is the Minimal model of Bergman and we also have personal experience with this approach [2,3].

2. Mathematical modelling related to metabolic syndrome

The minimal model is a calculation which is based on a 2 hours intravenous glucose tolerance test with frequent blood sampling (about 100 blood samples). It is time consuming for personnel and invasive for the patient. It is an important method used in research which cannot be used in practise. We have a personal experience in using this method in investigation of relationship of the adrenal hormone dehydroepiandrosterone an insulin [2]. We have also used another method of modelling in investigation of dynamic changes of glycated haemoglobin and protein [4]. Modelling approach was useful in teaching students and doctors being able to understand the dynamics of glycation process. The method of modelling is too complicated and too invasive for use in clinical practise.

3. Predictive calculation based on multiple linear regression

Since many years we are interested in long term treatment of obese patients (complex diet education, pharmacotherapy and surgical treatment). We have [5] evaluated an 8 years outcome (weight change) after hospitalisation with reduction regimen in 20 patients (group 1), 3 years after surgical gastric banding in 22 patients (group2) and 51 patients one year after surgical gastric banding (group 3). In all groups there was a part of diabetic patients which all were treated only by diet.

We have used basic metabolic data e.g. blood glucose, lipid, insulin, thyroid hormone, presence of diabetes, anthropometric data, and initial weight change in multiple linear regression approach. (BMI is universally used weight index /body mass index /: weight in kg divided by square height in meters)

We have derived following predictive calculations in these 3 groups of patients:

Group 1) BMI change in 8 years= 12.26- 2.28 xBMI change in 2 weeks hospitalisation.

Group 2) BMI change in 3 years= -7.88 + 2.39x BMI change in 3 months.

Group 3) BMI change in 3 months= 7.92- 1.74x(presence of diabetes)-0.697x log (insulin level) +0.79 x(triglycerides level).

Group 3) BMI change in 12 months = 0-4.07x log (T3-trijodothyroin /T4-thyroxin)-2.21 log (presence of diabetes)- 3.11 log (insulin level).

In group 1 and 2 no metabolic variables were able to fit the regression model and only early weight change could predict the outcome.

In group 3 only some basic variables were able to fit the regression and predict the long term outcome of the obesity surgery. Higher weight loss is present in patients without diabetes, with hypertriglyceridemia and with low insulin level. Lower weight loss was present in patients with diabetes, with high endogenous insulin (caused by insulin resistance), lower triglycerides (minimal reserve in diet treatment), lower ratio T3/T4 (adaptation to low caloric intake- low T3 syndrome).

4. One day starvation test

Obesity treatment is very expensive treatment especially in indicating obesity surgery. We are trying to develop some test which could identify patients who are able to change their insulin resistant state and so to change the fixation of metabolic syndrome.

We have started with a new type of simple investigation of patients with one day starvation test. This test is easy to perform taking only 2 blood samples in the beginning and at the end of starvation. We have found in a group of 17 patients after one day starvation change of insulin level -28%, T3 -12%, T4 0%, betahydroxybutyrate (keton production) + 117%, glucose -11%, cholesterol -1%, triglycerides -26% uric acid +11%, BMI -2%. The variance change of this patient group was highest in betahdroxybutyrate- change in variance +84%. The group of patients will be followed to find out the predictive importance of these dynamic changes of metabolic and hormone levels.

5. Discussion

The severity of metabolic syndrome is usually determined according to static variables (blood glucose, insulin level, BMI etc.) Dynamic parameters are perhaps telling more about the functional changes (like insulin resistance) which are important for patient description and description of the severity disease. The most important classification is dynamic and prognostic classification which can be used to determine the ability to decrease elevated metabolic levels or to lose weight.

Mathematical modelling is a precise method being able to quantify functional changes. This is often used in research (e.g. in drug testing). It is impossible to perform this investigation in daily practise because of invasiveness for patient and time and money consuming investigation.

Predictive calculations using multiple regression are able to identify simple basic data which are able to quantify the prognosis of patient. Static parameters have some importance e.g. presence of diabetes or high insulin level in metabolic syndrome.

There are 4 types of information in metabolic syndrome patients:

1) static describing of the severity of disease (describing how many components of this disease are present)
2) basic metabolic describing of the disease (metabolites and hormone levels)
3) functional description of disease (calculating model based parameters e.g. insulin resistance)
4) dynamic ability of patients to change parameters 1), 2) and3).

Prognosis of patient can be determined using the information 1), 2) and3) but prognosis of therapy could be determined only classifying the dynamic ability to change the metabolic state.

6. Conclusion

It is necessary to develop methods which are able to classify patients according to therapy effectiveness. The determination of the ability to change the fixed bad metabolic state is to be measured. This feature has to be measured by simple and cheap methods which could be used in large groups of patients. In the European population the percentage of people having genetic predisposition to metabolic X syndrome is about 30%. Epidemiological studies are bringing complex information about prevalence of this disease. Predictive importance have some basic and also repeated measured metabolic data which are able to classify the stability (fixation) of metabolic state in the concrete patient. Good cost effectiveness of the treatment of metabolic X syndrome is dependent on finding good dynamic information about patients and classifying patients according to potential therapy result.

References

[1] G. Reaven, Role of Insulin Resistance in Human Disease (syndrome X) *Ann Med Rev* **44,** (1993), 121-131.

[2] S. Svacina , M. Kvapil, T.Haas, D. Wichterle, B. Bendlova, P. Stolba, J. Sonka, Dynamics of Dehydroepiadnrosterone During Intravenous Glucose tolerance test *Diabetologia Croatica,* **27**, (1998) 23-26.

[3] R.N. Bergman, I.D. Hope, Y.L. Yung, Assessment of insulin sensitivity in vivo: Critical reviews *Diab Metab. rev.* **5,** (1989), 411-429.

[4] S. Svacina, R. Hovorka, J. Skrha, Computer Models of Albumin and Heamoglobin Glycation, *Comp.Meth Progr Biomed* **32,**(1990), 259-263).

[5] S. Svacina, T.Haas, J. Sonka M. Fried, Calculations Predicting Weight Loss in Diabetes and Obesity.*Diab Nutr. Metab.* **11,** (1998), 73.

Medical Informatics Europe '99
P. Kokol et al. (Eds.)
IOS Press, 1999

Computer-Aided Diagnostic System In Dentistry

D. Grošelj, M. Malus[1], I. Grabec[2]
Faculty of Medicine,
[2]Faculty of Mechanical Engineering,
University of Ljubljana, Ljubljana, Slovenia
[1]B.I.D.M.C., Boston, USA

Abstract. A dental diagnostic system for patient database management, automated measurements, diagnostics and statistical estimation of health conditions is described. To increase the diagnosis quality various diagnostic tools are developed using several statistical methods. The analysis provides information about the importance of particular general, dental, and periodontal data which are further used in quantitative modeling of healing process in the oral cavity. The system supports clinician's diagnostic process and leads to improvement of decisions obtained by a conventional routine. Increased control and evaluation of different therapy types is enabled.

1. Introduction

The role of adequate medical documentation has always been of the upmost importance for data analysis which is needed as a support for conclusions about patient health state. In the last 20 years there were many attempts to introduce different dentistry chart systems in Slovenia. Beside recording the settlement of dental treatment it is of importance for clinicians in research studies to store biomedical data and to perform data analysis. The resulting quantitative parameters are especially needed as a support for current patient diagnosis as well as epidemiological and clinical research.

Let us consider what a clinically oriented therapist mainly uses nowadays: extensive hand written database about patients, clinical oral examination with visual estimation of tooth mobility using manual loading, results of various laboratory tests and mainly subjective diagnostics supported by reviewing of manually prepared database. Such conventional methods make diagonsis and reviewing cumbersome and suggest introduction of modern computer supported techniques. In order to follow this suggestions we developed a new medical diagnostic system STOMSYS which is adapted to dentistry. Our intention is to provide efficient solution for dentistry supporting activites by the following actions:

- Computarization of databases and their adaptation to registration, reviewing, printout and exchange of clinical or laboratory parameters. An additional aim is to include telemedical capabilities that could enable clinicians consultation and opinion exchange via internet with colleagues world wide.
- Automatization of manual measurements of tooth mobility and parameter estimation from measured data.
- Changing of diagnostic process from mainly subjective to objective one by application of integrated tools such as statistical analysis and prediction by learning procedures.

Our main goal was to provide clinicians with a computerized system that would help to improve the diagnostic process.

2. System description

STOMSYS is a windows based diagnostic software that incorporates patient database and toolboxes for automated measurements, optimization, statistics and prediction of healing process. All parts of the system are accessible through user friendly menus, predefined shortcuts and button bars. Figure 2.1. shows information flow in STOMSYS while Figure 2.2. presents hardware interaction scheme.

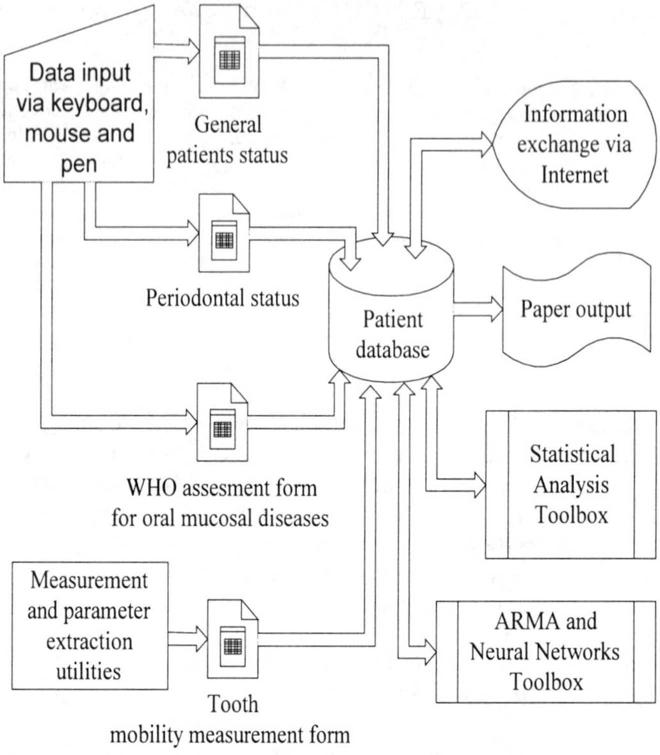

Figure 2.1.

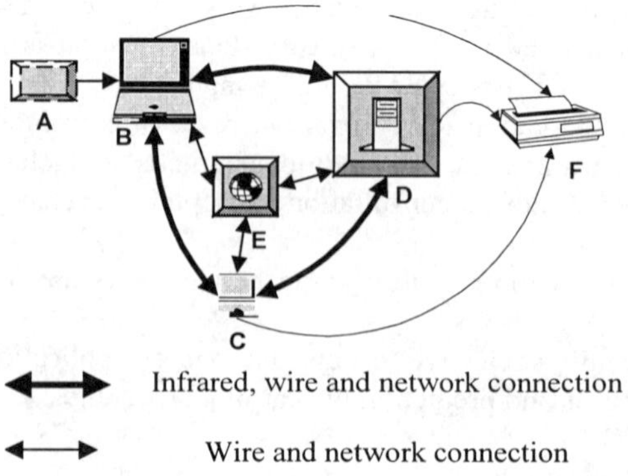

Figure 2.2.

A - Biomechanical measurement unit
B - Notebook computer
C – Handheld personal computer
D – Server
E – Internet socket
F – Printer

2.1. Patient database

Central part of STOMSYS is a relational computer database that includes general, dental and periodontal data of patients. There are twenty-one forms for patient data management including:

- general patient data,
- case history with health questionnaire (FDI 1989),
- 6 different views of general dental status,
- records of dental examinations (DMF values) with 5 different views of each tooth,
- data about therapist,
- tooth mobility logg,
- periodontal status with: gingival fluid flow rate, plaque index, gingival index, retention index, dark field microscopy, probing depth, clinical attachment level, bleeding on probing, width of keratinized gingiva, debris index, calculus index, furcation involvement, manual tooth mobility, Periotest and registration of mucogingival problems.
- WHO assessment form for oral mucosal diseases.

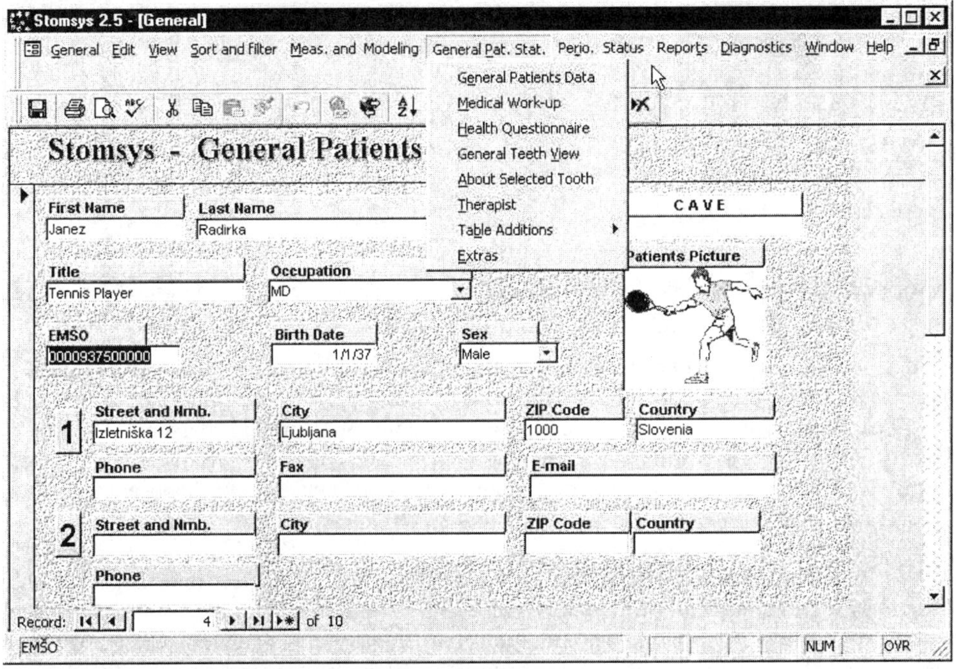

Figure 2.1.1. presents part of a general patient form with open general patient's status menu.

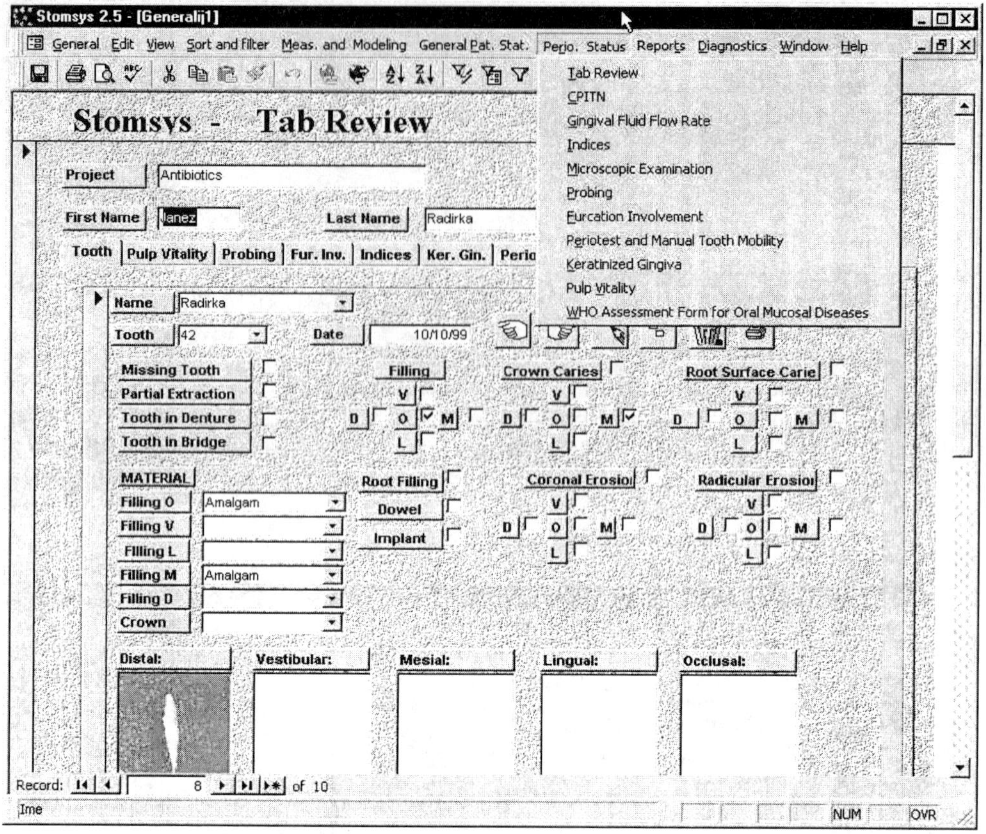

Figure 2.1.2. presents tab review of several patient forms with a currently active tooth status form and periodontal status menu.

We describe the tooth and periodontal status thoroughly with parameters which are widely applied in dentistry. These data are included in the forms that are residing and availabe in the STOMSYS. For convenience reason we introduced Handheld Personal Computer (HPC) reduced version of STOMSYS which includes only the most frequently employed forms. Hand held unit enables us to have a transportable data base at our disposal and it also allows simple operations of the system without disturbing the patient-clinician interaction.

Data are input via keyboard and on HPC also with convenient electronic pen. The PC version is also equiped with utilities for system control via voice and dictation using voice recognition facility. Databases on both units are completely synchronized via several networking links. All forms can be sent to various other applications such as: MS Word, MS Excel, SPSS, and others. We can distribute encrypted forms via E-mail and present them on World Wide Web for cilincial purposes such as second opinion as well as for research activities. Using included audio/video internet conferencing options we can also consult online colleagues world wide.

2.2. Measurement and parameter extraction utilities

Another significant part of STOMSYS are various software utilities for automated measurements of tooth mobility. The tooth mobility is one of the most important clinical indicators of patient periodontal status. With especially designed bio-mechanical apparatus we register accurate and repeatable mobility parameters. The apparatus which was designed in the Faculty of Mechanical Engineering laboratory (Grošelj and al.1996) is comprised of four components: dynamometer, force generating unit, a moveable system for fixation and positioning and signal processing unit. With integration of this instrument into STOMSYS we render possibile automatic execution of tooth mobility, recording of corresponding data, and estimation of important parameters. The tooth mobility is measurable on incisors in vestibulo-oral direction as function of applied force. STOMSYS connects this instrument to the computer via termination panel and A/D data acquisition card. The software helps to perform experiments, to save and review data, as well as to estimate parameters from measured signals. After performing measurements a clinician compares the tooth mobility diagram with stored ones and those of other patients. To simplify the comparison we incorporated two parameter estimation options. The first one has already been presented elsewhere (Grošelj and al.1990) and describes the force displacement diagram by two lines whose parameters represent a compressed information about the mobility process. In the second option the mobility curve is described by a more general visco-elastic model of Eq.2.1.

$$l = b*F+(1-\exp*(-c*F))*a \quad \text{eq. 2.1}$$

Where : l = tooth displacement , F = force applied to tooth, a,b,c = model parameters

The curve is described in a compressed form only by three coefficients a, b and c that characterize the adaptation of periodontal ligaments to the external loading. These coefficients are estimated from the empirical data by the least square optimization method called Marquardt-Levenberg algorithm (Press and al. 1992).

2.3. Multivariate Analysis Toolbox

When using extensive patient database the therapist has to decide which data in the diagnostic process are significant. In order to enable objective diagnostic process we have included multivariate statistical and discriminant analysis into STOMSYS. By this we estimate the significance of particular database parameters which are then applied as an aid in the diagnostic process.

2.4. Prediction of tooth mobility process

STOMSYS is also capable of performing prediction of the healing process. For this purpose it includes a non-parametric regression performed by incorporated artificial neural network and an ARMA modeling system (Grabec & Sachse 1997), The figure 2.4.1. shows the quality of prediction for a single patient from database with antibiotic treatment after surgery followed by treatment descriptor. With its help we evaluate the quality of treatment as well as the shift from one treatment to the other in case of worse predictions.

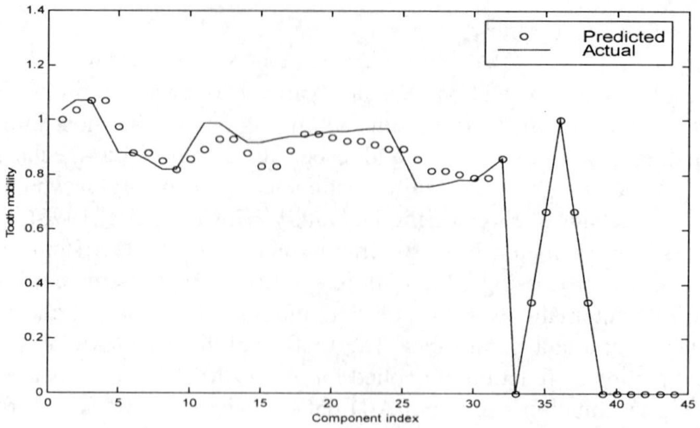

Figure 2.4.1.

3. Conclusions

STOMSYS is a diagnostic system for patient database management, automated measurements, diagnostic and statistical research of different oral condition. This opens new possibilities for systematic epidemiological studies and scientific research of different dental and periodontal phenomena. This software could also be used for teaching purposes because it makes feasible simple presentation of databeses to the audithory. After the completion of software development phase we are successfuly testing all posibilities of STOMSYS on clinical cases at the Department of Dentistry, Faculty of Medicine,University of Ljubljana.

References

[1] Grošelj D, Grabec I, Müller J. Loss of Marginal Alveolar Bone and Tooth Mobility. Zobozdrav Vestn 1990; 45: 88-92.

[2] Grabec I, Sachse W: Synergetics of Measurement, Prediction and Control. Springer - Verlag Berlin, Heidelberg, New York, 1997, 237-242.

[3] Grošelj D, Mužič P, Grabec I. A Technical Device for Measurement of Tooth Mobility using Small Loads. Zobozdrav Vestn 1996; 51: 155-61.

[4] Press William H., Teukolsky Saul A., Vetterling William T., Flannery Brian P.; Numerical Recepies in C, The Art of Scientific Computing, Second Edition, Cambridge Press, 1992; 683.

Medical Informatics Europe '99
P. Kokol et al. (Eds.)
IOS Press, 1999

Supporting decisions in diabetic patients management through Case-Based retrieval

S. Montani, R. Bellazzi, L. Portinale[1], S. Fiocchi[2], G. d'Annunzio[2], and M. Stefanelli
Dipartimento di Informatica e Sistemistica, Università di Pavia, Italy
[1] *Dipartimento di Scienze e Tecnologie Avanzate, Università del Piemonte Orientale, Alessandria, Italy*
[2] *IRCCS Policlinico S. Matteo, Pavia, Italy*

Abstract. In this paper we present a tool for the intelligent retrieval of past cases to support Insulin Dependent Diabetes Mellitus patients therapy revision. This tool was designed for assisting physicians during periodical monitoring visits. Each case is represented through i) a collection of features that describe the patient's clinical state at the decision time, i.e. the control visit, ii) the decision taken in terms of therapy revision and iii) the outcome obtained on the metabolic control during the following monitoring period. A new case is first classified into a protypical monitoring situation, and then similar cases are retrieved and shown to the user. This tool is fully integrated in a Web-based distributed system for Diabetes Management, developed within in the EU project T-IDDM.

1. Introduction

Current Information Technologies (IT) can provide physicians with a collection of tools for decision support, that integrate methods from several research areas in a comprehensive service to be applied "at the point of use". Following this perspective, we are working at the definition and implementation of distributed services for the management of chronic diseases. In particular, we are dealing with the management of Insulin Dependent Diabetes Mellitus (IDDM). The interest in the use of IT for IDDM management has grown up after the results of the Diabetes Control and Complications Trial [1], that showed how Intensive Insulin Treatment may delay or prevent the development of long-term complications caused by the disease. Since the same study has also assessed that the intensive therapy leads to the increase in the risk of severe hypoglycaemias and in the cost of diabetes management, IT applications may represent a valuable solution to the trade-offs underlying the therapy optimisation. In this context, we are carrying on a project, called T-IDDM (Telematic Management of IDDM), devoted to the implementation of an intelligent telemedicine system. In this project, physicians can exploit a Medical Workstation, that provides them with a number of IT services: an information system for data handling, a data analysis and visualisation system, a decision support system and a communication tool for data exchange with the patients' house; all of this subsystems are integrated in a Web-based service. Details on the T-IDDM project can be found in [2]. In this paper we describe a new tool we have made available for managing IDDM patients, based on a Case-based (CB) retrieval method, derived from Case-based Reasoning (CBR) technologies [3,4]. CBR is a problem solving paradigm that utilises the specific knowledge of previously experienced situations, called cases. Each case is usually described by a set of features, and is associated to a solution (or decision) and to an outcome. CBR basically consists in retrieving past cases that are similar to the current one and in reusing (by, if necessary, adapting) past successful solutions; the current case can be retained and put into the base of cases. CBR can hence be viewed as a method able to combine reasoning and learning steps and to produce solutions to problems by taking into account past experience. In current medical practice, diabetic patients are visited several times a year. During these visits the metabolic state of the patient is assessed by evaluating self-monitoring data and additional parameters coming from physical examination and blood analysis, in order to revise the therapeutic protocol. In the control visits, physicians are interested in detecting if the same metabolic behaviour has already occurred to the patient or to a similar patient, and, in such case, in seeing what decision has been taken and what was the outcome of that decision. This kind of support may be particularly interesting, considering that each diabetologist may visit more than a hundred patients every month; in this context, keeping track of the history of all patients is quite complex. For these reasons we have introduced in our system a CB retrieval tool, able to select in the data-base past cases that are in some sense similar to the current one; the result of the search is shown to physicians for comparison and further adaptation to the current case. A crucial capability of the proposed tool is the possibility of analysing the overall history related to the retrieved cases, showing the sequence of decision steps that precede and follow each situation. Moreover, our tool can be viewed as an instrument for the knowledge management of hospital institutions: the know-how expertise that guides the diabetologist's actions is stored in the case-base and can be re-used by other physicians. In such a way, both the general practice knowledge and the accumulated experience over a specific patient can be shared and exploited over years. The proposed CBR tool is fully integrated within the Hospital Information System and with the other services provided in the Medical workstation of the T-IDDM project.

2. Representing cases

Our CB retrieval system is based on the analysis of the decision making process involved in the periodical control visits. During these visits, three sources of information are considered: (i) historical characterisation, summarised by variables that generically describe the patient, such as sex, age, distance from diabetes onset; (ii) mid-term metabolic control, expressed through variables collected during the visits, like weight and Glycated Hemoglobin (HbA1c) values; (iii) short term (day-by-day) metabolic control, derived by the collection of home monitoring data, like Blood Glucose Level and insulin doses data. On the basis of this information, the physician decides the therapeutic protocol to be applied, as well as the diet and/or some recommendations about the patient's life-style. The outcome of the therapeutic decision is then evaluated at the following visit, usually considering HbA1c and the number of hypoglycaemic events. Following this analysis, and assuming that the control visit is the basic decision stage of the patients monitoring process, we define a case as the collection of the patients features and the decision taken during a visit, together with the outcome obtained, measured at the next visit.

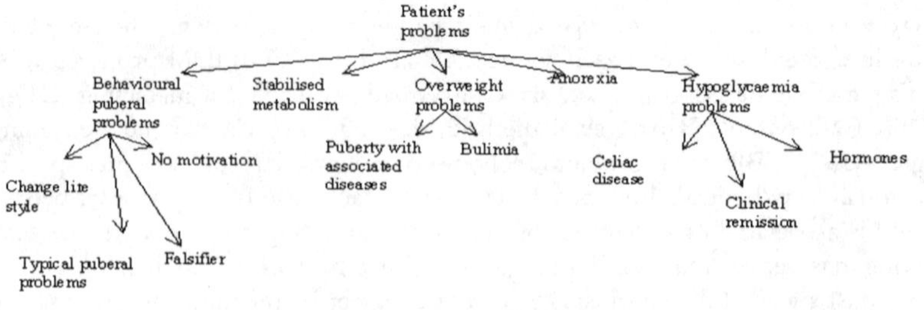

Figure 1: Taxonomy of classes of prototypical situations that may happen during monitoring of paediatric IDDM patients.

Physicians are allowed to retrieve cases of the same patient (intra-patient retrieval) and of different patients (inter-patients retrieval). The case library structure strongly influences the case search; to make retrieval more flexible we have structured it by resorting to a taxonomy of mutually exclusive prototypical classes (see figure 1), that express typical problems that may occur to patients in the age of infancy and puberty. A more complete taxonomy will be defined before testing the system in adult patients' clinics. The CB decision support procedure is splitted into two contributes: first, the system identifies the prototypical situation (class) that better describes the current case (classification step), then it retrieves the most similar cases belonging to the chosen class (retrieval step).

3. Retrieving similar cases

3.1 Classification

Various approaches are available for coping with the classification task [5]. Among them, we have chosen a Bayesian classification method that allowed us in explicitly considering the available prior knowledge, thus making up for reduced training data sets. In particular, we have used a Naive Bayes strategy [5], that makes the hypothesis of conditional independence among the different features given a certain class. Although this approach makes such a strong assumption, it is known to be quite robust in a variety of situations [6]. Prior probabilities have been derived through the collaboration with the diabetologists of the Pediatric Department of Policlinico S. Matteo in Pavia, while posterior probabilities were learnt from the available case base (145 cases from the histories of 29 pediatric patients) by using a standard Bayesian updating technique [7].

3.2 Retrieval

Once the case has been classified, similar cases belonging to the selected class (intra-class retrieval) can be found by applying a nearest-neighbour technique, that implements the Euclidean-Overlap Metric (HEOM) [8]; the search can also be extended to the set of most probable classes (inter-class retrieval) by using the Heterogeneous Value Difference Metric (HVDM) formula [8]. The two methods are able to deal both with numeric and with symbolic features, and to cope with the problem of missing data. When the data-base becomes very large, retrieval can be carried out by applying a non-exhaustive search algorithm, that implements a Pivoting strategy [9].

4. Implementation and Results

The CB retrieval tool is integrated in the T-IDDM Web-based environment, managed by **lispweb**, an HTML/HTTP server written in Common Lisp (see [2] for further details). The interaction between the CBR reasoning tool and the user (definition of a new case, classification and retrieval) takes place through a set of HTML pages, containing dynamically generated information, such as multicolumn tables and forms. The search space for retrieval is the collection of cases stored in an Oracle data-base, whose table structure mirrors the classes taxonomy; each leaf of the taxonomy tree matches a table, whose columns correspond to the case features, and whose rows are instances of the class at hand. An analysis of the system performances has been carried out on a data set that was made available by the Pediatric department of Policlinico S.Matteo. 3 physicians were interviewed for defining the prior probability distributions. In order to validate our classification approach, we have first applied a cross-validation technique to the data-base. Each case has been removed from its class and re-classified, relying only on the cases belonging to different patients, to maintain the hypothesis of conditional independence required by the classification technique; the probability distributions have been updated every time, so that the case at hand was not taken into account. Classification proved to be correct in the 83% of the cases, while in the 98% the correct class was one of the most probable ones. The result was improvable by excluding the class "falsifier", that identifies young patients who report wrong values of Blood Glucose Levels, in order to avoid complaints by parents and physicians on their life-style. It is hence clear that the classification step is quite difficult in this situation, even for physicians. As a second step, we have automatically generated more then 10000 random cases, starting from the probability distribution of the case-base. The results of validation on this expanded data-base proved to be encouraging as well: an error of less than 10% occurred in the validation of each class, excluding again class "falsifier" where the error rate reached 14%. Classification time was of the order of milliseconds, while retrieval ranged from 5 seconds (on about 20 cases) to 500 seconds (on the whole 10000 cases data-base) when adopting the HVDM formula, but was reduced to 170 seconds on 10000 cases when applying the Pivoting algorithm. The system hence proved to be really efficient in producing retrieval results to the user, when resorting to the most suitable technique.

5. Conclusions and Future Research Directions

Building Hospital Information Systems (HIS) does not only help in optimising the health care information flows, but also improves the quality of decisions in several clinical contexts. The use of CBR technologies, embedded in the HIS, bridges towards an intelligent use of the collected information, keeping track of past experiences and proposing solutions that are learnt from the cultural heritage of the care providers. We believe that CBR solutions, integrated with medical knowledge, may represent a valuable instrument for decision support, that should be more acceptable at the point of use that the classical expert systems. The physician, instead of being provided with a pre-compiled solution, is guided in mining past experience by intelligently navigating into the data-base of cases. In this paper we have studied the application of CBR methods to the problem of revising therapy during diabetic patients monitoring. This problem presents a collection of interesting characteristic: i) the patients evolve over time and similar situations may happen several times to the same patient; ii) the patient's features are summaries of time-dependent data that change with different velocity: for example, age changes from year to year, HbA1c is measured every two months and Blood Glucose Level varies from minute to minute; iii) the effect of the therapy may be delayed, due to some external reasons, like concurrent diseases (e.g. a flu). In the future we plan to investigate more deeply the time-dependency problem, retrieving not only similar cases, but also similar patients' histories, intended as the sequence of transitions between the different classes. Moreover, we are analysing the possibility of integrating the CB retrieval tool with other decision support tools, and in particular with a Rule-Based system, already operating in the T-IDDM architecture. More in detail, the classification and retrieval steps would be used to define the context into which the current patient's situation should be interpreted, and would therefore reduce the search space of the Rule-Based system through the application of some context-based meta-rules. In this way the integrated tool would not just produce a generically suitable solution, but would provide the physician with a therapy suggestion which is properly tailored on the single patient's peculiar needs.

Acknowledgments

We thank Alberto Riva for his contribute in the system implementation. This work is part of the project T-IDDM (HC 1047), funded by the European Commission

References

[1] The Diabetes Control and Complication Trial Research Group. The effect of intensive treatment of diabetes on the development and progression of long-term complications in insulin-dependent diabetes mellitus. The New England Journal of Medicine, 1993; 14-329: 977-86.

[2] Riva A, Bellazzi R, Stefanelli M. A Web-based System for the Intelligent Management of Diabetic Patients. MD Computing. 1997; 14: 360-64.

[3] Kolodner J. Improving Human Decision Making through Case-Based Decision Aiding. AI Magazine. 1991; Summer: 52-67.

[4] Aamodt A, Plaza E. Case-Based Reasoning: Foundational Issues, Methodological Variations and System Approaches. AI Communications. 1994; 7:39-59.

[5] Mitchell T. Machine Learning. New York: Mc Graw Hill. 1997.

[6] Zelic I, Kononenko I, Lavrac N, Vuga V. Induction of decision trees and Bayesian classification applied to diagnosis of sport injuries. Proceedings of IDAMAP 97 workshop, IJCAI 97, Nagoya, Japan: 1997; 61-67.

[7] Montani S, Bellazzi R, Portinale L, Fiocchi S, Stefanelli M. A case-based retrieval system for diabetic patients therapy. *Proceedings of IDAMAP 98 workshop, ECAI 98*. Brighton, 1998; 64-70.

[8] Wilson DR, Martinez TR. Improved Heterogeneous Distance Functions. Journal of Artificial Intelligence Research. 1997; 6:1-34.

[9] Portinale L, Torasso P, Magro D. Selecting most Adaptable Diagnostic Solutions through Pivoting-Based Retrieval. Lecture Notes in Artificial Intelligence 1266, 1997; 277-88.

Medical Informatics Europe '99
P. Kokol et al. (Eds.)
IOS Press, 1999

An integration system to rapidly identify aquatic bacteria

[1,2]M. Giacomini, [3]S. Bertone, [1,2]C. Ruggiero, [3]F. Caneva Soumetz, [2]A. Bisio, [2]G. Odino, [3]L. Calegari
[1]*DIST - Dept. of Communication Computer and System Sciences, University of Genova, Via Opera Pia 13, 16145 Genova – Italy. E-mail: giacomin@dist.unige.it*
[2]*DIST laboratory, Advanced Biotechnology Center - ABC, Genova - Italy*
[3]*Institute of Microbiology, University of Genova - Italy*

Abstract. An identification system for aquatic bacteria which would be useful for aspects ranging from pollution monitoring to health care, is described. It contains relevant information concerning the nature, taxonomy and activity of aquatic bacteria and allows to identify fresh isolates by means of their chemotaxonomic profiles. The system is simple and user friendly, so that it can be used by people not familiar with computers and has a modular interface that allows an easy interaction with laboratory instruments. The system is also connected with artificial neural network based programs to identify strains starting from the considered chemotaxonomic features.

1. Introduction

In the last few years environmental microbiology has become more and more important from several points of view. A huge range of micro-organisms, including bacteria, filamentous fungi, yeasts, micro-algae and protozoa, are considered the true inhabitants of the aquatic environment. As far as marine bacteria are concerned, representatives of more than 100 prokaryotic genera may be considered marine inhabitants. In the water column the majority of Gram-negative rods are located, while in the sediments there are higher proportions of Gram-positive bacteria. Many of these organisms have common traits, such as production of pigmented colonies on solid media, requirement of NaCl, exo-enzyme production and the preferential requirement of amino acids to sugar for growth [1]. A wide variety of micro-organisms can be isolated from fresh water. Since fresh waters are an important source of drinking water, bacteria which survive the common potabilization procedures have received special attention. Chlorination, the mainly used one, produces high amounts of chloroderivates which not only make waters less suitable for drinking for their uncomfortable taste and smell, but also could be mutagenic and cancerogenic [2]. The use of UV, on the other hand, reduces the previous problems, but produces high quantities of organic matter that cause the bacterial re-growth in the network [3]. Commonly used procedures in drinking plants as quality control are based on the recovery of index micro-organisms which can be linked to the presence of pathogens. However, the reliability of these determinations is poor, it would therefore be worthwhile to know which micro-organisms are present, in order to plan the minimal possible decontamination procedure required to asses quality. It is usually difficult to characterise fresh isolates from aquatic environment. There are several reasons such as the common phenotypic traits, but more importantly the poor diagnostic schemes available for environmental bacteria. The reason is

that taxonomy is continuously rearranged and many novel groups remain to be characterised, specially for environmental micro-organisms. The continuous changes of taxonomy and the identification of new groups bring about the need of a constant up dating from several sources. Moreover, these changes often produce modification of the routinely used identification protocols.
It is therefore felt that a complete, reliable and up to date system that integrates several chemotaxonomic methods to identify aquatic micro-organisms would be very useful. A data base providing a complete and reliable information about the nature, taxonomy and activity of aquatic bacteria can be very useful in order to help the operator to find the most relevant information about the types of bacteria commonly isolated from samples, and could be the first tool in order to start a deeper investigation. Moreover, a database containing chemotaxonomic data connected to pattern analyser system could be helpful in the identification of fresh isolates or as a check of preliminary biochemical identification.

We present a relational database which has been designed in order to provide relevant biochemical and chemotaxonomic information concerning the identification of aquatic bacteria. This database has been connected to a user friendly modular interface, that allows an easy interaction with both laboratory instruments and non technical users. Moreover, the modular and object oriented structure of the system, allows for connection with knowledge acquisition systems [4], which can maintain the database tuned with each taxonomic achievements appearing in the literature.

2. Methods

The system consists of a data base which collects and organises all significant data; a set of interfaces with laboratory instruments; a set of data elaboration procedures.

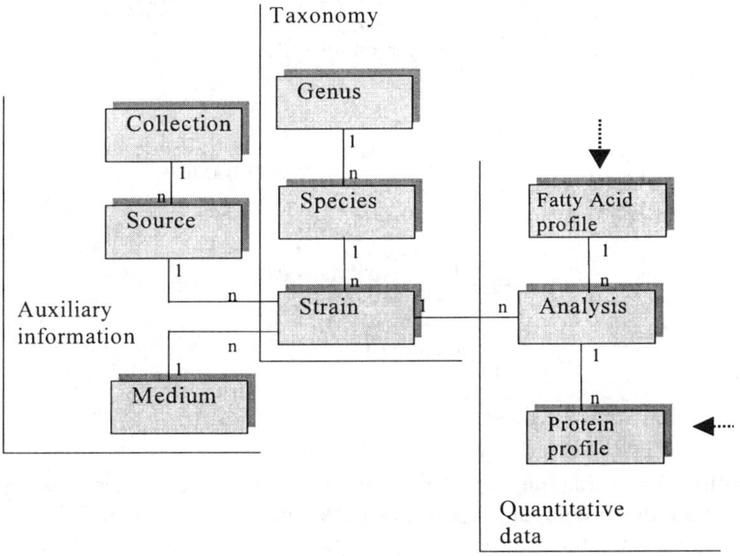

Fig. 1 E-R Level 0

We designed this database for us by non specialized people, so most choices were made aiming to obtain user friendly features. The Windows 95 environment was chosen, due to its wide circulation with workers in the field of biology and environment. The database structure has been developed with the mixed approach [5], starting form both the hierarchical taxonomic structure and the features of the quantitative data to be collected to implement bacteria identification procedures. Fig. 1 shows the level 0 of the Entity-Relation description.

The database has been implemented using Ms Office Access as data base management system, whereas the user interface has been implemented using the Ms Visual Basic programming Language. Fig. 2 shows the main actions which can be performed by the system.

To enhance the user friendly features of the system we used a standard mask. Each mask has three parts: the top part contains information coming from previous taxonomic levels, these information cannot be modified; the medium part contains interaction fields to collect/modify information on the current topic; the bottom part is the sensitive part of the mask with the command buttons and a grid to select the record to display in the medium part of the mask.

The system allows the automatic input of laboratory data coming from different sources. In the present version two interfaces are present: one connects the data base with a gas-chromatograph to record the pattern of whole cellular fatty acids; the other connects our system with a first level image analysis program which produces densitometric curves of the whole cellular protein pattern obtained by electrophoresis.

The system is also connected with artificial neural network based programs to identify strains starting from the considered quantitative features [6,7].

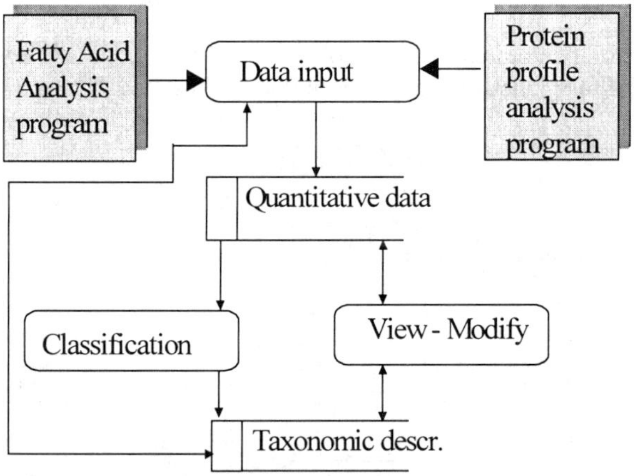

Fig. 2 DFD level 0

3. Results

During the first validation period the data base was used by biologists without any specific preparation in computer science. After a short training period they were able to input rather great amounts of data without any particular problem. Specifically, at this time within the data base there are data on: 35 genera, 141 species, 155 strains, 425 fatty acid profiles, 55 total protein profile. The times of response for any type of interrogations are below one second.

We test the identification system both using fatty acid profiles and protein profiles. In particular, we used a unsupervised neural network to identify genera of 155 strains starting from 425 fatty acid profiles. We used a 20x20 Kohonen neural network implemented in Matlab 4.2. All 10 genera considered, *Alteromonas, Cytophaga, Flavobacterium, Halomonas, Listonella, Marinomonas, Oceanospirillum, Pseudomonas, Shewanella* and *Vibrio*, were distinguishable and overlappings were limited to a few profiles. The same procedure was used to identify species of 16 strains belonging to *Halomonas* genus starting from 55 protein profiles. Using a 8x8 neural network all 6 species, *aquamarina, cupida, halophila, marina, pacifica* and *venusta*, were separated with the exception of only one output neuron containing 1 *H.aquamarina* and 2 *H.marina* profiles.

4. Discussion and Conclusions

The need of a complete, up to date and reliable identification system for environmental and in particular aquatic bacteria, has been pointed out for several years, since this field has gained more and more interest from the scientific community point of view.

The main goals of the present system are:

- to provide a complete and reliable information about the nature, taxonomy and activity of aquatic bacteria
- to contain chemotaxonomic data connected to pattern analyser system for the identification of fresh isolates
- to be simple and user friendly for people with no background in computing
- to allow a connection with knowledge acquisition systems which can update the database according to current literature.

The system is versatile and can be used at different levels. It could be useful in the first place as a simple data base to be consulted for rapid information about the nature, classification and metabolism of aquatic bacteria, and subsequently as a powerful tool for identification of fresh isolates based on their chemotaxonomic features.

Acknowledgement

This study was supported by a grant of the 'Parco Scientifico e Tecnologico della Liguria' within the project: "Sperimentazione di un sistema per il riconoscimento rapido di batteri viventi in acqua".

References

[1] B. Austin, "Taxonomy of marine micro-organisms", in *Marine Microbiology*, B. Austin Ed., Cambridge, Cambridge University Press, 1988, pp. 45-78

[2] G.R. Dyehdala, "Chlorine and chlorine compounds", in *Disinfection, sterilisation and preservation*, S.S. Block Ed., Philadelphia, Lea and Febiger, 1991, pp. 131-151

[3] I.L. Shechmeister, "Sterilisation by ultraviolet irradiation" in *Disinfection, sterilisation and preservation*, S.S. Block Ed., Philadelphia, Lea and Febiger, 1991, pp. 553-565

[4] G. Schreiber, B. Wielinga, H. Akkermas, W. Van de Welde, and A. Anjewierden "CML: the CommonKADS Conceptual Modelling Language", in A future for knowledge acquisition. Proceedings of the 8th European Knowledge Acquisition Worshop, EKAW'94, 1994, pp. 1-25

[5] C. Batini, S. Ceri, S.B. Navathe: "Conceptual database design". 1992, The Benjamin/Cummings Publishing Company, Inc. (Redwood City, CA – USA)

[6] S. Bertone, M. Giacomini, C. Ruggiero, C. Piccarolo, L. Calegari: "Automated systems for identification of heterotrophic marine bacteria by using their fatty acid composition". Applied and environmental microbiology, 1996, vol. 62, n° 6, pp. 2122-2132

[7] M. Giacomini, C. Ruggiero, S. Bertone, L. Calegari: "Artificial neural network identification of heterotrophic marine bacteria based on their fatty acid composition". IEEE Transactions on Biomedical Engineering, 1997, vol. 44, n° 12, pp. 1185-1191

Medical Informatics Europe '99
P. Kokol et al. (Eds.)
IOS Press, 1999

A Diagnostic Advice System based on Pathophysiological Models of Diseases*

Willem Jan ter Burg
Department of Medical Informatics
Academic Medical Centre, University of Amsterdam
Meibergdreef 15, 1105 AZ Amsterdam, The Netherlands
E-mail: W.J.ter Burg@amc.uva.nl

Peter Lucas
Department of Computer Science, Utrecht University
Padualaan 14, 3584 CH Utrecht, The Netherlands
E-mail: lucas@cs.uu.nl

Edith ter Braak
Department of Internal Medicine, University Medical Centre
Heidelberglaan 100, 3584 CX Utrecht, The Netherlands
E-mail: E.terBraak@digd.azu.nl

Abstract

Medical decision-support systems in which uncertainty plays an essential role are increasingly based on the formalism of probabilistic networks. Although this formalism is very powerful, the construction of actual networks is not straightforward, and requires the availability of clearly structured medical domain models as a starting point. In this paper it is argued that medical pathophysiological knowledge constitutes a good start for the development of such models, even though pathophysiological knowledge is semantically different from probabilistic knowledge. Two models concerning anaemia, which are part of a broad system covering the domain of anaemia, are discussed to illustrate the general approach.

Keywords: medical decision support, probabilistic networks, Bayesian networks.

1 Introduction

The proper clinical management of diseases in patients requires the handling of large quantities of uncertain medical knowledge. It is, therefore, not surprising that the representation and manipulation of uncertainty has been one of the key issues in the development of systems for medical decision support. Although a large number of different approaches to the representation of uncertain medical knowledge has been proposed in the past, it is increasingly believed by researchers that probability theory offers one of the best foundations for building medical decision-support systems [3, 4]. A major advantage of the probabilistic approach is the seamless integration with

*This research is supported by the Technology Foundation STW, applied science division of NWO, and the technology programme of the Ministre of Economic Affairs.

conventional medical statistics, such as the possibility to use clinical data for assessing uncertainty.

However, it is well-known that the construction of probabilistic models may impose unrealistic demands with respect to the amount of patient data required, a problem that is even more significant when dealing with rare disorders [3]. Such disorders are usually sparsely represented in clinical databases. The general problem of probability assessment may, in principle, be alleviated by adopting simplifying probabilistic independence assumptions, thus relaxing the requirements with respect to the number of patients needed. However, gathering relevant probabilistic independence information from various sources is a problem in itself.

In this paper, we investigate whether pathophysiological knowledge, as found in the medical literature, offers a sufficient basis to guide the development of probabilistic models. Moreover, we show how separately developed disease models can be integrated to obtain larger models. Pathophysiological models of two causes of anaemia, vitamin B_{12} and folic acid deficiency, have been designed for this purpose. The formalism of probabilistic networks (Bayesian networks) [2, 4] has been used for the representation of the resulting probabilistic models.

The structure of this paper is as follows. In the following section, the problem of diagnosing anaemia in patients is briefly reviewed. In Section 3, the theory of probabilistic networks is introduced, and models of anaemia are described from various perspectives. In Section 4, the results of a preliminary evaluation of the resulting model are presented, and finally in Section 5, we discuss future research.

2 Clinical diagnosis of disease resulting in anaemia

In the context of this research, *anaemia* was defined as a blood hemoglobin level below the lower bound of the reference values, considered clinically relevant and prompting further diagnostic procedures. This condition may give rise to a variety of general symptoms and signs, like fatigue, paleness, palpitations, exercise-related shortness of breath, and dizziness. Anaemia in general may be due to: (1) impaired production of red blood cells, (2) loss of red blood cells, or (3) increased degradation of red blood cells. The processes of production and degradation of red blood cells have been unravelled the last century up to the molecular level. The same is true for many forms of anaemia for which the pathophysiology is described quite detailed in the medical literature.

Examples of causes of anaemia are vitamin B_{12} and folic acid deficiency. Vitamin B_{12} and folic acid are both essential elements in DNA synthesis. Impaired DNA synthesis results in disturbed, ineffective formation of large red blood cells with certain features (megaloblastic cells), and in anaemia. Two diseases that may cause vitamin B_{12} deficiency are pernicious anaemia and atrophic gastritis.

Information from the patient history and physical examination, as well as results of laboratory tests, and sometimes imaging techniques, are required for making a diagnosis in the domain of anaemia. It is not always clear which tests are most informative for effective diagnosis making; a decision-support system could be very helpful in this respect.

3 A probabilistic model of anaemia

The central question was how pathophysiological knowledge from the literature could be used as a basis for the representation of the uncertainty underlying diagnosis of anaemia. This meant that we had to look for a mapping of pathophysiological knowledge to the formalism of probabilistic networks. The formalism of probabilistic networks is first briefly introduced. Next, we discuss how designed pathophysiological models can be mapped to probabilistic networks.

3.1 Probabilistic networks

A *probabilistic network*, also call Bayesian (belief) network, is a directed acyclic graph $G = (V_G, A_G)$, consisting of a set of vertices $V_G = \{V_1, \ldots, V_n\}$, representing discrete stochastic variables, and a set of arcs $A_G \subseteq V_G \times V_G$, representing stochastic influences among variables [3]. If a binary variable V assumes the value *true*, this is denoted by v; if it assumes the value *false*, this is denoted by $\neg v$. Assigning a value to a variable is called *instantiating* the variable.

On the set of vertices V_G is defined a joint probability distribution P that can be factorised according to the topology of the graph as follows:

$$P(V_1, \ldots, V_n) = \prod_{i=1}^{n} P(V_i | \pi(V_i))$$

where $\pi(V_i)$ denotes the set of parent vertices of vertex V_i. As this equation indicates, it is only necessary to represent local probabilistic information $P(V_i|\pi(V_i))$ to obtain the joint probability distribution P, because the variable V_i is assumed conditionally independent of all predecessors with the exception of the parents, given the parents.

A probabilistic network not only offers a compact representation of uncertain knowledge; it can also be viewed as an architecture for probabilistic inference. To determine the effects of evidence on the probabilistic information, several algorithms have been proposed that take a probabilistic network and a set of evidence E as input, and produce as a result an updated joint probability distribution [2, 4]. It appears that the marginal probability of a variable V_i in the Boolean algebra that results when evidence E is given, denoted by $P'(V_i)$, is exactly the same as the posterior probability distribution given the evidence, i.e. $P(V_i|E)$: $P'(V_i) = P(V_i|E)$. When the variable V_i represents a diagnostic category, the probability $P'(V_i)$ represents the updated, marginal probability distribution after processing evidence. It can be compared to the prior marginal probability $P(V_i)$, and this will indicate to what extent a diagnosis is (dis)confirmed by this evidence E.

3.2 Design of pathophysiological models

Although the medical literature on anaemia includes elaborate descriptions of the mechanisms underlying diseases causing anaemia, no complete *pathophysiological models* are available. Such models were designed from scratch, using directed acyclic graphs as the main modelling tool; in the graphs, arcs had the meaning of cause-effect relationships, and vertices were used to represent disease states, test results and disease categories. A small part of a large pathophysiological model of vitamin B_{12} deficiency is shown in Figure 1. Ellipses indicate test results, single boxes indicate states, and the double box represents a diagnostic category. The resulting graphs may be seen as *qualitative, causal models* of anaemia.

3.3 Mapping pathophysiological to probabilistic models

Although causal knowledge is not the same as probabilistic knowledge, notions of causality may guide the development of probabilistic models [1]. Let $c_1 \Rightarrow e, \ldots, c_m \Rightarrow e$

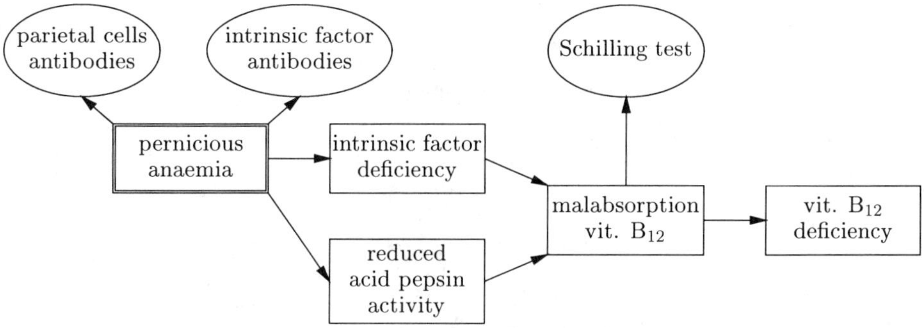

Figure 1: Small part of a qualitative model of vitamin B_{12} deficiency with disease category pernicious anaemia.

represent multiple causes $c_1, \ldots, c_m$ for a given effect e, such as '*pernicious anaemia* $\Rightarrow$ *intrinsic factor deficiency*'. The first step in the transformation concerns viewing a cause c_j and effect e as the stochastic variable V_{c_j} and V_e, respectively, with associated value domain. For most variables, the adopted value domain was binary.

Since a causal relation $\Rightarrow$ induces a stochastic dependency, causal direction can be employed as a heuristic in the modelling process. The main difficulty in the modelling process lies in the representation of possible interactions among the various causes; for the situation described above we would have to assess the probability distribution $P(V_e|V_{c_1}, \ldots, V_{c_m})$, which means assessing to what extent the causes $c_1, \ldots, c_m$ augment or weaken each other. As an example, consider the interaction between the causes *intrinsic factor deficiency* and *reduced acid pepsin activity* and the effect *malabsorption vit.* B_{12}. These variables, which are conditionally independent given *pernicious anaemia*, augment each other. In this way, the design of local interactions was guided by knowledge of pathophysiological interactions.

Besides such local interactions, which model the combined (probabilistic) effect of several causes, there are also interactions among causes which arise when combining separate disease models. Medical experts tend to devide knowledge concerning a medical domain into subdomains with relatively little overlap. When each subdomain is represented as a probabilistic network, the resulting combined model will have a *modular structure*, with some shared variables. The connection between the modules is accomplished by different types of shared variables. The possible situations are schematically depicted in Figure 2, where two modules describing separate disease mechanisms are shown. Each module contains one or more diagnostic categories, like *pernicious anaemia*. Note that we do not assume disorders to be mutually exclusive, because they have not been represented as values of a single stochastic variable.

The vertex with label C conditions the modules on particular evidence; in medicine, usually evidence concerning age or sex. The amount of probabilistic information to be specified is limited, because only prior probabilistic information $P(C)$ has to be specified. Propagation of this evidence through the modules can be done efficiently, if the module content is not too complex (i.e. the module graph is sparse). Note that the modules A and B can be developed separately, provided that the variable C is always instantiated, and that the variables T, G and all variables within the common mechanism are not instantiated. Under these conditions, the modules are independent. After separate constructions, the modules can be put together.

A major problem in putting modules together lies in the exponential number of

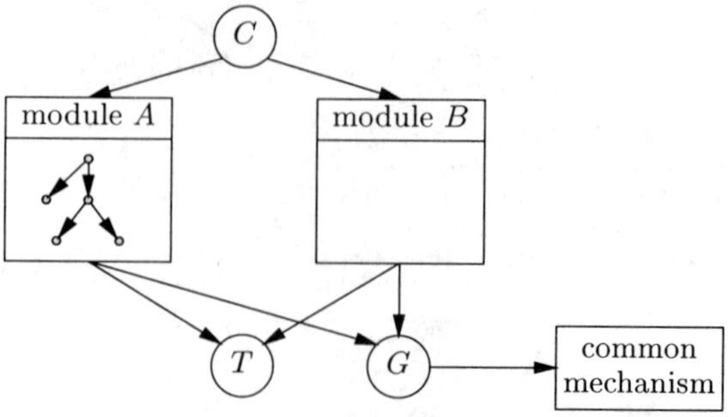

Figure 2: Modularisation of anaemia domain.

probabilities that must be specified for vertices like T and G. Vertex T represent a test result; since many tests are shared by different diseases causing anaemia, there may be many incoming arcs to T. By using a logical OR operator for combining probabilistic influence, a quite compact representation can be obtained. The resulting probabilistic behaviour is called a *noisy-OR gate* [4]. A noisy-OR gate saves in the number of probabilities to be specified, which is linear in the number of incoming arcs instead of exponential, and also in the time complexity of probabilistic inference.

The variable G is as T a shared variable, but since this variable concerns a common mechanism, and only few mechanisms among various modules are identical, the number of incoming arcs will not be very large. Rather, there will be a number of different common mechanisms shared by various modules, and there will be no need for use of the noisy-OR gate here.

The module structure shown in Figure 2 actually reflects the structure of the probabilistic model of two causes of anaemia, vitamin B_{12} and folic acid deficiency. Variables T are for example platelets and leucocytes counts; the variable G in this case stands for megaloblastic erythropoiesis, i.e. the production of megaloblastic cells, which occurs in both deficiencies.

4 Evaluation

Above, we have described the process of designing a probabilistic model, based on pathophysiological, qualitative knowledge from the medical literature. The constructed qualitative models provide strong support for the correctness of the structure of the resulting network model. However, by carrying out simulation experiments with patient cases, we have also investigated whether the actual probabilistic influences were as expected. Moreover, the posterior probabilities have been compared to frequency information (such as frequency of positive and negative test results, i.e. sensitivity and specificity, for certain diseases) from the literature. Based on the results of these experiments, the probabilistic model was slightly adjusted.

Furthermore, we have done a number of experiments with patient data, where in particular the effects of the systematic gathering of evidence, as is common practice in medicine, has been studied. The results for two patients are shown in Table 1. As can be seen, during three subsequent visits of a patient to the clinic, additional test results become available. For patient A the evidence slowly moves in the direction of pernicious anaemia when more specific information becomes available. In patient B, gastroscopy is the final test demonstrating atrophic gastritis. The results for both patients illustrate the capability of the system to guide the medical decision-making process.

Table 1: Results of the probabilistic model for two patients.

Patient A			**Patient B**		
Visit 1			*Visit 1*		
Hb	7.8	decreased	Hb	7.2	decreased
MCV	118	increased	MCV	104	increased
platelets	160	normal	reticulocytes	0.4 %	increased
leukocytes	4.1	normal	gastrointestinal symptoms		present
			neuropsychological symptoms		present
$P(pernicious\ anaemia)$	0.01			0.04	
$P(atrophic\ gastritis)$	0.01			0.03	
Visit 2			*Visit 2*		
haptoglobin	< 0.1	decreased	pentagastrin test		positive
LDH	667	increased	serum gastrin		increased
serum folate	21.1	normal	serum folate	17	normal
serum vit. B_{12}	59	decreased	serum vit. B_{12}	72	decreased
$P(pernicious\ anaemia)$	0.04			0.07	
$P(atrophic\ gastritis)$	0.03			0.07	
Visit 3			*Visit 3*		
TSH	1.4	normal	gastroscopy		atrophic gastritis
parietal cells antibodies	+++	yes			
intrinsic factor antibod.	+	yes			
$P(pernicious\ anaemia)$	0.82			0.00	
$P(atrophic\ gastritis)$	0.01			1.00	

5 Discussion

In this paper, we have shown that pathophysiological knowledge from the literature can be used to support the process of making a medical diagnosis. We have also discussed how separate models of subdomains can be integrated to obtain larger models. Obviously, this approach will only work when elaborate pathophysiological descriptions are available in the literature. Clearly, this does not hold for medicine in general, but there are many medical domains where this approach will work.

References

[1] M. Korver and P.J.F. Lucas, Converting a rule-based expert system into a belief network, Medical Informatics, 18(3) (1993) 219–241.

[2] S.L. Lauritzen and D.J. Spiegelhalter, Local computations with probabilities on graphical structures and their application to expert systems, Journal of the Royal Statistical Society (Series B), 50 (1987) 157–224.

[3] P.J.F. Lucas and L.C. van der Gaag, Principles of Expert Systems, Addison-Wesley, Wokingham, 1991.

[4] J. Pearl, Probabilistic Reasoning in Intelligent Systems, Morgan Kaufman, San Mateo, California, 1988.

Medical Informatics Europe '99
P. Kokol et al. (Eds.)
IOS Press, 1999

Modelling Oculomotor Data with Decision Tree Induction

Kati VIIKKI[a], Elina ISOTALO[b], Martti JUHOLA[a], Ilmari PYYKKÖ[c]
[a]*Department of Computer Science, University of Tampere, P.O.Box 607, FIN-33101 Tampere, Finland. Email: kv@cs.uta.fi*
[b]*Department of Otorhinolaryngology, Helsinki University Hospital, Helsinki, Finland*
[c]*Department of Otorhinolaryngology, Karolinska Hospital, Stockholm, Sweden*

Abstract. We studied relationships between oculomotor test results and the site of lesion in the data set containing patient cases with operated cerebello-pontine angle tumour, operated hemangioblastoma, infarction of cerebello-brainstem or Meniere's disease and control subjects. Several classification models were generated by decision tree induction to find parameter combinations which are efficient in classification. The studied data were characterised by missing values and scarcity of example cases. This study suggested that decision tree induction can be a useful method even in problematic real world classification tasks. Models generated by decision tree induction and evaluated by an expert physician may give information that is beneficial for research.
Keywords: Decision trees; Modelling; Otoneurology; Dizziness

1. Introduction

Decision tree induction [1] is one of the most popular machine learning methods used to generate classification models from a set of example cases. Generated models may give new information about the data set, and if the data are representative, these models can be expected to classify unseen cases correctly. Various medical decision making problems can be transformed into classification tasks, and decision tree induction has been employed widely in medical domains. Decision trees offer not only a decision, but also an explanation and their symbolic representation makes them intelligible and easily scrutinised.

In our earlier work [2,3], we applied decision tree induction to extract relevant parameters from the database of an otoneurologic expert system ONE [4] that is aimed to assist in decision making process for both peripheral and central diseases involving vertigo. In this study, we wanted to examine relationships between oculomotor test parameters and the site of lesion in the data set containing patient cases with operated cerebello-pontine angle (CPA) tumour, operated hemangioblastoma (HAB), infarction of cerebello-brainstem or Meniere's disease and control subjects. We constructed decision trees aiming to find parameter combinations, which are useful in classifying cases to the groups, based on the site of lesion.

2. Material and Methods

The data were gathered in the Department of Otorhinolaryngology at Helsinki University Hospital during the years 1990 – 1996. It contained 137 patient cases and 78 control subjects (Table 1). To study relationships between the voluntary eye movements and the site of lesion, the data were rearranged in classes according to the site of lesion [5] (Table 1). The groups of brainstem lesion, cerebellar lesion and cerebello-brainstem lesion were further combined in the group of central lesion. In the decision tree tests, both classification systems based on the site of lesion were used.

Table 1 - Data set

Diagnosis	N	Site of lesion	N
Control subject	78	Control subject	78
Cerebello-pontine angle (CPA) tumour	35	Brainstem	25
Hemangioblastoma (HAB)	20	Cerebello	17
Infarction of cerebello-brainstem	20	Cerebello-brainstem	13
Meniere's disease	62	Peripheral	70
		Non-classified	12
Total	215		215

The eye movement parameters used to describe cases are listed in Table 2. All eye movement signals were electro-oculographically recorded with skin electrodes in a common way [6-8]. The frequency combinations employed for stimulating random pursuit eye movements (RPEMs) were 0.15 and 0.35 Hz, 0.25 and 0.425 Hz, 0.3 and 0.7 Hz, and 0.45 and 0.7 Hz [5]. For constant amplitude saccades, saccades of 60° amplitude were studied, and for random amplitude saccades, saccades of 20° and 60° amplitudes were studied [5]. Totally there were 66 parameters of which all were continuous.

Table 2 - Parameters

Random pursuit eye movements	Saccadic eye movements
Best gain (gain value closest to 1) Minimum, mean and maximum gain by amplitude Minimum, mean and maximum gain by integration Minimum, mean and maximum phase shift Gain by Fast Fourier Transform Usage percent (signal duration decreased by sum of all saccades detected)	Ipsilateral and contralateral accuracy Ipsilateral and contralateral latency Ipsilateral and contralateral maximum velocity

With this data set, we encountered a problem that is typical for real world classification tasks: incompleteness of data. Only 70 from 215 cases were complete. Because of the great number of missing values and the missing value patterns within the diagnosis groups, any imputation method could not be used to fill in missing values. By discarding attributes and cases, we made 11 complete training sets of which two sets contained only RPEMs, three sets contained only saccades and six sets contained both RPEMs and saccades. The number of cases in these sets varied from 70 to 142.

We studied the data sets containing RPEMs to find the best frequency combination for RPEMs. Decision trees were first constructed using all the frequency combinations at the same time and then using one frequency combination at a time. From this part of the study all the patients with Meniere's disease were excluded, because they had test results only for the frequency combination 0.25 and 0.425 Hz.

According to preliminary studies [5], the mean gain by amplitude (GA) and the mean phase shift seemed to be the most important parameters in the group of RPEMs. We constructed decision trees using first all RPEM parameters and then using only the mean GA and the mean phase shift.

For saccadic eye movements, we examined whether the mean values calculated for ipsilateral and contralateral test values would yield better classification results. Decision trees were constructed using original values, mean values and finally, both original and mean values.

Decision trees were constructed using Quinlan's See5 [9] classifier generator, a descendant of C4.5 [10]. See5 takes, as its input, a set of cases with attribute values and class information and generates a decision tree in which inner nodes are tests based on attributes and leaf nodes are class labels. Decision trees are usually evaluated with a separate test set or cross-validation. Because of the small size of data sets we used neither way, but constructed decision trees using all the cases of each data set as a training set and the expert physician evaluated constructed trees by examining them branch by branch.

3. Results

For each decision tree, classification accuracy was calculated as a ratio of correctly classified cases to all cases used in the tree construction. Although the classification accuracy values were over-optimistic because decision trees were tailored for training sets, we used them to examine differences in accuracy between different attribute combinations. No statistically significant differences were found between the frequency combinations used for stimulating RPEMs. From this comparison all the Meniere patients were excluded. The difference between the results for the group of all RPEMs and the results for the combination of the mean GA and the mean phase shift was not statistically significant. In the comparison of the original saccade parameters and the calculated mean parameters, no statistically significant differences were found.

In decision tree construction, two classification systems based on the site of lesion were employed. There was a statistically significant difference (p=.000) in classification accuracy between these systems. For the system with the three classes (control subject, central lesion and peripheral lesion), the mean classification accuracy was 91%, and for the system with the five classes (control subject, brainstem lesion, cerebellar lesion, cerebello-brainstem lesion and peripheral lesion), the mean classification accuracy was 88%.

Table 3 – Results for training sets

Site of lesion	**Mean true positive rate (%) (±SD)**	
	3 classes	5 classes
Control subjects	93 (±11)	96 (±5)
Central	93 (±11)	
Brainstem		88 (±11)
Cerebello		84 (±14)
Cerebello-brainstem		83 (±14)
Peripheral	72 (±25)	77 (±18)

For each class, true positive rate was calculated as a ratio of correctly classified cases to the total number of cases in the class. Mean true positive rates for the classes of both classification systems are seen in Table 3. For the control subjects and the patients with peripheral lesion, better results were achieved with the 5 classes. For the patients with brainstem lesion, cerebellar lesion or cerebello-brainstem lesion, better results were reached when the patient cases were combined into the group of central lesion. The control subjects and the patients with central lesion were the easiest groups to model. The group of peripheral lesion was the most difficult one to distinguish. This result was expected because the group of peripheral lesion contains the Meniere patients, and the Meniere patients have been difficult to classify in our earlier studies [2,3].

4. Discussion

Numerous decision trees were generated from the oculomotor data to examine relationships between oculomotor test parameters and the site of lesion. Our aim was to find effective attribute combinations that yield accurate classification models.

None of the frequency combinations used to stimulate RPEMs appeared to be better than other combinations, and using all the frequency combinations at the same time did not yield better results. When saccade parameters were employed in decision tree construction with the RPEM parameters, the mean gain by amplitude and the mean phase shift were adequate from the group of RPEMs. The usage of mean values calculated for saccadic values did not yield better classification results. These results confirmed the expectations of the expert physician based on previous studies [5].

Best results were achieved when the ability of performance of the subjects was taken into account; i.e. both RPEMs and saccadic eye movements were included in decision tree construction. This result is reasonable because results of different tests and their parameters vary according to the site of lesion: some patients may have good results in some test for some parameters and weak results for other parameters or in other tests [5]. Decision trees were constructed using two classification systems based on the site of lesion. The classification system with the three classes (control subject, central lesion and peripheral lesion) yielded better results, and the difference between the systems was statistically significant.

According to the expert physician's opinion, generated decision trees were reasonable although there were trees with some "strange" branches. Decision trees found general patterns from the data and, furthermore, they were able to classify rare cases [5]. Classification paths from roots to leaves gave adequate explanations for decisions [5].

Because of the scarcity of the data and the great number of missing values, these results cannot be generalised. To get more reliable results, tests should be performed with an augmented data set. Even though the generated decision tree models cannot be used in diagnostic work, they are beneficial giving new information that physicians can utilise in their research work.

References

[1] J.R. Quinlan, Induction of decision trees, *Machine Learning* **1** (1986) 81-106.

[2] E. Kentala, K. Viikki, I. Pyykkö and M. Juhola, Production of diagnostic rules from a neurotologic database with decision trees. Accepted to *Annals of Otology, Rhinology & Laryngology*.

[3] K. Viikki, E. Kentala, M. Juhola and I. Pyykkö, Decision tree induction in the diagnosis of oto-neurologic diseases. Submitted to *Medical Informatics*.

[4] E. Kentala, I. Pyykkö, Y. Auramo and M. Juhola, Otoneurological expert system, *Annals of Otology, Rhinology & Laryngology* **105** (1996) 654-658.

[5] E. Isotalo, The human oculomotor system. A clinical, physiological and methodological study of voluntary eye movements. Doctoral Thesis, Manuscript. University of Helsinki, 1999.

[6] M. Juhola, I. Pyykkö and H. Aalto, A microcomputer system for clinical signal analysis of vestibular laboratory, *Journal of Medical Systems* **13** (1989) 205-213.

[7] M. Juhola, A syntactic analysis method for sinusoidal tracking eye movements, *Computers and Biomedical Research* **24** (1991) 222-233.

[8] H. Aalto, M. Juhola and I. Pyykkö, Visual stimulator system using laser beam for eye movement studies, *Medical & Biological Engineering & Computing* **27** (1989) 332-335.

[9] J.R. Quinlan, *See5, version 1.07a,* http://www.rulequest.com/, 1998.

[10] J.R. Quinlan, *C4.5: Programs for machine learning*. Morgan Kaufmann Publishers, San Mateo, 1993.

Medical Informatics Europe '99
P. Kokol et al. (Eds.)
IOS Press, 1999

A Decision Support System for Cholinesterase Genotyping

Richards B[a], Cadman J[a], France M[b]
a. Dept of Medical Informatics, UMIST, Manchester, England
b. Biochemistry Dept, Manchester Royal Infirmary, England

Abstract. Cholinesterase is a naturally occurring enzyme in the human body. Its importance became apparent when it was recognised that patients undergoing surgery and carrying abnormal genes for this enzyme were unable to recover from a dose of muscle-relaxant. It is therefore important to know the Genotype (the pair of genes) of a patient who might undergo surgery. The computer programme takes laboratory measurements and applies mathematical techniques and clinical judgements to determine the two genes present.

1. Introduction

Cholinesterase, more correctly called "acetyl cholinesterase", is an enzyme which occurs in human muscles, in the red blood cells, and in the serum. Its exact composition is governed by genes on each of the two chromosomes. An adult with normal cholinesterase can be regarded as having two normal genes UU, one on each of the chromosomes. This person will be homozygous (UU) for cholinesterase activity and will be classed as "normal". Some individuals will have a deficient gene (g) on one of their chromosomes and will therefore be heterozygous (Ug). Such individuals will have a somewhat reduced level of cholinesterase. The true abnormal homozygote (gg) will have a considerably reduced level of cholinesterase in their serum. These latter individuals will have a serum cholinesterase level of around 1 iu/L as compared with the serum from a normal homozygote (2 to 5 iu/L). Only 0.3% of the population have the homozygous abnormal genotype.

Why is cholinesterase deemed to be so important? When patients in hospital have to undergo a general anaesthetic, it is necessary for the anaesthetist to administer a muscle-relaxant in order to pass the intubation tube down the throat and into the trachea. To achieve this the patient must first of all be put to sleep and then a muscle-relaxant administered so that the muscles of the throat and trachea relax to permit the passage of the intubation tube.

Now the muscle relaxant used is generally the drug Suxamethonium. This drug has a very short active life (half-life) when administered to "normal" subjects. That is because the cholinesterase reacts with the Suxamethonium and metabolises it very rapidly. A dose of 0.6mg/kg of Suxamethonium will relax an adult in 30 to 60 seconds and the effect will last from 2 to 6 minutes. This is because the Suxamethonium will be broken down by the cholinesterase so then little remains after this time period. However, in the case of the homozygous abnormal patient, the levels of cholinesterase are anything up to 5 times lower than in the normal patient. The result of this is that the muscle relaxant does not metabolise, therefore the effect does not wear off and hence the patient is immobilised whether conscious or unconscious. Hence, without muscle contractility, the patient cannot breath and should this happen, the patient would have to be put on a ventilator until the effect of the muscle relaxant wears off, which may be several hours. This condition, of the patient being unable to breath unaided, is termed "Choline Apnoea".

Serum levels of cholinesterase are reduced in patients with Liver Disease, Anaemia, in pernicious anaemia, in the abnormal homozygous patient, and in patients suffering poisoning from organo-phosphorous compounds.

2. The Laboratory Practice

Hospital Biochemistry Departments will measure the activity level of cholinesterase in a patient's serum. [This "activity level" is the same as the serum level quoted above; the reason for this additional, more usual, terminology is that one can only measure the presence of an enzyme by measuring its "activity"]. The laboratory will then re-measure this activity in the presence of various "inhibitors" eg Dibucaine, Fluoride, Scoline, and RO. These latter reduce the activity in the cholinesterase but the reduction is non-uniform, the extent of the reduction will depend on the genes in the two chromosomes. As has been stated, the normal cholinesterase gene is U, and the abnormal genes are A, F, J, K and S. So individuals can present with various genotypes, those being the permutations of the genes quoted above. The combinations of clinical interest are: UU (normal), UF, FF, UA, AK, AF, AJ, AA, AS, SS. So when one measures the reduced activity in the presence of, say, Dibucaine, one will attempt to identify the genotype according to the measure of the "activity removed by the inhibitor". This latter is, mathematically, (Level without inhibitor - level with inhibitor) ie Level of activity removed = Level without inhibitor - level with inhibitor. This is usually scaled by division by the un-inhibited level and multiplied by 100 to give a "percentage removed", so:-

$$\text{percentage removed} = \frac{\text{activity without - activity with}}{\text{activity without}} \times 100$$

This calculation is performed for every different inhibitor. So, for Dibucaine, the percentage removed, expressed as the nearest integer, is referred to as the Dibucaine Number. To identify the genotype it is then necessary to "pattern-match" the Dibucaine Number against the current laboratory values for the various genotypes. Thus typically one might find the following:-

	SS	AS	AA	AJ	AF	AK	AU	FF	UF	UU
DN	0	16	21	42	45	54	62	67	74	80

So a patient with a DN of 72 would be thought of as having a genotype of UF. Alas these DN numbers for the genotypes are not "fixed" but only represent a mid-point or a median of a range of values in patients known to be UF through chromosome or other studies. So the range of DN numbers for a patient with a Genotype of UF is 67 to 80! Likewise for FF the range is 66-74 and for UU it is 73 to 89. So the question arises "If the DN number is 70 what is the Genotype?" "If the DN number is 77 what is the Genotype?"

In situations like this, one must invoke all the known data. So one would compare the diagnosis based on the DN number, with that based on the Fluoride Number FN, and on the Scoline Number SN.

Then one must also take into account the frequencies of the various Genotypes observed in the population. Thus 96% of the population will be UU; less than 4% will be UA, and the rest will be quite rare, eg AF will be 1/20,000.

The Decision Support System will analyse the Laboratory results obtained for DN, FN, SN, and RO and will attempt to discover the Genotype. Probabilities will be assigned to the diagnosis based on the closeness of the measured values to the median values and taking into account the frequency of occurrence of the various genotypes in the general population. This will then provide the doctor with all the information which can be gleaned from the laboratory data. He will merge this with other information from the family history, particularly studies of the family pedigree.

3. The Database

For reasons which should be obvious to any clinical informaticist, it was prudent to create a Database for use in the Laboratory which deals with the Cholinesterase Analysis. The reason for the Database is two fold, viz to aid in the administration and record keeping in the laboratory and to form part of the Electronic Patient Record (EPR). Given the existence of the Laboratory results in this Record, the Decision Support System can then make its suggested alternative diagnoses.

The Database, constructed around the ACCESS system, comprises four essential modules, viz Patient ID and data input, Genotype Analysis, Database Analysis Reporting, and Result Letters to the source of the referral.

Figure 1 below shows the ID screen and indicates the Reason for Referreal. Figure 2 shows the Laboratory Results. In this latter one can see recorded the Total (cholinesterase) Enzyme Activity, viz 0.9807, and <u>two</u> laboratory assays using, in turn, each of the inhibitors Dibucaine, Fluoride, Scholine, and RO20688. These values comprise the raw data. The computer then calculates the mean of the two laboratory measurements on each inhibitor and works out the percentage activity removed according to the formula given above which can be re-written as

Percent = [(T-D)/D] x 100

This formula produces the result shown in the right hand column of Figure 2

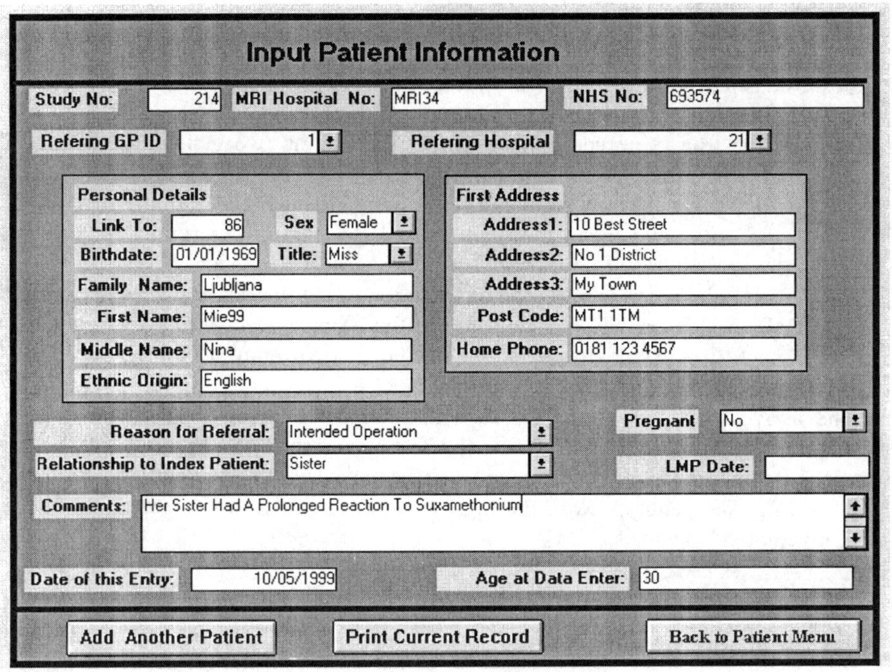

Figure 1. Input of Patient data

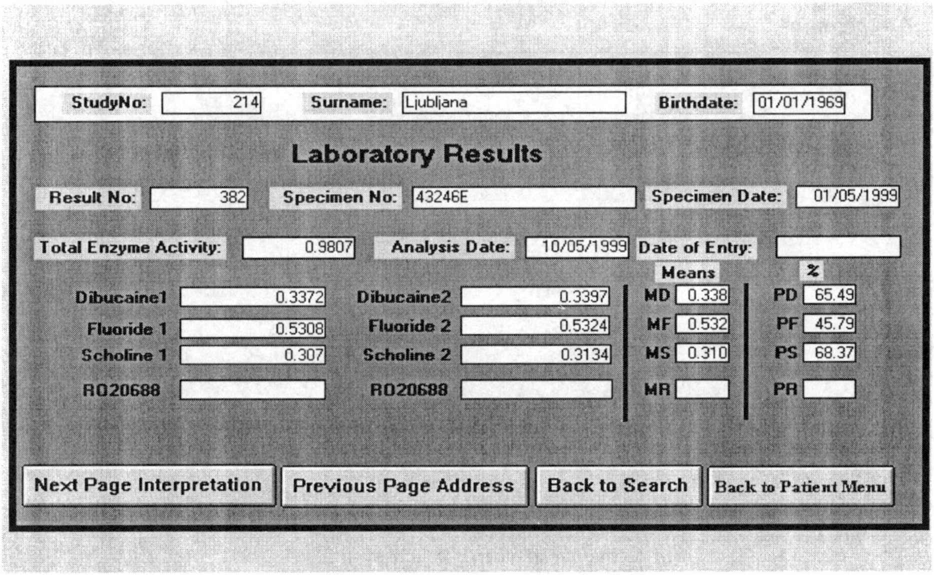

Figure 2. Input of Laboratory Analyses

4. The Decision-Support-System

Figure 3 shows some of the workings within the Decision Support System. For each inhibitor, eg Dibucaine, the Percentage is placed on the Genotype scale in relation to the probabilities of the true Genotype belonging to either of the two genotypes flanking the occurring value. For example, in Figure 3, one sees the Percentage Dibucaine as 65.49. The two "flanking" genotypes would therefore be UA(62) and FF(67). In the first Method, Method One, the arithmetic mean between those latter two is determined in the ratios (65.49 - 62) to (67-65.49) resulting in "probabilities" of 30.2%(UA) and 69.8% respectively. This calculation is based on an assumption that the Standard Deviation of the genotype UA about its Mean (62) is the same as the Standard Deviation for the genotype FF. In actual fact, these standard deviations are not known more accurately: new values will emerge from the present database.

The above procedures are then carried out for the Fluoride, Scholine, and RO determinations, and the results entered into the Tableau as shown in Figure 3. The figures of each genotype column are then summed, with equal weighting, to give the Probability Array as shown. The genotype with the highest result is chosen and entered into the box marked Unweighted Diagnosis.

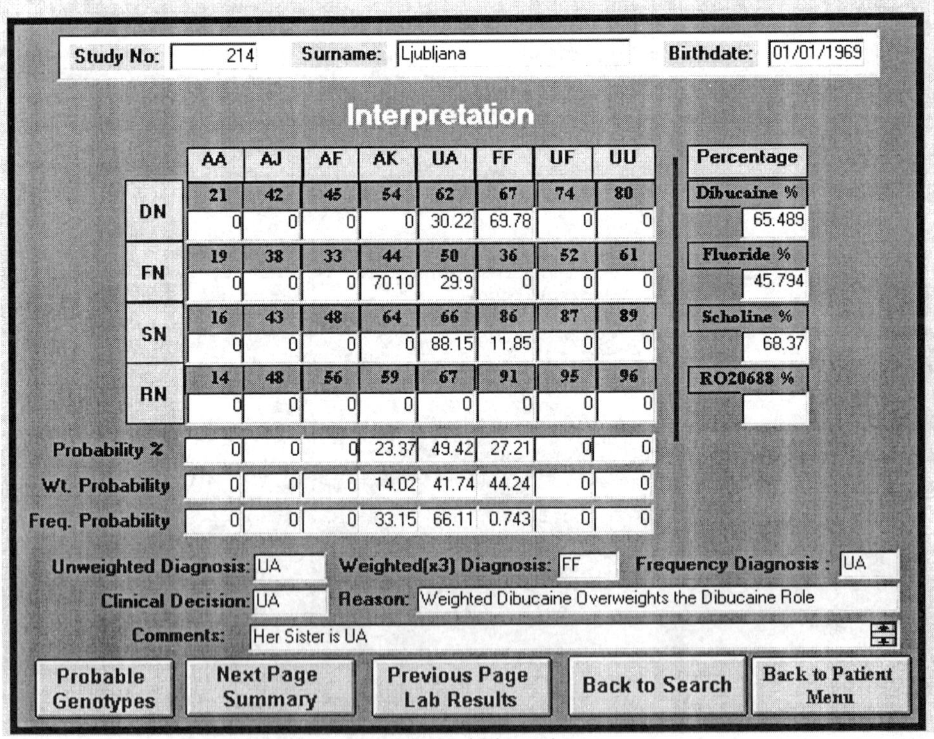

Figure 3. Interpretation and Diagnosis

The "logic" often used by the clinician is to give primary weighting to the Dibucaine values and to use the other three Inhibitors as confirmation. This logic was encapsulated into Method Two wherein the Dibucaine values were weighted in the performance of the summation referred to earlier. Such weighting gives rise to the Weighted(x3) Diagnois FF as shown in Figure 3

In Method Three, genotype frequencies are used. These vary from one ethnic group to another. The outcome of using the Genotype Frequency will be entered into the Dibucaine, Fluoride, Scholine, and RO rows as two percentages as in the previous manner. The unweighted results will then produce the Probability Array, and the Genotype corresponding to the highest value (UA) will be displayed in the Frequency Diagnosis box.

5. Evaluation

This system has proved to be of immense value to the clinicians - the Clinical Biochemists - as it provides a range of results in some of the difficult cases or a unique result in others. The clinician then has to evaluate these results in the light of other information such as family pedigree for this condition and other information. Cf Figure 3, where the Sister was UA.

6. Conclusion

The system has proved to be of enormous value firstly as an Administrative Database for improving the efficiency in the tracking of specimens and reporting thereof; and secondly as an aid to the biochemist who knows how to make an informed choice, the System having done all the calculations. The System is now in routine use.

Despite extensive searches on the WWW and in the medical journals, of the thousands of papers written on Cholinesterase, many refer to biological experiments on animals, some on the reactions of humans, but none has been found which reports on aids to Genotyping.

Medical Informatics Europe '99
P. Kokol et al. (Eds.)
IOS Press, 1999

Hierarchical Multi-Attribute Decision Models and Their Application in Health Care

Marko Bohanec(1), Blaž Zupan(2,1), Vladislav Rajkovič(3,1)
(1) *Jožef Stefan Institute, Jamova 39, SI-1000 Ljubljana, Slovenia*
(2) *University of Ljubljana, Faculty of Computer and Information Sciences*
(3) *University of Maribor, Faculty of Organisational Sciences, Kranj*

Abstract. Hierarchical decision models are developed through decomposition of complex decision problems into smaller and less complex subproblems. They are aimed at the classification or evaluation of options and can be used for analysis, simulation and explanation. This paper presents a set of methods for the construction and application of qualitative hierarchical decision models in health care. We present the results of four ongoing projects in oncology, radiology, community nursing and diabetic foot treatment.

1. Introduction

Hierarchical multi-attribute decision models are aimed at the classification and/or evaluation of objects defined in attribute-value space [1,2]. They are based on decomposition of a complex decision problem into smaller and less complex subproblems. Subproblems are represented by variables, which are organized into a hierarchy.

Hierarchical decision models are extensively applied in decision support [3]. There, the problem is to choose an option from a set of available options so as to best satisfy the goals of decision maker. A decision model is designed to evaluate the options, and can also be used for the analysis, simulation, and explanation of decisions. In practice, this approach is most often used for technical or economical decision making, such as project or investment evaluation, portfolio management, strategic planning, and personnel management. In Slovenia, we have contributed to these fields by developing an expert system shell for multi-attribute decision support DEX [4] and applying it in several tens of real-world decision problems [5,6].

Some recent developments of hierarchical decision models have made them very attractive also for medicine and health care. In particular, some new methods facilitate the design of qualitative (or symbolic) decision models. In contrast with traditional quantitative (numeric) models, the qualitative ones are better suited for dealing with "soft" decision problems, which are typical for medicine in health care: less structured and less formalized problems that involve a great deal of expert judgement.

In this paper we present an approach to the development and application of qualitative hierarchical decision models based on the DEX shell. Section 2 defines basic concepts of hierarchical decision models. In section 3, these are illustrated by a case study of breast cancer risk assessment. Section 4 presents three other ongoing Slovenian projects that involve hierarchical models. The paper is concluded by a summary and proposals for further work.

2. Hierarchical Decision Models

In general, a *hierarchical decision model* is composed of attributes X_i and utility functions F_i (Figure 1). *Attributes* (sometimes also referred to as *performance variables* or *parameters*) are variables that represent decision subproblems. They are organized hierarchically so that the attributes that occur on higher levels of the hierarchy depend on lower-level attributes.

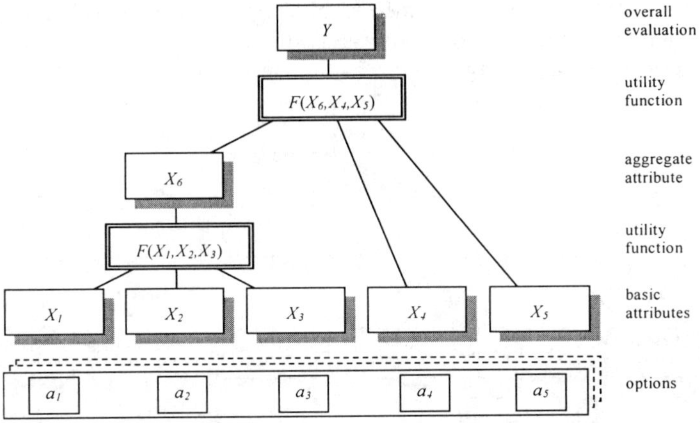

Figure 1: Components of a hierarchical decision model

In general, a hierarchy can be represented by a directed acyclic graph, but in practice it is usually simplified to a tree. According to their position in the hierarchy, we distinguish between *basic* attributes (leaves or terminal nodes) and *aggregate* attributes (internal nodes, including the roots of the hierarchy). In Figure 1, there are five basic attributes labeled from X_1 to X_5, and two aggregate attributes, X_6 and Y. For each aggregate attribute there is defined a corresponding *utility function F* that determines the dependence of that attribute on its immediate descendants in the hierarchy.

Options are described by values a_i of basic attributes. The *evaluation* of options is performed from bottom to the top by gradually aggregating their values according to model structure and utility functions. The overall evaluation (also called *utility*) of an option is finally obtained as the value of root attribute (Y in Figure 1).

A majority of contemporary multi-attribute decision methods is aimed at the development of *quantitative* decision models, in which all the attributes are continuous, and utility functions are typically defined in terms of attributes' weights, such as a weighted average of the lower-level attributes. In this paper we focus on *qualitative* decision models that are utilized by the DEX system. These models consist of *discrete* attributes, whose values are words rather than numbers, and utility functions that are represented by *decision rules* (see section 3 for examples of these).

Decision models are primarily developed for *option evaluation*: each option, described by values of basic attributes, is evaluated according to the model. By this, an overall evaluation is obtained for each option. On this basis the options are compared and ranked, and the best one is finally chosen.

However, this basic principle is insufficient for most practical applications. Decision models can become very complex, so they have to be thoroughly verified to reduce the chance of error. There is a need for an analysis and explanation of both the decision process and evaluation results. In the following case study, we highlight DEX's analysis and explanation methods that are particularly interesting for applications in medicine and health care.

3. Application in Oncology: Breast Cancer Risk Assessment

Breast cancer is a dangerous and unpredictable disease, where an early detection is of outmost importance [7]. To facilitate an early cancer detection, a screening procedure is often used where women of certain age or disease history in the family are invited for routine examination or mammography, if necessary.

In collaboration with the specialists from the Institute of Oncology in Ljubljana we developed a prototype model to assess the risk of breast cancer. The structure of the model is shown in Figure 2. Cancer risk, which is assessed using a four-valued scale, is derived by the model from features such as age, regularity of menstruation and fertility duration.

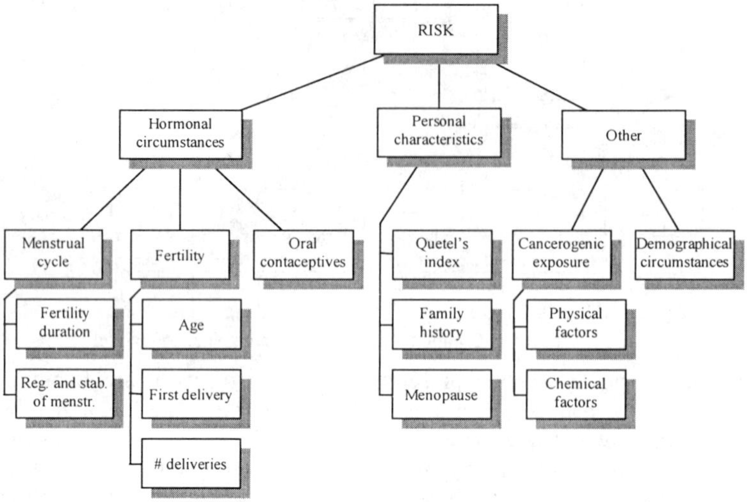

Figure 2: The structure of breast cancer risk assessment model

The risk of cancer is evaluated by decision rules defined by the experts. As an example, consider Table 1 that shows the rule that assesses the risk from the perspective of menstrual cycle and derives it from duration of fertility and regularity/stability of menstruation. Here, fertility duration can be either short (up to 30 years of menstrual period), average (30 to 40 years) and long (longer than 40 years), and menstruation either regular with a period of less than 28 days (R-28), regular with period longer than 29 days (R29+) or irregular (N).

This model was verified by the experts and tested on a small set of cases. A more exhaustive testing based on larger set of cases and comparison with independent examination of physicians is planned for the future.

Table 1: Decision rule to assess the risk specific to menstrual cycle

	Fertility duration	Reg. and stabil. of menstr.	Menstrual cycle
1	average	R-28	high risk
2	long	R-28	high risk
3	long	R29+	high risk
4	long	N	high risk
5	short	R-28	moderate risk
6	average	R29+	moderate risk
7	short	R29+	low risk
8	short	N	low risk
9	average	N	low risk

Knowledge representation and analysis of the model. The methods that support the analysis of model and provide different means for knowledge representation are primarily used to verify the model and detect potential errors. These methods either consider the model as a whole, or separately investigate a single utility function. A decision rule (such as the one in Table 1) may, for example, be interpreted as a training set given to some machine learning algorithm to devise a semantically equivalent representation. For example, consider Table 2 that was derived from Table 1 using the algorithm for induction of *complex rules* [8]. The resulting rule is more compact and in general easier to understand than its original.

Table 2: Complex rule as derived from Table 1

	Fertility duration	Reg. and stab. of menstr.	Menstrual cycle
1	≥ average	R-28	high risk
2	long	*	high risk
3	short	R-28	moderate risk
4	average	R29+	moderate risk
5	short	R29+, N	low risk
6	≤ average	N	low risk

Table 3: Attributes from breast cancer risk assessment model by their index of importance. Three different importance estimation methods were used. The indices of most important attributes are printed in bold

BREAST CANCER RISK	Regression	Informativity	Gini Index
Hormonal circumstances	**158**	**202**	**234**
Menstrual cycle	**125**	**123**	**130**
Fertility duration	**125**	**128**	**138**
Regularity and stability of menstruation	75	72	62
Fertility	111	99	130
Age	97	145	126
First delivery	**145**	**128**	**145**
# deliveries	58	27	29
Oral contraceptives	65	78	41
Personal characteristics	88	56	39
Quetel's index	29	5	11
Family history	**197**	**183**	**236**
Menopause	74	112	53
Other	55	42	27
Cancerogenic exposure	100	100	100
Physical factors	**160**	**166**	**179**
Chemical factors	40	34	21
Demographical circumstances	100	100	100

For a less detailed representation of utility functions we can use weights. These are derived by either a method based on regression [8], or by employing some measure to estimate the quality of attributes as used in machine learning [9]. For example, the rules in Table 1 determine the average weights of the attributes "Fertility duration" and "Regularity and stability of menstruation", which are, as computed by regression, 64% and 36%, respectively. That is, the first attribute is on average about twice as important as the second one.

Representation with weights is particularly interesting when we consider a model as a whole. Although it provides only a rough representation of utility functions, it may allow a quick verification of the model. Table 3 shows such weights for the breast cancer risk model. To ease the interpretation, the weights are represented as indices of importance, which are defined as a ratio between the actual attribute weight and the weight that would be obtained assuming all the attributes in the model were equally important. The index of 100 denotes that utility functions neither lower nor raise the importance of the attribute. Table 3 shows that the group of attributes "Hormonal circumstances" most influences the outcome of the model. Other important attributes include the presence of disease in the family, exposure to physical cancerogenic factors, and age at first delivery.

Evaluation and analysis of options. To demonstrate the utilization of the model, consider a woman aged 42, having two children, regular menstruation, and increased body weight (high Quetel's index). She does not use oral contraceptives and works in the environment that by its physical and demographical characteristics increases the risk of cancer. There was no cancer disease in her mother or sister. The results of risk assessment are given in the first column of Table 4. She obtained grade 3: an increased but not critical breast cancer risk. An explanation for such a risk can be found by the inspection of intermediate results in Table 4. Alternatively, a method of *selective explanation* can be used, which finds the subtrees of attributes that indicate particularly positive or negative influence to the risk. Such explanation is given in Table 5 and shows that the most important factors that contributed to the increased breast cancer risk are the age, increased body weight and environmental circumstances.

Table 4: Examples of evaluation and analysis of breast cancer risk

	Basic evaluation	Missing data	What-if analysis
BREAST CANCER RISK	**3**	**3**	**2**
Hormonal circumstances	2	3/0,5,2/0,5	2
Menstrual cycle	moderate risk	moderate risk	moderate risk
Fertility duration	average	average	average
Regularity and stability of menstruation	R29+	R29+	R29+
Fertility	moderate risk	moderate risk	moderate risk
Age	over 40	over 40	over 40
First delivery	29 or younger	29 or younger	29 or younger
# deliveries	up to 4	up to 4	up to 4
Oral contraceptives	no	*	no
Personal characteristics	1	1	1
Quetel's index	29+	29+	29+
Family history	no	no	no
Menopause	no	no	no
Other	high risk	high risk	moderate risk
Cancerogenic exposure	high risk	high risk	moderate risk
Physical factors	higher	higher	*lower*
Chemical factors	no	*	no
Demographical circumstances	high risk	high risk	*moderate risk*

Table 5: Selective explanation of evaluation

Reasons FOR higher risk		Reasons AGAINST higher risk	
Age	over 40	Personal characteristics	1
Quetel's index	29+	Family history	no
Other	high risk	Menopause	no
Cancerogenic exposure	high risk	First delivery	29 or younger
Physical factors	higher	Oral contraceptives	no
Demographical circumstances	high risk	Chemical factors	no

DEX incorporates mechanisms to handle missing and non-exact data. For example, assume that for the case considered we do not have data on chemical factors and oral contraceptives. For such case, the results of the evaluation are shown in the second column of Table 4. The final risk grade is the same as originally, while the only difference is in the less exact assessment of hormonal circumstances which is now expressed with probability distribution.

Another useful feature of DEX is "what-if" analysis. Here, we are interested in the effects of changing one or more attribute values. In the case examined so far, we may be interested what would happen if the risk from physical factors and demographical circumstances were reduced. The third column in Table 4 shows that this leads to the reduction of breast cancer risk, as it evaluates to grade 2. Similarly, we can use our model and DEX to answer, for example, what would happen if the woman would reduce her body weight, or what risk is she going to have while in menopause.

4. Other Applications

In Slovenia, there are three other ongoing projects that in one way or another employ hierarchical decision models:

1. *Radiology: Technical analysis of errors for lung roentgenogram*: For the purposes of education and systematizing the knowledge and for purposes, a model to assess the

quality of lung roentgenogram was developed. It includes 25 basic criteria that belong to two principal groups: the quality of equipment and recording procedure.

2. *Community nursing: Assessment of basic life activities*: In nursing, there are 14 basic life activities, which need to be properly assessed and recorded at every visit of the nurse. The aim is to develop models for all these activities; several prototype ones have already been developed, such as the one for patient's secretion [10] and physical activity [11].
3. *Risk assessment for diabetic foot syndrome*: With a long-term goal to reduce the number of amputations in diabetic patients, we recently launched the development of a model for assessing risk factors for developing foot pathology.

5. Conclusion

Hierarchical decision models are increasingly used within health care. For practical applications, it is particularly important that these models and supporting decision making tools allow the structuring of domain knowledge, can utilize qualitative variables and utility functions, and provide means for model and data analysis, evaluation in the presence of missing or inaccurate values, and explanation of evaluation.

The cases presented in this paper are based on a manual development of models. Recently, a new data mining method that supports structure and utility function development from pre-classified data called HINT was developed [12]. There is a growing number of such data bases and repositories within health care and medicine, and therefore an increased potential for these to enable an easier and better synthesis of decision models.

Acknowledgement

The authors are thankful to the oncologists Prof. Dr. Maja Primic-Žakelj, M.D., and Prof. Dr. Jurij Lindtner, M.D., radiology technician Mrs. Majda Budna and R.N. M. Sc. Olga Šušteršič for their initiative and help in developing the hierarchical decision models presented in this paper.

References

[1] Chankong, V., Haimes, Y.Y. (1983): *Multiobjective decision making*. North-Holland.
[2] Vincke, P. (1992): *Multicriteria decision-aid*. John Wiley & Sons.
[3] Nagel, S. (ed.) (1993): *Computer-aided decision analysis: Theory and application*. Quorum Books.
[4] Bohanec, M., Rajkovič, V. (1990): DEX: An expert system shell for decision support. *Sistemica* 1, 145–157.
[5] Urbančič, T., Kononenko, I., Križman, V. (1991): *Review of applications by Ljubljana Artificial Intelligence Laboratories*. Institut Jožef Stefan, delovno poročilo DP-6218.
[6] Bohanec, M., Cestnik, B., Rajkovič, V. (1998): Evaluation models for housing loan allocation in the context of floats, in *Context sensitive decision support systems* (eds. Berkeley,D., Widmeyer,G.R., Brezillon,P., Rajkovič,V.), Chapman & Hall, 174–189.
[7] Primic-Žakelj, M., Evstifeeva, T., Ravnihar, B., Boyle, P. (1995): Breast-cancer risk and oral contraceptive use in Slovenian women aged 25 to 54. *Int. J. Cancer* 62, 414–420.
[8] Rajkovič, V., Bohanec, M. (1991): Decision support by knowledge explanation. *Environments for supporting decision processes* (eds. Sol, H.G., Vecsenyi, J.), North-Holland, 47–57.
[9] Mingers, J. (1989): An empirical comparison of selection measures for decision-tree induction. *Machine Learning* 3, 319–342.
[10] Šušteršič, O., Rajkovič, V. (1996): An Information system for community nursing, Medical Informatics Europe 96 (eds.: J. Brender et al.), IOS Press, 665–669.
[11] Šušteršič, O., Rajkovič, V., Kljajić, M. (1998): An evaluation of community nursing process in the frame of the International Classification for Nursing Practice, 2nd European Telenurse Conference. Sesimbra.
[12] Zupan, B., Bohanec, M., Demšar, J., Bratko, I. (1998): Feature transformation by function decomposition. *IEEE Intelligent Systems* 13(2): 38–43.

Medical Informatics Europe '99
P. Kokol et al. (Eds.)
IOS Press, 1999

The influence of class discretization to attribute hierarchy of decision trees

Špela Hleb Babič, Peter Kokol, Milan Zorman, Vili Podgorelec
Faculty of Electrical Engineering and Computer Science, University of Maribor
Laboratory for System Design
Smetanova 17, 2000 Maribor, Slovenia

Abstract. Decision support systems that help physicians are becoming very important part of medical decision making. They are based on different models and the best of them are providing an explanation together with an accurate, reliable and quick response. One of the most viable among decision-making models is the concept of decision trees, already successfully used for many medical decision making purposes.

Although effective and reliable, the traditional decision tree construction approach still contains several deficiencies. Therefore we decided to develop and compare several decision supporting models, each of them built with different discretization of attributes and decision classes. For the construction of decision trees we used **MtDeciT**, in our laboratory developed tool for building decision trees using the classical induction method.

All solutions were evolved for determining the influence of basic properties of child and his/her parents to length of successful breastfeeding. A comparison between developed models and obtained results has shown that the way of discretization obviously plays a great role in the reliable and accurate real-world medical decision making.

1. Introduction

As in many other areas, decision making plays an important role also in medicine, especially in the medical diagnostic processes. Decision support systems (DSS) for helping physicians are becoming a very important part in medical decision making, particularly in those areas where decision must be made effectively and reliably [1,2]. Since conceptual simple decision making models with the possibility of automatic learning should be considered for performing such tasks [3], according to recent reviews [1,4,5,9] decision trees are a very suitable candidate. They have been already successfully used in DSS for many decision-making purposes, but some problems still persist. One of the most evident is the discretization: first of the attributes and second what is less known of the decision classes. In present study we built several decision trees with different discretizations of decision classes in order to compare the hierarchy of so obtained decision trees. The results have shown that wise discretization can affect the final decision making so far that it is worth of particular attention.

For our study the available real-world data were collected at regular monthly check-ups of infants in their first year of life. The structure of the data was determined by participating medical experts. The described research work is joint in the latest project[1] of our Laboratory for system design.

1.1. Background of the research

For the purpose of qualifying the influence of feeding the baby to his/her mental and physical development we have measured and collected data in form of precisely defined protocols. For 187

[1] The project is supported by Slovenian Ministry of science and technology by Grant No. L2-1640-0796-99.

infants who were present at the preventive monthly check-ups in their first twelve months of life we assembled basic and specific information about their habits and behavior [10]. Some data like birth weight and birth length is based on maternity's records while the rest was gained from the parents of checked children. The whole process was performed very carefully, in order to prevent mistakes. Notwithstanding, there were only 69 infants with all attribute values that were then included into our study.

1.2. The Approach and Aims of the Research

First we considered the relevant attributes among all available ones. We took all basic measurements of the baby and that of the parents, which describe their characteristics in the widest acceptable way. While the decision attribute was numeric; namely months of duration of breastfeeding, we had to determine possible classes as results of the decision tree. We decided for two possibilities; one composites of three while the other of seven different classes.
Upon so derived data we built several decision trees. For all we used a **MtDeciT**, in our laboratory developed tool for building decision trees with the classical induction method. The trees differ in tolerance for building final decision tree (0%,10%), where tolerance means the threshold of the incorrect classified instances, in discretization of numerical attributes (quartiles, octiles) and in applying instances to two sets of classes (3 classes, 7 classes).
For comparing all the results we have chosen six most representative decision trees. In that way we are able to show how the different trees evaluate the importance of attributes. Then we compare the complexity of the trees and discus the results.
In the paper the used method will be introduced first. Next the classes discretization problem will be introduced and following the results obtained with the described models for the breastfeeding-success prediction will be presented. A discussion about important findings, problems and analysis of the results will follow after which the paper will conclude with a short summary of achievements and directives for further research work.

2. Method

2.1. Decision trees

Inductive inference is the process of moving from concrete examples to general models, where the goal is to learn how to classify objects by analyzing a set of instances (already solved cases) whose classes are known. Instances are typically represented as attribute-value vectors. Learning input consists of a set of such vectors, each belonging to a known class, and the output consists of a mapping from attribute values to classes. This mapping should accurately classify both the given instances and other unseen instances. Inductive inference is often the basis for artificial intelligence techniques use of which is a common practice in various medical applications. Especially machine learning deals with the discovery of hidden knowledge, unexpected patterns and new rules. Therefore decision trees have been and are still being used to extract knowledge from data, in order to make decisions in cases, where explicit human knowledge cannot be used efficiently [11,12].
The algorithm for learning a decision tree is trivial and the representation of accumulated knowledge can be easily understood. Namely, the decision trees don't give us just the decision in a previously unseen case. They also give us the explanation of the decision, and that is essential in medical applications.
A decision tree is induced on a training set, which consists of training objects (instances). Each training object is completely described by a set of attributes and a class label (category, outcome). Classes are mutually exclusive, what means that the training object can belong to only one class. Attributes can be continuous (numeric) or discrete [7, 8]. A decision tree contains nodes and edges (links). There are two types of nodes. Each internal node (non-terminal node) has a split, which tests the value of the attributes, that have come into this node and with that splits the training set. External nodes, also called leaves or terminal nodes, are labeled with outcomes. The procedure of constructing a decision tree from a set of training objects is called induction of the tree. In

induction of a decision tree, we start with an empty tree and an entire training set. At every step an 'unused' attribute is chosen with the help of a heuristic evaluation function and the training set is divided, according to the values of the chosen attribute.
This decision tree characterization becomes next a basis for:

- the hierarchical representation of the importancy of attributes of the concept being investigated,
- forecasting in which class an object previously unseen belongs.

2.2. MtDeciT Decision Support Tool

MtDeciT is written in Visual C++ language and runs under the Windows environment. Supported are all phases from preparing the training data, automatic learning, and pruning, to decision making. Very friendly user-interface enables even the novice users to exploit all tool's capabilities. It also enables settings of various building properties and with that influences the form of extracted knowledge.

3. Application and results

3.1. Gathering and preparing data

Our aim in the study presented was to determine the influence of parents' and child's basic properties to successful breastfeeding. With the approval of parents we carefully observed each child from the day he/she was born. The data was collected from maternity hospitals and at regular monthly check-ups of infants in their first year of life. In that time we recorded almost 200 attributes. So we built a database, which contained data about 187 children but unfortunately only 69 records were complete and useful for final use. The structure of the data was determined by participating medical experts.
From the obtained data we have chosen the basic properties of child and his/her parents in order to find out how the selected attributes influence the success of breastfeeding. We selected 45 attributes and defined the possible solutions - classes. Classes were defined in following way: in the basic set of attributes we have found six attributes ***is_the_child_breastfed_at_month_x***, where x stays for the month of age of the child and has possible values between 1 and 6. From these attributes it is easy to figure out the length of breastfeeding period for each baby. The results were validated in order the longer child was breastfed the more successful the breastfeeding relationship was. We decided for two possibilities of instance classification. First is determined by seven classes: 0_months, 1_month, 2_months,...6_months, where baby was breastfed 0 months, 1 month, 2 months, ...6 months respectively. While distribution of instances to seven classes might be too fine, we considered the second classification using three classes: 0_months, 1-3_months, 4-6_months, where baby was breastfed 0 months, 1-3 months and 4-6 months respectively.

3.2. Building decision trees using MtDeciT method

Above described database was the groundwork for building decision trees. For the purpose of determining a hierarchy of attributes in case of successful breastfeeding, we generated numerous trees, each with different discretization of attributes, different discretization of classes or outcomes and different tolerance. To depict and compare the results, we took six decision trees. We considered the combination of: two ways of discretization of the classes (3 and 7 classes), two kinds of discretization of attributes (quartiles, octiles) and two levels of tolerance (0%, 10%). We designated the trees with:

- DT-3C-0%-Q (Decision tree-3 classes-0% tolerance-quartiles)
- DT-3C-10%-Q (Decision tree-3 classes-10% tolerance-quartiles)
- DT-3C-10%-O (Decision tree-3 classes-0% tolerance-octiles)
- DT-7C-0%-Q (Decision tree-7 classes-0% tolerance-quartiles)
- DT-7C-10%-Q (Decision tree-7 classes-10% tolerance-quartiles)
- DT-7C-10%-Q (Decision tree-7 classes-10% tolerance-octiles)

```
[] years_of_education_mother
|____[8 .. 10.5] years_of_education_father
|    |____[8 .. 10.5] weight_mother
|    |    |____[48 .. 63.5] 0_months
|    |    |____[63.5 .. 94.5] 6_months
|    |____[10.5 .. 13] weight_father
|    |    |____[60 .. 73.7] age_mother
|    |    |    |____[20 .. 24.7] 6_months
|    |    |    |____[24.7 .. 29.5] 1_month
|    |    |____[73.7 .. 87.5] 0_months
|    |    |____[87.5 .. 101.2] 1_month
|    |____[13 .. 15.5] 6_months
|    |____[15.5 .. 18] 1_month
|____[10.5 .. 13] age_mother
|    |____[20 .. 24.7] height_mother
|    |    |____[157 .. 164] 2_months
|    |    |____[164 .. 171] age_father
|    |    |    |____[21 .. 28.7] 6_months
|    |    |    |____[28.7 .. 36.5] sex
```

Figure 1: A first part of decision tree DT-7C-0%-Q

Trees are drawn hierarchically; lines connect levels. Figure 1 shows due to the large dimension only the first half of the hierarchy of decision tree DT-7C-0%-Q. According to the way of building the decision trees, more significant attributes occur higher in the hierarchy. Since our decision trees are drawn hierarchically from left to right, more important attributes occur more to the left side of the figures. For instance, if we look at Figure 1, the most important attribute or root of the tree is ***years_of_education_mother***, at the second level ***years_of_education_father*** and ***age_mother*** etc.

4. Results

4.1. *Importance of attributes*

For comparison of importance of attributes we took first three levels of each decision tree, what is fine enough to show the similarities and differences. The root of the tree was numbered as level one. From attribute hierarchy yield from different decision trees we can observe that similar attributes were chosen as the most important. For saying that we have to consider that only 15 of total 45 attributes contributed in upper three levels of the decision trees.

Table 1 shows the important attributes for each decision tree.

We can realize that in our case tolerance has little influence to the hierarchy (differences occur in lower levels) while the discretization of the numerical attributes (quartiles or octiles) and of the outcomes affects it a lot.

Table 1. The comparison of importance of attributes obtained by different discretization of classes and attributes, where single x means root or 1st level, double x (xx) means 2nd level and triple x (xxx) means 3rd level in the hierarchy.

	DT-7C-0%-Q	DT-7C-10%-Q	DT-7C-10%-O	DT-3C-0%-Q	DT-3C-10%-Q	DT-3C-10%-O
birth_head_circumference	xxx	xxx		x	x	
age_mother	xx	xx	xx	xx	xx	xxx
height_father			x	xx	xx	xx
years_of_education_mother	x	x				
years_of_education_father	xx	xx				
weight_father	xx	xx	xxx			xx
height_mother	xxx	xxx	xx	xxx	xxx	xx
age_father				xx	xx	x
days_of_ rooming_in						
weight_mother	xxx	xxx	xx			xx
birth_lenght	xxx	xxx		xxx	xxx	
birth_no	xxx	xxx				
sex			xxx	xxx	xxx	
consuming_alcohol_mother				xxx	xxx	
employment_mother						xxx

4.2. Complexity of decision trees

For estimating complexity of decision trees we have measured: the number of attribute nodes, the number of decision nodes or leaves of the tree and the maximum depth of the tree what means number of steps needed for the classification. The results show again that tolerance has no important influence, while discretization of numerical attributes (quartiles, octiles) and of the classes has evident impact on the construction of the trees. A look at the Table 2 offers us the logical explanation of the complexity of the trees. If we decide for less subsets of the attributes and divide the intervals to quartiles we yield the tree with more attribute nodes, less decision nodes and major max. depth and vice-versa: finer division of attributes domain with octiles gives us a tree with more decision nodes, less attribute nodes and minor max. depth. Interesting observations we got from comparison of different discretization of outcomes. The less classes we presume, the less complex the tree is but consequently gives less information. Final decision for choosing the right tree must be made according to desired accuracy and gained information of the final decision making.

Table 2. A comparison of the complexity between six characteristic decision trees

	DT-7C-0%-Q	**DT-7C-10%-Q**	**DT-7C-10%-O**	**DT-3C-0%-Q**	**DT-3C-10%-Q**	**DT-3C-10%-O**
Num. of attribute nodes	15	15	7	12	12	8
Num. of decision nodes	40	40	55	31	31	42
Maximum depth	6	6	4	6	6	4

5. Discussion

Several interesting discoveries have been made while comparing different decision trees. Note the relatively small size of training set; it may influence the quality of the obtained solutions. Since the real problem of tracing child's development is very extensive and is not easy to collect data we have done our best with available set of instances.

A very significant observation is definitely the influence of discretization of numerical attributes. Although decision trees are a decision-making method where the unexpected but very helpful results could be obtained, the human estimation of the results must not be disproved. When contemplating the above described decision trees we cannot oversight some unreasonable attributes being considered as most important. For instance: father's role in successful breastfeeding relationship is undoubtedly great but father's height could not influence breastfeeding so much that it is determined as the most important attribute of the decision tree. This gives us a hint that equable discretization of attributes isn't always very appropriate. Therefore our future research will focus on human predetermined discretization – fuzzy discretization.

When comparing the decision trees obtained by different classification we can see that "seven classes" discretization gave us results that are – on the first sight of course – more logical and natural. Here we can continue our thinking in two ways. First we can conclude that for specific problem of length of breastfeeding finer discretization is more appropriate what proves us that it is not adequate to determine the kind of discretization in advance. It must be stated according to nature of the real-world problem the decision model is built for.

Second we can see that it is not number of the classes what gives us a reliable decision model but proper division the domains into subintervals. What is the proper division for the specific problem isn't always good for the next one. Again we have to conclude that fuzzy determination of possible decision values might be the solution while some simple words can sometimes tell us more then vast amount of numbers.

6. Conclusion

In the paper we present the comparison study of effectiveness of decision trees based DSS. Several different models – decision trees were constructed with emphasis on influence of class discretization to attribute hierarchy of decision trees. All trees were built upon same set of data, which was obtained from regular monthly check-ups of infants in their first year of life. From the large amount of data we have chosen the subset which describes the problem of influence the basic properties of baby and baby's parents on length of breastfeeding.

The trees differ in tolerance for building final decision tree, in discretization of numerical attributes and in applying instances to two sets of classes. We determined the possible classification considering two cases: finer classification with seven classes and rougher with three classes. Then six characteristic representatives of decision trees were picked out in order to compare the results, show the findings and suggest possible guidelines.

Analysis of the results has shown that discretization of classes has a great influence on hierarchy of attributes in decision tree and therefore deserves a lot of attention. Discretization of numerical attributes has no minor importance than discretization of the classes and we made some suggestions for dividing the numerical attributes' domain into subsets. According to that our further research will focus on human predicted division of attribute domain and classes to proper intervals, what will result in so called fuzzy decision trees

Since present paper proved that division of numerical attributes' and outcomes' domain is very important and has great influence to quality of decision making we expect from our further research great improvements and a step forward in supporting general decision making processes with intelligent tools.

References

[1] Kokol P, et al: Decision Trees and Automatic Learning and Their Use in Cardiology, Journal of Medical Systems 19(4), 1994.

[2] Kokol P, Podgorelec V, Malcic I: Diagnostic Process Optimisation with Evolutionary Programming, Proceedings of the 11th IEEE Symposium on Computer-based Medical Systems CBMS'98, pp. 62-67, Lubbock, Texas, USA, June 1998.

[3] Kokol P, Stiglic B, Zumer V: Metaparadigm: a soft and situation oriented MIS design approach, International Journal of Bio-Medical Computing, 39:243-256, 1995.

[4] Kokol P, et al: Spreadsheet Software and Decision making in Nursing, Nursing Informatics'91, (Honvenga E J S et al. eds.), Springer Verlag, 1991.

[5] Quinlan J R: Decision Trees and Decision making, IEEE Trans System, Man and Cybernetics 20(2)339-346, 1990.

[6] Quinlan J R: C4.5: Programs for Machine Learning, Morgan Kaufmann, 1993.

[7] Quinlan JR, Decision Trees and Instance-Based Classifiers. In: Allen B Tucker jr, ed. *CRC Computer science and engineering handbook*. CRC Press, ch. 22, pp. 521-535, 1997.

[8] Zorman M, Molan Štiglic M, Kokol P, Malčić I: The Limitations of Decision Trees and Automatic Learning in Real World Medical Decision Making, *Journal of Medical Systems*, no. 6, pp. 403-415, 1997.

[9] Podgorelec V, Hleb Babič Š, Kokol P, Zorman M: The Art of building decision trees; sent for publication, IDA'99 Amsterdam, 1999.

[10] prof.dr. Mičetić Turk D.: Vpliv prehrane na razvoj otroka od prvega do šestega meseca starosti, 1998 (in Slovene).

[11] Kokol P, Završnik J, Zorman M, Malčić I, Kancler K: Participative design, decision trees, automatic learning and medical decision making. In: Brender J… (ed.). Medical Informatics Europe'96, (Studies in health technology and informatics, Vol.34). Amsterdam (etc.): IOS Press; Tokyo:Ohmsha,1996,pp./A 501-505.

[12] Stuart J. Russel, Peter Norvig, et al: Artificial intelligence: a modern approach, Englewood çliffs, Prentice _Hall, ch.18, pp.525-562,1995.

Medical Informatics Europe '99
P. Kokol et al. (Eds.)
IOS Press, 1999

A micropopulational modelling of a viral epidemic by using a special neural network

C.N. Zaharia, Al. Cristea
Institute of Virology, Str. Mihai Bravu nr. 285, 79650 Bucharest, Romania

Abstract. A general forward neural network was adapted for a simulation of viral epidemics. This involves the introduction of a strongly dependence upon history, upon the cumulated values of the corresponding neuron (individual) activations (states of infection) specifying the activation (health) states of the contaminated individuals, represented by the activated neurons and the dynamic parameters of the neural network: the matrix of the synaptic connection and the vector of the activation thresholds (corresponding to the matrix of the viral transfers between the various individuals and to the vector of the minimal individual contamination doses of virus). The recurrence relations and the learning procedures were also adapted to these processes. This methodology was used for the study of the micropopulational spreading of viral epidemics in various epidemiological situations.

1. Introduction

The forward neural network introduced must specify the detailed spreading mechanisms and the dynamical parameters of some simple viral epidemics ((Ac), (He)).

2. The micropopulational modelling of a simple viral epidemic by using a simple forward neural network

2.1 Significance - in this modeling - of the neural network elements

The essential epidemiological (usual) processes correspond to the contamination (at the time $\mathbf{n_{0i}}$) of an individual **i**, passing from the "receptive" (inactive) state $\mathbf{S_{0i}}$ to a contagious (active) state $\mathbf{S_{+i}}$ (by a virus transfer from $\mathbf{S_{+j}}$ to $\mathbf{S_{0i}}$); the time unit t.u. corresponds to the passage from contamination to S_{+i}; after **m** t.u., S_{+i} passes into the immune state S_{-i} (a definitive inactive state). In epidemic simulation, the following set of rules characterizes the new neural network:
a) the individuals were represented by the neurons N_i of a **NN;**
b) the state of $\mathbf{N_i}$, for the time **n**, is described by the binary variables $\mathbf{S_i(n)}$, **1** for $\mathbf{S_{+i}}$, **0** for $\mathbf{S_{0,-i}}$. The cumulated value of $\mathbf{S_i(k)}$ for **k<n** is $\mathbf{SC_i(n)}$, discriminating the $\mathbf{S_a}$:
- $\mathbf{S_{0i}}$ corresponds to $\mathbf{n < n_{0i}}$, to $\mathbf{SC_i(n) = 0}$;
- $\mathbf{S_{+i}}$ corresponds to **n = noi + k, 1=<k=<m**, for which $\mathbf{SC_i(n) = k}$;
- S_{-i} appears, when $\mathbf{n > n_{0i}+m}$ and $\mathbf{SC_i(n)}$ is equal to **m**;

2.2 Significance of the dynamical parameters in the special neural network

The elements $\mathbf{J_{ij}}$ of the synaptic connection matrix **J** represent the average quantity of "the specific viral material" transferred - during a t.u. - between $\mathbf{S_{+j}}$ and $\mathbf{S_{0i}}$. The variable $\mathbf{T_i(n)}$ is the average viral transfer (in a t.u.) from all the other $\mathbf{S_j}$ to $\mathbf{S_i}$ (the sum of the products of $\mathbf{J_{ij}}$ by $\mathbf{S_j(n)}$ on all the **N** neurons **j**). $\mathbf{S_i(n+1)}$ is a Heavyside function of the $\mathbf{T_i(n) - P_i(n)}$, an activation threshold:

$$\mathbf{S_i(n+1) = H[T_i(n) - P_i(n)]} \quad \mathbf{(1)}$$

The specific featuresof the viral spreading impose some neural network functioning rules:
A) Firstly, we should take into account $\mathbf{P_i(n)}$, during the infection:
a) for $\mathbf{S_{0i}}$, $\mathbf{P_i(n)}$ has a moderate positive value $\mathbf{P_1}$: if $\mathbf{T_i > P_{1i}}$, $\mathbf{S_{+i}}$ must appear.
b) for S_{+i}, for $\mathbf{n = n_{0i}+k\ (1=<k = m - 1)}$, $\mathbf{S_{ia}(n+1)} = S_{+i}$; thus $\mathbf{T_i - P_i > 0}$ for each $\mathbf{T_i}$ and $\mathbf{P_i(n)}$ must be $\mathbf{P_{2i}<0}$;
c) for $\mathbf{I_{-i}}$ ($\mathbf{n >= n_{0i} + m}$), the unit **i** remains inactive and $\mathbf{T_i(n)-P_i(n)<0}$ for all $\mathbf{T_i(n)}$; $\mathbf{P_i(n) = P_{3i}}$ should exceed $\mathbf{max[T_i(n)]}$ (the $\mathbf{maxU_i}$ of sums of $\mathbf{J_{ij}}$ for all **j**).
The correlation between $\mathbf{P_i(n)}$ and $\mathbf{SC_i(n)}$ can express $\mathbf{P_i(n)}$ analytically, as a $\mathbf{P_{1i}*Q_m}$, with $\mathbf{Q_m}$ an **m** degree polynomial in $\mathbf{SC_i(n)}$, dependent upon **m** and $\mathbf{P_{ki}}$ (**k=1,.,3**).
B) Secondly, we should take into account the decrease of the "viral" transfer $\mathbf{S_{+j}}$ and $\mathbf{S_{0i}}$, when $\mathbf{n-n_{0j}}$ is increasing: $\mathbf{J_{ij}=J_{0,ij}*D(n-n_{0j})}$, with a decreasing function **D**.
C) Thirdly, we must consider other non-epidemiological intervening processes:
a) the demographic processes increasing the number of $\mathbf{S_{0i}}$, by the appearance of susceptible newborns, in a number given by the birth rate **NT** (per t.u);
b) the anti-epidemic measures taken by the sanitary institutions: for ex. **VC** vaccinations, transforming some $\mathbf{S_{0i}}$ in $\mathbf{S_{ni}}$, by the increase of their $\mathbf{P_i(n)}$, from $\mathbf{P_{1i}}$ to $\mathbf{P_{3i}}$.

2.3 The obtained recurrence relations for the special neural network

The definition of $\mathbf{SC_i(n)}$, **(1)**, and the above mentioned considerations lead to the recurrence relations:

$$\mathbf{SC_i(n+1) = SC_i(n) + S_i(n+1)} \qquad (2)$$

$$\mathbf{S_i(n+1) = H[T_i(n) - P_{1i}*Q_m(SC_i(n))]}$$

$$\mathbf{SC_i(n+1) = SC_i(n) + D_{OP,ia}(n);\ D_{VC},\ S_{ia}(n)=+m} \text{ for } \mathbf{a=0}; \qquad (3)$$

H can be approximated with a continuous $\mathbf{H_u(x) = exp(ux)/(1+exp(ux))}$,with a great **u**.

2.4 The training algorithm for the special neural network

Our adapted backpropagation algorithms for training our neural network use as input and output activations the couples of successive states of the individuals.
For all the **(i,n)** couples, not related to the non-epidemiological processes, $\mathbf{x_{k,obs}(n) = S_{k,obs}(n)}$ and $\mathbf{y_{i,obs}(n) = S_{i,obs}(n+1)}$ are the observed inputs and outputs and $\mathbf{y_{i,calc}(n) = S_{i,calc}(n+1) = H_u(i;..,x_k,..)}$ the output vectors obtained by simulation.
The relations improving the neural network dynamical parameters by the gradient back-propagation method (acting by a minimization of the Euclidean norm of the vector $\mathbf{\{y_{i,obs}(n) - y_{i,calc}(n)\}}$, considered for the mentioned **(i,n)** components) are:

$$\mathbf{J_{0,ik}(p+1)=J_{0,ik}(p)+ n^2*s*A_i\ ;\ A_{ik} =(y_{i,obs}(n)- y_{i,calc}(n))*D*H_u'(p;.)*x_{k.obs}(n)} \qquad (4)$$

$$\mathbf{P_{1i}(p+1)=P_{1i}(p)+ n\ 2*s*B_{ik};\ B_{ik} = (y_{i,obs}(n) - y_{i,calc}(n))*Q_m(Y_{i,obs})} \qquad (5)$$

where **s** is a subunitary correction coefficient; $\mathbf{H_u'}$ is the derivative of $\mathbf{H_u}$; $\mathbf{Y_{i,calc}}$ is the cumulated value corresponding to $\mathbf{y_{i,calc}}$; **p** is the iteration stage.

2.5 The neurocomputing program used for the special neural network

We use a home made program, written in **C++** language on a PC.

3. Results of the simulation of viral epidemics in closed communities by using the above described metodology

The essential results of these simulations consisted in the time evolutions of the cumulated numbers of neurons in various activation states for **24** neurons.A theoretical example is given in **Table 1.**

Using - for training - the various viral epidemics observed, with similar **J** and **P**, these parameter were calculated for the usual viral epidemics in a kindergarten community with **30** children, using the backpropagation method, after which the calculated versions of the epidemics were obtained and compared with those observed from the training set **(Table 2)**

TABLE 1. SIMULATION OF THE MICROPOPULATIONAL EVOLUTION OF A SIMPLE VIRAL EPIDEMIC BY USING A SPECIAL NEURAL NETWORK

EPIDEM. PARAMETERS J_{kj} (=1 for some k,j) AND P_j k=1,..,24

The couples k,j for which J_{kj} = 1, for k,j = 1,.., 24

(1,2); (1,23); (2,3); (2,5); (2,24); (3,1); (3,4); (4,3); (4,6); (5,3); (5,7); (5,8); (6,2);(6,8); (7,9); (7,10); (7,12); (8,6); (8,7); (8,11); (9,6); (9,11); (10,8); (10,11); (10,13);(11,9); (11.13); (12,8); (12,13); (12,15); (13,10); (13,15); (14,10); (14,12); (14,17);(15,13); (15,20); (16,12); (16,18); (16,20); (17,16); (17,18); (17,19); (18,17); (18,21); (19,17); (19, 21); (20,16); (20,18); (20,21); (20,23); (21,17); (21,24); (22,2); (22,3); (22,24); (23,2); (23,24); (24,22); (24,4).

Pj values for j = 1,.., 24

0.82 0.89 1.14 1.28 0.85 1.18 0.93 0.78 1.06 1.18 1.23 0.90
0.87 1.19 0.93 0.88 1.06 1.1 1.17 0.91 0.89 1.11 0.94 1.1

THE HEALTH STATE H OF k INDIVIDUALS AT THE TIMES
n =1, .. , 10 ; (H, k), k = 1,.., 24

H: S= Susceptible Indiv. C=Contaminated Indiv., B = Contagious Indiv.,
I = Immunized Indiv.

n=1: (B,1), (C,2); (C,23);
n=2: (I,1), (B,2), (C,5), (B,23);
n=3: (I,1), (I,2), (B,5), (C,7), (C,8), (I,23);
n=4: (I,1), (I,2), (I,5), (B,7), (B,8), (C,12), (I,23);
n=5: (I,1), (I,2), (I,5), (I,7), (I,8), (B,12), (C,13), (C,15), (I,23);
n=6: (I,1), (I,2), (I,5). (I,7), (I,8), (I,12), (B,13), (B,15), (C,16), (C,21), (I,23);
n=7; (I,1), (I,2), (I,5), (I,7), (I,8), (I,12), (I,13), (I,15), (B,16), (B,21), (C,22), (I,23);
n=8: (I,1), (I,2); (I,5), (I,7), (I,8), (I,12), (I,13), (I,15), (I,16), (I,21), (B,22), (I,23);
n=9; (I,1), (I,2), (I,5), (I,7), (I,8), (I,12), (I,13), (I,15), (I,16), (I,21), (I,22), (I,23).

CUMULATED EPIDEMIC

n	S(n)	C(n)	B(n)	I(n)
1	21	2	1	0
2	20	1	2	1
3	18	2	1	3
4	17	1	2	4
5	25	2	1	6
6	14	2	1	7
7	10	1	2	9
8	12	0	1	11
9	12	0	0	12

4. Discussions

Table 1 shous the course of a viral epidemic for a given set of parameters of the neural work, for a specified inter-individual possible viral transmission and for given minimal infective doses. The overall indicators of the epidemic state, the number of susceptible **S**, of contagious persons **B** and of immunized subjects **I** are calculated. For a closed community, **S** decreases continuously, **B**

has an intermediate maximum before the epidemic extinction and **I** increases continuously till the maximal number of contaminated persons, for this epidemic.

In **Table 2** we specify a neural network for describing all usual simple viroses of a child, starting

TABLE 2. SUCCESSIVELY ACTIVATED NEURONS IN A TRAINING SET

1,3,5 -->11,12,13 ; 1,2,4,6,7,9 --> 11,14,17,19 --> 21,25 ; 4,6,7 --> 17
1,3,4,7,8,10 --> 11,12,13,15,18,20 --> 23,30;3,4,6-->13;2,8,9-> 2,3,4,7-> 11,13,14,18 --> 23, 25 ;4,5,6,9 -> 19; 3,4,6,7,9 --> 13,18,19 -->29;
3,4,7,9 --> 13,18,19 --> 29; 2,4,9-> 11,14,19--> 25; 7,8,10 --> 20 --> 30

MATRIX J = M ESTIMATED BY MEANS OF THE BACKPROPAGATION METHOD

M(1,11) = 1.2 ; M(1,12) = 0.6 ; M(2,14) = 0.8 ; M(3,12) = 0.7 ;
M(3,13) = 1.1 ; M(4,14) = 0.7 ; M(4,15) = 0.7 ; M(4,18) = 0.8 ;
M(6,17) = 0.6 ; M(7,17) = 0.5 ; M(7,18) = 0.4 ; M(7,20) = 0.4 ;
M(8,4) = 0.4 ; M(8,20) = 0.3 ; M(9,19) = 1.3 ; M(10,20) = 0.3 ;
M(11,21)= 0.7 ; M(12,23) = 0.5 ; M(12,29) = 0.8 ; M(14,25) =1.2
M(17,21) = 0.5 ; M(18,23) = 0.6 ; M(19,28) = 0.3 ; M(19, 29) = 0.3 ;
M(20,30) = 1.2

ACTIVATION TRANSFERS IN THE FORWARD NEURAL NETWORK RESULTING FROM THIS NEURAL NETWORK AND CORRESPONDING EXACTLY TO THE TRAINING SET

1 --> 11 ; 3 ---> 13 ; 9 --> 19; 2, 4 --> 14 ; 4, 8-->15 ; 6, 7 --> 17
4, 7 ---> 18 ; 7, 8 , 10 ---> 20 ;
14 --> 25; 20 --> 30 ; 13, 19 --> 29
11, 17 ---> 21 ; 12, 18 --> 23

from the hypothesis that the dynamical epidemiological parameters for the various viroses are similar. That means that the parameters of the representative neural network will also be similar. Using the data regarding the various viroses, considered as a variant of an "universal virosis", we have a sufficiently larger training set for specifying the dynamical parameters of the unique representative neural network.

Calculating, as in the case of **Table 1**, the epidemiological course by means of this neural network, we obtain a satisfactory correspondence between the observed and the calculated micropopulational course of the various viral diseases, indicating correctly the contaminated individuals and the order or their contamination.

5. Conclusions

For a micropopulational modeling of the viral epidemics, we introduce some special neural networks **NN**, strongly dependent on history, considering an adequate influence of the cumulated neuronal activation on the dynamic parameters of **NN**. Simulations of the **NN** activation, for different **J** types, give results very similar to the micropopulational observations of the modelled viral epidemics.

References

[1] E. Ackerman, Simulation of micropopulations in epidemiology Tutorial 1,2,3. Intern. Journal of Bio-Medical Research, **36** (1994) 229-238, **37,** 139-149, 195-204.

[2] J. Hertz and coll., Introduction to the Theory of Neural Computation, Santa Fe Institute, Addison - Wesley, Redwood City, 1991.

[3] Al. Cristea, C.N. Zaharia, Special neural networks for modeling of viral epidemics, Proc. 96 Roman. Conf. on Neur. Netw. Nat. Symp, Bucharest, 1995, pp. 136-145.

Medical Informatics Europe '99
P. Kokol et al. (Eds.)
IOS Press, 1999

Computer-Assisted Planning and Simulation of Hip Operations using Virtual Three-Dimensional Models

H. Handels[a], J. Ehrhardt[a], W. Plötz[b], S.J. Pöppl[a]
[a]Institute for Medical Informatics and [b]Department of Orthopaedic Surgery
Medical University of Lübeck, Ratzeburger Allee 160, 23538 Lübeck, Germany
Email: handels@medinf.mu-luebeck.de

Abstract. In this paper a new software system for virtual preoperative planning and simulation of hip operations is presented. The system simulates the endoprosthetic reconstruction of the hip joint with hemipelvic replacement for bone tumor patients and supports the individual design of anatomically adaptable, modular prostheses. Three-dimensional models of the patient's hip are generated based on CT data. The surgeon simulates the operation and defines the position and shape of the custom-made endoprosthesis. Stereoscopic visualization and 3D input devices facilitate the navigation and interaction in the virtual environment. Special visualization techniques like texture mapping, color coding of quantitative parameters or transparency support the determination of the correct position and shape of the prosthesis. Furthermore, the system can be used for patient information or educational tasks.

1. Introduction

For the treatment of bone tumors of the hip and pelvis an endoprosthetic reconstruction is often necessary. During the surgical operation the tumorous part of the pelvic bone is resected and replaced by a custom-made, modular manufactured prosthesis. Up to now solid anatomical models have been used for the planning of these hip operations and the design of individual prostheses in our department of orthopaedic surgery [1].

Computer assisted planning and simulation systems for orthopaedic surgery gain in importance more and more, especially with regards to quality control and cost reduction. In contrast to systems as described in [2,3], the presented software system supports the virtual planning of the endoprosthetic reconstruction of the hip joint with hemipelvic replacement. The intention of this system is to facilitate the precise planning of these hip operations as well as the positioning and design of the prosthesis without the manufacturing of an expensive solid model of the patient's hip.

2. Methods

Three-dimensional surface models of the hip bones are generated based on three-dimensional CT image sequences with a typical resolution of 0.75mm × 0.75mm × 4mm. The segmentation of the hip bones is done with commonly used intensity thresholding techniques. In a post-processing step, morphological operators reduce segmentation errors.

Finally, an interactive step to correct the segmentation results and to separate the different parts of the hip is needed.

Based on the segmented data surface-oriented, three-dimensional models are reconstructed using „The Visualization Toolkit“ (VTK) [4] implementation of the marching cubes algorithm [5]. In the virtual bone model the following objects are labeled: sacrum, left and right hip bone, left and right femur. After application of a triangle reduction algorithm [6] the surface models consist of 80.000 triangles, typically. The rendering of the three-dimensional models is based on the VTK as well (fig. 1, left). Interactive determined landmarks are used to reorient the surface models into a patient independent coordinate system.

For tumor patients often MR data have been acquired additionally. In this case a rigid body image registration of CT and MR data is performed to enable a simultaneous visualization of bone and tumor [7]. While the hip bone can be segmented in CT images, MR images give improved information about the bone tumor's position.

2.1 Simulation of the Operation

In the virtual environment the surgeon is able to interact with the three-dimensional models by translation, rotation and zooming operations and to measure distances, angles and volumes. Slices of original CT or MR data can be displayed in combination with the three-dimensional bone models. Furthermore, the virtual environment permits the interactive positioning of cutting planes and to cut the surface models (fig. 1, right). Stereoscopic visualization techniques and 3D input devices support the 3D interaction with the model, especially the precise positioning of cutting planes. After the cutting plane is chosen, the hip bone is resected and the tumorous part of the bone is removed. The resulting surface model consists of two or more disjoint segments.

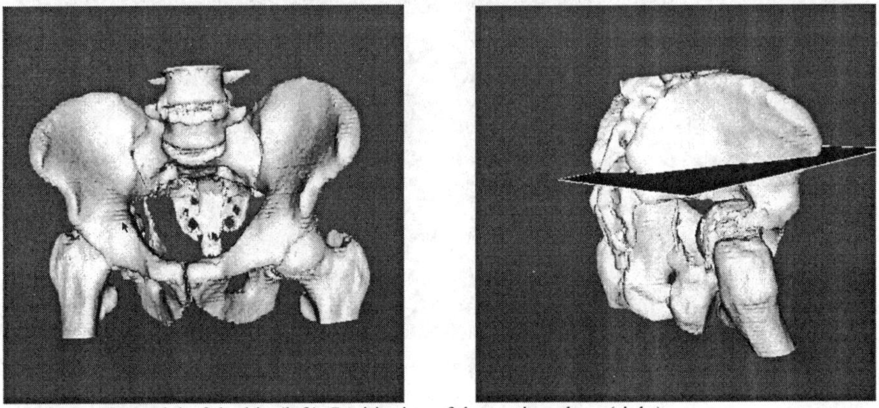

Fig. 1: 3D-model of the hip (left). Positioning of the cutting plane (right)

2.2 Virtual Positioning and Design of the Endoprostheses

Furthermore, the system supports the custom-made design of the implant as well as the positioning of the prosthesis and screws. The central task is the design and positioning of the upper part of the prosthesis, that consists of four main parts: central intramedullary stem, ground plane, fixation plate for the screws and artificial hip joint (Fig. 2). Therefore, the generated cut surface and the shape and geometric parameters of the implant are computed resulting in a CAD-model of the anatomically adaptable prosthesis.

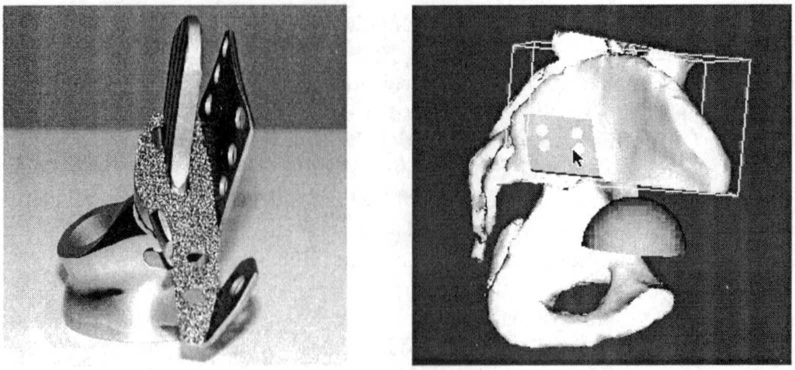

Fig. 2. Upper part of the endoprosthesis with central intramedullary stem, ground plane, fixation plate for the screws and artificial hip joint (left). Positioning of the CAD-model of the fixation plate (right).

The CAD-model of the individual prosthesis is created in several steps. While the ground plane of the prosthesis is given by the cutting plane of hip, the positions of the stem, the screws as well as the artificial hip joint have to be determined. After the fixation plate for the screws has been positioned interactively by the mouse pointer, the plate takes the particular shape of the individual hip (Fig. 1 right). The positioning of the intramedullary stem is supported by two visualization techniques: The distances between bone and the stem of the CAD-model are computed and visualized on the bone surface using color maps (fig. 3). Furthermore, the stem's position can be visualized within the hip in a transparent mode.

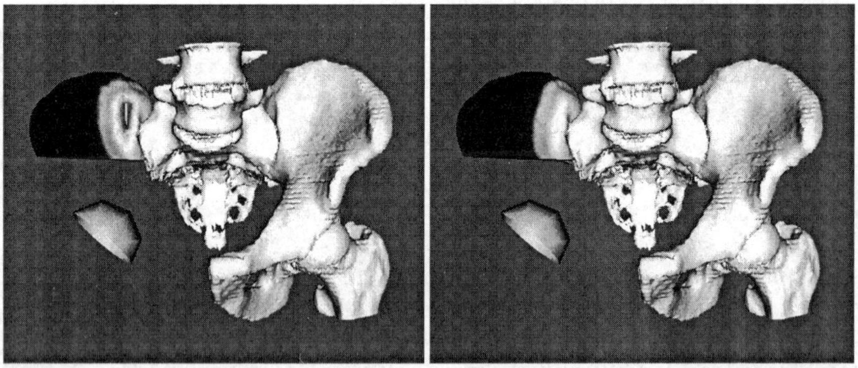

Fig. 3: Colored display of distances between bone and the intramedullary stem in an unsuitable (left) and a suitable position (right).

The position of the artificial hip joint is chosen in correspondence to the healthy hip part (fig. 4). The center of the artificial hip joint is calculated as the mirrored center of the femoral head of the healthy body side (fig. 4, right). Points on the border of the healthy hip joint are marked interactively as landmarks. The landmarks are approximated by a plane using the least square criterion (fig. 4, left). The resulting plane is mirrored to the other hip side and used as a reference plane to determine the orientation of the artificial hip joint (fig. 4 right). Alternatively, standard values for the orientation of the artificial hip joint can be used.

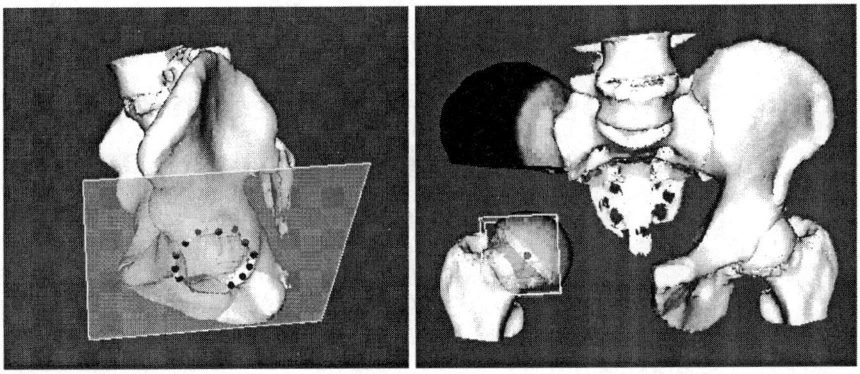

Fig. 4: Left: The marked points on the hip joint border and the approximated plane are shown. Right: Resulting position of the artificial hip joint in correspondence to the left, healthy hip part.

3. Conclusions

The use of the system makes possible a virtual planning of hip operations without the need to generate a time and cost intensive, individual solid hip model. In contrast to the planning procedure using solid 3D models of the hip the computer based operation planning enables the surgeon to compare different operation strategies given by varying cutting planes. Additionally, original CT and MR data can be displayed in combination with 3D models using texture mapping techniques. Furthermore, the system can be used for pre-operative patient information or educational tasks.

References

[1] Gradinger R, Rechl H, Ascherl R, Plötz W, Hipp E: Endoprothetischer Teilersatz des Beckens bei malignen Tumoren, *Orthopäde* **22** (1993) 167-173.

[2] Richolt JA, Teschner M, Everett P, Girod B, Millis MB, Kikinis R: Planning and Evaluation of Reorienting Osteotomis of the Proximal Femur in Cases of SCFE Using Virtual Three-Dimensional Models. In: Wells WM, Colchester A, Delp S, eds. Medical Image Computing and Computer-Assisted Intervention - MICCAI 98. Springer Verlag, Berlin, 1998, pp. 1-8.

[3] Tso CY, Ellis RE, Rudan J, Harrison MM: A Surgical Planning and Guidance System for High Tibial Osteotomies. In: Wells WM, Colchester A, Delp S (eds.), Medical Image Computing and Computer-Assisted Intervention - MICCAI 98, Springer Verlag, Berlin,1998, pp. 39-50.

[4] Schroeder W, Martin K, Lorensen B: The Visualization Toolkit - An Object-Oriented Approach To 3D Graphics. Prentice Hall, New Jersey, 1998

[5] Lorensen WE, Cline HE: Marching Cubes: A High Resolution 3-D Surface Construction Algorithm, *Computer Graphics*, **21** ,4 (1987) 163-169.

[6] Schroeder WJ, Zarge JA, Lorensen WE: Decimation of Triangle Meshes. In: SIGGRAPH92, Chicago, 1992, pp.163-169.

[7] W. Wells, P. Viola, H. Atsumi, S. Nakajima, and R. Kikinis, Multi-modal Volume Registration by Maximization of Mutual Information, *Medical Image Analysis* **1**, (1996) 35-51.

Medical Informatics Europe '99
P. Kokol et al. (Eds.)
IOS Press, 1999

A Probabilistic Approach to Improved Antibiotic Therapy

Nicolette de Bruijn and Peter Lucas
Department of Computer Science, Utrecht University
Padualaan 14, 3584 CH Utrecht, The Netherlands
E-mail: {nbruijn,lucas}@cs.uu.nl

Karin Schurink and Andy Hoepelman
Department of Internal Medicine, Utrecht University Hospital
Heidelberglaan 100, 3584 CX Utrecht, The Netherlands
E-mail: k.schurink@digd.azu.nl

Abstract

PTA is a decision-theoretic expert system that aims to assist clinicians in diagnosing and treating patients with pneumonia in the intensive care unit. Its underlying probabilistic network model includes knowledge for diagnosing pneumonia on the basis of the likelihood of tracheobronchial-tree colonisation by pathogens, and symptoms and signs actually present in the patient. Optimal antibiotic therapy is selected by balancing the expected efficacy of treatment, which is related to the likelihood of pathogen-specific pneumonias, against costs and side effects of treatment. In this article, the model underlying the system and results of a preliminary evaluation are described.

Keywords: medical decision support, probabilistic networks, Bayesian networks

1 Introduction

The medical community is presently in a state of transition from a situation dominated by the paper medical record to a future situation where all patient data will be available on-line by an electronic clinical information system. In many hospitals, laboratory data have already been stored and distributed by a hospital information system for some time. In technically more advanced hospitals, a number of wards in which the amount of data collected for a patient is huge, such as intensive care units (ICUs), have their clinical patient data already fully managed by a local clinical information system. The local system is usually capable of exchanging information with an available traditional hospital-wide information system.

However, it is not enough to provide facilities for storing and retrieving patient data to the clinician; clinical information systems should also offer facilities to assist clinicians in dealing with hard clinical problems, such as provided by facilities for decision support. In this paper, we describe the development of a decision-theoretic expert system [3], i.e. a system based on a combination of the theory of probabilistic networks (Bayesian belief networks) and decision theory [5], called *PTA* (Pneumonia Therapy Advisor), that is aimed at providing advice about the administration of appropriate antibiotic therapy to patients with pneumonia in the ICU.

2 Management of pneumonia at the ICU

Pneumonia is a frequently occurring clinical problem at the ICU. Many patients admitted to an ICU need respiratory support by a mechanical ventilator; in addition, many of these patients are affected by severe diseases which may result in depression of their immune system. Both conditions promote the development of bacterial pneumonia.

Ventilator-associated pneumonia (VAP) is a form of pneumonia that may arise in patients whom are mechanically ventilated [1]. The occurrence of VAP in a patient during a stay in the hospital is seen as a significant problem due to the presence of multi-resistant bacteria in clinical wards, in particular in the ICU.

Choosing an appropriate therapy for pneumonia not only involves the issue of susceptibility of pathogens to antibiotic drugs, but also of possible side effects and of future development of resistance to drugs. In the case of antibiotic therapy possible side effects are: renal failure, diminished hearing, epileptic seizures and allergic reactions varying from skin rash to anaphylactic shock. Clearly, the decisions about appropriate antibiotic therapy must be made on the grounds of a lot of uncertain medical knowledge. In particular, making decisions concerning the initial therapy, called *empirical therapy*, for these patients is difficult because it takes at least 48 hours before the results of sputum cultures become available. Sputum cultures yield information of the identity and antibiotic susceptibility of pathogens. Hence, empirical antibiotic therapy, the subject on which PTA focusses, is usually prescribed without actually knowing the identity of the causative pathogens.

3 A probabilistic model of pneumonia

3.1 *The probabilistic network formalism*

A natural representation of the uncertainties involved in dealing with treatment of pneumonia is offered by the probabilistic-network formalism [4, 5]. A *probabilistic network* is an acyclic directed graph $G = (V(G), A(G))$, with a set of vertices $V(G) = \{V_1, \ldots, V_n\}$, where each vertex $V_i \in V(G)$ represents a discrete stochastic variable; a set of arcs $A(G) \subseteq V(G) \times V(G)$ reflects all stochastic (conditional) independencies in the domain concerned. Arcs are often informally seen as to mirror causal or correlational influences among variables. On the set of variables $\{V_1, \ldots, V_n\}$ is defined a joint probability distribution Pr that can be factorised according to the topology of the graph as follows:

$$\Pr(V_1, \ldots, V_n) = \prod_{i=1}^{n} \Pr(V_i | \pi(V_i))$$

where $\pi(V_i)$ represents the set of variables associated with the parent vertices of V_i. This means that the joint probability distribution $\Pr(V_1, \ldots, V_n)$ can be defined in terms of 'local' probability tables $\Pr(V_i|\pi(V_i))$ by assuming the variable V_i to be conditionally independent of all predecessors of the associated vertex V_i given the parents $\pi(V_i)$.

3.2 *The VAP model*

The probabilistic network model was developed with the help of a number of infectious disease experts and by consultation of the medical literature. Figure 1 gives an overview of the structure of the model. Boxes indicate processes that can be (partially) observed,

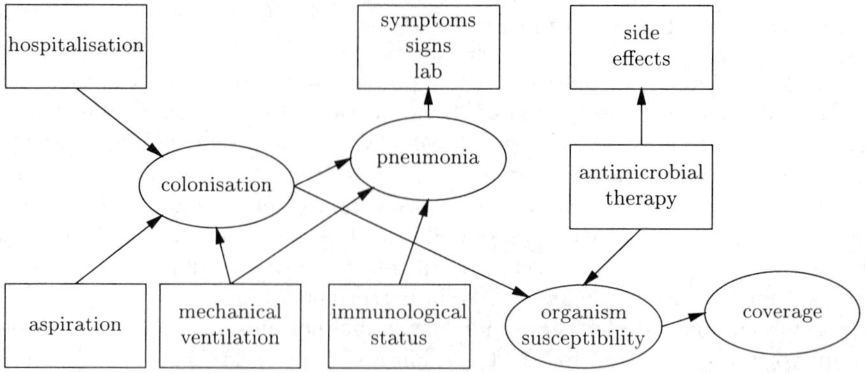

Figure 1: Global structure of probabilistic model.

or decisions that can be made by the clinician at the time of empirical therapy; ellipses indicate processes that cannot be observed at the time of empirical therapy selection.

Central to the model is the temporal process of *colonisation* of the laryngotracheobronchial tree by pathogens. The temporal nature of the process is expressed by the interaction between duration of stay at the ICU (*hospitalisation*) and the duration of *mechanical ventilation*: both duration of stay at the ICU and duration of mechanical ventilation are positively correlated to colonisation by pathogens. *Aspiration* of stomach content is another factor positively correlated to colonisation by certain pathogens (*Enterobacteriaceae*). When a patient is colonised by specific pathogens, there is a certain probability that *pneumonia* will develop. This is expressed in the graph by an arc from *colonisation* to *pneumonia*. Duration of mechanical ventilation and immunological status influence the probability that pneumonia develops as well; hence, an arc from these vertices to the *pneumonia* vertex is included in the model. When the patient is affected by pneumonia, certain symptoms, signs or laboratory abnormalities can be observed, as summarised in a corresponding vertex in the graph. Finally, the *susceptibility* of pathogens to particular antibiotic treatment is determined by the choice of medical treatment and the actually present pathogens causing infection. Some antibiotic drugs may give rise to certain side effects.

Some of the vertices shown in the graph in Figure 1 actually comprise a number of separate, but similar vertices. For example, colonisation by pathogens was modelled as a biological process, in which it was assumed that pathogens occur independently. Note that this representation allows for the presence in the patient of a pulmonary infection due to *multiple* organisms. Colonisation by 11 of the most frequently occurring pathogens, such as *Pseudomonas aeruginosa* and *Neisseria meningitidis*, is represented in the current model; similarly, the vertex *organism susceptibility* concerns the effects of antibiotic treatment on each of these 11 pathogens. In Figure 2, a small part of the model, only involving the vertices *hospitalisation*, *mechanical ventilation*, *colonisation* (e.g. `COL_P.AERUGINOSA`, i.e. colonisation by *Pseudomonas aeruginosa*), and *pneumonia* (e.g. `P.AERUGINOSA_Pneumonia`), *susceptibility* of pathogens to antimicrobial drugs, and *medication* is shown, restricted to 4 of the 11 included pathogens. Vertices with captial `I` are *instantiation vertices* (see below). The single vertex *coverage* represents the overall effect of the antibiotic drugs on the pathogens.

Antibiotic treatment consists of the selection of one or two different antibiotics – possibly also none – modelled by two identical therapy vertices; each therapy vertex

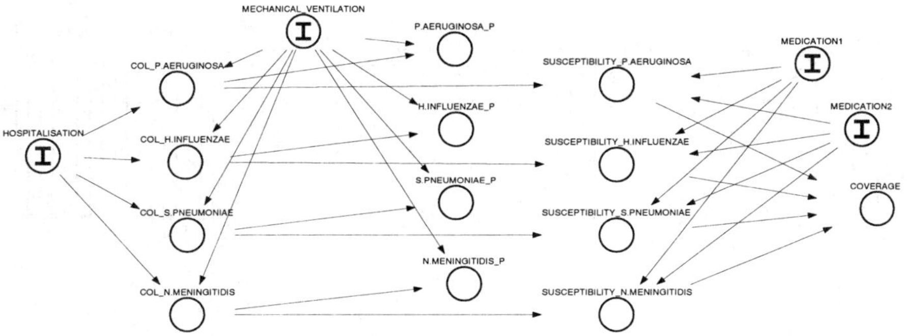

Figure 2: Part of a probabilistic VAP model.

includes 24 different antibiotic drugs (including none), yielding $24^2 = 576$ possible combinations, of which $\binom{23}{2} = 253$ (excluding 'none') are different, yielding a total of $253 + 24 = 277$ (now including 'none' and single drugs) different therapies.

3.3 Decision-making capabilities

The efficacy of treatment for a patient can be examined by entering observed symptoms and signs in the patient, duration of hospitalisation, mechanical ventilation, previously experienced side effects of antibiotic therapy, and laboratory data. Treatment selection is flexible in the sense that only data concerning vertices that are denoted as instantiation vertices must be supplied always; although entering more patient data may provide additional evidence concerning the cause of pneumonia, the model can be used even when most other findings are unknown. Using the probabilistic inference algorithm as described in [2], the probability distribution defined on the *coverage* variable can be updated, yielding a posterior probability of coverage of all possible pathogens $\Pr^*$ reflecting knowledge concerning all entered evidence (*Evidence*), i.e.

$$\Pr^*(coverage) = \Pr(coverage|Evidence)$$

Particular vertices without parents were indicated as instantiation vertices. This means that a value for the corresponding variable must always be supplied, yielding additional stochastic independence information. In this way, the speed of probabilistic inference could be dramatically improved.

By defining a utility measure in terms of coverage, it is possible, in principle, to automatically determine the treatment that gives optimal coverage by computation of the maximum expected utility. However, since the number of possible drug combinations was 576, computation of optimal therapy was practically infeasible. As a practical solution to this problem, we have restricted the 277 different therapies to the 32 different therapies considered adequate for most patients; this therapy choice is then represented as a single vertex.

4 Evaluation

The present structure of the network has a strong logical foundation, and we therefore believe it to be basically correct. There may be particular arcs missing due to gaps in the medical knowledge concerning pneumonia. However, correlations due to missing

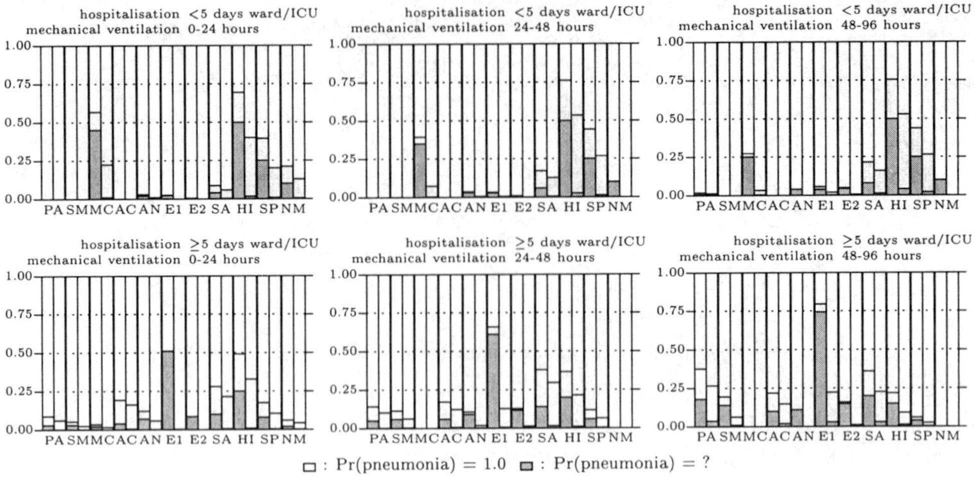

Figure 3: Obtained predictions after entering information concerning duration of hospitalisation and mechanical ventilation. Names of pathogens have been abbreviated. For each pathogen, the probability of colonisation and pneumonia are depicted, in that order.

medical knowledge are likely to be weak, and hence have little effect on the probability distribution.

In addition to the structure of a probabilistic network, the accuracy of the represented probabilistic information is an issue that requires attention. This has been investigated in two ways. First, some of the vertices in the model were instantiated (i.e. a specific value was chosen), and the resulting posterior probability distribution was compared with frequency of occurrence information available from the ICU; see Figure 3. It appears that the patterns of frequency of colonisation and pneumonia for particular pathogens changes with duration of stay at the hospital. For example, the relative frequency of colonisation and pneumonia by *Moraxella catharrhalis* (MC in the figure), which is high when entering the hospital, decreases during the first 96 hours of mechanical ventilation (upper three graphs), to become nearly absent when the patient has stayed more than five days in hospital. This frequency decreases to nearly zero for patients whom are mechanically ventilated during the next 96 hours (lower graph). In contrast, the relative frequency of colonisation and pneumonia with *Pseudomonas aeruginosa* rises after a stay of more than five days in the ICU, which is increased even further due to mechanical ventilation. These observations did agree with expert opinion.

Furthermore, the conclusions obtained with the model were examined for a group of 12 patients, drawn from the files of the ICU. For these patients, the system selected the therapy that best covered suspected pathogens. Similarly, a specialist in infectious disease was requested to select the best antibiotic therapy, and also to classify recommendations made by the system as being either acceptable, unacceptable or second best choice. The results are shown in Table 1. It appears that in 8 cases the model prescribed a therapy that covers more pathogens than the therapy prescribed by the expert. This is caused by the fact that the present model does not take broadness of antimicrobial spectrum into account. All 12 prescriptions were considered acceptable

Table 1: Results for 12 patients. Meaning of abbreviations: Hosp: Hospitalisation stay and location; ≥5daysW/IC: ≥5 days in hospital (at ward or ICU); Vent: duration of mechanical ventilation in hours; colonisation HI: colonisation by *H. influenzae*; Diff x/y: position x out of y different groups of drugs, ordered according to probability (from high to low) and grouped when probabilities were equal; Aug+Gen: Augmentin + Gentamycin; acceptable: advice of PTA is acceptable according to the expert; 2nd best: advice of PTA is second best choice of expert; Cov: coverage of recommendation by PTA; <: less broad spectrum; =: similar spectrum; >: broader spectrum.

n	Hosp	Vent	Extra Info	Expert Advice	Diff	PTA	Assessment	Cov
1	<5days	24-48	colonisation HI	Augmentin	3/21	Aug+Gen	acceptable	>
2	<5days	48-96	colonisation HI+SA	Augmentin	8/19	Aug+Gen	acceptable	>
3	<5days	48-96	colonisation SA	Augmentin	8/21	Aug+Gen	acceptable	>
4	<5days	48-96	-	Augmentin	3/21	Aug+Gen	acceptable	>
5	<5days	48-96	-	Augmentin	4/22	Aug+Gen	2nd best	>
6	<5days	48-96	-	Augmentin	5/21	Aug+Gen	acceptable	>
7	<5days	48-96	-	Augmentin	4/23	Aug+Gen	acceptable	>
8	<5days	24-48	COPD	Cefta+Tobra	5/23	Aug+Gen	2nd best	<
9	≥5dW/IC	0-24	aspiration	Aug+Gen	7/28	Tazocin	acceptable	>
10	≥5dIC	96-144	-	Cefta+Tobra	8/24	Tazocin	2nd best	=
11	≥5dIC	>144	phagocyts dys	Cefta+Tobra	7/19	Tazocin	2nd best	=
12	≥5dIC	>144	colonisation E1+E2	Imipenem	1/12	Imipenem	acceptable	=

or second best choice; none of the recommendations was considered unacceptable.

5 Discussion

Above, we have discussed the development of a decision-theoretic expert system that assists in exploring the diagnosis and treatment of ventilator-associated pneumonia. In the near future, we will design additional utility models, for example models that take into account antimicrobial spectrum and financial costs of antibiotics, to obtain a system that balances different costs and benefits of antibiotic drugs to reach optimal treatment. We intend to embed the resulting system in the clinical information system of the ICU.

References

[1] J.G. Bartlett, Management of Respiratory Tract Infections, Williams & Wilkins, Baltimore, 1997.

[2] S.L. Lauritzen and D.J. Spiegelhalter, Local computations with probabilities on graphical structures and their application to expert systems, Journal of the Royal Statistical Society (Series B), 50 (1987) 157–224.

[3] P.J.F. Lucas, H. Boot and B.G. Taal, Computer-based decision-support in the management of primary gastric non-Hodgkin lymphoma, *Methods of Information in Medicine* 37 (1998) 206–219.

[4] P.J.F. Lucas and L.C. van der Gaag, Principles of Expert Systems, Addison-Wesley, Wokingham, 1991.

[5] J. Pearl, Probabilistic Reasoning in Intelligent Systems, Morgan Kaufman, San Mateo, California, 1988.

Medical Informatics Europe '99
P. Kokol et al. (Eds.)
IOS Press, 1999

Possibilities of See5 software in forecasting of life expectancy not achieving

Silvije Vuletić, Josipa Kern, Zdenko Sonicki, Davor Ivanković
Andrija Štampar School of Public Health, Medical School, University of Zagreb, Rockefellerova 4, 10000 Zagreb, Croatia, e-mail:svuletic@snz.hr

Abstract. Results of application of See5 to epidemiological domain were presented. The aim of this paper is to find out if See5 can be used for forecasting whether life expectancy will be achieved or not. The basis for forecasting are data - attributes, predictors (anthropological data, living habits, laboratory data, blood pressure measured in years 1970/71, and the status of examinee - class (alive or dead) in 1990. Data were split at random into 10 blocks with approximately the same number of cases and the same distribution of classes. Results were given in the form of decision trees and rulesets, and tested through crossvalidation. The most interesting question - what are prediction-candidates for not achieving life expectancy estimated in the year of examination - did not give a satisfactory result: the accuracy of classification was about 70%. However, a very interesting fact is that each rule consists of at least one candidate predictor, usually considered as risk factor (e.g. high diastolic blood pressure and animal fat consumption).

1. Introduction

Life expectancy depends on many factors. The questions "which factors can be considered as predictors of life expectancy" or "which factors can reduce mortality" could be challenging for an epidemiologist [1]. The epidemiological domain is characterised by its complexity which can be considered as something: (1) having many varied interrelated parts, patterns, or elements and consequently hard to understand fully, or (2) marked by an involvement of many parts, aspects, details, notions, and necessitating earnest study or examination to understand or cope with. It means that epidemiology is a soft domain, and any methods for prediction or classification in that field should be of assistance.

The aim of this paper is to find out if See5, applied on epidemiological data, can be used for forecasting whether the life expectancy will be achieved or not according to a number of data measured many years ago. The database consists of results of the epidemiological investigation performed in Croatia in years 1970/71 (anthropological data, living habits, laboratory data, blood pressure and the status of examinee (alive or dead) in 1990.

2. Material and methods

A sample of 1888 examinees was taken into consideration. Each examinee was described by age, gender, smoking habits, systolic blood pressure - SBP, diastolic blood pressure - DBP, glucose, cholesterol, triglycerides, oil/fat consumption, alcohol consumption and body mass index - BMI, as well as by his/her status (alive or dead) after 20 years. All data mentioned above were described in detail elsewhere [2]. According to the status, age, and life expectancy data for this population, the new outcome variable was constructed. The values were: 'achieved life expectancy' - doesn't matter if he/she was alive or dead in 1990 (1317 cases), 'did not achieve life expectancy' - died before (571 cases). These outcomes should be predicted by using See5 algorithm and data described above. The examinees, who were alive in 1990 but who were too young to achieve their life expectancy, were excluded from the study.

The See5, successor of C4.5 [3,4], is a program for analysing data and generating classifiers in the form of decision trees and/or rulesets. It can use continuous and/or discrete attributes, and allows existence of unknown data. There are several options that can be used to influence the process of constructing the classifier. The Crossvalidate option can be used to estimate the accuracy of the classifier constructed by See5 even when there are no separate test cases. So, our data were split at random into 10 blocks with approximately the same number of cases and the same distribution of classes. For each block in turn, See5 constructed a classifier using the cases in all the other blocks (learning set) and then tested its accuracy on the cases in the hold-out block (testing set). In this way, there were 10 experiments, and each case in the data was used just once as a test case. The error rate of the classifier produced from all the cases was estimated as the ratio of the total number of errors on the hold-out cases (testing objects) to the total number of cases. The See5 could not give accuracy for the learning objects. No application of the See5 we found in recent literature.

3. Results

The See5 generated decision trees as well as the corresponding rulesets. The option "more than 10 items/examinees are required for rule generating" was set up in each of the ten folds (experiments) used for crossvalidation. General results on a number of rules in each of the ten folds, and the corresponding classification or prediction errors are shown in Table 1.

Table 1. Summary results of See5 procedure

Fold	Decision Tree		Rules		Rules for 'Not achieving LE' Number (%)
	Size	Errors	Number	Errors	
0	21.0	33.0%	12	29.8%	7 (58%)
1	18.0	27.7%	10	28.2%	5 (50%)
2	3.0	30.2%	3	30.2%	1 (33%)
3	3.0	29.1%	3	29.1%	1 (33%)
4	31.0	34.4%	21	32.8%	11 (52%)
5	20.0	32.3%	5	30.7%	3 (60%)
6	16.0	28.0%	7	28.0%	5 (71%)
7	10.0	31.2%	6	30.7%	3 (50%)
8	6.0	31.7%	3	30.2%	1 (33%)
9	15.0	29.6%	8	30.7%	4 (50%)
Mean	14.3	30.7%	7.8	30.0%	
SE	2.8	0.7%	1.8	0.4%	

Frequency of attributes, predictor-candidates, included in any of set of rules is shown in Table 2.

Table 2. Frequency and ranks of attributes included in the rules

Attribute	Frequency	Rank
Systolic blood pressure	12	4
Diastolic blood pressure	23	2
Fasting glucose	7	7
Postload glucose	4	10
Cholesterol	3	11.5
Triglycerides	3	11.5
Animal fat consumption	36	1
Smoking	5	9
Alcohol consumption	8	6
BMI	6	8
Age (beginning of the study)	13	3
Gender	9	5

Table 3. Rules covering most items/examinees (more than 100)

Rule 12: (cover 127)	Rule 21: (cover 243)
Animal_fat_consumption > 26448 (a lot)	*Diastolic_blood_pressure > 85*
Alcohol_consumption <= 20093 (low or moderate)	*Animal fat consumption > 24437 (a lot)*
-> class N [0.574]	*-> class N [0.531]*

The rule, combining Diastolic_blood_pressure and Animal_fat_consumption, is the most frequent one. It appears in 8 out of 10 folds (experiments). Numeric boundaries/limits of both attributes are changing from one to another fold (experiment) – e.g. diastolic blood pressure has the boundary of 106 mm Hg (6 times), 109 mm Hg (once) and 85 mm Hg (once). In spite of not being the clinical boundary of normal/abnormal diastolic blood pressure, the last value of 85 mm Hg appears in the recent literature as something reducing mortality [1]. The rules with the most frequent combination of attributes (DBP and Animal fat consumption) are as follows:

Table 4. Rules with the most frequent combination of attributes

	Diastolic blood pressure	Animal fat consumption	
Rule 9: (cover 26)	> 109	> 24437 (a lot)	-> class N [0.750]
Rule 8: (cover 39)	> 106	> 21662 (a lot)	-> class N [0.659]
Rule 3: (cover 41)	> 106	> 20707 (a lot)	-> class N [0.698]
Rule 3: (cover 39)	> 106	> 21662 (a lot)	-> class N [0.683]
Rule 21: (cover 243)	> 85	> 24437 (a lot)	-> class N [0.531]
Rule 5: (cover 40)	> 106	> 20707 (a lot)	-> class N [0.690]
Rule 6: (cover 34)	> 106	> 24437 (a lot)	-> class N [0.750]
Rule 3: (cover 36)	> 106	> 24437 (a lot)	-> class N [0.711]

4. Discussion

The most interesting question - what are prediction-candidates for not achieving life expectancy estimated in the year of examination – has not given a satisfactory result: the accuracy of classification (measured on testing set) is about 70%. However a very interesting fact may be noticed. Each rule consists of at least one candidate- predictor, usually considered as a risk factor. Those are excessive consumption of animal fat, high diastolic and/or systolic blood pressure, high glucose (fasting or postload), high blood lipids, extreme BMI, etc. Some of the rules seem to be trustworthy, especially those combining diastolic blood pressure and animal fat consumption. Age and gender seem not to be relevant for whether life expectancy will be achieved or not but they enter the rules in order to give better specification of population subgroups. For example, the rule (covering 14 examinees):

Age <= 64
Systolic_blood_pressure > 164
Diastolic_blood_pressure > 90
Animal_fat_consumption <= 9480.5 (low)
-> class N [0.813]

specifies the younger people, with low animal fat consumption but abnormal both systolic and diastolic blood pressure.

Acknowledgement

This project was in part supported by a Grant from the Foundation Open Society Institute.

References

[1] A. Schieppati, G. Remuzzi, Reducing mortality and increasing awareness, *Lancet* **352**(suppl IV) (1998); 352(suppl) 20.
[2] S. Vuletić, Ž. Jakšić, B. Kesić, B (Eds.), The Study of Fat and Carbohydrate Metabolism Indicators Correlated with the Occurrence of Diabetes in Animal Fat and Oil Consuming Population Groups. Final Report, Andrija Štampar School of Public Health, Zagreb, 1972.
[3] J.R.Quinlan, C4.5:Programs for Machine Learning, Morgan Kaufman Publishers, San Mateo, CA, 1993.
[4] See5 (ver. 1.06) on-line manual at http://www.rulequest.com/see5-win.html

Medical Informatics Europe '99
P. Kokol et al. (Eds.)
IOS Press, 1999

Intelligent systems in medical diagnosis

Bojan Novak
University of Maribor, Faculty of Electrical Engineering and Computer Science, Smetanova 17, 2000 Maribor, novakb@uni-mb.si

Abstract: From an intelligent system for a computer supported medical diagnosis it is expected to achieve high accuracy and ability to draw conclusions from a small data sets. Medical practice could takes many years to generate a large database. A new mathematical method that is able to learn on a small data set is presented.

1. Introduction

Recent development in the field of intelligent systems has greatly improved the ability and reliability of different methodologies and techniques for computer supported medical diagnosis. The reason for the use of the computer is mainly the following. In the case of the mass scale prevention against diseases such as different sorts of cancers: breast cancer, melanoma etc. medical treatment is effective only in the cases where the disease is detected in the early stages [1]. Today a lot of different technologies are available and the question is how to make a diagnosis from numerous laboratory examinations. With the application of learning methods based on different mathematical theories new steps can be taken towards computer supported medical diagnosis. This can be useful particularly in the cases where there are insufficient specialists and when immediate diagnosis is the critical factor.

In this paper an advanced method of classification is described with the ability to manage the cases with small data sets and nonlinear mutual relations.

2. Basic algorithm

The idea of the algorithm is to find some small subset of training data called support vectors (SV) and find for them optimal separation that is equivalent to optimal separation of the entire data set. Where optimal separation means that the minimal distance for the closest point to the separating hyperplane between the two different classes is maximal. If the hyperplane has equation $y = \mathbf{w}\mathbf{x}_i + b$ then finding optimal hyperplane means minimizing $||\mathbf{w}||^2$ .Details are described in [2,3,4]. For the nonlinear tasks such as regression, identification, control, fuzzy system modeling, the non-linear support vector approach is applied. A non-linear mapping is applied to map the data into the higher dimensional feature space where the linear regression is possible. This transformation is possible when applying the kernel functions. They have their origin in theory of Reproducing Kernel Hilbert Spaces [2,3,4]

3. Application in diagnosis

The performance of the described method was tested on well-known breast cancer databases obtained from the University of Wisconsin Hospitals, Madison from Dr. William H. Wolberg [6,7,8].. It has 699 cases (as of 15 July 1992) and 10 attributes plus the class attribute benign or malignant. The problem is not linearly separable, so different authors have extensively studied this data set [9]. In our case two different problems were considered. To generate such a base many years are necessary. At the beginning only a few examples are available and the question is what precision can be reached in this case. The normal procedures for testing the quality of diagnosis prediction are cross-validation methods. The data is split into three parts: the learning data set, the testing data set and the validation data set. In our case only about 50 examples were available during each year. In such cases in one or two years there is not enough data for cross validation. A test was made taking only the first 50 data and to construct a learning machine according to the structural risk minimization principle. In this case, without any cross-validation (because all data were used for learning), a 90% precision was achieved on the rest of the data set. Also an experiment was done with 67% data in the learning set and tested on the remaining data without validation error checking. The 97% accuracy is even slightly better than the extensive and time consuming cross-validation with the ANN resulting 96.6%. Some further tests will be done in the future on other medical problems to check and confirm the good performances of the proposed method.

4. Conclusion

Recent development in the field of intelligent, systems has greatly improved the ability and reliability of different methodologies and techniques for computer supported medical diagnosis. Particularly interesting are cases where linearization of the problem deteriorates the accuracy of diagnosis. Different methodologies have been developed for nonlinear modeling. Application of ANN has shown that these methods are sensitive to number and types of neurons in layers and weight initialization. Also a large data set is needed for good accuracy. In medicine this is not often available because it could take many years to generate a large database. The development of learning theory on small data set has overcome the problem to a great extent. A short theoretical description is presented. Its applicability is presented the on well-known breast cancer databases obtained from the University of Wisconsin Hospitals, Madison. In the first test accuracy of diagnosis based on only 50 patients records was tested. Such a small data set is generated in one year and the question is what accuracy can be expected. The normal procedure for testing the quality of diagnosis prediction is cross-validation methods. The data are split into three parts: the learning data set, the testing data set and the validation data set. Only 50 examples are not enough for cross validation. The structural risk minimization method was applied to set an optimal structure of network. Testing was done on the rest of the data set. Excellent 90% accuracy was achieved. In the second test 67% of the data was used for learning and remaining for testing. No validation was applied. The resulting 97% accuracy is even slightly better than extensive and time consuming cross-validation with the ANN. Some further tests will be done in the future on other medical problems to check and confirm the good performances of the proposed method.

References

[1] A. Kjoelen, M. J. Thompson, S. E. Umbaugh, R. H. Moss and W. V. Stoecker: Performance of AI Methods in Detecting Melanoma, *Engineering in Medicine and Biology, IEEE,* Vol. 14 No. 4. July/August 1995.

[2] B. Schölkopf, C. Burges, V. Vapnik: Extracting Support Data for a Given Task, in U. M. Fayyad and R. Uthurusamy, eds., First International Conference on Knowledge Discovery and Data Mining, *Proceedings, AAAI Press*, Menlo Park, CA, 1995.

[3] V. N. Vapnik, S. E. Golowich and A. Smola, Support vector method for function approximation, regression and signal processing in *Advances in Neural Information Processing Systems. Vol. 9 MIT Press*, Cambridge MA., USA.

[4] V. N. Vapnik, Statistical Learning Theory, *John Wiley and Sons*, 1998.

[5] O. L. Mangasarian and W. H. Wolberg: Cancer diagnosis via linear programming", *SIAM News*, Volume 23, Number 5, September 1990, pp 1 & 18.

[6] William H. Wolberg and O.L. Mangasarian: Multisurface method of pattern separation for medical diagnosis applied to breast cytology, *Proceedings of the National Academy of Sciences, U.S.A.*, Volume 87, December 1990, pp 9193-9196.

[7] O. L. Mangasarian, R. Setiono, and W.H. Wolberg: Pattern recognition via linear programming: Theory and application to medical diagnosis, in: Large-scale numerical optimization, Thomas F. Coleman and Yuying Li, editors, *SIAM Publications*, Philadelphia 1990, pp 22-30.

[8] K. P. Bennett & O. L. Mangasarian: "Robust linear programming discrimination of two linearly inseparable sets", Optimization Methods and Software 1, 1992, 23-34 (*Gordon & Breach Science Publishers*).

[9] B. Ster and A. Dobnikar: Neural networks in medical diagnosis: comparision with other methods, *Proceedings of the International Conference EANN 96*, p. 427-430, 1996.

Medical Informatics Europe '99
P. Kokol et al. (Eds.)
IOS Press, 1999

Power of Heterogeneous Computing as a Vehicle for Implementing E^3 Medical Decision Support Systems

Vili PODGORELEC, Janez BREST, Peter KOKOL
University of Maribor, FERI, Smetanova 17, 2000 Maribor, Slovenia

Abstract. A computer system of PCs, workstations, minicomputers etc., connected together via a local area network or wide area network represents a large pool of computational power. Our aim is to use this power for the implementation of E^3 (efficiency, effectiveness, efficacy) medical decision support system, which can be based on different models; the best of them are providing an explanation together with an accurate and reliable response. One of the most viable among models are decision trees, already used for many medical decision making purposes. In this paper we would like to present a heterogeneous implementation of genetic algorithm for the induction of decision trees with emphasis on solving the mitral valve prolapse syndrome.

1. Introduction

As in many other areas, decisions play an important role also in medicine, especially in medical diagnostic processes. Decision support systems (DSS) helping physicians are becoming a very important part in medical decision making, particularly in those where decision must be made effectively and reliably [1,2]. Since conceptual simple decision making models with the possibility of automatic learning should be considered for performing such tasks [3], according to recent reviews [1,4,5] decision trees are a very suitable candidate. They have been already successfully used in DSS for many decision making purposes, but some problems still persist in their traditional way of induction, which has not changed much since their introduction. Considering the advantages of the evolutionary methods in performing complex tasks, we decided to overcome these problems by inducing decision trees with genetic algorithms. A problem with evolutionary approach is the computational time, which is much higher than with the traditional induction approach. To reduce the required computation time we implemented the heterogeneous algorithm, which we will discuss later on.

2. Decision trees

The decision trees approach [5-7], which falls into wider range of inductive learning, a subset of learning from examples, is very simple and efficient. First the decisions and learning process can be presented with an easily visualised two-dimensional model, thus decision trees are straightforward to build and interpret. Decision trees use different object attributes to classify different subsets of objects (their great advantage is that they don't use a fixed number of predetermined attributes). Usually the members of a set of objects are classified as either positive or negative instances (patients with MVP Syndrome or without it). We extended this approach with multi-class decision making, enabling one to differentiate between patient with prolapse, silent prolapse and no prolapse at all.

3. Genetic algorithms

Genetic algorithms are adaptive heuristic search methods which may be used to solve all kinds of complex search and optimisation problems [8-10]. They are based on the evolutionary ideas of natural selection and genetic processes of biological organisms. As the natural populations evolve according to the principles of natural selection and "survival of the fittest", first laid down by Charles Darwin, so by simulating this process, genetic algorithms are able to evolve solutions to real-world problems, if they have been suitably encoded [10]. They are often capable of finding optimal solutions even in the most complex of search spaces or at least they offer significant benefits over other search and optimisation techniques.

4. Heterogeneous computing

A computer system of PCs, workstations, minicomputers etc., connected together via a local area network or wide area network represents a large pool of computational power. The use of parallel processing as a mean of providing high-performance computational facilities for large-scale and grand-challenge applications has been investigated widely. Until recently, however, the benefits of this research were confined to the individuals who had access to such systems. The trend is to move away from specialised platforms, such as the Cray/SGI T3E and IBM SP2 to cheaper, general purpose systems consisting of loosely coupled components built up from single or multi-processor platforms. This approach has a number of advantages including that of being able to build a system for a given budget, which is suitable for certain types of applications and workloads.

A cluster can be a network of PCs or UNIX workstations connected via network (Fig. 1). For parallel computing purposes a cluster will generally comprise of high-performance workstations inter-connected by a high-speed network. A cluster works as an integrated collection of resources and can have a single system image spanning all its nodes [11].

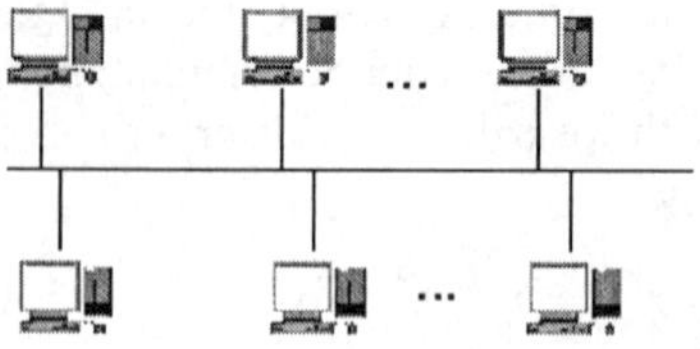

Figure 1. An example of a heterogeneous computing system.

A computer node can be a single or multiprocessor system with memory, I/O facilities, and an operating system. A cluster generally refers to two or more computers (nodes) connected together. The nodes can exist in a single cabinet or be physically separate and connected via a LAN. An interconnected (LAN-based) cluster of computers can appear as a single system to users and applications. Such a system can provide a cost-effective way to gain features and benefits (fast and reliable services) that have historically only been found on more expensive propriety shared memory systems.

5. Mitral valve prolapse

Prolapse is defined as the displacement of a bodily part from its normal position. The term mitral valve prolapse (MVP) [14,15], therefore, implies that the mitral leaflets are displaced relative to some structure, generally taken to be the mitral annulus. The silent prolapse is the prolapse which can not be heard with the auscultation diagnosis and is especially hard to diagnose. The implications of the MVP are the following: disturbed normal laminar blood flow, turbulence of the blood flow, injury of the chordae tendinae, the possibility of thrombus' composition, bacterial endocarditis and finally hemodynamic changes defined as mitral insufficiency and mitral regurgitation.

Mitral valve prolapse is one of the most prevalent cardiac conditions, which may affect up to five to ten percent of normal population and one of the most controversial one. The commonest cause is probably myxomatous change in the connective tissue of the valvar liflets that makes them excessively pliable and allows them to prolapse into the left atrium during ventricular systole. The clinical manifestations of the Syndrome are multiple. The great majority of patients are asymptomatic. Other patients, however may present atypical chest-pain or supraventricular tachyarrhythmyas. Rarely, patients develop significant mitral regurgitation and, as with any valvar lesions, bacterial andocarditis is a risk.

Uncertainty persists about how it should be diagnosed and about its clinical importance. Historically, MVP was first recognized by auscultation of mid systolic "click" and late systolic murmur, and its presence is still usually suggested by auscultatory findings. However, the recognition of the variability of the auscultatory findings and of the high level of skill needed to perform such an examination has prompted a search for reliable laboratory methods of diagnosis. M-mod echocardiography and 2D echocardiography have played an important part in the diagnosis of mitral valve prolapse because of the comprehensive information they provide about the structure and function of the mitral valve.

Medical experts propose [14,15] that echocardiography enables properly trained experts armed with proper criteria to evaluate mitral valve prolapse (MVP) almost 100%. Unfortunately however, there are some problems concerned with the use of echocardiography. The first problem is that current MVP evaluation criteria are not strict enough [private communication and 1]. The second problem is the incidence of the MVP in the general population and the unavailability of the expensive ECHO - machines to general practitioners. According to above problems we have decided to develop a decision support system enabling the general practitioner to evaluate the MVP using conventional methods and to identify potential patients from the general population.

6. Implementation of the algorithm

One significant disadvantage of our evolutionary approach [17,18], when considered the traditional induction method, is the time, spent for the solution to be evolved. Although evolutionary algorithms in general are used to reduce computation time significantly [9], in this case the traditional induction method is much faster. Sometimes, when only a few decision trees have to be induced, which are then used for a longer time, this disadvantage is not very serious, but there are several cases, when a larger number of decision trees are required. For example, in medical decision making based on the medical history and status praesens of a patient a new decision tree is required for each patient. To reduce the computation time of our method, we implemented our evolutionary approach [17,18] on a heterogeneous computer system.

Local Area Multicomputer (LAM) [13] is a parallel environment development system of independent computers. It features the message passing interface (MPI) programming standard, supported by extensive monitoring and debugging tools. We used MPI/LAM environment and 41 PCs connected in ATM network to implement the genetic algorithm for the induction of decision trees.

We decided to partition the whole population to several sub-populations. The number of sub-populations was determined by the number of computers in the heterogeneous system; the individuals were uniformly distributed to sub-populations. Each sub-population has been evolved in accordance with the described evolutionary process, but some important parameters, like crossover and mutation probability, weights for the evaluation function, etc. were different. The parameters for each sub-population were determined by a small random alteration of initial parameter values, which were defined experimentally. After a predefined number of generations all evolved individuals from all sub-populations are compared. The best individuals are stored as the current general solutions and some individuals are then randomly exchanged between sub-populations, after which the evolutionary process continues. The whole process is stopped when the best solution overall does not change significantly in the last few cycles.

7. Application and results

Using the Monte Carlo sampling method we have selected 900 children and adolescents representing the whole population under eighteen years of life. All of them were born in the Maribor region and all were white. Routinely they were called for an echocardiography with no prior findings. We examined 631 volunteers.

They all had an examination of their health state in the form of a carefully prepared protocol specially made for the Syndrome of MVP. The protocol consisted of general data, mothers' health, fathers' health, pregnancy, delivery, post-natal period, injuries of chest or any other kind, cronical diseases, sports, physical examination, subjective difficulties like headaches, chest-pain, palpitation, perspiring, dizziness etc., auscultation, phonocardiography, EKG and finally ECHO. In that manner, we gathered 103 parameters that can possibly indicate the presence of MVP.

All 631 patients were divided into a learning and a testing set, 500 patients were selected for the learning and the rest, 131, for the testing set. First we constructed decision trees traditionally with 0, 5 and 10 percent tolerance, without and with post-pruning upon the testing set. Then a few decision trees were evolved through our new evolutionary approach for the same learning and testing sets. A comparison of the best traditionally constructed decision tree (Table 1.a), with an evolutionary constructed solution (Table 1.b). A significant improvement has been achieved with our new model, both regarding the classification of prolapse (4 instead of 3 correct classifications mean improvement of 33 percent) and no prolapse, when considering all the advantages of our evolutionary approach over the traditional one beside the accuracy of classification.

A comparison of the decision trees has shown that similar attributes were chosen as the most important (nearer to the root of a decision tree), but the less important ones (deeper in tree, near to decision attributes) were quite different. This gives us a hint that the presence of MVP can be determined in several ways, with help of different examinations and data - the same opinion is shared by some medical experts who have tried to predict the MVP in different ways. This result favors our evolutionary approach that is able to find those different solutions as opposed to the traditional approach.

Table 1. The results of MVP classification by a) a traditionally constructed decision tree, and b) an evolutionary constructed decision tree.

	Classified as prolapse	Classified as silent prolapse	Classified as no prolapse
prolapse	3	0	4
silent prolapse	0	4	0
no prolapse	8	4	108

	Classified as prolapse	Classified as silent prolapse	Classified as no prolapse
prolapse	4	0	3
silent prolapse	0	4	0
no prolapse	5	3	112

Figure 2 shows an example of heterogeneous program execution under the XMPI environment which runs under several UNIX operating systems. We run the algorithm on the cluster of 41 workstations for approximately 6 hours; in that time over 21 million generations were evolved. A single computer would require approximately 10 days to perform the same task.

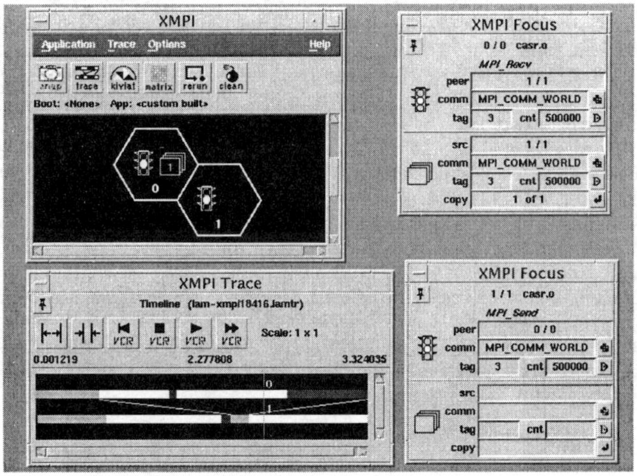

Figure 2. An example of a heterogeneous program execution in XMPI interface.

8. Conclusion

In the paper we present a heterogeneous implementation of decision trees induction used for the medical DSS. We applied it to the prediction of MVP in children, but it can be easily used for different kinds of medical decision making purposes. The whole evolution process is described: seeding of initial population, selection, crossover, mutation, and evaluation function, as well as the parallelization of the evolutionary process. Results of MVP classification by evolutionary constructed decision trees are compared with those obtained by traditionally constructed ones. Because of the advantages of our model and the quality of the obtained results, in our opinion this approach can be successfully used for different kinds of real-world decision making.

References

[1] Kokol P, et al, Decision Trees and Automatic Learning and Their Use in Cardiology, in *Journal of Medical Systems*, 19(4), 1994.

[2] Kokol P, Podgorelec V, Malcic I, Diagnostic Process Optimisation with Evolutionary Programming, in *Proceedings of the 11th IEEE Symposium on Computer-based Medical Systems CBMS'98*, pp. 62-67, Lubbock, Texas, USA, June 1998.

[3] Kokol P, Stiglic B, Zumer V, Metaparadigm: a soft and situation oriented MIS design approach, in *International Journal of Bio-Medical Computing*, 39:243 - 256, 1995.

[4] Kokol P, et al, Spreadsheet Software and Decision making in Nursing, in *Nursing Informatics'91*, (Honvenga E J S et al., eds.), Springer Verlag, 1991.

[5] Quinlan J R, Decision Trees and Decision making, in *IEEE Trans System, Man and Cybernetics*, 20(2)339-346, 1990.

[6] Quinlan J R, Induction of decision trees, in *Machine learning*, No. 1, pp. 81-106, 1986.

[7] Quinlan J R, *C4.5: Programs for Machine Learning.* Morgan Kaufmann publishers, San Mateo, CA, 1993.

[8] Baeck T, *Evolutionary Algorithms in Theory and Practice.* Oxford University Press, Inc., 1996.

[9] Goldberg D E, *Genetic Algorithms in Search, Optimization, and Machine Learning.* Addison Wesley, Reading MA, 1989.

[10] Holland J H, *Adaptation in natural and artificial systems.* MIT Press, Cambridge MA, 1975.

[11] Hwang K, Xu Z, *Scalable Parallel Computing: Technology, Architecture, Programming*, WCB/McGraw-Hill, New York, 1998.

[12] Buyya R (ed.), *High Performance Cluster Computing: The System Issues*, Prentice Hall PTR, NJ, 1998.

[13] Burns G D, Daoud R B, Vaigl J R, Lam: An Open Cluster Environment for MPI, *Proceedings of Supercomputing Symposium '94*, Toronto, Canada, June 1994.

[14] Anderson H R, et al, *Clinicians Illustrated Dictionary of Cardiology.* Science Press, London, 1991.

[15] Devereoux R, Diagnosis and Prognosis of Mitral Valve Prolaps, in *The New England Journal of Medicine*, 320(16)1077-1079, 1989.

[16] Podgorelec V, Kokol P, Genetic Algorithm Based System for Patient Scheduling in Highly Constrained Situations, in *Journal of Medical Systems*, Plenum Press, vol. 21, num. 6, pp. 417-427, December 1997.

[17] Podgorelec V, Kokol P, Evolutionary Construction of Medical Decision Trees, in *Proceedings of the 20th Annual International Conference of the IEEE Engineering in Medicine and Biology Society EMBS'98*, Hong Kong, 1998.

[18] Podgorelec V, Kokol P, Induction of Medical Decision Trees with Genetic Algorithms, in *Proceedings of the International ICSC Symposium on Computational Intelligence: Methods and Applications CIMA'99*, Rochester, USA, June 1999.

Medical Informatics Europe '99
P. Kokol et al. (Eds.)
IOS Press, 1999

Neural Network in Communication with Medical Computer System

Edward KĄCKI[a] Joanna STEMPCZYŃSKA[b] Rafał WAWRZYNIAK[a]
[a]*Institute of Computer Science, Technical University, ul.Sterlinga 16, 90-217 Łódź, Poland*
[b]*Department of Oncology, Medical University, ul.Paderewskiego 4, 93-548 Łódź, Poland*

Abstract. The paper presents a concept of an experimental module designed to recognise spoken utterances that cover a limited range of words indispensable in dialogues with computer medical systems. Research into the recognition of spoken words by a module based on artificial neural network is described. Usefulness of the obtained results for surgery-assisting multimedia systems and for a patient simulator supporting medical education of students in case history-taking and diagnosing is also discussed.

1. Introduction

One of the basic conditions for efficient computer assistance of medical education or physician's work is comfort in user-system communication. Multimedia make it possible to communicate with the system by means of a natural spoken language. However, while producing utterances through a computer loudspeaker during a man-computer dialogue cause no significant problem at the moment, the computer recognition of uttered commands still remains to be solved.

The paper presents investigations into pronounced utterances recognition by medical systems with the use of artificial neural networks, followed by the discussion of the obtained results. Usefulness of those results for multimedia systems designed to support physician's work as well as for the systems assisting medical education is evaluated. In order to carry out the investigations an experimental module of spoken language recognition (MSLR) with easy-to-change parameters has been designed. Its operation under different conditions has been examined, and some possibilities of the MSLR application to multimedia software of a patient simulator [3] and to a surgery-assisting multimedia system [1] have been preliminarily examined.

The work on algorithms and software for the MSLR has been carried out by a team of researchers under the supervision of the authors within a co-operation agreement between the Institute of Computer Science of the Technical University of Łódź and the Oncology Department of the Łódź Medical Academy.

2. Module of spoken language recognition

Experimental module of spoken language recognition (MSLR) was built with the use of artificial neural network in the form of perceptron taught with the error backpropagation method. The software operates in the DOS environment and uses sound cards compatible with Sound Blaster. It is written in C++ using the Easy Blaster Library, and compiled by Borland compiler 3.1. When applied to pronounced words, the program enables performance of four types of time analyses: a) intensity depending on time; b) density of zero passages; c) maximal time intervals between zero passages; d) time interval distribution between zero passages.

The configuration in which the above analyses are performed is entirely arrangeable by the user, which enables the selection of the extraction parameters for pronounced words to be close to optimal. Modular artificial neural network is composed of the following two blocks: a) classifying block; b) approximating block.

Speech recognition requires a variety of speech signal analyses and extraction of suitable parameters. What makes the process more difficult is the fact that each utterance can be pronounced differently, i.e. with different speed, sound intensity, accent or intonation. The way an utterance is pronounced is partly an individual characteristic of a speaker, but it is also subject to a temporary emotional, psychological or physical condition of the speaker. There are numerous external parameters on which an utterance depends. Thus it is clear that the choice of a suitable set of parameters that would describe speech is of essential importance.

In the investigations that have been carried out the following stages can be distinguished: 1) experimental selection of structural model parameters close to optimal; 2) creation of sets of; 3) one- or multi-word expressions; 4) classification of the elements of the expression sets; 5) analysis of the neural network learning and an expression recognition procedure; 6) selection of parameters for recognition criteria.

Tools in the form of designed applications enable examination of the impact that a structure of an artificial neural network has on the identification accuracy of the human speech by the MSLR. To this aim, a dictionary of some scores of patterns, like for instance: "good morning", "good bye", "pulse", "heart", "liver", "kidney", "pressure", "scalpel", has been built. For each pattern, 16 utterances, different in speed, accent and timbre, have been recorded. The goal has been to examine the behaviour of the system in the situation of slight differences in utterances resulting from psychological or physical changes on the part of speaker. All utterances have been processed by means of sound.exe. program. In this way learning sets that are used later at the first stage of neural network operation as well as testing sets applied then to estimation of working efficiency of the MSLR, have been created. For the sake of these analyses optimal parameters are determined experimentally, which is to improve the working efficiency of the artificial neural networkTests have been carried out for different sizes of the dictionary and for different network structures (different number of neurons in the hidden layer). The results have been obtained for a prescribed maximal error equal to 0.001, which means that an admissible error is 0.005.

3. Symulator pacjenta

The presented system is designed for medical students to assist them in learning oncological diagnosing [5]. It enables the student to make diagnosis on the basis of conversation with the system simulating a patient. The conversation consists in selecting appropriate questions and medical examinations from a list presented by the computer. The computer answers the questions displaying randomly chosen answers on the monitor. The student's task is also to decide each time whether the examination results are within the norm. After the case history taking, the student should make a diagnosis, which he does by choosing one item from the list of ninety-five oncological diseases.

The way in which a given case history is taken, additional examinations suggested by the student, qualification of given examination results, and the final diagnosis are all evaluated with points. At the end of the procedure the student learns his total score as well as the number of points he has received for particular steps in the procedure. In this way he is informed which of his choices have not been the proper ones. The conversational part

(TEST option in the main menu) constitutes the key element of the program which is designed to train the student in case history taking and diagnosing. However, to make it possible for medical specialists to complete the data with new cases, another part of the program, called SERVICE, has been constructed. This option enables not only introduction of new data but also checking and correcting of those already stored, which certainly makes the work with the program easier. Thus, the SERVICE option enables the academic teacher to modify the existing data, to update information and to extend the range of the system.

The system has two main options: TEST and SERVICE. Selection of the TEST option, designed for students, makes the program choose randomly one of the diseases and display the data corresponding to the chosen illness. The data cover ordered answers to the questions in the standard case history taking and examination results. Each question is assigned five different answers and each examination - five versions of results. Then, from the list of questions and examinations the student chooses those that he would ask the patient, and the system chooses one of the corresponding answers at random. The questions and examinations are divided into two main groups.

The first one covers introductory talk with the patient during his first visit and contains questions about age, profession, general health troubles, and the like. The other covers all kinds of examinations which can be made on the spot by the physician during the patient's visit, e.g. percussion, auscultation of particular systems and parts of the patient's body as well as all additional examinations to which the patient can be directed (morphology, urine analysis, X-ray, bone marrow examination, etc.). Each selection of a question is followed by the patient's answer displayed on the monitor, and each selection of an examination - by the description of result. Both answers of the system are chosen randomly from the set of the answers admissible for the kind of the disease selected earlier (at the beginning of the test) also at random; the disease should be indicated by the student as the result of his diagnostic procedure.

The second of the main options - SERVICE, is designed only for medical specialists who are concerned with the data edition in the program and who know the password. It enables addition of descriptions of new illnesses, checking and correction of the descriptions already stored, and the change of the password. Addition consists in introduction of connections between answers to questions and results "on the spot" examinations, assignment of points to questions and examinations, and then introduction of their contents.

On each level of the program, there is a help line at the bottom of the screen with information which keys should be used. Assessment of usefulness of the MSLR for the patient simulator involved: a) separation of dialogues in student-patient simulator communication; b) modification and selection of utterances subject to the MSLR operation; c) elaboration of learning sets; d) elaboration of testing sets;e) program linking of the MSLR with the patient simulator; f) experiments.

4. Multimedia system for surgery

The system consists of three main blocks named: description, communication, and expert. The first block covers patient's personal data, records of patient's condition before operation (e.g. description, scanned roentgenogram, microphotogram, tomogram, electrocardiogram, etc.), brief description of the operation and of convalescence. The communication block includes a collection of statements and dialogues necessary for the operating surgeon's communication with the group assisting him in the operation as well as graphic signs and sounds needed in this communication. The third block is an expert system in the area of the surgeon's specialisation. The software of the mentioned blocks is immersed in a multimedia environment.

Assessment of usefulness of the MSLR for the multimedia surgery-assisting system involved operations analogous to those listed at the end of the previous chapter, all of which were preceded by numerous discussions with surgeons.

5. Conclusions and final remarks

The SLR module can co-operate with systems designed to support different kinds of activity, like for example diagnosis, therapy, drug information, education, research or hospital management.

The preliminary decision to employ a three-layer network (with one hidden layer) did not promise high level of speech identification accuracy. Using networks with a greater number of hidden layers one can expect more complex mappings to be realised. Impossibility of changing the number of layers was partly made up for by the variable number of neurons in the hidden layer. However, identification quality need not improve with the increase of the number of neurons. The test for a dictionary consisting of 4 patterns can be a good example here. Too few neurons may make the network unable to learn a pattern rule. Too many neurons on the other hand leads to a long and quite ineffective learning process. There is no deterministic dependence between the identification process complexity and the complexity of a network structure. Thus the choice of structure is carried out with the use of the trial-and-error method.

The investigations have been carried out for a very small group of patterns. Although the network structure was limited to only one hidden layer, which excluded expectation of very promising results for more developed dictionaries, the accuracy level that was achieved (76%) turned out quite satisfactory. To a great extent this good result was due to a proper selection of pattern signals.

For the sets consisting of 16 randomly chosen words there were 75% of those correctly recognised, while in specially selected sets the result was 100%.

The results obtained in the systems in which selection of sets of utterances does not make the application of the system more complicated, like e.g. an educational system or a multimedia system of drug information, can be considered satisfactory. However in the present situation, when in order for accurate recognition results to be achieved a special selection of words that can be uttered must be first made, the proposed module cannot be applied to surgery-assisting systems. Instead of facilitating the surgeon's work such a system would be burdensome and cause much inconvenience to the user. Creation of better possibilities of exploitation of the MSLR in systems that would assist the work of physicians needs further research into development and improvement of the MSLR algorithms. Such research is presently being carried out by the authors.

The investigations were carried out within grant no. 8T11E02813 financed by the State Committee of Research (1997 – 2000).

References

[1] Kącki E., Stempczyńska J.: Artificial Intelligence Elements in Multimedia System for Surgery. *Studies in Helth Technology and Informatics,* Vol.43, IOS Press Ohmsha, Washington,1997, (pp.475-477).

[2] Stempczyńska J., Kącki E.: STUD2 System for Computer Assistence in Oncology Education. Proceed. of MedInfo'95 Congress, Vancouver, 1995, Vol.2, pp.1233-1237

[3] Stempczyńska J., Kącki E.: Multimedia Simulator of Patient. *Studies in Helth Technology and Informatics*, Vol.43, IOS Press Ohmsha, Washington,1997, (pp.722-725).

Medical Informatics Europe '99
P. Kokol et al. (Eds.)
IOS Press, 1999

Concepts, Contexts and Expert Systems

Daniel Karlsson[1], Olle Aspevall[2] and Urban Forsum[3]

1. Medical Informatics, Linköpings Universitet, Sweden

2. Department of Immunology, Microbiology, Pathology and Infectious Diseases, Karolinska Institutet, Huddinge University Hospital, Stockholm, Sweden

3. Division of Clinical Microbiology, Linköpings Universitet, Sweden

Abstract. This paper describes problems identified in our attempts to develop an expert system for management of urinary tract infections. We found three aspects which we believe are important to consider when developing such systems. The objective of our future work will be to evaluate the impact of these problems on expert system development and usage.

1. Introduction

Expert systems are inter-contextual entities. Expert systems are used to transfer knowledge from a domain expert context into an end-user context. The end user is a non-expert in the domain of the domain expert, but may be an expert in another domain. The end user would benefit in performing his or her assigned tasks from having access to knowledge of the expert. This is the rationale for using expert systems: the benefit of knowledge transfer. Obstacles in this knowledge transfer are, among many other things, differences in end user and expert conceptual contexts. These differences include the dimensions along which concepts are defined and the level of granularity within these dimensions. These dimensions and levels of granularity are in turn given by what knowledge is needed to perform the users' and the experts' individual tasks successfully as well as knowledge gained from various levels of education, etc. To add further complexity, the granularity and dimensions change over time as the area of medicine evolves.

The formalisation of medical concepts for use in medical information systems has been thoroughly examined from a terminological point of view. Our belief is though that there are fundamental epistemological issues which have not yet been fully addressed in the area of medical informatics.

2. Aspects of Medical Concepts

2.1 Conceptual Dimensions

In different contexts different dimensions will be used to specify and to state concepts more precisely. In the area of Urinary Tract Infections (UTI) classes of dimensions may e.g. be patho-physiology, diagnostic procedures, laboratory methods and analyses, specimen collection, the request-report procedure, the patient's symptoms, the patient's way of life and coping abilities. The set of relevant dimensions vary among contexts. The laboratory methods

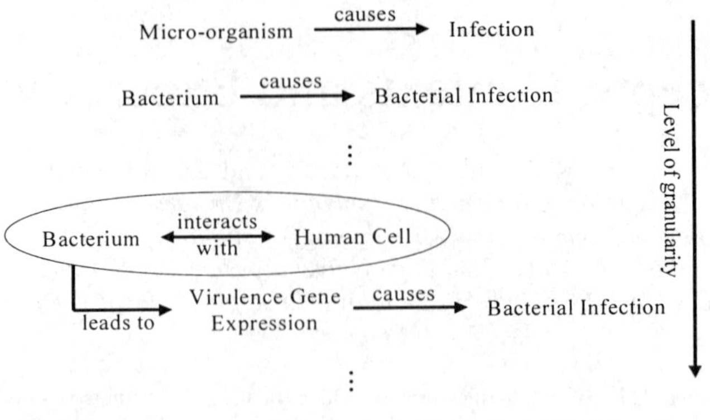

Figure 1. Granularity in the patho-physiology dimension

and analysis dimensions may not be relevant in a primary care context and the dimensions regarding the patient's way of life and coping abilities may not be relevant in a laboratory context. The set of diagnostic procedures vary greatly between the two contexts as does the significance of the patient's symptoms. In the laboratory much of the focus is on the specimen where as in primary care a more holistic view of the patient is needed. These differences can be seen with even greater contrast when comparing different provider categories.

2.2 Granularity of Knowledge

Knowledge within a dimension can be stated in a continuum of granularity. The level of granularity is chosen for a specific task in a specific situation and a specific context. As an example, the patho-physiology of micro-organisms causing infectious diseases can be detailed as in Figure 1.

The knowledge that a certain class of diseases are caused by micro-organisms is one of the great discoveries of mankind. This in turn led to the discovery of antibiotics, use of vaccine and improved sanitation. Although this kind of unspecific knowledge is clearly insufficient in many situations, it cannot be ruled out as false. The knowledge that infections are caused by micro-organisms together with the knowledge that anti-microbial agents kill or inhibate micro-organisms is sufficient for establishing treatment for most infected patients. Some more complicated cases may though require more extensive knowledge on the patho-physiology of the infection. Also, current research indicates that the pathogenicity of bacteria is dependant on an interaction between the bacterium and the human cell, the "bacterial–host cell cross-talk." [1] The characteristics of this interaction vary greatly among bacteria and among human beings. The causal relation between micro-organisms and infections in the top statement is an abstraction of a very complicated process.

Terminologically, the relation between the first two statements is analytical, i.e. holds by definition, because the statements 'Bacterium is a Micro-organism' and 'Bacterial Infection is an Infection' are analytical. The relation between the second and the last statements, and the relations between statements which could be placed in-between, are however non-analytical. This relation holds only according to theories of bacterial pathogenicity based on empirical knowledge developed throughout the years and will probably change as medicine evolves.

The second statement is a specification[1] of the first one. Both makes statements about the direct relationship between micro-organisms and infections, although the second one is

---

[1] Having a 'generic' or 'subset' relation

more specific. The last statement is not a specification of the first two. The last statement says more than the first two and thus something else, although the same relationship between micro-organisms and infections is described. The last statement is *stated more precisely* than the second one.

In different contexts different levels of granularity will be needed. This is especially true when comparing expert system end user and domain expert contexts. Thus, the expert system must support both the precise concepts of the expert domain as well as the more imprecise concepts of the end-user domain.

2.3 Changes Over Time

The area of medicine currently has a doubling time of about 19 years [2]. Still, medicine is an inert system and often new discoveries fail to penetrate routine practice [3, 4]. Thus, expert systems would be an attractive way of disseminating new findings, but end-user contexts will with high probability consist of a mixture of dated as well as updated knowledge based on a wide range of possible dimensions.

As the area of medicine evolves granularity as well as new dimensions are added and focus shift from dimensions to other dimensions. New dimensions are added as our understanding of pathologic and non-pathologic processes increase. New dimensions may also be added for non-professional reasons, e.g. the cost and cost-utility dimensions added due to the strained economic situation. The development in medicine also cause change in focus, e.g. the shift from symptom dimensions to patho-physiology dimensions when new explaining theories evolve.

3. Objective

The objective of this work is to further investigate the effects of the epistemological issues discussed above in the use and development of expert systems. To focus on inter-contextual issues we have initiated a pilot study regarding the concepts and terms used to describe UTI in primary health care [5]. The pilot study will be followed by a narrative analysis of the professional debate of UTI in the Swedish health-care community. This will allow us to build a model of the UTI domain. This model will be used in an expert system in the field of UTI, a system which we are currently developing. The system will be built using methods based on previous research by our group [6, 7] as well as lessons learned in other terminology and expert systems related projects were our group has been involved. Finally, the system will be made available to primary care physicians and the usage of the system will be evaluated using both quantitative and qualitative methods.

References

[1] Falkow S. What is a pathogen? ASM News 1998; 63(7): 359-365.

[2] Wyatt J. Use and sources of medical knowledge. Lancet 1991; 338: 1368-73.

[3] Williamson JW, German PS, Weiss R, Skinner EA, Bowes F. Health science information managment and continuing education of physicians. Ann Intern Med 1989; 110(2): 151-60.

[4] Evans CE, Haynes RB, Gilbert JR, Taylor DW, Sackett DL, Johnston M. Eduactional package on hypertension for primary care physicians. Can Med Assoc J 1984; 130(6): 719-22.

[5] Aspevall O, Forsum U, Karlsson D. Concepts and Terms used to describe Urinary Tract Infection (UTI) in Primary Health Care and in the Clinical Microbiology Laboratory. Submitted to MIE'99.

[6] Karlsson D, Ekdahl C, Wigertz O, Shahsavar N, Gill H, Forsum U. Extended telemedical consultation using Arden Syntax based decision support, Hypertext and WWW technique. Meth Inform Med 1997; 36(2): 108-14.

[7] Ekdahl C, Karlsson D, Wigertz O, Forsum U. A Study of the Usage of a WWW-based Decision-Support System. Submitted to Medical Informatics.

Medical Informatics Europe '99
P. Kokol et al. (Eds.)
IOS Press, 1999

Availability humanization expert model

Marija Molan[1], Gregor Molan[2]
[1]*Institute for occupational health, Korytkova 7, SI-1000 Ljubljana, Slovenia*
[2]*HERMES SoftLab research group, Litijska 51, SI-1000 Ljubljana, Slovenia*

Abstract: AH model as a tool for estimation in the occupational health care is presented. This is an expert model connecting data from the working environment with human availability and health status data. In this paper the idea of model and its components are presented.

Key words: expert model, humanization, availability, cost benefits, work load, working environment

1. Introduction

A high proportion of the same health problems in some categories of workers excited a lot of research activities with the same goal: reduction of work load and elimination of causes initiating the health problems. These reductions should be enforced whenever possible and they should assure adequate levels of human performance. All activities are oriented toward the reduction of work load to the level, which will assure less human related problems, and stable performance of the facility.

A system's performance is shaped by the level of human actual availability [1]. Trials to reduce work loads to the level which should assure higher availability are so called "*humanization measures*". Humanization measures are determined by the state of knowledge in the area of occupational health and ergonomics. There are particular researches focused to one or a few work loads. Suggestions as the result of these researches are specialized, focused to some particular improvements at the working environment [2]. It is difficult to eliminate all the problems at the working place and to reduce work loads to the level with minimal negative impact on workers performance and health.

2. Research goal

Particular improvements of working place are results of identified unhealthy effects of the working environment. According to the demand of safety and health legislation causes of health problems at the working environment should be eliminated by intervention in the working environment. Environmental hazards should be eliminated. This elimination's demands investments in the working environment and changes of technology. This means costs. For all the time in the reality there are negotiations between costs and profits.

Implementations of humanization measures are often results of workers demands and pressure of trade union. There are no systematic evaluations of implemented humanization measures and health problems. Connections between working place and health's problems are not systematic evaluated. There are focused researches and evaluations and there are particular limited changes in the working environment. Issues of all activities are determined by researches focused to defined health problems and diagnoses, there are researches focused to the measured values of environmental parameters.

In our research we focused on the human actual availability. This is a central part of our researches. According to our results [1] [3] human availability shaped the level of human performance. We have developed methods for estimating the level of human availability. Work loads shape the level of human availability, which determines the level of human performance. All changes in the work environment are reflected on the level of human availability. For this changes we use the term "*humanization*".

The goal of our present research work is focused to the development of a general model of work humanization. Focused on the human actual availability our model is named "***A**vailability **H**umanization model*" - AH model.

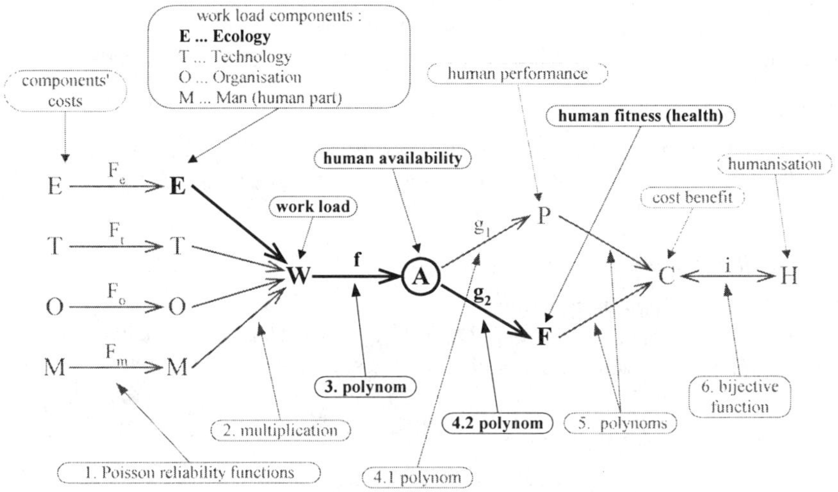

Figure 1. ***Availability Humanization model*" - AH model**

3. Method

Step 1: Identification of problems, determination of experts' groups, and identification of representative working places.
Step 2: Estimative analyses of working places, determination of critical work load's components.
Step 3: Modeling of human performance and human availability connections.
Step 4: Modeling of work load component's impacts on human availability.
Step 5: Modeling of human fitness and human availability connections.
Step 6: Modeling of human performance's and human fitness' costs benefits.
Step 7: Evaluation of humanization measures via cost benefits.
Step 8: Determination of the AH model.
Step 9: Collections of data in the field studies for AH model verification.
Step 10: Computer supported evaluation of the data and verification of the AH model.
Step 11: Evaluation of the AH model from the aspects of mathematical analyses and from the human factor aspect.
Step 12: Suggestions of changes and modification of model in the real working environment on the basis of research results.

4. Results

Steps 1,2, and 3 were performed as a part of research work in Nuclear and Thermal plant [1].

A step 4 was developed as a part of research work in the project "Development of the program for complex health care for workers working with ionizing radiation [5]. Steps 5 to 12 should be defined and performed in the present and future research work.

The essential part of this paper is a formal determination of the AH model, step 8.The formal definition of the AH model

Proposition 1 : $F_e : \mathcal{E} \rightarrow E$, $F_t : \mathcal{T} \rightarrow T$, $F_o : \mathcal{O} \rightarrow O$, and $F_m : \mathcal{M} \rightarrow M$ are Poisson reliability functions.

Proposition 2 : $W = E \cup T \cup O \cup M$ and $E \cap T \cap O \cap M = \emptyset$

Proposition 3 : $f : W \rightarrow A$, $g_1 : A \rightarrow P$, and $g_2 : A \rightarrow F$ are continuos functions.

Proposition 4 : $\iota : C \rightarrow H$ and the function ι is a continuos function and bijection.

4.1 Finding extremes

Our goal is: *Find the maximal human availability for given investments resources.*

In our mathematical model this means: *Find the extreme (maximum) of the continuos function.*

4.2 Additional explanation of connections

Ad. 1. Poisson reliability functions

This type of data has a Poisson distribution, so the connections between costs and work load components are modeled by Poisson reliability functions:

$$F_\Psi(x) = \sum_{k=0}^{x} \frac{\lambda^k}{k!} e^{-k}, \text{ where } x \in \mathbb{N}, \text{ and } \Psi \in \{e,t,o,m\}$$

Here it is assumed that costs can not be changed continuously. So, costs are presented with natural numbers $\mathbb{N} = \{0,1,2,3,...\}$.

Ad. 2. Multiplication

From the basic probability theory [4] it has been assumed that the lifetimes of the disjunct components are independent (Proposition 2):

$$P(E \cdot T \cdot O \cdot M) = P(E) \cdot P(T) \cdot P(O) \cdot P(M)$$

Ad. 4. Model

Connection between human availability and human performance has been described in our earlier work [3]. There was used a model, where human performance base was modeled with pairs from human availability items. Human performance in the night shift was best modeled with pair (well being, vigilance):

$$g_{night\ shift}(A) = 20\ a_{well\ bing} - 38\ a_{vigilance} - 25.96$$

5. Discussion

Humanization means investments and changes activity, adaptation and accommodation. In modern complex system humanization is a broad conception. It demands global approach of different experts and integration of their work in a unique general model. Presented AH model is our suggestion.

The AH model is a possible suggestion for implementing humanization measures at the working environment. It offers a clear description of connections between the work place, human performance and human fitness to the cost benefits. The center of the model is a self-estimated level of actual availability. This is approved by ours previous research work.

Work loads are important as far as they influence the human availability. It is not necessary to wait for work impacts on human health. We have to react earlier immediately when we get information that work load affects human availability. The decrease of human related mistakes and stable system performance is management's interest. The suggested AH model is based on the following issues:

- Workers are able to perceive work load influence on their availability. Perceived self estimated level of human availability is shaped by the work components' influence.
- Human performance depends on the level of human availability. Connections have been modeled.
- People are able to perceive unfitness and fatigue before they have health problems.
- Collected data in the field studies will offer precise component data for the further use of the model and its validation.
- Permanent collection of data in occupational health routine activities offers possibility to get enough data for analyses, modeling and evaluations of suggested model.
- Development of expert model connecting human availability, health status human performance and working environment data offers a tool occupational health staff, organization specialists and engineers for their work

All the interventions and changes have their own price. Also health should be economically evaluated. Humanization suggestions will be realized if they are economically justified.

In reality humanization goes as far as it is economically justified and not a bit more. This is the crucial element of all humanization efforts and suggestions - it is a reality.

References

[1] Škof, M. and Molan, G., 1992, Human availability and system's performance in systems of high technologies. In Organization and information systems 2 by Z. Kaltneker (eds.) (Moderna organizacija, Kranj), pp. 237-248.

[2] Costa, G., 1992, A seven-point program to reduce stress in air traffic controllers in Italy. In Conditions of work digest by M. B. Jankanish (eds.) (International labour office, Geneva), pp. 172-183.

[3] Škof, M. and Molan, G., Human potential capacity, real capacity, and performance : models and connections. In Use of probabilistic safety assessment for operational safety by IAEA (IAEA, Vienna), pp. 766-770.

[4] Feller, W., 1968, An introduction to probability theory and its applications. (J. Wiley, New York)

[5] MOLAN, Marija, MOLAN, Gregor, 1998, Estimations of actual availability in the hospital. In: V: VINK, Peter (ur.), KONINGSVELD, Ernst A.P. (ur.), DHONDT, Steven (ur.). Human factors in organizational design and management - VI: proceedings of the sixth international symposium on human factors in organizational design and management held in the Hague, the Netherlands, august 19-22, 1998. Amsterdam: Elsevier science, 1998, pp. 257-262.

Medical Informatics Europe '99
P. Kokol et al. (Eds.)
IOS Press, 1999

TIDE: An Intelligent Home-Based Healthcare Information & Diagnostic Environment

Syed Sibte Raza ABIDI
Health Informatics Research Group, School of Computer Sciences, Universiti Sains Malaysia, 11800 Penang, Malaysia.

Abstract. The 21st century promises to usher in an era of Internet based healthcare services—*Tele-Healthcare*. Such services augur well with the on-going paradigm shift in healthcare delivery patterns, i.e. patient centred services as opposed to provider centred services and wellness maintenance as opposed to illness management. This paper presents a Tele-Healthcare info-structure *TIDE*—an 'intelligent' wellness-oriented healthcare delivery environment. TIDE incorporates two WWW-based healthcare systems: (1) *AIMS* (Automated Health Monitoring System) for wellness maintenance and (2) *IDEAS* (Illness Diagnostic & Advisory System) for illness management. Our proposal comes from an attempt to rethink the sources of possible leverage in improving healthcare; vis-à-vis the provision of a continuum of personalised home-based healthcare services that emphasise the role of the individual in self health maintenance.

1. Introduction

Healthcare in the 21st century is deemed as an 'extended enterprise'—a global enterprise that is experiencing a paradigm shift towards a preventative, managed and self-care, client-focused approach to the delivery of healthcare services [1] [2]. Emerging healthcare concepts and philosophies are reflective of innovative Information Technologies (IT)—Innovations such as computer-based patient records, hospital information systems, computer-based decision support tools, image processing, data compression, community health information networks, Telemedicine and new ways of distributing health information to consumers are beginning to affect the cost, quality and expanded access to healthcare information and services. Whilst this paradigm shift in the definition of healthcare is due in part to the powerful functionality of available IT technologies, it can be argued that IT, for our case the field of Artificial Intelligence (AI), is both being pulled by and helping to draw a new agenda about how healthcare will be practised in the future. Here, concepts and technologies are impacting on each other.

This paper discusses the synergy between AI and the new trends in the healthcare delivery system [3] [4], i.e. the delivery of healthcare via the Internet/WWW. The efficacy of AI towards healthcare is demonstrated by discussing an on-going in-house Tele-Healthcare project *TIDE—Tele-Healthcare Information and Diagnostic Environment*. TIDE aims to ensure a continuum of healthcare throughout the life-time of the individual. This is to be achieved by the delivery of *Personalised, Pro-active, Persistent, Perpetual* and *Present* healthcare maintenance *Information* services, coupled with *Diagnostic* services to the community via the Internet. Technical realisation of TIDE involves a confluence of information technologies—AI (expert systems, case-based and common-sense reasoning), medical informatics, multimedia, Internet and database technologies. This unique confluence of technologies within TIDE gives rise to an efficacious 'intelligent' info-structure that has the potential to re-think the modalities and mediums in which medical information is retrieved, disseminated and exploited.

2. TIDE: An Overview

TIDE is a manifestation of the emerging trends in modern healthcare practices, i.e. more person-centred as opposed to provider-centred together with an emphasis on wellness maintenance as opposed to illness management [5] [6] [7].

In the realm of TIDE we present two AI-based healthcare systems: (1) *AiMS (Automated Health Monitoring System)* and (2) *IDEAS (Illness Diagnostic & Advisory System)*. During the lifetime of an individual, he/she is likely to remain in the wellness cycle for most of the time yet there would be instances when the individual will fall in the illness cycle. To cater for the above two eventualities, TIDE aims to provide individuals an opportunity to maintain their own health and respond to illness episodes on a day-to-day basis from the confines of their home/workplace.

The objective of AiMS is to promote wellness maintenance, ensuring individuals remain healthy for prolonged periods of time. AiMS will provide personalised healthcare services, i.e. simplified *Personalised Lifetime Health Plans (PLHP)*, to assist individuals to manage and interpret their own healthcare needs. Put simply, a PLHP 'intelligently' integrates existing illness records (the past health perspective) with wellness plans (the future health perspective) to guide the individual in healthcare planning. A PLHP comprises a merged set of *Health Expectations* and *Health Tips*. Health expectations are evidence based health events that require planning. Health tips are lifestyle recommendations to ensure a healthy life.

The focus of IDEAS is illness management—to provide timely medical advice whenever an individuals fall in the illness cycle. IDEAS is an AI-based consultation package that is adept to provide primary health-care for non-critical illnesses: it would make a diagnosis, prescribe a treatment plan and direct the patient to the nearest pharmacy.

When an individual is in the wellness state, his/her health will be regularly monitored by AiMS so as to ensure that the individual remains healthy for prolonged periods. Whenever the individual falls ill, control of the PLHP is passed to IDEAS—IDEAS will conduct a 'virtual consultation session' with the patient, perform a diagnosis based on the patient's current symptoms/signs and finally prescribe a treatment plan.

3. The Wellness Perspective: Automated Health Monitoring Services (AiMS)

AiMS is a personalised health monitoring system that helps to keep track, manage, interpret an individual's health history and offer health maintenance advice. Each session with AiMS entails several important functions: (a) it collects an individual's current health data—a dynamic and pro-active web-based questionnaire is generated to acquire specialised information; (b) it interprets the acquired information and explains to the individual medically relevant facts; (c) it monitors the individual's health status based on his/her personalised health plans and it subsequently renders medically-relevant advice to maintain a healthy lifestyle; (d) it provides reminders for scheduled therapy and appointments and can electronically schedule medical appointments; (e) it also alerts healthcare agencies whenever an emergency situation is detected. Being in the prototype stage, AiMS currently provides monitoring services for depression, hypertension, diabetes and cardio-vascular related diseases. Functionally, AiMS comprises two main components:

Personalised Health Monitoring: AiMS incorporates personalised health monitoring routines that are formulated based on an individual's current health profile. For each 'virtual consultation session', AiMS extracts the medical history of an individual from the centralised EMR database. Next, AiMS proceeds to 'intelligently' ask pertinent questions to the user to determine the user's current health profile (as shown in Figure 1). Intelligence derives from the fact that the questions posted to the user are dynamically generated (on the fly) after analysing the answers furnished by the user to previous questions. Typical responses of AiMS are shown in Figure 2 and are:

- An advice in the form of a list of *do and don't* activities.
- An advice to monitor certain health indicators such as cholesterol and glucose levels and perhaps suggest procedures to monitor these indicators.
- An advice for a detailed medical examination or to see a healthcare professional.
- An advice for a particular therapy or treatment programme.

General 'Personalised' Health Tips and Facts (PHTF): To ensure a continuum of healthcare and dissemination of health information, AiMS incorporates the PHTF module that provides general health tips, customised to an individual's health requirements. PHTF builds on the individuals PLHP to provide a variety of WWW-based services such as: an *immunisation planner*, a *dietary guide* , an *exercise/fitness monitor,* a *stress level indicator, body mass index (BMI) guides, personalised health information.*

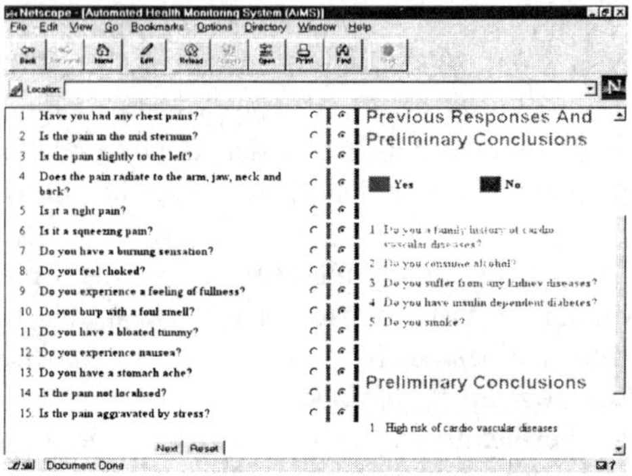

Figure 1: A typical screen for a consultation session with AiMS for monitoring diabetes

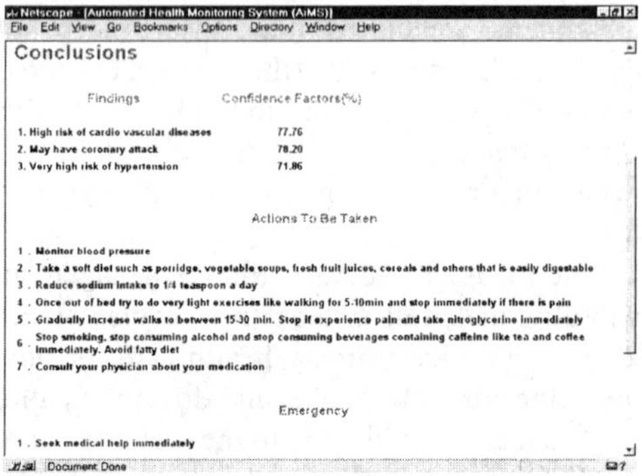

Figure 2: Suggestions rendered by AiMS at the conclusion of the consultation session

4. The Illness Perspective: 'Intelligent' Diagnostic & Treatment Advisory Services (IDEAS)

IDEAS aims to provide the community quality 'virtual' medical consultation for non-critical illnesses over the WWW. IDEAS, being in the prototyping stage, minimally covers the following medical conditions: cough, cold, sore throat, diarrhoea, abdominal pain, chest pain, dizziness and earache.

Functionally, IDEAS will conduct a web-based 'virtual consultation session' comprising *dynamically* generated questionnaires for the collection of relevant patient's health information (see Figure 3). Next, based on the collected information and the patient's health record (i.e. centralised EMR), IDEAS would come up with a diagnosis and treatment plan (see Figure 4). In a Tele-healthcare environment, IDEAS serves as a patient screening agent—screening patients in need of just primary healthcare as opposed to patients in need of tertiary health-care. IDEAS is intended to be the community's initial point of contact for non-critical diagnostic and treatment services.

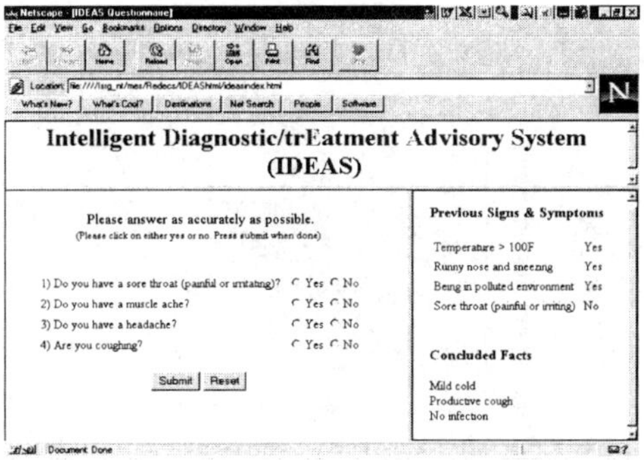

Figure 3: Snapshot of an IDEAS screen used for the collection of signs from patients

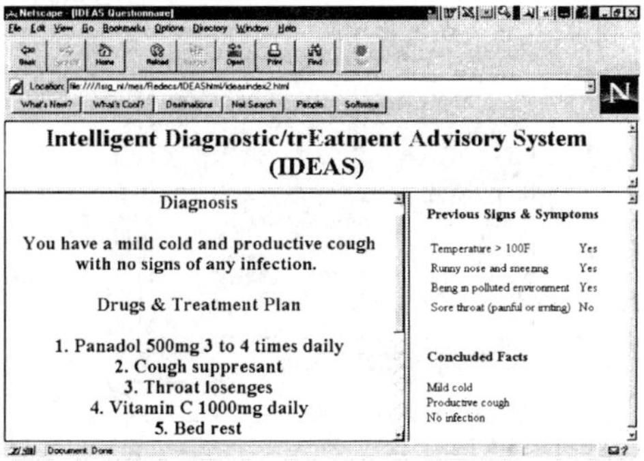

Figure 4: Snapshot of the IDEAS diagnosis screen, depicting both the diagnosis and the treatment plan.

5. TIDE: Design and Implementation Issues

TIDE manifests an info-structure that provides a seamless synthesis of AI-based decision-making systems (the expert systems embedded within AiMS and IDEAS), databases storing the EMRs and web-based programs and protocols.

At the heart of AiMS and IDEAS are two individual expert systems, encapsulating medical knowledge and reasoning techniques. For inferencing purposes we have devised a hybrid of forward and backward chaining strategies. In addition, the inference engine is also responsible for the 'intelligent' generation of subsequent questionnaires (i.e. web-pages) that may contain only the next set of pertinent questions—questions derived from the previous responses and in support of the multiple hypothesis active at that stage of the consultation and accompanying information. Both AiMS and IDEAS feature a friendly web-based interface for the collection of platform-independent person/patient data.

Expert medical knowledge, in particular the Malaysian medical procedures, is represented using typical *if ...then ... else* statements, with additional HTML text to output. TIDE's knowledge base—referred as the Decision Guide—partitions the rules into various modules, each addressing a particular scenario. Conceptually, the rule structure itself is divided into three constructs: *Question Constructs* address the questions to ask the user for a value for a fact; *Rule Constructs* represent pure knowledge that can be inferred over during the reasoning cycle; and finally *Rule-Answer Constructs* representing HTML-based information that is presented to the user (as part of the output) when the rule is satisfied (shown in Figure 5). Operationally, the rules combine in a dynamic manner, during inferencing, to address the defined diagnostic scope of TIDE. Dynamic web-pages are prepared to present the conclusions of the expert systems, together with hyperlinks to various information-related Web documents (as shown in Figure 6).

TIDE has been implemented using the Prolog, more specifically *LPA Prolog 3.5*. Both the TIDE expert systems reside on a server. Interactions between the client (the users) and TIDE is conducted over the WWW and is accomplished by using *ProWeb*—a Prolog-Web interface toolkit supplied by LPA. The web-based user-interface is developed using HTML and Java Script and the graphical charts are derived from Java applets. The functionality of TIDE demands frequent access to patient's EMR that may be stored in a centralised server-based database. Database connectivity is implemented by using the *ProData* (supplied by LPA) toolkit that provides a tight coupling between LPA Prolog and all DBMS which support ODBC. Here, we will like to point out that TIDE is one of the few successful Prolog based AI applications that reside on the WWW.

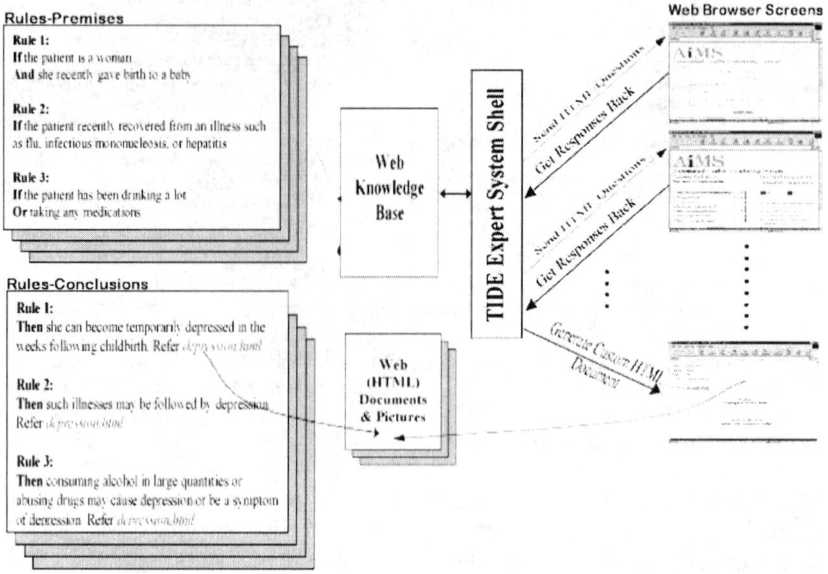

Figure 5: Illustrating the Rule Constructs—The top box shows the question construct and the bottom one the rule-answer construct. The right hand-side of the diagram shows the transactions involved in the generation of the dynamic HTML pages during the consultation session.

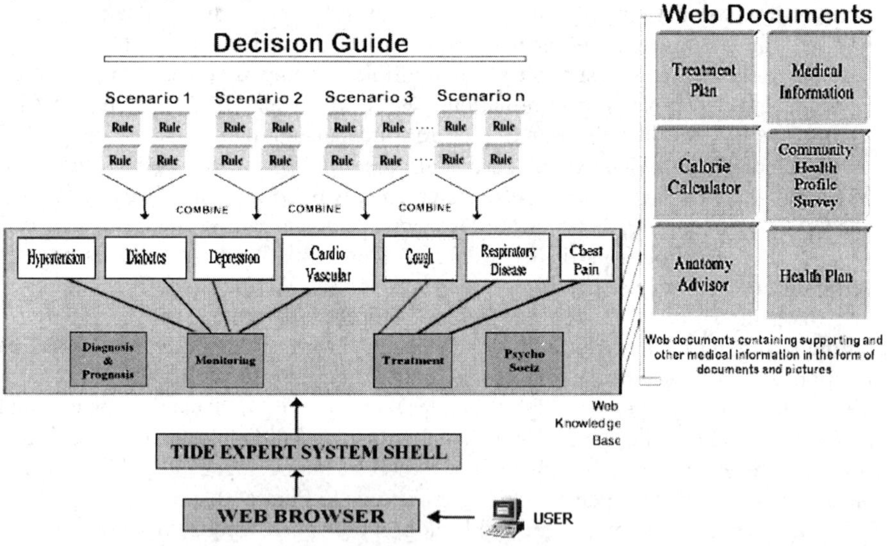

Figure 6: The functional architecture of TIDE.

5.1. Generation of Dynamic Web-Based Questionnaires

User's interaction with the TIDE applications is via a *Dynamically* generated HTML user interface comprising highly pertinent questions. This strategy is a step forward from the 'static' web user-interfaces in which pre-determined, yet at times irrelevant, questions are presented to the user.

Dynamic generation of web-based questionnaires is achieved by first designing a layout of the questionnaire and storing it in a template file. Throughout the consultation session, this template file is repeatedly modified and posted by the expert systems to the user. After every interaction with the user, the expert system modifies the contents of the template file as per the earlier answers, i.e. it writes the next set of questions to the template file. The updated template file is then posted to the user as the next web pages. The response of the user is passed via the web-pages back to the expert system for the updating of the template file. This process is transparent to the user as it is repeated throughout the web-based consultation session. Figure 7 shows a simple functional diagram to elucidate process of dynamically generating web pages.

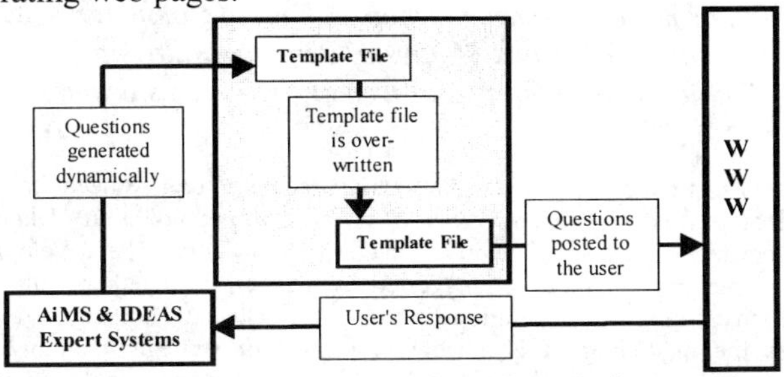

Figure 7: Functional diagram depicting the process of dynamically generating web-pages.

6. Concluding Remarks

In conclusion, we emphasise that the conception of TIDE has identified opportunities to improve healthcare delivery through increased use of information technology, in particular AI. Each interaction with TIDE is an active process, with an intelligence bias, that performs several important functions: it collects patient data; it checks, interprets, and explains to the subject medically-relevant facts and plans; it adapts its advice based on the subject's prior experiences and stated preferences; it performs "sanity checks" on both medical efficacy and cost-effectiveness of diagnostic conclusions and therapeutic plans; it monitors wellness progress and it helps to educate and encourage individuals towards health maintenance.

Finally, the TIDE info-structure is a showcase application demonstrating the efficacy of AI concepts and functionality on the WWW. The TIDE project is still in progress and more sophisticated and extended services are expected to evolve.

References

[1] J. Flower, The Future of Healthcare. Encyclopaedia of the Future, Macmillan & Co., Indianapolis (1995).

[2] S.S.R. Abidi, A. Goh & Z. Yusoff, Telemedicine and Medical Informatics in the Multimedia Super Corridor: The Malaysian Vision. 9th World Congress on Medical Informatics (MedInfo'98), Seoul. (1998).

[3] E.W. Coiera, Artificial Intelligence in Medicine: The Challenges Ahead. Journal of American Medical Informatics Association, 3 (6), (1996), pp. 363-366.

[4] E.H. Shortliffe, "The Adolescence of AI in Medicine: Will the Field Come of Age in the 90's?". Artificial Intelligence in Medicine, **5** (1993), pp. 93-106.

[5] E. Rogers, AI and the Changing Face of Healthcare. IEEE Intelligent Systems, Jan/Feb (1998).

[6] J.E. Larsson & B. Hayes-Roth, Guardian: An Intelligent Autonomous Agent for Medical Monitoring and Diagnosis. IEEE Intelligent Systems, Jan/Feb, (1998).

[7] B. Hayes-Roth, Guardian: A Prototype Intelligent Agent for Intensive-Care Monitoring. Artificial Intelligence in Medicine, 4 (2) (1992) 165-185.

Medical Informatics Europe '99
P. Kokol et al. (Eds.)
IOS Press, 1999

Healthcare Knowledge Management Through Building and Operationalising Healthcare Enterprise Memory

CHEAH Yu-N & Syed Sibte Raza ABIDI
Health Informatics Research Group, School of Computer Sciences,
Universiti Sains Malaysia, Penang, Malaysia.
Email: yncheah@insys.cs.usm.my, sraza@cs.usm.my

Abstract. In this paper we suggest that the healthcare enterprise needs to be more conscious of its vast knowledge resources vis-à-vis the exploitation of knowledge management techniques to efficiently manage its knowledge. The development of healthcare enterprise memory is suggested as a solution, together with a novel approach advocating the operationalisation of healthcare enterprise memories leading to the modelling of healthcare processes for strategic planning. As an example, we present a simulation of Service Delivery Time in a hospital's OPD.

1. Introduction

The role of information technology in healthcare is well-established, yet the practice of medicine is becoming so complex that it is consistently pushing the sophistication of information technology tools and techniques to newer frontiers. Lately, there is a growing demand from the healthcare community to leverage upon and transform the vast quantities of healthcare data and information into value-added, 'decision-quality' knowledge. Indeed, the healthcare enterprise is coming to terms with the prevailing sentiment that in an IT-driven world, knowledge is one of the enterprise's most significant asset.

The task at hand now is to identify a knowledge environment that supports mechanisms to not only create or even capture viable healthcare knowledge and experiences but also to operationalise them to positively impact the healthcare enterprise. This brings into relief the need to establish the role and significance of the emerging methodology/technology of *Knowledge Management* in healthcare.

In this paper, we present a case for the possible synergy of knowledge management techniques in the healthcare domain. Capitalising on knowledge management services and processes, we propose the concept of the *healthcare enterprise memory*—akin to organisational memories—that can support the sharing and reuse of individual and enterprise-wide knowledge, experience, and lessons learned. We show that a healthcare enterprise memory can provide a number of knowledge-oriented services, such as automatic dissemination of knowledge, reuse of knowledge and experience, support of intelligent knowledge management services, timely provision of knowledge and experience, transforming information to action, connecting and converting knowledge and above all *healthcare modelling*. We conclude that the synergy between healthcare enterprises and knowledge management brings about a win-win situation, thereby realising a knowledge-theoretic healthcare environment.

2. Understanding Knowledge Management in a Healthcare Context

In a healthcare context, *Knowledge Management (KM)* is the formal management of knowledge for facilitating the creation, identification, acquisition, development, dissemination, utilisation, and preservation of a healthcare enterprise's knowledge using advanced technology [1, 2]. KM also involves converting knowledge from a healthcare enterprise's sources (individuals, groups, data and text) and connecting healthcare participants (healthcare professionals, management and patients) with that knowledge [3].

A typical KM framework [4] consists of a number of processes in a cyclic arrangement. For our discussion, we regard *creation* as the initial process of the KM framework:

1. *Create*: Responsible for the creation of healthcare knowledge, possibly through trial-and-error or blind variation and selective retention methods.
2. *Identify*: Determines the existence of useful healthcare knowledge from the knowledge created in the earlier process. This can be achieved through mining efforts similar to that of data mining and knowledge discovery.
3. *Collect/Acquire*: Once useful knowledge has been identified, next follows the process of acquiring the knowledge.
4. *Organise/Develop/Preserve*: This can be viewed as a form of 'knowledge processing' whereby the knowledge is transformed, represented, and organised in a defined format.
5. *Share/Disseminate*: Provides the mechanisms to disseminate the stored knowledge to all participants of the healthcare enterprise and possibly to other healthcare enterprises.
6. *Adapt*: This process is typically the responsibility of healthcare professionals in their practice. Upon introspection of the 'created' knowledge healthcare professionals may then need to tailor it to ensure appropriateness, currency and accuracy.
7. *Apply/Utilise*: This process is, again, the responsibility of healthcare professionals. The success of a healthcare KM framework depends on its success in providing knowledge that is effective in meeting the demands of the healthcare enterprise.

In order to face various internal and external challenges in the healthcare environment, KM-based applications, such as healthcare enterprise memories, could be mobilised to facilitate the management of healthcare knowledge.

3. Healthcare Knowledge Management Using Healthcare Enterprise Memory

Central to most practical, context-sensitive KM solutions is the *Healthcare Enterprise Memory (HEM)*—a structure similar to an organisational memory [5]. HEM can be envisaged as a systematic confluence of various knowledge bases, managed by a common infra- and info-structure that can be operationalised to deliver a variety of knowledge-driven strategic services. HEM provides the functionality to store, share and re-use individual and organisational knowledge, experience, and lessons learnt [6].

Effective healthcare knowledge management is achieved by the HEM in a number of ways such as through automatic dissemination of knowledge, reuse of knowledge and experience, support of intelligent knowledge management services, timely provision of knowledge and experience, and the transformation from information to action. [2, 7, 8]

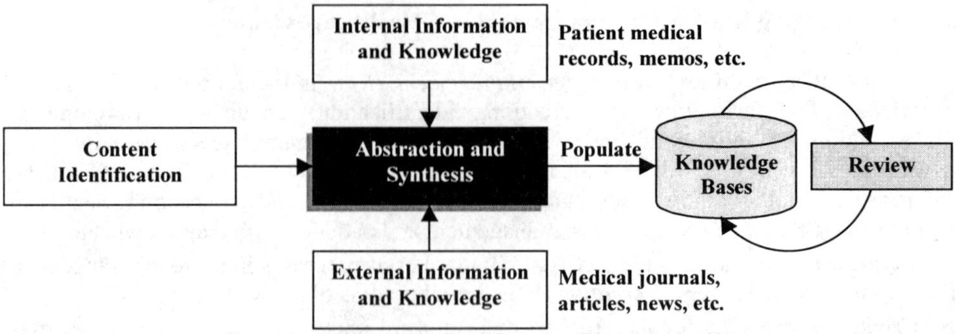

Figure 1. A Knowledge Base Creation Environment [1]

4. Building a Healthcare Enterprise Memory: A Model

The term 'building' here refers to the modelling of an HEM with emphasis on knowledge representation, ontologies and creation of knowledge bases. In simple functional terms, an HEM can be created through the process of identifying, capturing and leveraging formal (e.g. texts and documents) and informal (e.g. experience and lessons learnt) medical knowledge from internal and external sources (see Figure 1).

According to Figure 1, the healthcare knowledge bases are to be populated by the abstraction of internal and external healthcare information/knowledge based on certain content identification criteria. The synthesis process transforms the abstracted knowledge into a formal representation scheme that renders it operable by computer systems. Finally, the emergent knowledge bases undergo a process of review or update to ensure the validity and consistency of the extracted knowledge.

For our purposes, we propose a four-layer HEM model:

1. *Object Layer*: Consists of various healthcare information and knowledge sources. The sources may be formal (machine-readable) and/or informal (human-readable).
2. *Knowledge Description Layer*: Enables uniform and intelligent access to object-level resources. The main purpose of this layer is to facilitate accurate selection and efficient access to relevant healthcare knowledge in a given task context and situation.
3. *Application Layer*: Models and executes processes and tasks. The HEM's services can be realised in different ways, ranging from dedicated programs (which perform a well-defined task) to flexible query interfaces. These include medical protocol models and healthcare work process management systems [9].
4. *Services Layer*: Providing specialised services to healthcare professionals or the public through the use of various applications.

Figure 2 illustrates a complete scheme of an HEM with a mapping of its four layers to KM processes, to KM technologies and to various AI technologies.

5. Operationalising Healthcare Enterprise Memory

Traditionally, healthcare policies are derived by taking into account on-the-ground information, resource constraints, lessons learnt and domain knowledge. However, the effects of any devised policy cannot be ascertained until it is applied and data (spanning over a considerable period of time) concerning its effects is obtained and analysed. We propose a novel and knowledge-driven approach to healthcare policy making whereby the

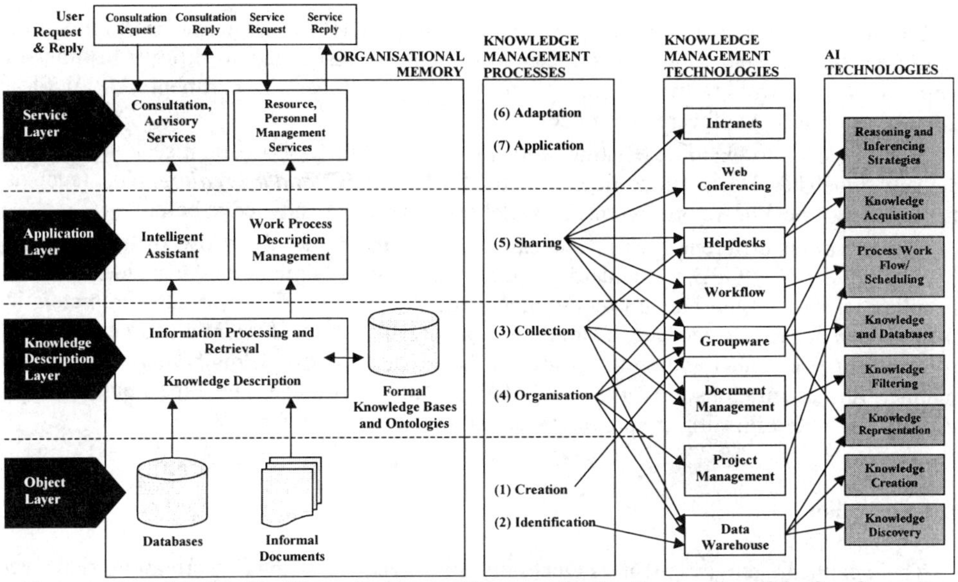

Figure 2. A model of the Healthcare Enterprise Memory, showing the mapping of the four-layers to KM Processes to KM Technologies and finally to AI Technologies

knowledge encapsulated within the HEM is operationalised to simulate specific scenarios and to analyse the effects of under-study 'policies' with respect to the simulated scenarios.

Healthcare modelling entails the development of a *healthcare process model* (addressing a specific goal or task). The modelling aspect entails the submission of different (experimental) values to the various parameters of the healthcare model and noting the influence of the parameter values towards the efficacy of the task/process being modelled. This strategy is akin, to some extent, to traditional simulation and modelling activities. However, the value-added aspect of our approach is that the healthcare model is derived from the manipulation of vast medical knowledge and outcome data contained within the HEM. Hence, it can be argued that healthcare modelling involving HEM is more informed, context sensitive, aware of relationships between disparate knowledge entities and realistic. Figure 3 identifies the process of healthcare modelling by operationalising healthcare knowledge, i.e. an HEM.

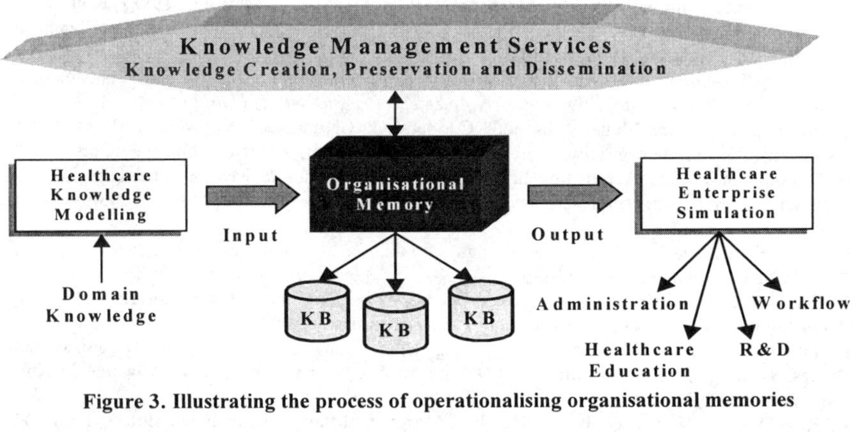

Figure 3. Illustrating the process of operationalising organisational memories

To substantiate our proposal for operationalising an HEM, we describe a modelling exercise with the evaluation of resources allocation and associated workflows in order to improve the *Service Delivery Time (SDT)* at an Out-Patient Department (OPD) of a government-based healthcare enterprise:

First, we need to examine existing workflows of the OPD for a patient seeking medical consultation. The SDT is a consequence of the fulfilment of *standard requirements* (such as the number of healthcare professionals available) in the OPD knowledge base.

To determine different SDTs, one can simulate the OPD workflow by varying the parameters in the OPD's standard requirements. Such simulations can identify the peculiarities of various standard requirements and the bearing of the various parameters in the eventual SDT. For instance, a simulation may yield that insufficient resources in terms of healthcare personnel and facilities are the main causes of *workflow bottlenecks*. In this manner, further solutions to workflow bottlenecks can be simulated by experimenting with different number of healthcare providers and noting the estimated SDTs.

6. Conclusion

The healthcare environment is generally perceived as being 'information rich' yet 'knowledge poor'. With advances in the domain of KM and the effectiveness of organisational memories, healthcare professionals and knowledge management experts could join efforts to venture towards the realisation of a 'knowledge rich' healthcare environment to enhance the effectiveness and efficiency of healthcare enterprises.

Indeed, this paper has identified the possible role of knowledge management technology in healthcare. Subsequent efforts need to focus on in-depth practical issues and applications of knowledge management techniques for meeting the ever-growing healthcare delivery demands. It is our contention that the healthcare domain can gain a lot by leveraging on existing and up-coming KM tools and techniques, and by working towards a synergy between healthcare enterprises and KM, leading to a win-win situation [10].

References

[1] D. O'Leary, Using AI in Knowledge Management: Knowledge Bases and Ontologies, *IEEE Intelligent Systems*, Vol. 13, No. 3, May/June 1998, pp. 34-39.

[2] A. Abecker, A. Bernardi, K. Hinkelmann, O. Kühn, and M. Sintek, Toward a Technology for Organisational Memories, *IEEE Intelligent Systems*, Vol. 13, No. 3, May/June 1998, pp. 40-48.

[3] D. O'Leary, Knowledge Management Systems: Converting and Connecting, *IEEE Intelligent Systems*, Vol. 13, No. 3, May/June 1998, pp. 30-33.

[4] C. O'Dell, C.J. Grayson, If We Only Knew What We Know: Identification and Transfer of Internal Best Practices, *Best Practices White Paper, American Productivity & Quality Center*, 1997.

[5] J. Euzenat, Corporate Memory through Cooperative Creation of Knowledge Bases and Hyper-documents, *10th Knowledge Acquisition Workshop, Banff (CA)*, 9-14 November 1996, pp. (36) 1-18.

[6] G. Simon, Knowledge Acquisition and Modelling for Corporate Memory: Lessons Learned from Experience, *Proceedings of Tenth Knowledge Acquisition for Knowledge-Based Systems Workshop*, 1996.

[7] G. van Geijst, R. van der Spek, E Kruizinga, Organizing Corporate Memories, *Proceedings of Tenth Knowledge Acquisition for Knowledge-Based Systems Workshop*, 1996.

[8] M. Negendra Prasad, E. Plaza, Corporate Memories as Distributed Case Libraries, *Proceedings of Tenth Knowledge Acquisition for Knowledge-Based Systems Workshop*, 1996.

[9] D. Fridsma, J. Gennari, M. Musen, Acquiring, Maintaining, and Customising Organisational Work Process Descriptions, *Proceedings of AAAI Spring Symposium, Artificial Intelligence in Knowledge Management*, 1997, pp. 40-46.

[10] R. Ruggles, Knowledge Tools - Using Technology to Manage Knowledge Better, *Ernst & Young Working Paper*, 1997.

Health Guidelines and Protocols

Medical Informatics Europe '99
P. Kokol et al. (Eds.)
IOS Press, 1999

Guidelines in Healthcare: the experience of the *Prestige* project

Colin Gordon[1], Mario Veloso[2] and the PRESTIGE Consortium
[1] *Information Services, Royal Brompton & Harefield NHS Trust, Sydney Street, London SW3 6NP, UK*
[2] *CENTIS, Rua dos Industriais, 7-2°-Dt., P-1200 Lisboa, Portugal*

Abstract. The paper reports the work and results of PRESTIGE: **Guidelines in Healthcare**, a large EU project designed to applying ICT to assist the application of clinical practice guidelines.

PRESTIGE: Guidelines in Healthcare [a project in the EC's Telematics Application Programme (DG XIII C4), December 1995-May 1999] is one of the most extensive initiatives yet undertaken worldwide to apply information and communication technology to assist healthcare professionals in the daily application of evidence-based guidelines of best practice. The project has been a collaboration of 30 organizations from eight countries, representing all the key players whose contribution is essential to this initiative: national and international bodies which are authors of standard clinical guidelines, health authorities, associations of clinical professionals, commercial system suppliers in primary and secondary care, academic centres, hospitals and health centres. The project has created clinical applications in six countries, linked to established clinical IT environments, with programmes for validation in routine practice. The aim of the project is "an installed and sustainable healthcare telematics infrastructure that supports dissemination and application of research based and consensus based guidelines, that in turn supports best practice for routine clinical care".

This undertaking involves a challenging combination of cultural, technical and organizational change. European health services are, however, increasingly accepting the goals as essential and committing themselves to mobilising the necessary policies and resources to carry them through.[1]

Some of the component tasks in this agenda for which PRESTIGE sets out to prove workable solutions are:

- The need to add new modules of functionality to a range of existing clinical IT environments in existing healthcare settings;
- The need to raise the existing level of implementations of the Electronic Patient Record, to provide a data infrastructure able to support patient specific application of guideline recommendations through individualised care planning over time;
- The need to incorporate new person-machine interactions within the process of the patient consultation in a workable and acceptable manner, and to fit the process of applying evidence in practice;
- The need for a shared methodology to convert the text of published clinical guidelines, and the intentions of their authors, into a formal, machine-readable semantic structure capable of being reliably combined with computerised clinical data to generate recommendations for action;

- The need for a sound, sustainable process for maintaining, disseminating and locally adapting electronic versions of clinical guidelines.

The PRESTIGE Consortium

CENTIS	WHO DiabCare, Munich
Hospital de Egas Moniz	Mainz University Heart Centre
Anestesia, Reanimação e Nurologia	OSE
UNINOVA	SAPHIS
Health Region of Lisbon and Tejo Valley	Bull France
Royal Brompton & Harefield NHS Trust	Danish Institute for Health Services
MIG, University of Manchester	County of Funen
UK WHO DiabCare Office	Gentofte Hospital
NHS IMC, UK	LHV
Sowerby Unit, Newcastle University	SMS Cendata
Siemens Nixdorf Healthcare Solutions	NHG
Royal College of Radiologists	MIE, University of Nijmegen
AAH Meditel Ltd.	Modena Local Health Unit
Bromley Hospitals NHS Trust	THETA
	SIMG
	Linkoping University Hospital

The rationale for a European collaborative initiative of this kind is both industrial and clinical.

Industrially, the development of common reusable components of technology provides vendors of clinical practice systems in national markets with an affordable path to adding major functionality and added value to their product in areas where national healthcare providers and users demand continuous improvements in its support for delivery of healthcare quality.

Clinically, the creation of a common electronic format for protocols provides international and national professional consensus bodies with a route for more effective dissemination and implementation of best practice standards which can 'plug and play' on a variety of clinical software platforms at the point of care. PRESTIGE's results should accelerate movement towards sound and workable European standards to make this vision a reality.

In the following we set out some key points in the technical results achieved to date.

- PRESTIGE technology functions with local and existing **patient record database** structures. Each application has linked generic PRESTIGE technology to a locally designed implementation of the electronic patient record.
- All applications contain a common **Protocol Manager** (the software component which identifies clinical guideline recommendation relevant to a specific patient). The Protocol Manager is being used in all the project's applications, and is supplied in the form of a developer's source code kit and as an ActiveX control. Its external interfaces have been successfully used to connect it to each application's Operational Front End, Patient Record and Knowledge Server.
- The project has a set of shared and local services for creating and storing **protocol knowledge**. The project has a common conceptual model of protocol knowledge; some applications are sharing database implementations to represent protocol knowledge in the runtime system. Several applications have used the tools **GAUDI (Guideline AUthoring and DIssemination Tool),** which incorporates a terminology server and

model (GRAIL) developed by the GALEN organization. Some applications use the tool **GLEAM (Guideline Editing and Authoring Module)** which has the capability to directly edit the knowledge base of an application. A project-wide Interchange Format for protocols and their associated terminology has been defined and is being used as a common transfer medium between GAUDI, GLEAM and the various project application platforms (see diagram and illustrations below). Partners in one application (THETA I.T.; Modena Local Health Unit, Italy) implemented its own tool (PAT: Protocol Authoring Tool) to edit its protocol knowledgebase.

- The project has produced a suite of generic **Act Management** software (that is, tools for managing shared information on requested and performed activities in a cooperative healthcare environment) and which implements the same conceptual model as the Protocol, Manager and Authoring Tools. These servers have been validated in a HIS environment at Hospital Egas Moniz, Lisbon. Other applications have implemented equivalent, appropriate forms of act management support for the primary care environment.

Guidelines implemented
Cervical Screening (primary care - NL, IT)
Influenza vaccination (primary care - NL, IT)
Diabetes Management (primary care - UK, PT)
Angina Management (primary care, hospital care - UK, DE)
Asthma Management (primary care, UK)
Epilepsy Care Planning (primary care, hospital care - PT, DK)
Anticoagulant Therapy (primary care, hospital care - DK)

Approach to Knowledge Modelling

In its initial phase, *PRESTIGE* developed a suite of object-oriented conceptual model definitions of the healthcare enterprise, the patient healthcare record and the protocol. The model was used to derive a set of shared component interface definitions, authoring tools and an Interchange Format (IF) for exchange of guidelines between authors and application in a standard BNF-defined text file format.

The approach to knowledge representation is declarative, based on the separation of knowledge structure from knowledge use. A protocol is basically conceived as a compositional hierarchy in which a main protocol (with its entry and exclusion criteria) is composed of a number of component protocols, which may themselves have further components. A leaf node protocol always contains a specification of an act recommended by the guideline. The logic of the protocol - what should be done when - is given by the compositional structure together with *lifecycle criteria* which can be specified for the component protocols and (if required) for the act which they specify.

A practical issue which demanded close attention and consistent handling in the project application was the correct coordination of the protocol model with the local application EPR, its coding system(s), and the working and technical environment of the user healthcare enterprise. This enables a clear division of tasks between:

- **the Protocol Manager,** which uses the standard constructs of the Protocol Model criterion grammar to logically evaluate the criteria specified in a protocol for recommended actions,
- **the Application EPR**, invoked by the Protocol Manager to evaluate a *Subject Phenomenon* expression which may be constructed using coded terminology constructs local to that EPR

- **the host clinical management system,** which can be invoked to assist in performing a recommended class of act specified in a protocol, by activating a corresponding functional service (e.g. communicate a booking request, enable generation of a drug prescription).

The adoption of this layered and partitioned modelling approach thus enables two key architectural and organizational benefits:

- The smooth functional coupling of new generic technology and existing, legacy technology functions;
- A clear framework for adapting and customising a shared (national or international) guideline to use with a locally specified dataset, technical infrastructure and service structure.

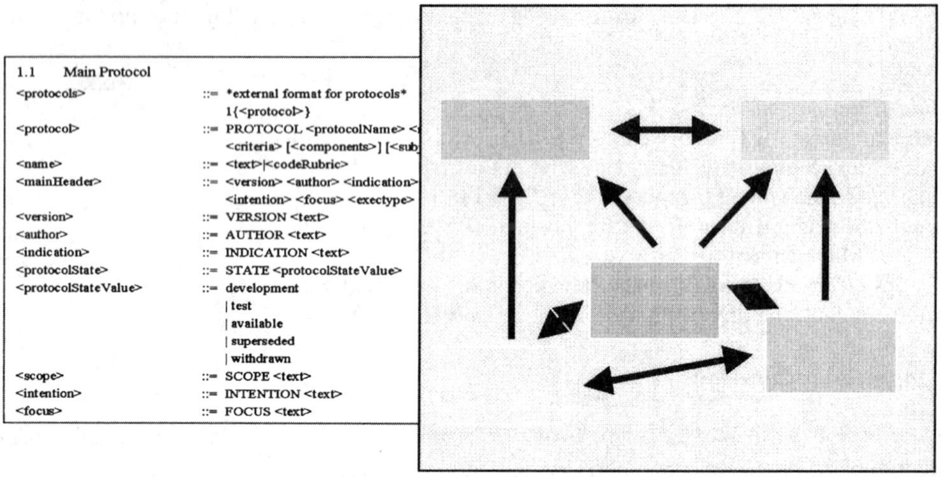

```
1.1     Main Protocol
<protocols>               ::= *external format for protocols*
                              1{<protocol>}
<protocol>                ::= PROTOCOL <protocolName> <
                              <criteria> [<components>] [<sub
<name>                    ::= <text>|<codeRubric>
<mainHeader>              ::= <version> <author> <indication>
                              <intention> <focus> <exectype>
<version>                 ::= VERSION <text>
<author>                  ::= AUTHOR <text>
<indication>              ::= INDICATION <text>
<protocolState>           ::= STATE <protocolStateValue>
<protocolStateValue>      ::= development
                              | test
                              | available
                              | superseded
                              | withdrawn
<scope>                   ::= SCOPE <text>
<intention>               ::= INTENTION <text>
<focus>                   ::= FOCUS <text>
```

Figure 1. The PRESTIGE Guideline Interchange Format

Lessons and further steps

A major part of the clinical activity in any protocol is collecting datasets (e.g. patient history, current medication, family history, physical examination, test results, etc.) Our model envisaged providing a fully declarative definition of the data capture mechanisms required for such activities (specifying which data items are mandatory or optional, whether existing data items should be displayed and whether these need to be systematically reconfirmed). To date it has not yet been practicable to use such a declarative specification to automatically generate and drive specific data entry dialogue for each act. Our current applications thus comprise either coded dialogs for each act class (a common approach in a hospital clinic) or generic system functions, not tailored to the specific protocol (a common approach in GP systems).

The EC's auditors reported in November 1998 that *PRESTIGE* had set itself "an ambitious goal" but "demonstrated solutions convincingly". Remarking that the results had "theoretical huge potential" but pointed to two potential bottlenecks: the availability of a supply of guidelines processed into the required format, and the achievement of compatibility and integration between *PRESTIGE*'s technology and existing and used software for the EPR.

We agree these are two key areas where much work remains to be done and a high level of effort will be required. There are still significant conceptual, cultural and clinical lessons to be learned before guideline working groups are routinely able to convert their product in computer-intelligible forms.

Indeed the very agenda of patient-specific application of guidelines in the consultation, although well justified by existing research results, sometimes demands greater explicitness and definition of guideline content than the cautious and nuanced wordings, evolved through consensus and compromise, currently provided in published guidelines. We anticipate that the availability of computer-aided implementation pathways will impact on and feedback into the guideline definition process, and it is desirable and necessary that this should occur.

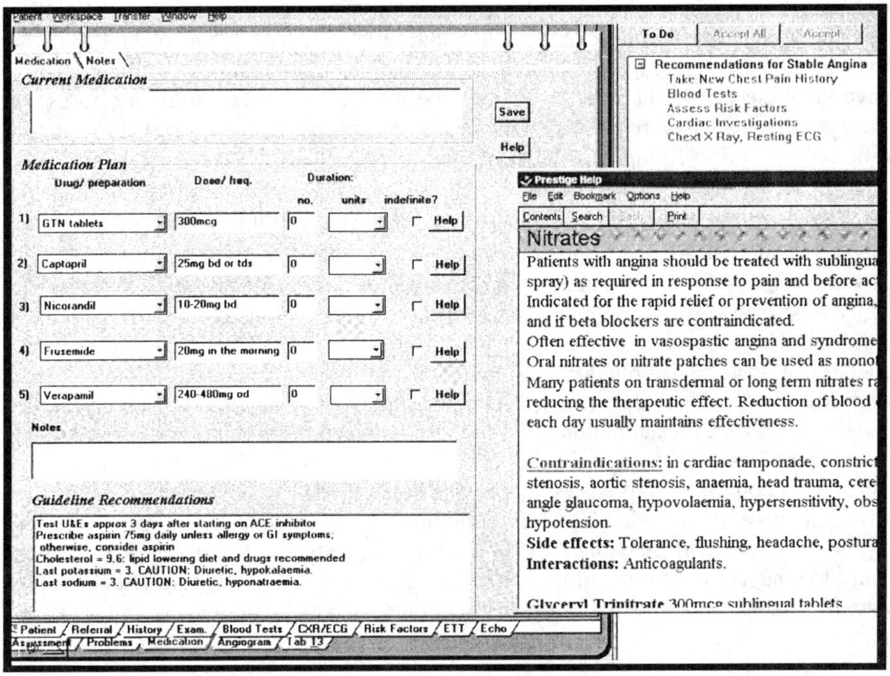

Figure 2. Assistance for medication planning using a guideline for managing Stable Angina

Web technologies can now provide major supports and intermediate steps in progress towards electronic dissemination of guideline knowledge in computer-intelligible form. Some organizations like the USA's Agency for Health Care Policy Research (AHCPR) already make their guidelines available as web documents, although with as yet limited exploitation of the full power of hypertext. The release by the WWW Consortium in 1998 of the Extensible Markup Language (XML) and Resource Description Framework (RDF) standards promise to greatly enhance the capabilities of the Web as a medium for communication of structured clinical knowledge and data.[2] The accumulation of experience from initiatives like PRESTIGE in 'full content' guideline knowledge representation should within the next few years provide a solid basis for a fuller standardised structuring of electronic health service knowledge resources in both document and knowledge base formats. In the short term the PRESTIGE Association may shortly investigate establishing an XML/RDF version of its existing guidelines Interchange Format.

The second key bottleneck identified by our auditors relates to the cost and difficulty of connecting new functional components based on a common data and knowledge standard to the multiplicity of existing commercial platforms for clinical management in European healthcare. PRESTIGE has gained ground-breaking experience by working on this problem with leading commercial GP system suppliers in four EC States (UK, NL, DK, IT), with close technical consultation with engineers developing next-generation versions of these companies' products. Our project was based on the premise that this exercise is unavoidable and necessary. Support for the practice of evidence-based medicine is a service to the clinician which supplements and must build on the more basic services provided by existing products for practice management and patient data management. The complexity of this existing market and product type precludes any realistic prospect of implementing common services across Europe for guideline implementation through a common new product which would supplant the less advanced approaches currently in use. On the other hand, the progress made by the existing suppliers in developing a more complete, structured and expressive database for the patient record, and the maturing of modular architectures for client PC applications, have meant that some of the systems are now well suited to support the additional level of functionality PRESTIGE can offer.

In an initiative explicitly supported by the European Commission and its auditors, the PRESTIGE consortium launched in March 1999 (at a public meeting in Lisbon, sponsored by Portugal TELECOM, Siemens Portugal and Portuguese health services), the PRESTIGE **Association**, an ongoing, open-membership organization designed to build and extend the community of shared experience and consensus in the domain of technology for guidelines in healthcare. The Association will provide an umbrella for practical collaborations between clinical systems suppliers in different national markets, working along parallel lines to extend the capabilities of their products for supporting evidence-based medicine. It will also act as a forum for the building of alliances between the communities of guideline authors, evidence-based medicine initiatives (such as the Cochrane Collaboration), and the health telematics community, to ensure that in the future guideline developers are aware of and fully able to exploit technology for structured representation and computer-aided implementation of clinical guidelines.[3] It will cooperate with the health service research community to study in further detail the critical success factors and ongoing effectiveness, in terms of process and outcome, of the computer-assisted use of clinical practice guidelines.

---

[1] NHS Executive, *Information for Health. An Information Strategy for the Modern NHS 1998-2005.* London 1998.

[2] Cf. the keynote address by Tim Berners-Lee at AMIA98: *Web Phase II: Evolution or Revolution?* [http://www.w3.org/Talks/1998/1108-amia-tbl/slide1-1.htm]

[3] C Gordon, 'Practice Guidelines and Healthcare Telematics: Towards an Alliance', in C Gordon and J P Christensen eds., Health Telematics for Clinical Guidelines and Protocols, IOS Press 1995.

Medical Informatics Europe '99
P. Kokol et al. (Eds.)
IOS Press, 1999

The RITHME Inter-Mediation Platform for data exchanges between Healthcare Professionals

Régis Beuscart[a,b], Marie-Catherine Beuscart-Zéphir[a], Jean-Marie Renard[a], David Delerue[a], Alexandre Souf[b]

[a] *Université Lille2 - Faculté de Médecine - CERIM - 1 Place Verdun 59045 Lille Cedex (F)*
[b] *CHRU de Lille - DIM - 2 Avenue Oscar Lambret - 59037 Lille Cedex (F)*

Abstract. Data Exchanges between Healthcare Professionals are always limited to paper. For letters, reports, results, the physicians and hospitals are yet using the classical post-office mailing system. With the growing development of Medical Informatics within the Hospital Information Systems and the GPs offices, the way to exchange medical data will be more and more oriented towards the Telematics procedures. If Tele-consultation, video-conferencing applications appear as routine procedures, a safe, protected, and rapid transmission of medical data and records through electronic mailing systems is not yet really available.The Rithme* Inter-mediation Platform is an experimental product, tested in the town of Armentières (in the City of Lille) in the North of France to allow a better, safer, more rapid electronic communication between all the professionals of a geographical sector. One of the mail component of this platform is the "Events Server" which collects and displays all the available information concerning a dedicated patient to the medical authorised correspondents. To realise this task the Rithme* Platform takes charge of 4 main functions: formatting the messages, assuring the security, managing the directories, notifying emergencies. Currently experimented with success in the City of Lille, this Platform will be soon customised and commercialised.

Key words : Healthcare Networks, Telemedicine, Intermediation, Communication platforms.

1 Introduction

New Information Technologies are introduced in all the dimensions of life: Tele-commerce, Tele-training, Tele- or video-conferencing, Electronic mails are today regularly used not only by computer scientists, or by information professionals, but by a growing part of the population. In the Healthcare domain, the electronic communication becomes a striking challenge for hospitals, organisations, doctors and patients. It is also a commercial challenge as the number of Healthcare professionals (3 million of people in France, more than 10 millions in Europe) is extremely high, and their communication flows increasing. Some countries try to apply Telecommunication policies in the Healthcare Sector; one characteristic example is the "Réseau Santé Social" in France, described as an Intranet for the communication between doctors and the Reimbursement system of the Social Security.

Too often, Telemedicine is considered only for co-diagnosis [1], Tele-education and Tele-training [2], Tel-radiology and Tele-treatment [3]. A new domain is emerging, concerning Tele-care networks for data exchanges between hospitals, between hospitals and

G.P.s, between laboratories and other Healthcare professionals…and for a better, more rapid transmission of information. This information includes administrative, medical, biological and therapeutic data of dedicated patients. This may also concern general information about the way to obtain appointments, facilities provided by the hospital as well as quality indicators. Some experiences demonstrate the possible benefits of such professional networks within a geographical sector or even a region: the Coco project and the Fyncom experience in Denmark, The Medibridge network in Belgium. But these experiences are not easily transferable as the technical solutions are mainly dependant upon the security procedures allowed by the legislation of the countries, and upon the organisation of the Healthcare system in the country.

We present here the experience of the Inter-Mediation Platform in the area of Lille in the North of France (1 million of people). This experience includes the University Hospital of Lille, and two general Hospitals: the Hospital of Tourcoing, and the Hospital of Armentières, in a small town (26 000 habitants), plus 55 G.P.s, 3 private biological laboratories, and the therapeutic accommodations for HIV-infected patients. This platform named RITHME* was designed to allow a better, best organized communication of information between all the medical actors of the sector. Currently under evaluation, the objective is the packaging and customisation of the product for a large dissemination in the region and throughout Europe.

2 Material and Methods

2.1 Objectives of the Project

A complete analysis of the Users Requirements involving all the parties was organised with General Practitioners, Specialist Physicians (cardiologists, dermatologists, radiologists), laboratories, hospitals physicians and administrative directors. At the end of this first phase, we obtained a rather complete description of the potential users needs and expectations that are summarised and ordered below:

GPs Requirements

Requirement 1: To inform the GP that a patient is hospitalised. The GP will receive relevant information concerning the patient's hospitalisation : entry (emergency or not), discharge, movements of the patient between different medical units, eventually death. For each GP, the complete list of the hospitalised patients he is responsible for, should be available.

Requirement 2 To receive as soon as possible a relevant information after the patient's discharge (liaison letter) including: diagnosis, prescribed treatments and therapies (order), instruction and recommendations for the follow-up

Requirement 3: Transmission of relevant information from the emergency unit : diagnosis, treatment, follow-up, surveillance ...

Requirement 4: To receive information from the hospital in case of significant event of change in the patient's status.

Requirement 5: When a patient leaves the hospital on Saturday , the GP or the Homecare Nurse must be informed before the discharge

Requirement 6: When a patient leaves the hospital, the labs results, liaison letters and discharge letters are available.

Hospital Doctors Requirements

Requirement 1: Hospitals must be equipped with Hospital Information Systems for : Medical record, Integration of results (labs, consultations, hospitalisations), Connection with other hospitals and GPs.

Requirement 2: To receive short, relevant, and concise patients' information from the GPs (as the GPs can afford short summary of their computerised medical record.)

Requirement 3: Appointment Systems : To share agendas between different hospitals.

*2.2 The Inter-Mediation platform: Rithme**

The platform provides basic and specific services to make possible the data exchanges between Hospitals, GPs and other practitioners (labs, specialists…).

Basic services.

The platform provides four main functions to permit the connection of Healthcare actors. These basic services are described below:

- Directory of the physicians, organisations, laboratories, and hospitals included in the network
- Security of the transactions. To make safe the transmission of data, we encipher the messages with a "tunnelling" procedure.
- Formatting the messages. As there is no standardisation of the documents the platform receives documents and messages under different formats (Word6, Word97, RTF, Hprim, …). To send the documents in a format understandable by the receiver's application, it is necessary to translate the document in a comprehensible format. To do so, each received message is deciphered and then re-formatted in XML. And the XML format is re-translated under the receiver's format according to a table contained in the directory.
- Notification. In case of a doctor's absence, or network disturbances, or machine unavailability, it is indispensable to route the messages under different ways. In case of emergency, a message can be displayed on the phone of the doctor or even on his portable phone if available.

Specific Services. The Inter-Mediation Platform Rithme* is not only a secure E-Mail. It organises the communication between physicians to make it safer productive and more efficient. Based on a data Base (Oracle*), the main component of the Platform is the "Events Server"

- The "Events Server" is the most original part of the Rithme* Inter-Mediation platform.. For one patient i, the platform can receive several documents from diverse origins and directed towards one unique address: Labs Results LR(i), Report R(i), Letter L(i), or administrative information A(i). In case of an hospitalised patient, movements, reports, letters are provided within a common short period of time. The Events server packages the different documents LR(i), R(i), L(i), A(i) in a common "Event" Event (i) for the patient i.). So, for one patient, this database collects, gathers and organises the data in the relevant format,

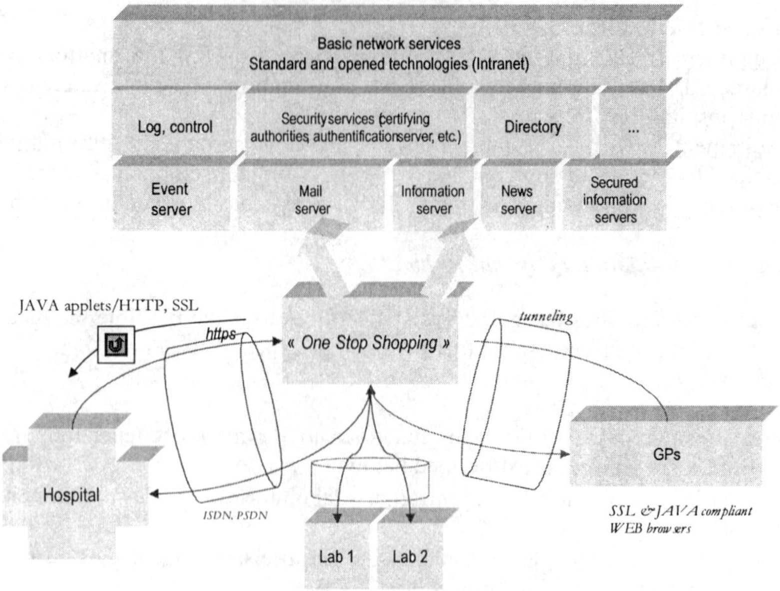

Figure 1. General functions of the Inter-Mediation Platform

in one "event". In the database, for one patient, there are as many events as packages. For the moment, these events are destroyed when read by the receiver but in the next future it could be possible to aggregate these events under a comprehensible format for statistical analysis or to keep archives on the patient's history.

- Access to medical databases and medical Internet services.
- Protected E-Mail throughout the network for the actors participating to the experiment.

2.3 *Other services and applications*

This project was developed to be integrated in the French national medical network dedicated to the Healthcare professionals and organisations. This network called "Réseau Santé Social" (RSS) is under construction and will provide the actors of the domain with a professional Extranet assuring three main functions for routage, security, and directory maintenance, plus a safe access to Internet.

3 Results

3.1 *Usage of the Inter-mediation Platform*

After a first experimental phase in summer 98, all the physicians are currently connected to the Platform to receive messages and data from the Hospitals as well as from the labs. In this validation phase we register all the comments, remarks and suggestions of the GPs and of the Hospital to provide a better and more efficient service.

A recent statistical analysis of the logs gives us interesting elements on the way the server is used by the partners. (Table 1). The maximum number of messages are rather short messages of 100 bytes to 100 Kbytes, corresponding to administrative messages (movements of the patients) or short letters or reports (cardiology reports, X-Ray reports, liaison letters). Large messages greater than 100 kbytes are quite unusual.

Table 1. Length of the messages transmitted through the platform.

Size of the message	Percentage of messages	Percentage of Bytes
0-1b	0,9	-
1b - 10b	1.7	-
11b – 100b	5.5	0.16%
101b – 1kb	48.4	7.61%
1kb – 10kb	39.2	38.84%
11kb – 100kb	4.1	42.45%
101kb – 1Mb	0.2	10.94%

As the use of the Platform is growing, the number of calls and connected physicians is also growing rapidly. 29/55 physicians use daily the platform, only one month after installation. Nevertheless, the real success of the network will be confirmed only after several months of utilisation.

3.2 *Qualitative Results*

The Inter-Mediation Platform RITHME has proven to be a safe means for communication between the Healthcare Professional of a geographic area. It allows a real-time communication system, a service availability 24 hours per day, and the possibility of transferring all types of documents daily used by the Healthcare professionals: texts, labs numerical results, schemas, even images.

But the service is also providing other services that are useful for every actor in the network: a safe E-Mail system allowing the transmission of confidential messages concerning patients or Public Health, and an access to information services and servers, epidemiological alert systems.

The most positive aspects of the contribution of hospitals physicians and GPs can be summarized as: increasing benefits in time and travels (most efficient visits to the hospital), easy access to a rich source of relevant data concerning the commonly followed patients, and a renewed quality of the presentation of the documents.

4 Discussion

The Inter-Mediation Platform named Rithme* was designed during the ISAR-Telematics project of the European Union Fourth Framework Program. It was finalised and experienced during the IRISI Project of the European Union Programme for the development of the Information Society in the European regions.

This platform is currently running in the town of Armentières in the Region Nord-Pas-de-Calais in France. The main exchanges concern administrative information (entry/ outcome / movements/ death of a patient) and medical information as letters, results of biological tests, reports from different sources. The current follow-up of the rates of exchanges indicates a rapid growth of the number of regular users and of the number of messages.

Organisational and human constraints [4] are important to take into account for estimating the success of such applications. On one hand, the majority of the healthcare professionals of the area must have computers, and moreover software applications to manage their patients records. Even if the use of computers is growing in all the regions of Europe, only a limited percentage of them utilise the capabilities of the electronic patients records. On the other hand, if the labs are all equipped, it is not the case for the hospitals where Hospital Information Systems are not in routine use everywhere. As a consequence, the installation of Inter-mediation Platforms will require the equipment, training, maintenance of many professionals. This new way of working will introduce new methods for treating documents and letters and will have huge organisational impacts [5].

The management of such a platform focuses also on security procedures, confidentiality respect, identification, authentication and signature procedures. Some of these problems can be technically solved but the technicians and the physicians must stay aware that it is an essential point for the success of Telematics in healthcare.

The platform is currently installed in a limited geographical sector. One question is the dimension of the area that must be covered to optimise the size and costs of the material. From Health Geography studies, it appears that the exchanges are mainly concentrated in a sanitary sector (400 000 to 1 million people). Inter-regional exchanges are rare and concern a small population of patients, if we exclude the holidays seasons.

5 Conclusion

Asynchronous communication between physicians, hospitals and other professionals is an important factor of quality of care as this quality is depending upon a good communication of the relevant information between all the parties. Health Telematics can improve this communication by improving the rapidity, the security and the availability of the right data in the right place at the right time.

The Inter-mediation Platform RITHME* allows the safe transmission of data and messages within the network of participating professionals. The success of these applications will also depend upon organisational changes in the work process and improvement of Human Computer Interfaces to improve their utilisation by the end-users.

Acknowledgements

This project was granted by the European Union during the Research Project ISAR-Telematics from the Health Telematics Program (from the 4th framework Program) and from the European Program for regions IRISI. It was also sustained directly by the Region Nord-Pas-de-Calais in the Research Contract "Ganymède".

References

[1] V. Kopsacheilis, I. Kamilatos, M.G. Strinzis, and L. Makris, Design of CSCW Applications for Medical teleconsultation and remote diagnosis support, Med Informat. J., 1997 ; 22 ; pp. 121-132.

[2] Internet Update, M.D. Computing , 1998, 1 ; pp. 10-28.

[3] E.R. Carson, D.G. Cramp, A. Morgan, and A.V. Roudsari, Clinical decision Support, Systems Methodology, and Telemedicine : Their Role in the Management of Chronic Disease, IEEE Transactions on Information Technology in Biomedicine, 1998, 2 ; pp. 80-88.

[4] A.W. Kushniruk, D.R. Kaufman, V.L. Patel, Y. Levesque, P. Lottin. Assessment of a computerized patient record system: a cognitive approach to evaluating medical technology, M.D. Computing 3 (1996) ; pp. 406-415.

[5] M.C. Beuscart-Zéphir, J. Brender, R. Beuscart, I. Menager-Depriester, How to access the usability of information technology in Healthcare, Computer Methods and Programs in BioMedicine, 1997 ; pp. 19-28.

Medical Informatics Europe '99
P. Kokol et al. (Eds.)
IOS Press, 1999

Development of a reminder system for General Practitioners

R. Bindels[1], A. Hasman[1] and R.A.G.Winkens[2,3]
[1]*Dept. Medical Informatics, Maastricht University, Maastricht, the Netherlands*
[2]*Transmural & Diagnostic Centre, AzM, Maastricht, the Netherlands*
[1]*Dept. of General Practice, Maastricht University, Maastricht, the Netherlands*

Abstract. In this contribution we describe a prototype reminder system that has been developed to influence General Practitioners' (GP) test request behaviour. It is intended to substitute conventional written feedback by human experts. The system generates critical comments about the rationality of the test request at the moment the GP requests a test that is not in line with national or regional guidelines.

1. Introduction

Over the last 20 years there has been an increase in the consumption of diagnostic tests and there is a growing awareness that the use of diagnostic tests should be reduced [1]. In the past, various strategies have been developed to change GPs' test-ordering behaviour, for example education, redesigning the request form and feedback on number, rationality or costs of the requested tests. To prevent a further increase in test consumption in the Maastricht region, the Maastricht Transmural & Diagnostic Centre (T&DC) has been giving personal feedback to GPs in the Maastricht region since 1985. Twice a year each individual GP in the Maastricht region (±85 GPs) receives structured feedback reports with critical comments on his/her test requests in a previous month. The individual written biannual feedback is based on a comparison between requests (including provided clinical data) on the one hand, and information contained in accepted regional guidelines or the Dutch College of General Practitioners (NHG) standards, on the other hand. Earlier studies focused on the effects of feedback on GPs' test ordering behaviour [2, 3]. Although the feedback procedure described above was effective and was appreciated by the GPs, the T&DC was looking for more efficient intervention techniques. Consequently, we have tried to develop a less laborious way to provide information on diagnostic tests to GPs and to give them insight into their own test-ordering behaviour. We chose to develop a reminder system that has to substitute the conventional written feedback.

2. Design criteria

Currently GPs in the Maastricht region indicate on a pre-printed request form, developed by the T&DC, which tests they want to order. They have to check off boxes on a paper form and voluntary enter some relevant patient data. These data consist of: (1) patient registration data such as name, address, gender and date of birth; (2) medical data: working hypotheses, signs and complaints, existing problems, physical examination and medication and (3) reason for test request.

In daily practice the GP has about 8 minutes for the consultation of one patient. For this reason the reminder systems' most important requirement is to work fast. To accomplish this goal the system must be easy to use, has to be fast and has to prevent that the GP has to enter data twice.

We decided that the reminder system should provide feedback concerning incorrect or redundant requests and the adequateness of the provided patient information. Another important requirement was that the GP receives the feedback at the time the investigations are requested. Finally we wanted to limit the use of free text concerning working hypotheses, existing problems and complaints to enable the reminder system to better respond to the medical data entered in the reminder system.

3. Development of the system

The main goal of the reminder system is to reduce the number of non-rational test requests as well as the total number of test requests through influencing GPs' behaviour. Before it is possible to implement the national and regional guidelines into the reminder system, the guidelines, written in natural language, have to be properly translated into a formal language. Guidelines that are used by intelligent humans need not to be fully consistent or complete. For computer use the guidelines need to be complete, free of contradictions and sufficiently detailed to avoid that only the most trivial reminders are given. After studying the guidelines it was concluded that if-then rules could be used as a knowledge representation. In total 273 if-then rules were extracted from the national and regional guidelines. Only 65 of the above-mentioned total of 273 rules were useful. The other 208 rules were either not clearly formulated, lacked well-defined conditions or were found not relevant. Of the useful rules reminders, each consisting of an if-then rule and a remindertext, were made. The expressions of the rules consist of logical propositions combined with Boolean operators, such as AND, OR or NOT.

Two clinicians and the researcher checked the formalised reminders for errors, inconsistencies, and clinical relevance. Since one if-then rule can result in more than one reminder, finally 113 reminders resulted.

4. System description

To use the reminder system, the GP will have to enter the data that (s)he thinks are sufficient to support the test request. The reminder system has an on-line connection with the EPR via an intermediate database. When the GP starts the reminder system the data will be transferred automatically from the intermediate database into the corresponding fields of the reminder system. Request specific data may be entered directly into the reminder system. These data consist of: (1) medical data: working hypothesis, signs and complaints and physical examination; (2) reason for test request. On the paper request form the diagnostic tests are divided into clusters. These clusters represent tests that are conducted by different laboratories. In our program we use tabs to separate these different clusters of tests. Contrary to the paper form, the GP has to fill in a separate form for each working hypothesis.

In addition, we added a list, containing all International Classification of Primary Care (ICPC) terms [4] and a thesaurus with synonyms of the terms used in the ICPC list so the GP can select medical terms for complaints and diagnoses. With this tool we can standardise the medical data the GP enters into the system and therefore our if-then rules can now be based on ICPC coding only.

The second part of the reminder system provides the active support, i.e. generates the actual reminders. The if-then rules are entered via a KBE, a graphical knowledge acquisition tool that stores the rules into a knowledge base. The knowledge base is compiled into a DLL-file that is used by the reminder system [5]. This part of the system reads the patient data and checks whether any of the if-then rules will fire. If a rule fires it means that an inconsistency is found and consequently the corresponding reminder is generated immediately and presented by means of a pop-up window, overlaying the interface of the request form (fig. 1).

The reminder contains critical comments about the requested tests. In addition to the reminder text, the pop-up window contains three buttons. The GP presses 'accept' to indicate that (s)he accepts the reminder and 'reject' to indicate that (s)he does not agree. In both cases it is still possible for the GP to make changes in the request form after (s)he has seen the reminder. Moreover the reminder window contains a button to request more information that may contain hyperlinks to the appropriate guidelines and/or references to the literature.

Another option in the reminder system allows the GP to ask for additional background information about the guidelines. With this option textbook information about the regional and national guidelines is presented in a web-based environment by means of an internal web browser. The web-based environment enables the user to browse quickly through the available information.

The information on the request form, the reminder(s) the GP has received as well as the additional information (s)he has used are recorded in a database. Finally, the request form is printed using the same layout as the conventional paper form.

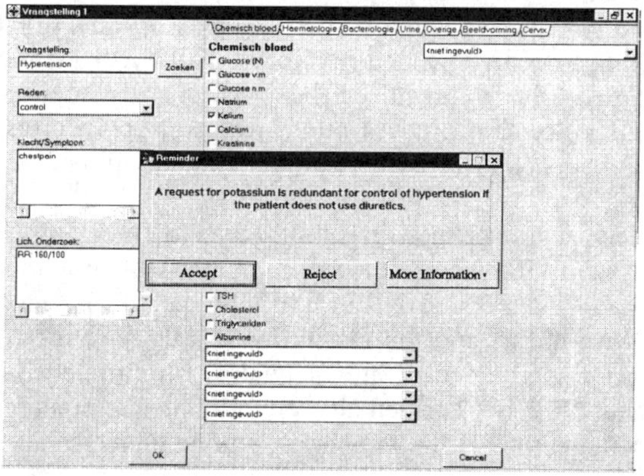

Figure 1: If a request is not according the guidelines, the reminder system generates and displays a reminder that overlays the normal user interface of the request form.

5. Results

The first reactions of the GPs on the actual reminder system were positive. At present, the actual reminder system contains 113 reminders concerning various medical problems. The 78 tests that are dealt with in the reminder system cover about 75 % of the total amount of the requested tests and most of the frequently requested tests are included in the rules.

The conditions of the if-then rules can contain a requested test, medical patient information, personal information (age and gender) or a combination of these types of information. The majority of the conditions of the if-then rules (78%) contain a requested test in combination with medical information about the patient. For example: IF working hypothesis is glandular fever AND ESR (erythrocyte sedimentation rate) is requested THEN give reminder text: "Requesting an ESR for the working hypothesis glandular fever is unnecessary."

A first validation of the medical information in the reminder system has been carried out. Ten request forms, from the archive of the T&DC, were selected and both an internist and the reminder system assessed the rationality of the requested tests. There were 26 different tests or test combinations on the 10 forms. Two independent reviewers judged the reminders. In 12 situations the reminder system gave the same feedback as the internist. In three of the remaining 14 situations, the feedback of the internist was outside the domain of the reminder system (feedback was not about missing medical data or not based on the guidelines). In five situations, according to the reviewers, the reaction of the reminder system was correct. The remaining six situations were errors in the formalisation process, the translation from the written guidelines into the IF-THEN rules (3) and lacking reminders in the knowledge base (2). The last discrepancy concerned a less detailed reminder that was given in addition to a more detailed correct reminder (belonging to the first 12). The less detailed reminder should not be presented. A larger study to validate the medical information will be carried out to analyse the reactions of the reminder system.

6. Discussion

It is clear that the feedback given by the reminder system has several advantages compared with written feedback. First, reminders can be produced whenever necessary and continuously (after every request), while written feedback can only be given in a selection of cases, due to the effort needed. Second, reminders will act at the moment the GP needs the information, namely the moment he/she performs the request. This immediate intervention in the GP's decision process might result in another response than the one following the manual feedback. Third, the reminder system will be less labour intensive on the long run.

An important disadvantage of the current system is the fact that there is no integration with the GP's EPR system. Further, the current reminder system is more dependent on the amount and the quality of the medical data provided by the GP. To make sure the GP enters at least the working hypothesis and the reason for request into the reminder system, the system alerts the user that these data are mandatory. A problem is the quality of the provided medical data. If a GP accidentally provides the reminder system with wrong information, he/she will get the wrong reminders or no reminders at all.

References

[1] J. P. Kassirer, Our stubborn quest for diagnostic certainty. *N. Engl. J. Med.*, **320** (1989) 1489-1491.

[2] R. A. G. Winkens *et al.*, Effects of routine individual feedback over nine years on general practitioners' requests for tests. *BMJ*, **312** (1996) 490.

[3] P. Pop and R. A. Winkens, A diagnostic centre for general practitioners: results of individual feedback on diagnostic actions. *J. R. Coll. Gen. Pract.*, **39** (1989) 507-8.

[4] H. Lamberts and M. Wood, International Classification of Primary Care, in International Classification of Primary Care, eds. pp. (Oxford University Press, Oxford, 1987).

[5] P. A. de Clercq *et al.*, A strategy for developing practice guidelines for the ICU using automated knowledge aquisition techniques. *Int. J. Clin. Monit. Comput.*, **In press.** (1999)

Medical Informatics Europe '99
P. Kokol et al. (Eds.)
IOS Press, 1999

Quantitative Collagen as a Golden Standard in Differential Diagnosing of Fibrotic Changes in Liver Tissue

Jens JONSSON[1], Ankica BABIC[1,2]
1. Linköpings universitet, Department of Biomedical Engineering, Medical Informatics S-581 85 Linköping, SWEDEN
2. Faculty of Electrical Engineering, University of Ljubljana, Slovenia

Abstract. Determining a presence and degree of liver fibrosis provides means for diagnosing disease related processes. We have used two data mining methods, discriminant and regression analyses, to acquire knowledge from the data of 211 patients. We have shown and discussed that quantitative collagen has a distinguished discriminating power and can serve as a golden standard. We have additionally succeeded to obtain a formula consisting of standardised blood tests that can replace quantitative collagen. Practical implications of this is a non-invasive and cost efficient patient examination. All the results are now left for clinical evaluation and so is the current way of histopathological classifications.

1 Motivations and methods

The purpose of this research was to verify the hypothesis that quantitative collagen, qcoll, can serve as a golden standard in diagnosing liver disease. Secondary objective was to replace the variable qcoll, with convenient blood laboratory tests that are less invasive for patients than biopsy performed in liver. In our previous research [1,2] we have proven how powerful multivariate statistical methods can be in the field of asymptomatic liver disease. By means of the same methods we have shown benefits of blood laboratory tests to monitor viral hepatitis C.

The quantity of collagen, qcoll, is measured by staining a sample from a liver biopsy with a hematoxyline-eosin and hematoxyline-van Gieson. After staining the samples they are scanned into a computer and image analysis is used to determine a percentage of collagen [3]. It is known that measurable substances are passed into the blood as a result of developing fibrosis in liver.

We have used multivariate discriminant analysis to verify quantitative collagen being a golden standard and regression analysis to find its replacement using other variables such as convenient laboratory tests. The statistical package used was SPSS version 8.0 for Windows.

The patient material contained 211 cases of reasonable quality, which meant that some cases with missing values had to be dealt with. The problem of missing data is that all conventional computer programs are implemented without considering missing data. When a multivariate model is used, the corresponding records are dropped from the analysis [4].

Cases were classified using the Knodell scoring system [5] ranging from 0 to 4, where 4 represents a case of cirrhosis and 0 represents no fibrotic scarring found in liver.

2 Statistical background

2.1 Multivariate discrimination

Discriminant analysis is used to classify data into groups based on a nominal or non-metric categorical variable, where the independent variables are metric [6]. Categorical variables are e.g. man/woman, low/high or as in this case "having a severe illness"/"having a moderate illness". This way of representation could make the latest definition quite a "soft" variable especially in comparison to more clear cut definition of groups. Conditions for successful discriminant analysis are that data should have a natural variance, equal and unknown dispersion and a priori group membership being equal. For each case a discriminant score is calculated using the following formula $Z = W_1X_1 + W_2X_2 + \ldots + W_nX_n$ where Z is the discriminant score, W is a discriminant weight and the X:s are the independent variables.

Figure 1a – Representation of Z-scores, well separated groupings

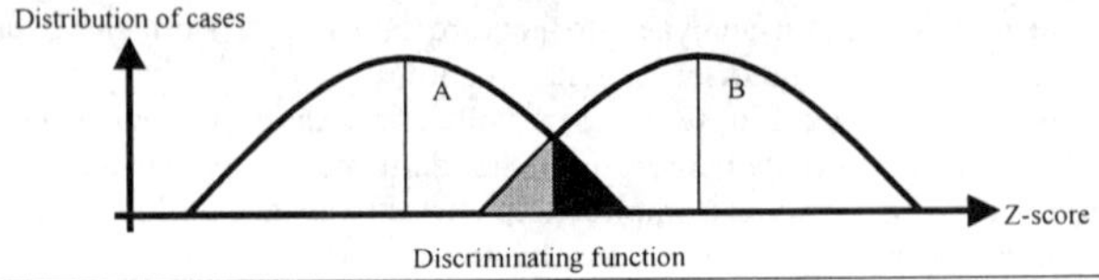

Figure 1b - Representation of Z-scores, groupings almost identical

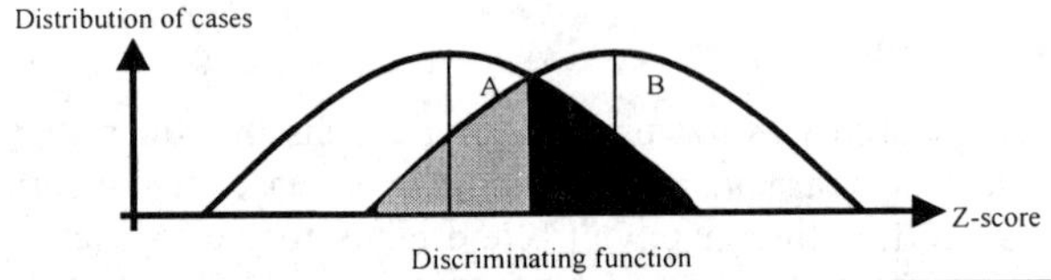

The two examples of Figures 1a and 1b, based on the same data, are different due to the usage two different discriminant functions resulting in different Z-scores. The discriminant function of Figure 1a separates the groups well whilst the same can not be said for the function of Figure 1b. There it is shown that the Z-scores for the two groups are similar which prevents an accurate classification. The shaded regions represent the cases not correctly classified, i.e. cases belonging to group A classified into group B, and vice versa. Starting from this presumption our goal was to find a function that could successfully distinguish between diseased and healthy subgroups of examined patients.

Figure 2 – Graphical illustration of two-group discriminant analysis

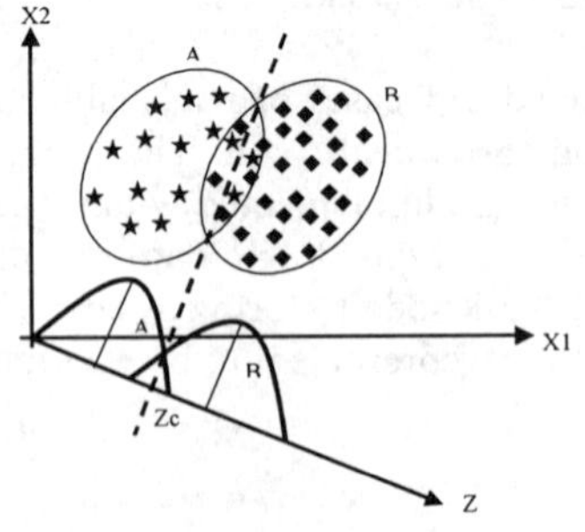

Figure 2 shows an example of a two group discriminant analysis. Stars and diamonds belong to two different groups. Two independent parameters, X1 and X2, are used to calculate the discriminant function, Z. It can be seen that the variable X1 has a greater discriminating power since the Z axis is more closely aligned to the X1 axis than the X2 axis. The dashed line shows discriminating score used for classification, Zc, which is calculated from the different group centres and number of cases belonging to them. Cases with a Z-score below Zc will be classified into group A and those with Z-scores greater than Zc will be classified into group B, respectively.

Results are represented in classification tables, Table 1, showing the accuracy. The overall number of correct classifications, appearing in bold, should be further evaluated by considering the cost of misclassification. *"Can we accept missing a few ill patients?", "What is the cost of treating/examining a healthy patient?"*.

Table 1

		Predicted group membership	
		Not having fibrosis	Having fibrosis
True group membership	Not having fibrosis	**38**	5
	Having fibrosis	12	**28**
	Not having fibrosis (%)	**88.4%**	11.6%
	Having fibrosis (%)	30.0%	**70.0%**
	79.5% of all cases correctly diagnosed.		

2. 2 Multivariate regression

We intended to use regression analysis to replace the verified golden standard, quantitative collagen, with a set of a few statistically significant variables.

Basic linear regression analysis relies on the assumption that one variable can be expressed as a linear combination of other variables: $Y = B_0+B_1X_1+B_2X_2+\ldots+B_nX_n$ [6]. Here Y is our new fabricated variable and X_1 through X_n are our set of variables with a power to describe the same qualities as the original variable.

Coefficients B are corresponding to a variable X which is precisely expressed through value of the correlation. The coefficients are calculated using the mean-square method to minimise each case's distance to the resulting regression function. The function is built in a stepwise process where variables entered at each step updates the function and a measure of information gain is calculated.

The stop criteria is no variation of R^2-value, which expresses the amount of new information added. Analogously, a significantly smaller change of R^2 means a minimal or no information gain obtained by adding a particular variable.

3 Results

3.1 Discriminating power of quantitative collagen

The clinical goal that motivated the data analysis was to distinguish between the cases of severe illness from cases of mild or no illness. The variable used is a diagnosis of fibrosis on a scale ranging from 0 to 4, where 0 is a case where no fibrosis is found and 4 is a case of cirrhosis. Four analyses are presented here with respect to different groupings/histopathological classifications.

1. Cases with fibrosis = 0 form one group and cases with fibrosis between 1 and 4 form the other. The parameter qcoll is not used here.
2. Cases with fibrosis = 0 or 1 form one group and cases with fibrosis between 2 and 4 form the other. The parameter qcoll is not used here.

3. Cases with fibrosis = 0 form one group and cases with fibrosis between 2 and 4 form the other. All cases of fibrosis = 1 are removed. The parameter qcoll is not used here.
4. Cases with fibrosis = 0 form one group and cases with fibrosis between 2 and 4 form the other. All cases of fibrosis = 1 are removed. The parameter qcoll is used in this case.

Respective classification matrices are following. Cases correctly classified are marked in bold.
Variables: PREALB = Prealbumin, FERRITIN = Ferritin, CHEN = Chenodeoxycholic acid , K = Potassium, PIIINP = Procollagen III N-terminal Peptide.

Table 2

Analysis 1 Qcoll not used		Predicted group membership	
		Having fibrosis = 0	Having fibrosis Between 1 and 4
True group membership	Not having fibrosis	**7**	36
	Having fibrosis	4	**142**
	Not having fibrosis (%)	**16.3%**	83.7%
	Having fibrosis (%)	2.7%	**97.3%**
	78.8% of all cases correctly diagnosed. Variables used: PREALB, FERRITIN, CHEN, K		

Table 3

Analysis 2 Qcoll not used		Predicted group membership	
		Having fibrosis Between 0 and 1	Having fibrosis Between 2 and 4
True group membership	Not having fibrosis	**144**	6
	Having fibrosis	31	**9**
	Not having fibrosis (%)	**96.0%**	4.0%
	Having fibrosis (%)	77.5%	**22.5%**
	80.5% of all cases correctly diagnosed. Variables used: FERRITIN, CHEN, PIIINP		

Table 4

Analysis 3 Qcoll not used		Predicted group membership	
		Having fibrosis = 0	Having fibrosis Between 2 and 4
True group membership	Not having fibrosis	**38**	5
	Having fibrosis	12	**28**
	Not having fibrosis (%)	**88.4%**	11.6%
	Having fibrosis (%)	30.0%	**70.0%**
	79.5% of all cases correctly diagnosed. Variables used: PREALB, FERRITIN, CHEN, K		

Table 5

Analysis 4 Qcoll used		Predicted group membership	
		Having fibrosis = 0	Having fibrosis between 2 and 4
True group membership	Not having fibrosis	**42**	2
	Having fibrosis	11	**34**
	Not having fibrosis (%)	**95.5%**	4.5%
	Having fibrosis (%)	24.4%	**75.6%**
	85.4% of all cases correctly diagnosed. Variables used: QCOLL, PREALB, FERRITIN		

These classification tables reflect differentiating diagnosis of liver diseases where identifying different stages of fibrosis can be of confounding nature. This means that patients with fibrosis=0 are not automatically healthy, they can still suffer from an infection without having developed liver fibrosis.

Perhaps this explains the results from the first analysis, Table 2, which are not satisfactory. The model tends to classify 36 cases out of 43 of false fibrosis. The situation is best described by the Figure 1b but with the only difference that the group of patients not having fibrosis is almost completely covered by the group of patients having fibrosis. The cutting Z-score, Zc, lies more close to the group of healthy patients causing many of the healthy patients fall into the group of sick by clinical definition. Discriminating cases of no or mild fibrosis from the others gave the opposite results (analysis 2, Table 3). The model classifies almost all cases as having mild or no fibrosis. The ability to detect fibrosis is too low to adjust for the overall ability to correctly diagnose 80.5% of all cases. Thus the results are not to be accepted unreservedly.

In the third analysis, Table 4, all cases with fibrosis=1 are removed to increase the spread between the different groups. Now the difference between the two groups became more obvious. The balance between correctly and incorrectly classified cased is improved and thus the percentage of correctly classified cases is more relevant than in the first two analyses.

The fourth analysis, Table 5, is identical to the third, but with the variable qcoll included. The percentage of correctly classified cases is now even better than in any of the previous analyses. Qcoll was used here barely to increase the discriminative power and to reach the classification pictured in Figure 1a, which is a sought goal of knowledge extraction in our case.

3.2 Applications of regression analysis to replace quantitative collagen

Regression analysis was applied to replace the qcoll variable by employing criteria of information gain practically expressed as changes in value of R^2.

Variables: IGG = Immunoglobulin class G, CHEN = Chenodeoxycholic acid, PREALB = Prealbumin

Model	B-coefficients	Standard deviation	Significance	Change in R^2
1) (Constant, B0)	-4.720	0.960	0.000	
IGG	0.615	0.074	0.000	–
2) (Constant, B0)	-4.586	0.858	0.000	
IGG	0.493	0.069	0.000	
CHEN	0.645	0.096	0.000	0.145
3) (Constant, B0)	-1.786	1.542	0.249	
IGG	0.431	0.073	0.000	
CHEN	0.613	0.097	0.000	
PREALB	-6.782	3.118	0.031	0.013

The result is a function describing qcoll as a function of two other variables.

Qcoll = -4.586 + 0.493 * IGG + 0.645 * CHEN

A discriminant analysis, shown in Table 6, was made to test a discriminative power of the new variable. The intention was to prove its capacity the previously used variable, qcoll. In the case that its discriminative power is too weak to add knew knowledge, it ought to be ruled out.

Table 6

Analysis 5 Qcoll replaced with the new substitute variable used. Otherwise the same premises as analysis 4.		Predicted group membership	
		Having fibrosis = 0	Having fibrosis Between 2 and 4
Real group membership	Not having fibrosis	**36**	3
	Having fibrosis	11	**26**
	Not having fibrosis (%)	**92.3%**	7.7%
	Having fibrosis (%)	29.7%	**70.3%**
	81.6% of all cases correctly diagnosed. Used variables: QCOLL-Substitute, FERRITIN, K		

4 Discussion

The use of a manufactured variable, qcoll-substitute, is here shown to be useful in improving the discrimination between studied patient groups. Since qcoll is not available in everyday treatment, formulating the substitute variable by using routine laboratory tests could be utilised in everyday diagnosing of liver diseases. From the patient's point of view, the fact that diagnosis can be established using blood tests and avoiding biopsy is a great improvement in reducing suffering. The blood tests that were found significant represent a new clinical knowledge. Procolagen III N-terminal Peptide (PIIINP) and hyaluronic acid have not proven their discriminative power which goes in line with the knowledge extracted by means of bivariate statistical analysis [3]. Therefore, a throughout analytical comparison should be conducted to figure out why these tests failed to mark fibrosis in spite of their efficiency in the field of chronic viral hepatitis C [7,8].

5 Conclusions

In the presented research we identified a set of the routine blood laboratory findings efficient to trace fibrosis in the liver. We have discussed how and why, from the methodological point of view, these findings might be taken as a sign of the disease. We have used powerful multivariate statistical methods to, firstly, open several classification layers of the laboratory tests and, secondly, to formulate a minimal laboratory set with a potential to replace quantitative collagen, which is accepted as a golden standard of the kind. We have done all this work with great respect to the detailed pathological classification of the patient material. The results of the analyses are now to be evaluated by the clinicians that had initiated our investigation in the first place.

Acknowledgements

The authors would like to thank Associate Professor G. Bodemar, MD, Ph.D., Prof. L. Franzén, MD, Ph.D., and H. Aaselious, MD, for the research initiative and encouragement to conduct here presented investigation

References

[1] Babic A, Bodemar G, Mathiesen U, Ahlfeldt H, Franzén L, Wigertz O. Machine Learning to Support Diagnostics in the Domain of Asymptomatic Liver Disease. In R.A. Greeneset al. (Eds) MEDINFO'95 Proceedings, IMIA, 8th Wrold Congress on Medical Informatics, Vancouver, Canada, pp 809-813, 1995

[2] Babic A, K Hedin, U Mathiesen, L Franzén, A Frydén, G Bodemar, O Wigertz. Decision support for monitoring of chronic hepatitis C: Can blood laboratory test help? In Proc MIE'96, Human Facets in Information Technologies. J Brender, J P Christensen, J-R Scherrer, P McNair, ed:s, IOS Press, Netherlands. pp 551- 554, 1996.

[3] Aaselius H., Bodemar G., Mathiesen U., Fryden A., Hedin K, Franzén L., Estimation of Liver Fibrosis with Image Analysis. Comparison to Knodell scores and associations to serum markers of fibrosis, Journal of Hepatology, Submitted, 1998

[4] Marshall G, Hendersson WG, Moritz TE, Et al., Statistical Methods and Strategies for Working with Large Data Bases, Medical Care, 1995, Vol. 33, Number 10, pp OS35-OS42

[5] Knodell R.G., Ishak K.G., Black W.C. et al. Formulation and application of a numerical scoring system for assessing histological activity in asymptomate chronic active hepatitis. Hepatology 1:431-435, 1981.

[6] SPSSX, Statistical Algorithms, SPSS Inc., Chicago, 1993, McGraw-Hill

[7] Guechot J, Loria A., Sarfraty L., Giral P., Giboudeau J., Poupon R., Serum hyaluronon as a marker of fibrosis in chronic viral hepatitis C: effect of alfa.interferon therapy, Journal of Hepatology, 1995;pp 22:22-6

[8] Trinchet JC, Hartman DJ, Pateron D. Et al., Serum type I collagen and N-terminal peptide of type III procollagen in chronic hepaptis C. Relations to liver histology and conventional liver tests. Jorunal of Hepatology, 1991, pp 17:390-6

[9] Verbaan H., Bondenson L., Eriksson S., Non-invasive assessment of inflammatory activity and fibrosis (grade and stage) in chronic hepatitis C infection, Scand J Gastronetrol, 1997:11:pp 447-55

Medical Informatics Europe '99
P. Kokol et al. (Eds.)
IOS Press, 1999

A Development Protocol for a Diagnostic DSS

Ying-Lie O[1], W.J.P.P. ter Burg, E.W.M.T. ter Braak, J.P. Neijt
University Medical Centre, Utrecht, The Netherlands

W.A.J.J. Wiegerinck, M.J. Nijman, H.J. Kappen
Stichting Neurale Netwerken, University of Nijmegen, The Netherlands

Abstract. A diagnostic decision support system (DSS) in medicine is an expert system that aids the physician in the determination of the diagnosis based on findings and test results. The DSS can be divided into 2 different types of components: the knowledge component and the information system component. Methods from software engineering, knowledge engineering and management are combined into a dynamic development cycle that allows stepwise update and refinement. The development of the knowledge component is based on knowledge engineering. In the starting phases, rapid prototyping is convenient to determine and evaluate the specification. The content of the knowledge base is frequently updated during its life time. For this purpose, a knowledge modelling protocol is supplied.

1. Introduction

A diagnostic decision support system (DSS) in medicine is an expert system that aids the physician in the determination of the diagnosis based on findings and test results. An expert system consists of a knowledge base and an inference engine [5]. The domain knowledge is stored in the knowledge base according to a *probabilistic network* that is built of nodes and links between related nodes. The nodes represent variables that are relevant in the chosen medical domain such as diagnoses, tests, underlying pathofysiological causes, and other findings. The directed link between nodes represent the causal relation and a conditional probability. For each node, information about the node and references to literature are stored, thus supplying relevant information [7]. It is also beneficial for collection and dissemination of knowledge, thus contributing to one of the desirable improvements in health information systems [6].

The DSS contains domain knowledge, decision support functionality, and a user interface that is comparable to that of information systems. Decision is based on domain knowledge and patient data. The utilisation using an integrated workstation [1] is therefore desirable. Most of the functionality of the workstation are provided by the information system (IS) that contains patient data. Generally, the DSS is developed separately from the IS. Also, the DSS is generally extended with additional medical domains during its life-time. To assure consistency, a development procedure and a knowledge modelling protocol is composed.

---

[1] Julius Centre for Health Sciences, Email: y.o@jc.azu.nl

2. The development protocol

Knowledge engineering and management [8,9] comprises modelling of processes for knowledge representation and inference algorithms, including evaluation [10, 2].

Software engineering is a discipline that provides methods to produce good software with quality assurance. The utilisation of a development cycle and established standards is of common practice. Methods from software engineering, knowledge engineering, and knowledge management are combined into a *dynamic development cycle* that allows stepwise refinement. The DSS is divided into 2 different types of components: the *knowledge component* and the *information system component*.

Table 1: The dynamic development cycle

knowledge component		**IS component**
	0. preliminary exploration	
0.1 identification		
domain, main parameters		
0.2 modelling and evaluation	early prototype	
structure of model		
	1. initial specification	
1.1 identification		1.1 identification
(sub)domains, parameters		user requirements
1.2 modelling and evaluation	initial prototype	
knowledge model test and case validation		
	2. framework design	
2.1 modular design		2.1 component-based design
knowledge base inference engine		application functions database
2.2 methods & techniques		2.2 methods & techniques
knowledge engineering		software engineering
	3. functional model iteration	
3.1 identification		3.1 identification
(sub)domain, parameters decision support		functionality, user interface data
3.2 modelling		3.2 modelling
qualitative model information on model quantitative: educated guess		application functions user interface information model
3.3 evaluation	“good”, rapid prototype	3.3 evaluation
verification and validation test and case validation		functionality user interface
	4. design and build iteration	
4.1 identification		4.1 identification
refinement		refinement
4.2 modelling		4.2 modelling
qualitative model quantitative: evidence		application, help function data(base) model
4.3 evaluation	“good” prototype	4.3 evaluation
verification and validation case (cross-)validation		integration, flow control functionality
	5. implementation iteration	
…	pilot sites	…
5.3 evaluation		5.3 evaluation
real case validation		usability

The main development life-cycle is based on DSDM [4]. In the iterations, prototyping is used to demonstrate the functionality and to evaluate intermediate results. "Good" prototypes are intended to evolve to the final product.

The development of the knowledge component is based on knowledge engineering. Activities on knowledge identification, modelling, and evaluation are guided by the *knowledge modelling protocol*.

Table 2: The knowledge modelling protocol

1. Identification	
Knowledge sources	Summary of knowledge sources: books, papers, experts, common practice.
Domains and subdomains	Classification and choice of the domain and sub-domains for instance based on diagnoses according to a classification system.
Parameter types	Determination of the type of parameters the knowledge model, possible extension, and further refinement.
2. Modelling	
Knowledge elicitation	Elicitation of knowledge from sources on the domain, standard taxonomy and concepts.
Qualitative model	Design of the qualitative knowledge model: the nodes and causal relations by links.
Information	Information and references on the nodes.
Quantitative model	Design of the quantitative model: the conditional probabilities, either based on references, evidence, or "educated" guess, and the inference algorithm.
3. Evaluation	
Model verification	Verification of the links for "false" relations.
Model validation	Validation of the qualitative knowledge model: nodes and links.
Test validation	Validation using (composed) test cases, for instance by "leave one out" strategy.
Case validation	Validation using "standard cases", and cross-validation.

3. Case example: a pathofysiological model of anaemia

A detailed description of the modelling is presented in a separate paper [3]. Here only the remarks in relation with several parts of the development cycle are presented.

Table 3: Part of the development cycle of a pathofysiological model of anaemia

knowledge component	IS component
1. initial specification	
1.1 identification (sub)domains: according to classification of diagnoses and a research database parameters: laboratory tests, additional findings data: patient data with anaemia from the HIS	1.1 identification user interface: list of parameters and results
1.2 modelling and evaluation knowledge model: neural net test validation: leave one out using cases in the research database; using patient data with and without additional rules; statistical analysis of patient data case validation: prototype is compared to experts and users using cases in the research database	
initial prototype for cases in research database show good evaluation results initial prototype for patient data show better evaluation results using additional rules statistical analysis of patient data show missing values, thus inappropriate as cases	
decision based on evaluation knowledge model: probabilistic network, parameters: pathofysiological and tests	
2. framework design	
2.1 modular design knowledge base: divided into (sub)domains inference engine: able to handle (sub)domains	2.1 component-based design application functions: as a 4GL-based IS database: possible connection to the HIS

knowledge component	IS component
2.2 methods & techniques flexible modelling tool that allows evaluation	2.2 methods & techniques must run on a stand-alone PC platform
3. functional model iteration	
3.1 identification (sub)domains: according to classification of diagnoses and pathofysiological model parameters: tests, findings, pathofysiological decision support: list of probable diagnoses, list of tests to confirm a diagnosis	3.1 identification functionality: mainly decision support, presentation and input/output of parameters, and modelling user interface: user friendly data: input data, decision support results
3.2 modelling qualitative model: elicited from textbooks and references information on model: for important nodes quantitative: mainly educated guesses	3.2 modelling application functions: modelling, and use user interface: large lists of information information model
3.3 evaluation verification and validation: using the modelling tool test and case validation: using assembled cases	3.3 evaluation functionality, user interface: using rapid prototype and good prototype
rapid prototype: to demonstrate the user interface good prototype: initially for the evaluation of the knowledge component, gradually modelling functions and IS functionality are added	

4. Conclusion

The development of a complex and ever growing DSS requires adequate life-cycle management and supporting protocols. Verification and validation is an important part that is integrated in the development cycle. The importance is illustrated by the case example, in which a rather drastic decision to change the knowledge model has been made. The proposed development cycle and knowledge modelling protocol provide a convenient and structured method. Unfortunately, such a development environment is currently not available.

References

[1] B. Brigl, P. Ringleb, T. Steiner, P. Knaup, W. Hacke, and R. Haux. An integrated approach for a knowledge-based clinical workstation: architecture and experience. Meth. Inf. Med., 37:16-25, 1998.

[2] B. Buchanan et al. Evaluation of Knowledge-based Systems. US National Library of Medicine, (USA), 1995.

[3] W.J.P.P. ter Burg, P.J.F. Lucas, E.W.M.T. ter Braak. A diagnostic advisory system based on pathofysiological models of disease, this conf, 1999.

[4] Dynamic system development method. DSDM Server, www.dsdm.org, 1997.

[5] P.J.F. Lucas and L.C. van der Gaag. Principles of Expert Systems. Addison-Wesley, 1991.

[6] J.R. Moehr. Informatics in the service of health, a look to the future. Meth. Inf. Med., 37:165-170, 1998.

[7] J.A. Muir Gray. Where is the chief knowledge officer? British Medical J., 317:832-840, 1998.

[8] A.Th. Schreiber, H. Akkermans, A.A. Anjewierden, R. de Hoog, N.R. Hadbolt, W. van de Velde, and B.J. Wielinga. Knowledge Engineering and Management. The CommonKADS Methodology. MIT Press, 1999.

[9] R. Studer, V.R. Benjamins, and D. Fensel. Knowledge engineering: Principles and methods. Data and Knowledge Engineering, 25(1-2):161-197, 1998.

[10] J. Wyatt and D. Spiegelhalter. Evaluating medical expert systems: what to test and how ? Med. Informatics, 15:205--217, 1990.

Medical Informatics Europe '99
P. Kokol et al. (Eds.)
IOS Press, 1999

A protocol building software tool for medical device Quality Control tests

Y. Theodorakos, K. Gueorguieva, J. Bliznakov, Z. Kolitsi and N. Pallikarakis
University of Patras, School of Medicine, Department of Medical Physics Laboratory, 26500 Patras, Greece

Abstract. Q-Pro is an application for Quality Control and Inspection of Medical Devices. General system requirements include friendly and comprehensive graphical environment and proper, quick, easy and intuitive user interface. Functions such as, a tool library for protocol design widely used multimedia, as well as, a support of a local database for protocol and inventory data archiving are provided by the system. In order to serve the different categories of users, involved in Quality Control procedures, the system has been split into three modules of different functionality and complexity, each of which can work as a stand–alone application. The implementation of protocols and use of the software functions, as well as, the user interface itself have been proved by the evaluators to be clear and intuitive. The software seems to adapt easily to different kinds of Quality Control procedures and objectives. Q-Pro effectively supports and enhances the processes to attain a highly tuned, professional, responsive and effective quality control and preventive maintenance procedures for biomedical equipment management.

1. Introduction

Health care is a complex environment consisting of a multitude of continuously running procedures, that share a wide range of data and engage an extended variety of professionals of diverse expertise. Recent technological advancements have improved considerably the efficiency and the efficacy of the medical procedures and the management strategies in health care. This improvement has introduced complex and sophisticated technologies, increasing thus the demands on the users and shifting the focus for quality improvement to a safe and efficient use of this technology [1].

Quality Control data provides information about the functional condition of equipment. Traceability of performance of equipment is necessary for regulatory and legal purposes. Data compiled over a period of time also contains valuable information for predicting anticipating failures, needs for replacement etc., of much value to the administration of the clinical engineering department and the hospital.

Quality Control (QC) in the hospitals is always performed on the basis of protocols, by authorized personnel and at scheduled intervals. The complexity of the procedures to be carried out may vary from very simple recording on a checklist, to complex experimentation. Similarly, the persons carrying out QC may be experienced engineers that routinely perform the relevant tasks, or less experienced staff that needs increased guidance and support to carry out the job [2, 3].

Q-Pro is an application that has been designed to provide the necessary flexibility to accommodate the different degrees of difficulty and specialization in carrying out the Quality Control sessions and to store all necessary information to meet the above requirements.

2. System Description

Q-Pro is an application for QC and Inspection of Medical Devices. QC sessions are performed periodically, on a planned basis, using specific measuring instruments and phantoms. Their outcome is a set of data, reflecting the functional status of equipment. Evaluation of this data, leads to decisions on the suitability of equipment for further use and may initiate other actions (e.g. repair).
General system requirements include friendly and comprehensive graphical environment and proper, quick, easy and intuitive user interface. A tool library containing the most commonly used tools for protocol design, widely used multimedia features available at any time and a support of a local database for protocol and inventory data archiving, tests scheduling, daily plans and data records have been implemented.
The different categories of users, implicated in the QC procedure, impose a functional differentiation of the application. For that reason the system is designed of three modules of different functionality and complexity, each one possessing the property to work as a stand–alone application as well as to have good and coherent interactive connection with the rest of the modules.

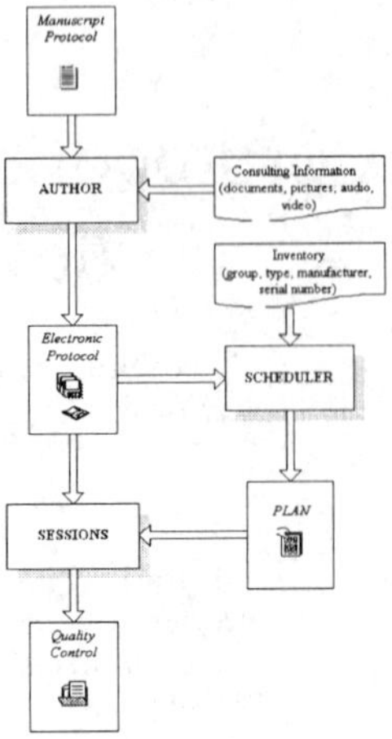

Figure 1. *Q-Pro modules relation.*

The first module, the AUTHOR, is used to create new or edit existing protocols. The second one, the SCHEDULER, provides the basic functionality for establishing the QC programme in the clinical engineering departments. The third module, the SESSIONS, is used to perform the sessions, record data and make analysis. Schematically, the interaction of the three modules is shown on Figure 1. Multimedia presentations are essential key components of the system, presenting full descriptions of the relevant quality procedures and the respective quality measures.

2.1. The AUTHOR module

The functionality of the Author module encompasses the process of creation of a protocol and the customization of existing ones. The protocol development approach is facilitated by means of a number of functions for defining sub-processes and activities (infoelements). Each infoelement is linked with supporting information and is associated with a number of further infoelements that originate from it.
The protocols can be represented by trees, flowcharts or both. This is simply a different way of protocol presentation, a choice decision made by the author himself.
The tree mode is built by breaking down a protocol in logical groups of tests and procedures (mechanical tests, safety tests, image quality tests, calibrations, etc.). The main process is then broken into a number of sub-processes and for each of them the necessary attributes and supporting information is provided. As many levels as necessary may be used. Process trees are easy to navigate, in order to arrive at the neighborhood of any group of tests with measurements that share the same principles (equipment, frequency etc).

Often, it is easier to follow a written document and describe procedures in a serial manner, as they take place in a time sequence, rather than try to create logical sets of measurements or tests leading to the creation of a flowchart. It is also here possible to analyze any sub-process into another flowchart sheet and repeat this to any required depth. This multi sheet property allows a good arrangement of the designed protocol. Flowcharts constitute valuable guidance for the execution of the QC sessions. They also provide the possibility to indicate decisions, not possible with trees.

When the flow analysis is completed all sub-processes and activities can be exported into a tree and sorted into groups, in order to assign to them the measurement parameters. The export carries also the information contained in each sub-process or activity.

For protocol customization, a procedure that facilitates the easy and quick protocol reusability has been created. The user may copy any part of an already existing protocol - along with all information related to it - and place it in an arbitrary place in his own protocol.

The process documentation is supported by means of multimedia presentation of the infoelements. Individual processes can be described by text, images and recorded audio passages or short video sequences. For this purpose the system interacts with broadly available and commonly used software, to provide aids and guidance to those that will carry out the sessions. Moreover, flags to draw the attention to particular items may be also created as 'tips', in any one of the infoelements' boxes.

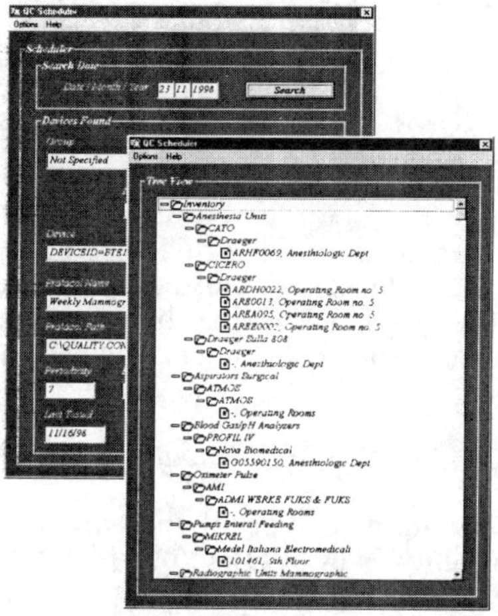

Figure 3. An example of medical equipment inventory is being browsed using the tree-view technique. Date search provides all the information, needed to perform the daily QC sessions

The Author module possesses its own graphical environment for flowchart and tree designing. The design of the Author module includes four parts: worksheet, tool library, properties window and navigation tree. The design area is comprised of a set of worksheets, where the protocol is described. The protocol is realized with the help of the tool library, containing a complete set of tools for the two different modes. Using simple drag and drop of the objects from the tool library window, the author composes easily and quickly the outline of the protocol. The details in the form of links to information (images, text, video, audio) and graphical aesthetics are handled by the properties window. For the case of constructing a quality indicator (measurement), the properties window includes the additional required information (measurement units, upper and lower limits).

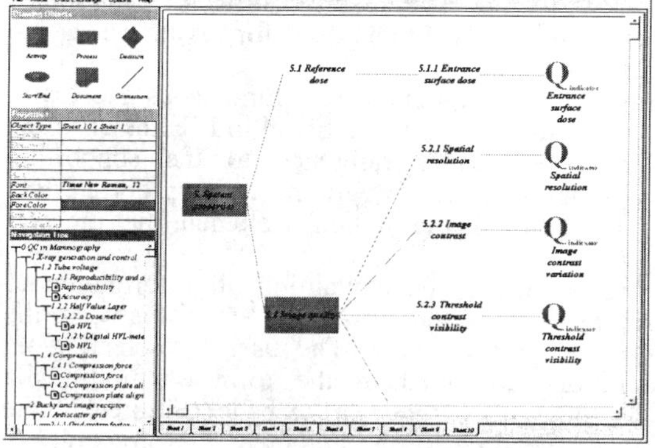

Figure 2. Design AUTHOR module overview. Tool library and object properties windows are displayed on the top left. Expanding the process tree in different working sheets provides better rearrangement. The navigation tree on the down left assures the easy navigation between them.

The navigation tree plays the role of a compass for the protocol creator, displaying the whole map of the process tree being created. It is two-way selectable meaning that a selection of a branch will highlight the corresponding object in the working area (worksheet) and vice-versa.

2.2. The SCHEDULER module

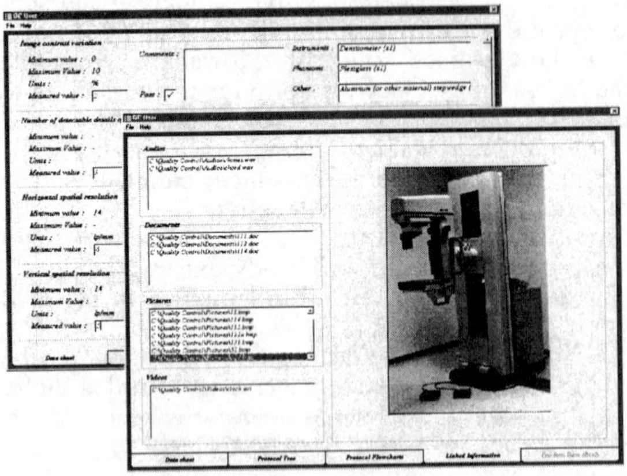

Figure 4. SESSIONS module overview. While performing the measurement procedure the user has available the necessary instruments and all the information related to the specific process.

The process of Quality Control in the hospitals is accomplished by authorized personnel at pre-scheduled intervals. The SCHEDULER is the connection between the AUTHOR and SESSIONS modules. It provides the basic functionality for creating an inventory of equipment undergoing inspection, systematic QC or preventive maintenance, but moreover it can import an external inventory from specific inventory software (e.g. Medical Equipment Management System - MEMS). Its main task is to link a created protocol with a given equipment item and create schedules, daily job lists and human resource assignments for the QC sessions.
Taking into account that the functionality of the SCHEDULER is mainly related to data manipulation, an inventory database has been created.
The SCHEDULER has been designed as a comprehensive application of one main window, dynamically changing its contents, according to the functions carried out (Figure 3).

2.3. The SESSIONS module

The third module of the software package, the SESSIONS, is addresses to the actual Quality Control tests to be performed. The SESSIONS module supports the process of the QC data report generation, providing information for the functional and technical condition of the biomedical equipment subjected to the tests. The results of the measurements accomplished and the data itself are included in a final report used for taking decisions, concerning its working condition and its reliability.
An easy task would simply involve recording of data and entering comments as necessary. In the end, a report on the session is generated, in order to be archived in MEMS or in the department's files. More complex tasks may require reference to the supporting information, which may then be done by bringing to the foreground the appropriate tab. Tabs are always updated with information available for the particular element that the user is working on (i.e., subprocess or quality indicator).
The SESSIONS module is organized in five tab sheets, containing all information to perform a given test. The protocols presented as trees and flowcharts are available in the panels *Protocol Tree* and *Protocol Flowchart,* respectively. The user by selecting an infoelement receives all relevant information, displayed in the form of multimedia (documents, pictures, audio or videos) on the *Linked Information* panel (Figure 4). The *Data Sheet* panel allocates the measurements specified by the author of the protocol and subjected to tests. Each measurement field consists of a measured value, its upper and lower limit, a flag indicating its success, comments marked by the person accomplishing the tests and information on the instruments and the materials needed to perform the test. The success of the test is automatically indicated based on the limits but it can be overridden by the user. The results of the tests are saved in a local database. All the tests performed on the device are available in the *Previous Data Sheets* panel of the application. Automatic acquisition of a measured value is accomplished by using special devices designed for performing specific tests.

3. Implementation of the system

The application was developed for Microsoft Windows (all versions) and its computer system requirements are minimal. Microsoft Visual Basic 5.0, which offers the latest achievements of object-oriented programming and a wide variety of graphical user-interface tools was chosen as the programming language. The databases of the software were developed in Microsoft Access 7.0.

4. Evaluation

The Q-Pro has been integrated in the BEAM II project and was evaluated in the clinical engineering departments of 8 European countries. Q-Pro was assessed by clinical engineers in Portugal (INSA-LEMES), Italy (ITAL-TBS) and Greece (PSP) in September 1998 for a period of two weeks.
The implementation of protocols and utilization of the software functions was found by all evaluators to be clear and intuitive. The user interface was judged to be friendly and easy to learn. The software seems to adapt easily to different kinds of Quality Control procedures and objectives (specific or general, done by a hospital or a central organization). The recommendations received concern the possibility to export the measured values of the history for statistical manipulation with external software and the generation of reports with a user defined layout.
Plans for the future development of the program also include the implementation of a new customized mode for editing protocols, that will combine the tree and flowchart mode, support of graphical tools for data presentation (e.g. pie, graphs etc.) and different types of measurements units (not only numerical ones).

5. Conclusions

The Q-Pro application is used to get the list of jobs, open the data files, obtain print outs of the data collection forms and input data post priori. It gives logical, easy and intuitively to use tools, which support and enhance the efforts to attain a highly tuned, professional, responsive and effective quality control and preventive maintenance in the clinical engineering departments. The Q-Pro includes specific modules providing different facilities for creating protocols, proper scheduling and quality control implementation and functions for quality control and preventive maintenance. It provides better utilization of the staff needed for preparing a protocol, as well as the less time consuming and more efficient communication with other clinical departments.

References

[1] Kolitsi Z., Griva V. and Pallikarakis N., *Computer assisted process management for health care: the IBIS tool.* Med. Inform. 1997; 22/3: 215-225

[2] Griva V., Kolitsi Z., Panayiotakis G. and Pallikarakis N. *The use of an Interactive browser for documentation of quality control in mammography.* In proceedings: Roentgen Gedaechtmis Kongress, Wurzburg, Germany, 1995

[3] Gikas Panousis S., Malataras P., Patelodimou C., Kolitsi Z., Pallikarakis N., *Development of a new Clinical Engineering Management Tool & Information System (CLE-MANTIS),* Journal of Clinical Engineering, 22(5):342-349, 1997

Medical Informatics Europe '99
P. Kokol et al. (Eds.)
IOS Press, 1999

Telematics applications to support the role of the community pharmacists as self-medication advisors

Ferran SANZ[1], Claudio SILVEIRA[1], Albert ALONSO[1], Carles DIAZ[1], Maria Isabel LOZA[2], Luis CORDERO[2], Fernando FERNANDEZ-LLIMÓS[2], Lisette TIDDENS[3], Flora GIORGIO[3], Hubertus CRANZ[4], Jasmina MIRCHEVA[4] and the TESEMED Consortium[‡]
[1]*R.G. on Medical Informatics, IMIM/UPF, Dr. Aiguader 80, E-08003 Barcelona (Spain)*
[2]*Dep. of Pharmacology, University of Santiago de Compostela (Spain)*
[3]*Pharmaceutical Group of the European Union, Brussels (Belgium)*
[4]*Association of the European Self-Medication Industry (AESGP), Brussels (Belgium)*

Abstract. One of the applications developed within the EU-funded projects TESEMED and TESEMED-II is a program for the information and continuous training of community pharmacists, with the aim to empower them as advisors of the citizens about self-medication topics. Several programs are being developed on the basis of ad-hoc developed protocols about minor ailments (currently, cold and flu, haemorrhoids, constipation and cough). Each program includes three modules: a hypertextual version of the protocol, an interactive scheme of it, and an educational tool called Encounter Simulator, that trains the pharmacist about the protocol by means of simulated pharmacist-customer interactions. The testing of these applications with 84 community pharmacists offers positive results in terms of expectations, program characteristics and perceived usefulness.

The current trends towards self-medication should be accompanied by the strengthening of information measures [1]. As stated by a document adopted by the European Commission [2], community pharmacies have a key role to play in providing assistance, information and advise to the public about self-medication products and the circumstances in which a doctor should be consulted. There are more than 115,000 in the European Union and consequently they are easily accessible to the citizens. To help the pharmacies to play the mentioned role, they require specially tailored information means. The distribution of this information could benefit from electronic means. This possibility

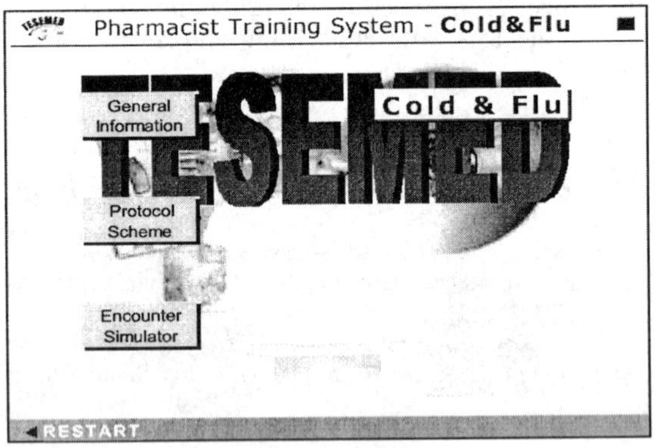

Fig. 1. Main menu of the TESEMED application for information and continuous training of community pharmacists.

‡ In addition to the mentioned institutions, the TESEMED Consortium is also constituted by Arakne Srl and EMA Group.

seems especially appropriate because community pharmacies are geographically disperse and the information on medicines needs to be permanently updated.

TESEMED and TESEMED-II are research projects funded by the European Commission (TAP HC1114 and TAP HC4022). Their objectives are the development, testing and implementation of telematics applications in the European community pharmacies in order to disseminate information and education about the correct management of minor ailments that could be treated with OTC medicines.

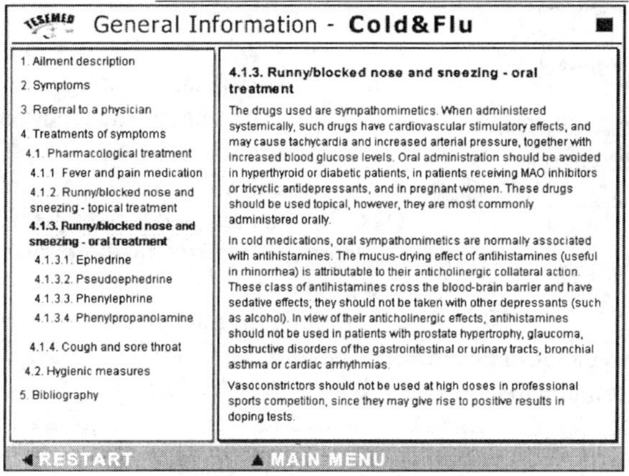

Fig. 2. Hypertext describing an ailment, its symptoms, the circumstances that require the referral to a physician and the relevant treatments.

One of the applications developed within the TESEMED projects is a program for the information and continuous training of community pharmacists, in order to empower them as advisors of the citizens about self-medication topics. Several applications are being developed on the basis of ad-hoc developed protocols about minor ailments (currently, cold and flu, haemorrhoids, constipation and cough). Each application includes three modules (Fig. 1). The first one is a hypertextual description of the considered ailment and its symptoms, the circumstances that require referral to a physician, the relevant treatments and a selection of bibliographic references (Fig. 2). The second module of the application is an interactive scheme that summarises the issues that have to be examined during the pharmacist-customer interaction, as well as the appropriate order to make them. Such questions aim at the collection of the following information: 1) Age of the patient, 2) Symptoms and their duration, 3) Chronic diseases and medications, and 4) Special situations like pregnancy (Fig. 3). Finally, the third module of the application is an educational tool called Encounter Simulator, that trains the pharmacist about the above mentioned questions and their relevant order, as well as about the advice to be given in each particular situation.

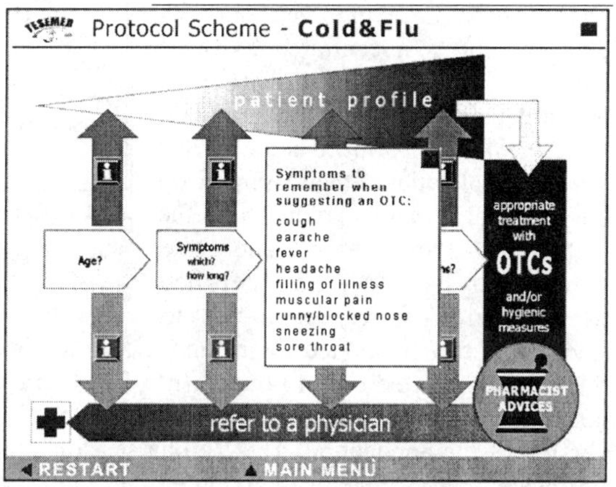

Fig. 3. Protocol scheme showing the questions that should be asked and their appropriate order. The reminders that can be visualised by clicking in the buttons are also shown.

The Encounter Simulator is the most innovative part of the TESEMED application for community pharmacists and it has the following characteristics:

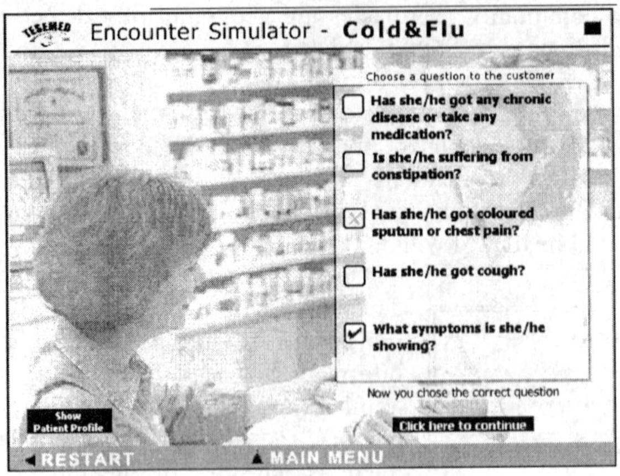

Fig. 4. A sample screen of the Encounter Simulator.

- It is based in dialogues between the pharmacist and automatically generated citizens.
- The pharmacist is asked to choose questions or advises from menus that are offered step-by-step (Fig. 4)
- Menus change at each simulation.
- Answers to the right questions change with each simulation.
- Subsequent menus depend on the previous answers.
- The possible final advises are OTC medicines and/or hygienic measures, or referral of the patient to a physician.
- If the appropriate final advice is the use of OTC medicines and/or hygienic measures, the pharmacist is invited to select the ones that are relevant for the automatically generated patient profile (Fig. 5).

The TESEMED application for pharmacists runs in personal computers with Pentium processor and Windows 95 (or higher) and is disseminated, downloaded and updated through the TESEMED Web site (http://www.imim.es/tesemed).

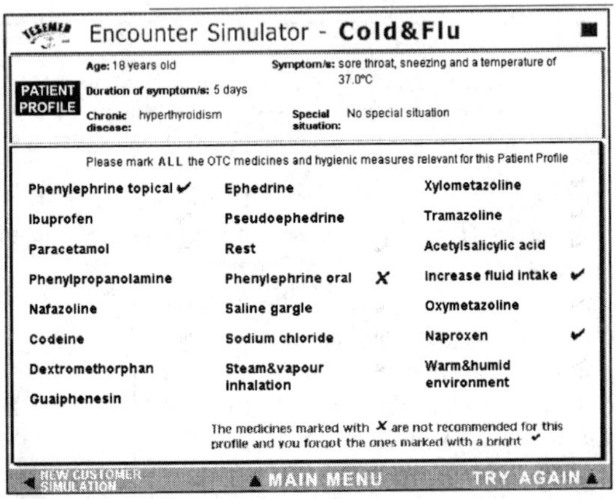

Fig. 5. Encounter Simulator facility to remind the relevant treatment for a particular patient profile.

The testing of the application by pharmacists not involved in its development is a central activity of the TESEMED projects. The main investigated topics are: the general opinion of the pharmacists about this kind of applications, their opinion on the structure and layout of the TESEMED application and the opinion on its usefulness. Ad hoc questionnaires were developed to investigate the mentioned topics and they have been administered after demo sessions of the program carried out in London (n = 14 pharmacists), Almeria (n = 31), Barcelona (n = 23) and Verona (n = 16). The three first demo sessions were carried out using the initial version of the application. The Verona session was carried out using an improved version of the application developed taking into account the answers to the questionnaires collected in the previous sessions. The 84 interviewed pharmacists had an age mean of 41.2 years (SD = 11.6 years) and a balanced gender distribution (34 men, 48 women, 2 not recorded).

One of the items of the questionnaire asks about the opinion on the use of Internet for the information and continuous training of community pharmacists. It uses a scale with scores from a 0 (worst opinion) to 10 (best opinion). The answers to this question were very high: 8.5 ± 1.5 (mean ± SD).

On the other hand, six items of the questionnaire investigate the opinions about the application for pharmacists developed within the TESEMED project. These items use scales ranging from 1 (worst opinion) to 5 (best opinion). These items and a statistical summary of their answers are shown in Table 1.

Table 1. TESEMED application testing results

Investigated issue	mean±SD (n) (initial version)	mean±SD (n) (improved version)
Overall opinion on the TESEMED application	3.60±0.68 (67)	4.50±0.63 (16)
General structure of the program: description, protocol scheme and encounter simulator	3.79±0.69 (66)	4.50±0.73 (16)
Style/appearance of the ailment description	3.31±0.76 (62)	4.44±0.63 (16)
Layout of the protocol scheme	3.42±0.72 (66)	4.19±0.66 (16)
Structure of the simulator	3.33±0.71 (66)	4.06±0.85 (16)
Appearance of the simulator	3.31±0.87 (64)	4.44±0.63 (16)

It has to be noted that all the means shown in table 1 are above 3 (the neutral opinion), and they clearly reflect the improvements introduced before the Verona session. The changes in such means from the initial to the improved versions are statistically significant in all the items ($p \leq 0.003$). These comparisons were carried out by means of non-parametric Mann-Whitney tests.

Finally, it has to pointed out that a high percent (81%) of the respondents answered “probably” or “for sure” to the question: "Do you think that a program like this would improve your knowledge and skills in treating the minor ailment covered?".

All the above mentioned positive results envisage a high users' acceptance of the TESEMED applications for community pharmacists.

References

[1] Bond CM, Bradley C. The interface between the community pharmacist and patients. *BMJ* 1996; 312: 758-760.
[2] Communication from the European Commission adopted on 1 June 1994

Medical Informatics Europe '99
P. Kokol et al. (Eds.)
IOS Press, 1999

The "Mediator Service", a component to ease the integration of medical applications in the SynEx framework

Yigang Xu, Dominique Sauquet,
Eric Zapletal, David Lemaitre, Patrice Degoulet
Medical Informatics Department, Broussais University Hospital,
96 Rue Didot, 75014 Paris, France
Tel: (+33) 1 43 95 91 66; Fax: (+33) 1 43 95 92 09
e-mail: xu@hbroussais.fr, sauquet@hbroussais.fr

Abstract: Interoperability is a key issue and a long-term domain of research for distributed healthcare information systems. The European project SynEx provides an open and standard integration platform for both new and legacy medical applications. It allows the collaboration of distributed and heterogeneous healthcare records and services. It aims to provide access to Hospital Information Services, to remote sources of medical data and to medical knowledge, in a seamless way, hiding the distribution aspects and the heterogeneity of systems.

In this project, the Medical Informatics Department of the Broussais University Hospital is responsible for the development of the "Mediator Service". It is a software component of the SynEx platform which is used as a "glue" mechanism to provide a flexible way to facilitate the interchange between any pair of systems, with different nomenclatures and data structures.

The Mediator Service uses a generic model of mediators to create, through specialisation, specific mediators for practical cases. Based on this model, it offers a C++ library to be used as the tool case by the programmers, to reduce the development effort. The use of XML as a powerful data interchange format and as a data structure descriptor is proposed and evaluated.

Keywords: Integration Platform, Distributed Information Systems, Interoperability, Semantic Heterogeneity, Middleware, Mediator, Mapping, XML.

1 Introduction

In the today's medical informatics domain, numbers of different medical information systems have been developed in different places with different technologies. To improve the patients' healthcare, the co-operation among different medical information applications is required. These applications need to connect to an increasing number of information resources, which are hosted by different data management systems on different sites, and need to exchange and share those resources. Rather than the heavy and complex re-developments, the integration of such systems into an open architecture is proposed. This architecture provides the end-users with the ability to access the required information transparently whatever its nature or localisation. Quite a lot of projects have aimed to build this kind of architecture, such as HELIOS [[1]], HERMES [[2]], TeleMed, HANSA or TSIMMIS [[3]]. The SynEx project intends to bring a standard and flexible way to build an integration platform with several application components which integrates different legacy medical systems, federates electronic healthcare records and provides services.

However, integrating distributed legacy applications is always a challenge. These applications, which either manage data or knowledge, are developed in different places and with different technologies. They can rely on file systems, databases, object stores, electronic mail systems... Some are only close applications without API (Application Programming Interface) or implement a legacy API. They use multiple operating systems, different types of inter-process communication mechanisms or different communication protocols [[4]]. Different paradigms of exchange co-exist: one represented by the family of Objects Brokers, such as CORBA, coming from the RPC technology, another one where the exchange is achieved through messages with a possible set of standards (e.g. HL7, ASN.1, ASTM, DICOM, UN/EDIFACT, etc.).

Moreover, the information used by these distributed systems are represented differently:

- They can be non coded or coded in different ways (e.g. The "sex" can be coded in one system as "Male-1" and "Female-2" but in another system as "Male-M" and "Female-F").
- They might be represented by different data structures and with different granularities.
- They can reference different dictionaries. Multiple nomenclatures or classifications coexist in Health Information Systems (e.g. ICD9-CM, ICD10, Mesh, SNOMED International, UMLS, etc.) and none of these classifications is able to capture all the concepts in a living health institution [[5]].

These problems concerning syntactic, structural and semantic mismatches must be managed in a flexible and extensible manner. It is why, to ease the construction of an integration platform, a mechanism which manages the various connections and exchanges of information, taking heterogeneity into account, is greatly required.

Wiederhold has proposed a mediator approach years ago [[6]] and in the TSIMMIS project [[3]] both "Wrapper" and "Mediator" are used. Several other approaches are based on a "meta-model", such as the "Medical Connection Services" [[7], [8]] of the HELIOS project. In the SynEx integration platform, "mediators" are proposed to be the communication mechanism to manage various connections and exchanges of information. The "Mediator Service" is an application component which facilitates the creations of such mediators. This component must take into account the syntactic and semantic aspects to ensure that the exchange is not only possible but also meaningful.

This paper will introduce first the context of our work on the Mediator Service and, after a summary of our development strategy, will detail the modelling, the implementation and the current results. It will then present how the emerging XML technology [[9]] has been applied to enhance the flexibility and the genericity of the Mediator Service. At the end of this paper, the semantic aspects will be discussed as well as several necessary improvements.

2 Background and issues

Both in hospitals and in primary care, healthcare information is electronically collected within distributed sites on heterogeneous systems[[7]]. Then, there is a great need to provide the physician a federated and shared view of the distributed health records. The lack of open systems is the main obstacle.

SynEx addresses issues inherent to multimedia patient records distributed across large enterprise-wide networks. It brings together the knowledge and use of appropriate technologies from GALEN (terminology server) [[10], [11]], I4C (integrated platform for cardiology), the Synapses Federated Healthcare Record server or FHCR [[12]], and TeleNurse for nursing care. It is conformant to the CEN/TC 251 European pre-standards prENV12967-1 or HISA (Healthcare Information System Architecture) and to prENV 12265 or Healthcare Record Architecture. The basic SynEx integration platform relies on the DHE (Distributed Healthcare Environment) [[13]], a middleware implementation of HISA. Complex services, such as the FHCR module or the Mediator Service, complements this platform. Finally, SynEx aims to provide access to Hospital Information Services, to remote sources of medical data and to medical knowledge, in a seamless way, hiding the distribution aspects and the heterogeneity of systems.

To bring the interoperability among all the components and medical information systems, the SynEx integration platform implies great needs for communication services [[14]]. In this context, we propose to specify, design and implement a component, the "Mediator Service Component", to facilitate the implementation of the connection mechanisms, to reduce development time and to foster re-use.

3 The Mediator Service

3.1 *Strategy*

Mediators can be used as the "glue" to integrate the various legacy systems and to hide their heterogeneity. For a federating model such as the SynEx FHCR server, mediators allow to integrate into it new data sources without knowing in advance their APIs. The main functions of a mediator to be used between 2 systems (a Source and a Target) are:

- to receive "any kind" of information (messages, objects, etc...) from a *Source* system;
- to filter the information, keeping only what is useful for the *Target* system;
- to send the filtered and adapted information to the *Target* system by using the communication API of the latter.

The Mediator Service Component is a software component that facilitates the development process of such "glue". It is designed to act in a flexible and extensible way in order to manage the interchange between any pair of systems (a *Source* and a *Target*) such as legacy systems, application components, client systems, ... It provides:

- a generic model of mediator that can be specialised, thanks to the Object Oriented paradigm, to create specific mediators for practical cases;
- a set of implementation tools provided as a C++ library;
- several ready-to-use specialisations for well defined use cases to simplify the development process (ODBC specialisation, XML specialisation, ...).

3.2 *Design*

The communication between two systems or applications is modelled in Figure 1 :

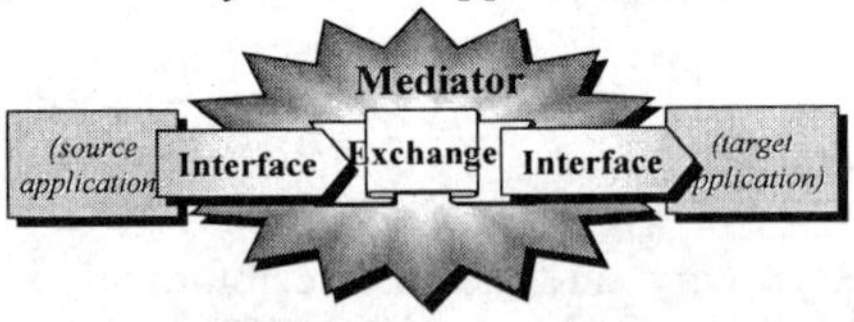

Figure 1 The general model of exchange between two systems

The *Mediator* gets information from a *Source Application* by the means of *a (Source) Interface*, models it as an *Exchange*, passes it to a *Target Application* by the means of a *(Target) Interface*. This model can be applied to different application contexts. The main task of a programmer is to develop the two interfaces: *Source Interface* and *Target Interface*. The development of an interface is done by specialising the abstract class ApplicationInterface of the C++ library of the Mediator Service. The object oriented approach allows this model to be generic and easily extended.

3.3 Implementation

Inside a mediator

From an implementation point of view, the generic model of mediators can be translated into
the following scheme (Figure 2) which shows the different modules of a mediator:

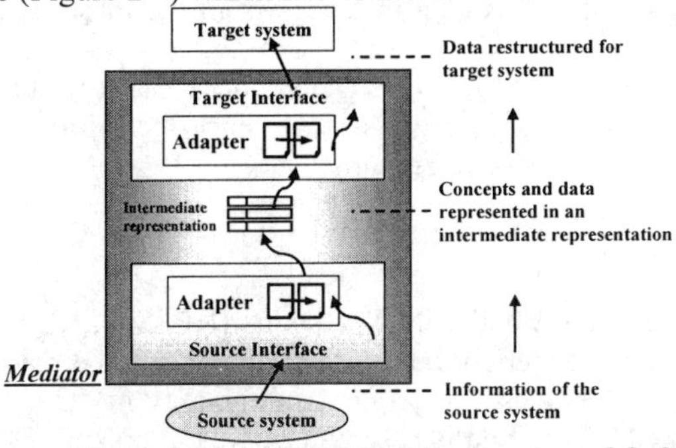

Figure 2 The implementation view of the generic model of the mediator

The *Source* and *Target* interfaces take in charge the communication protocols with both the Source and Target systems. It is up to the Source Interface to decode the information (if it is coded) by associating a specific decoding process. The Target Interface may need to restructure the adapted information in a way comprehensive for the Target and use the system specific methods to send the adapted information to the Target system.

To manage syntactic and semantic, the concepts of *Intermediate Representation* and *Adapter* are used. The *Intermediate Representation* models, inside the mediator, as a flattened list of Attribute-Value, the information exchanged between a Source and a Target system. Adapters, which contains a *Mapper* (for concepts and data structures) and a *Converter* (for data formats), can be used in both the Source and Target interfaces to transform information from a Source Representation into the Intermediate Representation with intermediate concepts, structures and data formats and then from the Intermediate Representation into a Target Representation. The concepts used in the Intermediate Representation can reference to a classification specific of the domain.

The ready-to-use XML specialisation

To enhance the flexibility of the Mediator Service, the emerging XML technology is applied to find out a possible way to reach the maximum independence of the Mediator model. XML has here been used not only as a document structure format, but as an interchange format and as a powerful data structure descriptor to ease the conversion between data structures of different systems.

A specialisation using the XML technology is ready to use for any XML compliant Target system whatever their data structure. A class XMLInterface, derived from the class ApplicationInterface, is provided. An *XML Messages Generator* is integrated to inform the mediator about the data structure descriptions of the Target systems. This generator creates XML messages representing the data of the Source system modelled with the data structure of the Target system. This generator requires 3 inputs:

- An XML **DTD** (***Document Type Definition***) representing the structure of the data model of the Target system. It allows to separate the structure of data from the data.
- The **Mapping Information** used to find out the correspondence among concepts. These information are stored in a database and in the current version the description is done manually during configuration.
- The **Intermediate Representation** which contains the exchange.

When the *Intermediate Representation* is passed to the XMLInterface, the *XML Messages Generator* analyses the *DTD*, generates an image of the object model of the Target system, and then fills this image with the data represented in the *Intermediate Representation* by using the *Mapping Information*. Finally, the result is transformed into an XML message and sent to the Target system. Since XML is self-descriptive, a Target system based on an object model can easily construct its data instances from the information contained in this message.

The main advantage of our XML Messages Generator is that it is completely generic and independent to any XML compliant Target system, since the information concerning data model, mapping and conversion is stored externally.

4 Results

The Mediator Service exists on both UNIX systems (HP, Sun,...) and on Windows NT. The C++ library contains the generic model of a mediator and the ready-to-use specialised Interfaces. The XML Messages Generator integrated in the ready-to-use XML specialisation is developed in Java and is based on Microsoft msxml [[16]].

The Mediator Service component has been tested, in the Broussais University Hospital, to support the following protocols: file sharing through NFS, messages transfer using X400 and access to an ORACLE database. An EDIFACT decode process has been associated in a Source Interface to manage EDIFACT messages from both a patient identity server and a laboratory results server. A ward legacy application has been used as the Target system. The XML specialisation has been tested with different Targets based on different object models. We are now testing it with the FHCR server of the Department of Electrical Engineering of Dublin Institute of Technology, as a Target system.

The next version of the Mediator Service will provide ready-to-use specialisations such as an XML compliant Source Interface, a connection to a CORBA broker and a DHE [[13]] Interface. It will have extended functionalities such as the possibility to manage multiple Sources or multiple Targets within a single mediator. Audit trail or monitoring tools are also greatly required. Besides, since the Mediator Service does not completely automate the development process, automation or configuration tools will be designed.

5 Discussion and Conclusion

A "glue" mechanism is required on a SynEx platform which federates the medical information from distributed legacy systems. Mediators can be considered as this glue. The Mediator Service is an application component on the SynEx platform to facilitate the creation of such mediators. The described approach does not spare a developer from writing code (except if he uses the ready-to-use specialisations). However, it helps the development process by offering both a methodology and a framework or architecture of mediators and can hence foster re-usability.

This component has taken into account both syntactic and semantic mismatches of different systems. It separates on one side the syntactic coding and decoding process and on the other side the semantic mapping and conversion process. The XML technology integrated in the Mediator Service can manage the data model and structural conflicts as well as descriptive conflicts in an independent and flexible way.

In the open distributed medical applications development context, it is known that total interoperability will not be reached without semantics sharing [[8]], but in the current development, it is not completely managed. We used several mapping processes to handle the semantic issues. However, the manual creation of the mapping information can be a painful process. Moreover, the structure of the Intermediate Representation and the mapping information is not standard and may not be suitable for those more complex cases.

Several proposed solutions in other compatible projects concerning the semantic conflicts that can be adopted in the Mediator Service. The Medical Connection Service in the HELIOS project uses a meta-model as its internal representation to declare explicitly the semantic correspondences [[7], [8]]. In the TSIMMIS project, a tagged object exchange model (OEM) in which object have labels, types, values and an optional identifier also acts as an intermediate representation [[3]].

The "Computer-based Patient Record Reference Model" of the HELIOS project proposes to use the characteristics of the medical data to handle different medical vocabularies [[1], [17]]. Several medical data dictionaries with updating facilities are developed as references, where medical concepts are described with their labels, synonyms and definitions. Hence, the medical concepts are given their medical meaning. Furthermore, Medical concepts can also described by their codes in several nomenclatures and classifications [[18]]. We argue that the use a semantic network or the access to a generic terminology server such as GALEN could provide more comprehensive semantic matching to the Mediator Service Component [[5]].

Acknowledgments

The authors would like to thank all the members of the SynEx Consortium for their contribution to this research. The financial support of the European Commission is also gratefully acknowledged.

References

[1] Lavril M, Doré L, Zapletal E, Jean FC, Degoulet P, A Reuse Oriented Development Database: The HELIOS Object Information System, *Comput Methods Programs Biomed.* 1994; 45, Suppl.: S35-S45.

[2] van Mulligen EM, Timmers T, van Bemmel JH, A new architecture for integration of heterogeneous software components, *Meth Inform Med*, 1993; 32: 292-301.

[3] Papakonstantinou Y, Garcia-Molina H, Object Exchange Across Heterogeneous Information Sources, in : Proc Data Engineering Conference, Taipei, Taiwan, March, 1995.

[4] Hoffert J, Resolving Design Problems in Distributed Programming Environments. *C++ Report*, 1998; July-August: 33-42.

[5] Degoulet P, Sauquet S, Jaulent MC, Zapletal E, Lavril M, Rational and Design Considerations for a Semantic Mediator in Health Information Systems, *Meth Inform Med.* 1998; 37: 518-526.

[6] Wiederhold G, Mediators in the architecture of future information systems. *IEEE Computor,* 1992; 25 (3): 38-49.

[7] Jean FC, Engelmann U, Sauquet D, Lavril M, Schröter A, Degoulet P, The HELIOS Medical Connection Services, *Comput. Methods Programs Biomed.* 1994; 45, Suppl.: S117-S126.

[8] Jean FC, Mascart JJ, Codaccioni A, Lavril M, Sauquet D, Degoulet P, Using a meta-model to build a Connection Service in an object oriented medical application development environment, *Proc Annu Symp Comput Appl Med Care.* 1994: 483-487.

[9] XML: http://www.w3c.org/xml

[10] http://www.cs.man.ac.uk/mig/galen

[11] http://www.cs.man.ac.uk/mig/giu/

[12] Kalra D (ed). Synapses Federated Healthcare Record Server-Object Model and Object Dictionary version2. London: University College, December 1996.

[13] Ferrara FM. The middleware-based architectural approach for opening and evolving healthcare information systems. *Medical Informatics Europe* '96. IOS Press, 1996: 264-270.

[14] Graeber S, Communication services for a distributed hospital information system. *Meth Inform Med* 1996; 35: 230-241.

[15] Ben-Shaul I, Gish JW, Robinson W, An Integrated Network Component Architecture, *IEEE Software*, 1998; September/October: 79-87.

[16] http://www.microsoft.com/workshop/xml/

[17] Doré L, Lavril M, Jean FC, Degoulet P, An Object Oriented Computer-Based Patient Record Reference Model, *Proc Annu Symp Comput Appl Med Care.* 1995: 377-381.

[18] Barrows Jr R, Cimino J, Clayton P, Mapping Clinically Useful Terminology to a Controlled Medical Vocabulary, *Proc Annu Symp Comput Appl Med Care.* 1994: 211-215.

Medical Informatics Europe '99
P. Kokol et al. (Eds.)
IOS Press, 1999

Emergency Protocols in Prehospital Emergency Medicine in Slovenia

Jožica Leskovšek[1], Andrej Žmavc[2]
Vizija d.o.o., Ljubljanska 42, Celje, Slovenia[1]
Javni zavod ZD Celje, Gregorčičeva 5, Celje, Slovenia[2]

Abstract. Emergency medicine is a branch of medicine in which prompt and accurate information is of crucial importance, because a patient's survival and the final outcome of a treatment very often depends on it. Therefore the standardization of prehospital emergency service administration with uniform documentation, methods of annotation of technical data as well as uniform gathering and data analysis are necessary. Wanting to process a fair amount of data and specially to disburden personnel, a need for computer aided processing is evident. Application that was developed in strong collaboration with EMS project team and information science engineers definitely improves data quality. Firstly when team members, especially physicians, are constrained to fulfill paper forms and secondly when data are entered into the computer, because all inconsistencies are being reconsidered and corrected if necessary. The developed application also gave the opportunity to the emergency team for prompt and accurate information.

Keywords. Emergency medicine, Emergency administration, Emergency medical service system, Medical informatics applications, Information system, Emergency documentation

1. Introduction

A nationwide project of establishing a prehospital emergency medical service (EMS) system is currently in progress in Slovenia. The project is lead by the Ministry of Health. In some parts of the country the EMS system is already well developed, while in the other parts it is only in a nascent stage or there is no EMS system at all. EMS in such areas depends mostly on general practitioners if they are reachable at that moment. A fully developed prehospital EMS system established at fifteen to twenty locations around Slovenia, should encompass a medical triage facility, an emergency team consisting of a physician and two emergency technicians on a round-the-clock stand-by duty and a fully equipped ambulance car for emergency purpose only.

One of the crucial elements for the whole project is how to get relevant and comparable data. Emergency medicine is a branch of medicine in which prompt and accurate information is of crucial importance, because a patient's survival and the final outcome of a treatment very often depends on it. Retrieving correct information is particularly difficult in a prehospital environment, where we are very often faced with difficult rescue circumstances combined with a severe patient's condition besides the lack of personnel and time that are always present.

2. Standardization of prehospital emergency service administration

Therefore standardization of prehospital emergency service administration was an essential part of the project. A uniform documentation and methods of annotation of technical data as well as uniform gathering and data analysis were required. A special paper form - the emergency protocol - has been designed for gathering all necessary data related to intervention circumstances, patient condition and medical procedures at the site of the incident and during the transport. The emergency protocols are of tree types - *the dispatching protocol, the emergency intervention protocol and the prehospital cardiopulmonary resuscitation protocol.* These forms have to be fulfilled at each intervention and represent the basic data by means of which the system performance as a whole as well as the performance of each single unit can be assessed and analyzed. On the other hand these protocols enable assessment of quality care of each single emergency patient. The protocol of emergency intervention is also designed to inform a hospital physician at the time of admission about the course of events before acceptance in a hospital.

3. Software development

The amount of data in all three forms is not negligible and additionally burdens emergency personnel with administration. To process all this standardized data and specially to disburden personnel, a need for computer aided processing was evident. Therefore we developed an application called **Urgenca Ver. 1.0** (Emergency). It was developed in a strong collaboration with EMS project team and information science engineers.

The application is written for Windows operating systems (Microsoft® Windows© 95+, Microsoft® Windows© NT) with programming language Inprise Delphi 3.0. Microsoft® Access 97 is the supporting database. The program can be simultaneously used by several users via network or as a single user program.

Working with the application is rather easy for an average user of Windows environment/programs and, despite of the amount of data to be entered, it does not require too much time. The program includes a help file and frequently asked questions. In original package a user gets a user guide and free on-line help by e-mail or by helpdesk software system (bug reporting system). New versions of program are planned to be delivered through Internet or by e-mail.

The application fully supports all three emergency protocols because what we see on the screen is practically the copy of the paper form (see Picture 1). Program can be used in two ways: interactive mode, for writing data directly into the program at the time of receiving an emergency call, or in so called off-line mode, for entering data later after the intervention is completed. The first mode is appropriate for dispatch service and prehospital emergency units in lager centers, while the second one is suitable for all other locations, especially for smaller emergency units in semi urban and rural areas. A complete interactive mode is feasible only on the dispatch protocol form. The other two forms can be fully completed only after the intervention.

Most of the data on protocols is in a preset or closed form (like YES or NO) so it doesn't take additional time to mark it. The order of rubrics follows the natural order of diagnostic and therapeutic intervention procedures, so it serves as an emergency checkout list as well. There are only three fields in protocols into which a free form text can be entered - the field for anamnesis, the field for observation remarks and comments and the field for a descriptive diagnosis. The last one is also supported by the complete international classification of diseases, included into the software, so the statistics can be more accurate and uniform.

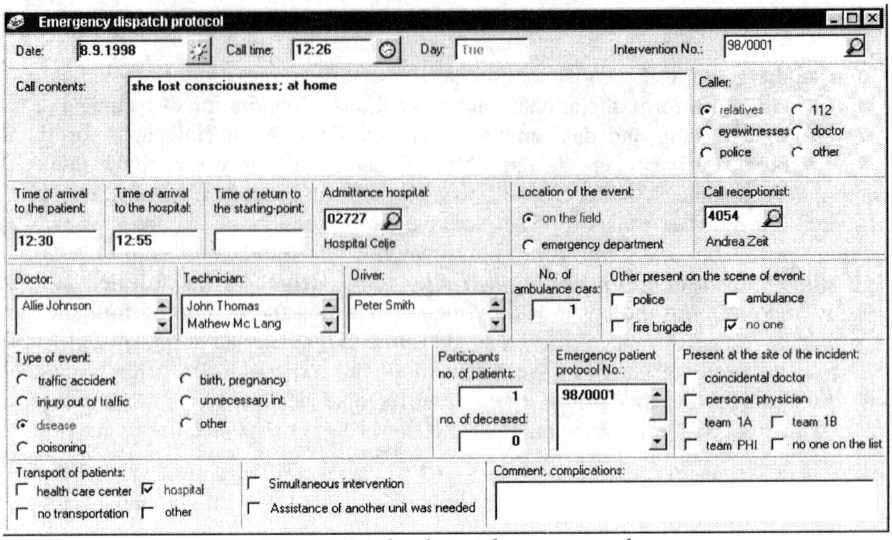

Picture 1: The dispatching protocol

For more accurate assessment of patient's condition two emergency scoring calculations are included - the Mainz emergency evaluation score for all patients and the Revised trauma score for trauma patients. The calculation is made instantly when all the required physiologic parameters are entered.

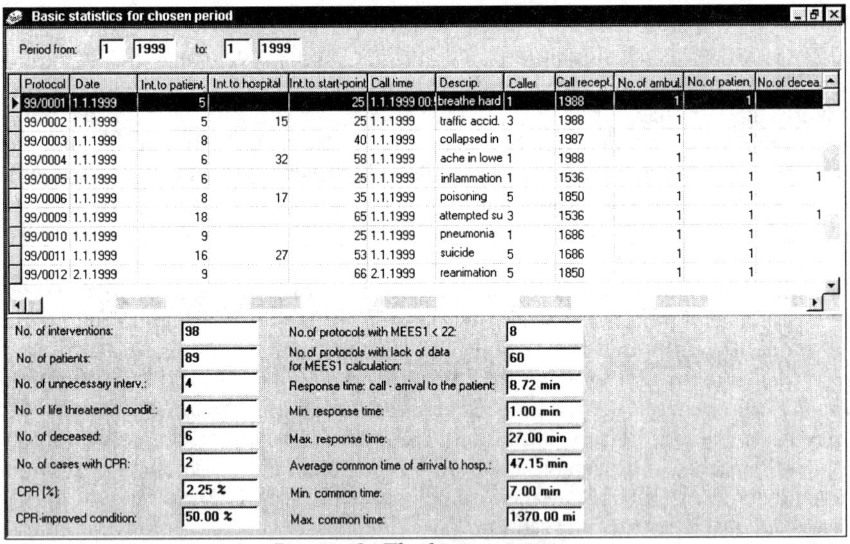

Picture 2: The basic statistics

Once all necessary data have been entered a whole spectrum of statistical calculations and data presentations is available. Some statistics are prepared in advance and serve as a comparison tool on a nationwide level. The basic statistics (see Picture 2) comprehend data such as a number of interventions, a number of patients, a number of deaths before the emergency team arrives, average response times, percentage of cases where CPR was needed, percentage of CPRs with satisfactory outcome, etc.

Similar statistics can also be calculated for a special emergency team. Other statistics the program supports are: statistics based on the main diagnosis, anamnesis, given medications, detailed statistics of CPR cases (number and percentage of successful CPRs, cardiac arrests in front of eyewitnesses, the number and percentage of correctly reanimated patients by eyewitnesses, average Δ MEES ...), response times etc.

There is also a tool available for user inquiry for further, more detailed, analysis. It includes the selection of data for display, record selection conditions, sorting and grouping of data by different criteria and data summation.

All the statistics, pre-prepared and user-defined, can be presented. There are also some special charts (graphs) for intervention frequency, response time, Mainz emergency evaluation scores, etc. (see Picture 3 and Picture 4).

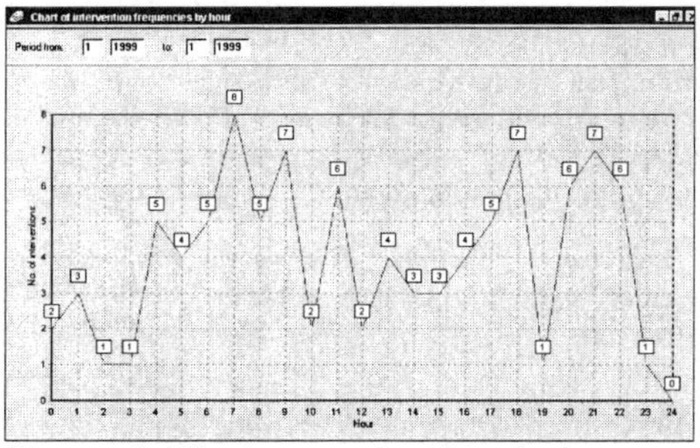

Picture 3: The intervention freq. by hour

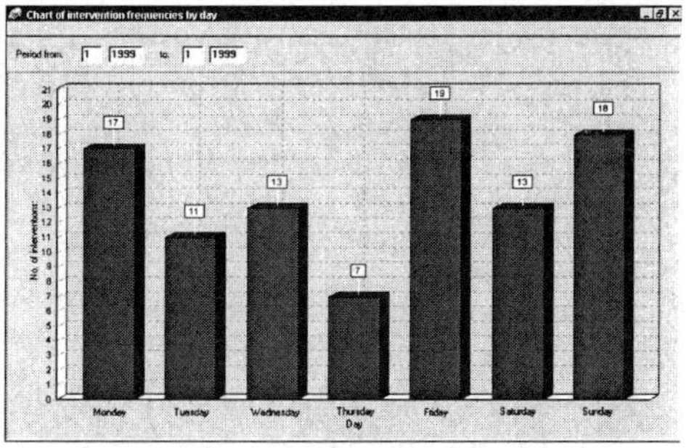

Picture 4: The intervention freq. by day

An element of extreme importance in each EMS system, also supported by the software, is the possibility to access patient data (at any time), of any previous treatment in EMS.

As mentioned before, this application works in Windows environment but nevertheless it is integrated with other almost standardized programs like MS Word and MS Excel and special programs like Vizija's medical information system called SOVA. All the statistics made by the program Emergency can be exported to Word or Excel where they can be used as any other independent data. The integration with SOVA is even more interesting, since it is DOS based and works with dBase DBF files and NTX indexes. So we had to solve the problem of indexes with built-in user defined function. This problem was solved with the help of Halcyon 6 software, so that a user will not notice the difference between working with Access or dBase database.

4. Conclusion

How does the new way of work influence the quality of work in EMS system?
It definitely heightens data quality. Firstly when team members (especially physicians) are constrained to fulfill paper forms and secondly when data are entered into the computer, because all inconsistencies are being reconsidered and corrected if necessary. Therefore an overall EMS data quality is improved significantly.

As planned, the software ameliorates work quality. Accurate data are always available almost instantly. Therefore, we can presume that emergency personnel would consequently do their work better, knowing that it will be systematically checked out afterwards. This last statement of course needs further assessment.

What are the perspectives of program evolution?
Although the program is carefully designed with lots of mechanisms to accelerate data entry we have to focus on finding better ways for entering data. We are considering automatic data reading from paper forms using OCR technology as well as voice-recognition system where administrator would dictate data from paper form into the computer. This would accelerate data entry and disencumbrance emergency personnel of additional administrative work that is required by computer data collection.

In the near future the program will also support multimedia. This involves saving electrocardiograms, X-ray photographs, etc.

References

[1] Pravilnik o službi nujne medicinske pomoči. Uradni list Republike Slovenije, 77; 1996: 8452 - 60.
[2] Skupina za prehospitalno dejavnost Projekta NMP pri ministrstvu za zdravstvo - obrazci za NMP.
[3] Žmavc A. Ocenjevanje prizadetosti in ogroženosti bolnikov in poškodovancev v NMP s pomočjo ocenjevalnih lestvic. Zdravstveno varstvo 1998; 37: 275-8.
[4] Hennes HJ, Reinhardt T, Dick W., Beurteilung des Notfallpatienten mit dem MEES Mainz emergency evaluation score. Notfallmed. 1992; 18: 130-6.
[5] Virginia Howlett, Visual interface design for Windows: effective user interfaces for Windows 95, Windows NT, and Windows 3.1, John Wiley & Sons, cop., New York, 1996.
[6] Halcyon Ver. 6.0, Griffin Solutions, Inc., Georgia, 1998.

Medical Informatics Europe '99
P. Kokol et al. (Eds.)
IOS Press, 1999

A system for the description of healthcare guidelines

Patrizia Grifoni, Daniela Luzi, Fabrizio L. Ricci
Istituto di studi sulla ricerca e documentazione scientifica,
Consiglio Nazionale delle Ricerche,
Via Cesare De Lollis 12, 00185 Roma, Italy
e-mail: {grifoni,luzi}@www.isrds.rm.cnr.it; ricci@iasi.rm.cnr.it

Abstract. Contained costs and quality of treatment are two elements which have to be considered when planning and controlling both clinical and managerial activities of healthcare structures (HCSs). Each structure has to be marked by a high level of quality of treatment and by specific professional competencies and skills of its operators. It is therefore fundamental to provide a system which supports the management of processes and of guidelines which characterise an healthcare structure. In this paper we present a system able to describe processes of an HCS and in particular clinical guidelines. This system is based on a workflow conceptual model, able to represent clinical and managerial activities carried out in HCSs (the Atreus model).

1. Introduction

Within heathcare treatment we can distinguish among clinical, managerial and communication activities [1]. The complexity of the activities carried out in healthcare structures requires a conceptual description which uses administration and ad hoc workflows (WFs) [2]. The Atreus model [3] makes it possible to link dynamically the different types of WFs: clinical, managerial and communication WFs. With the Atreus model it is possible to construct a WF using subsequent refinement processes through the top-down development [4]. The clinical guideline of a new patient refers to guidelines described by a very generic WF schema (WF template). This schema is detailed gradually taking into consideration the patient's characteristics, as well as the managerial aspects (resources and actors available and temporal constraints). The definition of the WF schema is therefore based on predefined WFs stored in a library or on WFs developed *ad hoc*. In addition to facilitating and speeding up the process of WF construction, library collects guidelines and descriptions of standard processes as well as guidelines used within each structure.

2. Characteristics of the Atreus model

The model provides a graphic and textual representation of the information contained in guidelines. A set of possible states of each activity of the guideline is associated to these representations in order to describe the evolution of the WF. The three representations are complementary among themselves.

- *The graphic representation* describes the activities and the events that activate them.

- *The textual representation* describes the data and constraints connected to each activity.
- *The representation of the activity execution* describes and controls the functioning of the WF.

In order to design a guideline model at different level of description and to simplify the design by a refinement process and by a re-use of WFs collected in libraries, the Atreus model is based on an algebra for the WF manipulation. The algebra operators are used for: a) cancelling activities and events; b) inserting activities and events; c) substituting a part of WF; d) making a comparison between two WFs in order to cancel the parts in common; and e) defining a new WF obtained from the combination of two different Wfs.

3. Feature of the interface

The system has been designed and developed according to a WYSIWYG approach associated to a user interface, which provides commands from both menu and keyboard in order to speed up the interaction with the system (duplicated commands). The interaction approach chosen is that of "object-verb". This allows to: a) select the object of interest; and b) specify the command on the selected object. When the object has been selected, the system makes available only those actions associated to each object. This removes a whole set of syntactic mistakes and avoids the confusion between operators and their values.

Typically the construction of a guideline is undertaken following two subsequent steps: a) definition of an activity; and b) definition of the events which connect the activity to other activities of the guideline.

From the point of view of human-computer interaction, the definition of an activity implies the definition of the object which represents the activity, the input of the information, proprieties and constraints which define the activity as well as the identification of all possible states which characterise the activity. In the definition of an activity it is necessary to indicate if this is simple or a complex one. Then the user selects one of the graphic primitives corresponding to the primitives of the Atreus model which are [3] (fig. 1): a) simple activity; b) sequence of simple/complex activities; c) parallelism of simple/complex activities ; d) multitasking, that is the parallelism of different instances of the same activity; and e) iteration of a simple/complex activity repeated until a condition has been verified. Moreover it is possible to combine these primitives (for example, iteration of parallel activities). Each activity has to be identified by: a name, a set of descriptors and constraints. These constraints and the attribution of values to the descriptors (resources, actors, etc.) are filled in using the form associated to the activity (Fig. 2).

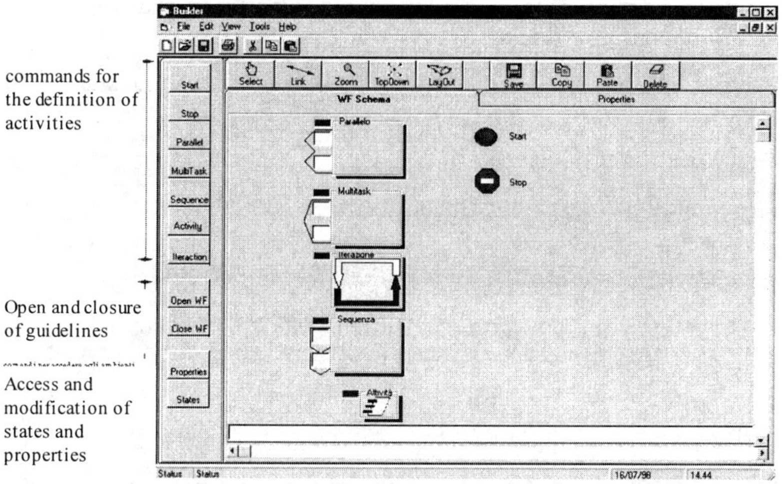

Fig. 1 Structural primitives of the simple and complex activities of a guideline

In order to verify the enactment of an activity, the Atreus model uses the following constraints; pre-conditions, post-conditions, temporal constraints and exceptions. The pre-conditions are necessary in order to establish when the activity has to be executed. In the case in which an activity can end with more events, post-conditions make it possible to identify which event makes the next activity start. Temporal constraints are considered during the execution of the complex activity: they have a control function in order to define the temporal links between start, duration and conclusion of the component activities. Exceptions are considered during the execution of the activity. They are linked to a state diagram associated to each activity. The state diagram editing allows to change the execution of the current activity (e.g., by interrupting it and subsequently resuming it normally). The states which express exceptions are the following: suspended, aborted, cancelled and re-assigned.

The system allows to link the graphic representation, the textual representation and the state diagram among themselves.

When the user begins to describe the guideline using the graphic module, the system fills automatically the textual representation with the related information. The presence of exceptions in the textual representation implies the existence of at least one state expressing an exception in the state diagram and vice-versa.

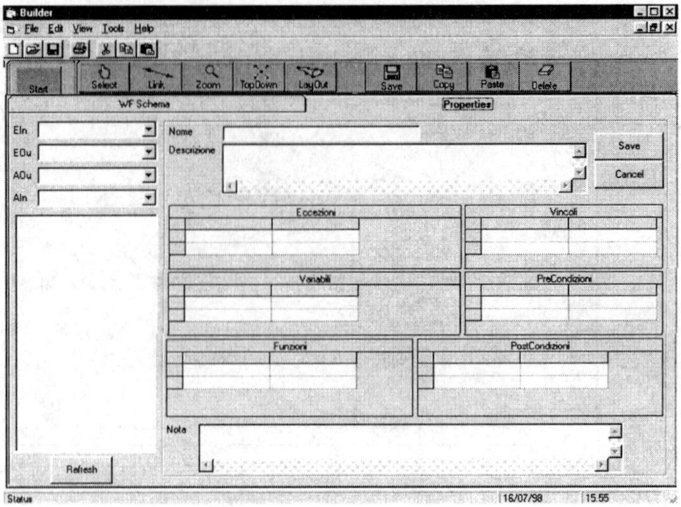

Fig. 2 Form for the definition of the proprieties associated to each activity

4. Conclusion

The use of systems which support the guideline management has a key role to promote co-operation within and among healthcare structures in order to improve the quality of treatment without increasing costs. In this paper we have presented the editing module of guidelines, which allows to: a) define one or more activities and their graphic connection; b) identify for each process the component processes, which can be collected in a library; c) define the information which characterise each activity through the use of pre-conditions; d) post-conditions, temporal constraints and other data associated to each activity; and e) define the evolution of the activity execution through the state diagram.

References

[1] A. Rossi Mori, et al.,"A model for structured description of healthcare activities and related data", in C. Gordon, J.P. Christensen (eds), "Health telematics for clinical guidelines and protocols", IOS Press, 1995.

[2] P.D. Gearglopoulos, et al., “An overview of workflow management: from process modeling to workflow”, Journal of Distributed and Parallel databases, (3), 1995.

[3] P. Grifoni, et al.,"ATREUS: a model for the conceptual representation of a workflow", Proc. of 8th International Conference and Workshop on Database and expert Systems Applications, DEXA'97, 1997.

[4] P. Grifoni, et al.,"A conceptual representation of clinical and managerial guidelines: the Atreus workflow model", Proc.9th World Congress on Medical Informatics, MEDINFO'98, 1998.

Medical Informatics Europe '99
P. Kokol et al. (Eds.)
IOS Press, 1999

Take Care: Guidelines for Patients with Chronic Hepatitis C

Kristina Hedin[1], MD, Ankica Babic,Ph.D.[2,3] , Aril Frydén, MD, Ph.D.[1]
1 Department of Infectious Diseases, Faculty of Health Sciences, Linkoping University, Sweden
2 Medical Informatics, Department of Biomedical Engineering, Linkoping University, Sweden
3 Faculty of Electrical Engineering, University of Ljubljana, Slovenia

Abstract. Alcohol consumption has significant impact on the condition of the liver, by itself, and even more in conjunction with other liver diseases such as chronic hepatitis C. Drinking habits might be delicate issues to address and could harm otherwise satisfying communication. Therefore, we intended to outline guidelines for advising hepatitis C patients concerning alcohol consumption.

Analysis of a relatively limited knowledge base revealed the complexity of the disease rather than statistically significant findings regarding consumption. Thus, we instead chose to suggest a set of patient educational guidelines, which could be implemented on the Internet, hypothesizing that a better informed patient will be more able to comply with restrictions concerning alcohol consumption. A brief ad hoc evaluation pointed out Internet as a favourable media to present the information. We also suggest a tentative algorithm for further development of clinical decision support systems addressing monitoring of chronic hepatitis C patients.

1. Introduction

Understanding of Hepatitis C, outlining its treatment regimes and predicting immediate, as well as long term patient outcomes has been a distinguished subject of clinical studies over the last decade. In 1989, the genome of the hepatitis C virus (HCV) was completely outlined by molecular biology techniques. This virus was shown to be responsible for approximately 90 % of cases previously diagnosed as "non-A non-B hepatitis". The virus is mainly spread by the parenteral route, i.e. blood to blood contact, with blood transfusion and intravenous drug use (IVDU) as the main routes of transmission. The infection is most often asymptomatic for many years, but can still lead to significant damage of the liver and a considerable risk of liver cirrhosis and primary liver cancer [1]. HCV infection is now one of the leading causes of liver transplantation in the western world [2]. The virus has several subtypes with differing prognoses and different geographical distribution [3,4]. Given the slow and insidious nature of the disease, scientific publications, among other things, discuss ways of identifying and relating important findings, in order to disclose if the virus is likely to lead to a more or less severe liver inflammation in the individual patient. At present, antiviral treatment with alpha-interferon alone or in combination with ribavirine can lead to resolution of the disease in 10-70 % of treated patients, depending e.g. on virus subtype and viral load [5,6]. Treatment can be demanding, with side effects as fatigue and depression, and is also rather costly. It is thus important to consider the advantages and disadvantages of treatment in relation to stage and grade of the liver disease, and in relation to the patients somatic and psychological status which might influence compliance. The treatment should be evaluated with respect to established diagnosis, expected outcome and the patient's ability of self-care and maintaining a healthy life style. Negative consequences of the latter, such as excessive use of alcohol might hamper the patients' recovery [7,8]. It is, therefore, important to make patients aware of risk they might be taking.

The main goal was to get insights into patterns of laboratory and histological findings and, within them, check if alcohol was significantly connected to the disease-related changes. The next step was to outline a graphical presentation of algorithms based on the results of knowledge discovery. Their purpose is to explain the complexity of the liver disease with respect to causes, clinical development, and factors that influence outcome of HCV infection. Such presentation of disease scenarios is not by itself normative, but it does reflect the patient material and gives a patient points of identification. Having an established diagnosis, and being aware of their own alcohol intake, patients would be able to estimate a predisposition for an eventual long-term outcome. Paradigm “Take Care” suggests physicians' recommendations and gives an impulse to patients to take control over their situation.

Several sites dealing with viral hepatitis already exist on the Internet, such as “Hepnet” and the American Liver Foundation Homepage [9,10]. These are very large information systems, addressing both physicians and patients, and they are most often supported by large institutions such as universities or pharmaceutical companies. To our knowledge, no such site exists in Swedish. Since approximately 40.000 Swedes could be affected by HCV, one could assume a need for a local Internet based information system for those who are not fluent in English. “Take Care” would be an attempt to develop this kind of site in a more local setting. A strong interactive component in a software application aims at developing a more active understanding of the patient’s position both with respect to the disease and its treatments. During a visit to an outpatient clinic, the patient might not be able to ask all questions, or digest all the information the physician provides. Time constraints and demands for an efficient cost-benefit patient management might force a patient to be more responsible for his or her own health giving them an active role in getting informed.

2. Material and methods

58 patients with chronic hepatitis C, who between 1989 and 1993 underwent liver biopsy at the Linkoping University hospital and Oskarshamn hospital, Sweden, were included in the study. The patients could be divided into several groups according to HCV subtypes: 1a (n=21), 1b (n=5), 2b (n=9) and 3a (n=23). This distribution of subtypes is similar to that in other Scandinavian materials [11]. The liver biopsies were evaluated according to the Knodell score, a score which grades different types of inflammation in the liver, and also stages the extent of liver fibrosis [12]. In addition, the amount of steatosis (fatty change) was evaluated, since this is a prominent feature of hepatitis C [12]. A large number of blood laboratory tests were performed on the day of biopsy. The results of the tests were analyzed in the search of relations between easily obtainable blood tests and findings in the liver biopsy. Furthermore, the patients were interviewed concerning alcohol consumption. They were divided into three groups; group 1: no or minimal consumption (n= 35), group 2: moderate (70-420 g of absolute alcohol/month, n=17), and group 3: higher consumption (> 420 g/month, n=6). The mean age of the population was 42 years, range 18-75. There were 39 men and 19 women in the study.

3. Results and discussion

In this preliminary study, we analyzed only a few findings associated with alcohol consumption and / or hepatitis C, i.e. presence of steatosis and periportal inflammation of the liver, liver enzymes in blood (AST and ALT) and HCV subtype.

Discriminant analysis according to virus subtype showed that the only significantly different factor was amount of periportal inflammation in the liver. Patient classification according to self-reported alcohol consumption was done using the above mentioned variables. The only significant finding was steatosis of the liver, which was more pronounced in alcohol consumption group 3. A potential problem with that finding was that a confounding factor might be the HCV which itself can induce liver steatosis [13]. HCV subtype 3a is associated with IVDU [11], but further testing in the patient group which reported highest alcohol consumption, showed no statistically valid connection between subtype of virus and heavy drinking. A confounding factor in this case could, however, be age, which was lower in the 3 a subgroup.

We thus conclude that the patient material and the amount of variables examined were not sufficient for constructing valid guidelines for professional monitoring of chronic hepatitis C patients. However, our findings elucidated the complexity of this disease in respect to interaction between e.g. viral factors, host factors and environmental factors (alcohol). It is possible that studies of a larger patient material and / or more groups of data could lead to the development of more statistically valid decision support systems, as we have shown in previous articles [14,15].

"Take care" is intended to address three different aspects of the information background. First, as illustrated in Figure 1, is a schematic representation of the natural course of the disease. It shows in sequential steps how the disease can be acquired, and what the possible outcomes are. It introduces a notion of potentially severe disease. By clicking on the circles one could get detailed explanations and updated statistical findings concerning e.g. which path of disease development is most likely in the general population. The end of the algorithm corresponds to the end stage of the disease, and could provide further information of risk factors for this development. It should be noted that only a small proportion of patients are at risk of finally reaching this stage.

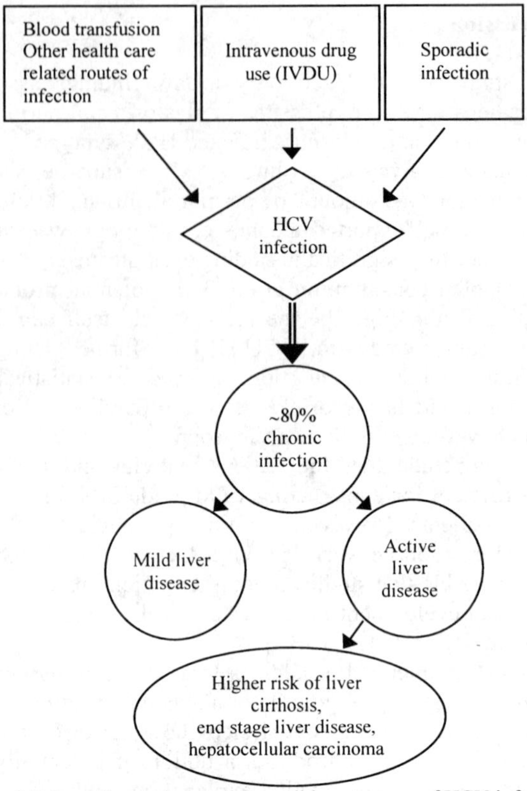

Figure 1 Schematic graph over the possible outcomes of HCV infection.

Secondly, we wanted to present factors that can influence the course of the disease both positively and negatively (Figure 2). The purpose of this is both to inform and inspire the patient to make possible changes in lifestyle, which with our present knowledge mainly concerns abstinence from alcohol and other liver toxic drugs. Furthermore we introduce the possibilities of treatment, which could be further explored by clicking on the circle. We also wanted to illustrate the complex nature of the disease, with multiple interacting factors that could modulate the disease process.

The ambition is to create several specialized algorithmic graphs of this basic one. In that way we would capture a complex interaction between all the factors, available treatments relating it to the outcome.

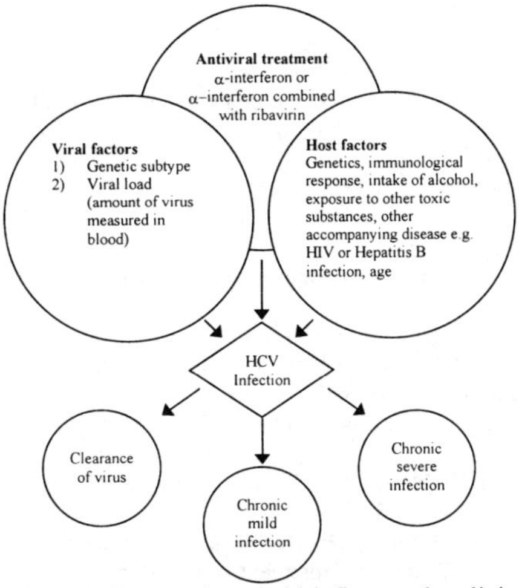

Figure 2. Factors that could influence the clinical course of the disease

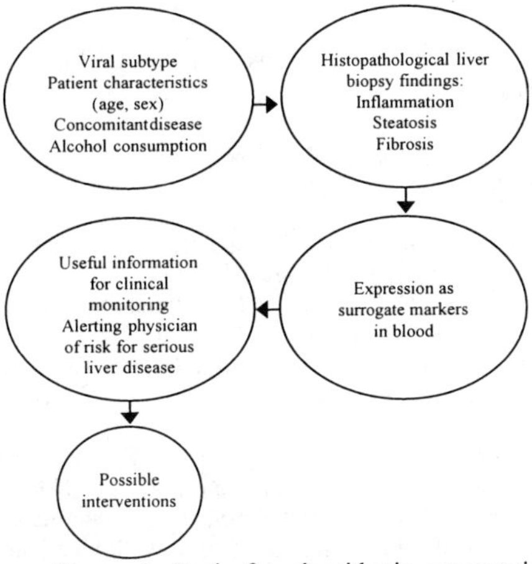

Figure 3. Basis for algorithmic presentation for development of professional guidelines.

At last, we also present an algorithm (Figure 3) which could illustrate how the physician can obtain and process data in order to make treatment and other management decisions.

This algorithm could in the future be further developed into a more comprehensive clinical decision support system. Clinical data could be a valuable source of precise knowledge needed to differentiate patients with respect to the disease severity, interventions and outcomes.

4. Conclusions

"Take Care" offers a fairly specialized knowledge, which is reflective of the clinical competence lying behind this work. However, we believe easily accessible instruments for patient information concerning chronic hepatitis C, could be a valuable complement to straightforward advice concerning e.g. alcohol abstinence. A better compliance to advice would be expected if the patient has a larger understanding of the nature of the disease.

In comparison with other systems on the Internet, our system is smaller and directed to a selected population. We followed the philosophy of Scott et al [16] to redirect information from general to more individually oriented patient viewpoints. Maintenance of the prototype system is not going to be normative, nor with a large knowledge base in the background. Instead, physicians who work with patients would be able to contribute their own empirical knowledge as well as updated information on ongoing research. Software routines for updating the systems are prioritized as well as personal responsibilities for keeping the system up to date. Knowledge based decision support with a basis in the presented algorithms is feasible, but is likely to demand significant efforts.

The concern of the future is evaluation, where the main question to the users (patients) would be whether this system makes it easier to deal with the task of living with a chronic disease, and to "take care" of themselves.

Acknowledgements

The authors would like to thank Jens Jonsson, M.Sc., for valuable help with the graphical outlay of the guidelines.

References

[1] Tong MJ, El-Farra NS, Reikes AR, Co RL, Clinical outcomes after transfusion-associated hepatitis C. N E J Med 1995;332:1463-66.
[2] Hoofnagle, JH, Hepatitis C: The Clinical Spectrum of Disease. Hepatology 1997;26: Suppl.1.
[3] Zein NN, Rakela J, Krawitt EL et al, Hepatitis C Virus Genotypes in the United States: Epidemiology, Pathogenicity, and Response to Interferon Therapy. Ann Intern Med. 1996;125:634-639.
[4] Smith DB, Pathirana S, Davidson F Et al, The Origin of Hepatitis C Virus Genotypes. J Gen Virol, 1997, 78, 321-328.
[5] McHutchinson JG, Gordon SC, Schiff E, et al,Interferon alfa-2b Alone or in Combination with Ribavirin as Initial Treatment for Chronic Hepatitis C. N E J Med. 1998;339:1485-1492.
[6] Poynard T, Marcellin P, Lee SS, et al, Randomised Trial of Interferon alfa2b plus Ribavirin for 48 weeks or for 24 Weeks Versus Interferon alfa2b plus Placebo for 48 Weeks for Treatment of Chronic Infection with Hepatitis C Virus. Lancet 1998;352:1426-1432.
[7] Mochida S, Ohnishi K, Matsuo S, Kakihara K, Fujiwara K, Effect of Alcohol Intake on the Efficacy of Interferon Therapy in Patients with Chronic Hepatitis C as Evaluated by Multivariate Logistic Regression Analysis. Alcoholism, Clinical & Experimental research 1996; 20 (9Suppl):371A-377A.
[8] Shev S, Dhillon AP, Lindh M, Serleus Z, et al, The Importance of Cofactors in the Histologic Progression of Minimal and Mild Chronic Hepatitis C. Liver 1997;17(5):215-223.
[9] Schering Canada Inc. 1995-99, http://www.hepnet.com/.
[10] The American Liver Foundation 1998, http://gi.ucsf.edu/alf/infohep.html.
[11] Shev S, Widell A, Foberg U et al, HCV Genotypes in Swedish Blood Donors as Correlated to Epidemiology, Liver Disease and Hepatitis C Virus Antibody Profile. Infection 1995;23:253-257.
[12] Knodell RG, Ishak KG, Blac WC et al, Formulation and Application of a Numerical Scoring System for Assessing Histological Activity in Asymptomatic Chronic Active Hepatitis. Hepatology 1981;1(5):431-435.
[13] Dhillon AP, Dusheiko GM, Pathology of Hepatitis C Virus Infection. Histopathology 1995;26:297-309.
[14] Babic A, Hedin K, Mathiesen U, et al, Decision Support for Monitoring of Chronic Hepatitis C: Can Blood Laboratory Tests Help? In J. Brender et al. (Eds.) Medical Informatics Europé '96 pp 551-554, IOS Press 1996.
[15] Babic A, Mathiesen U, Hedin K, Bodemar G, Wigertz O, Assessing an AI Knowledge Base for Asymptomatic Liver Disease. In JAMIA Proceedings of AMIA'98, pp 513-517.
[16] Scott GC, Lenert LA, Extending Contemporary Support System Designs to Patient-Oriented Systems. In Chute (Eds), Proceedings of the AMIA98 Annual Symposium, 1998, pp376-38.

Electronic Patient Encounter, Card Technology, Electronic Data Interchange

Medical Informatics Europe '99
P. Kokol et al. (Eds.)
IOS Press, 1999

C3: Java-based Medical Record System for Cardiology

Alessandro TADDEI, Stefano DALMIANI*, Gabriele CECCHETTI,
Alberto MACERATA, Clara CARPEGGIANI,
Lia CHELOZZI, Carlo MARCHESI^
CNR Institute of Clinical Physiology, via Trieste 41, Pisa, Italy
** MS-Informatica, Massa, Italy*
^Department of Systems and Computer Engineering, University of Florence, Italy

Abstract. This paper describes a system for electronic medical record (EMR) we have developed for use in our health care institution, mainly dealing with diagnosis and treatment of cardiovascular pathologies. This activity is part of the project SPERIGEST, supported by Health Ministry of Italy, for the management of health care delivery, as concerns both clinical and administrative aspects. A networked computer-based information system was realized to integrate the different heterogeneous sources of patient information. Both clinical and administrative patient relevant data are provided from the various systems and stored into a central database. The EMR system was designed using World Wide Web (WWW) technology (Java, HTML). The system is currently under clinical evaluation.

1. Introduction

The information system, developed at our institute, is aimed at the integration of different architectures (both existing and new installations), applications and health care services. It integrates clinical, administration and management systems [1,2]. Administration is enabled to derive healthcare costs directly from data provided by clinical system. The outstanding feature of this system is the full data access allowing design of a comprehensive patient record and playback consultation for both patient care and clinical research. The core is the clinical information system (SIC-C), which integrates the different sources of information related to the single patient. Diagnostic units (e.g. Clinical Chemistry, ECG labs, Imaging labs) and cardiosurgery units have been integrated in the SIC-C. These units (called Functional Islands), which autonomously provide to local data processing and archiving, take care of storing structured patient reports into the database of SIC-C (ARCA) (Figure 1). Excerpts of signals and significant images are possibly added to these reports for better documentation of test findings or procedural results. Even though many patient data are provided in electronic form and stored automatically into the database, there still remains the need for health care personnel to enter manually much information (e.g., medical history, physical examination, reports of external tests). A viewer/editor of EMR was developed addressing friendliness and communication capability.

2. The Electronic Medical Record

All data of interest for medical record are stored in ARCA, the clinical repository of SIC-C (DB2 database) (Figure 1), either collected automatically from the functional islands or manually entered by health care personnel. Patient data are structured according to the

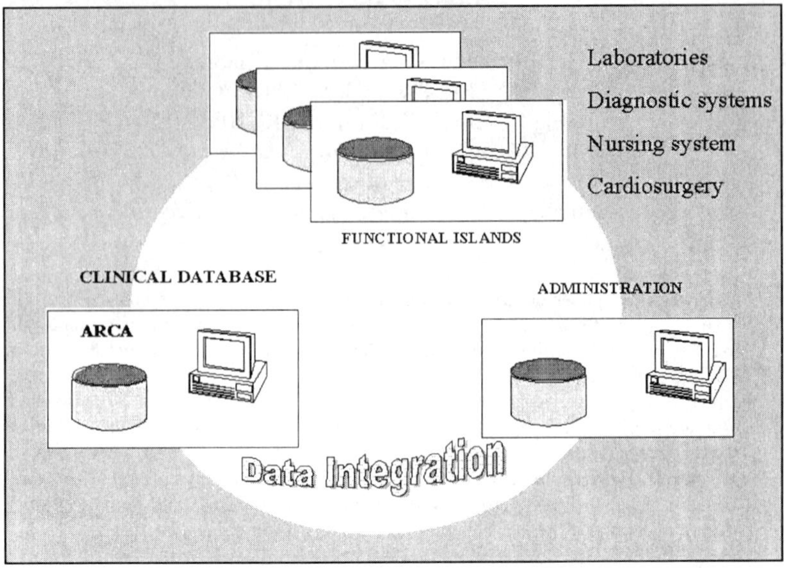

Figure 1 Integration of patient information (SIC-C)

specific aspects of information (i.e. demographic data, medical history, laboratory tests, diagnostic tests) and are associated with the single patient.

WWW technology was applied to develop the EMR system in such a way that any authorized user can access patient data from every workstation within the Intranet hospital infrastructure or outside through Internet, using proper confidentiality and security safeguards [3]. A Java application was developed, accessing ARCA by JDBC standard and allowing patient data entry and consultation through graphical user interface (windows style). HTML documents, produced on the WWW server of the clinical database, were used to represent multimedia patient reports by the use of standard browsers. Use of Java allowed to execute this EMR application, originally developed for MS-Windows platform, on other common platforms (e.g. IBM-OS2, Apple Mac-OS) [4].

The time interval since admission to discharge represents a single "session" of the patient diagnostic-therapeutic process. A new session is opened each time the patient is again admitted (Figure 2). A medical record describes, session by session, patient events as a function of time (e.g. patient history, hospital admission, visit, diagnostic test, surgical operation).

The EMR application is started by a password-based login procedure which allows the identification of the user and the authorization to access patient information. The single patient is selected from the list of the patients currently admitted in the care department under the care of administration, with the exception of emergency situations or network faults when patients need to be admitted directly through EMR session using provisional identifiers. Data concerning medical history or physical examination of patients, who previously accessed to the health care institution, can be retrieved from the database and used in the current patient session after proper editing or updating.

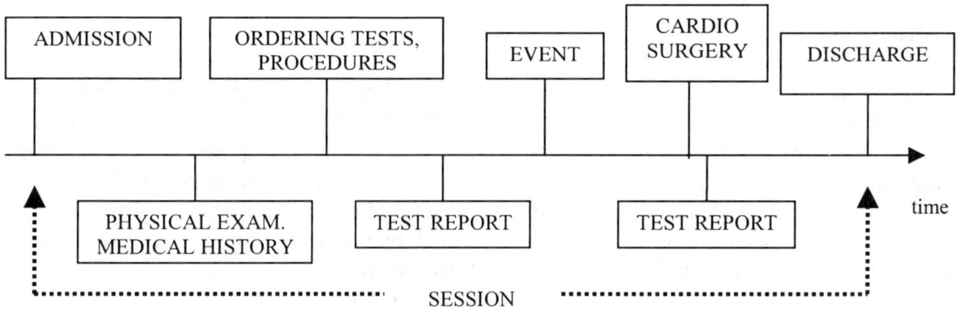

Figure 2 Typical operations of the in-patient "session"

Through the main page of the single patient all the system functions are accessed: data entry, view, editing and consultation (Figure 3). Data entry is made mainly in structured form. Anamnesis is inserted through four sections: physiological, metabolism and hypertension, familiar, pathological. For each pathology or procedure the corresponding ICD9-CM code is stored. Similarly physical examination concerns: general, nervous, cardiovascular, respiratory, abdomen, cutaneous, muscular, urinary. During structured data entry of both anamnesis and physical examination text summaries are automatically generated from structured data and their editing is allowed. These summaries are included in printouts of both medical record and discharge letter.

Most of diagnostic tests are executed in the Functional Islands, which are integrated in the SIC. So, reports are transferred into the database automatically, as soon as they are ready, in two forms: structured records of heterogeneous data (text, signals, images), describing test details, and short text summaries. On the other hand, a number of tests is also executed by external or not yet integrated laboratories and only summary reports can be manually entered. Anyway, in case of breakdown of the SIC system reports need to be inserted manually. Thus, manual data entry of reports has been provided through the EMR interface. Standard classification codes (ICD-9-CM) were associated with pathologies and procedures throughout the EMR in such a way that cost analysis by administration is made possible. Any information acquired on patient during the session is stored into the database and listed in the main page (Figure 3). Pointing and clicking on the list the synthetic view is first obtained (i.e. text summary of the test report); next, the analytic view can be required. The latter is obtained starting the WEB browser for representation of HTML document including, possibly, signals or images.

Information on patient conditions and test scheduling, therapy and diet plans are provided automatically by the Nursing system to the ARCA database. A time-oriented color graphical interface is provided to summarize chronologically (weekly or daily) the patient care events and conditions. Biohumoral parameters (i.e. temperature, weight, blood pressure, pulse rate, liquid balance), provided from Nursing system, are plotted. Patient events (e.g. pain episodes, symptoms), visits, diagnostic and laboratory tests are represented on the time diagram by specific symbols. Pointing and clicking synthetic and analytic views are obtained. Therapy and nutrition plans are also reported.

External data repositories as well as guidelines or knowledge resources can be consulted from EMR main page by the use of standard browsers and navigation through Internet allows to search information of interest from any WWW site.

3. Discussion

The information infrastructure, developed in SPERIGEST project, allowed the integration of the different sources of patient information in the department of Cardiology. Collection of all patient relevant data in the database was crucial to set up the EMR, aimed at supporting healthcare personnel in patient care, but also allowing playback data consultation for clinical research. Use of Java through the Intranet, protected by a firewall system, allowed secure access to patient medical record from almost any workstation equipped with standard browser. Remote EMR consultation through Internet will need to apply special techniques for protecting security and confidentiality. Particular attention was

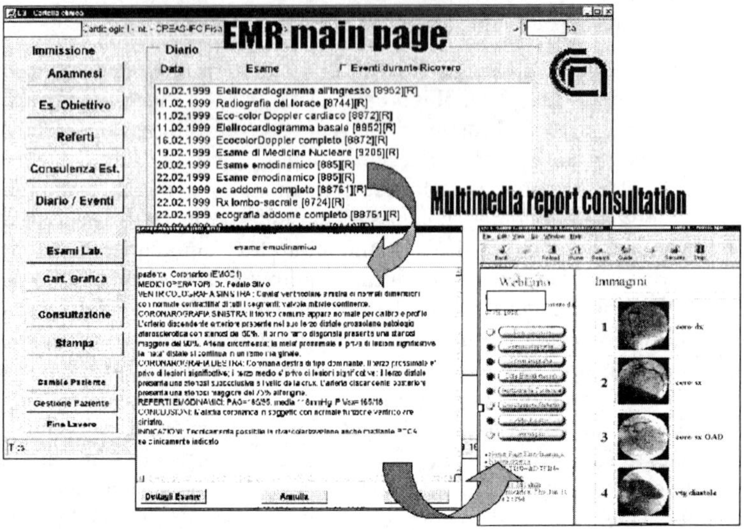

Figure 3 Screen capture showing the main patient page (data entry and consultation functions on the left). The user has selected a report to view (from the report titles list): first text summary report is represented and secondly analytic multimedia report (by WWW browser).

dedicated to the design of the user interface through interaction of health care personnel. The developed model of EMR is currently under clinical evaluation in the Cardiology department.

Acknowledgements. This work was supported by the Special Program of National Health Ministry (project SPERIGEST: art.12 D.Lgs 502/92).

References

[1] Dick R.S., Steen E.B. and Detmer D.E. The computer-based patient record. (revised edition) Washington D.C.: National Academy Press, 1997.

[2] Macerata A., Landucci L., et al. Networking for health care administration and delivery: the information system at the CNR Institute of Clinical Physiology. In: Proceedings of Health Telematics '95. Pisa: Area di Ricerca CNR, 1995, 113-18.

[3] Computer Science and Telecommunication Board. For the record: protecting electronic health information. Washington D.C.: National Academy Press, 1997.

[4] Sittig D.F., Kuperman G.J. and Teich J.M. WWW-based interfaces to clinical information systems: the state of the art. In: Proceedings of 1996 AMIA Annual Fall Symposium. Philadelphia: Hanley & Belfus, 1996, 694-8.

Medical Informatics Europe '99
P. Kokol et al. (Eds.)
IOS Press, 1999

An experimental electronic patient record for stroke patients

M.J. van der Meijden[1], H.J. Tange[1], J.Boiten[2], J.Troost[2], A.Hasman[1]
[1] *Department of Medical Informatics, University of Maastricht, Maastricht, the Netherlands*
[2] *Department of Neurology, Maastricht University Hospital, Maastricht, the Netherlands*

Abstract. This contribution describes an electronic patient record for stroke patients at the neurology ward of the Maastricht University Hospital. Daily practice at the ward will be supported with the developed electronic patient record that integrates both the medical and the nursing record, that will provide decision support and it will be connected to the hospital information system. In an evaluation project we will study the effects of the usage of the electronic patient record and additional effects of providing decision support.

1. Introduction

Time is critically important for the treatment of stroke patients. A patient should be transferred to the hospital as soon as possible after a stroke event. Preferably to a hospital with a special unit, a so-called stroke unit, where patients can receive intensive care and be monitored carefully.[1] The neurology department of the academic hospital in Maastricht participates in a special project to improve the treatment of stroke patients. Upon admission, patients are transferred immediately to the medium care unit, part of the stroke unit of the department. At the ward, a multidisciplinary team takes responsibility for the treatment and care of every admitted stroke patient. In this team neurologists and nurses collaborate with physical therapists, social workers, ergotherapists and speech therapists to optimise (diagnostic) treatment and care for each patient. Adequate and timely information exchange is of high importance here. Currently, nurses and physicians document their findings in separate records. Also other care providers maintain their own records. Moreover, they report in the nursing or the medical record on separate forms.

Generally, it is recognised that paper record keeping does not suffice in the complex environment of modern medicine. It is believed that many of the objections of paper record keeping can be overcome by electronic record keeping. Therefore, we developed an electronic patient record (EPR) to study how the usage of an EPR will affect the treatment of stroke patients, and to study what the effects of the addition of decision support.

This contribution describes the EPR that was developed to facilitate the information exchange between all care providers involved. The decision to develop this system is based on the belief that the multidisciplinary team can collaborate better when using electronic record keeping and that the combined EPR can serve better as a means of communication than the separate paper records can. A connection with the hospital information system (HIS) will be established, so all patient data will be accessible at one spot. The EPR will provide reminders and clinical decision support specifically for neurologists and nurses and it will have a connection to the HIS. The latter elements, however, are not discussed in this paper.

2. Design considerations

Our main concern was to develop a system that would support daily practice at the ward of the neurology department of the Maastricht University Hospital. Therefore, we defined what functionality the EPR should offer. In the first place, it should provide a multi-user environment, since all care providers need access to the same records, probably simultaneously. Second, access rights need to differ between different disciplines. Third, information must be presented from different user perspectives. A fourth requirement is ease of use. In an academic setting residents often change and student-nurses come and go. Therefore, an EPR needs to be easy to learn for novice (computer) users. Clear presentation of data is a fifth requirement. A final aspect that deserves attention is the intended integration of our EPR with the HIS.

The Maastricht University Hospital is adapting its HIS to a more up-to-date system. A new user interface in a Windows 95 environment, Mirador (trademark of Hiscom), will give us the opportunity to connect with the HIS to present all patient data, including laboratory results, in one record.

A crucial element of an EPR is the user interface. [2] As far as possible we adapted our system to the Windows 95 standards in terms of lay-out, screen handling, the usage of right mouse buttons, etc. Since data need to be entered by care providers themselves, data entry forms have a recognisable format. Furthermore, predefined (multiple) choices are presented wherever possible. Recently, both the medical record and the nursing record were investigated thoroughly to create structured paper forms. Those forms were implemented with only slight lay-out changes.

Presentation of patient data is an important element of the EPR user interface. In a previous research project conducted at our department, presentation of patient data was studied. The contents of the records were ordered in a treestructure according to source and data were presented in a matrix. Physicians were asked to browse the medical narratives that were offered in more or less detailed paragraphs, also described as differences in granularity of data. The results pointed out that both too large and too small paragraphs slowed retrieving relevant information. [3] We based our system on the experimental electronic medical record, developed in that study.

In the design phase of the system we communicated intensively with the future users to obtain their information needs and wishes. In close cooperation with them, we formulated several criteria for the system and its user interface. These criteria were: a) simple data entry forms with predefined (multiple) choices and only limited free text entries, b) data entry forms based on the structured paper record forms, c) clear overview of patient data in data retrieval forms, d) integration of the nursing and medical record. Patient data are oftentimes registered more than once. Integration of the nursing and medical records resolves this inconvenience and eliminates a potential source of errors. Furthermore, discharge summaries and a nursing working list should be easy to compose and print.

3. System Description

We developed an electronic patient record (EPR), consisting of a database containing information about both the structure and the content of de patient record, a user interface, several programming modules, and a research module with a logging function. The system was implemented in a Windows 95 environment. We used a MS Access 97 database and MS Visual Basic 5.0 for developing the system.

3.1. *Data entry*

Most data entry forms were based on the paper forms already in use at the ward. The medical record captures many data in a structured format, while in the nursing record the daily report was completely structured. At admission, results of medical history and physical examination are registered on one data entry form. Tabs are used to distinguish three different sections. Many questions were formulated as multiple choice items, with an option to add remarks in free text. Figure 1 shows one section of that form. Medical progress notes are divided into eight sections. Three sections (medication, complications and diagnostic tests) support structured data entry. The assessment notes, reports of talks with the patient and his/her family and the notes of consulting physicians are composed of free text entries. All entries are presented chronologically, the most recent entry first. In addition, the list of vital signs filled in by the nurses is presented in a separate section.

Nursing history is registered on a data entry form, presenting some patient data already filled in by the neurologist on medical data entry forms. Most of the remaining entries can be made by choosing from predefined lists. The medium care unit of the ward reports vital signs, motor and sensory functions, consciousness etc. on a 24 hour form.

As mentioned above, the nurses' daily report was already structured in its paper form. Several aspects of the patient's health status are scored on a predefined list and presented in a one week view. In one glimpse a patient's health status can be assessed.

Order communication between nurses and physicians is registered a special form. Unanswered questions and not (yet) completed orders are marked blue and yellow respectively.

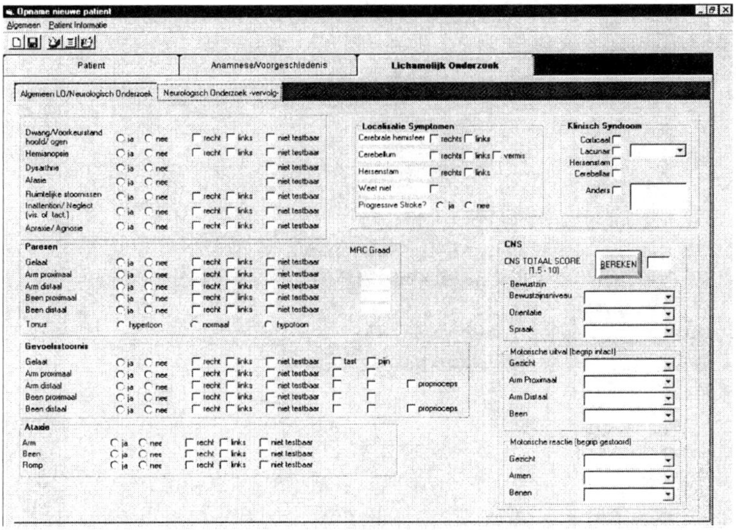

Figure 1. Example of structured data entry form of the EPR. The physical examination (motor and sensibility dysfunctions) is reported in a structured format.

Not only nurses and physicians need access to patient data, also the physical therapist, the social worker etc do. In the current situation they report on a special form adhered to the nursing record. In addition to the nursing and medical record we offer free text entries for other disciplines with separate sections for different disciplines.

3.2. *Presentation of patient data*

The main data retrieval form contains three sections (figure 2). A left pane with a hierarchical list of the content of the medical and nursing records, comparable with the left pane of the windows explorer containing the folders. The list can described as a tree with branches and leaves. By clicking, branches can be expanded to show subbranches or to show the leaves, called endnodes. Clicking the endnodes presents the patient data in the top section of the right pane. The top section of the right pane shows an overview of the selected data in a day by day or week by week view. Data in the top section can be selected column-wise and row-wise and the complete data are presented in the lower section of the right pane.

4. Future plans

At the moment the EPR is still under construction. Although it does not yet contain all of the required functionality, the system has been assessed positively by the future users. We expect to start the evaluation in daily practice in September 1999. The evaluation will be conducted to answer our research questions. Our principal research question is how the use of an electronic patient record will affect record keeping and the process of care and what effects the addition of decision support will have. In a pre/post designed study we will study several aspects of the patient record itself as well as the process of care. First of all, completeness of the record will be evaluated. We expect a more complete record with electronic record keeping. Secondly, the communication at the ward as a part of the process of care will be evaluated in a qualitative way. [4]

Finally, since the success of the system will depend heavily on the acceptance by its users, user satisfaction and user attitudes will be measured in every phase. For this reason, we developed a questionnaire, based on questionnaires described in the literature. [5-11] Users' navigation through patient data will be recorded in a research database.

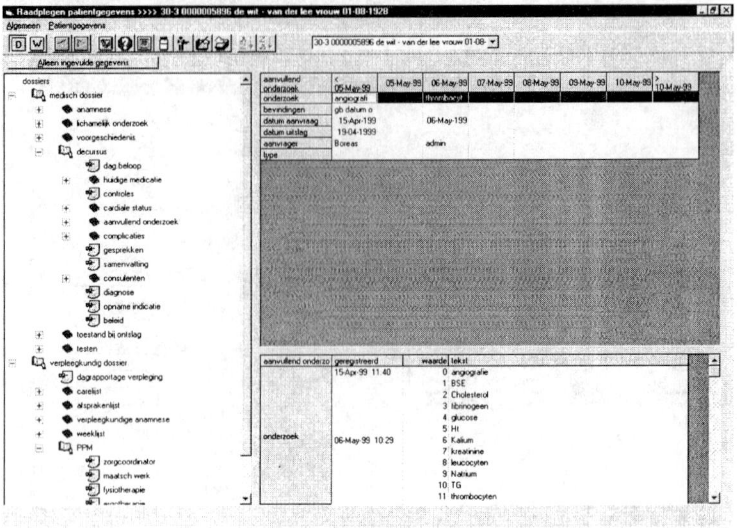

Figure 2. The main data retrieval form. View of both the medical (=medisch dossier) and the nursing records (=verpleegkundig dossier) in the left pane. The upper right section presents an overview of this patient's medical, vascular history. The lower right section presents the complete content of selected items.

References

[1] P. Langhorne, B. O. Williams, W. Gilchrist, K. Howie. Do stroke units save lives? Lancet, **342** (1993) 395-398.

[2] P. C. Tang, V. L. Patel. Major issues in user interface design for health professional workstations: summary and recommendations. Int J Biomed Comput, **34** (1994) 139-48.

[3] H. J. Tange, H. C. Schouten, A. D. M. Kester, A. Hasman. The granularity of medical narratives and its effect on the speed and completeness of information retrieval. JAMIA, **5** (1998) 571-582.

[4] C. P. Friedman, J. G. Wyatt. Evaluation methods in medical informatics in Evaluation methods in medical informatics, eds. H. F. Orthner, pp. 311 (Springer-Verlag, New York, 1997).

[5] T. S. Startsman, R. E. Robinson. The attitudes of medical and paramedical personnel toward computers. Comput Biomed Res, **5** (1972) 218-227.

[6] R. L. Teach, E. H. Shortliffe. An analysis of physician attitudes regarding computer-based clinical consultation systems. Comp Biomed Res, **14** (1981) 542-558.

[7] J. E. Bailey, S. W. Pearson. Development of a tool for measuring and analyzing computer user satisfaction. Mangement Science, **29** (1983) 530-545.

[8] S. H. Brown, R. D. Coney. Changes in physicians' computer anxiety and attitudes related to clinical information system use. JAMIA, **1** (1994) 381-394.

[9] J. R. Lewis. IBM computer usability satisfaction questionnaires: psychometric evaluation and instructions for use. Int J Human-Comput Interact, **7** (1995) 57-78.

[10] H. J. Tange. The paper-based medical record - Is it really obsolete? Comput Methods Programs Biomed, **48** (1995) 127-131.

[11] R. D. Cork, W. M. Detmer, C. P. Friedman. Development and initial validation of an instrument to measure physician's use of, knowledge about, and attitudes towards computers. JAMIA, **5** (1998) 164-176.

Medical Informatics Europe '99
P. Kokol et al. (Eds.)
IOS Press, 1999

QUALIDIAB: Implementation of the Diabcare project in the french-speaking environment: regional, national and international issues

R. Beuscart (1), M.P. VanHoecke (2), P. Devos (1), R.Allouche (3), L. Kleinebreil (3), and the Qualidiab Group (3).
1 - CERIM – Faculté de Médecine, Université de Lille II, 1, Place Verdun, 59045 Lille Cedex (F)
2 – LIFL –USTL – 59650 Villeneuve d'Ascq (F)
3 – Qualidiab Group

Abstract. Diabcare is an international Project devoted to the evaluation of the Quality of Care [1] in the population of diabetic patients. As Diabetes is one of the most frequent chronic illnesses, the management of its treatment has a strong impact on the public health policy both regional and national [2]. Funded by the European Commission, initiated by WHO and the International Diabetes Federation (IDF), this Project is now recognised as a Pilot Project throughout the world as an example of a large international collaboration for the surveillance of quality of care in a typical chronic disease.

1 Objective

The objectives of the project are (1): To collect relevant, coherent and valid information from different practices (hospitals / specialists / GPs), from different regions, from different countries in Europe for use in the assessment of the quality of care management in Diabetes. These data are coherent as the patient's file was designed according to the St Vincent's Declaration, so the format of the record is quite identical from one site to another. (2) To aggregate these data for extensive statistical analysis (figure 1). (3) To give access to these information through the easiest telematics procedures. (4) To use state-of-the-art security procedures and make the system compatible with the implementation of professional cards at the doctor's office.

2 Methods

Similar paper forms were designed to collect data concerning the diabetic patients management. These forms are filled by doctors in the hospitals or in their offices during or after a regular consultation. Campaigns are organised once a year in November or in January. The paper forms are then gathered and transmitted to the central office where they are collected and computerised for further exploitation. Statistical analyses are performed to identify similarities and differences in the ways diabetic people are treated and followed, and to analyse the objective results of this management. Results are obtained through paper reports but are now reachable through the internet, thus giving every participant a secure and personalised access to the relevant information.

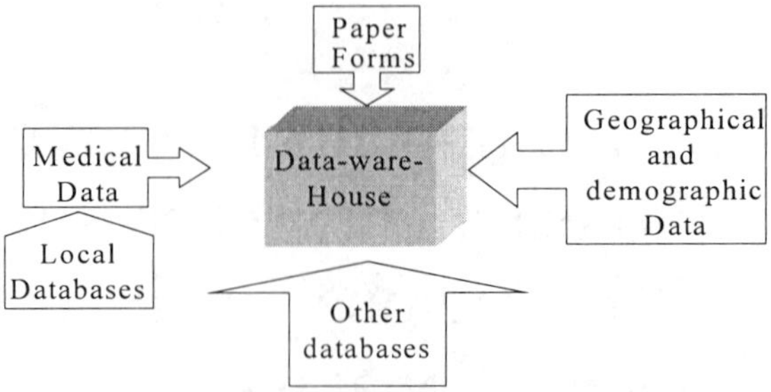

Figure 1 : QUALIDIAB : An international network sending Data to a common Warehouse for exploitation.

3 Results

A large Oracle™ DataBase was designed to gather all the files collected in different places, regions, countries and nations. This DataBase, situated in Lille (France) allows for the management of all the items included in the St Vincent Protocol. A Data Mining System using Oracle Express™ and SAS™ tools permits a rapid and interactive exploitation of the DataBase. Results can be obtained at different levels: doctor level, organisation level, regional level, national level. Geographical analyses can be performed. Comparative analyses are made easy through this process.

As the access to the results is essential for the doctors as well as for the Healthcare authorities, the World Wide Web access was designed to allow two types of interactions: (1) for every healthcare professional, access to fixed quantitative descriptive results describing the modalities of treatments of Diabetic patients throughout Europe; and (2) for the providers of information, an interactive access to the Data-warehouse allowing on-line data analyses for refinements of statistical investigations.

4 Discussion

In 1997, 4145 patients records were collected and analysed, giving a comprehensive view of the diversity in the treatment, management and follow-up of diabetic patients with striking consequences on the pathologic complications of the disease. In 1998, the campaign will include new refinements with exhaustive data collection in some regions for a better epidemiological survey. Computer patient records are also being experimented to collect data more easily and for their telematics transmission through internet.

5 Conclusion

Diabcare campaigns are now routine in Europe for thousands of doctors and medical organisations. The extensive statistical analysis of the patients database gives relevant information to professionals and Healthcare authorities so they can have a better comparative knowledge of the medical status of patients in a dedicated area. Correction of routine dysfunctions and improvements in patient management are expected from this large dissemination of information.

References

[1] M. Angell, J.. Kassirer, Quality and the medical Marketplace – following elephants. N.Engl J Med., 1996; 335: pp. 883-885.

[2] C.D. Naylor, What is appropriate Care ? N. Engl. J. med., 1998; 338: pp. 1918-1920.

Medical Informatics Europe '99
P. Kokol et al. (Eds.)
IOS Press, 1999

The Electronic Patient Records of the Hannover Medical School

A. J. PORTH, C. NIEHOFF, H. K. MATTHIES
Medical Computing Center, Hannover Medical School, D-30623 Hannover, Germany

Abstract. In this paper, the succesfull introduction of a commercially available electronic patient record archiving system at the Hannover Medical School is described. Since 1996, more than 11 million document sheets of 130.000 patient records have been stored electronically. Currently, 100.000 sheets are stored each week.

1. The Hospital Network is the Electronic Patient Record

In the 1970s and 1980s several computer-based medical record systems were introduced that evolved to systems used in many medical disciplines, completely integrated with the hospital information system, and extended with various kinds of decision support [1]. Since 1990, many electronic patient record systems have been developed world-wide [2, 3]. The increasing importance of the electronic patient record is dramatically changing the workflow in healthcare organisations. In conjunction with this gradual progression from a distributed, mostly paperbased record to its electronic equivalent, many requirements arise, especially regarding confidentiality. In todays healthcare institutions, systems for electronic medical records tend to be implemented with proprietary interfaces on various operating systems and a variety of methods for storage of data. This aggravates sharing of medical data not only between different institutions, but in many cases already between different departments in an institution. These interconnected departments include administration, clinical departments, laboratories, imaging, medical record archiving systems. The incorporation of data management technologies in such clinical communication networks (e.g. communication server DataGate [4]) allows data transmission between all distributed systems which contain patient's administrative and medical data. Therefore one can say: *The hospital network is the electronic patient record.*

Access to medical data is an aggregation of many distinct aspects, such as identification and authentication of the user, access rights for consultation, modification and completion of data, storage, backup, archiving of data, encryption and transmission, data integrity and audatibility [5].

Another point is that almost all medical records have to be stored for a fixed period of time, depending on contents and the legal situation in the respective countries. Therefore, in addition to making sure that there is no breach in security concerning access to and storage of data, one has to take care that the chosen storage method does not prohibit future use of the data due to advances in technology. Electronic patient records should not only be considered as an electronic extension of the conventional paper form, but as an enhanced way of storing all health information. The ideal implementation of a system for electronic medical records would include not only the actual information recorded about a patient, but also offer context sensitive background information, e.g. access to online medical databases or, when feasible, record systems of other health care providers to support clinical problem solving when necessary [6].

Special care has to be taken when it comes to the way the data are to be entered into the system. Whenever the desired data have to be expressed in words instead of values, the question is what vocabulary to use. In many cases, it would be the easiest way for medical personnel to input the data in the traditional free text form that is used in todays paper records.

2. The Medical Record Archiving System ALIDA

An even simpler way to store medical data is realized by using the commercially [7] medical record archiving system ALIDA (Arzt und Leistungsstellen unterstuetzendes Informationssystem der digitalen Dokumenten-Archivierung) that is employed for storage and retrieval of medical records at the Medical School Hannover [8, 9]. This is not only an electronic patient record in the traditional sense, but offers more possibilities than a pure storage system. The data are still primarily being recorded on the traditional paper forms. In addition to micro-filming everything, the records are digitized at 200 dpi using a scanner camera and then stored on WORMs. This has proven sufficient for later retrieval over a client PC and is being accepted by the medical staff. The system has a real capacity for digitalization of about 5,000 pages per hour. Because the contents of the records are categorized before digitalization, retrieval of data is more efficient than the traditional storage on microfiche. The high availability by using client server technology is another advantage. Client systems are simply placed wherever necessary and allow access to patient data 24h a day, provided that there is sufficient authorization for retrieval. Access to data is allowed using a role based model to manage the access rights. Authentication of users can be achieved using many different technologies.

For example, a screen shot of the ALIDA query mask (Fig. 1) for retrieval of electronic patient records shows various search criteria: patient (identification) id-number, surname, first name, admission number.

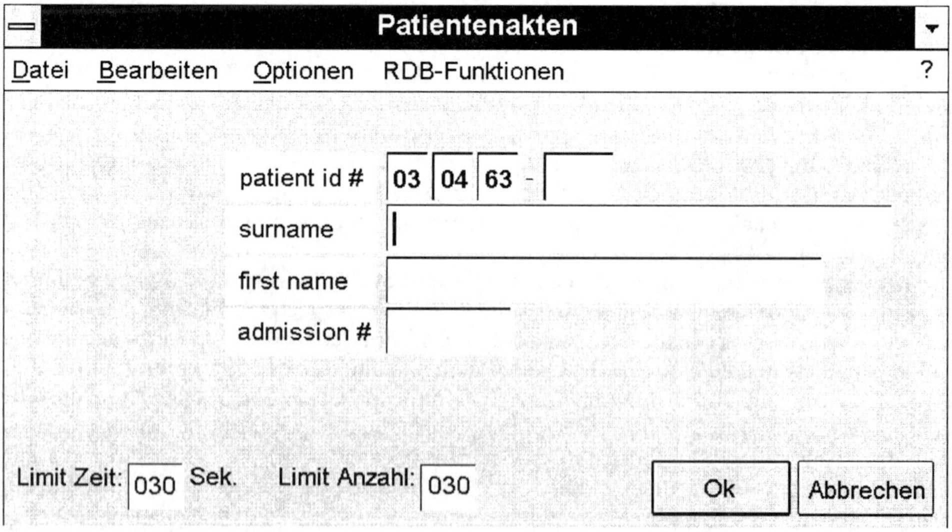

Figure 1: ALIDA query mask for retrieval of electronic patient records

The unambiguous patient identification criterium is the **patient id-number** (10 digits structure **dd.mm.yy-nnso**: birth date, class of birth name, sex, ordinal) which is created at the Hannover Medical School. This number is consistently used in patient administration and all clinical department systems since 1972. Today are more than 1 million different patient id-numbers processed. In figure 2, the result list for the above query is shown. Detailed information for each line record is possible via "mouse-click".

Patientendokumente 11/0/11

I-Zahl patient id-number	Name	Uorname	A S	Aufn. nummer	Entl. datum	Entl. Stat.	Archiu datum	Typ	Sei- ten
03.04.63-5710	MÜ [redacted] w	Gert	S	96025132	15.03.96	33	26.10.96	A	14
03.04.63-5710	MÜ [redacted] w	Gert	S	96025132	15.03.96	33	26.10.96	B	58
03.04.63-5710	MÜ [redacted] w	Gert	S	96025132	15.03.96	33	26.10.96	D	2
03.04.63-5710	MÜ [redacted] w	Gert	S	96025132	15.03.96	33	26.10.96	S	28
03.04.63-5710	MÜ [redacted] w	Gert	S	96025132	15.03.96	33	26.10.96	U	12

Anzeige weitere Daten Abbrechen

Figure 2: Result list

The medical record archiving system ALIDA is powerful. Figure 3 shows that in the last two years more than 130.000 patient records with over 11 million patient document sheets have been digitally recorded. Approximately 100.000 new patient document sheets are being scanned and stored into the ALIDA system each week. The ALIDA search possibilities are used for healthcare (60%) and scientific research (40%), approximately 20.000 patient document sheets are being retrieved each week.

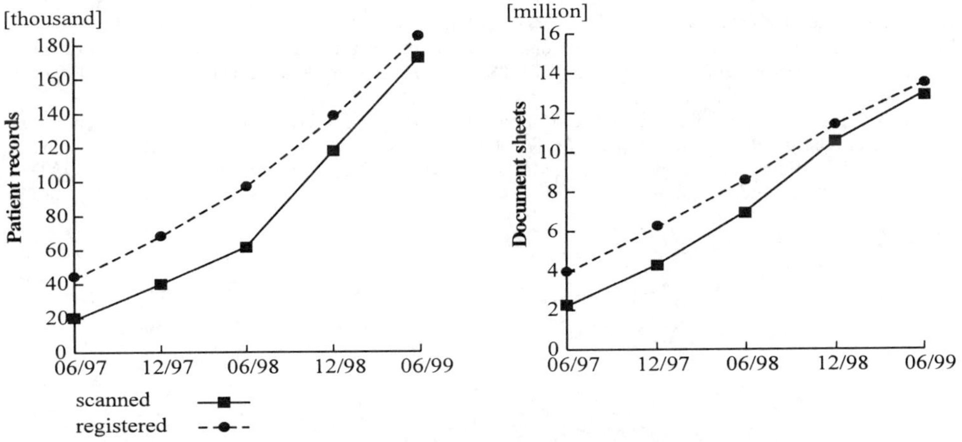

Figure 3: Number of patient records (left) and number of document sheets (right)

3. Results

The implementation of an electronic patient record system is a long and difficult process. Its introduction involves major personnel, organizational and technological changes. In addition to a modified network infrastructure, it requires continuous sharing of new concepts, approaches, experiences, technologies, facilities and services.

The functional requirements of an information system, security aspects of the system and a model of possible threats all influence a security policy. Users must be especially sensitized about security concerns and the consequences of carelessness (e.g. handling of passwords) when it comes to managing data in modern information systems to eliminate possible security holes due to ignorance. Transmitting data securely is another aspect that has to be taken under consideration. In todays information systems, asymmetric cryptographic algorithms are generally used to negotiate so called session keys while symmetric methods are employed for the actual encryption and decryption.

In the future, a multimedia patient record will make it possible to compile an electronic p.o. box that contains findings and records from a patient's history as well as records about a patient from other departmental systems or digital archives (e.g. neuroradiology). The use of modern telematics allows for secure, worldwide transmission of the contents of an electronic p.o. box. The authenticity of the documents may be determinded by examination of a digital signature.

References

[1] H.J. Tange, A. hasman, P.F. de Vries Robbe, H.C. Schouten, Medical narratives in electronic medical records. In: J. van Bemmel, A.T. McCray (Eds.), Yearbook of Medical Informatics 1998, Stuttgart, pp. 230-252.

[2] P. Waegemann (Ed.), Proceedings Toward an Electronic Health Record Europe'96. London: CAEHR 1996.

[3] C.J. Atkinson, V.J. Peel, Transforming a Hospital through Growing, not Building, an Electronic Patient Record System. In: *Meth. Inform. Med.* **37**, 1998, pp. 285-293.

[4] http://www.stc.com

[5] T. Fiers, F. de Meyer, Confidentiality and Accessibility in the EHCR. In: P.W. Moorman, J. van der Lei, M.A. Musen (Eds.), Electronic Patient Records in Medical Practice. Rotterdam, 1998, pp. 245-247.

[6] H.K. Matthies, U. v. Jan, A.J. Porth, General Aspects of Electronic Medical Records in a Clinical Environment. In: P.W. Moorman, J. van der Lei, M.A. Musen (Eds.), Electronic Patient Records in Medical Practice. Rotterdam, 1998, pp. 245-247.

[7] CE datronic Medical Services GmbH, Kurzes Gelaend 6, D-86156 Augsburg, Germany

[8] A.J. Porth, C. Niehoff, ALIDA, das digitale Dokumentenarchivierungssystem der Medizinischen Hochschule Hannover. In: C. Hartung (Ed): TK '97 – Technik im Krankenhaus. Hannover, 1997, pp. 224-238.

[9] A.J. Porth, C. Niehoff, R. Weiss, H.K. Matthies, Das Pilotprojekt ALIDA – erste Erfahrungen bei der Einfuehrung digitaler Patientenakten. In: R. Muche, G. Buechele, D. Harder, W. Gaus, Medizinische Informatik, Biometrie und Epidemiologie GMDS '97. MMV Medizin, Muenchen, 1997, pp. 284-289.

Medical Informatics Europe '99
P. Kokol et al. (Eds.)
IOS Press, 1999

DIABCARD Core System - A Chip Card Medical Information System For Diabetes Care

G. Gogou[a], A. Mavromatis[a], N. Maglaveras[a], C. Pappas[a], R. Engelbrecht[b]
[a] *Laboratory of Medical Informatics, Aristotelian University of Thessaloniki, Greece*
[b] *GSF Research Center, Medis-Institute, Munich, Neuherberg, Germany*

Abstract: A chip card based medical information system was developed as a good possibility to create a portable electronic patient record. The produced software module provides an on-line, portable diabetes medical record information system. In particular the patient data card makes the up-to-date patient's record available whenever needed. The developed Core System includes a patient record management system that has the ability to handle topics such as medical anamnesis, administrative, medical and physical examination data. Issues tackled were simplicity, data security and reporting. Customization and internationalization were also covered by presenting a novel approach using native initialization files. Proper care has been addressed during the development of the software modules for matters of security, data integrity and confidentiality.

1. Introduction

Effective patient treatment requires the healthcare personnel to know the patient's accurate and complete (as possible) medical history. Patients may be put at risk if additional treatment is unknown. The use of a smart card for storing part of the Computer-based Patient Record (CPR) renders this information available when and where it is needed. The long-term goal of the DIABCARD project is to improve the quality of care in chronic diseases by applying state-of-the-art technology for documentation and communication [1]. The DIABCARD installation is based on the improvement of inter-hospital communication, communication between diabetes centers and between diabetes centers and GPs. The architecture of the DIABCARD is flexible and adaptable to technological advance of the chip card [2]. The medical documentation of the Chip Card based Medical Information System (CCMIS) is based on a common set of terms and definitions compliant to the EU/G7 specification and DIABCARD Data Set. These definitions were also used in other projects such as EURODIABETA, DIABCARE, and DIABCARD and agreed upon by the medical partners of the DIABCARD-3 project [1,3,4]. The St. Vincent Declaration includes a commitment to improve the quality in diabetes care on a continuous basis [5]. Databases for diabetes management can be administered in two ways: (a) as a population register and (b) as a clinical management system. The first approach is designed for people living in a particular place and is mainly used for annual medical review, like the Dialog system [6]. The second one (clinical management system) is incorporated into the clinical process and the main target is the improved function of the administration of care.

The success of any database system for diabetes care is dependent upon several critical factors like the co-operation and continuing involvement of physicians, the acceptance and use by them of a standard data set, user friendliness and the ability to modify the system [7]. These factors can be accomplished by object-oriented approach, which has received increased attention recently especially in medical computer environments [8,9]. One reason, is that it seeks to mimic the way that models of the real world (entities) are formed, constrains are put on them and relationships among objects are defined [10]. In contrast to the procedural way of thinking, it de-emphasises the underlying computer representation by handling *objects*, which are used to symbolise real-world entities and their interaction [11, 12]. Every object can encapsulate a state (attribute) and a behaviour (method) and allow only a pre-specified set of operations to act upon itself.

2. Methods

A CCMIS was used as a good possibility to replace paper records. The Patient Data Card (PDC) makes the up-to-date patient's record available whenever it is needed. The analysis stage was centralized in the development of a patient record management system that can handle topics such as administrative, medical anamnesis and physical examination data. Proper care has been paid during the development of the software modules for the following matters: **(a) Simplicity:** The system has to deal with a large amount of data fields of various types and also it was a prerequisite that the program should be user friendly. So the MS-Windows'95 environment was chosen for the development of user friendly forms and functions that the software had to cover. **(b) Customization and Internationalization:** These are two other issues that are handled by the program through the use of external "table set-up files" (TBL files) which contain data field descriptions and form properties. During the form creation stage of the software, the above files are used to dynamically produce the final output of the form on the screen. The customization of the TBL files allows the system to have a multilingual dimension and offers the ability for each site to setup the system environment parameters according to local terms that are used in routine procedures. **(c) Data security:** In order to achieve data security, a user management system was developed to prevent unauthorized persons from accessing the patients' data. **(d) Reporting:** A flexible reporting system was developed giving the end-users the ability to create and customize their own reports according to their needs using Structured Data Entry (SDE).

The CPR handles the following functionalities: administrative, patient record administration, document administration, data import/export, CPR dynamic browsing, user defined reporting, Chip card input/output and user management.

2.1. Analysis and Design

The medical record of the DIABCARD Core System is *Document Oriented.* Every record of medical data items is linked to a record in a document table, the document is linked to a table of patient visits and every visit is linked to a patient. This means that for every patient's visit the user has to fill out documents as in every routine of a paper based medical record system. Each document can have one of the following states: "created", "in-work", "signed" or "rejected". Once a document is "created" it can be edited ("in-work") until it is "signed". Signed documents can only be "rejected" and they can not be deleted from the medical record.

The data structure of the DIABCARD Core System was based on the DIABCARD Data Set version 2.2. To enforce interoperability the Data Set took into account the data and existing data sets from other projects related to the DIABCARD, like CHIC for the socio-demographic data [13], the EUROCARDS Working Group 3 for administrative data [14], the approved EURODIABETA Diabetes Data Set [4] and the DiabCare Basic Information Sheet (i.e. the implementation of the St Vincent Declaration) for medical data [15].

The database system manages data tables of patient data, patient visits, documents and lookup tables. The field names for the EU/G7 data (administrative and emergency data) and the Medical data match the ID of the corresponding item in the data set so that they can be easily accessed in the future from other applications. Every type of document has a corresponding TBL control file that defines which items will be included in the document. These TBL files can be altered through an included tool that guides the administrator through user-friendly dialogs and multi-choice selections. So each site can customize the program according to language and local terms that are used in routine procedures.

2.2. Chip Card Access

The file structuring on the DIABCARD chip card implements an ISO-7816 file system. EU/G7 interoperable data, ensuring interoperability with other similar projects, are stored in three distinct Elementary Files (EF): (a) EU/G7 card data, (b) EU/G7 administrative data, (c) EU/G7 medical emergency data. The contents of these data sets are defined within the DIABCARD DataSet. While the DIABCARD Data Interface provides access to the contents of these files via predefined tags. DIABCARD medical data, not contained within the three interoperability data sets, are stored in one single EF.

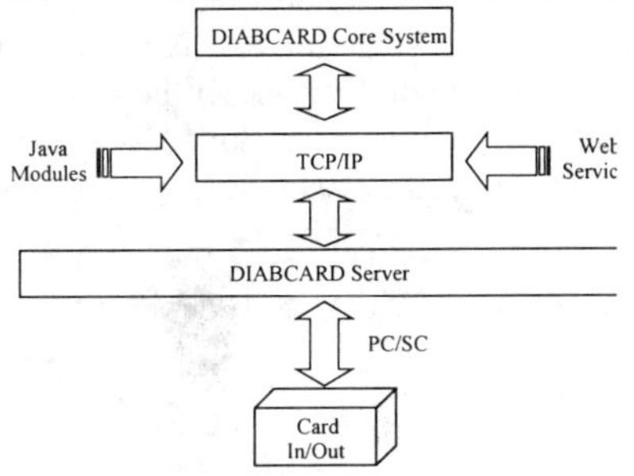

Figure 1: The DIABCARD Core System/DIABCARD Server interface

The DIABCARD Core System is using the DIABCARD Server developed by ACG SmartGate for accessing the chip card through a TCP/IP Interface (figure 1). This Interface can be integrated into existing medical information systems, allowing access to the chip card data through PC/SC interface. Also, the DIABCARD Server (not described in this paper) ensures that application programs are independent of the used chip card reader, chip card operating system, security algorithms and of details concerning data location and file structure on the card.

The data structures for the communication with the DIABCARD Server are coded in the form Tag-Length-Value (TLV). The tag contains of 1-4 bytes and is the indication of the data object. The length indicates the length of the bytes and of the value field and contains of 1-4 bytes. The value field contains the necessary data in byte coding or in TLV coding, when the data objects are put together. The field length determines the size of the necessary data.

3. Results

The system is currently being tested by clinicians in Greece, Spain, Italy, Germany and Austria. The environment is proven to be user friendly and was initially accepted by the clinicians. Complexity of the DIABCARD data set seems difficult to be handled by the users that prefer to deal with smaller amounts of data. Thus two general documents, the B.I.S. (Basic Information Sheet) and D.P. (Diabetes Passport), that can be filled in or created automatically from the common data of other documents, are the only data subsets that are for the moment agreed to be stored on the chip card.

Also the Custom Document Creation Wizard tool and the Document Customization tool that give the end-users the ability to create custom documents in their own language was another advantage that proved to be very important for the system users. Moreover, the reporting functionality was well accepted by the physicians, because it follows a well organised structured data entry through a field tree of possible user choices with the combination of free text input.

4. Discussion

In conclusion, the produced system can provide an on-line, secure and portable diabetes medical record that uses the advanced technology of chip cards. It offers extensive management of large amount of data fields in a user friendly multilingual man machine interface, user manageable reporting system with the ability to dynamically expand the internal data structure and functionalities. Because of the object-oriented design of the Core System the application can be easily upgraded and extended taking advantage of the work that has already been done. New Document objects can be derived from existing ones to satisfy special needs that may come up in the future.

References

[1] Bohm V et al. *DIABCARD: Specification of data structures formats and communication protocols. Diabcard Report*: GSF Medis Institut, 1997.
[2] Engelbrecht R, Hildebrand C, Jung E. The smart card: an ideal tool for a computer-based patient record. *Medinfo* 1995; 8: 344-348.
[3] Engelbrecht R, Hildebrand C, Brugues E, De Leiva A, Corcoy R. "DIABCARD – an application of a portable medical record for persons with diabetes", *Medical Informatics* 1996; 21 (4): 273-282.
[4] EURODIABETA, Information Technology for diabetes care in Europe: the EURODIABETA initiative. *Diabetic Medicine*, 1990; 7:536-560.
[5] World Health Organisation (Europe) and International Diabetes Federation (Europe). Diabetes Care and Research in Europe: The St Vincent Declaration. *Diabetic Medicine*, 1990; 7, 360.
[6] Vaughan N.J.A, Shaw M, Boer F, Billett D, Martin C. Creation of a District Diabetes Register Using the DIALOG System. *Diabetic Medicine*, 1996; 13: 175-181.
[7] Kopelman P.G, Sanderson A.J. Application of Database Systems in Diabetes Care. *Medical Informatics* 1996; 21 (4): 259-271.
[8] Pappas C, Mavromatis A, Maglaveras N, Tsikotis A, Pangalos G, Ambrosiadou V. Cardiological database management system as a mediator to clinical decision support. *Methods Inf Med* 1996 Mar;35(1):52-58
[9] Pappas C, Tsikotis A, Mavromatis A, Pashalouthi V, Pangalos G, Maglaveras N. Cardiological database management using object-oriented analysis. In: *MIE Proceedings* 1993; 758-61.
[10] Coad P, Yourdon E. *Object-Oriented Analysis*. Yourdon Press, New Jersey 1990.
[11] Deux O. The Story of O_2. *IEEE Trans Knowl and Data Eng* 1990; 2(1):91-108.
[12] Kim W. Object-Oriented: Definition and research directions. *IEEE Trans. Knowl. Data Eng.* 1990;2 (3):327-41.
[13] CHIC, The Chic Project – Project Summary. Advanced Informatics in Medicine DG XIII, 1990.
[14] Markwell D.C. Administrative uses of patient data cards. In *Health Cards 1995* (Amsterdam: IOS Press) 1995 : 284-287.
[15] Piwernetz K, et al. Monitoring the targets of the St Vincent Declaration and the implementation of quality management in diabetes care: the DiabCare initiative. *Diabetic Medicine*, 1995; 10:371-377.

Medical Informatics Europe '99
P. Kokol et al. (Eds.)
IOS Press, 1999

Electronic Patient Record for N.N.Burdenko Neurosurgical Institute: on the Verge of Implementation

M.A.Shifrin, E.E.Kalinina
Medical informatics laboratory,
N.N.Burdenko Neurosurgical Institute,
Moscow, Russia

Abstract. This presentation is the first report about development of Electronic Patient Record System (EPRS) for N.N.Burdenko Neurosurgical Institute (NSI). This EPR system is the core of Integrated Automatic Information System intended to support all buisness processes running in the Institute. A new technology for developing information systems in poorly formalized subject domains, named IBS/Records, was was created.

1. Basic theses

The aim of developing of EPRS – implementation of computer technology of documenting of diagnostic and treatment process.

Context of developing of EPRS – EPRS is a component of Integrated Automatic Information System (IAIS) which is intended to support all business processes running in NSI. The main goal of developing and implementing IAIS is *to create integrated information environment of the Institute using modern computer technologies as the basis.* EPRS may be considered as the forepart and the core of IAIS at one time. It's important to emphasize that IAIS as a whole and EPRS as a part are treated as integrated systems from the very beginning. Developing of EPRS isn't integrating of existing working places, on the contrary, working places are designed as functional and interface solutions based on the unique platform.

NSI possess 300 neurosurgical beds, 40 beds in ICU, outpatient department, full set of diagnostic equipment (including several MRI and CT devices, digital angiografy device, devices for nuclear diagnostics and therapy) and, in near future, 30 beds for reabilitaion and 30 beds for nuclear therapy. About 3000 patients with all kinds of neurosurgical pathology are treated every year.

Hardware. NSI possess modern LAN built as a star with collapsed backbone. The central switching node has two CELLplex 7000 – ATM-devices of 3Com. Structured cable system consists of fiber cables for vertical traces and UTP Cat.5 for horizontal ones. There are about 600 sockets for PC and the same number of phone sockets.

The cluster consisting of two IBM RS600 Model J40 is used as a database server, IBM PC-servers work as NT-domain, file and other servers.

System software. The main network OS is Windows NT, working stations of IAIS will run under Windows 95/98/NT. Oracle 7 under AIX is chosen as DBMS for EPRS.

Developers. Network infrastructure and special software for EPRS are designed and mounted by Moscow company IBS, one of the leading system integrators in Russia. Working places and system functions of EPRS are actualized by NSI medical informatics laboratory.

2. Subject domain dependence

At the very beginning of the EPRS' designing developers stated that many of architectural and interface solutions will be specified by particularities of the basic subject domain, which has it's own traditional information technologies, and by characteristic features of information environment in which EPRS will run.

Specific features of subject domain and information technologies. In our case dealing with clinical medicine next basic statements may be accentuated:

- any patient record – paper or electronic – is intended to make sure of integrity of diagnostic and treatment process in space and time;
- many specialists are involved in generating of patient record and they observe patients in asynchronous mode;
- traditional paper patient records (PPR) have many serious disadvantages, and eliminating of them is one of principal goals of ERP implementation; at the same time the structure of PPR is the result of longterm evolution and is in many cases adequate to actual medical technologies – so EPR has to inherit and enhance best features of PPR;
- medical knowledge is poorly formalized and at the same time has extremely complicated structure;
- neurosurgical diseases may provoke or be combined with pathology of almost any system of human organism, so we have to deal with clinical medicine in whole as subject domain, but not with neurosurgery only; it means very serious uncertainty in patient description;
- neurosurgeons use many different images in their practice, so EPRS must have tools to access to image storage and to visualize images;
- the everyday activity of NSI staff consists of two essential parts: diagnostic and treatment at one hand, and scientific researches at another; these kinds of activity demand different organization of data; at a first approximation one can say that treatment process demands to gather as much data as is possible for single patient and to store them in patient record, and scientific research demands to gather fixed amount of data for as many patients as is possible.

Specific features of information environment of EPRS. We'll point out next features as basic ones:

- large and indefinite number of "information nodes", points where data are generated and analyzed;
- diversity of sources of data and ways of data processing;
- dynamism of information environment;
- arbitrary demands for data presentation;
- users of EPRS are medical persons who have very different level of special and common knowledge, they are not in all cases ready to use information technologies.

3. Basic features of IBS software solution

Analysis of listed above features of subject domain together with the results of analytical survey of NSI business processes forced developers to work at new program solution – IBS/Records, an universal tool for building information systems in poorly formalized subject domains. We can point out following features as basic for IBS/Records:

- IBS/Records provides information support of observation processes with multiple asynchronous observers and multiple objects of observation;
- there are no a priori requirements to data structures; in particular, the logical model of results of observation process is not necessarily relational; briefly saying, IBS/Records deals with a collection of minimally organized data, and necessary structarization is dynamically defined accordingly to the needs of the viewing person;
- all patients data are stored in unique database, what guaranties welltimed access to data for multiple users;
- IBS/Records includes tools for developing working places for users;
- the system has tools to organize teamwork for multiple users;
- IBS/Records has advanced tools for data exchange with other program systems;
- built-in expert system may be used for both representation of pre-formalized knowledge and investigation for eliciting and formalization of implicit expert knowledge.

4. Learned lessons

Standing on the verge of implementation of IBS/Records in everyday activity of Neurosurgical Institute it's possible to say a few important statements which are results of almost three year long intensive work.

"Philosophical" lessons are most important and at the same time most manifest:

Information system is a man-program-machine complex.

Sophisticated information system is an alive system.

Developing of information system is a process of searching compromise solutions to satisfy conflicting requirements of numerous groups of designers and users.

Management lessons. The work management for developing EPRS was influenced by many factors, most important of which are following:

- IBS/Records is a new solution;
- IBS/Records is sophisticated universal tool system for developing different information systems; so developing of EPRS or any other particular system requires work of "IBS/Records-designers" – persons knowing design tools of IBS/Records in all details;
- developing of information system for so complex and nonstandard medical institution as NSI is requires especially much work of designers;
- there is a group of qualified IT professionals working for long time in NSI and knowing it "from the inside".

These factors and process of developing EPR allowed us to say following about management of developing medical information systems which are large-scale like EPR is.

Specialists of following domains have to be involved in developing process: network technologies, information systems, medicine.

It is be the best situation for developing medical information system, when medical informatics professionals are employees of medical institution where the system is intended to run.

Medical informatics professionals have to play role of "interface" between medical stuff and other participants of the work. They have to help medics to represent their requirements on the language of information systems and to help programmers and developers to reach solutions adequate to medical goals.

Uncertainty principle. As it was noticed above professionals in many different domains take part in developing and operating of information systems. This fact results in several collisions, which have be resolved during design process and implementation. We shall formulate some of them in the form of "uncertainty principle".

The less a priori demands are made from data structures -
the more complex is developing of particular version of information system.

The more flexible are basic design tools -
the more hard must be technological discipline.

The more comfortable is the system for users -
the more difficult is the work of administrator.

5. Conclusion

All stated above is only the beginning of long – as we hope – story of EPR for N.N.Burdenko neurosurgical institute. In the time of MIE'99 we shall be able to speak not only about experience in design, but also about first steps of implementation.

Medical Informatics Europe '99
P. Kokol et al. (Eds.)
IOS Press, 1999

Towards a multi-professional patient record – a study of the use of headings

Hans Åhlfeldt PhD [1], Margareta Ehnfors, RN, PhD [2], Lisa Ridderstolpe RN [1]
[1]*Medical Informatics, Linköping University, Sweden*
[2]*Department of Caring Sciences, Örebro University, Sweden*

Abstract. This paper reports on the differences and similarities of used headings among Swedish health care professionals; nurses, occupational therapists, physiotherapists, dietetics, logopedics, welfare officers and general practitioners. The background of the study is a national project where representatives of the different health care professionals compiled used headings from clinical practice. Based on that survey, a hierarchical system of headings was constructed in accordance with the notion of record items and record item complexes described in the European Health Care Record Architecture (EHCRA). The work was done separately by the different health care professionals, leading to separate lists of headings. The current study reports on an analysis of these multi-professional lists of headings with respect to structure, degree of specialization, synonyms and homonyms. The study is descriptive in nature, giving a status report of the variety of used headings in clinical practice, providing necessary material for a normative approach with focus on a truly multi-professional patient record in the future.

1. Introduction

The content and structure of the electronic patient record (EPR) has been one of the major research topics of medical informatics during the 80s and 90s [1], and it will probably remain as a major challenge also in the next decade. The EPR has to face the requirements of quality assurance and evidence-based medicine, but at the same time preserve the richness of the patient-centered story, the so-called narratological function of the patient record [2, 3]. The requirements of quality assurance has generated several EPRs based on terminological models for structured data entry, as presented by van Ginneken in a review paper [1], but there is still a long way to go before these systems have come into any wide spread clinical use. Sweden has together with The Netherlands and England the highest percentage of EPRs in use in general practice in Europe, but there are only a few large installations in the major hospitals.

Information about individual patients is normally kept in a variety of records, which usually are profession specific, e.g., the medical record, the nursing record and the physiotherapist record. This paper reports on the current process in Sweden with respect to analysis of headings for the establishment of a multi-professional patient record. Several factors acts as driving forces; there is a growing need for common infrastructures facilitating information exchange between health care professionals, information systems and different levels of the health care organization, there is a wish to reduce the amount of redundant information in the profession specific information, and there are the requirements for evidence-based medicine which highlights the problems with unstructured free text in the clinical documentation. Clinical records are normally organized into groups of items of information, which share a common context. In the Swedish tradition these groups of information items have names such as anamnesis, status, diagnosis, procedures etc. These groups of information items are in this paper referred to as record headings. In agreement with EHCRA [4], it is natural to see these information items as a hierarchical structure, where main headings such as diagnosis and procedures correspond to record item complexes in the EHCRA terminology.

2 Material and method

Spri, the Swedish Institute for Health Services Development, is an independent research and development institute committed to advancing healthcare delivery in Sweden. The current work is based on a collaborative effort between Spri, Linköping and Örebro University and the different health care professional organizations in Sweden. The material used is hierarchical lists of headings with textual descriptions as compiled through the professional organizations. The material has been analyzed in a series of meetings with representatives from all professions, where synonyms, homonyms, similarities and differences in structure have been identified. The results presented should be seen as a status report from an ongoing work towards a multi-professional patient record, a process which will include several phases and still take several years to implement in full scale clinical practice.

3. Results

The result from the inventory of used heading by the different health care professionals is summarized in table 1. The table shows the number of headings and the number of hierarchical levels, and it can be seen that both these numbers varies substantially between the professions. Despite these differences, all professions share six main headings (see table 2), namely *anamnesis or patient history, status, analysis, goals, actions* and *results*, as well as administrative information about the patient.

The use of the heading 'anamnesis' or 'patient history' has a long tradition in the Swedish medical record, but there are differences in the interpretation among the professionals. The subheadings used reflect a content of personal history, past (medical, nursing, physiotherapeutic etc.) problems, reasons for contact, and symptoms. One of the differences concerns the use of the SOAP structure which is a common way to structure clinical notes into Subjective, Objective, Analysis, and Planing, where in the nursing tradition the 'anamnesis' part only contain facts about the past, whereas the heading 'status' is used to capture description of the current situation of the patient, without the distinction of subjective and objective information. The alternative way of using 'status' is to restrict the information to what can be measured "objectively" through physical examination and to use 'anamnesis' for symptoms and the patients description of the current situation. Two major dimensions in the traditions concerning 'anamnesis' and 'status' can be identified; the information source and the temporal aspect. The information could be categorized as objective or subjective depending on the source and method used for information gathering, and the time dimension could be divided into past, present, and future. In the traditions of e.g. the physicians, the physiotherapists and the dietitians, the division between 'anamnesis' and 'status' follows the objective / subjective categorization rather than the temporal aspect as in the nursing tradition. There are also examples of traditions with a mix of the two dimensions in both 'anamnesis' and 'status'. It seems as if the use of these terms varies along a continuum with the extreme on one side with very strict limitation to one type of information and on the other a deliberate mix of subjective and objective data.

The 'analysis', 'goal', 'action' and 'result' headings (see table 2) are used uniformly without any major differences in interpretation, although the naming and the levels of subheadings differs substantially. Although differences among the professions on the use of 'status' and 'anamnesis' with respect to objective and subjective information and past and current problems, there is a consensus on the usability of a common set of main record headings for the multi-professional patient record referring to the so called caring process. There is also a high degree of similarities between the profession specific lists, leading to redundant information, specially in the 'anamnesis' where social facts about the patient is recorded by all professions and large parts of the medical history could be shared.

Table 1. Number of record headings and number of levels by different health care professionals.

Profession	No. of headings	No. of levels
Nurse	56	3
Occupational therapist	94	3
Medical social worker	108	3
Dietetics	134	4
Physician (GP)	140	2
Logopedics	194	4
Physiotherapist	480	5

The present hierarchical lists of headings are enumerative in nature, explaining the large number of sub-headings for the physiotherapists, where e.g. in the status section 'physical examination' of joints is exploded with respect to location and a series of tests where each combination of joint and test has generated its own subheading. The enumerated approach, which is common in all professions, is a general problem, which seeks a solution for the future. If the lists of the physiotherapists should be collapsed into a structure allowing multiple attributes or aspects to be associated with an entry in the record, the nursing list need to be further specified. The fifty headings in the nursing list are too broad to allow for any clear semantic comparison with e.g. the lists of the physiotherapists which is broken down into five levels. The GP list also need to be further decomposed to allow for a more precise semantic analysis, and such expanded lists exist in several EPRs within general practice, but they are locally extended without any harmonization across systems or without any nationwide consensus.

Table 2. Common record headings with example of content.

Main heading	Example of content
Anamnesis / Patient history	Personal and medical history, current problems, symptoms.
Status / Physical examination	Physical examination with respect to the different professions. Subjective and/or objective information.
Analysis / Assessment	Assessment of patient problems including specific classifications of patient problem and diseases.
Treatment goals	Goals of health care actions as formulated by the patient and the professional expressed as sub-goals and desired final outcome.
Actions / Procedures	Procedures such as diagnostic, therapeutic, preventive, rehabilitation, information, compensatory, administrative etc.
Result	Final judgement of outcome in relation to treatment goals, discharge summary.

There are also examples of misleading similarities, where the terms used indicate a common concept when they indeed are homonyms, that is the same term or subheading is associated with completely or slightly different concepts. Examples of homonyms found are 'activity', 'ADL', 'social facts', 'nutrition', and 'communication'. 'Activity' is used by the Occupational therapists to record the patients working ability, by the Dietetics as an advice concerning physical activity, by the Medical social worker as a container for the patients spare-time occupations, and by the Physiotherapist to record the patients degree of full-time work. The heading 'ADL' is also used differently. 'Social facts' include for some professions personal and family history whereas the medical social worker use it as a specialized rubric for the patients social network of relatives and friends. 'Nutrition' and 'food / diet' are also used in different contexts and with different levels of specialization among e.g. Nurses and Dietetics.

Different traditions exist for recording assessment of diagnostic procedures under either subheadings of 'actions/procedures' or 'analysis'. 'Progress notes' or 'daily notes' are used differently; by some it is not used at all since the information can be captured under 'physical examination' or 'analysis' whereas others use it for a variety of unstructured information which do not fit well into any other main heading.

4. Discussion

To proceed towards a common multi-professional patient record, several limitations in the current situation need to be addressed. The process of analyzing the different traditions of clinical documentation need to be continued, with the aim to clearly identify similarities and differences in the use of record headings among the different health care professionals.

The paper gives a status report from an ongoing work which have both a short and a long term objective. In the short term perspective, the existing lists of hierarchical record headings could be harmonized into a unified list. Such a unified lists of headings would limit the amount of redundant information and would ideally promote the delivery of care by the team of health care professionals. In a long term perspective, the work need to be guided by the development in international projects trying to bring together issues from patient record architecture and concept models, as expressed e.g. by the ToMeLo workshops [5, 6]. The record headings need to be analyzed and modeled within the context of a common medical concept system [7, 8] to allow system developers to derive data entry applications for the EPR based on terminology models as described in the review paper by van Ginnecken [1].

The reported results and conclusions of this work is limited with respect to technical issues of the EPR, but we believe that this kind of basic descriptive work is necessary and in accordance with ongoing international projects [9-12], and that the reported work form the basis for further development towards the multi-professional patient record.

Acknowledgement

This work has been part of the Spriterm project funded by the Swedish Foundation for Knowledge and Competence Development. The project leaders at Spri, the Swedish Institute for Health Services Development, together with the project leaders of the Swedish health care professionals are acknowledged for their invaluable work.

References

[1] Van Ginneken A. Review paper: the structure of data in medical records. Yearbook of Medical Informatics 1995:61-70

[2] Kay S, Purves IN. Medical records and other stories: a narratological framework. Methods Inform Med 1996; 35:72-87.

[3] Rector A. Literature and logbook – art or science. Methods Inform Med 1996; 35:101-103.

[4] EHCRA – The Electronic Health Care Record Architecture, PT-011, prENV 12265, CEN TC251, 1996.

[5] ToMeLo worhshop on the Electronic Health Care Record Architecture and Terminology 1998, Internet www.kun.nl/tomelo.

[6] Mori AR, Consorti F, Galeazzi E. A system of semantic tags to mediate between terminology and structure of patient records. EPRiMP - IMIA conference on Electronic Patient Records in Medical Practice 1998, pp.260-263.

[7] Junfors A, Wallin SB, Thurin A, Carlsson M. A conceptual model for a terminological system for healthcare in Sweden. MIE 1996, pp.203-207.

[8] Rector A, Rogers J, Pole P. The GALEN high level ontology. MIE 1996, pp.174-178.

[9] Leiner F, Haux R. Systematic planning of clinical documentation. Methods Inform Med 1996; 35: 25-34.

[10] Bakken Henry S, Warren J, Lange L, Button P. A review of major nursing vocabularies and the extent to which they have characteristics required for implementation in computer-based systems. JAMIA 1998; 5: 321-328.

[11] Aronsky D, Merkley K, Haug P, James B. Reducing free text entries: a continuous quality improvement project. AMIA Fall Conference 1998.

[12] Severs M. Headings for communicating clinical information from the personal health record. NHS report (UK), IMG ref.C3231, April 1998.

Medical Informatics Europe '99
P. Kokol et al. (Eds.)
IOS Press, 1999

Validation of a European Message Standard for Electronic Health Records

David MARKWELL [1], Leo FOGARTY [2], Andrew HINCHLEY [3]
[1] *The Clinical Information Consultancy, Reading, UK*
[2] *Clinical Informatics Consultant, York, UK*
[3] *Communications Planning Ltd, Bury St Edmunds, UK*

Abstract. A European Standard message for communication of the contents of Electronic Health Records is currently at a late stage in development and is due to be adopted during 1999. This paper reports on the development and content of this message and on current work to clinically validate this message. The validation process involves a new method based on an instantiation of the proposed message in the Extensible Markup Language. This method allows the message to be viewed and compared with the same record on the source system.

1. Introduction

The Health Informatics Technical Committee of the European Standardization Committee (CEN TC251) recently completed a draft four part prestandard on Electronic Health Care Records (EHCR). One of the four parts is a message designed to convey all or part of the EHCR between heterogeneous clinical information systems. This message is designed to be applicable to a wide range of situations in which the EHCR needs to be transferred. However, the initial focus for validation of the message has been on primary care. This paper reports the first of the validation activities in the UK. This activity has been jointly supported by the European Commission's ISIS XML/EDI project, the National Health Service in England (NHS) and the UK Royal College of General Practitioners (RCGP).

2. Objectives

Information systems that store and process clinical information are now widespread in several European countries. In the UK 90% of general practitioners have computers and the majority of these record some clinical information in these GP systems. Clinicians have become increasingly dependent on the patient records stored in these systems. However, to transfer or share care effectively, it is important to be able to transfer or share relevant information from the electronic health record. Shared access to a common or distributed health record is a future possibility but currently this approach does not meet known requirements in a cost-effective manner. The most frequent way of transferring records between systems is as a printed copy. This is unsatisfactory as it forces a parallel paper system on clinicians who have adopted paperless record systems.

The proposed EHCR message standard is intended to be a standard pragmatic solution that enables communication of all or part of the patient record within an electronic message. To ensure the safety and completeness of this message, an initial validation has been undertaken. This involved four leading suppliers of GP systems, who populated instances of the message, and a group of clinical professionals, who acted as scrutineers.

3. Message development

The proposed EHCR message prestandard was developed using methods for the developing clinical messages that have evolved over the last six years. This evolutionary process began with messages for laboratory requests and reports [1] which now form the basis of implementations in several European countries. Further work resulted in a formally adopted technical report describing the method [2]. A more recent revision of the method adopted the Unified Modelling Language (UML) in place of earlier modelling methods.

Several healthcare messages have already been accepted as formal European Prestandards. These cover laboratory requests and reports [1], diagnostic service requests and reports [3], referral and discharge [4] and healthcare administration [5]. Messages for prescribing and blood transfusion are also due for completion this year. There are overlaps between the content of these messages and the EHCR message. Where possible, the same structures are used to convey the same type of information in all these messages. However, in some cases an information structure that was sufficient to support a service request or report needed elaboration for EHCR communication. Furthermore, work on other parts of the EHCR prestandard indicated many areas in which generalisations could be applied rather than using the specialised data structures used in request and report messages.

A general high-level EHCR architecture was adopted as a prestandard in 1996 [6]. This is being revised and extended as one of the other parts of the current EHCR standard. This architecture is a key reference point for the message. The message is designed to support communication between systems whether or not they are formally aligned with the architectural standards. However, communication will be most effective between systems that are based on or closely aligned with the architecture.

Another parallel activity is addressing the issues of term-lists that can be used to provide common semantic references to particular parts of the EHCR. The EHCR message uses a set of high-level document names, section titles and annotation labels specified in this part of the prestandard. These are particularly important when used to disambiguate qualifications that fundamentally alter the meaning of record items.

The third part of the EHCR prestandard defines structures for representing distribution rules. The message can convey these rules and can associate them with components parts of the EHCR. Thus it is possible to inform a recipient of EHCR information about constraints on access to all or part of this information that have been specified by the author or sender.

The EHCR standardisation work drew on practical experience from several European countries, materials produced by a range of European R&D activities [7,8] and consideration of the work of HL7. In respect of the application of this work to support the care of diabetic patients, the team are also working closely with the *Diabetes care Optimization through Information Technology* (DOIT) study group of the European Association of Specialists in Diabetes (EASD).

4. The proposed message

4.1. Status

At the time of writing this paper, all four parts of the proposed EHCR prestandard [9] have been submitted to CEN for a formal ballot. The results of these ballots will be reported to the conference. The document includes a summary of the communication scenarios to be supported, an information model, and general message descriptions covering communication requirements derived from the scenarios.

4.2. Scenarios and requirements

The messages will allow information from an EHCR held by one clinician to be transferred to a heterogeneous system used by another clinician who is taking over responsibility for the care of the patient. The messages will also allow occasional or regular transfers of patient medical record information between health professionals with a transient or continuing role in the care of an individual patient. The main purpose of the communications supported by these messages is the provision of care to individual patients.

To meet the requirements identified in a study of these scenarios the message should be able to convey the information from the sending system in a form that:

1. Allows any receiving system, as a minimum, to present that information in a human-readable form within or as an annotation from the locally held EHCR.
2. Allows a receiving system that supports an equivalent or higher level of structure to store, retrieve and process received information to support functions such as analysis and decision support in a manner that is consistent with processing of locally recorded information.
3. Ensure that qualifications fundamentally altering the meaning of an item of information are represented unambiguously.
4. Refers to distribution rules that should be applied to limit viewing or further distribution of all or part of the communicated clinical information.
5. Appropriately attributes the time and party responsible for originating the message as a whole or where possible and necessary individual items within that message.
6. Enables information to be integrated with an existing EHCR for the same patient without duplicating or inappropriately superseding existing information.

4.3. Information Models and levels of EHCR structure

The proposed information model consists of four distinct parts:

- Message structure, communicating partners and matching messages to patients.
- The overall EHCR structure, based on the EHCR architectural standard.
- Structure of essential types of data items that form part of the EHCR.
- Representation of relationships between, and views of, EHCR content.

The message supports different levels of structure to accommodate communication between systems that are unable to represent the full richness of the EHCR. The lowest structural level allows information to be communicated either as a single text block or as a set of text blocks associated with different dated encounters or events. These text blocks will support presentation enhancement using markup such as HTML. This level provides minimal functionality, allowing transferred information to be presented as part of (or as an attachment to) the record held by the receiving system. The higher levels will support communication of structured coded clinical information, with appropriate contextual information and with the ability to convey relationships between items.

The message also permits the addition of enterprise extensions that facilitate communication of structures specific to a communicating community or system supplier.

4.4. General Message Descriptions and implementation

The final step of the development of a CEN standard message is to produce General Message Descriptions (GMDs). A GMD is a hierarchical subset of the information models designed to meet the requirements of a particular scenario or a set of related scenarios. A GMD is not syntax dependent and can be mapped into any messaging syntax. Previous messages have been implemented in EDIFACT and ASN.1.

Recent experiments have shown that automatic mapping into implementable Extensible Markup Language (XML) is possible whereas mapping to EDIFACT was a labour intensive activity. The end results of this mapping process are Document Type Definitions (DTD) which outline the content and constraints applicable to instances of a message. There is considerable interest in using Extensible Markup Language (XML) as a messaging syntax in healthcare [10] and this is the approach that was used for validation of the message.

5. Method of clinical validation

5.1. *The need for clinical validation*

The clinical profession in the UK has given great emphasis to the need for clinical validation to ensure that messages are safe. This is particularly important for messages that transfer all or part of the patient record. Therefore the NHS in consultation with the RCGP decided to support an activity to provide this validation prior to the final acceptance of the proposed EHCR message Prestandard.

5.2. *Selecting a format for validation*

Clinical validation of a message for transfer of the EHCR requires informed clinical professionals to compare the content of a message with the information stored in the source system. Therefore a representation of the message that could readily and faithfully be displayed and reviewed was a prerequisite for progress. Implementation of the message in XML offered several advantages in terms of availability of viewers and programming interfaces. This made early validation feasible without waiting for a final version of the message standard.

5.3. *An outline of the process*

The process of validation involved the production of message instances by exporting several patient records from four different commercially available GP systems. The information was exported in the form of XML documents that complied with the DTD for the draft version of the EHCR message. These messages were then viewed through one or more of a selection of the available XML browsers or viewers. The available viewers included freely distributed products such as Microsoft's XML Notepad and Internet Explorer as well as plain text viewers and a special viewer developed within the project. Clinicians compared views of the record within the original application with the content and structure of information in the message. Comments on discrepancies, inadequacies and ambiguities were linked to the relevant part of the message using the specialised viewer developed in the project. These comments were fed back to technical experts to determine the cause and appropriate action for resolution. Figure 1 illustrates this process.

6. Results

The final report of the validation of the message [11] is publicly available with other related materials. The conclusion was that as a result of the clinical scrutiny process of the XMLEPR project, it is clear that, provided that some additional attributes are included in the message definition, the message would be able to carry the information present on the GP systems that took part. Those additions have been made. The system suppliers involved together represented between 70-80% of the market in England and Wales. Accordingly the scrutiny team assert that the revised message is able to convey the information present in the majority of existing GP systems in England and Wales.

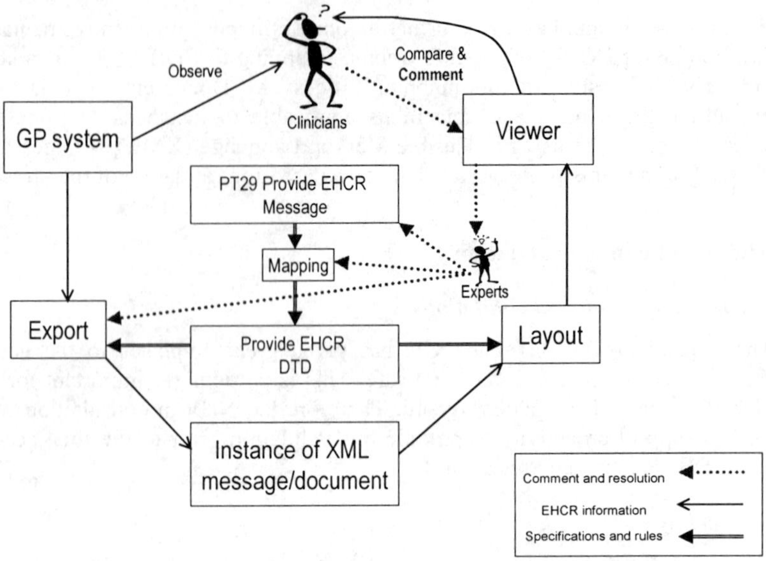

Figure 1. Illustration of the process of message development and validation

The final report also made several recommendations for further action. These included the development of specific implementation guidelines for use of the message in UK GP to GP communications and further validation as a prelude to widespread implementation. The next stage of validation is likely to be a brief repeat of the original process using the final version of the message. However, the critical step will be to demonstrate safe reconstitution of records from message information. Trials of this process are planned and should take place in the next six months.

Further work on mapping rules from message models to XML is proceeding within the EU funded ISIS XML/EDI project. This work will be fed back to CEN TC251 and together with the experiences of the HL7 community it will also be a key input to a work item on this use of XML in healthcare messaging that has recently started in the ISO TC215 Health Informatics group.

7. Conclusion

The successful use of clinical information systems requires effective and safe methods for communicating the content of the electronic healthcare record. Standards are essential if the communications requirements are to be met in a generally applicable manner. The work of CEN TC251 in developing EHCR architecture and message standards is thus an important contribution to realisation of the potential benefits from the application of information technology to clinical record. However, if a standard for EHCR communication needs to be validated by clinicians as well as by technical experts.

References

[1] European Committee for Standardization, ENV 1613:1995, Medical Informatics - Messages for exchange of laboratory information.

[2] European Committee for Standardization, CR 12587:1996, CEN Report: Medical Informatics - Methodology for the development of healthcare messages.

[3] European Committee for Standardization, ENV 12539:1997, Medical Informatics - Request and report messages for diagnostic service departments.

[4] European Committee for Standardization, ENV 12538:1997, Medical Informatics - Messages for patient referral and discharge.

[5] European Committee for Standardization, ENV 12612:1997, Medical Informatics - Messages for the exchange of healthcare administrative information.

[6] European Committee for Standardization, ENV 12265, Medical Informatics - Electronic healthcare record architecture.

[7] Kalra D, Ingram D. The good European health record, Conference proceedings, Healthcare Computing 93, BJHC Books 1993: 543-549

[8] Synapses, From http://www.chime.ucl.ac.uk/HealthI/SYNAPSES.

[9] European Committee for Standardization, ENV 13608 parts 1-4, Health Informatics - Electronic Healthcare Record Communication.

[10] World-Wide-Web Consortium, Extensible Markup Language, From URL http://www.w3.org/XML/Activity.

[11] Fogarty et al, Scrutiny study of GP-GP Electronic Healthcare Record transfer, From URL http://www.communicationsplanning.ltd.uk/infopages

Medical Informatics Europe '99
P. Kokol et al. (Eds.)
IOS Press, 1999

Clinicians must invest resources when implementing Electronic Patient Records

Nikula, Rolf E. [a], Elberg, Pia B. [a], Svedberg, Helena B. [b]
[a] *Virtual Centre for Health Informatics, Aalborg University, Denmark*
[b] *Enator Medical AB, Lund, Sweden*

Abstract. Most often the investment in Electronic Patient Records (EPR) is decided upon on the basis of descriptions of all the advantages this new technology will bring. However, most of these advantages from EPR's are only obtainable if the clinicians are motivated to invest their knowledge and resources in this implementation process. This paper proposes a simple method to qualify the decision making process by introducing the "price to pay" concept.

Keywords. Health Care, Information Technology, Electronic Patient Record, and Organisational Change.

1. Problem domain

How would you explain the functions and possibilities of the Internet to somebody who has never encountered it? Would it be any different to explain the functions and the possibilities of the Electronic Patient Record (EPR) to clinicians or Health Care Managers? Today's systems for documentation are complex and the clinicians have different understanding of the existing systems depending on their profession, professional experience and experience with information technology (IT). Nevertheless, EPR's are promoted by comparing the possibilities of existing paper-based patient records (PPR) and newly developed EPR applications or EPR's existing only on the vendors blueprint. The assumptions underlying these comparisons are that we have clear-cut definitions of as well PPR's as EPR's. This in mind, it is thought-provoking that when promoting EPR in strategies, literature and conferences there is a tendency to simplify the task and only focus on possible advantages of the new technology. An example of this is found in Argument 2.7 in the NHS Strategy [1]:

"The arguments for a move towards an electronic record are compelling. Such records are more likely to be legible, accurate, safe, secure, and available when required, and they can be more readily and rapidly retrieved and communicated. They better integrate the latest information about a patient's care, for example from different "departmental" clinical systems in a hospital. In addition, they can be more readily analysed for audit, research and quality assurance purposes."

Also when reviewing the literature regarding EPR in general expressions like "improved, increased, better, faster, easier" appears frequently where advantages of *the* EPR are compared to the disadvantages of *the* PPR. Hence, focus is mainly on the change of tool, i.e. the shift from paper-based technology to computer- and network-based technology. However, introducing information technology at hospitals also implies a discussion on quality aspects of the record as information and communication medium. The Swedish Institute for Health Services Development (SPRI) has for many years played a major role in the development and implementation of EPR by providing information and know-how and they state very clearly that EPR is about sharing knowledge and not about computers [2]. This is why it is so important that clinicians invest knowledge and resources in the implementation of EPR.

2. The Price to Pay concept

To effectuate the advantages of EPR there is a "price to pay" i.e. actions have to be taken before and during the implementation and later on when the application is used in the everyday clinical setting. Textbooks on Medical Informatics present lists of potential advantages of EPR and describe prerequsites for obtaining all these advantages in general terms [3,4,5]. This paper will not argue that *all* advantages have a "price tag" fixed to them, but merely point out that in most cases there is a certain amount of effort, inconvenience, or compromise "to pay" before each of the advantages can be effectuated. The authors state the need to be very explicit and precise in order not to confuse "price to pay" with disadvantages. To exemplify what we mean by "price to pay", we have inserted two supplementary columns in the list of advantages of the PPR as presented in the Handbook of Medical Informatics by van Bemmel et al [5]. The example is shown in table 1.

Table 1. Advantages, the "price to pay", and disadvantages of paper-based records.

Advantages (v Bemmel et al.[5])	**The price to pay (authors)**	**Disadvantages (authors)**
They can easily be carried around	Collecting; sorting; filing; copying information	Only available in one place at a time
Much freedom in reporting style	A quantity of different charts and forms etc.	Medical risk due to lack of standards
Easy data browsing	Legible writing; order; discipline	Lack of confidentiality; requires space
Requires no special training		No structure; risk of miscoding; medical risk due to misunderstandings
Never 'down' as computers sometimes are	All records in place all the time	Lost; misplaced; not updated

To create a broader foundation for assessment and discussion of the effects of an EPR, we must clarify the arguments related to advantages and disadvantages. One way to do this is to discuss the necessary prerequisites and actions to obtain the advantages. Van Bemmel et al also lists seven advantages of computer-based patient records in a table [5, p114], but they use the expression "7 principle strength" in the text explaining the table, which emphasise that the advantages depend on how the application is implemented and used. The seven advantages and the authors' proposal of the price to pay to obtain these advantages are commented beneath and summarised in table 2.

1. *Simultaneous access* to the patient data in the clinical setting also implies that the process of adding new data to the EPR has to be accelerated compared to existing practise. The EPR cannot, any more than the paper record, present data that is still in a manuscript or on tape waiting to be entered. The concept "simultaneous" also contains expectancy of getting access to the record from everywhere within the hospital. Today, the PPR allows the clinician to bring the record to reception, pharmacy room, bedside and so on. A large number of workstations or handheld computers connected to the network is required if this workflow is to be continued with EPR. Alternatively, the workflow may be changed and consequently affect the hardware dependency.
2. *Legibility* is an important aspect in PPR as well as EPR, but it is difficult to control whether legal rules are followed or not in the PPR. An EPR may be designed to automate a given set of rules, which may restrict clinicians access to and use of patient data.

3. *Variety of views on data* appears to be a very attractive advantage. The clinician may decide to read the record as he read the PPR or to adjust the presentation to his need in the clinical situation, but this feature requires structured data entry, common terminology and that the clinician learns how to retrieve the information he needs.
4. *The structure of data* is important if data is to be re-used and presented in several different ways. All data (tests, notes, nursing diagnoses, physical findings etc.) entered into the system has to be clearly "marked", the terminology has to be agreed upon and the clinicians' discipline when entering data rigid. An EPR application may be designed to support this behaviour e.g. by providing on-line guidelines.
5. *Decision support* is advantageous if the clinician enters the data. What is the use of a sophisticated alert system proposing e.g. clinical paths or pointing out a potential risk for medication interaction, if a medical record clerk enters the record? Decision support facilities also demand structured data entry if data should be automatically recognised and responded to by the EPR system. Systems able to analyse free text and propose actions are not to be found in clinical use for a long time to come.
6. *Support of other data analysis* may prove an important feature for quality control, quality improvement and resource management. This feature may enable rapid information retrieval. However, without restrictions on data entry structure and terminology a data analysis would be difficult or even impossible to perform or interpret.
7. *Electronic data exchange and sharing care support* assumes re-use of data i.e. data is only entered once. When this feature is applied to already structured data like name, date of birth or addresses it is simple. It would though be more interesting to share clinical information between professions e.g. when the nurse has entered information about the patients social situation (family, type of housing, profession/job etc) the physician could use this as part of his notes. This form of cross-clinician sharing of patient information demands an agreement between clinicians on rules, standards and most of all on common terminology.

Table 2. Seven main advantages and the "price to pay" of electronic patient records.

	Advantages (v Bemmel et al. [5])	**Price to pay (authors)**
1	Simultaneous access	All data registered at once Infrastructure
2	Legibility	Rules become automated Access control
3	Variety of views on data	Structured data entry Common Terminology Search for - not look up - information Education
4	Support of structured data entry (SDE)	Structured data entry Common terminology Data entry by clinicians Agreements on and maintenance of e.g. guidelines
5	Decision support	Structured data entry Common terminology Data entry by clinicians Agreements on and maintenance of e.g. guidelines
6	Support of other data analysis	Structured data entry Common terminology Agreements on and maintenance of e.g. guidelines Legal issues e.g. patient consent
7	Electronic data exchange and sharing care support	Common terminology Standards (semantic, technical) Legal issues e.g. patient consent

3. Conclusion

If we accept the idea that almost no person can describe and ask for functionality that they never encountered, the Medical Informatics Society should help provide a better foundation to those who must decide on new technology despite uncertainty. We have proposed a fairly simple concept to be used by hospital management as well as clinicians involved in EPR projects to make the objectives of EPR implementation explicit. Clinicians and management could derive the "price to pay" of a specific technology from discussing the prerequisites of possible advantages. Merely supplementing the expected advantages related to EPR with the "price to pay" for each function provides a broader foundation for discussions on how to invest the given resources in EPR implementation.

The advantages of EPR derived from strategies are primarily related to the potentials of a new tool, i.e. information technology in general. If potential advantages of EPR were the starting point of the process of developing the requirements for an EPR system, the clinicians would naturally expect these advantages to be the result of implementation of an EPR application. It is common knowledge that habits and existing routines are difficult to change and not necessarily changed just because a new tool is introduced. However, the "price to pay" in order to achieve the expected benefits are issues primarily related to re-design of the way clinicians use patient information and how they co-operate. Whether the promising visions of the strategies for EPR becomes reality or shelf-ware thus depend on how many resources the clinicians are willing to invest in redesign of their practise.

In this study we have found that most often the "price to pay" in order to make EPR advantageous to PPR is (table 2): Structured data entry, Common terminology, Maintenance of e.g. guidelines, and Data entry by clinicians. Advantages of EPR demand co-operation between clinicians from different categories (e.g. doctors, nurses, physiotherapists) and different specialities (e.g. orthopaedic, internal medicine or psychiatry) because EPR demands consensus on matters like patient record structure, which terminology to use, normal values etc. Our experience from implementing EPR's in hospitals within Skåne Region in Sweden confirms that these four issues are the most important and problematic in the clinical setting, and they must be dealt with if we want the EPR to become advantageous to PPR. Implementing EPR is a continuous process and most of the features mentioned above will need maintenance in terms of adding new terms and altering rules or normal values. This work has to be carried out by clinicians and this further emphasises how important it is that clinicians are sufficiently informed about and prepared for EPR. The authors advocate that the "price to pay" concept will qualify the discussions related to both EPR and PPR and thus make it feasible for the clinicians to invest their scarce resources in implementing patient record systems to support improved patient care.

References

[1] Information for Health: An information strategy for the modern NHS. NHS Executive. 1999. http://www.imt4nhs.exec.nhs.uk/strategy/

[2] Introducing Computer-based Patient Records. Prerequisites and Requirements. ISSN 0586-1691. Spris Förlagstjänst. 1998; Spri Report 477.

[3] Petersson G and Rydmark M (ed.). Medicinsk Informatik. ISBN 91-634-1384-1. Falköping: Liber Utbildning AB; 1996.

[4] McDonald CJ, Barnett GO. Medical-Record Systems. In: Shortliffe EH, Perreault LE, Wiederhold G, Fagan LM (ed.), Medical Informatics. Computer applications in health care. ISBN 0-201-06741-2. Massachusetts: Addison-Wesley Publishing Company; 1990; ch. 6, p. 181-219.

[5] van Bemmel JH and Musen MA, editors. Handbook of Medical Informatics. ISBN 3-540-63351-0. Springer; 1997.

[6] Nikula, R.E. and Svedberg, H.B. Vårdpersonalens uppfatning av datorjournalen - en förändringsprocess? Virtual Centre for Health Informatics. ISSN 1397-9507. Aalborg, Denmark. 1998; 98-4.

Medical Informatics Europe '99
P. Kokol et al. (Eds.)
IOS Press, 1999

Constructing Scenarios for validating the Electronic Health Care Record Architecture

Dr. Stephen Kay[1], Tom Marley[1], Per Arne Lundgren[2], Helen Broberg[2] and Dr. Hanne Prytz[3]

1. *Medical Informatics Group, University of Manchester, UK, M13 9PL*
2. *Information Technology, University Hospital Lund, SWE*
3. *Department of Gastroenterology, University Hospital Lund, SWE*

Abstract. The CEN TC 251 Electronic Health Care Record Architecture is the first part of a four part communication prestandard intended to facilitate the safe communication of clinical information, irrespective of circumstances related to time, distance, and responsibility. The work has important implications for a diversity of stakeholders and must embody clinical principles if it is to succeed. The issue at hand is how to enable clinicians to validate the reference architecture, which is necessarily a technical document, so that they have confidence that it can meet the clinical requirement for safe communication. A model of communication that has been used to ground the architecture is shown to be useful in creating relevant clinical scenarios to permit the first steps towards coherent validation in a systematic way.

1. Introduction

In 1995 the prestandard ENV12265 for the electronic health care record architecture (EHCRA) was approved by CEN. The prime purpose of EHCRA being to facilitate the safe and effective communication of the health care record by enabling 'healthcare record information of any sort to be recognizable and understandable when displaced from its origin, through faithful preservation of its content and context' [1]. ENV12265 was intended to be a foundation for further versions, each moving a little closer towards that goal.

In 1998 TC 251 initiated a new work item to take the architecture forward. It considered the prestandard to be a firm foundation for communicating part or whole of a health care record between heterogeneous systems, and thus suitable for extending. The new extended ECHRA is now to replace the previous prestandard. This paper considers the use of scenarios for testing the appropriateness of the new EHCRA, which is a more formal architecture than its predecessor.

2. Validation and Verification of a Reference Architecture

The new reference architecture [2] is a set of principled design decisions that must be validated by clinical consensus despite its technical nature. The prestandard, however, is a document that will be read mainly by technicians, e.g. suppliers and designers of clinical record systems. For these stakeholders, it embodies clinical principles expressed as concepts and associations, both abstract and concrete. It is not merely a design; rather it is a set of constraints on any design to ensure that safe communication of clinical information, in a diversity of circumstances, can be implemented to the highest standard.

Before a prestandard can be formally accepted in Europe it has to have achieved a consensus based upon a measure of confidence that it satisfies the requirements as detailed in its scope. The task facing the architects is to show that the proposed prestandard satisfies the requirement by demonstrating its qualities to both the technical and lay stakeholders. This task is difficult with respect to a reference architecture, for its description is necessarily both abstract and complex, modelled in formalisms for the essential rigour of technical specification but at the cost of being esoteric and difficult for clinicians or non-technical healthcare personnel to understand.

It is common for software engineering practice to distinguish between 'verification' and 'validation', i.e. 'doing something right', and ' doing the right thing' respectively. The technical verification of the prestandard is concerned with the correctness of the models, its conventions and terminology. It must also be concerned with the tenor of the guidance given, i.e. the prestandard must be descriptive and permissive, and must not deliberately rule out a particular product, if that product can achieve the same clinical requirement by some other means. The over riding concern is that the prestandard is technically sound and 'fair', i.e. it does not discriminate against one or more vendors due to error or intent. Verification is the main concern of the technical stakeholder.

Validation, however, is concerned with fitness of purpose in the specified domain; in this instance, the domain of communicating clinical information. Validation is therefore primarily something that the clinical community must do, as the principles in this prestandard must support clinical record usage. Some means is required of permitting clinicians to express their requirements in a way that does not require them to be fully cognisant with the technical document, yet will provide some confidence that the architecture does support such a requirement. The way that this has been traditionally done is to use the notion of a scenario. One major problem with the use of scenarios for this purpose, however, is that they are relatively unstructured, and each scenario is couched in a way which does not make it easy to see what principle is being tested nor how an architecture such as EHCRA can support the principle. The following is a framework for ensuring that the scenarios to be used for validating the record architecture can be readily checked against the constructs of the architecture.

3. Scenarios: Generation and Customisation

The development of appropriate scenarios is a non-trivial exercise. Generating new scenarios according to a specified model is probably the most straightforward approach. The model, however, must be relevant to the domain and, in effect, this approach puts the problem one stage back, i.e. there is a need to develop an appropriate model before work on constructing the scenarios can begin. Assuming such a model can be developed then it would be prudent to maximise its benefit. In particular, as well as using it to generate new scenarios, it would also be efficient if it could re-use some part, if not all, of the many existing scenarios that have been developed prior to the model. Re-use of existing scenarios has three other principal benefits in addition to efficiency:

- first, it recognises the former construction experience, often attended with much effort and care, protecting the investment spent in deriving the original scenarios;

- second, it provides a ready resource rather than requiring unnecessary, costly re-invention; and
- last, but by no means least, it brings confidence in the product from using proven scenarios that have already been tried and tested over a period of time.

4. The Architecture's Communication Model

The model is the key to both the generation and customisation of scenarios. For it to be useful, the model has to be specific and, furthermore, be specific to the domain under test. Simultaneously, it also has to provide a structure that can accommodate a wide diversity of scenarios if it is not to be too limited in its application and usefulness. These two constraints of specificity and diversity are potentially in conflict with one another. It is therefore necessary to provide guidelines as to how the model can be used effectively. The general domain under consideration by the CEN architecture is of 'communication', specialised to clinical information as found in electronic health care records.

Re-use acknowledges the debt owed to the originator, showing the general relevance of the original idea, often extending it beyond the original scope and intention of use. The communication model used in the architecture is derived from two sources, one of which, it is claimed, is derivative of the other. The model that came to our attention was by Jakobson [3] one that had been used in Narratology [4] to consider how the message within a narrative was communicated between an author (or addresser) and a reader (or addressee). Hawthorn [5] points out that it is generally believed that Jakobson himself was influenced by Shannon and Weaver [6] who developed a more technical, mathematical model of communication. The Shannon and Weaver model was developed to address the communication of a signal across a noisy channel. The point of considering the history of its derivation, is simply to emphasize that the model under consideration has been found to be applicable to scientific and 'artistic' forms of communication, involving a variety of written, verbal and electronic media prior to being adopted by Kay for the Architecture. It has therefore been shown to accommodate multi-media communication in a number of different settings.

4.1 What the model is and how it is used in the Architecture

The term, 'communication', is interpreted in the prestandard in its broadest sense; as an act or an instance of imparting or exchanging information. The term, 'context', speaks of the circumstances and conditions that are relevant to that act, and for clinical communication in an electronic environment a primary concern is that the information is safely exchanged. The Architecture's communication model has seven constituents, i.e. the extended Jakobson's model, which have been renamed to emphasize context and to avoid terms commonly used in the Health Informatics domain (see figure 1).

Setting
Topic
Originator (s) --------------------------------- Recipient (s)
Impression
Engagement
Standards

Figure 1: The Context Model corresponding to the seven constituents of communication

In a previous paper [7], it was argued that each constituent of the communication model could be considered as being relevant to considering the implications for 'context'. 'Context' as a principle is not found in just one component of EHCRA, an isolated box in a model, but rather is diffused throughout the architecture. It was therefore appropriate to consider each of the constituents of the communication model and to see what implications they had for managing context in the communicative act.

The second use of the model with respect to the architecture builds upon the first and is considered here. It is used here to generate and customise scenarios for the purpose of validating the architecture. As a worked example, we take an existing scenario provided by stakeholders in Skåne, Sweden. At an invited workshop, the stakeholders used the scenario to test their own understanding of the architecture. We show how this scenario, which was actually developed for a number of different but allied purposes (e.g. system architecture, messaging, as well as record architecture), was decomposed according to our model and made more relevant to the validation of the architecture.

5. The Arthur Scenario

The scenario provided was 12 pages in detail of which only an outline is given here. It was developed by a group of healthcare professionals led by Dr. Hanne Prytz and its purpose was intended for exercising requirements for the development of a healthcare record system. Spri too have been very active in this area [8]. In particular it was given to the architects to validate and communicate the architecture in a concrete way. The Scenario, in outline form, is as follows:

Arthur [id no] is a 69 year old widower who has lived alone for the past two years. He is a retired Chief Buyer for a medium sized company. Arthur lives in [address], 4th floor with a lift. Arthur has 3 children. The eldest, Kerstin, lives close by [telephone no.]. On August 1st, Arthur incurred a fracture to his right hip when he fell in his home ... was operated at the Orthopaedic Clinic and came home on the 15th. ... Arthur rejects home help. Kirsten has recently become concerned about him: "he seems to have changed and I suspect him of not eating properly." ... Kerstin decides to ring the Health Centre for advice. ... Dr Sunden reviews the case and decides to book an earlier appointment. ... [later, Arthur attends the health centre, the casualty department, is admitted to a medical clinic, transferred to Gastroenterology Department, and is finally discharged after seeing a variety of health care professionals for different purposes in several different institutions]

From the architect's point of view it was a rich description but much too big to be of immediate use. We therefore devised a way of decomposing the scenario into a set of communicative acts that could then be related to the communication model. Each communicative act would need to be satisfied by the architecture. Some of the material would not be about communication per se, but may well provide resource to be used in the communication. Such detail can be reintroduced later to ensure that the architecture has captured the richness. In brief, the method used in the workshop was:

1. Analyse the input scenario as given.
2. Identify the communicative act(s). For Arthur, we identified multiple distinct acts.
3. Express each act as a brief passage (perhaps just a sentence); in effect a new small scenario.
4. Classify the scenario features with respect to the seven constituents (i.e. S,T,O,R,I,E,S).
5. For each constituent, ask questions as to how the architecture supports the necessary 'context'.

6. At this point, it becomes the architect/technician responsibility to show how the architecture can accommodate the requirement, identifying what architectural constructs can be used or whether the scenario has exposed a short-coming in the architecture.

In step 4, STORIES is derived from taking the first letter of each model constituent, reading top down, left to right in Figure 1. It is merely an aide memoir device for remembering the constituents. Details about what each constituent represents are given in the architectural prestandard in an informative annex [2]. The model becomes a simple template in which the various features of the scenario can be slotted in. Some features may be implicit. For example, 'Standards, slot 7' will usually be implicit, yet common to a number of scenarios. Due to lack of space, only one of the many communicative acts identified in the Arthur Scenario is presented in Table 1.

6. Communication Scenario Generation Method as Process

We have mentioned the different sources of scenarios. At the same time, any scenario intended to validate the architecture, be it new or customised, will be derived by various means and to define just one way of doing it will probably be counter productive. The process as outlined is intended to be helpful, but the important output is the product, not the process, and if scenario authors find alternative means of producing the same product then that is what matters. It is also of interest to the architects, should scenario authors find examples that are unable to be decomposed in the way that we suggest. Evidence of any such scenarios would be most welcome.

Table 1: Communicative Act scenario for framing architectural questions.

	Setting	Topic	Originator(s)	Recipient(s)	Impression	Engagement	Standards
scenario1	Dr Sunden reviews Arthur's existing record whilst giving advice to Kerstin over phone.						
feature:	Phone consult ation	Assess- ing Arthur	Past record details entered by some other clinician (s)	Dr. Sunden of record, also Kerstin of advice	Previous medical history in case notes. Assesment	Telephone call is the medium; Duration of contact	Health Centre rules for phone advice
Example questions	S	When was the call made? Details such as date, time, and other attributes considered relevant should be able to be documented.					
	T	How does Dr. Sunden establish who the phone call is about? Identity details of Arthur? Demographics? Is Dr Sunden familiar with Arthur's case? Has this patient been seen at this centre before? When is his next appointment?					
	O	Who wrote the original notes? How confident/senior were the original authors? Is the record composed of multiple entries from health care professionals and can they be identified? Can Dr. Sunden seek more detail?					
	R	Does the record permit/ exclude access to Dr. Sunden? Is Dr Sunden's access recorded? Is the purpose of access and his role recorded? Can he enter Kerstin's comments verbatim about her father? Can they be attributed to her?					
	I	What data is required for the assessment? How is the data presented? How is it ordered, organised, managed? What is kept or linked together, e.g. can we link 4th floor flat- lift available- fractured hip & elderly- home help rejected?					
	E	Is the duration of the contact recorded? A log? Can it be noted that the fact that it is advice by phone, from a relative, rather than face to face with patient?					
	S	What institutional rules exist in the Health Centre to govern what can, and what can not, be said over the phone and recorded? Ethical constraints?					

7. Conformance and Compliance to a Reference Architecture

Standards in general cannot demand conformance. Again, in general, adherence to any standard is voluntary. Customers may demand such adherence as part of their own contractual requirements; suppliers may claim conformance to the standard to gain competitive advantage. Standards are thought to work best if they are adopted rather than imposed. This is self evident for de facto standards, if not always for de jure standards. The assumption here is that the strength of the standard lies in its usefulness rather than in a legal binding. Of paramount importance then, is whether the stakeholders can understand it sufficiently well to be able to judge whether it is relevant to their needs.

Kona [9] usefully distinguishes between Conformance and Compliance. Compliance is a policy that can be met and expressed in the applicable conformant schema. The community of interest can specify the policy. The objective is to 'make the technology transparent to policy-makers in the same manner as existed when information was exchanged on paper.' The separation of conformance from compliance is useful and fits with our requirements for different stakeholders. Here we suggest that the use of clinical scenarios developed according to the model of communication go some way to enabling stakeholders to judge whether or not the architecture is relevant to their needs and policy.

8. Conclusion

We have shown that the model of communication underpinning the new architecture can be used to construct tightly focused scenarios. We have shown further, how it was possible to re-use an existing, large and complex scenario. This was a realistic clinical scenario, developed for a variety of purposes, but made useful for the purpose of validating the reference architecture. Finally we have provided a simple method, which can be used to generate specific scenarios to validate the EHCRA prestandard for clinical communication.

Acknowledgements

We wish to thank the Skåne participants for organising and contributing to the validation workshop and for permission to use the Arthur Scenario. Also to Siemens Health Services for being our host in Malmö and CEN TC 251 for funding the new EHCRA multipart prestandard.

References

[1] Medical Informatics – Electronic Healthcare Record Architecture. Brussels: CEN, 1995.
[2] TC 251. EHCRA-EA. FFV, June 29th, 1999.
[3] Jakobson R. *Closing Statement: Linguistics and Poetics.* In: Sebeok, TA ed. Style in Language. New York: Wiley. 1960:350-77
[4] Kay S, Purves I. *The Electronic Medical Record And The "Story Stuff": A Narrativistic Model* In: Greenhalgh T, Hurwitz B eds. Narrative Based Medicine. .BMJ, 1998, London.
[5] Hawthorn J. Contemporary Literary Theory. Edward Arnold. 1994:186-187
[6] Shannon CE, Weaver W. *The mathematical theory of communication.* Urbana, IL: University of Illinois Press. 1949.
[7] Kay S. *Contextualising the Record Architecture along Story Lines.* Proceedings Of The IMIA working group 17, EPRIMP, Rotterdam, 1998;.137-141
[8] Spri Report. Introducing Computer-based Patient Records. ISSN 0586-1691
[9] KONA . Website on 24/04/98

Medical Informatics Europe '99
P. Kokol et al. (Eds.)
IOS Press, 1999

Realization of a CPR Using HL7 Queries From Communication Server to Information Server

U. Schrader[1], A. W. Zaiss[2], S. Büchele[2], M. Binder[2] U. Leupolz[2], R. Klar[2]
[1]*University of Applied Sciences Frankfurt a. M., Nibelungenplatz 1, D-60318 Frankfurt a. M., Germany*
[2]*Dept. of Med. Informatics, University Hospital Freiburg, Stefan-Meier-Str. 26, D-79104 Freiburg, Germany*

Abstract. A communication server is often used in Germany to interface legacy systems. It handles the translation, duplication, and transmission of messages to all systems that might need this information. Based on the principles of "for every data there is only one master" and "information on demand" we have built an information server that reduces the messages required and simplifies the handling of messages, the update of data already sent compared to a communication server. It also allows to implement a security policy as required by the German data privacy legislature.

1. Introduction

Freiburg university hospital has about 1,700 beds, over 50,000 inpatients, and about 300,000 outpatient visits per year. Like most German hospitals the information infrastructure has been developed incrementally with the result of many independently coexisting legacy systems. Their interfaces are mostly proprietary. Only recently built systems use standard interfaces, as defined by Health Level Seven (HL7)[1]. Communication servers are used to connect to proprietary interfaces. HL7 messages are then sent to all systems that might need the information. If necessary they are converted again to suit proprietary interfaces of the receiver [2]. In principle, the communication server is only a message handling system that rarely does any information handling or interpretation. A communication server centralizes the message handling tasks, and so the task of interfacing the different systems is simplified. The responsibility for the information is not touched and lies with the legacy systems. This will create problems as will be shown. They can be solved if the responsibility for the information is centralized too. Especially the problem of access control can then be delegated to one system and has not to be solved individually for each system.

2. The Communication Server

On of the main tasks of a communication server is to serve as a *message hub*. Every message is only send to one system and will only come from one system. This reduces the number of interfaces needed for each message generating or receiving system. Most commercially available communication servers offer a wide range of tools for *message translation* to the HL7 standard. The obvious advantage of a communication server is then that any proprietary interfaces or HL7 "dialects" are hidden and only "standard" HL7 messages are visible. The servers are used to implement a *message store and forward* mechanism to make the sending system independent of the state of the receiving system if an asynchronous transfer is selected. Another important feature discussed in depth by Simonic and Gell [3] is *message flow supervision* e.g. the replication of incoming messages to systems that

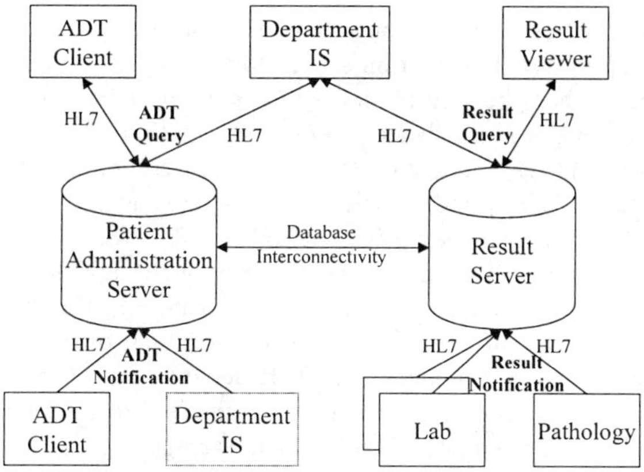

Figure 1 Information server architecture

might have an interest in the message. So organisational aspects only have to be maintained in the communication server. As they point out, even data privacy can be enforced this way. When sending the duplicated messages data can be omitted depending on the receiving system.

If it is assumed that the communication server will send copies of an incoming message to only systems that need this information at that time (data privacy), there has to be a query mechanism to get the information, if the need will arise at a later time, perhaps after a patient has been transferred. This has two possible implications: either a query mechanism has to be implemented for each system sending messages. This will greatly expand the interfaces to be implemented. Their cost will increase. Or to avoid the need to query, all messages are copied to each system that might have an interest in the contents either now or in the future. This unnecessarily adds to the message traffic since messages are transmitted without any need. While it might not be of importance considering the capacity of modern networks, it also means that information is being made available without any need. This creates a conflict with German data privacy laws stating that information should only be made available if it is needed in the clinical context.

Another problem concerns the *update of message contents*. If messages are only send to systems that have a need as determined by a time variant clinical context the communication server has to keep track of each message being sent. Only then can it deliver updates to all systems that have received the original message. This problem will increase if some systems have originally queried the possibly erroneous data.

The advantage of the store and forward capabilities of the communication server has been described above. But problems can arise due to a *partial store and forward* in combination with the duplication of messages. If one of the receiving systems that has been offline might discover an error in the original message hours later, all systems that have already acknowledged must have a rollback mechanism. It is obvious that one of the reasons causing the inconsistencies is the distributed storage of redundant information. A purely event-driven messaging paradigm often will lead to redundant storage and precautions have to be taken to prevent inconsistencies. This means increasing the functionality of the interfaces, making them more expensive to implement. So we decided to develop an information server rather then using a communication server.

3. Information server

The information server is based on three principles:

1. For every type of data there is only one storage place accessible.
2. Data will be transmitted "on demand" rather than "to whom it may concern".
3. Redundant storage of data is not encouraged.

Since the information server is positioned between the information sources and the sinks, it acts as an *information hub*. The information sources transmit their data once they are available or need to be updated to the appropriate information server where they are stored. Any request for the data by systems other than the information sources themselves is fulfilled by the information server. This concept is not restricted to one information server as long as each stores its own types of data and they do not have any types in common. The second principle *data on demand* can be easily fulfilled if the information sink will always query for the data when they are needed. There will be no unsolicited transmission to any information sink. Thus the problems of communication servers concerning the update of data already sent is eliminated. The drawback of this restriction is that alerting must be realised by a polling mechanism. Precautions have to be taken to prevent to much overhead for the information server. The third principle is a matter of trust. It depends on the performance and the availability of the information server. As long as the queries are fast and the expected downtime will be acceptable there is no need for redundant storage.

If access is restricted to querying, the access rights at the time of the query can be easily checked even if they are defined on the basis of the clinical context. The *security policy* at the hospital is based mainly on five rules [4]:

1. Access by an information sink is restricted to read-only access.
2. Patient data are visible by the unit that ordered them and the unit that filled the order.
3. The unit directly taking care of the patient has *temporary access* to all patient data. This access is denied after the patient's care is completed.
4. Units indirectly involved in the diagnostic or the treatment process of a patient by being the filler of orders for this patient also have *temporary* access to all patient data.
5. Each data object can be individually hidden either rule-based or on demand. (This is used for hiding stigmatizing diagnoses, inpatient stays at specific clinics, etc.).

Upon receipt of a query the information server checks all data objects of the type requested whether any of the four rules allowing access do apply. Since access is only by way of the information servers, only they have to implement the security policy. So three advantages are gained: 1. the security policy can be easily implemented or changed; 2. compliance with the security policy can be enforced since only a few centrally controlled systems are involved; 3. the information sources do not have to offer a query interface or enough computer capacity to fulfill all queries without loss in performance even during peak hours.

4. Experiences

Two information servers are currently implemented. One is a *patient administration data server (PADS)* as supplied by the administration system, the other is a *result and report server* used to integrate the different laboratory systems, pathology, microbiology, ECG, radiology, department systems, etc. as illustrated in fig 1, that will be described in more detail. They are both used in daily routine. As information sinks department systems and client systems are connected to the two servers in a typical client-server architecture as described by Sinha [5]. To simplify the design every system uses HL7 queries to access the servers as described by Ohe and Kaihara [6]. On purpose there is no additional SQL layer for data retrieval as done by Willard, Sielaff et. al. [7]. The downside of this is that queries are restricted to a set of predefined types needed for daily routine. But this way we can assure that only queries are allowed that will not hinder the performance of the information server in total. This could be the case if queries can be defined freely that make very poor use of the data model of the information server. The same reasoning does also apply to the approach to integrate SQL logic into the HL7 syntax as described by Ohe and Kaihara [7].

MIRAplus, the central result and report server, is an information server based on the above principles. Its concept is that any result or report source will transfer asynchronously their data upon availability as unsolicited observation messages according to the HL7 standard. MIRAplus stores the data in its database. All information sinks will use HL7 queries to get the data using synchronous communication. Several department systems and individual clinical workstations using a specially developed viewer are currently accessing this server. MIRAplus has been developed by the department of medical informatics using an ADABAS C database. It runs on a Sun Ultra II Twin Processor (2x300 MHz) under Solaris 2.6 (640 MB memory, 50 GB hard disk capacity) connected to the FDDI backbone of the hospital network. Weekly downtime is less than 15 minutes. December 1998 there were stored about 17 million lab values increasing by 15,000 values per day. More than 100.000 textual reports are available. Since preliminary lab results are transmitted also, the server handles about 36,000 unsolicited HL7 messages sent by the result sources daily. More than 100,000 laboratory values and other medical reports are transmitted as the result of HL7 queries to department systems or clinical workstations. This number is constantly increasing. The report and result data are not stored locally in the clients. Mean response time to a query is 1.4 seconds with a median of 1.0 second ($q_{25\%}$ = 0.7 seconds, $q_{75\%}$ = 1.5 seconds) and a maximum below 30 seconds. It must be taken into account that a query usually is quite complex like "give me all recent lab values for all patients on my ward". Currently the main effort is put into creating HL7 interfaces for the other result and report sources and to integrate them in MIRAplus to complete a computerised patient record (CPR).

5. Conclusions

Using the concept of an information server we were able to integrate existing legacy information sources like laboratory systems etc. with minimal requirements for the interface. The information servers act as a hub thus reducing the number of interfaces required for integration of information sources and sinks. Since each information server is the one trusted server for its specific type of information, the need for redundant storage is minimized. Thus the problems with update of information as can be experienced with communication servers is eliminated. The restriction of access to only queries turned out not to be a problem. So a very simply HL7 interface for connecting the information sinks to the information server could be realized. It also allowed for a centralized implementation of the security policy as defined by our hospital and the German data privacy laws.

References

[1] HL7 Standard Version 2.3. Ann Arbor, Michigan: Health Level Seven, 1997.

[2] Jostes C, Pacskowski J, Schröder J. Ganzheitliche Medizin - HL7 - Schnittstelle für Klinikanwendungen. IX 1993; (7):92-6.

[3] Simonic K.-M., Gell G. A General Approach to the Strategy of Integrating Healthcare Applications using HL7. in: Lun KCetal, Editors. MEDINFO 92. Elsevier Science Publishers B. V., 1992: 1432-6.

[4] Schrader U, Kotter E, Pelikan E, Zaiß A, Timmermann U, Klar R. Critical Success Factors for a Hospital-wide PACS. in: Masys DR, Editor. The Emergence of "Internetable" Health Care - Systems that Really Work. JAMIA - Journal of the American Medical Informatics Association, 1997: 439-43.

[5] Sinha A. Client-server computing. Communications of the ACM 1992; 35:77-98.

[6] Ohe K, Kaihara S. Implementation of HL7 to Client-Server Hospital Information System (HIS) in the University of Tokyo Hospital. J Med Syst 1996; 20(4):197-205.

[7] Willard E, Sielaff BH, Connely P. Integrating Legacy Laboratory Information Systems into a Client-Server World: The University of Minnesoty Clinical Workstation (CWS) Project. Methods Inf Med 1995; 34:289-96.

Medical Informatics Europe '99
P. Kokol et al. (Eds.)
IOS Press, 1999

Design of the SGML-based electronic patient record system with the use of object-oriented analysis methods

Eila KUIKKA, Anne EEROLA, Jari PORRASMAA, Ari MIETTINEN
Department of Computer Science and Applied Mathematics,
University of Kuopio, P.O.Box 1627, 70211 Kuopio, Finland
Jorma KOMULAINEN
Department of Pediatrics, Kuopio University Hospital
P.O.Box 1777, 70211 Kuopio, Finland

Abstract. Since a patient record is typically a document updated by many users, required to be represented in many different layouts, and transfered from place to place, it is a good candidate to be represented structured and coded using the SGML document standard. The use of the SGML requires that the structure of the document is defined in advance by a Document Type Definition (DTD) and the document follows it. This paper represents a method which derives an SGML DTD by starting from the description of the usage of the patient record in medical care and nursing.

1. Introduction

The electronic patient record (EPR) is an answer for the well-known difficulties in the use of the paper patient record. Numerous electronic patient record systems [2, 3, 4] have been implemented in particular environments with the use of some predefined techniques. An opposite approach to these specific implementations is taken in a set of systems or prototypes which represent the patient record as a structured document containing the standardized markup [7, 11]. SGML (Standard Generalized Markup Language)[5] is an international standard to define the markup notation used in structured documents. An SGML document follows the structure which is defined with the use of a Document Type Definition (DTD). The DTD can be designed by considering the paper patient record and by defining the potential semantic elements and their relationships [6, 10]. The derived structure may, however, conflict with what doctors and nurses actually require in their everyday practices. The problem here is that the necessity of information is not considered, new information requirements may not be found, and the possibilities to evaluate the medical care and nursing routines may not be discovered.

The aim of the paper is to develop a method for the derivation of an SGML DTD by starting from the description of the utilization of the patient record in medical care and nursing. The method has the following steps:

1. The flow of the data in the clinic is considered from the patient records point of view.

2. The conceptual modeling is done using the Unified Modeling Language (UML) [1] to describe the medical treatment in a natural way.
3. The tree diagram [6] of the SGML DTD is created from the UML class diagram using a set of rules presented in Section 4.

2. Analysis and design

Our target was to analyze carefully where in the organization the information of the EPR is utilized and in which order, what is the importance of the information and when, where and why the information about the patient is gathered to the EPR. Therefore we made a careful analysis with doctors, nurses and secretaries of the Department of Pediatrics of the Kuopio University Hospital. We felt the UML [1] insufficient for the description of the flow of the information in the organization. Hence we utilized the traditional data flows [12].

According to the object-oriented approach the concepts of the real world are *objects*, for example patient record, clinic, blood test, etc. Each object possesses an *identity*, a *state* (consisting of the values of its *attributes*), and a *behavior* (methods). An attribute of an object can be an object. This leads to the *aggregation relationship* between objects. The objects are defined in *classes* which form a class hierarchy. The class hierarchy allows subclasses to inherit properties from superclasses. The superclass is a *generalization* of it's subclasses. *Concrete classes* define objects. *Abstract classes* are used for the definition of the properties that subclasses inherit. These concepts are usually described using UML class diagram [1].

Our work has similarities with the work of Salminen *et al.* [8] who appied the metodology of Shlaer and Mellor [9] for document analysis.

3. SGML DTD

According to the SGML standard, a structured document consists named elements whose identifiers and hierarchical relationships are defined in the DTD. All the documents of a type have to follow the same DTD. The DTD defines for each element *a content model.* It specifies the subelements, their order and existence conditions. The following sample DTD defines that the `patient` element consists of the name of the patient (`name`) and zero or more visits (`visit*`) in the clinic. The patient name is a sequence of characters (`#PCDATA`) defining a *content element.* The `day`, `clinic`, `doctor?` and `problem` elements are contained in the `visit` element, in this order and by the condition, that the `doctor` element is optional.

```
<!ELEMENT patient          - - (name, visit*)>
<!ELEMENT (name)           - - (#PCDATA)>
<!ELEMENT visit            - - (day,clinic,doctor?,problem)>
```

A document instance according to this DTD would start, for example, as follows

```
<patient><name>John Hui</name><visit><day>21.12.1998</day><clinic>...
</clinic><doctor>...</doctor><problem>...</problem></visit><visit>...
</visit>...</patient>
```

If the same content model exists in many places of the DTD, it is possible to define a *parameter entity* to shorten the DTD. The parameter entity is used like an element in the DTD, but the names of parameter entities are not used in the document instance.

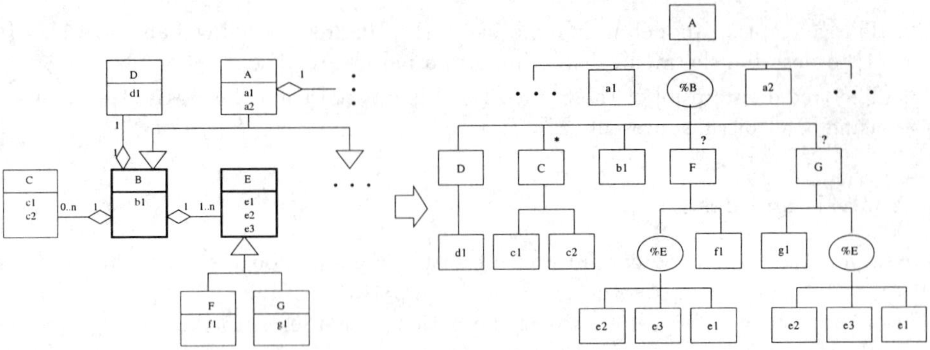

Figure 1: An UML class diagram and the corresponding DTD tree representation

4. From the UML class diagram to the SGML DTD

The potential semantic components are designed in the UML class diagram. The following two sets of rules can be used by the analyst to generate from it the DTD tree representation. Examples in parentheses refer to Figure 1. The rules 1–4 are *transformation rules* and 5–7 *placement rules.*

Rule 1: The concrete class generates an element. (Classes `A`, `C`, `D`, and `F`, `G`)

Rule 2: The abstract class generates a parameter entity. (Classes `B`, and `E`)

Rule 3: The attribute generates a content element (Attributes `a1`, `a2` of `A`)

Rule 4: The parameter entity may be divided into many parameter entities.

Rule 5: The parameter entity corresponding to the super class in the generalization relationship is placed into the content model of the element or parameter entity corresponding to the subclass. (The super class `E` of the subclasses `F` and `G`)

Rule 6: The part in the aggregate relationship is placed as an element or a parameter entity of the content model of the element corresponding to the aggregate. (The aggregation between the class `B` and classes `C`, `D` and `E`)

Rule 7: The element corresponding to the attribute is placed into the content model of the element or the parameter entity corresponding to its class. (The attributes `e1`, `e2` and `e3` of the class `E`)

When we applied the rules to the class hierarchy on the left side of Figure 1 the tree diagram of the DTD on the right side was produced. The UML class diagram does not, however, define all the information needed to generate the DTD. First, the order of the attributes or parts is not fixed. Orders were defined by discussing with the users and examing the paper patient record. Second, elements corresponding attributes of the abstract class may be grouped in various ways when they are placed into the content models of the subclasses.

The relationship between the aggregate and the part defines how many elements are generated into the content model. If a part may exist many times there are two possibilities. If the relationship is `0..n`, then the repeating element is marked by a star character $*$ (for example, the class `C`). If the relationship is `1..n`, then the repeating elements is marked by a plus character $+$. If the repeating part is abstract it generates a parameter entity into the content model of the element of its subclasses. This situation exists in our example for the class `E`.

5. Results and conclusions

We applied the method to define the SGML DTD for the patient record of the Department of Pediatrics in the Kuopio University Hospital.

First, we made a careful analysis with the staff of the outpatient ward of the Department of Pediatrics. We utilized the traditional data flows in describing how the EPR would be used and transfered in the department. We noticed that the doctors and nurses felt the data flow analysis as a natural way to describe their work.

Second, we modeled the content of the EPR with UML class diagrams. Here we tried to increase uniformity, reusability and comprehensibility of the system. At the same time we took into the consideration the queries that the doctors and nurses desired to ask from the EPR data.

Third, we applied the rules represented in Section 4 to the UML class diagrams to generate the SGML DTD of the EPR. The rules produced the tree diagram almost automatically without requiring "too much intuitive design".

The method produces a DTD which is very suitable to be used by the users. Since the classes and attributes in the UML diagram have very content-based names the DTD also uses the specific identifier names. The SGML editor programs use these names to advice the user. However, we are convinced that using a slightly modified set of rules to the same UML diagrams, also a DTD more flexible for queries can be generated. This will be the next step in our work. To get more material to test the method we are currently analyzing the work flows in the inpatient ward of the Department of Pediatrics. The interesting point will be whether the generated DTD differs from the DTD generated for the outpatient word.

Acknowledgments

This work was financed by the University of Kuopio. The authors would like to thank the persons of the ELSA (electronic patient record) project of the Kuopio University Hospital and the Department of Pediatrics for their help.

References

[1] G. Booch. *UML Users Guide*. Addison Wesley, Chicago, Il, 1998.

[2] V. Bradley. Innovative informatics CPR: Computerized patient record. *Journal of Emergency Nursing* **20** (1994) 230–232.

[3] T. Bürkle, H.-U. Prokosch, and J. Dodeck. Steps towards integration of knowledge based functions into a hospital system. In J. Brender *et al.* (ed), *MIE'96*. IOS Press, 1996, pp. 286–290.

[4] P.C. Carpenter. The electronic medical record: perspective from Mayo Clinic. *International Journal of Bio-Medical Computing* **34** (1994) 159–171.

[5] ISO 8879. *Information Processing – Text and Office Systems – Standard Generalized Markup Language (SGML)*. ISO, Geneva, 1986.

[6] E. Maler and J. El Andaloussi. *Developing SGML DTDs from Text to Model to Markup*. Prentice Hall, Upper Saddle River, New Jersey, 1996.

[7] D. Pitty, C. Gordon, P. Reeves, A. Capey, P. Vieyra, and T. Rickards. The place of SGML and HTML in building electronic patient records. In C. Pappas *et al.* (ed), *MIE'97*. IOS Press, 1997, pp. 329–333.

[8] A. Salminen, K. Kauppinen, and M. Lehtovaara. Towards a methodology for document analysis. *Journal of the American Society for Information Science* **48(7)** (1997) 644–655.

[9] S. Shlaer and S.J. Mellor. *Object Lifestyles – Modeling the World in States*. Yourdon Press, Englewood Cliffs, NJ, 1992.

[10] B. Travis and D. Waldt. *The SGML Implementation Guide*. Springer-Verlag, Berlin, 1996.

[11] H. Yoshihara, K. Obe, K. Ohashi, R. Yamamoto, S. Yamazaki, Y. Hirose, K. Matsui, T. Hishiki, Y. Yamashita, M. Kimura, K. Minagawa, and H. Oyama. Standardization of exchange procedures of clinical information using Medical Markup Language (MML). In B. Cesnik *et al.* (ed), *MEDINFO 98 Proceedings*. IOS, Press, 1998, pp. 129.

[12] E. Yourdon. *Modern Structured Analysis*. Yourdon Press, Englewood Cliffs, NJ, 1989.

Medical Informatics Europe '99
P. Kokol et al. (Eds.)
IOS Press, 1999

Computerised Patient Record with Distributed Objects

Tomaž GORNIK, Andrej OREL, Dominik ROBLEK, Roman VERHOVŠEK
Marand d.o.o., Cesta v Mestni log 55, SI – 1000 Ljubljana, Slovenia

Abstract. The vast spectrum of information and functionality requirements imposed on a Computerised Patient Record (CPR), fuelled by an ever changing and expanding business model demands information system interoperability. The management of information, created across the continuum of care, and associated information system functionality, can not be provided by data interchange to and from monolithic applications. WebDoctor is a Computerised Patient Record (CPR) which is fully used at the Institute of Oncology in Ljubljana, Slovenia – a hospital with 500 beds and more than 200 users, all of them medical professionals. The data are stored in an underlying Oracle hospital data base. For logging the username and password security is used. WebDoctor uses Internationalisation APIs. Currently GUI is currently written in Slovenian language, but can be easily adapted to any other language. It is available in either Metal or Windows look. Search for patients is based on CPR No. or partial data from demographics. All the available patients data can be found on a single screen divided into several tab sections. The tab sections cover general and speciality data. The general data include demographics, admissions and diagnoses, meanwhile the speciality data are divided into Labs where data are represented numerically by date or by type and graphically with the ability of detailed view in separate window, Radiology where results are represented in textual form as well as pictures together with a special viewer to provide detailed analyses and Radioisotopes where results are also being represented in textual form together with a graphical representation. WebDoctor is running on virtually any platform. It achieved the 100% Java Certification which places the application among the firsts if not the first of this kind in the healthcare industry. It excels with a small and light client which doesn't exceed the 150K.

1. Electronic Insight into Patient Data

Electronic media are increasingly superseding paper medical records. The well-designed and easy-to-use Electronic Patient Record (EPR), including text, pictures, graphic display of findings, and in some cases even audio and video clips, provides doctors with complete information on the patient's treatment history. One does not need to be a computer expert to use this information: user-friendly web browsers enable users to retrieve various types of information, regardless of its location. The data is linked and displayed on a full-screen window; it is available to doctors in outpatient clinics while making decisions on further treatment, in hospitals while monitoring hospitalised patients, and in their research chambers while examining different cases. Furthermore, they can also use this information when treating emergency cases and during home visits.

2. WebDoctor, the Web-Based Physician

The Computerised Electronic Patient Record is the result of joint efforts between MARAND d.o.o. company and experts from the Institute of Oncology both based in Ljubljana, Slovenia. WebDoctor, as the EPR has been named, is adjusted to the particular healthcare situations in different countries, including a non-uniform database, user requirements, and current conditions at the time of its introduction.

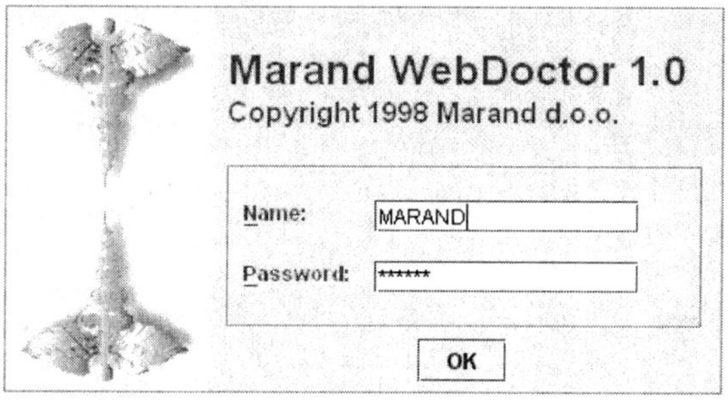

Figure 1: The login applet

3. Three-Level System

WebDoctor's three-level structure is based primarily on Java technologies. At the highest level the client is using his favourite web browser. It supports Java 1.1.5 or higher and can be used by PCs and Macintosh computers, UNIX and other work stations, network computers and smaller portable computers. The middle level is realised by means of a middleware server connected to users via the Internet or Intranet. Objects based on business logic contained in the server respond to inquiries submitted by users. They are linked to databases and other interfaces, which prepare and process data and see to its security. The lower level includes a relational database which encompasses all types of data: text, graphic and multimedia.

The middleware server, which uses its methods to prepare and process EPR data, is written entirely in Java. It is connected to clients via the RMI (Remote Method Invocation) or CORBA protocol. The data are stored in the database being accessible to the server by means of a JDBC driver.

The user interface is also written in Java. It was programmed using Java development tools. The interface was made using standard Swing components and enables simple browsing through EPR data.

The entire system is password-protected. Every user must log in by entering his or her user ID and password. By adding a special card reader, authorisation is also possible using a smart card (for example, Slovene Health Insurance Institute healthcare cards) or some other identification tool (for example Java ring).

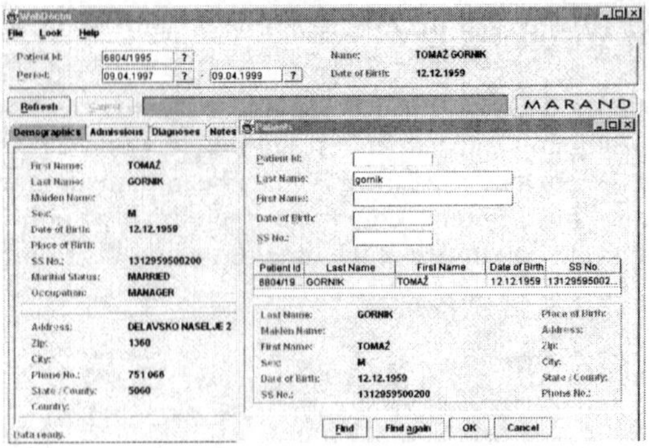

Figure 2: Demographics and patients search

4. Browsers in the Doctor's Office

The program has to be started using a browser. First, a system logon applet is displayed. Upon entering User ID and password the main EPR window is displayed. All the data are available in the same window, and depending on their contents they are divided into individual worksheets that can be selected using tabs. If required, the worksheet can include several pages, to be selected with lower-level tabs.

The data are arranged into seven groups, or data sheets. On the demographics sheet personal data are collected, and on the others followed by the admission to medical treatment data, diagnoses, physician's records, laboratory findings, isotopic examinations and radiology (X-ray, ultrasound and CT). The upper part including the patient's record number, his basic data, the period for which data should be displayed, and the display refreshing button is common to all the sheets. All the data on individual sheets are namely always referred to the same patient.

The patient is selected by entering his record number. If that number is unknown, it can be found in a separate window by means of part criteria (first name, family name, year of birth, and suchlike). The period for which data should be displayed has to be selected, too. The personal data also include data on relatives, employment and the authorised (personal) doctor.

Every patient's visit in the health-care institution is registered. In addition to the date the reason of treatment, summary of treatment, doctor and department the patient has visited are stated. At each episode the doctor prepares an entry. The records can be browsed on the corresponding CPR sheet. On a separate sheet all the patient's diagnoses are recorded, together with the corresponding classification, if it is available.

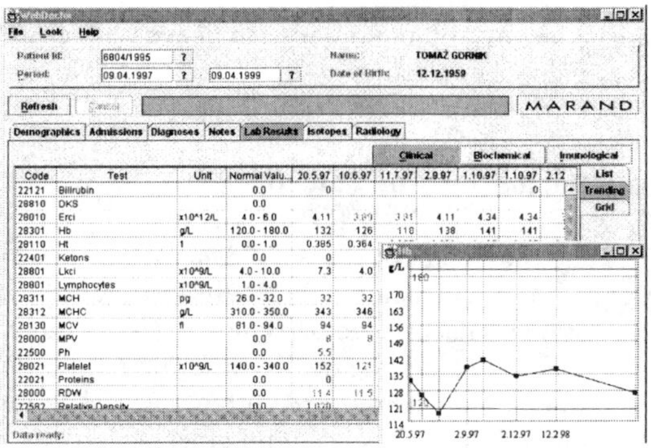

Figure 3: Laboratory results

The laboratory examinations are divided into clinical, biochemical and immunological ones being all arranged within the CPR. The results of all the examinations on a specific day, or the variation of the examination results within a specific period can be retrieved. As a help orientation values for individual examinations are used. A result lying within normal limits is written in blue colour, otherwise it is red. If the colour is black, this means that data could not be compared to the normal values. For graphic display one or several kinds of examinations can be selected. A corresponding number of graphs with the orientation values indicated, and the curve connecting individual examinations are displayed. By clicking an individual graph it can be enlarged (zoomed) and displayed within a separate full-screen window.

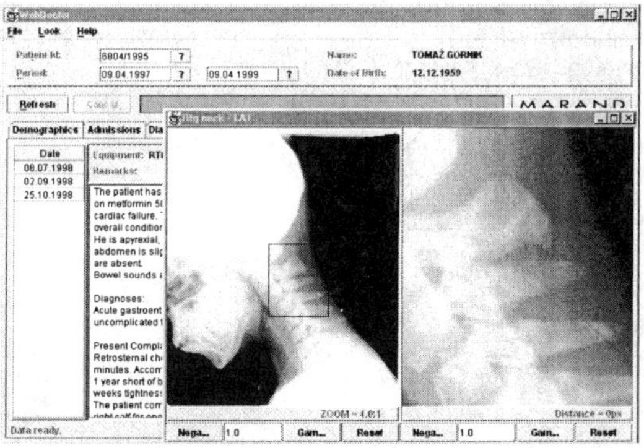

Figure 4: Radiology

For the isotopic examinations all the examinations, carried out within a single episode, together with the doctor's opinion and renogram are indicated. The similar situation is with the radiological examinations, only that pictures are added there. On the worksheet only a preview picture is available, which is, indeed, too small for more detailed examination. By mouse click a special viewer is started, and the whole picture is displayed in the left half of the window, while in the right half its selected enlarged part is displayed. If a X-ray radiogram is recorded with a good enough resolution, an ordinary monitor screen will do for the diagnostic needs. The radiogram can also be displayed in inverted (negative) view, or with a selected gamma correction.

5. Any Time, for Any Doctor, for Any Patient

The ease of use and the excellent access to data located in different databases are the two biggest advantages of WebDoctor. Personalisation opens up the possibility for individual users to access the data they actually need. The reliable network infrastructure with Intranet and Internet services and the quality information service maintain the site and see to its uninterrupted operation. Internet and Intranet access is no longer a rare thing in the world, and the Web-based interface is becoming increasingly user-friendly.

References

[1] O'Connor K., Information Technology Policies for Integrated Delivery Systems, Proc. HIMSS 1997, Healthcare Information and Management Systems Society, vol. 2, 24-31, 1977

[2] Lafrance S., Integrating the Electronic Health Record with Existing and New Hospital Systems", Proc. Toward An Electronic Patient '96, Medical Records Institute, vol. 1, 566-569, 1996

[3] Metzger J. and Marwaha S., Redefining the Patient Care Information System, in: Patient Care Information Systems - Successful Design and Implementation, ed. Hannah K. and Ball M.,Springer-Verlag, New York, NY, 187-212, 1996

[4] Ernst & Young, Information Technology for Integrated Health Systems - Positioning for the Future, ed. Kissinger K. and Borchardt S., John Wiley and Sons, New York, NY, 16 -17, 1996

[5] Jagannathan V., Reddy Y.V., Srinivas K., et al., An Overview of the CERC ARTEMIS Project, Proc. Symp. Comput. Appl. Med. Care, 19:12-16, 1995

[6] Kohane I.S., Greenspun P., Fackler J., Cimino C., Szolovits P., W3-EMRS: Access to Multi-institutional Electronic Medical Records via the World Wide Web, in: Hripsak G., ed. Proc. of the Spring Congress of American Medical Informatics Association, Boston, Mass., 1995

[7] Cimino J.J., Socratous S.A., Clayton P.D., Internet as Clinical Information System: Application Development Using the World Wide Web, J. Am. Med. Inform. Assoc., 2:273-284, 1995

Medical Informatics Europe '99
P. Kokol et al. (Eds.)
IOS Press, 1999

The holistic architectural approach to integrating the healthcare record in the overall information system

Fabrizio Massimo Ferrara, Pier Angelo Sottile, *GESI Gestione Sistemi per l'Informatica srl & Consorzio EDITH - Via Rodi, 32 - 00195 Roma*
William Grimson, *Dublin Institute of Technology, Dublin*

Abstract. The integration and evolution of existing systems represents one of the most urgent problems facing those responsible for healthcare information systems so that the needs of the whole organisation are addressed. The management of the healthcare record represents one of the major requirements in the overall process, however it is also necessary to ensure that the healthcare record and other healthcare information is integrated within the context of an overall healthcare information system. The CEN ENV 12967-1 'Healthcare Information Systems Architecture' standard defines a holistic architectural approach where the various, organisational, clinical, administrative and managerial requirements co-exist and cooperate, relying on a common heritage of information and services. This paper reviews the middleware-based approach adopted by CEN ENV 12967-1 and the specialisation necessary for the healthcare record based on CEN ENV 12265 'Electronic Healthcare Record Architecture'.

1. The Middleware-based architectural approach

The organisational structure of healthcare is distributed, being a geographical spread of centres at different levels of complexity - from general hospitals and clinics to individual GPs. From the information technology point of view, delivery of healthcare is usually supported by a number of different, heterogeneous and often mutually incompatible applications, which are installed and operational in individual centres, meeting the specific needs of particular groups of users. Generic middleware components like DCOM and CORBA provide solutions for the technological interconnection of distributed systems but do not address inter-operability and inter-working of the systems from the point of view of application-oriented support meeting a range of users' needs. Or put another way, the semantic aspects of inter-working needs to be the prime focus once the technical problem of distribution is solved. In passing it can also be noted that the exchanging of messages is not sufficient, since this approach can only lead to a loosely coupled inter-working among the different sectors in an organisation, without meeting the needs of the healthcare organisation as a whole.

As for other business scenarios, the overall healthcare organisation can be considered as a set of users, individually different and doing specific jobs, but all needing to rely on and to share a set of common fundamental data and exploiting a common set of business services. Such common data and facilities ideally should not be under the ownership of individual applications and/or suppliers, but must be accessible to all applications (under controlled conditions) through public and stable interfaces which should not depend on any specific technical characteristic or system configuration. These objectives and requirements may be effectively satisfied and supported by structuring the architecture as defined in the CEN ENV 12967-1 standard 'Healthcare information systems architecture' (HISA) [1]. In this standard the information system is modelled as three co-operative layers (applications, middleware, and bitways), individually responsible for addressing specific design and operational aspects of the information system, as shown in Figure 1. The three-layer structure can be interpreted in terms of the 7-layer OSI model [2], but for the purposes of this paper a few points can be made. The 'bitways' refer to the technical infrastructure providing distribution and connectivity in the generally heterogeneous environment and are not specific to the healthcare domain. The applications refer to the software components identified and associated directly with the user activities, and in very general terms includes data operations, the use of embedded knowledge and presentation of information on computer screens and other devices. It is the choice of splitting the location of these software applications that is crucial to the development of a middleware approach. The reasoning used is that applications providing services to more than one user or category of users points strongly to positioning such services where they can be made available to all users – and the middleware-layer is the appropriate location. In addition to these Common Services, other components offering generic support are ideally placed in the middleware-layer too, security being one example.

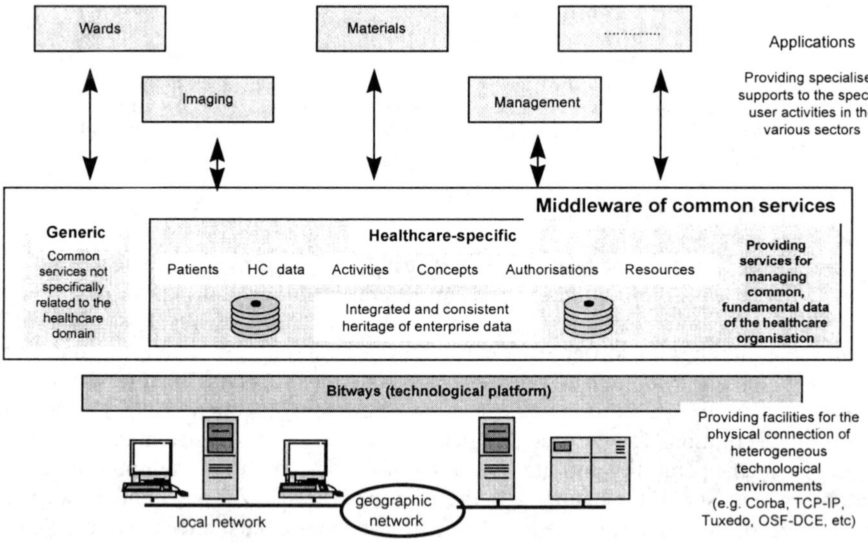

Figure 1. The 3-layers structure of the CEN architecture of health care information systems

The essence of the HISA standard is that **information represents a common heritage and must be clearly separated from the client applications;** and that the information should be made be available to other components of the information system.

The middleware-layer (usually just referred to as middleware) represents therefore the central element of the system, providing a holistic infrastructure where all applications may be connected, as shown in the Figure 2. This middleware, through its services, facilitates the management of the information common to the whole organisation through stable and technology-independent interfaces.

To illustrate the role of the HISA middleware and explain that it offers extensibility the inclusion of components providing **Clinical Coherence** is briefly explored. It is intended that a generic Galen Terminology Server resource will be positioned in the middleware [3]. The Galen Terminology Server encompasses, manages, and provides access to a large extensible formal model of clinical terminology, and it can be foreseen that such a service or set of services would be useful to a range of users in different clinical domains. There are three main aspects to be considered, each of which explains why a middleware approach is appropriate. First, *hiding complexity*: the GALEN Terminology Server provides a tool-set for local use to configure the server appropriately and to hide any complexities that are not required. Second, *mapping*: to provide a mapping between elements of the model held within the server, and elements of local or external coding schemes or data-sets. Third, *extending*: to extend the underlying model, perhaps to cope with specific complexities that are not covered by the model within the server. In each case the problems in providing support across organisations is manageable if these aspects are dealt with at the middleware level rather than within the desktop. In addition to the above configuration activities, the multilingual capabilities of the Galen Terminology Server providing generic support for a particular language, as well as cross-language support (such as providing the set of language annotations for the elements of the model) are by their very nature ideally placed in the middleware.

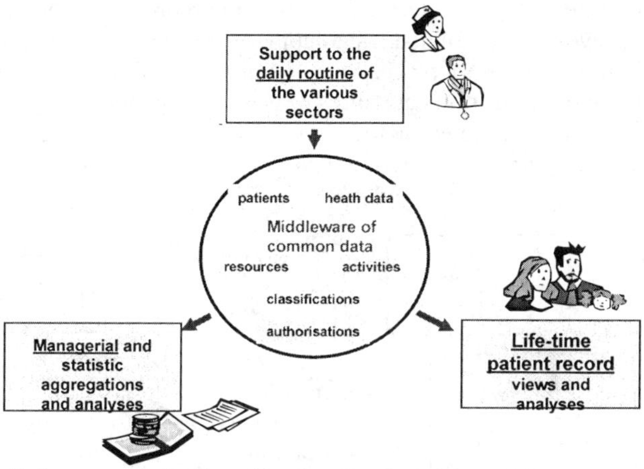

Figure 2. The holistic approach facilitated by the adoption of the middleware paradigm: data are common and may be accessed and used for supporting different needs and applications

2. The Healthcare Record in the middleware-based architecture

As defined in the CEN ENV 12265 'Electronic Healthcare Record Architecture', the healthcare record is an aggregation of information which *'may contain anything'* relating to the patient [4]. Each user is free to include the various types of information in the healthcare record of one patient, according to the specific needs, depending on reasons based on the clinical speciality, the health status of the patient, the organisational needs, etc. Because of this complexity, it is difficult to reach agreement on the precise definition of a healthcare record architecture that can lead to implementable record systems. Synapses addresses this problem in a pragmatic manner and the approach is outlined later in this paper [5],[6].

HISA currently addresses the issue of the Healthcare Record, fundamental in any healthcare community, through a homogeneous view, capable of integrating the various needs and ensuring the consistency of the whole information heritage of the organisation. And it must be noted that in most cases the information being included in the healthcare record is the result of some activities being carried out with respect to the patient. However, the same information, which might be present in the healthcare record also, represents fundamental data used to support a number of other processes in the organisation. For example, the same information in a request for a radiology examination (being part of the HCR of the patient) might also be necessary for planning purpose in the radiology department, for accounting reasons in the administrative department, and from the clinical point of view to the physicians/technicians actually performing the examination. This means that the way the data is made available needs to take into account the wide range of users of the data in addition to the principal clinical users of the HCR.

From this general perspective managing the healthcare record (HCR) as a completely separate entity in the information system would therefore be a strategic error, unavoidably leading to technical problems and even to organisational conflicts. And, the same information-centred perspective discussed for the whole organisation (see Figure 1), is also valid from the standpoint of the healthcare record information: in fact, we have a number of different users, different each from other and individually responsible for certain activities, but all of them needing to share a set of common data, fundamental for doing their daily work, as shown in the Figure 3. The question that then arises is what constraints need to be put in place to provide those elements of the common data that various users require without making every piece of data available to everyone: some control in addition to 'authorisation' needs to be in place. And the need to be able to construct meaningful aggregations of data to users and categories of users is dependent on the application of rules defined by the users and accepted by the organisation. For the HCR as a special aggregation of fundamental data Synapses and *SynEx* have proposed a solution [7].

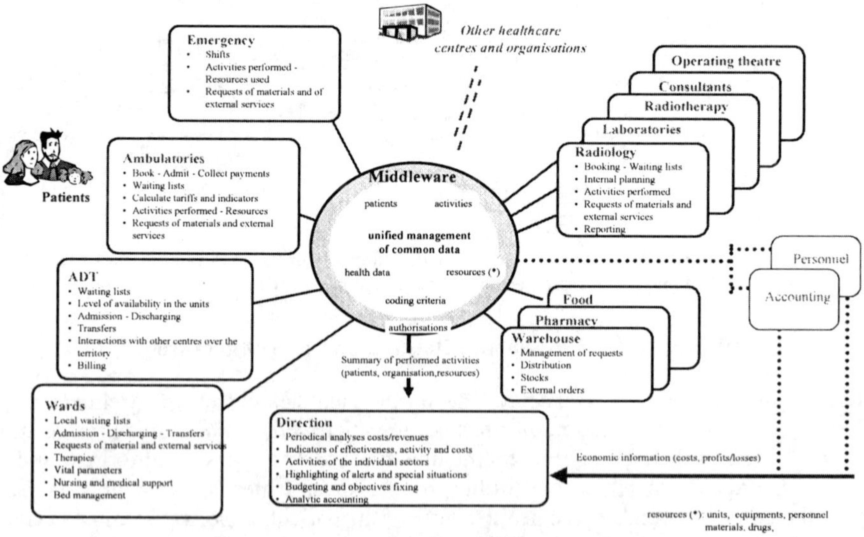

A set of users, performing individually specific activities, but sharing a common set of fundamental data

Figure 3. Categories of Users/Functional units having common access to fundamental data

Through such an approach, the HCR can be considered as an aggregation of (parts of) the information available in the information system, being clustered according to different views, criteria and perspectives according to the specific needs and characteristics of the individual users. Consequently each user is free to define the most suitable HCR (and to select the HCR application suiting their needs), and in addition multiple HCRs can co-exist in the (local or regional) organisation, ensuring nevertheless the integrity of all data as well as the facilitating the use of the data by other applications. As is outlined in section three of this paper each of these HCRs will however be subject to some constraints.

From the architectural point of view the relationships between the HCR and the common data and services may be schematised as shown in the Figure 4. A set of common services of the healthcare information system provides the facilities for accessing and manipulating the elementary common data. On top of these services, a set of more specialised services are responsible for allowing the manipulation and communication of the healthcare record concepts, by aggregating the elementary data and managing them according to the requirements, views and constraints of healthcare records.

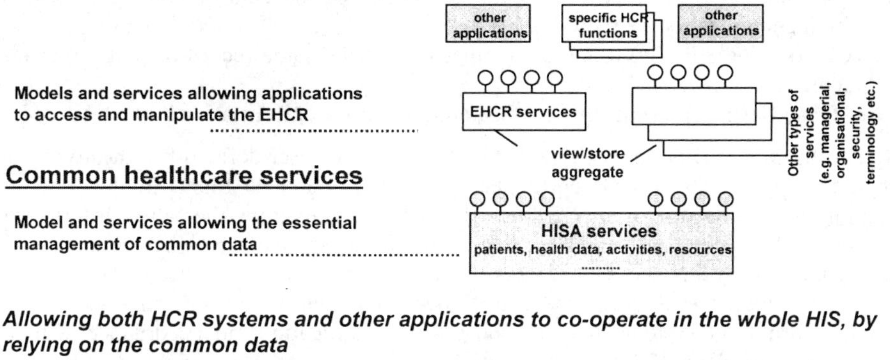

Figure 4. Complementarity and mutual positioning of services for the manipulation of the common data and for the management of healthcare records

This mutual positioning of the common and specialised services also provides the guidelines for facilitating the definition/evolution of common specifications (e.g. standards) in the different fields, nevertheless ensuring their mutual consistency and complementarity. The evolution of the HISA standard should focus mainly on the common services guaranteeing the support and the consistency of the overall information heritage of the healthcare organisation, by means of direct access to the elementary data, together with the more complex 'business objects' capable of implementing complete functionalities (e.g. admission of patients, identification of patients, requesting exams, etc.). HCR evolutions, on the other hand, should focus on the common services capable of supporting the specific (legal, clinical, communication) requirements of the various healthcare actors, regarding the retrieval, aggregation and manipulation of the various elementary data of interest, wherever they have been generated.

3. The Synapses/SynEx approach to the EHCR

The architecture of the EHCR initially proposed by Synapses, and being currently refined in the *SynEx* project, is based on the previously discussed considerations. By using the HISA services for the access and manipulation of the common elementary data, the *SynEx* EHCR server provides a set of services for managing the healthcare record, based on a well-defined object model (SynOM).

At one level the SynOM provides an aggregation mechanism for the record where the aggregation hierarchy contains the object classes in the model. In addition to their use in the exchange format, the classes of the SynOM form the basis for the Synapses object dictionary (SynOD). There are six concrete classes in the aggregation hierarchy which are derived from the Record Item Complex class. These classes perform the following functions:

Record Folder is the root of the aggregation hierarchy and forms the basis for identification of the patient and entry into a particular patient's EHCR.

FolderRIC is used for high level aggregation and may be used to split the record into organisational units.

ComRIC may be considered as the smallest autonomous set of ordered information in the record, which is permissible from an ethico-legal perspective. In other words it should be structured so that it contains sufficient data to make medical sense on its own.

DataRIC may be used to provide the primary context for record items containing medical data.

ViewRIC1 contains a query procedure for the source of the data or another part of the record which generates sets of record items.

ViewRIC2 contains a link to a RIC in another part of the same record or part of an other related record.

And the **RecordItem** represents the smallest atomic piece of information in the record.

The Synapses Object Dictionary (SynOD) contains a set of user defined healthcare objects, which are mapped to the data representations of these objects found in the 'common heritage' in the middleware or other information systems containing the patient information. The purpose of the SynOM becomes clearer now as these SynOD object definitions are expressed using **only** instances of classes derived from those which can be found in the SynOM. The records thus constructed are indeed aggregations of information available from the information systems but are constrained aggregations in accordance with the requirements of the ENV 12265.

4. Conclusions

One of the goals of *SynEx* is to bring together the work on EHCR from GEHR, CEN TC 251 and Synapses with the Information Systems perspective of HISA for the general reasons set out in this paper; surmounting the technical challenges is now well under way. As a possible extension to HISA, the possibility of defining additional data objects and services in the specification of the middleware is being considered with a view to providing a more specific and optimised support. To put it another way, extensions are being sought to provide additional support to the application functionalities responsible for manipulating the EHCR (e.g. to define templates for the various EHCR's used in the specific organisation, to simultaneously enter/retrieve groups of healthcare record items, etc.). And it can be remarked that one of the strengths of the HISA middleware architectural approach is that it facilitates such extensions and in principle allows information systems to evolve in an orderly fashion.

References

[1] CEN ENV 12967-1 "*Healthcare Information System Architecture*"

[2] S. Spahni, J.R Scherrer, D. Sauquet, P-A Sottile, *Consensual trends for optimizing the constitution of middleware*, ACM SIGCOMM Computer Communications Review, vol. 28 Number 5 (October 1998).

[3] A. Rector, W. Solomon, W. Nowlan and T. Rush, *A Terminology Server for Medical Language and Medical Information Systems,* Methods of Information in Medicine, Vol 34, pp.147-157.

[4] CEN ENV 12265 '*Electronic Healthcare Record Architecture'*

[5] J. Grimson *et al*, *Synapses - Federated Healthcare Record Server,* Procs. MIE 96, IOS Press, pp.695-699.

[6] J. Grimson *et al*, *A CORBA-based Integration of Distributed Electronic Healthcare Records Using the Synapses Approach*, IEEE Trans. Inform. Tech. In BioMedicine, vol 2, no 3, Sept 1998

[7] http://gesi/synex/

Medical Informatics Europe '99
P. Kokol et al. (Eds.)
IOS Press, 1999

Document versus Data Centred Approach to the EPR

Baud Robert PhD, Rassinoux Anne-Marie PhD, Lovis Christian MD
Medical Informatics Division
University Hospital of Geneva, Switzerland

Abstract. This paper presents the document centred Electronic Patient Record (EPR) as currently in production in a large university hospital and subject to multiple additional developments in the coming years. A number of basic hypothesis have been developed in order to reach the best medical practice and the success of this application. In addition, the alternative approach of data centred EPR is compared, and different benefits and pitfalls are highlighted. It is not easy to evaluate the consequences of such an initial trend, but changing one's mind after having a system in daily production is anyway costly and difficult. Therefore, the selection of the right orientation in a given hospital necessitates a scientific debate.

1. Possible contexts for an EPR

Strictly speaking, one can build a new EPR in two extreme contexts and therefore in any of the multiple intermediate contexts in-between. In the presence of an existing Information System (IS) in a given hospital, the EPR benefits from a source of information under the form of "photographs" of the patients at specific moments, corresponding to the actual state of the IS regarding this patient. Due to the multiplicity of IS in an hospital after many years of informatics solutions, it is clearly an advantage not to assume any standard about this information.

On the other hand, in a low computerised hospital where the existing IS are not really of interest for physicians and patients (because of a too strict administrative orientation), the EPR is without original medical sources. This presents the advantage of an open situation where nearly any new solution can be built upon. The freedom of developing new ideas is counter-balanced by the need to develop anything from scratch and this may be a heavy burden with high consumption of resources.

The reality generally lays somewhere between those two extreme situations. One can frequently take advantage of an existing ADT system (Admission Discharge Transfer) for patient identification. Laboratory results are quite often available as computer outputs. But drug orders are rarely available through a computer application. Follow-up medical notes generally are out of reach of a centralised word processing systems. They are good exceptions, but the ideal situation never exists. One is inevitably faced with some existing IS and the need to cope with them. If this would not be the case, one would observe duplication of information and basically such a situation is not acceptable by the medical community. One is definitely forced to interface existing systems when building the EPR. As a consequence, because interfaces are difficult and costly, the careful inventory of categories of existing IS is of major importance.

2. Basic prerequisites for an EPR

Some basic conditions which are more or less prerequisites for the success of the EPR [1]. Such conditions - considered as "axioms" - are generally set at initial design time, and they should not be modified; if this would be necessary, a broad consultation of all actors is necessary to prevent collapses between different parts of the system. Well designed axioms are the premises to guarantee the success of the system and lack of axioms may be a reason for failure. Axioms act as a contract between the physicians and the implementers of the EPR: good contracts give good results. In general a good contract should have the written form. This approach by axioms may be compared with the initiative of the Institute of Medicine [2].

When looking for the axioms of the EPR, the designers try to open the way to emerging key paradigms. Axioms may be just the confirmation of existing practice and solutions; hopefully, they are also the leading entities for the future application. Discovering the basic axioms is another way to push the new solutions and to define the new trends, according to today's technology [3].

The authors started an EPR system in 1996 at the Hospital of Geneva and the first discussions rapidly led to a couple of strong decisions. They soon wrote a document containing 22 axioms about functionalities and principles of implementation. This document has been left unmodified three years later and the axioms are still perfectly valid. The major ones are: EPR is made of read-only documents only; towards an ubiquitous paper-less EPR (on the long term); content-oriented browsing strategies for document access; linkage from in- to out-knowledge; strict control of accesses and log of all actions; implementation on a low-cost platform to insure large distribution of terminals; fast access time (below the second); horizontal increment of the system when facing heavier workload (N servers architecture).

3. Pros and cons of data centred and document centred approach

Multiple criteria can be considered in order to compare the situations of IS and EPR. They are enumerated hereafter.

3.1. Event driven or content dependent

The IS focus on daily activities with the ultimate goal to help and control the management of the patients; the IS is sensible to different events which act as triggers for a number of actions like entering an order in a list, printing laboratory results or noticing the need for patient transportation. Events are the starting point for actions, therefore the IS is mainly reactive. On the other hand, the EPR is more static. It represents the history of the patient and acts mainly as repository of documents; it provides views of the patient at different point in time. In the EPR, documents may be organised by content.

Access by content is desirable. Lexical browsers are clearly insufficient like many examples can demonstrate. On a lexical browser a query like “fracture of the lower extremity” may not retrieve a “fractured metatarsal bone”. There is a lack of inference capabilities. Another query like “eyelid” may miss “blepharitis” or “papebral ectropion”. There is a lack of conceptual representation. One can understand that the solution should be conceptual based on a model of the medical domain. Current researches are performed in this direction and new solutions are emerging elsewhere [4, 5] and by the authors [6, 7].

3.2. Chronological versus multiple views

Events in the IS occur chronologically; therefore, the IS is largely time-oriented. Such an organisation is visible in the deepest implementation of the data base. On the contrary, the EPR is most often organised according to the content of its documents, and not their chronology; this means that documents reporting on the same topic are grouped based on content similarities, typically laboratory results or follow up medical notes are grouped and chronological order is only a secondary sort key.

3.3 Data or patient history

The IS basically collects data about patients: name, ID, sex, laboratory data, diagnosis code, drug prescription with drug name, dose, route of administration, appointment, etc. The atoms on which transactions are based are data from 1 to a few bytes. Any single data may be changed according to given user request. The patient is represented through a rough model built on a couple of hundreds of fields in the best situations. In other words, only a small part of the medical reality is grasped by current IS even in the best hospitals. The clear advantage of this situation is that any data is well known in advance regarding its scope and variability. The coherence of any data pertaining to a set (generally called a record) is guaranteed; cross checks are the rule and in case of error different procedures are able to come back to a previously coherent state. An excellent review paper with numerous references considers this aspect [8].

The EPR handles documents in free text, and possibly images and other media; its capacity to represent the reality of the patient conditions is limited only by the author of the texts using natural language or the technical limits of the specified media (image resolution, etc). This unlimited power of expression comes with an evident drawback: the control of the document's content is left to the user and incoherence between one document and the next is evidently possible. Emerging techniques of natural language processing are not yet ready to change this situation, despite such a move will certainly be true during the next decade. Text representation and content dependent methods are future directions to explore [9].

3.4. Transaction on database or write once file system

IS are built on large transactional database. Different relational tables are developed and links between fields of tables are designed in order to allow cross relationships. Nevertheless, the authors have clearly advocated the solution of a file system to store the documents of the EPR. One directory is open for each patient and a hierarchy of directory is implemented on top to partition the whole set of more than 1 million documents today. The selected file system is NTFS under NT 4 on the Intel PC platform. This approach is simple, efficient and at lower cost than the database approach.

3.5. Frequent updates or read only

An on-line transactional system is characterised by frequent update. For example, to satisfy a laboratory request a number of actions are triggered in a short time frame between 30 minutes and 2 hours: entering the order, validating the order, editing sample labels, printing work lists, managing the lab analysers, controlling the workflow, validating the results, printing the results, just to mention the main ones. Each action is reported in some way in the computer system and some data are changed at each step. Frequent updates are the first characteristics of a transactional system.

On the other side, the EPR is document centred, and through those documents it provides the history of events for this patient as well as detailed reports on patient conditions. The history of the patient has to be considered as an established fact and most hospitals give a strong legal connotation to this aspect: nobody is allowed to modify the history, except some trivial situations. This means that basically there are no updates, except some particular situations. The main indication in favour of a database system is down.

3.6. Data oriented versus document centred

Considering now the needs of clinicians in front of their patients, looking for recent or older health episodes, what do they want? First, they ask for a fast retrieval; second they advocate the best rate of success for this retrieval; third they want an intelligent application and fourth they appreciate the conviviality of the interface, because they never have enough time to learn computer intricacies. They want to see the past of their patient like a story with text and images. They are looking for opinions of their colleagues, for status, for discussion of diagnosis and prognosis, and other information usually somewhere "between the lines"; they also want to have access to multiple media like images, sounds, etc. In other words they want documents and not data.

4. Conclusion

The decision of implementing a document centred EPR was not common, but it has shown a number of advantages, especially the ease to develop and to deploy new application and the concomitant low-cost. Read-only documents is a very strong early condition imposed to this system, but it is the right choice. In some way the EPR is part of the past, but conveying the future. The history should be read-only for the sake of its integrity. Another key to the success is the fast response time and there is no doubt that this is true in all countries for all physicians: do not make them wait more than a second if you want a long life for your system. Finally, intelligent browsing of documents is regarded as a key point, because this is the way to link internal knowledge about the patient to general knowledge of medicine in general.

In the present experiment, we have learned to make simple steps if possible one at a time. We are working with new technologies like document centred approach. Therefore, we need to discover what are the new dominant paradigms. No way is paved leading automatically to success. An approach by trials and successive evaluation is necessary. In those conditions, we have already found some leading features of the EPR, others are still to be discovered.

References

[1] AL Rector, WA Nowlan, S Kay. Foundations for an Electronic Medical Record. Meth. Inform. Med 1991; 30, pp 179-186.

[2] Institute of Medicine committee on improving the patient record. The computer-based patient record: an essential technology for health care. Washington DC, National Academy Press, 1991.

[3] C Lovis, RH Baud, AM Rassinoux, JR Scherrer. Value to add to the patient record when making the EPR. In proc Eprimp conference, IMIA working group 17, Rotterdam, Oct 1998, pp 225-227.
[4] YL Zieman, HL Bleich. Conceptual mapping of user's queries to medical subject headings. Proc of the 1997 AMIA Annual Fall Symposium, DR Masys (eds), pp 519-522.
[5] CA Sneiderman, TC Rindfleich, AR Aronson. Identification of findings in medical literature using restricted natural language processing. Proc of the 1996 AMIA Annual Fall Symposium, J Cimino (eds), pp 239-243
[6] RH Baud, C Lovis, AM Rassinoux, JR Scherrer. Morpho-semantic parsing of medical expressions. Proc of the 1998 AMIA Annual Fall Symposium, CG Chute (eds), Orlando FL, pp 760-764.
[7] A-M Rassinoux, JC Wagner, C Lovis, et al. Analysis of medical texts based on a sound medical model. Proc of SCAMC 95, RM Gardner (eds), pp 27-31.
[8] AM van Ginneken. The structure of data in medical records. IMIA yearbook of medical informatics 1995, Schattauer eds, pp 61-70.
[9] RH Baud, Present and Future Trends with NLP, Medical Informatics Europe conference (MIE 1997) in International Journal of Medical Informatics 52 (1998), pp133-139.

Medical Informatics Europe '99
P. Kokol et al. (Eds.)
IOS Press, 1999

Donor And The Health Insurance Card

Alenka Posega, dr.med., prim. Pleterski Rigler Dušica
Health Insurance Institute of Slovenia,
Miklošičeva 24, 1507 Ljubljana, Slovenia

Abstract. The health insurance card is a new electronic identification document of insured persons and facilitates smoother communication between the health insurance information system and the Slovene health care service provider information systems. The card stores the insured person's identification details as well as the information on the selected personal physician. Another procedure also to be hosted on the card, will be the card holder's personal decision about being voluntary donor of organs and tissues for transplant purposes. This data item will, supported by the enhancement of technological infrastructure, improve the control of the donorship information. In Slovenia, registering, recording and application of the organ and tissue donorship data is carried out, on a pilot basis, in the region of Posavje.

1. Introduction

The idea of introducing the card into our health insurance system raised high interest among the insured persons, physicians and other health care workers around Slovenia, as well as among the professional public outside the health care sector. In tune with the variance of particular group interests, as well as of theoretical background or familiarity with experiences elsewhere, the opinions and suggestions regarding the definition of the card role and functions varied widely. Some saw the card merely as a substitution for the obsolete health care booklet, while others had much higher expectations. The most part of discussions in the public were concentrated around the dilemma whether to apply the card only to administrative procedures in implementing the health insurance rights, or to apply it also as a carrier of certain medical data, or to apply it in both roles.

In the first phase, the card was designed to serve exclusively as the insured person's identification document and further, to improve communication between the health insurance information system and the health care service providers' information systems. The card chip memory also stores the details of the card holder's selected personal physician.

This first phase of implementation of the health insurance card system did not set final boundaries to the scope of card roles and functions in the health care system, but rather only opened the ways to enhancement. As early as in the health insurance card project start-up document, the second development phase was announced, to follow the first phase after a short interval. Consensus has been reached to enhance the card application range with the application of storing data on donorship of organs and tissues for transplant purposes (shortly denoted as "donorship" and "donor" here).

2. Regulation of the Field in Other European Countries

When approaching the introduction of donorship data, we examined the solutions in **European** countries; we encountered a variety of regulations of registering this information, however, not on the health insurance cards but rather on separate cards or appended as an extra entry in other documents.

In England, they practice the use of a donor's card, but nevertheless, consent from the family is still required (the donor's card sponsored by the Slovene Red Cross is very similar to the English donorship card).

In Spain, the law allows removal of organs, provided that the individual is not declared against it. Despite such regulations, the physicians still seek consent with the transplant procedure from the family. The data itself is not extra registered, neither in a card or any other document.

In Portugal, Hungary and Sweden, organs are removed without any preliminary inquiry. They have no donorship cards and the data is not registered in any explicit form.

In Austria, no cards are in circulation, however, a register of opponents to removal of organs and tissues for transplant purposes has been set up, and physicians are obliged to respect it. Verification of data in the register is not protected and can be carried out by phone.

In Belgium, organs may be removed, but here too, the register of opponents to removal of organs and tissues has to be respected.

Sweden is introducing a donorship register. The donorship information is maintained in a centralised manner. Data are accessible at the time of an insured person's death. There is no specific card to register donorship data. Verification of data in the register can be carried out by phone.

3. Regulation of "Donorship" in Slovenia

After the introduction of the new card application, **in Slovenia,** the card will store an invisible data item to tell whether the card holder is a voluntary donor. In this way, the card communication value will be enhanced. With this new project, we aim to achieve a better evidence of those insured persons having opted to sign the donorship document, to shorten the time required to establish the "donorship" information, to facilitate the achievement of all goals with observance of modern and statutorily provided principles of personal data security, to increase awareness among the public with the assistance of beneficent organisations, medical profession, media, etc. We may also expect that, by expanding the card data set with the "donorship" data will also result in a promotion of the activity itself.

In defining the "donorship" data, we had to observe the following legal bases:

- Law on Removal and Transplant of Human Body Organs for the Purposes of Healing
- Regulations on Precise Conditions of Conducting of the Removal and Transplant of Parts of Human Body
- Regulations on Conditions of Operation of Health Care Organisations Performing Removal, Transplanting, Processing (Typisation and Storage) of Parts of Human Body
- Regulations on Data Kept in Specialised Registers by Health Care Organisations, and on the Method and Terms of Reporting and Notifying

Considering the transfer of this data item to the health insurance card and the regulation of this field by the Law on Red Cross, we further established that the field is also in implicit ascendancy of the said law, since this law authorises the Red Cross to carry out the activity of recruiting voluntary donors of organs and tissues for the transplant purposes, and to issue the special donorship cards. To this end, the Red Cross organisation is also funded from the national budget.
In view of the delicacy of the field and of several legal and deontologic issues arisen in the process, the opinions regarding the expansion of the health insurance card with the data on organ and tissue donorship for transplant purposes have been sought from the following bodies:

- Extended Professional Collegium on Transplantation
- Chamber of Physicians of Slovenia
- Deontology Commission of the Ministry of Health Care
- Health Council of the Ministry of Health Care
- Red Cross of Slovenia

All of these bodies agreed with the initiative to enter the "donorship" data into the health insurance card, under strict observance of the rules of securing personal data.

After the completion of preparatory activities, the Institute, in September 1998, appointed the "Donor" project group, inviting the participation of the representatives of Extended Professional Collegium on Transplantation, Red Cross of Slovenia, Deontology Commission of the Ministry of Health Care, and the Caritas organisation. At its regular monthly sessions, the project group developed the "Donor" project, the primary guidelines of which are as follows:

- The "donors" declarations will be archived by the Health Insurance Institute, at its premises in Ljubljana, Mikloši~eva 24.
- The declaration in favour of donorship is a personal declaration, and can be effected exclusively applying the prescribed affiliation form. The insured person signs the statement, one copy of which is then sent to the Institute. In the case of the "donor's" subsequent changing of mind, he is to fill a withdrawal form, one copy of which is, again, sent to the Institute.
- By signing the affiliation statement, the "donor" expresses his consent to entering the data on such decision into the health insurance card in the form of an invisible data item. After entering the data in computer, the original copies of the affiliation and withdrawal forms are archived at the Health Insurance Institute of Slovenia. The archiving procedures will strictly adhere to the Law on Personal Data Security. The "donorship" data is stored in the health insurance card at the time of updating the card at the self-service terminal. To provide extended security, no indication of the status of the donorship data is shown on the SST screen. The status can only be examined by calling in person at the authorised Institute official.
- The "donorship" data can be read from the card only at ten locations of intensive care around Slovenia (so called "donorship" hospitals), where the hospital organ and tissue transplant coordination officers will have, at the time of establishment of the patient's clinical death, the right to read the organ and tissue donorship data item from the patient's HIC.
- In the cases the deceased does not carry on himself the "donor" document, the same terms apply as in the case of the person not having declared in favour of donorship.

- In the card memory, a data field is allocated to the donorship information, to store one of the following codes:
    - 0- no information
    - 1- donor (entered by SST)
    - 2- not a donor, withdrawal form submitted (entered by SST).
- The information on organ and tissue donorship for transplant purposes will be introduced into the health insurance card system in a progressive manner, hence, the Red Cross paper donor card will remain in use. The new method of transmitting the donorship information is introduced into the Slovene environment in a progressive manner. First, it will be tested in the region of Posavje, where the health insurance card has already been introduced.

4. Conclusions

According to statistical data, in Slovenia, 42 kidney, 4 heart and 3 liver transplants were performed in the period of first ten months of 1998. Those organs for which the transplant service could not find a suitable recipient in the country, were offered to the Eurotransplant organisation. This is a transplant network comprising the EU members Austria, Netherlands, Germany, Belgium and Luxembourg. The Slovene network Sloveniajtransplant is in the course of foundation and will be an affiliate member of the EU network.

The advantage of the introduction of the "donorship" information into the health insurance card stems from the assertion of order and evidence in the field of donorship. Up to now, there have been cases where an individual, after having declared as donor and received the Red Cross donor's card, subsequently discarded of that card or destroyed it at no consequence. Hence, in the event of his death, the hospital did not have confirmation whether the person is still a donor or not. By entering this data item onto the card, such situations will be avoided. Namely, the card is a mandatory instrument of access to the health care services. In addition to other insurance data, the card will also store the record stating whether the holder is a donor. Opposite to other data, the set of which is mandatory and provided statutorily, the donorship information will be based on an individual's personal decision to declare as donor and to enter this information onto the card, on an absolutely voluntary basis. This also observes the Law on Security of Personal Data and the principle of voluntary provided statutorily in this field.

It is obvious that the health insurance card and the introduction of the organ donorship in case of death can in no way resolve all the problems facing the field of transplantology in Slovenia. To promote and popularise the idea of the benefits of donorship of organs to preservation of life and health of co-citizens, further activities will be necessary in a variety of fields and performed by a variety of associations and organisations, not the least, among the ranks of the Slovene physicians.

References

[1] Health Card 97 Congress, L. van den Brock, A.J. Sikkel
[2] Martin Toth, Uporaba kartice in širitev nabora podatkov (Use of the Card and Expansion of its Dataset), Čatež 98
[3] Prim. Von~ina Jasna, dr. med., national coordinator of organ and tissue transplants, Data on transplants in European countries

Medical Informatics Europe '99
P. Kokol et al. (Eds.)
IOS Press, 1999

Structuring clinical information in Healthcare Records

A.Rossi Mori (1), F.Consorti (2)
(1) CNR-ITBM, Viale Marx 15, 00137 Roma, Italy (angelo@itbm.rm.cnr.it)
(2) IV Clinica Chirurgica, Università La Sapienza, Roma

Abstract. We carried out an analytical study about names of clinical documents, titles of generic sections, names of data elements, to prepare the European Prestandard CEN ENV13606-2 on "Health Informatics — Communication of Electronic Health Care Record — Part 2: Domain Termlist". The goal of the standard is to facilitate transmission and/or homogeneous browsing of clinical information from disparate patient records, without any preliminary agreement on coding systems, data elements, record organization.
With the assistance of the members of CEN/TC251/PT27 and under the control of CEN/TC251/WG I and WG II, we defined three layers to structure clinical information (structuring records into complexes, complexes into statements, statements into details) and we prepared many lists suitable to represent coarse-grained information about the different constructs used in the above layers.

1. Introduction

The Technical Committee TC251 "Health Informatics" of CEN (the European Standardization Body) [1] is preparing the European Prestandard ENV 13606, in 4 parts, about "Health Informatics — Communication of Electronic Health Care Record".
A standard cannot impose a particular organization to a record system, but it can facilitate the communication and the processing of clinical information by the receiving record system, by preserving as far as possible the structure of the information in the sending system by an appropriate markup. The topic is innovative and needs extensive field tests.
CEN procedures allow to approve a provisional version of the standard, as the basis for three years of distributed testing. The final standard (EN) is planned for the year 2003.

2. Materials and method

In order to prepare the "Part 2: Domain Termlist" of the CEN Prestandard ENV 13606, we carried out an analytical study of

- several lists of document names, e.g. Notes (progress notes), Requests (diagnostic request), Reports (discharge summary, report of diagnostic procedure), Notifications (infectious disease notification), Charts (observation chart);
- 700+ titles — e.g. Reason for contact, Family history, Treatments Plans — from 7 authoritative sources of section titles [11, 15, 16, 18, 19, 20, 22];
- several lists of names for data items, e.g. ocular reflexes, birth weight, drinking habits.

We used the approach for terminological modelling adopted by CEN/TC251 [4] and the methodology developed by GALEN project [2,5,6]. The integration between the perspectives of terminology and of information modelling within the patient record structures [8, 9] was the topic of three workshops of the European Project ToMeLo [3] in 1997 and 1998.

3. Results

We defined three major layers for structuring clinical information within a record system, and we produced a series of related lists. as described below.

3.1 Structuring the record into documents and sections (record complexes)

A record may be organized in nested complexes, i.e. documents or sections. Complexes convey to the receiver the original organization and may contain structured and/or unstructured clinical data (e.g. free text or multimedia not directly processable from a semantic point of view).
Even without using further structures, names of complexes (i.e. document names or titles of sections) may be useful, e.g. to build a table of content for manual browsing or to limit the search within complexes with a particular name in text-based information retrieval.
We prepared two classifications (one with 20 classes of document names and one with 30 classes of section titles), a taxonomy of 200 generic section titles, a system of 75 descriptors to annotate the above titles (41 descriptors in 8 primary annotation types, 34 descriptors in 7 secondary types).

3.2 Structuring a complex into clinical statements (data items)

Certain complexes may be organized into smaller processable units, called here clinical statements, each representing a "situation", e.g. a symptom, a laboratory result, a drug prescription. Clinical statements can be individually handled according to task-dependent criteria, e.g. to create dynamic views.

A clinical statement is made of two parts:

- the **clinical concept**, regarding the nature of the situation (e.g. surgical procedure) and the essential details (e.g. body part, approach, extent, instruments);
- the **status concept**, regarding circumstances in a particular patient record, as information about *subject of information* (e.g. patient or relative) or *actual status* (e.g. an activity may be "done" or "planned", a finding may be "goal" or "result" of observation).

According to the results of our experimental studies, we defined a taxonomy with the most relevant subtypes of situation:

situation

- condition or state
- - normal condition
- - abnormal condition
- - - allergy state
- - property
- - - constitutional features
- - - - vital signs
- - body process
- - family dynamics and relationships

- life features
- - activity of daily life
- - habits
- - education
- - occupation
- - marital status
- - residence status

- events
- - healthcare events
- - - acquiring information
- - - - history taking
- - - - physical examination
- - - investigation
- - - recording images and signals
- - - interpretation
- - - decision-making activity
- - - therapeutic activity

- - - - physical actions	- - - information and education activity
- - - - drug-related activity	- - - administrative activity
- - - - preventive activity	- - non-healthcare events
- - - - - immunization activity	- - - accidents
- - - - - screening	

3.3 Structuring the content of a statement

Certain statements may have an explicit internal structure, i.e. a record system may be able to handle the detail within a statement. For example, within the statements on laboratory tests, a system can handle name, sampling date, numeric value and units to draw a chart.
We defined the idea of "archetype", to describe the details that can appear in the internal structure of the various kinds of statements, e.g.:

therapeutic activity	
acts on	*body component, lesion, body process, device*
has location	*body component*
is performed according to	*method*
has means	*device*
has qualifier	*approach, route*

It is anticipated that the requirements about well-formed statements are satisfied by the most common coding systems. Developers and users of record systems can use archetypes to increase their awareness on the overlaps among details expressed within coded values, data element names, and section titles [7, 9].
Archetypes are also useful to design and use terminological services to extract specific details from entries of advanced terminological systems.
We prepared a provisional list of archetypes for various subtypes of situations.

3.4 Links between constructs

Finally we studied the relationships among the previous constructs. In fact, an important feature enabled by a proper markup of electronic record systems will be an extensive usage of links among record components.
We produced a tentative list of 30+ link names to allow for experimenting with this mechanism, e.g

healthcare activity	*is documented by*	*note*
situation	*is assigned to*	*problem*
condition	*is interpretation of*	*findings, report*
informing	*has topic*	*record component*

4. Conclusions

With our experimental studies on a reasonably wide and differentiated set of corpora, from different countries, we prepared a basic European Prestandard, that allows to process coarse grained information from different record systems without preliminary agreements on record organization, coding systems, data elements.
Our results should not be intended as a conclusive solution, but as the substrate for a formative evaluation of the various measures, to be consolidated in a final standard by the year 2003.
The measures described in the CEN European Prestandard ENV 13606-2 can be applied in data transmission from a record system to another, as well as for homogeneous browsing of different records of the same patient in different locations (i.e. the "virtual patient record", the "life-long patient record").

The above achievements are the basis to share a principled structure across heterogeneous healthcare records, that can be enforced by further standards by different organizations (e.g. HL7, CEN/TC251, ISO/TC215).

Acknowledgements

Work undertaken by CEN/TC251/PT27 on "Health Informatics — Electronic Health Care Record Communication — Part 2: Domain Termlist" under mandate of UE to CEN, with the contribution of the UE Projects GALEN-IN-USE and ToMeLo.

References

[1] CEN/ TC251 "Health Informatics", at http://www.centc251.org
[2] GALEN and GALEN-IN-USE. documentation (1992-99), available from AL Rector, Medical Informatics Group, Dept. Computer Science, Univ. Manchester, Manchester M13 9 PL, UK e-mail galen@cs.ac.man.uk; see also http://www.cs.man.ac.uk/mig/galen and http://www.cs.man.ac.uk/mig/giu
[3] ToMeLo (an European Project) see documentation at http://www.ehm.kun.nl/tomelo/#Workshops
[4] Rossi Mori A, Consorti F, Galeazzi E. Standards to support development of terminological systems for healthcare telematics. Meth Inform Med 1998 (in press)
[5] Galeazzi E, Rossi Mori A, Consorti F, Errera A. A cooperative methodology to build conceptual models in medicine. In: MIE 97, IOS Press 1997
[6] Galeazzi E, Rossi Mori A, Consorti F, Errera A. MEDITA: the reference methodology for cooperative production of dissections by terminological analysis. GALEN-IN-USE, internal report MET01/97, May 1997
[7] Rossi Mori A, Galeazzi E, Consorti F, Bidgood WD Conceptual schemata for terminology: a continuum from headings to values in patient records and messages JAMIA symp. suppl., 1997:650-4
[8] Rossi Mori A, Consorti F. Integration of clinical information across patient records: a comparison of mechanisms used to enforce semantic coherence. IEEE TITB, 1998 (in press)
[9] Rossi Mori A, Consorti F. Exploiting the terminological approach from CEN/TC251 and GALEN to support semantic interoperability of healthcare record systems. Int J Med Inform 1998; 48:111-124
[10] Alschuler L, Sokolowski R, Rossi Mori A, Dudeck J. SGML/XML in healthcare information exchange standards, in: Proceedings Conf. SGML/XML Europe, Paris, May 98
[11] HL7 SGML/XML Special Interest Group. The Kona architecture proposal. Draft available at http://www.mcis.duke.edu/standards/HL7/committees/sgml/kona.htm
[12] Rector AL, Nowlan WA, Kay S, Goble CA, Howkins TJ. A framework for modelling the Electronic Medical Record. Meth Inform Med 1993; 32:109-19
[13] Rector AL, Nowlan WA, Kay S. Foundations for an Electronic Medical Record. Meth Inform Med 1991;30:179-86
[14] ASTM E1384-91. Standard Guide for Description for Content and Structure of an Automated Primary Record of Care
[15] Severs M (on behalf of the Multi-professional Working Group). Headings for Communicating Clinical Information from the Personal Health Record, a position paper. IM&T training unit, Solihull (UK), September 1997
[16] AMA/HCFA, Documentation Guidelines for Evaluation and Management Services, 1998, available at http://www.hcfa.gov/medicare/mcarpti.htm
[17] Servers M. EPR Programme, Occasional Papers – paper 1: Headings for Communicating Clinical Information from the Personal Health Record. NHS Executive (UK), April 1998, IMG ref. C3231
[18] Severs M (on behalf of the Multi-professional Working Group). Headings for Communicating Clinical Information from the Personal Health Record, a position paper, revision 1998
[19] Pollock D. (ed) Data Elements for Emergency Department Systems (DEEDS). US Department of Health and Human Services, National center for injury prevention and control, Atlanta, Georgia, release 1.0 1997
[20] National Committee on Vital and Health Statistics (NCVHS). Core Health Data Elements, US Department of Health and Human Services, National Center for Health Statistics, August 1996
[21] SNOMED DICOM Microglossary (SDM), see http://www.snomed.org/sdm/sdm.htm
[22] Vaughan NJA, Home PD, Vermeij D, Sando SH, Cashman SJ (eds). The Development of a Generic Message for Use in Diabetes Care. from the "Fifth Gubbio Workshop of the EASD Study Group DO IT" held jointly with the European Union BIOMED Concerted Action project MFIT, GUBBIO, (PG-Italy) 16 -18 May 1997.

Medical Informatics Europe '99
P. Kokol et al. (Eds.)
IOS Press, 1999

Security for Electronic Patient Record Systems

M.A.Pronkin, M.A.Shifrin
Medical informatics laboratory,
N.N.Burdenko Neurosurgical Institute,
Moscow, Russia

Abstract. The presentation is devoted to the problem of security for Electronic patient record system with EPRS for N.N.Burdenko Neurosurgical Institute (NSI) as an example.

1. Introduction

Electronic Patient Record System (EPRS) is an object for application of numerous technologies. These are:

- system survival technologies, power supply first of all;
- common informatics technologies like network technology, database, application design;
- information technologies, specific for medical informatics like use of special standards HL7, DICOM, medical curves processing etc.;
- and last but not least, medical technology of treatment and diagnostic process, which determines most architectural and interface solutions for EPRS.

All these technologies set up specific claims to security, and security of EPRS as whole may be guaranteed only if all "partial" securities are guaranteed . We shall point out main security problems using EPRS for N.N.Burdenko Neurosurgical Institute as an example (NSI EPRS, Ref. [1], [2]).

2. Main features of NSI EPRS

NSI possess 300 neurosurgical beds, 40 beds in ICU, outpatient department, full set of diagnostic equipment (including several MRI and CT devices, digital angiografy device, devices for nuclear diagnostics and therapy). About 3000 patients with all kinds of neurosurgical pathology are treated every year.

EPRS is a component of Integrated Automatic Information System (IAIS) which is intended to support all business processes running in NSI. EPRS is the forepart and the core of IAIS at one time.

Hardware. NSI possess modern LAN built as a star with collapsed backbone. The central switching node has two CELLplex 7000 – ATM-devices of 3Com. Structured cable system consists of fibre cables for vertical traces and UTP Cat.5 for horizontal ones. There are about 600 sockets for PC and the same number of phone sockets.

The cluster consisting of two IBM RS600 Model J40 is used as a database server, IBM PC-servers work as NT-domain, file and other servers.

System software. The main network OS is Windows NT, working stations of IAIS will run under Windows 95/98/NT. Oracle 7 under AIX is chosen as DBMS for EPRS.

Developers. Network infrastructure and special software for EPRS are designed and mounted by Moscow company IBS, one of the leading system integrators in Russia. A new technology IBS/Records for developing information systems in poorly formalised subject domains was realised. Working places and system functions of EPRS are actualised by NSI medical informatics laboratory.

3. Technical facets of security

Technical security may be accomplished with common ways used for critical applications, working in 24/7 mode: uninterrupted power supply for most important devices, doubling of main network and server systems, etc. All these ways are realised (or will be realised in the nearest future) in NSI EPRS. As example we shall point out cluster architecture of the database server and use of two CELLplex 7000 in the central node of the network.

4. Network, database and application facets of security

EPRS is designed as two-level client-server system with DBMS Oracle 7 and "thick" clients. DBMS works on RS/6000 cluster under AIX, clients are work under Windows 95/98/NT. So we have next levels of network security:

- Windows NT security services,
- AIX security services,
- Oracle security services,
- security service of IBS/Records system.

These services deliver reliable defence of database as whole.

Let us say several words about specific IBS/Records security services. First of all, IBS/Records has standard Name/Password entry. Secondly, there are two categories of consumers of IBS/Records system: designers and users (see some details in ref. [2]), and they have different rights to retrieve and update data in database. User may retrieve and update only patient data, and only if they are involved in treatment process of that patients. These rights are managed by system administrators. Designers may also retrieve and update only that system data which are premised by system administrator. Every designer and user may have private data invisible for all other users and designers.

5. Medical technologies facets of security

Technology of TDP make various demands for security. First group of them deals with patient data and arises from the main goal of running any patient records: to ensure integrity of treatment diagnostic process "in space and time", i.e. patients data must be available to any person who needs them for the sake of TDP at any time. EPRS may meet this demand much better than traditional paper patient record (PPR), because use of modern information and communication technologies gives possibility to create integrated informational environment of the hospital (or even hospitals). We treat this demands as security ones because the lack of them jeopardise not only running or EPRS, but TDP itself and, in some cases, life of patient. Next basic features of IBS/Records technology show possible ways to satisfy demands of this kind:

- unique database to store all data: as soon as a user inputted data and saved them, they are available for any other user with proper rights;
- IBS/Records has special embedded mechanisms to put data in the scope of necessary person (doctor, laboratory researcher, etc.) as soon as they are stored in database;
- the high performance of database server and DBMS guarantee that data retrieving and update will take reasonable time so that users will not wait too long; if the access time will be too long, users will stop using EPRS very quickly;
- doctors may will to see patient data in almost any combination - IBS/Records allows to do it with little effort;
- data may be stored for unlimited time and will not be lost in archives.

Another group of security demands is connected with mandatory data, which must be present in patient record in any case. IBS/Records system gives possibility to meet such demands by programming interface items in simple embedded programming language.

6. Legal facets of security

A vast set of security demands are connected with legal facets of treatment and diagnostic process. First of all, no data stored in patient record may disappear. Following this demand designers of IBS/Records found such solutions, that only result of last correction of any item of patient data is visible on the screen, but there exists special mode to see full history of data correction. Deleting of data is available only in debug mode, but not during regular running of the system. Note that all stored data authorised and it is very easy to find out the author of any record and time of input.

Very important legal demand is to have paper copy of electronic patient record. There are several possibilities to meet this demand with IBS/Records system.

7. Conclusion

All said above demonstrate that security for EPRS is a complex problem, involving not only traditional questions of secure data storing, but many specific medical demands. Meeting of principal part of these demands is necessary to make EPRS really working system, capable to help doctors in their work.

References

[1] M.A.Shifrin, E.E.Kalinina, Electronic Patient Record for N.N.Burdenko Neurosurgical Institute: on the Verge of Implementation. This book.

[2] T.E.Pronkina, M.A.Shifrin, Professional Knowledge as the Basis of Electronic Patient Record Systems. This book.

Medical Informatics Europe '99
P. Kokol et al. (Eds.)
IOS Press, 1999

Professional Knowledge as the Basis of Electronic Patient Record Systems

T.E.Pronkina, M.A.Shifrin
Medical informatics laboratory,
N.N.Burdenko Neurosurgical Institute,
Moscow, Russia

Abstract. The presentation is devoted to the role of professional knowledge in the developing of Electronic Patient Record System (EPRS). The main example – EPRS for N.N.Burdenko Neurosurgical Institute (NSI).

1. The aim of presentation

The main aim of this presentation is to demonstrate numerous modes of use of professional knowledge in developing EPRS. The presentation is tightly connected with presentation [1], devoted to some specific features of EPRS for N.N.Burdenko Neurosurgical Institute. This EPRS was developed on the basis of new technology IBS/Records for building information systems in poorly formalised subject domains. The IBS/Records technology enables different ways to use professional knowledge in information system.

2. Transforming knowledge to data

Any program system intended to support professional activity in some subject domain is based on professional knowledge of its designers and users. In "ancient" times principal part of this knowledge was "dissolved" in different components of program systems: architectural solutions, numerous algorithms, interface solutions. If knowledge were changed or refined – programs have to be changed too. Such systems usually do not live without their creators.

General trends in programming, artificial intelligence (AI), cognitology and other related disciplines resulted *in transforming knowledge to data*: there were developed methods of knowledge elicitation and verbalisation, formats to store knowledge and procedures to process knowledge. For example, if we consider expert systems (ES), we shall find out at least two different ways to handle with professional knowledge. Knowledge of experts in subject domain for which ES is intended is stored in knowledge base, very often in the form of productions. These knowledge may be refined and extended with regular procedures of ES, with no programming. Knowledge of AI expert are fixed in architecture of deduction engine. These kind of knowledge may be parameterised, but any serious change leads to new programming. We see that some part of knowledge necessary for ES capacity for work is transformed to data, another one is still "dissolved" in the structure of program.

In general, the lager part of knowledge is transformed to data, the more flexible and multi-purpose becomes the programming system. Further we shall discuss some features of N.N.Burdenko Neurosurgical Institute EPRS from this point of view.

3. Several words about IBS/Records technology and its consumers

As was mentioned above IBS/Records is technology and a programming tool for building information systems in poorly formalised subject domains. At least three categories of persons deal with IBS/Records: programmers, designers – usually specialists in information technologies (IT), users – in our case medics, paramedics, medical administrators, etc.

Programmers deal with program code and we shall not consider representation of their professional knowledge in program system – this question is interesting, but not specific for information systems.

Similarly we shall not ***discuss*** representation of designers' professional knowledge because it is reflected in technology of IBS/Records design process and is not specific for medical information systems.

Professional knowledge of medics – this is the subject of further considerations.

4. Reflection of professional knowledge of medics in information systems designed using IBS/Records

Different kinds of medical professional knowledge are reflected in different structures of EPRS. All of them are transformed to data and may be changed at any moment of design process and other moments of life cycle EPRS.

Technological knowledge, i.e. knowledge related to technology of *treatment and diagnostic process* (TDP) is reflected in *operation model*. This model demonstrates processes in which patient is involved, their sequence and intercommunication. Operation model is designed with special tools of IBS/Records using standard for such models graphic notation and is stored in common database.

Standard medical classifications. All kinds of standard medical classifications (like ICD or drug classifications) may be stored as hierarchical classificators. The also may be changed at any moment. The only restriction is as follows: if any part of classicator was at least once used to describe patient's state, it cannot be deleted. It is result of standard integrity conditions for databases and with natural requirement to EPRS: information about patient may not disappear.

Description of patient state. Very important (maybe, most important for medical information systems) part of medical knowledge is knowledge about signs necessary to describe patient's state. Part of this knowledge is formalised to some degree, and this knowledge may be stored as signs in the sense of IBS/Records. Sings in IBS/Records looks like signs in any other information system with except of one extremely important property: set of signs as they are used in IBS/Records may be changed in any time without help of programmer or database administrator. This feature of IBS/Records technology allows to modify patients descriptions at any time, with no risk to loose any information. This feature is very important for scientific researches.

Non-formalized medical knowledge. It's well-known that very often most essential part of medical knowledge is not formalised and belongs to best experts in domain. Elicitation, formalisation and **dissem**ination of this knowledge is an important task of medical informatics (Ref. [2], [3]). IBS/Records has instrument for solving this problem – embedded expert system (EES). Medical knowledge may be represented in the form of productions. Important feature of EES is that it may use data already stored in information system and use them for refining formalisation of expert knowledge. And again we see that professional knowledge is transformed to data and may be changed at any moment.

5. Conclusion

All presented above shows, that a principal part of medical knowledge may be transformed to data in EPRS designed using IBS/Records technology. All these data may be changed and refined at any moment of life cycle of EPRS, so *the design process becomes continuous and evolutionary.* For example, the first version of the system may consist of demographic and main administrative data, installed on a little part of working places and only a little part of medical knowledge will be formalised. Patients' data will be stored as free text signs and the system will work. And already during its everyday running new working places and functions will be included in the system, new formalised data will appear in it. *The system will live and grow as a live creature.*

References

[1] M.A.Shifrin, E.E.Kalinina, Electronic Patient Record for N.N.Burdenko Neurosurgical Institute: on the Verge of Implementation. This book.

[2] Gelfand, I.M., Rozenfeld B.I., Shifrin M.A., Ocherki o Sovmestnoi Rabote Matematikov i Vrachei (Essays on Collaboration of Mathematicians and Physicians), Nauka, Moscow, 1989.

[3] A. V. Alekseevskii, M. L. Izvekova, I. M. Gelfand, M. A. Shifrin Capabilities and Applicability Range of Formal Methods in Solving Problems of Clinical Medicine. The Purpose of Research and Formal Statement of the Problem , Pattern Recognition And Image Analysis, Vol. 2 No. 3 1992

Terminology

Medical Informatics Europe '99
P. Kokol et al. (Eds.)
IOS Press, 1999

A method for an automated decomposition of a complex term into its conceptual components

BARAC'H V ., BURGUN A., DELAMARRE D., LE BEUX P.
Laboratoire d'Informatique Médicale, Faculté de Médecine, Université de Rennes 1
Avenue du Professeur Léon Bernard, 35043 Rennes cedex, France

Abstract. The paper deals with the improvement of the MAOUSSC model (Modèle d'Aide et d'Orientation d'un Utilisateur au Sein des Systèmes de Codage) and system. Its specific purpose is the automation of the description of medical and surgical procedures. We have developed an automatic decomposition method using a linguistic and conceptual approach based on the UMLS knowledge base. This work concerns the processing of 100 procedure wordings from the digestive surgery domain. We introduce a prototype of such a system automating the decomposition through a web interface.

Keywords : medical language - linguistics - semantics - user computer interface-digestive surgery procedures□ - UMLS.

1. Introduction

The MAOUSSC terminology server has been developed and dedicated to the multiaxial decomposition of the wordings of medico-surgical procedures into their elementary conceptual components [1]. It is based on Web technology and a relational Oracle data base [3]. The MAOUSSC system is associated with the 97 version of the UMLS knowledge base [2]. Multiaxial decomposition of medical procedures by the MAOUSSC system is carried out according to eight axes.

- Four axes are mandatory (Nature, Topography, Instrumentation and Approach).
- Four others are optional (Matter device, Additional topography, Body process, Disease).

It should be noted that the last four axes may depend on the content of the mandatory ones [2]. The first stage for the automation of the decomposition of procedure wordings takes into account only the mandatory axes. Moreover, this decomposition considers only elementary acts (also called MAOUSSC procedures). For example an elementary act is given in figure 1. In the previous system, to decompose a procedure into several axes, all the contents of the axes had to be filled in by the user. The aim of this work was automatic decomposition.

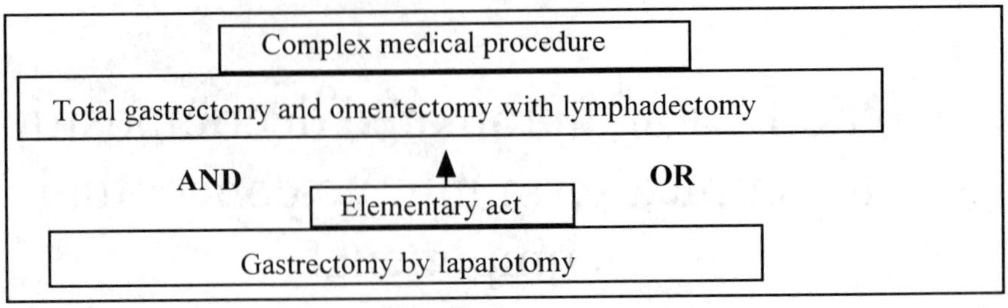

Figure 1: Different aspects of medico-surgical procedures

2. Materials and Methods

The material used for this study was :

- the UMLS knowledge base [4],
- the MAOUSSC data base [1] ,
- the terminology server [3].

The decomposition method of a procedure wording into the axes was done by the various facets of the MAOUSSC procedure. It was carried out in two stages. The figure 2 shows the methodology summary.

1st stage: typing of the wordings. It consists in classifying the items according to the number of words they contain. Three types were identified: «simple» built with only a single words, «compound» constituted of two word «aggregate » made up of more than two words.

2nd stage: automatic decomposition diagram expected for each category. For each category, a decomposition diagram proposes to fill in the four mandatory axes automatically. Three diagrams were exploited: a conceptual diagram for the «simple» type, a combination diagram for the «compound» type, a linguistic diagram for the «aggregate » type.

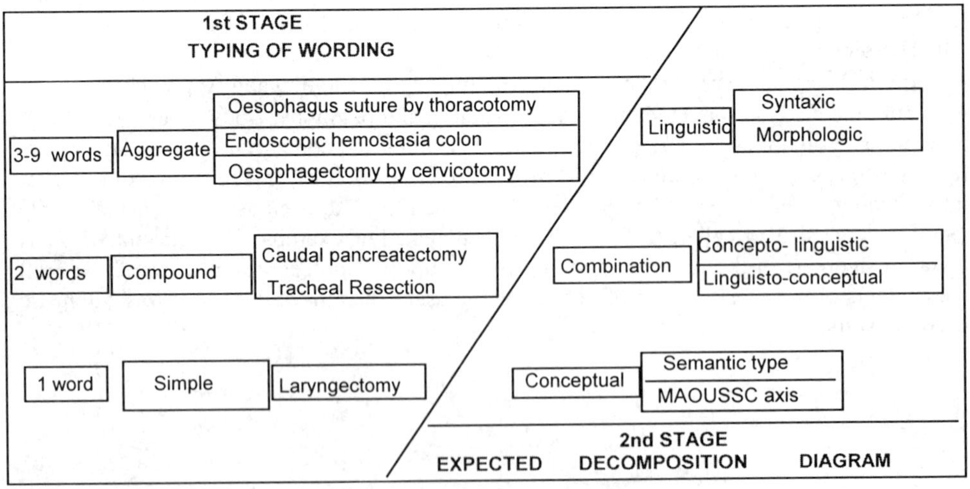

Figure 2: Methodology summary

2.1. Conceptual diagram

It was developed for the description of a «simple» act. The French wording was looked up in the UMLS Metathesaurus. This concept existed in the Metathesaurus or not. When it existed in the Metathesaurus: a correspondence between the MAOUSSC axes and the UMLS Semantic Types performed. This enabled us to establish links between the MAOUSSC axes and the UMLS Semantic Types. If it did not exist in the Metathesaurus: the root-word of the procedure label was extracted from the wording. The root was then looked up in Methathesaurus. The example is given in figure 3.

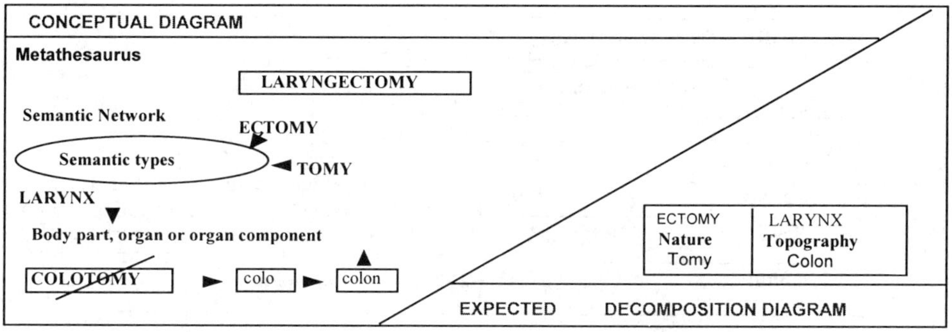

Figure 3: wording presence or not in the Metathesaurus

2.2. Linguistic diagram: syntaxico-morphological analysis

Two sub-stages were necessary for this case: the first one was a syntactic analysis [4]. It had to find in an univocal way the semantic contents of the words. The second one was based on a morphological analysis. Our purpose was to recognize the medical terms and the non medical terms in order to make them play a role. Then it is a question of solving the problem concerning the informational granularity brougth by each word. For example: «Suture» provides one element of information whereas «oesophagectomy» provides two elements. The example is shown in figure 4.

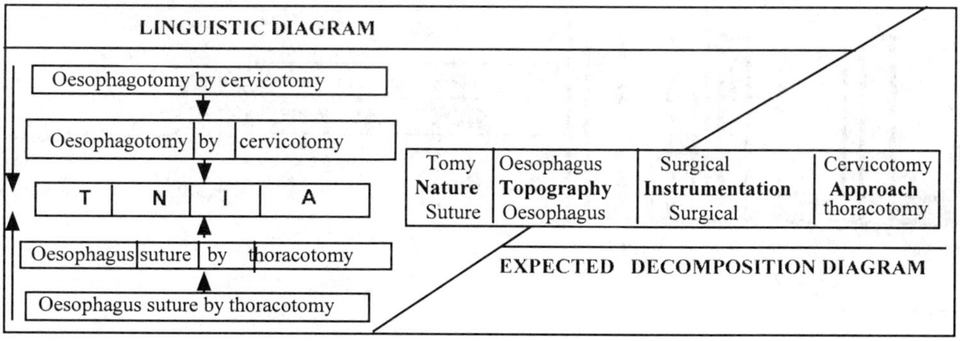

Figure 4: Decomposition diagram of an «aggregate» type

2.3. Combination diagram

There were two sub-types for the «compound» type: the wording of «compound» type and of «simple» sub-type when the first word evokes a «simple» type the wording of «compound» type and of «verbal» sub-type when the first word does not evoke a wording of «simple» type. A combination of two approaches was used for combination diagram is shown in figure 5.
If the word pointed to «simple» type wording, the decomposition diagram was first conceptual then linguistic. But if the first word does not refer to the «simple» type, the decomposition diagram was first linguistic then conceptual.

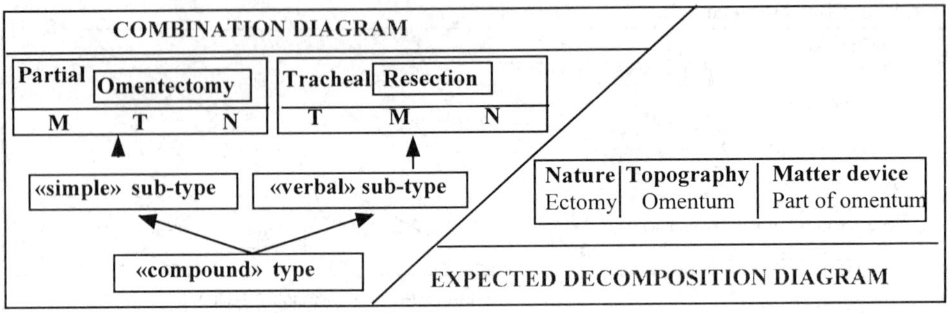

Figure 5: Decomposition diagram of a «compound» type

2.4. The prototype

The automatic decomposition model implementation was carried out on a Unix station. The development was based on Web technology using PERL language [3]. This system has the following functionalities: connection to the browser, data entry of the wordings, analysis of the wording. This last function ensures the analysis of the wording by the recognition of the wording type, the setting up of the decomposition diagram s corresponding to the type of the wording, the interfacing browser on the MAOUSSC server displays the result of the decomposition in an ergonomic way.

Table 1: Synthetic results for each type of wording

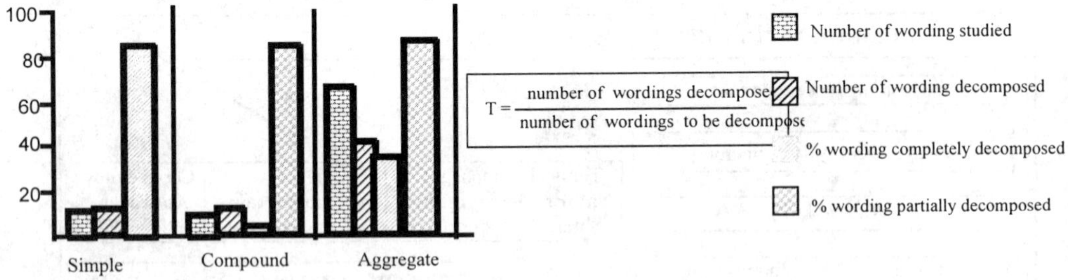

3. Results

100 wordings of the MAOUSSC elementary procedures were used in this method and subdivided into :

17 «simple» type, 14 «compound» type including 6 «simple» sub-type- 8 «verbal» sub-type and 69 «aggregate» type. The results are given in the table 1. Most of the simple «type» wordings were completely decomposed. Whereas the computer-assisted decomposition of «compound» and «aggregate» wording were often partial. The decomposition rate (T) is given in table 1.

4. Discussion

The results are satisfactory but three aspects must be discussed with regards to the previous results.

4.1. The importance of the implicit aspect in the wording of procedures

For the «simple» or «compound» type of the digestive surgery field: the Instrumentation axis could be indicated, in an implicit way as they are usually identical for most procedures [5]. This principle being allowed, an implicit value could be assigned for the Instrument and Approach axes to the wording of the «compound» type. These axes were often implicit but sometimes ambiguous. For example in the case of «appendicectomy» it is impossible to infer the way which was used (coelioscopy or laparotomy). This aspect raises the problem of implicit degree.

4.2. The importance of the conceptual UMLS base

The degree of medical concept coverage of the UMLS knowledge base was analysed and shows a coverage of: 82 % for the «simple» type, 89% for the «aggregate» type including 36% of the wording fully decomposed, 85% for the «compound» type with 6% of the wordings completely decomposed. These results consolidate the choice of the UMLS as the reference terminology. Nevertheless it would be interesting to follow the continuous effort of completing the Metathesaurus.

4.3. Partially decomposable wording

The various facets of the procedure label raised the problem of the multiplicity of formulations. This is why it is necessary to propose a «standard» or «canonical» forms for writing the wordings of procedures. This could be implemented by a linguistic preprocessing which would give these canonical forms and could be mainly automated. A solution for the wordings that are partially automatically decomposable is to reformulate it according to the model. The MAOUSSC system integrates in its model syntactic-semantic rules which are representative the comprehension of the procedure labels. The same is true for the GALEN-IN-USE project which uses a more linguistic approach [6]. The linguistic and conceptual approachs were permitted to decompose automatically the mandatory axes.

5. Conclusion

We have presented a methodology for an automatic decomposition of a complex medical term into its components through the MAOUSSC terminology server. This study lies within the scope of the improvement of the MAOUSSC system. Indeed, the estimates of production of the trained users of the MAOUSSC system have shown that a user could break up an average of 25-30 wordings of acts per day [7]. If the results can be extrapolated from the base of the 100 studied acts, it can be estimated that the prototype would make it possible to gain at least half of the time necessary for a manual decomposition. Recent work on ICD-10-PCS coding system has shown that such a semi-automatic decomposition could be extented to any natural language system [8].

References

[1] Burgun A., Denier P., Bodenreider O., Pouliquen B., Oberlin P., Leveque JM., Luckas B., Kohler F., Fieschi M., Le Beux P. Methodology for using the UMLS as a background knowledge for the description of surgical procedures. *Int -J-Biomed-Comput.* **43** (1996) 189-202.

[2] Burgun A., Delamarre D., Botti G., Luckacs B., Mayeux D., Bremond M., Kohler F., Fieschi M., Le Beux P. Designing a sub-set of the UMLS knowledge base applied to clinical a domain: methods and evaluation. *Proc- Annu- Symp-Comput-Appl-Med-Care.* (1994) 968-973.

[3] Burgun A., Denier P., Bodenreider O., Pouliquen B., Oberlin P., Leveque JM., Luckacs B.KohlerF., Fieschi M., Le Beux P. A web terminology Server using UMLS for the description of medical procedures. *JAMIA.* **4** (1997) 356-363.

[4] McCray AT., Razi A. The UMLS knowledge source server. *Medinfo.* **8** (1995) 75-79.

[5] Huntley M. Presupposition and implicature. *Semantikos.* (1976) 167-88.

[6] Rodrigues JM., Trombert Paviot B., Baud R., Wagner J., Rush P., Meusnier F. An EU Project Applied to the Development of a New National Coding System for Surgical Procedures : NCAM. *Medical Informatics Europe.* **43** (1997) 897-901.

[7] Bodenreider O., Burgun A., Botti G., Fieshi M., Le Beux P., Kohler F. Evaluation of the Unified Medical Language System as a Medical Knowledge Source. JAMIA. **5** (1998) 76-87.

[8] http://www.hcfa.gov/stats/idc10.html

Medical Informatics Europe '99
P. Kokol et al. (Eds.)
IOS Press, 1999

Automatic enrichment of the Unified Medical Language System starting from the ADM knowledge base

Franck LE DUFF, Anita BURGUN, Bruno POULIQUEN, Denis DELAMARRE, Pierre LE BEUX
LABORATOIRE D'INFORMATIQUE MÉDICALE, FACULTE DE MEDECINE, RENNES

ABSTRACT : The Unified Medical Language System (UMLS) project aims to provide a repository of terms, concepts and relationships from several medical classifications. This work describes the possibility to enrich automatically with meaningful links the UMLS database by using description of diseases from another knowledge base, in our case ADM (Aide au Diagnostic Medical). In spite of the constraints and the difficulties to qualify the interconcept links, the results show that it is possible to find and create new links from a french knowledge database to the UMLS one. One of the interests of this work is that the automated learning of the connections could be used with others knowledge databases like expert system databases.

1 - Introduction

Representing knowledge remains an essential problem for medical information systems and networks on account of the plethora of the documents produced. It is necessary to obtain reliable and powerful browsers to reach the most relevant information quickly. The work that we approach here is of interest in the construction of these tools for nomenclatures and in the exhaustivity of such tools. There exists many possibilities to carry out a medical nomenclature. According to the method, the result will be connected more with one catalogue or classification [1] i.e. with a tool more or less fixed, or it will give a 'compositional' system largely dependent on the data-processing tool [2] . Many authors [3, 4, 5, 6] show that these classifications instruments can be complementary from each other and that it is possible to enrich a system from another. This idea of re-usable lexicons has been described by [7]. Our choice was made on the analysis and the transposition of the conceptual links between two systems to try to answer the following question: Is it possible to enrich the inter-conceptual links of the UMLS language unified starting from another knowledge base? The ADM Base is a French base developed at the beginning of the Seventies by a team of intermist physicians [8] which currently contains the description of several thousands of diseases . The UMLS is a project of the American National Library of Medicine which has the goal to integrate information coming from different backgrounds. Although the Metathesaurus includes a lot of concepts, some authors remind the necessity to improve the quality and the structure of the database [9]. In our case, we wanted to see if it was possible to extract knowledge from the French ADM data base and then complete the UMLS data base by integrating this information as new relations between concepts rather than adding new concepts. The first goal and interest of this work lies in the creation of links between concepts which belong to different databases, indeed, each base included in the UMLS project, keeps its meaningful links between concepts but there is few relations between data bases. The second goal was to create and display new relations between signs or symptoms and diseases and then improve the requests to the UMLS database.

2 The interchange space

Acquisition of knowledge by accumulation of concepts in the base by automatic methods has been already described in the literature [3,5,6] More interesting for the subject that we treat in this paper, are the articles describing knowledge acquisition by accumulation of links or creations of links between concepts. [10] evokes on this subject the difficulty of updating the successive versions of the Metathesaurus and the possible conflicts between the original thesaurus and the thesauri locally improved by the teams. Acquisition of knowledge has been also discussed for the description of surgical procedures, [11] recalls the difficulty of exploiting information from the meaningful links on account of the richness of the labels (broader, narrower, other, " is_a ", " part_of " ...). [12] and his team proposes to create relevant associations between concepts by inheritance in the UMLS Semantic Network. The first step consists in defining 'views' that could be classes of network and the second step consists in defining rules of associations. The links between concepts are then represented with conceptual graphs and are functions of defined views and constraints between concepts. The ARIANE project is an example of this work. The purpose of this project consists in modelling and implementing an intelligent and ergonomic interfaces according to the kind of the biomedical information database [13].

2.1 - The UMLS Database

The Unified Medical Language System is a collection of concepts resulting from several data bases elaborated in various places with different languages and different logics. The UMLS knowledge base includes three parts : The Metathesaurus is a collection of terms and concepts from many different biomedical vocabularies and classifications. The Semantic Network is a structure for categorizing objects in a medical domain. The Information Source Map is intended to describe the computerized biomedical sources. Whereas the Metathesaurus contains many concepts, the number of relations between two concepts should be increased.

2.2 - Description of the ADM knowledge

The ADM knowledge base is a base covering most of the medical specialities [8]. It contains 15600 diseases or syndroms descriptions and a lexicon of about 110000 terms. The goals were, first to help physicians to find diagnosis and next to provide a quick access to the medical information by using telematics. Recently, ADM has been brought on the Internet network. The knowledge base uses a relational data base system and physicians can query it with a web natural language interface (by the end of 1998 october, morether 2000 users were registered and morether 50000 requests had been done since the beginning of the year). The reason why we choose the ADM database was the structure of the diseases descriptions. Indeed, by using this database, we made the hypothesis that it was possible to complete relations between signs, finding, symptoms and diseases into the UMLS Metathesaurus.

2.3 - Methods

As we have seen ADM is built mainly on a hierarchical semantic model and provides descriptions of diseases whereas UMLS carries out a grid between concepts and categories semantics. The hierarchical structure of the ADM base presents relations between several labels which were validated by experts. Our hypothesis is that it is possible to extract some meaningful links from the first database for integrating it in the UMLS metathesaurus similar meaningful links between concepts.

Stages

We decomposed the work in several process (Fig1). First of all, we sought compatible concepts of UMLS (noted U1n) with the labels of descriptions of the ADM database (noted A1n). This search consisted in finding the correspondences i.e. we searched a link between terms from the ADM labels and terms from the UMLS concepts to match terms from one database to another. The second stage consisted in searching all the labels attached to the first one that had been selected in the first stage and then extract all the symptoms from the ADM description. Next, we searched all the UMLS concepts corresponding to the labels found (an English-French translation of the found signs could allow an extension of the results). One by one, we took the labels of the signs (Sij) and symptoms of the ADM database and searched in the UMLS database if the concepts existed(Cij). The last stage consisted in seeking Lij links between the concept Ui and the signs Cij. If the link didn't exist, we created it (enrichment of UMLS base).

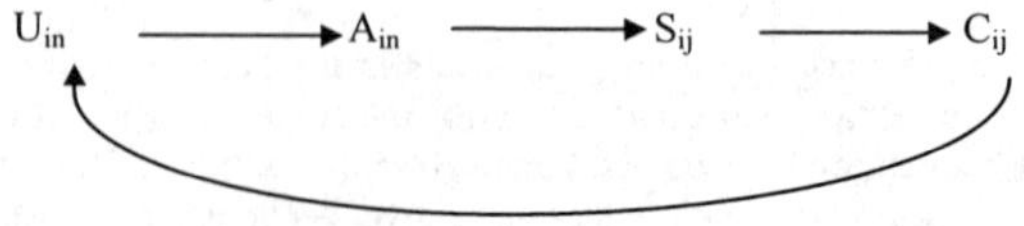

Fig 1 - Ring of search

Common space search
The fields covered by ADM and UMLS are not the same. This constraint forced us to work on the intersection of the fields covered by both databases. To expand this space, we have used an automaton to translate the english concepts terms into french concepts terms. Indeed, ADM strictly French-speaking leads us to work only on the French part of UMLS (this part concerns only the french MeSH, in the 1998 UMLS version). To be relevant and lead to a result, it is necessary and essential that the described labels and the signs attached to these labels, are all in French in the ADM/UMLS intersection. To enlarge the common space between the two bases, we needed to translate automatically all the UMLS preferred concepts and then we used an utility developped to translate english words in french words. The choice to translate UMLS from english to french rather than to translate ADM from french to english was made after analysis of the ADM labels. Whereas the Metathesaurus has a structured wording, the ADM wording is often expressed with many details shortened or not. In addition, there is no accent in the ADM labels and the translation from French to English can be ambiguous [14]. The few following examples illustrate this characteristics, particularly the French word 'FORCE' which can be translated into 'STRENGTH' with an accent or into 'FORCED' without an accent (example : S48271 MOUVEMENTS ARTICULAIRES ANORMAUX GENOU BAILLEMENT INT. EN VALGUS FORCE (FLEXION ROTATION EXT.)

Correspondences search
Once our translation is carried out, we finally built a table of correspondences between ADM codes and UMLS codes starting from the whole translated and not translated French wording (Fig. 2). At this level we had to use a last module for automatic processing of the wording, available in the development tools of ADM. The enrichment can be summed up in four steps. First, we take a concept from the UMLS Metathesaurus. Then we look for an equivalence in the ADM data base. Third, we glance through the ADM description disease and for each entity included in the description we look for an equivalence in the Metathesaurus. Fourth, if we find an equivalence, we take the code of the UMLS concept and we seek if there is a link between this code and the first one which we had started.

3 - Results

Identical french words in the databases
The bases are not similar. French wording are so different that the intersection between ADM and UMLS is a small percentage of the whole bases.

• Among the 354 579 concepts available in the UMLS base and the 96991 labels referred in the ADM base, we could only highlight 1988 identical concepts. This result corresponds to a very low rate of recovery (2,01 % on the ADM database ands 0,56 % on the UMLS).

• On the whole set of UMLS synonyms, we located the 785 identical wording between ADM base (96991) and the table of synonyms of the UMLS (168 629). The rate of recovery is lower than 1 % in both cases (0,80 % for ADM and 0,46 % for UMLS).

Translation
The translation let us double the quantity of concepts included into the common space. The totality of the wording automatically translated to extend the working area gave us the following results :

• 52 803 preferred terms (15 % of the total) and 31 334 synonyms or inflections were translated (that is to say 18,5 %). Once the correctly translated wording obtained, an automatic search on the present words was carried out.

• On the whole, 1415 occurrences (including 960 synonyms) among the 84 137 (52803+31334) were translated (1,7 %), i.e. which it was possible to us to bring closer 2830 codes (half ADM, half UMLS).

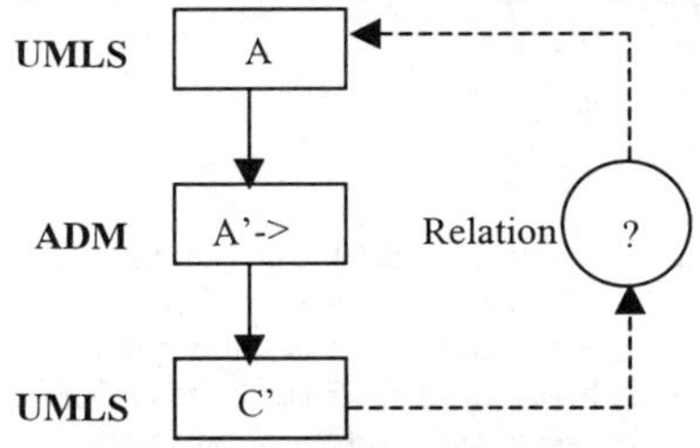

Fig. 2 – The matching Algorithm

New links proposals

Once correspondences between UMLS codes and ADM codes had been made up, we sought if there were missing links. On account of the small common space between the two bases, we did not wish to limit search to a particular nosology and we look up through all the table.

Our table of analysis included 4187 lines and allowed us to locate 14144 links not yet existing in UMLS base. In addition, it should be noted that about 100 % (99,97 %) of the codes processed by this work permits to create at least one additional link in the table of links M_REL of the UMLS table.

CCPT1	LCPT1	CCPT2	LCPT2
C0017658	GLOMERULONEPHRITIS	C0027712	NEPHROLOGY
C0017658	GLOMERULONEPHRITIS	C0018965	HEMATURIA
C0017658	GLOMERULONEPHRITIS	C0235220	ARTERIAL HYPERTENSION
C0017658	GLOMERULONEPHRITIS	C0013604	OEDEMA
C0017658	GLOMERULONEPHRITIS	C0028961	OLIGURIA
C0017658	GLOMERULONEPHRITIS	C0027726	NEPHROTIC SYNDROM

Table 1 : Example of correspondences between the code relating to 'GLOMERULONEPHRITIS' of the ADM description and the codes of the UMLS concepts where there is no relation in the Metathesaurus.

Knowing that UMLS proposes 1 711 054 links, the result of our work allowed an enrichment of the UMLS Metathesaurus from approximately 1 % (0,82 % exactly).

Semantic network

We examined the semantic categorisation of the concepts which help us to create new links.
Three points can be pointed out :

- Concerning the concepts at the origin of the new links, we can note that the semantic type T047 is the most important type compared to the others with 9650 occurences. We find next the semantic type T109 'Organic chemical', T121 'Pharmacologic substance', T033 'Finding', T019 'Congenital abnormality'.
- Concerning the concepts where the new links are pointed we can notice that it is also the semantic type T047 which is the most important type, just before the type T0 to 3 'Finding', T184 'Sign or symptom', T032 'Organic attribute' and T091 'Biomedical occupation or discipline'.
- If we study the T047 type and T033, we can see that the part of the concepts belonging to these semantic types which allowed us to create new links in the whole concept base represents about 30 per cent. 30887 concepts belong to the type T047 and we found 9650 new links with concepts of this type (that is 31,25% and 29,16% with the semantic type T033. These important results can be explained by the structure of the ADM data base).

Nosologies

If we analyse the nosologies related to the UMLS concerned with our work we notice that the links that could be created, are mainly concentrated in four fields : urology, orthopedy, oto-rhino-laringology, dermatology.
If we seek the origin fields of ADM from which these links were found, we find also four fields: Infectious diseases (bacteria, virus, mycoses) (N00006), constitutional diseases and/or congenital (N00007), metabolic diseases and nutrition (N00014), toxic diseases or diseases by chemical agents (N00022). The distribution of the concepts for which one or more links were located starting from ADM base shows that UMLS nosologies concerned with enrichment are not the same as the ADM ones. Cardiology for example, is sparsely concerned with an enrichment in the UMLS but if we look at cardiology (nosology N00003) of ADM database, we can see on the other hand that about 600 concepts contributed to the enrichment of the Metathesaurus. This nosology comes ninth on twenty nine.

4 - Discussion

According to [3], it appears clearly that the UMLS aims at integrating already existing thesauri, than create a standardized vocabulary. '*The UMLS is not intended to serve have as a standard vocabulary, but rather has a means of mapping between existing vocabularies*'. It is not a question to limit the richness of the medical vocabulary but on the contrary to gather in the same base the totality of the expressions and terms indicating the same object. From this point of view, the work what we carried out respects the philosophy that the researchers of the Medical Library of Medicine. Indeed, we sought to transfer and integrate into the UMLS, a knowledge acquired from the ADM data base. The construction of the UMLS initially aims to reach a high level of integration of most significant medical terms within a Metathesaurus and not to work out an exhaustive grid of links between concepts. This fact allowed other research in particular the inheritance of links by the semantic network as we saw with Joubert and coll. Locating and extracting links from ADM fit in the logical continuation of the construction of a concepts repository like UMLS. The other important point we have to approach relates to the automation of the task. Indeed, the work that we carried out concerned more than 1,7 million of links and several thousands of concepts. This quantity of information justified the development of a data-processing tool to obtain a result. An automatic data-processing is possible when data are homogeneous and standardized. Then we have to look at the quality of UMLS tables, the relevance of their construction and their composition.

Limits related to the structure of base ADM

The results we obtain should not however occult many skews and constraints which have limited our work in a significant way. Considering the quantity of information that we had to process, our work does not concern the majority of the UMLS database (less than 1% of the total) and it is legitimate to see if this work is representative of the database. Four limits must be stated here :

• *The linguistic barrier.*

Work that we carried out was possible after the translation of the UMLS concepts to widen the field of the concepts common to both bases. This constraint shows obvious the limits of search since we were subordinated to the performances of an automat. As we showed in the method, the choice to translate the UMLS from english to french rather than french to english does not seem to have an alternative because of the structure of ADM labels.

• *The lexical barrier.*

This second limit is inherent to the automatic translation and processing of the languages. The labels of the ADM data base do not always correspond to the terms of the diseases used in the Metathesaurus so that common diseases were not all located. The power of the specialized lexicon, completely in English could not help us. The reasons which explain the difficulties of working on the translation of the ADM labels are, on the one hand that ADM database has been existing since more than twenty years and same of terms seems to have aged, and on the other hand because ADM was not conceived so that the labels were reusable. Many links seem unusable or without interest.

• *The fields covered by the ADM labels.*

The descriptions integrated into the data base ADM do not cover the totality of medical knowledge. The maintenance of the base indeed requires time and efforts which are not always easy to mobilize. It results from that an inequality in the nosologies covered by the base and a delay or a lack of updating the data and information included in the descriptions. We can notice in addition that the knowledge of ADM base is the fruit of several participants over several years, which could be at the origin of a certain heterogeneity between descriptions suggested (we can find in the base as an example an entity for 'GLAUCOMA LEFT' and an entity for the disease 'GLAUCOMA RIGHT' and sometimes few descriptions have some English words). This heritage has probably limited the probability of matching between ADM labels and UMLS concepts.

Qualification of the links

Our work was restrained first to seek and second to show if it were possible to automatically create links in the UMLS, starting from another knowledge base. During this work, the problem of the qualification of the links arose quickly. According with the literature, we have been confronted ourselves mainly with two problems:

- the search for an automatic routine of qualification (implied standardized) of the links seems difficult to carry out because of the great quantity of combinations between links [11, 9]. A manual stage for confirmation seems necessary.

- the choice of the method of qualification does not appear obvious. Before adopting the heritage of a qualification via the semantic network like the one shown by Joubert and coll, we tried to see whether it was possible to deduce the new link starting from adjacent relations. It is as an example of what [Lehman 92] describes in a precise way when it presents the Cyc project and the algebra of Huhns and Stephens where the relation of the 'hypotenus' is deduced from the different relations.

5 - Conclusion

Our work has shown that it is possible to extract automatically information meaning as conceptual links from one knowledge data base in order to integrate it into another knowledge data base . Although many obstacles are opposed to match the information contained in each of the two bases, this enrichment of the UMLS starting from a knowledge base in French and which concerns a little more than 14000 links, and confirms in addition the possibility of integrating another knowledge and other languages that the English language into the UMLS and then increases the opportunities to use the Unified Medical Language System in other countries.
The difficulties and the constraints which we encountered persuade us on the one hand to pursue a reflexion on the ADM base and its contents and on the other hand to consider this same type of work on other knowledge bases. When [9] evokes the reinforcement of the UMLS structure ('More versus Better'), a similar analysis should be carried out on the ADM. This basic work will consist in taking again the entirety of the contents to model it, to purify it in order to eliminate ambiguities from descriptions. This work could finally extend at other French or English based knowledge bases. An extraction of knowledge of these bases could probably quickly enrich the grid between concepts in the Metathesaurus. Finally further work must be done to determine a powerful and relevant tool for the qualification of the links lately highlighted.

References

[1] Degoulet P., Fieschi M. Informatique médicale in : Masson (éd.) *Abrégés Paris* 1997 : 240 pages.
[2] Rector A., Nowlan W.A. The GALEN project *Comput Methods Progr* Octobre 1994; 45 (1-2) : pp. 75-78. [Salomon 94 - 1] Salomon D. Documentation overview *GALEN documentation* Novembre 1994; A : 5 pages.
[3] Cimino JJ, Octo Barnett G Automated translation between medical terminologies using semantic definitions *M D Computing* 1990; 7 (2) : pp. 104-9.
[4] Joubert M., Fieschi M., Botti G., et al. Représentation de concepts médicaux pour la recherche d'information : réalisation d'une maquette à partir d'UMLS in : Springer Verlag France (éd.) *Informatique et santé* 1992 (5) : pp. 3-17.
[5] Lindberg DAB._, Humphreys BL., Mc Cray AT., et al. The Unified Medical Language System *Meth Inform Med* 1993; 4 (32) : pp. 281-91.
[6] Mc_Cray AT., Srinivasan S., Browne A.C. Lexical methods for managing variation in biomedical terminologies in : Proceedings 18 Anual Symposium on medical applications in medical care (éd.) *J Am Med Informatics Assoc* 1994 : pp. 235-39.
[7] Musen MA Dimensions of knowledge sharing and reuse. Computer and Biomedical Research, 1994, **25**, pp 435-467.
[8] Lenoir P, Michel JR, Frangeul C, et al. Réalisation, développement et maintenance de la base de donées A.D.M. *Med. Inform.* 1981; 6 (1) : pp. 51-56.
[9] Bodenreider O, Burgun A, Botti G et al. Evaluation of the Unified Medical Language System as a Medical Knowledge Source *JAMIA* 1998; 1 (5) : pp. 76 - 87.
[10] Tuttle MS, Sherertz DD, Erlbaum MS, et al. Adding your terms and relationships to the UMLS Metathesaurus in : Hanley & Belfus, Inc (éd.) *AMIA* 1992 : pp. 219-33.
[11] Burgun A, Bodenreider O, Denier P, et al. Knowledge acquisition from the UMLS Sources : Application to the description of surgical procedures in : Greenes et al. (éd.) *Medinfo Proceedings* 1995 : pp. 75-79.
[12] Joubert M, Miton F, Fieschi M, Robert JJ A conceptual graphs modeling of UMLS components in : Greenes et al. (éd.) *IMIA Proceedings* 1995 : pp. 90-94.
[13] Joubert M., Fieschi M., Robert JJ, et al. UMLS-based Conceptual Queries to Biomedical Information Databases : an overview of the Project ARIANE *JAMIA* Jan/Fév 1998 (1) - 5 : pp. 52 - 61.
[14] Simard M Automatic Restoration of Accents in French Text, Centre d'innovation en technologies de l'information, Laval, Canada 1996 : 9 pages.

Maintenance of self-consistency of coding tables by statistical analysis of word co-occurrences

György Surján, Gergely Héja
Haynal Univ. for Health Sciences P.O.B 112 Budapest Hungary H-1389

Abstract. The author presents a method for maintaining the internal consistency of coding tables. The method was tested on a table used for assisting the daily work of indexing clinical cases to International Classification of Diseases. 300 item were tested selected randomly form a corpus of 3082 clinical diagnoses. The method discovered potential consistency problems in 39 cases, out of which 10 were false positive.

1. Introduction

Computer systems assisting the work of coding diseases usually contain some sort of coding tables, consisting of a list of clinical terms and the corresponding codes. Such tables are growing in size by time to time. The updating process usually leads to loss of the internal consistency. The correct semantic representation of all concepts would be necessary to solve the problem. There are promising ongoing works in this field. (Like in the GALEN-IN-USE project [1].) However it will be a long way, when the results of these projects can be used in the everyday practice. Therefore, it seems to be useful to search for more simple methods, which do not solve the problem in an exact way, but can be still helpful.

2. The method of word co- occurrence measurements

The word co-occurrence analysis is commonly used method in computational linguistics [2]. This usually based on so called *n*-grams, that is a window of *n* consecutive words. Instead of n-grams, our approach is sentence based. The code values are included in the text as if they where regular words. For example, the last item in the left table in Figure 1 can be considered as a sentence, consisting of three words: *aortic, vitium* and *I069.* In order to be able to discriminate from normal words, all code values are placed within $ signs: *$I069$ aortic vitium.* Now we can represent our table by a Sentence × Word matrix, in which the sentences form the columns, and the words appearing anywhere in the whole corpus form the rows. The value of the matrix cells is *1* when the corresponding word appears in the corresponding sentence, and *0* if not. (Figure 1.)

This vector space model is used in *latent semantic indexing* [3]. In this approach the cosine of the angle between the vector of two documents (sentences) represents their semantic similarity. We consider the Sentence × Word matrix as a set of word-vectors in the space of sentences. Then the cosine of the angle between the word vectors represents the "co-occurring tendency" of the corresponding word pairs. The formula that defines the cosine values is as follows:

$$\frac{\mathbf{w}_i \circ \mathbf{w}_j}{\|\mathbf{w}_i\| * \|\mathbf{w}_j\|}$$

where $\mathbf{w}_i$ and $\mathbf{w}_j$ the two Word vectors, ° represent their scalar product, and ‖ ‖ symbol means the Eucledian norm of the vector. The resulting Word × Word matrix is necessarily symmetric. If the presence of one of the words is obvious, another measure can be used, according to the following formula:

$$\frac{\mathbf{w}_i \circ \mathbf{w}_j}{\|\mathbf{w}_j\|^2}$$

Table 1 shows the result of this calculation for our demonstrating example. Clearly, this matrix is asymmetric. The word '*aorta*' appears whenever '*vitum*' appears, but the reverse is not true. (The 'given word' is represented by the columns.)

the original table → conversion into "sentences" → Sentence × Word matrix

ICD code	language expression
I.700	aorta atherosclerosis
I.069	aorta vitium

S1	$I700$ aorta atherosclerosis
S2	$I069$ aorta vitium

	S1	S2
$I700$	1	0
$I069$	0	1
aorta	1	1
atherosclerosis	0	1
vitium	1	0

Figure 1 The representation of tables by Sentence × Word matrix

A sufficiently large corpus of sentences can be considered as training set representing some kind of knowledge about word co-occurrences. Any expression consisting of the same set of words can be considered as testing sample. Now we define the 'environment' of a sentence. This is a set of all words of the training set, which have co-occurrence likelihood with any of the words of the analysed sentence above a given threshold. If any word (or code) is missing by mistake, it likely will appear in the environment. For all words in the environment the co-occurrence tendency to all words of the tested expression can be calculated. These values form the *environment matrix* (Figure 2.)

The conditional co-occurrence likelihood values

	$I700$	$I069$	aorta	atherosclerosis	vitium
$I700$	1	0	0.5	1	0
$I069$	0	1	0.5	0	1
aorta	1	1	1	1	1
atherosclerosis	1	0	0.5	1	0
vitium	0	1	0.5	0	1

Table 1

The geometric mean of the co-ordinates of the word vectors of the environment matrix can serve as a measure for how strongly belongs the corresponding word to the analysed sentence.

3. Application of co-occurrence measurements to the problem

The table, which is subject of the consistency analysis, has be used as training set. Then, all codes should be removed from all sentences, and the rest serves as testing set. Now we have two assumptions:

Assumption 1:The original code should appear in the environment, with non-zero co-occurrence likelihood to all words of the sentence. This is self-evident.

Assumption 2: When the training set contains ambiguity, then apart from the original code, some others will also appear in the environment.

Words	$K37H0$	Appendicitis	geometric mean
xxxxxxxx	xxxxxxxx	xxxxxxxx	xxxxxxxx
$K3500$	0.	0.25	0.
$K3590$	0.	0.25	0.
acuta	0.	0.5	0.
Consec.	0.5	0.25	0.3536
ulcero-phlegmonosa	0.	0.25	0.

Figure 2. The environment matrix of the expression "$K37H0$ Appendicitis".

The second assumption is the subject of our study. The experiment was performed by means of a special software was developed by the authors to analyse word co-occurrences. Technical details are not discussed here.

A table containing 3082 clinical diagnosis expressions was used as training set. The diagnoses were taken from discharge reports collected from five different departments of our hospital. They where assigned to International Classification of Diseases (ICD-10) by a physician. The 'sentences' contain the words of the diagnostic expression with one and only one ICD code. The test sample was 300 diagnosis randomly selected from the training set. The candidates for error according to assumption 2 were detected, and analysed in details. E.g. in the environment of "Art. scler. cerebri" (cerebral atherosclerosis) two codes were found: the original I6720 and I2510 with higher co-occurrence tendency. The training set was searched for occurrences of $I2510$. The expression shown in the rectangle in Figure 3 is a combination of two different diseases in a single diagnostic statement: 'arterioscleoris coronarium (I2510) and 'arteriosclerosis cerebri' (I6720). Such compound diagnoses should be split up to avoid ambiguity. (The essential difference between *diagnosis* and *disease* is described by us in a previous paper [4].)

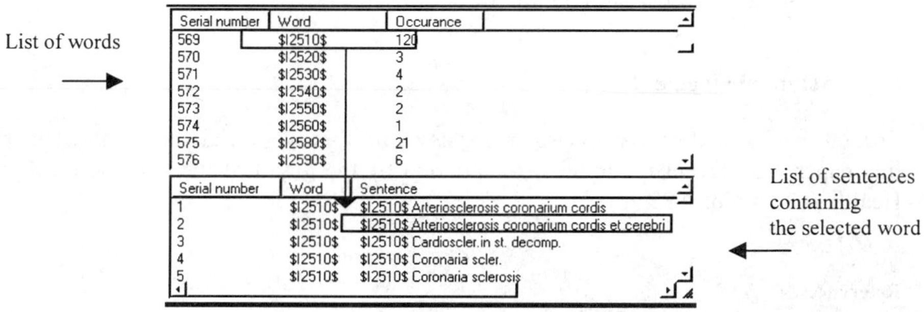

Figure 3 Occurrences of the code I2510

The different reasons why non-original codes emerge in the environment can be categorised in four main groups: 1) error or inconsistency of the training set; 2) inconsistency of the ICD; 3) false positive result. Group 3) can be divided into two subgroups: 3a) the emerging codes are alternatives of the original; 3b) true false positive result. A case belongs to 3a) only if all the emerging codes have lower co-occurrence tendency than the original and are semantic relatives of it.

4. Results

A) The original code always appeared in the environment. This is in accordance with Assumption 1, and proves that the software does not make serious errors.
B) No other codes appeared in the environment in 87% (261 cases). In these cases the method was not able to detect consistency problems in the coding table.
C) Other codes appeared with lower affinity than the original in 5.6% (17 cases)
D) Other codes appeared with equal or higher affinity than the original in 7.33% (22 cases)

The cases C) and D) were analysed manually and the reasons were categorised using the above described groups. The result is presented in Table 2. Note that one case might belong to more than one category. The most frequent error type was the ambiguous indexing of the same concept into different ICD category.

Causes of appearance of non-original codes in the environment

co-occurrence tendency of the other codes:	Number of cases	1) Error in reference sample		2) inconsistency of ICD		3a) alternative codes		3b) false positive cases	
C) lower	17	10	45.45%	3	13.64%	7	31.82%	0	0%
D) equal or higher	22	14	63.64%	7	31.82%	-	-	10	45.45%
Total	39	24	61.54%	10	25.64%	7	17.95%	10	25.64%

Table 2

5. Discussion

The presented result convinces us that it is possible to reduce but not eliminate inconsistency of the coding tables by this method. Considering the computational requirements, the cost benefit is questionable, but the same approach can be used for other purposes. We were able to detect inconsistencies in the ICD as well. The most typical problem was here the lack of generic concepts. Our approach with some modifications can be used also as a tool for assisting the work of encoders.

6. Acknowledgements

Special thanks to Prof. Arie Hasman for assisting this work and commenting the draft of this paper. The recent research was supported by the grand of the Hungarian Ministry of Health. (Grant No.: 155/98)

References

[1] Rector AL Compositional Models of Medical Concept: Towards Re-Usable Application - Independent Medical Terminologies in Knowledge and Decisions in Health Telematics, (Eds) P Barahona and J P Christensen, IOS Press 1994. pp 109 - 114
[2] J Allen Natural Language understanding Addison Wesley 1995
[3] Chute C G, Yang Y An overview of Statistical Methods for the Classification and Retrieval of Patient Events Methods of Information in Medicine (1995); 34:104-110
[4] Surján G Questions on validity of ICD coded diagnoses International Journal of Medical Informatics54 (1999) 77-95

Medical Informatics Europe '99
P. Kokol et al. (Eds.)
IOS Press, 1999

Towards a Multilingual Morpheme Thesaurus for Medical Free-Text Retrieval

Stefan SCHULZ[1,2], Martin ROMACKER[1,2], Pius FRANZ[2],
Albrecht ZAISS[2], Rüdiger KLAR[2], Udo HAHN[1]
[1]*Computational Linguistics Lab, Freiburg University, Germany*
[2]*Department of Medical Informatics, Freiburg University Hospital*

Abstract. We introduce a methodology for the segmentation of complex compounds into medically plausible morphemes. A tool for thesaurus compilation and management is presented, and design principles for a multilingual morpheme thesaurus are outlined. Our goal is to enhance the quality of medical free-text retrieval by replacing lexically based through morpheme-based search procedures.

1. Introduction

Modern clinical documentation systems and health-related electronic publications have swamped the physician's desktop with large amounts of computer-readable free text. Making full use of these resources is currently hampered by inadequate retrieval facilities. The string matching paradigm of today's information retrieval systems is based on the processing of complex lexical forms (words) as their basic unit. Such an approach does neither account for morphological regularities (inflection, derivation, composition), nor for semantic relations such as (quasi-)synonymy in a given language, nor does it support mappings between semantically equivalent terms from different languages. As an alternative, we propose to replace lexical items by morphemes as the basic unit for document retrieval procedures. This requires a procedure for the segmentation of inflectional (*leuk-o-cyt-es*), derivational (*leuk-o-cyt-ic*), and compositional (*leuk-em-ia*) lexical forms into their constituent morphemes. We may then enrich the emerging morpheme repositories by incorporating semantic relations among monolingual morphemes as well as multilingual morphemes from different European languages.

We conducted an experiment to find out whether morphological analysis of complex word forms is a desideratum for standard free-text retrieval systems at all. In a random sample of 100 German-language pathology reports, we found 895 occurrences of different domain-specific compounds. We then matched these compounds with all words contained in the electronic version of a comprehensive German-language medical dictionary, the *"Pschyrembel Klinisches Wörterbuch"*, whose entire text corpus contains more than 100,000 different words. 400 out of these 895 compounds were not found in the dictionary. This sheds light on the enormous productivity of medical language as evidenced by a large number of *ad hoc* compounds like *Lungenoberlappenbronchus, Weichteilresektionsfläche, Tubulusepithelveränderung*. Clearly, this productivity precludes to enumerate all possible derivational and compositional forms in a lexicalized thesaurus, since there is no finite upper bound to composition.

Morphological decomposition is a reasonable way out of this dilemma. A repository of morphemes as the smallest meaningful linguistic units is likely to be several orders of magnitude below the size of phrasal or fully lexicalized thesauri, at significantly smaller growth rates. Hence, such a repository should be much easier to compile and cheaper to maintain. This parsimony must, however, be traded off against the weaker semantic expressiveness of its entries (compared with lexicalized thesauri), and the increased computational costs of the algorithms needed for decomposition and disambiguation (compared with mere string matching).

2. A Pilot Study for the Construction of a Morpheme Thesaurus

In the following, we describe a pilot study for the construction of a German morpheme thesaurus. As lexical sources for morpheme extraction we selected the German versions of ICD-9, ICD-10 (tabular list and alphabetical list), SNOMED, and the German translation of the International Classification of Procedures in Medicine (OPS 301). The syntactic rules for morphological combinability within lexicalized forms were formally encoded in a finite-state automaton using the following *morpheme classes*:

- *Stems*, like {*gastr*, *hepat*, *diaphys*...}, can be prefixed, linked by infixes, and suffixed.
- *Prefixes*, like {*a*, *de*, *in*, *ent*, *ver*, *anti*, ...}, precede the word's stem(s).
- *Infixes* (e.g., *o* in *gastr-o-intestinal*) are only used as a formal glue between stems .
- *Derivational suffixes*, such as {*io*, *ion*, *ung*, ...}, usually follow the word's stem(s).
- *Inflectional suffixes*, like {*e*, *en*, *s*, *idis*, *ae*, *oris*, ...}, appear at the very end of a word.
- Eponyms (mostly proper names), digits and acronyms {*AIDS*, *ECG*, ...} are non-decomposable and do not undergo any morphological alteration, at all.

A purely linguistically motivated decomposition of a word into its smallest meaning-bearing units might not lead to a useful degree of atomicity from a retrieval point of view, since the composite semantic content of a complex word form might get lost. In Fig. 1, a linguistically motivated segmentation of *diaphysis* into *dia-phys-is* is contrasted with a medically plausible one into *diaphys-is*. Therefore, we enhanced the purely syntax-based description of word composition by semantic criteria for word *stem atomicity* in order to determine *plausible* entities for segmentation. As a rule of thumb, a subword is not further segmented into constituent morphemes when an atomic (quasi-) synonymous stem exists (in Fig. 1., *shaft* for *diaphys*).

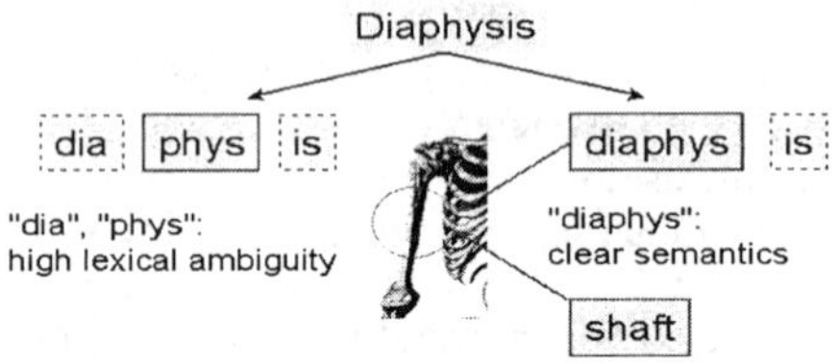

Fig. 1: Task-specific Atomicity: Linguistic vs. Medical Considerations

The problem of properly delimiting the length of word stems can also be considered as a trade-off between a higher degree of compactness (the number of morphemes is considerably smaller than the number of lexemes) and a lower degree of expressiveness (morphemes are semantically far less significant than lexemes). Further complications arise from the need to account for variants of word stems, so-called allomorphs (e.g., *leuko, leuco, leuk, leuc*). While the size of the morpheme thesaurus would certainly benefit from letting the word stem radically shrink to the longest common substring, here *leu*, an increased number of segmentation ambiguities and false positives would be encountered in an information retrieval environment. We refrain from such a solution and subscribe to a modest size growth of the thesaurus by the inclusion of allomorphs.

Accordingly, we developed a formalism covering German and Greco-Latin morphology. The corresponding tool, *MedSearch*, consists of a morphological parser that enumerates all possible parse trees for a lexical input based on a morpheme lexicon. Morphological segmentation ambiguities are ranked according to the following preference criteria: (1) longest match, (2) minimal number of stems per word, (3) relative weight of morphemes: W[stems] > W[most affixes] > W[infixes and inflection suffixes], (4) minimal number of consecutive affixes (this criterion penalizes utterly formal segmentations).

The *MedSearch* tools provide a graphical interface for interactive thesaurus management, the *MedSearch Morphology Workbench*. In the start-up phase, *MedSearch* was only supplied with German and Greco-Latin prefixes, suffixes and infixes. All terms contained

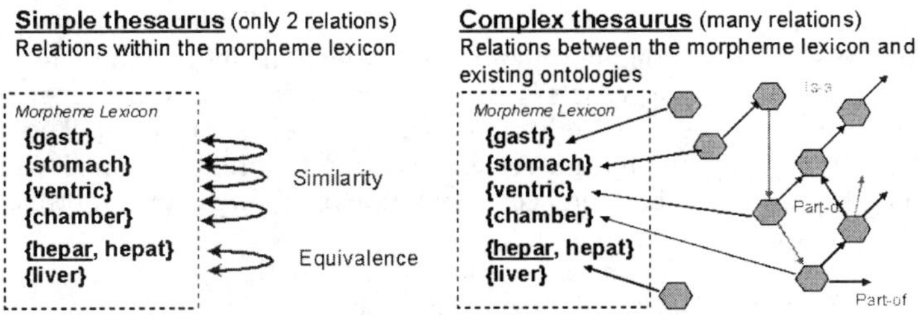

Fig.2: Two Approaches of Semantic Linkage within a Multilingual Morpheme Thesaurus

in our test corpus were then automatically segmented by the morphological analyzer using only this limited portion of initial morphological knowledge. Strings that could not be segmented were considered as unknown substrings and stored in a list ranked by frequency. The first 1,000 most frequent unknown substrings were then manually assigned appropriate morpheme classes using the *MedSearch Morphology Workbench.* Prior to entering a new morpheme into the repository, its morpheme class and language type always have to be specified. After a second semi-automatic training cycle, finally, 6,130 medical morphemes were obtained and included in the morpheme lexicon. The remainder, totaling 22,369 subwords, remained nonsegmented, because they (1) occurred only once in the sources, (2) were acronyms or proper names, or (3) did not belong to the medical domain.

During each additional training cycle, the workbench is supplied with complex word forms from the corpora under consideration. The system then performs segmentation on the basis of the morphemes already available, and displays the parsed results, weighted according to the above-mentioned criteria. The inclusion of new morphemes has continuously improved the segmentation capability of *MedSearch.*

3. Semantic Linkage and Multilinguality

The semantic linkage between morphemes is a main rationale for the development of the morpheme thesaurus. Fig. 2 sketches two alternatives how to proceed. The first approach ("Simple Thesaurus") is based on the explicit definition of semantic links *internal* to the morpheme thesaurus, without any reference to external terminologies. We deliberately restrict the types of relations to two very basic ones, viz. semantic equivalence and similarity. Both these relations are considered symmetric and reflexive, but only equivalence is transitive. As an example, semantic equivalence holds between the morpheme sets {*hepar, hepat*} and {*liver*}. In contrast, a similarity relationship is assumed to hold between {*gastr*} and {*stomach*}, {*stomach*} and {*ventric*}, as well as {*ventric*} and {*chamber*}, but not between {*gastr*} and {*chamber*}.

In the second approach ("Complex Thesaurus") each content-bearing morpheme is mapped to a set of elements of an existing terminology, e.g., the UMLS. Unlike the first approach, semantic relations are not defined internally at the level of the morpheme

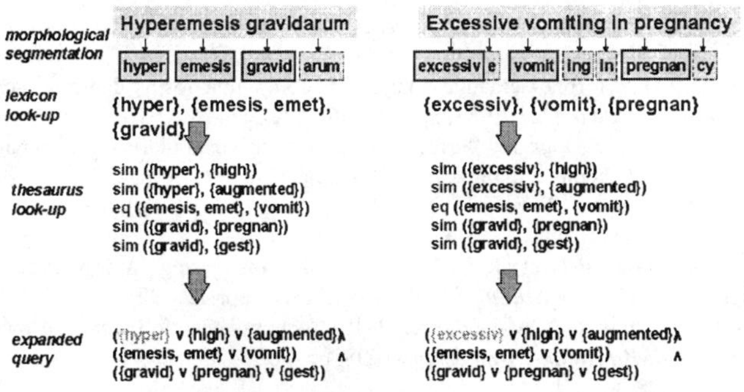

Fig.3: Query Obtained by Morpheme-supported Expansion of two Synonymous Surface Expressions

repository. Instead, they can be derived from a richer set of relations (e.g., part-of, is-a) defined for concepts in the external terminologies to which the morphemes are linked.

The advantage of the first approach is that all knowledge necessary for morphological analysis and efficient retrieval is directly available at the repository level. The value of the second approach lies in its potential for reusing existing terminologies with richer relation sets (and, possibly, powerful inference capabilities), though the morpheme-concept mapping might turn out to be nontrivial.

Considering the "Simple Thesaurus" approach, a scenario for information retrieval is outlined in Fig. 3. Nearly identical queries are obtained by the morpheme-supported expansion of two synonymous, though lexically entirely different surface expressions.

4. Related Work

The foundations for medical-morpheme decomposition were laid more than 20 years ago. Pacak et al. [1] and Norton & Pacak [2] extracted morphological rules, which were restricted to two domain-specific suffixes *–itis* and *–tomy*, using the SNOMED axis to encode typical patterns of word combinations. A generalization of this approach is presented by Wolff [3]. Wingert [4] used 255 cascading rules to capture the combinatorial regularities of the different morpheme classes. The corresponding word grammar was encoded in terms of augmented transition networks, a much more expressive formal device than finite-state automatons. Recently, Lovis and Baud [5, 6] developed a multilingual system for word decomposition that is linked to the GRAIL ontology. They propose basic semantic entities at the morpheme level, so-called morphosemantems, a notion conceptually much richer than medically plausible morphemes.

5. Conclusion

Given the developmental productivity of medical terminologies, it seems almost impossible to keep pace with their lexical growth rates. Our solution to cope with this problem requires automatic morphological segmentation. In order to support effective free-text retrieval, we propose here a language engineering methodology that builds on a repository of medically plausible morphemes that are used for automatic deflection, dederivation and decomposition. While we stressed the morphological segmentation aspect of our work, we have also outlined the next step required, viz. how to link these basic morphological units via conceptual relationships. As a consequence, the "flat" morpheme repository will have to grow for a morpheme thesaurus. While the currently available lexical inventory covers already Greek and Latin morphemes, in the future, emphasis will also be laid on integrating different modern European languages in order to meet the requirements of a truly multilingual morpheme thesaurus.

References

[1] Pacak, M.G., Pratt, A.W., White, W.C. Automated morphosyntactic analysis of medical language. *Information Processing & Management*, 12 (1), 1976, pp. 71 – 76.

[2] Norton, L.M., Pacak, M.G., Morpho-semantic analysis of compound forms denoting surgical procedures. *Methods of Information in Medicine*, 22, 1983, pp. 29 – 36.

[3] Wolff, S. The use of morphosemantic regularities in the medical vocabulary for automatic lexical coding. *Methods of Information in Medicine*, 23, 1984, pp. 195 – 203.

[4] Wingert, F. Morphologic analysis of compound words. *Methods of Information in Medicine*, 24 (3), 1985, pp. 155 – 162.

[5] Lovis, C., Michel, P.A., Baud, R.H et al. Word segmentation processing: A way to exponentially extend medical dictionaries. *Proceedings of MEDINFO '95*, 1995, IMIA, pp. 28 – 32.

[6] Baud, R.H., Lovis, C., Rassinoux, A. M., Scherrer, J.-R. Morpho-semantic parsing of medical expressions. *Proceedings of the 1998 AMIA Annual Symposium*, 1998, pp. 760 – 764.

Medical Informatics Europe '99
P. Kokol et al. (Eds.)
IOS Press, 1999

A Model for Integration and Continuous Development of Standards for Tumour Documentation Using Relational Database Techniques and Extensible Markup Language

Udo ALTMANN, Werner WÄCHTER, Ali Gerhard TAFAZZOLI,
Frank Rüdiger KATZ, Ralf SCHWEIGER, Joachim DUDECK
Institute of Medical Informatics, Justus-Liebig-University
Heinrich -Buff-Ring 44, 35392 Gießen, Germany

Abstract. In oncology various international and national standards exist for different aspects of a disease. These standards, maintained by different organisations, have multiple relationships with each other. A common data dictionary like UMLS would facilitate the reorganisation of such relationships when a new version of a standard is published. While the modelling of relationships usually is restricted to types having a relevant frequency, there are often relationships which are expressed in texts like definitions or explanations. Such texts are a very important supplement for the acceptance and the safe use of coding systems, but often are neglected when implementing coding systems in computerised systems, because they are costly to implement. This paper discusses potentials when integrating various sources in a common, database based dictionary enhanced by XML (Extensible Markup Language) techniques.

1. Introduction

In oncology various international and national standards exist for different aspects of a disease. These standards, maintained by different organisations, contain detailed descriptions of the usage of data items and have multiple relationships with each other. For Germany, the most important systems (among additional) are:

- WHO maintained International Classification of Diseases for Oncology (ICD-O) for topography and morphology, and their German translations and extensions
- TNM-Classification of Malignant Tumours (maintained by the UICC)
- a minimum basic data set of items for all tumour diseases "Basisdokumentation für Tumorkranke", defined for the Association of German Cancer Centres (ADT)
- a detailed organ specific data set, "Organspezifische Tumordokumentation", defined for the ADT

Several types of relationship within and between these standards can be found which are used for plausibility checks like in CHECKIT [1]. The "Basisdokumentation für Tumorkranke" is a subset of the "Organspezifische Dokumentation. Between topography and morphology codes inside the ICD-O and with the TNM-Classification exist also close relationships which have to be considered when modifying one of this coding standards.

2. Problems

The following problems can be identified when analysing the reasons for occuring inconsistencies between these documentation systems and classifications:

- update anomalies between different standards
- standards that don't reflect the current medical knowledge
- lack of reuse of data element in various contexts
- lack of electronic versions for the implementation in computer systems

The asynchronous publishing of the different coding systems is one particular reason of occuring inconsistencies. In other areas like, e.g., lymphomas or leukaemias, the dynamic of the development of the medical knowledge is so high, that data standards are often already at least partly out of date shortly after being published. Clinical trials and other investigations often build up their own documentation standards instead of reusing existing standards, e.g., as defined in the "Organspezifische Tumordokumentation". Incompatible data sets cause extra work in the daily routine of clinicians. Electronic versions are often not available or are implemented in proprietary programs. Developers of computer systems who want to use such systems for lists of values or for on-line-help have to retype them or to extract them from program files.

3. Proposed Methods

The various requirements can be met by a combined approach of a database based data dictionary and the use of Extensible Markup Language (XML), respectively its related techniques XML Linking Language (Xlink), XML Pointer Language (Xpointer), style sheet techniques (e.g., Extensible Stylesheet Language (XSL)), and query techniques (e.g., XQL or XML-QL), that are all described at the World Wide Web Consortium's web site.

The database contains objects of following types:

- items, characterising the information objects of diagnosis, treatment and follow-up.
- codes (including synonyms etc.) for item domain control
- bits of descriptive or explaining texts, stored as markup tagged and formatted texts
- dependencies, relationships and rules
- information about document structures
- comments from authors or readers, e.g.. for developing new versions of publications

Generally, version control is to be implemented for every object type to support development of standards and includes, e.g., status, source and author information. Every text can be structured using format or content markup for readability and for situations, in which formal substructuring is not sensible, e.g., narrative text containing definitions, references etc. Xlinks are used for relationships from inside a narrative text to another object. Every entry in the database has a unique ID which is used for linking and constructing XML-documents (e.g., using the IDREF-attribute). Relationships exist between items and the corresponding codes, for characterising dependencies between codes of different items, e.g., between topography, morphology and staging or conversions, and for Xlinks. Every relationship has, in conformity with the Xlink model, a name (content-role) characterising the nature of the relationship (e.g., is_code_for, occurs_in).

The example in table 1 is taken from the German version of the ICD-O Morphology "Tumorhistologieschlüssel" [2]. The preferred term for a code is typed in bold. Synonyms are written in normal type. The codes and words in round brackets refer to the topographies in which the terms are valid. The pointed brackets refer to explanatory remarks.

8080/2 **Erythroplasie Queyrat** (Haut, C44; Penis, C60) <Anm. 36>
8081/2 **Morbus Bowen** (Haut, C44; Penis, C60; Larynx, C32) <Anm. 36>
Intraepitheliales Plattenepithelkarzinom vom Bowen-Typ

<Anm. 36>
Dieser Tumor wurde von der International Society of Gynecological Pathology (Kurman et al. 1992) als Variante des Plattenepithelkarzinoms eingeführt. Die Kodierung erfolgt nach dem Vorschlag der OTD (1995).

```
<morphology classification="ICD-O-2">
    <code codesystem="ICD-O-2">8080/2</code>
    <preferred_term>Erythroplasie Queyrat</preferred_term>
    <occurs_in>
        <topography>
            <term>Haut</term>
            <code codesystem="ICD-O 2">C44</code>
        </topography>
        <topography>
            <term>Penis</term>
            <code codesystem="ICD-O 2">C60</code>
        </topography>
    </occurs_in>
    <remark>Anm. 36</remark>
</morphology>
<morphology classification="ICD-O-2">
    <code codesystem="ICD-O-2">8081/2</code>
    <preferred_term>Morbus Bowen</preferred_term>
    <synonymous_term>
        Intraepitheliales Plattenepithelkarz. vom Bowen-Typ
    </synonymous_term>
    <occurs_in>
        <topography>
            <term>Haut</term>
            <code codesystem="ICD-O 2">C44</code>
        </topography>
        <topography>
            <term>Penis</term>
            <code codesystem="ICD-O 2">C60</code>
        </topography>
        <topography>
            <term>Larynx</term>
            <code codesystem="ICD-O 2">C32</code>
        </topography>
    </occurs_in>
    <remark>Anm. 36</remark>
</morphology>
```

Table 1: Example of the printed version of the "Tumorhistologieschlüssel", the German version of the ICD-O Morphology (upper part), and its exemplary transformation to XML (lower part).

The structure of the book's accompanying software already realises typing and linking to comments in an HTML-like way, but does not realise additional relations (occurs_in, does_not_occur_in) that would have been necessary for expressing the relationship with topography concepts. Although pattern recognition tools sometimes are able to extract such relationships automatically, they fail in less structured texts. For example, if remarks refer to each other, the reference usually is somewhere in the text and it wouldn't be sensible to decompose the text in a highly structured way. In the data dictionary, item respectively code entries would be made for morphology, codes, terms, and remarks. Relationship entries would be made for occurs_in, has_remark, is_preferred_term_for, ...

Information about document structures is used for generating documents and publications. A modular construction system will allow to compose various documents with reduced efforts. The Xlink model with the link properties "show" (replace the link with the referred content or just as a link) and "actuate" (follow the link automatically or on request) offers a powerful design method for constructing and combining XML documents. The contents of the database are usually distributed as XML documents. Style sheet techniques, especially XSL, are a powerful tool for preparing such documents for printed or online-versions, which may even be capable of processing data in HTML-Forms. Query languages like XQL or XML-QL are, on the other hand, a way, in which generated XML documents can be reduced to a form, in which their contents may be imported into applications to fulfil specific functions (lists of values, consistency checks, etc.).

4. Results

Since the XML technique is rather new and still under development, there exists no prototype of the described model. In our tumour documentation system (GTDS) [3], we implemented the classifications and documentation systems mentioned earlier. Based on an earlier version of a dictionary for our non-graphic user interface [4] and system catalogues, we intend to construct a prototype version and use it as basis for integrating it in our

HTML-help system for the graphic version as a realisation of a document structure. Although this proceeding causes more efforts than generating HTML directly, we want to show, that for the future there will be benefits by reusing information, e.g., in the context of organ specific documentation. Issues that have not been addressed yet are questions of copyrights and funding. We hope, that by showing the potential of this approach, there will be willingness to support such a work in both areas.

5. Discussion

The idea to combine various sources (classifications) in a common source has a long tradition. The most outstanding system, UMLS, has some fundamental weaknesses for the purposes mentioned above. Since UMLS focuses on medical terms and concepts, there is a lack of definitions. E.g., although the major categories of the TNM-system are contained in the metathesaurus ("T1", "T2", "T3", etc.) there are no definitions for the usage of the categories for a specific organ ("size of tumour less than 2 cm"). The advantages of the presented approach are:

1. maintenance and development of multiple publications, especially documentation systems with reuse of items
2. various types of presentation (printed or online-publication, integration with applications)
3. awareness of the various contexts, in which an item or a code is used and assessment of consequences of changes
4. easier maintenance by generating multiple views with different levels of detail
5. consistent representation of items in any context, reduction of "update anomalies"
6. continuous development by enabling comments in online available versions of documents. (quicker feedback, provision of more concise definitions, better reflection of the medical knowledge, broader discussion of proposals)

6. Summary

This contribution shows with examples from tumour documentation, how the combination of classic dictionary techniques with emerging document processing techniques (XML) can enhance development, distribution and deployment of data standards by integrating and working up various documents for different purposes.

Acknowledgements: Parts of the work of our working group are funded by the German Ministry of Health in a joint project with the German Cancer Society (Information Centre for Standards in Oncology).

References

[1] Parkin, D.M., V.W. Chen, J. Ferlay, J. Galceran, H.H. Storm, S-L-Whelan. Comparability and Quality Control in Cancer Registration. IARC Technical Report No. 19, Lyon, 1994

[2] Grundmann, E. , G. Wagner, P. Hermanek, Tumorhistologieschlüssel, 2. Aufl., Springer Verlag Berlin Heidelberg New York etc. 1997

[3] Altmann, U., F. R. Katz, A. Tafazzoli, V. Haeberlin, J. Dudeck. GTDS - a Tool for Tumor Registries to Support Shared Patient Care.Proc AMIA Annu Fall Symp: 512-516 (1996)

[4] Altmann, U., F. Katz, V. Haeberlin, J. Dudeck. Entwicklung und Bedeutung eines Data Dictionaries für Funktionalität und Integration eines Anwendungssystems am Beispiel des Gießener Tumordokumentationssystems (GTDS).H.J. Trampisch, S. Lange (Hrsg.): Medizinische Forschung Ärztliches Handeln, 40. Jahrestagung der GMDS, pp 413-416

Medical Informatics Europe '99
P. Kokol et al. (Eds.)
IOS Press, 1999

Preliminary Report: Concepts and Terms used to describe Urinary Tract Infection in Primary Health Care and in the Clinical Microbiology Laboratory

Olle Aspevall[1,2], Urban Forsum[2] and Daniel Karlsson[2,3]
1) Department of Immunology, Microbiology, Pathology and Infectious Diseases, Karolinska Institutet, Stockholm, Sweden. Corresponding author.
E-mail: olle.aspevall@bactlab.hs.sll.se
2) Division of Clinical Microbiology, Linköpings universitet, Sweden
3) Medical Informatics, Linköpings universitet, Sweden

1. Objective

This pilot study is part of a project to develop a combined expert/ education computer programme for urinary tract infections (UTI). We study the difference between terms and concepts used in the context of a Primary Health Care (PHC) visit for urinary tract infection and those used in the setting of performing urinary culture in a Clinical Microbiology Laboratory.
The objective of this project is to find and select relevant and sufficiently unambiguous terms and map these terms to a conceptual model of the UTI domain, also being constructed within this project. This model will be used in an index module of the expert programme for UTI [1]. The computer programme will be WWW-based [2].
Much benefit can be gained from establishing a global (common, collective) system of well-defined concepts with meaningful relations and unambiguous terms. A common terminology system would prevent misunderstanding, may make machine operated search of electronic patient records more useful and could be used as a search and index module within computer programmes.

2. Material and methods

Thirty-six PHC-centres were asked to send us twenty consecutive patient records from visits for UTI, cystitis or pyelonephritis. Twenty-two of the centres were located in the south-western area of Stockholm and fourteen were in the central area of Östergötland.

Nine PHC-centres participated, two in Östergötland, seven in Stockholm. In total we received 198 patient records.

Terms relevant in UTI management (diagnostics and treatment) were selected from the patient records and compared to another set of terms obtained from a published Swedish reference method for diagnosis of UTI [3].

Recommended concepts and terms were those used in the reference publication [3] or those recommended by other authoritative bodies.

3. Results

From the collected patient records 4352 words were selected, these were sorted and found to be composed of 409 unique terms. When analysing the terms 285 corresponding concepts could be found.

From the Swedish national guideline [3] 283 concepts had been identified. Comparison of the two sets of concepts yielded 68 common concepts.

For some concepts there were an abundance of terms in use. Some examples: for *cystitis* five different terms were used, for *red cells in urine (recommended term U-erytrocytes, particle concentration)* seven terms were utilised, for *control specimen* six dissimilar terms were found in the patient records, for *white cells in urine (recommended term U-leucocytes, particle concentration)* thirteen different terms could be found, the *nitrite test* was referred to by six terms, *pyelonephritis* by six terms and *dipstick* by six dissimilar terms.

In some instances the terms were used so that the meaning of the sentence was vague or ambiguous, e.g. ”Dipstick was positive.”, ”The patient has typical symptoms of urinary tract infection.”. In the mentioned sentences the reader cannot know which analyses the writer refers to in the first and which symptoms he refers to in the latter.

4. Discussion

Different categories of health-care providers require different levels of explanation to successfully perform their tasks. E.g. for a GP to establish a treatment for a urinary tract infection it is sufficient for him/her to use a patho-physiologic model where infections are directly caused by microorganisms whereas an infectious diseases specialist establishing a treatment for a certain disease would require a more elaborate model [1]. The GP on the other hand as being a community medicine specialist requires other dimensions than patho-physiology, e.g. patient reported symptoms, patient's way of life etc.

The relatively low yield of common concepts in the two domains studied could thus be expected since there is a great difference between the two activities, which necessarily needs to be described with different concepts and terms. However when describing matters related to bacteriological diagnosis the same concepts were used in the patient records as in the laboratory, although in the laboratory more numerous concept and concepts with a greater granularity (i.e. more specific and detailed) were used.

In our future terminological work we will include reference publications dealing more with clinical picture, pathogenesis, management and treatment of urinary tract infection to achieve full coverage of concepts needed in primary health care. Our conceptual model will also be compared to existing classifications such as ICD-10 [4]and ICPC-2 [5].

References

[1] Karlsson D, Aspevall O, Forsum U. Concepts, contexts and expert systems. Submitted to MIE 1999.

[2] Karlsson D, Ekdahl C, Wigertz O, Forsum U. A qualitative study of clinicians ways of using a decision-support system. Proceedings/AMIA Annual Fall Symposium 1997:268-72.

[3] Aspevall O, Hallander H (Eds.). Referensmetodik för laboratoriediagnostik vid kliniskt bakteriologiska laboratorier. I 5. Urinvägsinfektioner/bakteriuri. (Reference methodology for laboratory diagnosis at clinical bacteriology laboratories. I5. Urinary Tract Infections/Bacteriuria) SBL-tryck nr 136-1993, Stockholm, 1993.

[4] World Health Organization. International statistical classification of diseases and related health problems : ICD-10. 10th Ed. Geneva : World Health Organization, 1992-1994.

[5] WONCA International Classification Committee. International classification of primary care, ICPC-2. 2nd Ed. Oxford: Oxford University Press, 1998.

Medical Informatics Europe '99
P. Kokol et al. (Eds.)
IOS Press, 1999

Galen : a third generation terminology tool to support a multipurpose national coding system for surgical procedures

B Trombert-Paviot*, JM Rodrigues*, JE Rogers**, R Baud***, E van der Haring****, AM Rassinoux***, V Abrial*, L Clavel*, H Idir*

**Department of Public Health and Medical Informatics Fac de Médecine University of Saint Etienne France*

***Medical Informatics Group Victoria University of Manchester United Kingdom*

****Department of Medical Informatics University Hospital of Geneva Switzerland*

*****Department of medical Informatics Catholic University of Nijmegen Netherlands*

Abstract. GALEN has developed a new generation of terminology tools based on a language independent concept reference model using a compositional formalism allowing computer processing and multiple reuses. During the 4th framework program project Galen-In-Use we applied the modelling and the tools to the development of a new multipurpose coding system for surgical procedures (CCAM) in France. On one hand we contributed to a language independent knowledge repository for multicultural Europe. On the other hand we support the traditional process for creating a new coding system in medicine which is very much labour consuming by artificial intelligence tools using a medically oriented recursive ontology and natural language processing. We used an integrated software named CLAW to process French professional medical language rubrics produced by the national colleges of surgeons into intermediate dissections and to the Grail reference ontology model representation. From this language independent concept model representation on one hand we generate controlled French natural language to support the finalisation of the linguistic labels in relation with the meanings of the conceptual system structure. On the other hand the classification manager of third generation proves to be very powerful to retrieve the initial professional rubrics with different categories of concepts within a semantic network.

Keywords. knowledge representation, knowledge acquisition, classification, natural language processing

1. Introduction

The Galen artificial intelligence technology has been used within the Galen-In-Use (HC 1018) Health Care Telematics project of the 4 Th. R § D framework program to support the development of a new French coding system named CCAM. The work is going on within a contract between the French department of health and GOL (Galen Organisation Limited). We have presented in [1] the initial works on the increased linguistic coherence for urology rubrics by using Galen tools and techniques and natural language processing. We stressed here the power of the classification tool based on the language independent common reference model as an example of a practical support given by the third generation terminology Galen.

2. Materials and methods

◆Materials

Galen stands for Generalised Architecture for Languages, Encyclopaedias and Nomenclatures in Medicine. The project has developed a scheme in which all and only sensible medical concepts are represented and which is accessible and processed by computers. This scheme is named CORE (for COncept REference model) [2]. It is based on an ontology (high level schemata) to model the categories within the universe of discourse and to classify them automatically being language independent and on a kernel of general medical knowledge. It is application independent and reusable for it uses a compositional formalism named GRAIL (for Galen Representation and Integration Language) [3]. The second outcome was the development of practical tools and techniques (the terminology server) for managing healthcare terminology including natural language processing. Galen-In-Use has been the application phase of Galen among nine national classification centres from Belgium, Finland, Germany, Greece, Italy, Sweden, United Kingdom, The Netherlands and France.

The French demonstrator is applying Galen tools to the development of a new coding system for surgical procedures initiated in 1994, named CCAM (for Classification Commune des Actes Médicaux) [4]. It is using an integrated set of tools named CLAW [5] for Classification workbench and ALN (for Atelier Langage Naturel) to generate controlled French natural language sentences [6]. It plans to merge two existing systems for billing the physician fees and for coding hospital discharge abstract in one only multipurpose coding system. The program is managed by a joint effort from the ministry of health and the national agency of the main mandatory health insurance system. CCAM is planned as part of a broader CCAP (Classification Commune des Actes Professionnels) for healthcare professionals. The initial work concerning surgery is planned for 15 parts of 500 rubrics each : 7 500 rubrics including combined interventions. To day 11 parts have reached step 3 and 6 step 4 with 3 000 rubrics. The final product is planned for 2001 for surgery and 2002 for an additional 15 parts of medical interventions.

◆Methods

There are four stages as described in [1] : an intermediate dissection, the validation of the compliance with CEN /ENV 1828, the representation with the Grail CORE model and the outputs.

Once the formal knowledge representation of each rubric of CCAM is built, there are a lot of opportunities for the outputs. First there is a strong need to come back to natural language expressions in French language for quality assurance : error detection, disambiguation or inconsistency [7] and to assess the process. The second opportunity is automatic indexing for retrieval and dynamic reclassification for cross reference to restructure an apparently first generation terminology (a flat list) in a de facto compositional (multi axial) second generation terminology [8] and with an unlimited range of possibilities. We are presenting some examples in the following part and more for the oral presentation.

3. Results

Overview

Tab 1 : Distribution of entities by classes by levels

Level 1	Level 2	Level 3	Level 4	Level 5	Level 6	Total
0.4 surgery in order to achieve repair	95	11	16	29	15	166
0.6 accompanying	8	44	105	6		163
0.7 closure	2	40	40	5	1	88
0.8 creation	32	7	16	7	4	66
0.9 destruction	2	28	7			37
0.10 cauterizing	0					0
0.11 fastening	5	36	32	8	2	83
0.12 freeing	14	11	1			26
0.13 tension	1					1
0.14 decompression	16	1				17
0.15 compression	1					1
0.16 installation	12	153	55	18	2	240
0.17 opening	9	120	66	16	4	215
0.18 manipulation	8	5	1	1		15
0.19 movement	29	26	13	1		69
0.20 removal	17	651	326	75	18	1087
Total	251	1133	678	166	46	2274

We are presenting the results for 3 clinical domains, Neurosurgery with 436 rubrics, Ear Nose and Throat surgery with 695 rubrics, oral surgery with 409 rubrics and a total of 1540 rubrics. They were mapped to 1926 different terminological phrases for some initial CCAM rubrics must be represented by more than a only dissection for ontology reason when for instance they describe different incompatible approaches within the same rubrics. Further on these 1926 different terminological phrases are classified in 2274 entities for the same sentence can have more than one parent and be classified in different classes. The granularity is summarised in Tab 1 where the 6 levels are presented starting from the 16 initial classes at level 1.

At level 1 they are 20 possible classes but only 16 are populated by our sample coming from only 3 clinical domains of surgical procedures. The classification is based first on the main deed, then on different concepts depending upon the main classes. There are 6 hierarchical levels clustering the 2274 entities. The main class (level 1) “removal” groups 47.8% of the entities with the most common surgical deed excising. The level 3 is the most frequent (49,8%) and the level 4 (29.81%) is more frequent than the level 2 (11.03%).

At level 2 the classes are based on different concepts. As an example :

- the deed, for class 0.11 “fastening” which is divided in 0.11.0 immobilization, 0.11.1 fixation, 0.11.2 fusion, 0.11.3 stabilization, 0.11.4 binding
- the object on which the deed is done e.g for 0.18 “manipulation”.

Automatic indexing and multiple parents (Tab 2)

The same entity can be automatically retrieved several times depending upon the position of the concept in the hierarchy of the typology and its relation with other concepts in anatomy, device or approach. This multiple criteria retrieval is very useful to cluster the rubrics by their meaning proximity. One example for “alignment” shows the power of the composite knowledge representation to generate automatically the meaning connections between elementary entities.

Tab 2 : multiple indexing

- 0.4.0 alignment in order to achieve repair
  - 0.4.0 alignment in order to achieve repair
    - 0.4.0.0 reduction
      - 0.4.0.0.0 reduction on fracture
        - 0.4.0.0.0.5 reduction on fracture involves of Orbit & Skull
        - 0.4.0.0.0.15 reduction on fracture of zygoma Transoral Approach
          - 0.4.0.0.0.15.0 reduct. on fract. of zygoma, Transoral Approach with Incising of face
        - 0.4.0.0.0.16 reduction on fracture of zygoma with Incising of Face
          - 0.4.0.0.0.15.0 reduct. on fract. of zygoma, Transoral Approach with Incising of face
      - 0.4.0.0.2 open reduction on bone of nose
      - 0.4.0.0.3 closed reduction during postpartum period on nose
      - 0.4.0.0.4 closed reduction on bone of nose
- 0.19 movement
  - 0.19.9 alignment
    - 0.4.0 alignment in order to achieve repair
    - 0.19.9.1 alignment on segment of nose
    - 0.19.9.2 primary bilateral alignment cartilagoalarismajor
    - 0.19.9.3 primary unilateral alignment cartilagoalarismajor
    - 0.19.9.4 alignment on orbit
      - 0.4.0.0.0.5 reduction on fracture involves of Orbit & Skull
      - 0.4.0.0.0.15 reduction on fracture of zygoma TransOralApproach
      - 0.4.0.0.0.16 reduction on fracture of zygoma with Incising of Face
  - 0.19.26 movement on nose
    - 0.4.0.0.3 closed reduction during postpartum period on nose
    - 0.19.9.1 alignment on segment of nose
    - 0.4.0.0.2 open reduction on bone of nose
    - 0.4.0.0.4 closed reduction on bone of nose

0.4.0 , 0.4.0.0.3 ,0.4.0.0.2 , 0.4.0.0.4 , 0.4.0.0.0.5 , 0.4.0.0.0.15 , 0.4.0.0.0.16 are classified within the level 1 class 0.4 "alignment to achieve repair" at levels ranging from 2 to 5 and reclassified within the level 1 class 0.19 "movement" at levels ranging from 3 to 4. This automatic indexing is very useful to show that the flat list first generation like CCAM coding system has a multiple parents structure which cannot be managed without computer processing.

Reclassification and multiple hierarchy

Another important opportunity with galen tools is to reclassify the coding system depending upon the different concepts categories which are represented with the core model. For instance within the 3 clinical domains there are 16 entities on oesophagus or 67 entities by endoscopy.

4. Discussion

The utilisation of a third generation terminology tool [8] like Galen for surgical procedure coding systems development must not be misinterpreted. Galen is not the new generation terminology to replace the existing coding systems in different countries but a set of tools and technique to support and to ease such developments at least on 3 points.

- to increase the coherence and the consistency of the linguistic (even in a minority language as French) expressions of the lists of rubrics (first generation terminology) which are still needed for some very important purposes (like the use for billing for CCAM). We have demonstrated in [1] the usefulness of generating controlled vocabulary based on all the sensible and only the sensible knowledge to increase the quality of such first generation terminology which will be kept in use.

- to allow the creation of a second generation terminology starting from the apparent flat list of rubrics produced by the traditional consensus method by the multiple concepts categories representation allowing reclassification by different concepts hierarchies and cross references.
- to open the way to third generation terminology by automatic indexing based on the semantic network and the multiple parents structure of the GALEN concept model .The availability of all the acquired knowledge on surgical procedures and later on other clinical domains on a computer accessible form is a major enabling factor to shift from the utilisation by national or regional coding centres to the broader utilisation within the electronic healthcare record.

5. Conclusion

All the recently developed coding systems for surgical procedures share some common features for the process which can be named a consensus method. The clinical input and the many reviews of the linguistic expressions are scattered among clinical consultants, coders and health care recorders. The CCAM French process has introduced and added the use of artificial intelligence tools allowing to transform an apparent first generation terminology in a second generation one and opening the way to the advanced third generation use.
On the other hand the so called consensus method results in underestimated invisible costs and constant high cost maintenance. On the contrary the use of the third generation terminology tools have a clear defined cost and allow decreasing cost maintenance. The increasing strategic use of coding systems is a strong support to the extended utilisation of such tools.

Acknowledgements

To Galen-in-Use (HC 1018) project, funded by E.U Fourth R § D framework program .

References

[1] Rodrigues JM, Trombert-Paviot B, Baud R, Wagner J, Meusnier-Carriot F. Galen-In-Use :Using artificial intelligence terminology tools to improve the linguistic coherence of a national coding system for surgical procedures. In : Cesnik B and all, Eds. Proceedings of the ninth World Congress on medical informatics - Medinfo'98 ; Seoul; IOS Press. 1998, pp 623-627
[2] Rector AL Compositional Models of Medical Concept : Towards Re-Usable Application -Independent Medical Terminologies. In: P Barahona and JP Christensen (eds) Knowledge and Decisions in Health Telematics, IOS Press. 1994, pp 133-142.
[3] Rector AL, Bechofer S, Goble C, Horrocks I, Nowlan W, Solomon W. The GRAIL Concept Modelling Language for Medical Terminology.In: Medical Informatics Group, Department of Computer Science, University of Manchester, 1996.
[4] NCAM.Structure technique NCAPS Paris 02/01/1997.
[5] Zanstra P The Galen project. Classification manager. CBV Niews 1993 ; (4).
[6] Baud RH, Alpay L, Lovis C. Let's Meet the Users with Natural Language Understanding; In P Barahona and JP Christensen (eds) Knowledge and Decisions in Health Telematics, IOS Press. 1994, pp103-108.
[7] Rector AL, Baud R, Ceusters W, Claassen W, Rodrigues J-M, Rogers J, Rossi Mori A, van der Haring E, Solomon WD, Zanstra P. A Comprehensive Approach to Developing and Integrating Multilingual Classifications: GALEN's Classification Workbench. Theater-Style Demonstration, AMIA 1998 Annual Symposium (AMIA'98). Lake Buena Vista, FL, November 9, 1998.
[8] Rossi Mori A. Towards a new generation of terminologies and coding systems..Proceeding MIE 96 IOS Press Copenhaguen 1996

Medical Informatics Europe '99
P. Kokol et al. (Eds.)
IOS Press, 1999

Synapses/SynEx goes XML

Benjamin JUNG [Benjamin.Jung@cs.tcd.ie]
Jane GRIMSON [Jane.Grimson@cs.tcd.ie]
Dept. of Computer Science, Trinity College Dublin, Dublin 2, Ireland
Tel. +353-1-608 1335/1594, Fax. +353-1-677 2204.

Abstract. This paper describes the first approach to use the Extensible Markup Language (XML) as a data interchange/delivery format in the Synapses and SynEx healthcare environment. It will ease the semantic mapping between healthcare systems (server-server, server-client) and make them more interoperable.

1. Introduction

The management of electronic patient data was relatively easy as long as the data was collected, stored and viewed in a closed environment like a hospital or doctor's practice. Heterogeneous and compatible IT systems were provided by one company and externally or internally employed, centralised system administrators were responsible for the smooth use of all installed components. No connection to the 'outside world' was established which eased the protection of patient data immensely. Data exchange was only possible by paper, mail, fax or telephone, which lead to extra work and unreliability: feedback and results had to be manually entered into a new system. Increased computerisation throughout the health sector has given rise to a proliferation of independent systems storing patient data. However, the growing trend towards shared care requires that these systems are able to share their data. This has led to the development of projects such as Synapses [1] and its follow-up, SynEx [2] that aim to provide healthcare professionals with integrated access to patient records and related data. The Synapses Federated Healthcare Record (FHCR) project exploited ideas from federated database technology [3] which provide client applications with an integrated view of data stored in heterogeneous, distributed database systems. At the heart of Synapses is the FHCR server which accepts request for data (in the form of clinical objects) from clients, decomposes them into queries against the connected "feeder" systems, where the data is actually stored and integrates the responses dynamically. Synapses was concerned with the specification of an open standard for the server and its interfaces and for pragmatic reasons used an *ad hoc* mechanism for exchanging clinical data between feeders, server and client. An obvious markup for such an exchange is the Extensible Markup Language (XML) [4] and this is being actively pursued in the SynEx project. This paper assesses how XML could be usefully incorporated into both Synapses and SynEx and the advantages of this.

XML, which was introduced in 1996 for the first time, has the power to become the independent data exchange format of the future. Hierarchical structured patient data, user defined tags and inclusion of machine-understandable assertions about FHCR objects for machine understanding (searching, reasoning and analysing) were goals for the use of XML in data exchange between non-heterogeneous systems.

2. Enterprise Viewpoint

This section describes the Synapses/SynEx project and summarises the user requirements for the introduction of XML as data interchange format in the SynEx environment. In its early days XML was often summarised as another hype on the Internet, but it increasingly became a general tool for data handling in a variety of different ways and areas and a common syntax for expressing structure in data. Corporate strong support from commercial companies as well as non-commercial consortia lead to a fast and dense development of first proposals and recommendations.

The Synapses Project is a three-year project funded under the EU 4th Framework Health Telematics Programme. The consortium consists of 26 partners from 14 different countries representing the health software industry sector, research institutes and universities, and end-users through the participation of several hospitals. Synapses sets out to solve problems of sharing data between autonomous information systems, by providing generic and open means to combine healthcare records or dossiers consistently, simply, comprehensibly and securely, whether the data passes within a single healthcare institution or between institutions [5, 6, 7]. The SynEx Project as a direct successor of Synapses Project is also funded under the EU 4th Framework Health Telematics Programme and assembles most of the previous partners and countries. The main goal of the two-year project is the integration of previously developed Synapses components with additional commercial modules into one Healthcare Information Systems Architecture (HISA) [8].

Requirement 1: Use of existing Synapses components: The re-use of existing Synapses components and code as well as the future use of Synapses in one HISA is the main task of the project. An already existing and working Dublin Synapses FHCR Server (DSFS) shall be extended and completed with general XML functionality. Simplicity and speed of implementation are given emphasis on the integration of the additional services.

Requirement 2: Platform/vendor independence: The World Wide Web Consortium (W3C) [16], the 'mother' of XML guarantees a platform and vendor neutral development and specification in the future. Incompatibility problems between data structures from different (e.g. database) applications, even between different versions of one application, will be a problem of the past. Support of XML is already implemented in a variety of existing applications and further announcements appear every week in the news.

Requirement 3: Easy access: The Document Object Model (DOM) [9] and Simple API for XML (SAX) [10], are platform- and language-neutral interfaces that will easily allow programs and scripts to dynamically access and update the content, structure and style of documents. Most of the current parsers support all specified methods of the DOM. The wide use and existence of Internet browsers and HTTP transfer technology strongly influences a Web-based interface to the Synapses FHCR Server.

Requirement 4: Use of Metadata: XML gives the possibility to include machine-understandable assertions ('Metadata', 'data about data') in the XML document itself. Metadata will help systems to describe their data structure in ways that search engines, browsers and other applications can understand. It preserves the source data structure, includes additional semantic information and leads to better document discovery services (searching, reasoning, analysing and evaluating).

Requirement 5: Increase of speed: FHCRs often contain many hundreds often even thousands of objects. One big problem in a Common Request Broker Architecture

(CORBA) client-server environment is the fact that CORBA establishes new connections for every object transmission/migration. This phenomenon increased the transmission time in the Dublin implementation of the Synapses Server in an unacceptable way. The use of XML must ensure a huge decrease in transmission time.

Requirement 6: No Loss of information: It must be guaranteed that neither patient data nor the data structure of the FHCR is lost while mapping from system A to B. Back and forth mapping should lead to the exact image of the original FHCR data and structure.

3. Information Viewpoint

The following section describes briefly the concept of the Synapses Record Architecture, the Synapses Object Model (SynOM) and the Synapses Object Dictionary (SynOD). It furthermore outlines in a short example the direct mapping from the Synapses Object Model (SynOM) into equivalent XML ELEMENTS, XPointer [11] or Xlinks [12].

The SynOM is a common object model and extends the model described in the pENV12265 from the Comité Européen de Normalisation Technical Committee 251 (CEN/TC251) [13, 14]. It contains a set of seven base classes, their attributes and hierarchical aggregation, which will be used as general building blocks to build up the SynOD (FHCR shape or skeleton).

The first step in building Synapses compliant system is the creation of a local set of definitions of healthcare objects, called the SynOD. In the next step, individual objects have to be mapped to the data representations within local storage systems (e.g. databases). This is the requirement for the DSFS to dynamically fill up the SynOD skeleton with real patient data from the feeder systems on request and therefore create the individual 'synapsed' patient record. It has to be mentioned that this procedure leads to totally different SynOD in different sites, but the SynOM is still common to all.

Together with the Dublin FHCR Synapses Server, the Record Structure Builder (RSB) will be available. This application's graphical user interface eases the process of SynOD building and supports the user with structural information from the SynOM.

SynOM class	XML equivalent
RecordFolder	ELEMENT
FolderRIC	ELEMENT
ComRIC	ELEMENT
DataRIC	ELEMENT
RecordItem	ELEMENT
ViewRIC1	ELEMENT
ViewRIC2	Xpointer, XLink

Figure 1: SynOM – XML mapping

The mapping from SynOD objects into XML ELEMENTS is a straight 1:1 process (see Figure 1). All SynOM baseclasses within the SynOD are equivalent to XML ELEMENTs, except the ViewRIC2, which compares to a Xpointer or XLink. SynOD class attributes are included as XML ATTRIBUTEs in the final XML document and the retrieved data from the feeder systems maps to XML ELEMENT content. This follows the CEN/TC251 XML Taskforce recommendation that all patient data that has to be signed by the responsible person will appear as XML ELEMENT content. Structural information is stored as XML ATTRIBUTEs in the related XML ELEMENT.

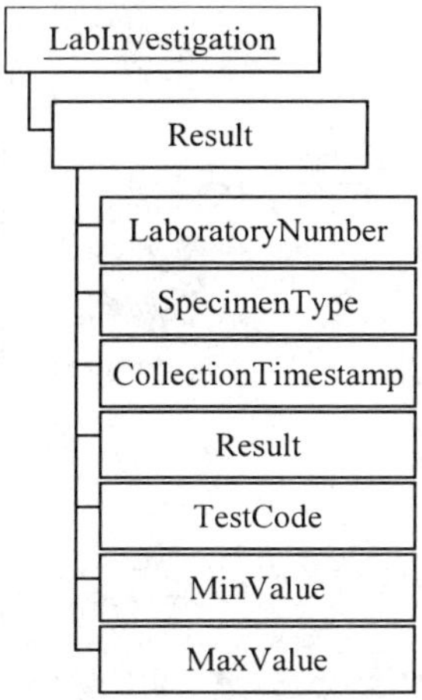


```
<LabInvestigationComRIC BC="ComRic" RCId="47" RecId="0123456">
    <Result BC="RecordItem" RCId="50" DT="EMPTY">
        <LaboratoryNumber BC="RecordItem" RCId="57">
            S,96.0110835.R
        </LaboratoryNumber>
        <SpecimenType BC="RecordItem" RCId="58">
            B
        </SpecimenType>
        <CollectionTimestamp BC="RecordItem" RCId="59">
            3/3/1996 10.15
        </CollectionTimestamp>
        <Result BC="RecordItem" RCId="60">
            29
        </Result>
        <TestCode BC="RecordItem" RCId="61">
            ALB
        </TestCode>
        <MinValue BC="RecordItem" RCId="62">
            35.00000
        </MinValue>
        <MaxValue BC="RecordItem" RCId="63">
            50.00000
        </MaxValue>
    </Result>
</LabInvestigationComRIC>
```


Figure 2: Example of a direct mapping from SynOD objects into XML ELEMENTS

4. Computation Viewpoint

This section describes the two additional methods that were included into the Synapses Server Kernel to serve patient data in XML format. It furthermore explains their counterparts within the Common Gateway Interface (CGI-scripts), which maps HTTP-requests into IIOP-requests and IIOP objects into XML documents.

Both methods cast the internal object-oriented record structure into one single CORBA object of type string (in XML format). The hierarchical structure and all attributes of each object are preserved and included into the XML document for later use. For each method exists a correlating CGI-script which will be invoked through the Webserver. The CGI-script names are exact copies of the DSFS methods.

RetrieveRecordShape: This method wraps all SynOM classes down to the level of ComRICs (i.e. RecordFolder » FolderRIC » ComRIC) and possible ViewRIC2s into one XML document. Afterwards, this document represents the skeleton or shape of the FHCR; 'real' data from the feeder systems is not included. This XML document allows the user to navigate through the structure of the FHCR on the client and select a specific part of the FHCR, which will be downloaded as large bulk of a single ComRIC data.

RetrieveXmlComRic: The second method collects all SynOM classes within a ComRIC as root node down to it's leaf nodes where the real data from the feeder systems is stored in RecordItems. The ComRIC indicates a perfect spot to split up the FHCR into smaller sub-sections, because of its intended representation of the smallest meaningful, autonomous set of medical information.

5. Engineering Viewpoint

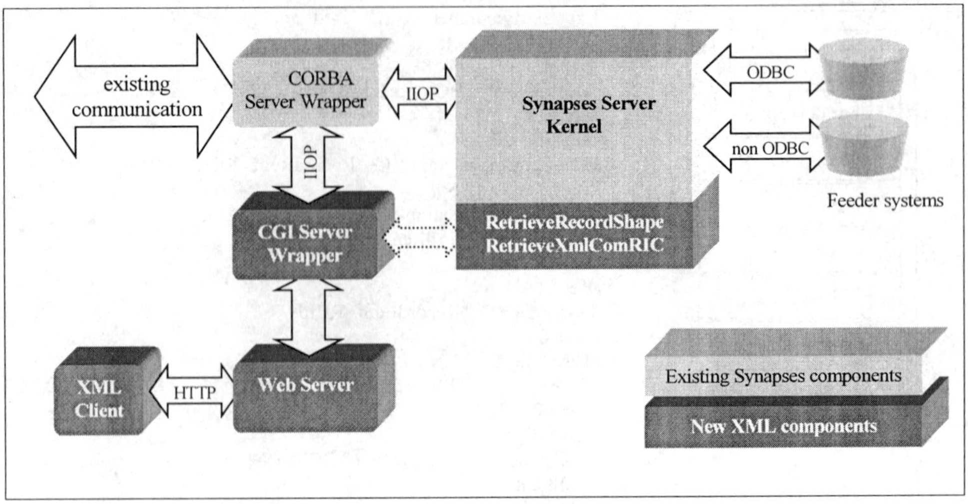

Figure 3: The elements of the Synapses XML Architecture

The Dublin XML solution preserves the full functionality of the pre-existing DSFS. Two additional methods in the Synapses Server Kernel are necessary to map the collection of SynOM classes and SynOD structure into a single XML document FHCR, which is immediately sent to the Webserver via CORBA Server Wrapper and CGI Server Wrapper. The use of XML as an interchange format is 'only' an additional feature of the DSFS. All existing functionality and communication architectures are preserved. Further evaluation has to show whether it will give the needed flexibility in data exchange.

6. Technology Viewpoint

This part describes the software and software tools that are necessary to make the DSFS XML compliant. All mentioned components were developed and tested on a Windows NT4.0 environment. Future migration to other platforms is not envisaged.

The Synapses Server Kernel itself was written in Microsoft Visual C++ and connects to various (existing) feeder systems by ODBC and SQL. The use of other (non-ODBC using) database engines is possible, practical and easy to complete, but additional software will be needed. The CORBA Server Wrapper is part of the Synapses Server Kernel and uses IONA's Orbix CORBA implementation. All CGI scripts are written and compiled in Microsoft Visual C++.

The actual implementation uses the Microsoft Personal. The use of CGI-scripts is always a security issue, which should be handled most carefully. They should be written with the most thoroughness especially in a medical environment where security is imperative.

7. Conclusions

As mentioned above, the XML functionality of the DSFS is only additional to the existing output format and communication technologies. At this stage of the research the implementation does not rely on XML as the only exchange format and further development is also done in all other existing components. We expect feedback from users as well as from implementers whether data in XML format is useful and can ease the process of data exchange.

It is also clear, that XML does not solve every problem without any adaptation of applications. Using XML does not mean data exchange at once without problems, but it helps and makes the whole process more transparent and easier.

References

[1] Synapses Homepage, http://www.cs.tcd.ie/synapses/public/.

[2] SynEx Homepage, http://www.gesi.it/synex/.

[3] Sheth, A.P., Larson, J.A., *Federated database systems for managing distributed, heterogeneous and autonomous databases,* ACM Computing Surveys, 22, 183-235, 1990.

[4] Bray, T., Paoli, J., Sperberg-McQueen, C. M., *Extensible Markup Language (XML) 1.0*, http://www.w3.org/TR/1998/REC-xml-19980210, W3C Recommendation 10-February-1998.

[5] Grimson, W., Berry, D., Grimson, J., Stephens, G., Felton, E., Given, P. and O'Moore, R., *Federated healthcare record server - the Synapses paradigm,* International Journal of Medical Informatics, 1998.

[6] Grimson, J. *et al*, *Synapses - Federated healthcare record server,* Procs. MIE 96, IOS Press, 695-699.

[7] Grimson, J., Grimson, W., Berry, D., Kalra, D., Toussaint, P. and Weier, O., *A CORBA-based integration of distributed electronic healthcare records using the Synapses approach*, IEEE Transactions on Information Technology in Biomedicine, 2, 124-138, September 1998.

[8] CEN/TC251 WG I, *Healthcare Information System Architecture Part 1 (HISA) Healthcare Middleware Layer*, Final Draft prENV 12967-1, not publicly available at the moment, March 1997.

[9] Wood, L. (chair), *Document Object Model (DOM) Level 1 Specification Version 1.0*, http://www.w3.org/TR/REC-DOM-Level-1/, W3C Recommendation 01-October-1998.

[10] Megginson, D., *SAX 1.0: The Simple API For XML*, http://www.megginson.com/SAX/.

[11] Maler, E., DeRose, S., *XML Pointer Language (XPointer)*, http://www.w3.org/TR/1998/WD-xptr-19980303, W3C Working Draft 03-March-1998.

[12] Maler, E., DeRose, S., *XML Linking Language (Xlink)*,http://www.w3.org/TR/1998/WD-xlink-19980303, World Wide Web Consortium Working Draft 03-March-1998.

[13] CEN/TC251 Homepage, http://www.centc251.org/.

[14] CEN/TC251 WG I, *Electronic Healthcare Record Architecture*, Final Draft 2 prENV12265, not publicly available at the moment, July 1995.

[15] Hurlen, P., Skifjeld, K., Andersen, E., *Synapses – Design and functional specification of FHCR server and interfaces*, not publicly available at the moment, 1998.

[16] World Wide Web Consortium Homepage, http://www.w3c.org/.

Medical Informatics Europe '99
P. Kokol et al. (Eds.)
IOS Press, 1999

German Adaptations of ICD-10

Bernd Graubner and Gerhard Brenner
Zentralinstitut für die kassenärztliche Versorgung in der Bundesrepublik Deutschland (ZI) (Central Research Institute of Ambulatory Health Care in Germany), Herbert-Lewin-Str. 5, D-50931 Köln, Germany

Abstract: The introduction of the ICD-10, published by WHO 1992–94 in English and by DIMDI 1994/95 in German, is a very slow process. Some states introduced ICD-10 for the preparation of statistics of mortality, but only few use it for morbidity. ICD-9 is in Germany only in hospitals still in use. Much effort was put into the improvement of the official ICD-10 and the development of additional aids for more simple and better encoding of diagnoses. Thus a revision especially for ambulatory health care (ICD-10-SGBV with the incorporated ICD-10-Basisschlüssel) and a collection of German terms and expressions of diagnoses that are not at all part of the official ICD-10 (ICD-10-Diagnosenthesaurus) were published. Three years ago a conversion table ICD-9/-10 was developed which can now be harmonised with WHO's Translator. The experiences with all these instruments are satisfying. The development of methods for automatic encoding of free-text phrases of diagnoses has now been started.

1. Introduction

The history of The International Statistical Classification of Diseases (ICD) goes back more than hundred years. It is the only world wide accepted universal classification of diseases and causes of death and represents the centre of the family of diseases and health-related classifications. But its wide distribution is also the cause of its weakness, because there are always contradictions between the demands for geographical and medical universality on the one hand, and the local, scientific and medicine-special requirements for a practicable and actual classification on the other hand. Nevertheless, all member countries of the World Health Organization (WHO) are obliged to provide by means of the currently valid version of ICD statistics on mortality and if possible also on morbidity.

The International Statistical Classification of Diseases and Related Health Problems, Tenth Revision (ICD-10), was published by the WHO in three volumes in the years 1992–1994. The German translation was performed by the German Institute of Medical Documentation and Information (Deutsches Institut für medizinische Information und Dokumentation [DIMDI]) in co-operation with the corresponding institutions in Austria and Switzerland. This was published 1994–1995 (version 1.0). Electronic updates were published in 1997 (version 1.1) and 1998 (version 1.2 [in accordance with the first WHO update]), however up to now only version 1.0 is available in a printed German version [3]. The next electronic update by DIMDI is expected for July 1999 (version 1.3).

Contrary to expectations by the WHO, the introduction of ICD-10 and the replacement of the old fashioned ICD-9 (1976) has been delayed in all countries. The situation in the three mainly German speaking countries is as follows:

- In the Federal Republic of Germany the ICD-10 has been in mandatory use for mortality statistics since 1998, and in voluntary use for medical documentation and morbidity statistics in ambulatory health care since 1997. The replacement of ICD-9 in hospital care, which has been used to encode the main diagnoses of all inpatients in East Germany since 1979 and in West Germany since 1986, is expected for the year 2000 or 2001.
- In the Federal Republic of Austria the ICD-10 has also been in mandatory use for mortality statistics since 1998, but in hospitals a special version of ICD-9 (ICD-9 BMAGS 1998) is still in use. The change to ICD-10 is being prepared by a comprehensive experiment in all hospitals of the province Carinthia (Kärnten) started in January 1999. Hospital doctors use only the "ICD-10 BMAGS 1999", while all administrative work is still done with ICD-9 codes, automatically translated from ICD-10 codes. The "ICD-10 BMAGS 1999" was developed on the basis of DIMDI version 1.2. Books and files with tabular list and alphabetical index were published too [1] [2].
- In Switzerland the ICD-10 (DIMDI version 1.0) has been in use for mortality statistics and in all hospitals since 1998.

2. Objectives, methods and results: Development of ICD-10 adaptations and similar products in Germany

In Germany, the replacement of ICD-9 in hospitals and in particular the introduction of any classification of diagnoses in ambulatory health care has been highly debated. Due to strong criticism of ICD-10 by physicians in ambulatory health care the three partners of medical self-government (Spitzenverbände der Krankenkassen [Central Organisations of Health Insurance Companies], Deutsche Krankenhausgesellschaft [DKG] [German Hospital Association] and Kassenärztliche Bundesvereinigung [KBV] [National Association of Statutory Health Insurance Physicians]) signed an agreement about a revision of the official ICD-10 version in 1996. An expert group worked out a proposal for the so-called *ICD-10-SGBV* (ICD-10 for the purpose of §§ 295 and 301 of Fünftes Buch Sozialgesetzbuch [SGB V]), that is reduced in extent and has simplified rules for use in ambulatory health care (see Fig. 1). This special adaptation has been available in the version 1.2 from the DIMDI server (http://www.dimdi.de) since 1998 [6]. The ZI published two special editions of the ICD-10-SGBV in 1997: *"ICD-10-Basisschlüssel"* with tabular list (see Fig. 2) and alphabetical index [4] and a complete tabular list of the ICD-10-SGBV without glossary descriptions, inclusion and exclusion terms (*"ICD-10 ZI-Spezialausgabe"*) [7]. The ZI also published a short manual with an introduction to the organisation and performance of the encoding of diagnoses in ambulatory health care (*"ICD-10-Verschlüsselungsanleitung"*) [8] – The ZI intends to publish an edition of the complete and reduced version of ICD-10 in one combined volume this year.

The ICD-10-SGBV was designed for more practicable use, especially in ambulatory health care. The basic principles for its development were set up according to legal demands for medical documentation and ensured the complete main structure of ICD-10.

- All three-character categories of chapters I–XIX can be used for encoding.
- Those four-character subcategories which are essential are marked. These are part of the "Basisschlüssel". All other four-character subcategories may also be used. Alternatively their superior three-character categories may be used instead. For that reason they are not part of the "Basisschlüssel". But this rule is only valid for general practitioners, for medical specialist outside of their speciality and within the emergency

medical service. Examples: A02.0 and A02.- (for A02.1, A02.2, A02.8 and A02.9). (See Fig. 1 and 2.)

- The chapters XXI (factors influencing health status and contact with health services) and especially XX (external causes of morbidity and mortality) can be used at a reduced extent only.
- Four-character subcategories for diseases that are very seldom in Middle Europe ("exotic") are shifted in an appendix (mainly from chapter I [certain infectious and parasitic diseases]). Examples: A00.0, A00.1 and A00.9.
- Some codes especially in the chapter XXI are not allowed as primary codes and have to be used similar to the asterisk-codes of ICD-10 only as secondary codes.
- Two groups of additional characters behind each code can (or shall) be used for the certainty of diagnosis ("V" = suspicion [Verdacht], "A" = exclusion [Ausschluß] or "Z" = condition after [Zustand nach]) and the side-location of a diagnosis ("L" = left [links], "R" = right [rechts], "B" = both [beiderseits]).

Complete official ICD-10, tabular list:
- 14,479 codes and groups of codes (chapters, blocks, categories and subcategories) within 21 chapters,
- among them 10,762 codes and groups of codes in chapters I–XIX and XXI,
- among them **8,757 codes for primary encoding:**
  240 three-character categories and 8,517 four-character subcategories

↓ *reduction of „exotic" diagnoses, nearly the total chapter XX (with the exception of 22 secondary codes) and parts of chapter XXI*

ICD-10-SGBV:
- **8.069 codes for primary encoding** (= 92 % of 8,757):
  229 three-character and 7,840 four-character codes (= relation 1:34)

↓ *reduction to important codes for the purposes of § 295 SGB V (encoding in ambulatory health care)*

ICD-10-Basisschlüssel (chapters I–XIX and XXI):
- **2.879 codes for primary encoding** (= 33 % of 8,757 respectively. 36 % of 8,069):
  1,461 three-character and 1,418 four-character codes (= relation 1:1)

Fig. 1: Quantitative comparison of official ICD-10 and the two new versions ICD-10-SGBV and ICD-10-Basisschlüssel. Only one third of codes of the official ICD-10 and ICD-10-SGBV is used in the Basisschlüssel, and among them fewer than on fifth of all four-character subcategories of ICD-10-SGBV. On the other hand, most of all three-character categories in the ICD-10 can be used for primary encoding with the Basisschlüssel according to its special rules. Only 36 % of these 1,461 categories are divided by subcategories. Encoding with the ICD-10-Basisschlüssel is comparable simple due to this reduction (see Fig. 2).

The Central Research Institute of Ambulatory Health Care in Germany (ZI) established a team of scientists of different medical institutions, headed by Prof. W. Giere, Johann-Wolfgang-Goethe-Universität Frankfurt/Main, to develop the so-called *"ICD-10-Diagnosenthesaurus"*. The target is a validated collection of terms and expressions of diagnoses in German language with ICD-10 codes (and not a real "thesaurus"!), whereby many of them are (up to now) supplements of the official ICD-10. The version 2.2 (1999) contains nearly 30,000 terms (phrases) and is available in two different forms: as a computer file and as a book file with an alphabetical index (nearly 60,000 entries). This work is going on, and version 3.0 is expected by the end of this year. These files are available from the DIMDI server [5].

Replacing the ICD-9 in hospitals while ensuring the continuation of the ICD deployment can be simplified by using a translation table between ICD-9 and ICD-10. This *"Überleitungstabelle ICD-9/10"* was 1996 written by Dr. A. Zaiß, Albert-Ludwigs-Universität Freiburg i. Br., with the support of the Deutscher Ärzte-Verlag (DÄV) and is now also available from the DIMDI server. Meanwhile also the WHO published a Translator. This table and the German table will be compared and combined in 1999. The translation table is also published as software by the DÄV (version 2.1 [12]) and is a component of DÄV's encoding software for diagnoses (ICD-9/-10) and medical procedures (OPS-301 [ICPM]) "ICD/ICPM professional" [9]. These tables are used for clinical research, statutory minimum basic data sets, epidemiological morbidity trends and public health statistics. They will be helpful for comparing data collected in ICD-10 with data formerly classified by ICD-9, and when using ICD-10 in documentation if there is the necessity of delivering still ICD-9-codes for legal purposes [11] [13] – *"Full-text versions"* of all these classifications with the complete text-formulation for each code are commercially available, e. g. [9], whereas the DIMDI server provides SGML, ASCII or WORD files with the data as printed in the books.

A00–B99	**I. Bestimmte infektiöse und parasitäre Krankheiten**
A00–A09	**Infektiöse Darmkrankheiten**
A01.-	**Typhus abdominalis und Paratyphus**
A02.-	**Sonstige Salmonelleninfektionen**
A02.0	Salmonellenenteritis
A03.-	**Shigellose [Bakterielle Ruhr]**
A04.-	**Sonstige bakterielle Darminfektionen**
A04.4	Sonstige Darminfektionen durch Escherichia coli
A05.-	**Sonstige bakteriell bedingte Lebensmittelvergiftungen**
A05.0	Lebensmittelvergiftung durch Staphylokokken
A06.-	**Amöbiasis [Amöbenruhr]**
A07.-	**Sonstige Darmkrankheiten durch Protozoen**
A07.1	Giardiasis [Lambliasis]
A08.-	**Virusbedingte und sonstige näher bezeichnete Darminfektionen**
A08.0	Enteritis durch Rotaviren
A09	**Diarrhoe und Gastroenteritis, vermutlich infektiösen Ursprungs**

Fig. 2: The first entries of the tabular list of the ICD-10-Basisschlüssel [4]. The block A00–A09 contains only 14 codes and all of them are primary codes. The same block in the complete official ICD-10 contains 59 primary codes and 8 three-character categories.

3. Discussion and conclusion

In 1997 the ZI performed a voluntary comprehensive field : More than 2,000 ambulatory physicians in the federal states of Lower Saxony (Niedersachsen) and Saxony-Anhalt

(Sachsen-Anhalt) applied the ICD-10 for encoding their diagnoses. In general, the ICD-10 was found to be practicable. The ambulant physicians made good use of the German adaptations of ICD-10 and particularly preferred the ICD-10-Diagnosenthesaurus for daily practice [10].

Similar positive experience had physicians of the hospitals in Carinthia, who use the ICD-10 BMAGS 1999 [1] and the Austrian version of the Diagnosenthesaurus [2] in an obligatory comprehensive test since January 1999. The automatic conversion of ICD-10 codes into ICD-9 codes does not cause any particular problems.

Because of the current unsteadiness in the German ICD-legislation, the ICD-10 is not really introduced in the ambulatory health care, but it is used on a voluntary basis by about 10 % of the physicians. The general use of ICD-10 in hospitals is still an exception (e. g. in the University hospital Heidelberg). Although so many adaptations of ICD-10 are now available and encoding in ICD-10 is easier than encoding in ICD-9, the ICD-10 is hardly in use in the daily operations.

In addition to the above mentioned special editions of ICD-10, in Germany there are also speciality-based adaptations available, e.g. for Dermatology, Oncology, Ophthalmology, Orthopaedics, Paediatrics and Psychiatry (see [10]). Currently, there are no plans to develop a German clinical modification of the ICD-10 comparable to ICD-10-CM, that is being prepared in the U.S.A. However, for all physicians, medical record officers and other people engaged in encoding of diagnoses useful aids have been developed. Work is in progress to encode the diagnoses of German ambulatory physicians in an automatic way. This is co-ordinated by the ZI.

We are convinced that a joint effort to improve the use of ICD by scientists in the German speaking countries as well as in the European Union and in the WHO will be successful.

References

[1] *Diagnosenschlüssel ICD-10 BMAGS 1999.* Internationale statistische Klassifikation der Krankheiten und verwandter Gesundheitsprobleme. 10. Revision, BMAGS-Version 1999. Erarbeitet auf der Grundlage der vom DIMDI hrsg. deutschsprach. Übersetzung in der Vers. 1.2, Stand Juli 1998. Projektleitung: G. Embacher, Erarbeitung: B. Graubner. Wien: Bundesministerium für Arbeit, Gesundheit u. Soziales (BMAGS). 1999. Band I: Syst. Verz., 792 S. Band III: Alphab. Verz. 840 S.

[2] *Diagnosenthesaurus ICD-10 BMAGS 1999.* Sammlung von Krankheitsbegriffen im deutschen Sprachraum, verschlüsselt nach der ICD-10. Erarbeitet auf der Grundlage der vom DIMDI hrsg. u. von einer Projektgruppe des ZI erstellten Fassung in der Vers. 2.2, Stand 11.2.1999. Projektleitung: G. Embacher, Erarbeitung: B. Graubner. Wien: BMAGS. 1999. 552 S.

[3] *ICD-10.* Internationale statistische Klassifikation der Krankheiten und verwandter Gesundheitsprobleme. 10. Revision. Hrsg. vom DIMDI im Auftrag des Bundesministeriums für Gesundheit (BMG). Band I: Syst. Verz.. *Version 1.0.* Stand Aug. 1994. Band II: Regelwerk. Vers. 1.0. Stand Juni 1995. Band III: Alphab. Verz.. Vers. 1.0. Stand Okt. 1995. – Complete editions were published 1994/96 by the following publishing houses: Bern, Göttingen etc.: Huber / München, Wien etc.: Urban & Schwarzenberg / Landsberg/Lech: ecomed. – *Version 1.2* of volumes I and III was published by DIMDI in July 1998 as data files and is available from its server (http://www.dimdi.de). *Version 1.3* is announced for July 1999.

[4] *ICD-10-Basisschlüssel.* Alphabetisches und systematisches Verzeichnis zur Verschlüsselung von Krankheiten und verwandten Gesundheitsproblemen. Überarbeitung auf der Grundlage der amtlichen deutschsprachigen Ausgabe des DIMDI. Hrsg. v. ZI. Bearb. v. B. Graubner u. G. Brenner. Köln: Deutscher Ärzte-Verlag. 1997. XIII, 415 S.

[5] *ICD-10-Diagnosenthesaurus.* Sammlung von Krankheitsbegriffen im deutschen Sprachraum, verschlüsselt nach der ICD-10 (Vers. 1.2 [Juli 1998]). Vers. 2.2, Stand 11.2.1999. Hrsg. vom DIMDI im Auftrag des BMG. Erarbeitet von einer Projektgruppe des ZI unter Leitung von W. Giere. Schlußredaktion: B. Graubner. 1999. 552 S. – Available from the DIMDI server (http://www.dimdi.de) as ASCII-file for use in computer programs and as PDF-file for outprints.

[6] *ICD-10-SGBV.* Internationale statistische Klassifikation der Krankheiten und verwandter Gesundheitsprobleme. 10. Revision. Vorläufige Ausgabe für die Zwecke des SGB V. Erarbeitet v. e. Expertenarbeitsgruppe unter Beteiligung d. Spitzenverbände d. Krankenkassen, d. Kassenärztlichen Bundesvereinigung u. d. Deutschen Krankenhausgesellschaft. Hrsg. v. DIMDI im Auftrag d. BMG. Band I: Syst. Verz.. Vers. 1.2, Stand Juli 1998. – Available from the DIMDI server (http://www.dimdi.de).

[7] *ICD-10 ZI-Spezialausgabe.* Systematisches Verzeichnis zur Verschlüsselung von Krankheiten und verwandten Gesundheitsproblemen. Überarbeitung auf der Grundlage der amtlichen deutschsprachigen Ausgabe des DIMDI. Hrsg. v. ZI. Bearb. v. B. Graubner u. G. Brenner. Vers. 1.2 (8.4.1997). Köln: ZI. 1997. X, 286 S.

[8] *ICD-10-Verschlüsselungsanleitung.* Hrsg. v. ZI. Bearb. v. B. Graubner. Köln: Deutscher Ärzte-Verlag. 1997. 19 S.

[9] *ICD/ICPM professional.* Verschlüsselungsprogramm für Diagnosen und Operationen (ICD-9, ICD-10 und OPS-301). Hrsg.: dr. ruffing & partner. Wissenschaftl. Bearbeitung: B. Graubner. Vers. 3.3. Köln: Deutscher Ärzte-Verlag. 1999. – Full-text versions of the used classifications are available.

[10] *Koch, H.; Graubner, B.; Brenner, G.: Erprobung der Diagnosenverschlüsselung mit der ICD-10 in der Praxis des niedergelassenen Arztes.* Ergebnisse der wissenschaftlichen Begleituntersuchung zum Modellversuch in Niedersachsen und Sachsen-Anhalt im Jahre 1997. Hrsg. v. ZI. Köln: Deutscher Ärzte-Verlag. 1998. 182 S. (Wissenschaftl. Reihe des ZI. 54.)

[11] *Schulz, S., A. Zaiß, R. Brunner, D. Spinner a. R. Klar: Conversion Problems Concerning Automated Mapping from ICD-10 to ICD-9.* Methods of Information in Medicine. 1998; 37: 254–259.

[12] *Zaiß, A., et al: Überleitungstabelle zwischen ICD-9 und ICD-10.* Vers. 2.1. Programmgestaltung: dr. ruffing & partner. Köln: Deutscher Ärzte-Verlag. 1997

[13] *Zaiß, A., S. Schulz, B. Graubner a. R. Klar: Conversion Table between ICD-9 and ICD-10.* In: Medical Informatics Europe '96. Ed. by J. Brender, J. P. Christensen, J.-R. Scherrer a. P. McNair. Amsterdam, Oxford etc.: IOS Press. 1996. 193–197.

Nursing Informatics

Medical Informatics Europe '99
P. Kokol et al. (Eds.)
IOS Press, 1999

SysTerN
A Nursing Terminology System based on ICNP

Simona ALECU[1], Ioana MOISIL[2], Elena JITARU[3]

1 *Software ITC, 167 Calea Floreasca, BUCURESTI, 72321 Romania, Phone: 40-1-2320030/133, Fax: 40-1-2305612, E-mail:sitc@.softnet.ro*

2 *CCSSDM - Center for Health Computing, Statistics and Medical Documentation, 9 George Vraca St. , 70706 BUCURESTI, Romania, Phone : 40-1-3147035, Fax: 40-1-3112998, E-mail: imoisil@sunu.rnc.ro*

3 *ICI - Research Institute for Informatics, 8-10 Averescu Avenue, 71316 BUCURESTI, Romania, Phone: 40-1-2241259/224, Fax: 40-1-2241030, E-mail: jitaru@u3.ici.ro*

Abstract. This paper is presenting a terminology system for nursing - SysTerN – that is based on the ICNP[1] classification. SysTerN has been developed using the framework of the TeleNurse ID - ENTITY Telematics for Health EU project as a support for the dissemination actions carried on by CCSSDM (Center for Health Computing Statistics and Medical Documentation of the Romanian Ministry of Health) for Romania and other Central Eastern European countries.
Currently, the terminology system uses the alpha version of ICNP, but this version is going to be replaced by the beta version.
SysTerN is designed primarily for Romanian users but an English version is also available for other partners from CEE countries.

1. Introduction

This paper presents a terminology system for nursing - SysTerN – that is based on the ICNP classification. SysTerN has been developed using the framework of the TeleNurse ID - ENTITY Telematics for Health EU project as a support for the dissemination actions carried on by CCSSDM for Romania and other CEE countries.

TeleNurse ID - ENTITY is coordinated by Randi Mortensen, director of the Danish Institute for Health and Nursing Research and CCSSDM is one of the partners. The main objective of the TeleNurse ID - ENTITY project is to strengthen and enlarge the European consensus on the use of the International Classification of Nursing Practices (ICNP) as a standard computerized nursing language. This will be achieved by promoting and disseminating the classification in CEE countries, including translation of ICNP in Central and Eastern European languages and by carrying through a demonstration phase the software tools that were designed and built to integrate nursing modules in the shared electronic patient record.

Currently, the terminology system is using the alpha version of ICNP; the Romanian translation being done by two nurses. ICN has now dynamically released the ICNP-

[1] Copyright 1996 by ICN – International Council of Nurses, 3, place Jean Marteau, CH-1201 Geneva (Switzerland)

Phenomenon Classification. The ICNP-Action Classification is coming soon. As part of TelenurseID, CCSSDM will provide a full translation of all terms, including definitions.

For the beta - ICNP the translation procedure will follow the next steps:

1. translation from English to Romanian by a certified translator
2. refinement of the translation from English into Romanian by a nurse
3. back translation from Romanian into English by another certified translator and another nurse
4. comparison of the original version with the back translation.

The evaluation procedure is that recommended by ICN. It should be mentioned that currently, practically no nursing classification is being used in Romanian hospitals. We hope that with the introduction of ICNP into the electronic file this deficiency will disappear.

2. System description

The classifications of nursing phenomena and nursing interventions are intended to facilitate documentation of nursing practice by providing a terminology or vocabulary for use in the description of the nursing process.

The Nursing Phenomena and also the Nursing Interventions are defined by means of a set of qualities or properties, which are used for their classifications. Characteristics are also indispensable.

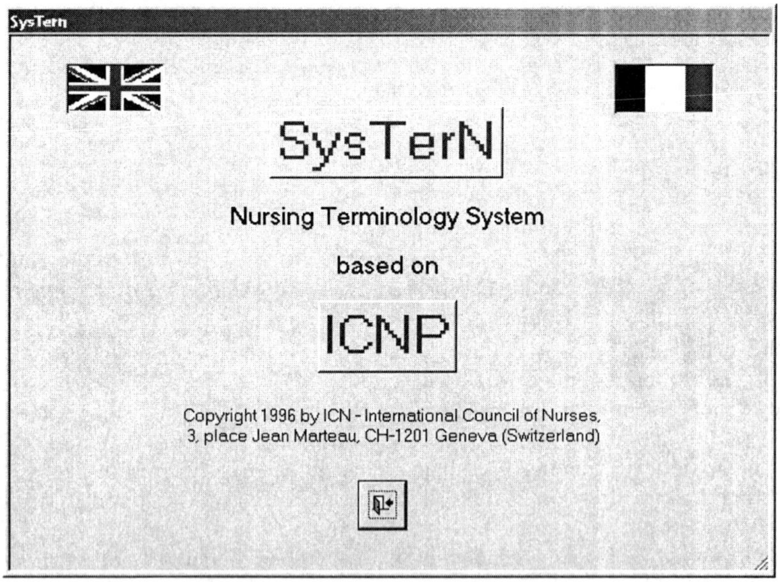

Figure 1. The main screen of the SysTerN

SysTerN is designed mainly for the Romanian users but an English version is also available for other partners from CEE countries. Therefore, on the main screen of the system (figure 1), the user can choose the language by clicking on the corresponding flag.

SysTerN is organized mainly as a dictionary, but also operates like a Thesaurus. For each of the terms it offers the users both the definition and also the corresponding synonyms.

There are three ways to select a term:

1. Use the four navigation buttons (|◄ , ◄ , ► , ►|) from the bottom of the screen;
2. Type the term's name or a part of it.
3. On a level by level basis: Select one of its subdivisions and click on the "next level" button; the selected term will be displayed. The "previous level" button allows the return to the previous term on the classification tree.

A term can also be selected by typing one of its synonyms.

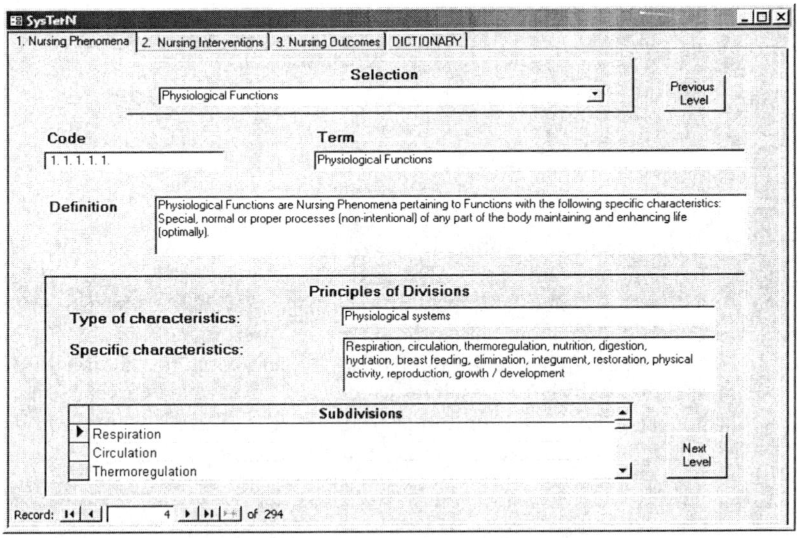

Figure 2. "Factors influencing health status. Nursing phenomena" screen

For each term (nursing phenomenon / nursing intervention) the following information is displayed (figure 2-3):

- code and name
- definition
- principles of division: type of characteristics, specific characteristics, subdivisions.

While accounting for the principle of subdivision, Nursing Interventions subdivide the following axes:

Axis A: Action Types in Nursing Practice
Axis B: Object Types in Nursing Practice
Axis C: Types of approaches in Nursing Practice
Axis D: Means in Nursing Practice
Axis E: Anatomical sites in Nursing Practice
Axis F: Time / Place in Nursing Practice

Thus, for the Nursing Interventions terms, SysTerN displays also the corresponding axis (A-F). (Figure 3). Axis can also serve as a selection criterion.

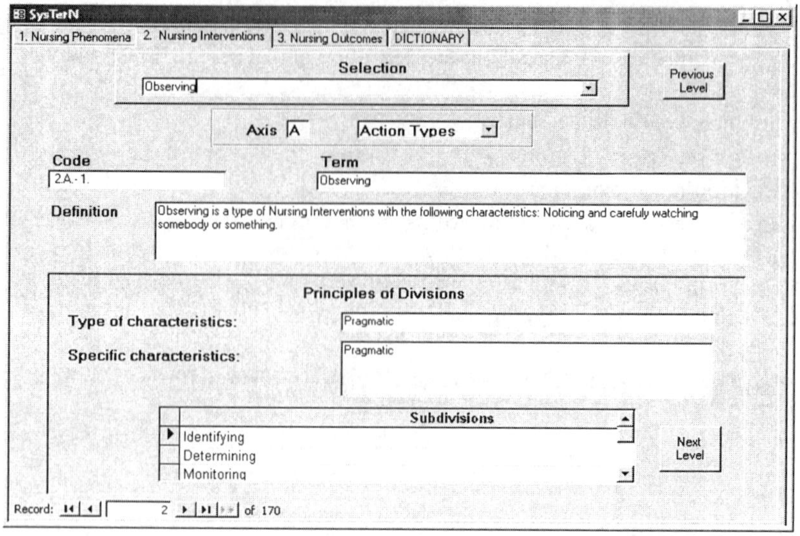

Figure 3. "Nursing intervention" screen

The SysTerN's database, containing the classification of nursing phenomena and the classification of nursing interventions, can be used when entering structured and coded data into nursing modules of the electronic patient record. A nurse will enter in the electronic patient healthcare record data about patient problems and preferences, a care plan and notes about patient's progresses. When entering Nursing Phenomena in relation to a patient, names and definitions will be accessible to consult. For the Nursing Interventions documentation, the nurse may pick up terms from a list displayed on request. There are several pick lists, one for each of the six axes of the classification.

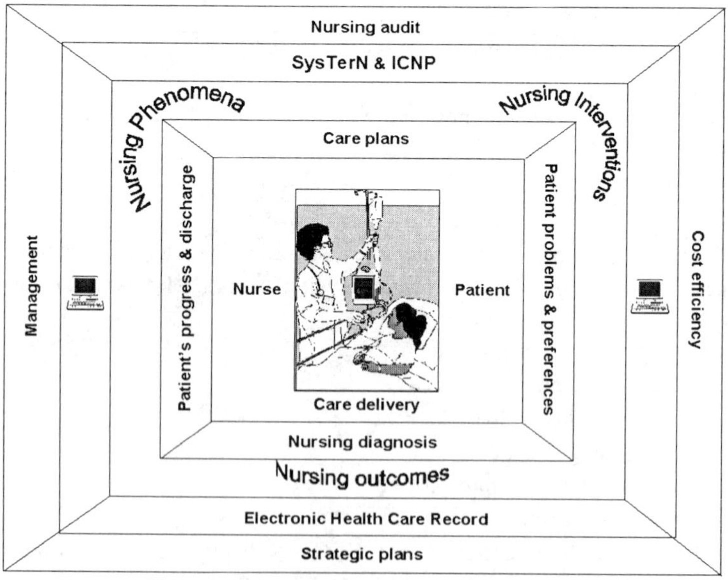

Figure 4. SysTerN in the Healthcare environment

3. Conclusions

1. SysTerN is easy to use, having a modern, friendly interface.
2. SysTerN is a valuable software tool that enables users (nurses, informaticians, decision-makers) to browse easily the ICNP classification and to evaluate it. Moreover SysTerN may be used for educational purposes achieving a double goal: training in the use of ICNP and bringing non-informaticians closer to the computer.
3. SysTerN will have a special place in the health care record. Based on the electronic format of the ICNP classification a nursing minimum data set will developed.
4. Moreover, a sound research project concerning the development of quality indicators of nursing practicing based on the ICNP classification cannot be carried on without a software tool as SysTerN.

References

[1] International Council of Nurses. *Nursing's Next Advance: An International Classification for Nursing Practice (ICNP)* A Working Paper (1993). Geneva International Council of Nurses Headquarters. Revised 1996

[2] *** *The International Classification for Nursing Practices ICNP Alpha version with TELENURSE Introduction*, Mortensen R.A. (ed), DIHNR, Copenhagen, 1996

[3] Nielsen, G.H., Mortensen, R.A., *The Architecture of ICNP: Time for Outcomes—Part I*, Int. Nurs.Rev.44, 6, 1997

[4] Moisil, I., Tieru, C., Telman, M., Cioara, E., *Strategic Plan for Promoting ICNP in Romania*, Medical Informatics Europe'97, IOS Press, Technology and Informatics, 43: 691-693,1997

[5] Moisil, I., *Preparing Nursing Information Systems through Education*, workshop at the 6th International Congress on Nursing Informatics NI'97 Stockholm Proceedings, IOS Press, 1997

[6] Nielsen, G.H., Mortensen, R.A., *The Architecture of ICNP: Time for Outcomes—Part II,* Int. Nurs.Rev.45, 1, 1998

[7] Moisil, I., *Communication in Medicine and Health Care. Information Sources on Internet*, Medical Informatics Course, EuroMISE , Prague, 1998

[8] *** *Handbook of Medical Informatics*, J.H. van Bemmel (ed), Bohn Stafleu Van Loghum, Houten, 1996

[9] *** *WHO – International Classification of Impairments, Activities and Participation (ICIDH-2)*, http://www.who.int/msa/mnh/ems/icidh/brochure/howuse.htm

[10] Jorgensen, H.D., Nielsen, T.M., *TELENURSE – Nursing Classifications, Quality Indicators and the Electronic Nursing Record*, Medical Informatics Europe'97, IOS Press, Technology and Informatics, 43: 133-137,1997

[11] Borst, F., *Computer-based -patient record. Synopsis*. Year Book of Medical Informatics *95 The Computer-based Patient Record,* Edts. Jan H. van Bemmel, Alexa T. McCray, Schattauer, IMIA, 1995

[12] Mortensen RA and Nielsen GH, *TELENURSING: European Classification of nursing practice with regard to patient problems, nursing interventions and patient outcomes, including educational measures.* Comput. Methods Programs Biomed 1994;45:171-3

Medical Informatics Europe '99
P. Kokol et al. (Eds.)
IOS Press, 1999

Electronic dissemination media for promoting ICNP in CEE countries

Ioana I. MOISIL[1], Elena JITARU[2], Ioana PERTACHE[1]
[1]*CCSSDM - Centre for Health Computing, Statistics and Medical Documentation*
9, George Vraca St., 70706 Bucuresti, Romania, Phone: 40-1-3147035, Fax: 40-1-3112998, E-mail: imoisil@sunu.rnc.ro
[2]*ICI - research Institute for Informatics, 8-10Averescu Avenue, 71316 Bucuresti, Romania*
Phone: 40-1-2241259/224, Fax: 40-1-2241030, E-mail: jitaru@u3.ici.ro

Abstract. The TeleNurse ID-ENTITY Inco-Copernicus project, co-ordinated by Randi A. Mortensen, director of the Danish Institute for Health and Nursing Research, is offering to the health informatics community of CEE countries a frame and an opportunity to determine nurses to become active actors in the development of the nursing language and terminology and to promote nursing informatics. This is of great importance, for these countries do not have yet a standard for the electronic patient record and the standard that will be proposed has to incorporate a nursing minimum data set. The ICNP[1](International Classification of Nursing Practices) classification of nursing phenomena and interventions is a poly-hierarchical, multi-axial classification system, allowing different concepts in nursing practice and from different classification systems, to be expressed as combinations of ICNP concepts, located on different axis. The features of ICNP are making it a sound candidate for a standard computerised nursing language. As part of the general strategy for promoting and disseminating ICNP in CEEC, CCSSDM has developed an electronic environment based on Internet and WWW facilities. The main composant and characteristics of this electronic dissemination environment are described in this paper.

1. Introduction

The cornerstone of health care telematics is the person-based clinical information system, from which will flow all the data needed for patients care and health managers. The data flows are expressed in the 'language of health', which consists of clinical and nursing terms, classifications and groupings. Nursing terms are words and phrases that nurses use to record and communicate their findings, impressions and management of patients. Each term in ICNP represents a nursing concept which can range from very general to highly detailed. Each concept is coded to make it easier for it to be electronically stored, retrieved and communicated.

Until now the developers of ICNP had monitored the way that the six key criteria for a standard computerised language, i.e. to be comprehensive, hierarchical, computerised, coded, cross-referenced and dynamic, are satisfied by the ICNP alpha version in the frame of the TELENURSE project. One of the objectives of the TeleNurse ID ENTITY project is to reach consensus on the above categories of terms in CEE countries. That means in the

---

[1] Copyright © 1996 by ICN - International Council of Nurses, 3, place Jean Marteau, CH-1201 Geneva

end that nursing terms need to be identified from different countries and from different cultures in natural language to produce a common standard language, from which we can define several categories of terms:

- preferred terms for each concept;
- true synonyms for preferred terms;
- terms with different meanings in different contexts (homonyms);
- terms that have been found inadequate (wrong description or not accepted by the nursing community).

The set of preferred terms will become then the infrastructure of nursing knowledge (the nomenclature).

The overall objectives of the work of the two CEE partners of TeleNurseID-ENTITY - Romania (CCSSDM) and Slovenia (PRIMCARE) are to create awareness about the development of an International Classification for Nursing Practices initiated by ICN representing 118 national nurses associations, to identify and involve relevant partners in CEEC that will make a sound contribution to the project by translating the beta version of ICNP and to encourage CEEC partners to implement ICNP in the healthcare patient record. Therefor a major concern of CCSSDM was to find out the best ways to disseminate ICNP and relate knowledge.

2. The electronic dissemination environment

One of the characteristics of CEE countries' nursing is its heterogeneity. That was one of the reasons we have thought that it is important to offer nurses the access not only to ICNP but to the knowledge needed for understanding and evaluating the classification

The designed electronic dissemination environment speculates at the maximum the facilities offered by Internet and WWW. A web page for ICNP has been designed and implemented on the Romanian EHTO site (http://atlas.ici.ro/ehto/telenurse). This page is hosting a general presentation of the project, news concerning the development of ICNP, other classifications for nursing practices, a short presentation of the electronic health record concept, a user guide and instructions for downloading the demonstration tool and also the TeleNurse ID-ENTITY project news release (figure 1). A discussion forum will be also created. Due to the fact that a great number of nurses do not have daily access to Internet, the former information will be accessible in hard copy in the Romanian Medical Informatics Society - Nursing Informatics Special Interest Group Newsletter. A diskette with the Romanian translation of ICNP beta version is also provided. The web page is bilingual, Romanian- English, in order to enlarge the discussion forum with members from other CEE (or Non-CEE) countries. The button " Other links" is offering to the user information about other sites related to ICNP, TeleNurseId-ENTITY , standards for terminology and health informatics and also access to a hypertext system - The Telenurse Assistant- for analysis of the Romanian version of ICNP.

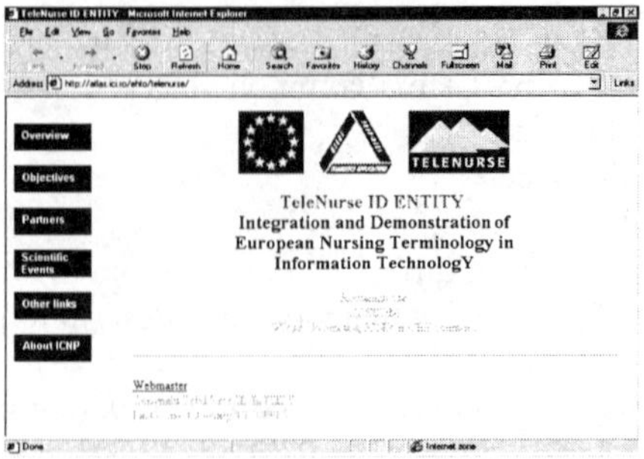

Figure 1. TeleNurseID-ENTITY Romanian Site

At present the textbook is in Romanian, but the English version will be loaded by the end of July. The textbook is periodically updated with relevant information. For example, we have included recently aspects related to the European standards for the development of terminology systems for healthcare telematics, with emphasis on the European Prestandard ENV 12264 developed by the European Committee for Standardisation (CEN) Technical Committee on 'Medical Informatics' TC 251 Working Group 2 (Terminology, Semantics and Knowledge Bases). The standard has been developed taking as granted that the idea of a universal coding system is obsolete and that the future belongs to coherent families of terminology systems, diversified according to tasks. The central idea of this standard is that the content of a large terminology system can be synthetically described by a small semantic network, made of semantic categories and links. Semantics links and categories and other relevant structural patterns for a subject field are described by a categorial structure. Another concept introduced by the standard is the one of "cross-thesaurus" , which is a system of descriptors for building a systematic representation (called "dissection") of a terminological phrase, coherent across different terminologies on a given subject field. The objective of the standard is to provide support for the development and maintenance of terminology systems and at the same time to enable the coexistence and interoperability of three generations of systems: traditional paper-based (first generation), compositional systems build according to a categorial structure and a cross-thesaurus (second generation) and formal models (third generation). According to this classification, ICNP is a second generation, compositional system.

The translation evaluation form is a dynamic document, linked to a relational data base containing ICNP (terms, concepts and definitions) and evaluation results. For generating the dynamic document we used the ASP technology. In our opinion ASP is a powerful tool, with a large set of programming services for data access, management of the session, form input retrieval and HTML output. Moreover ASP supports both client-side and server-side programming using scripting languages as JavaScript or Visual Basic Script.

3. Discussion

In developing the strategy for disseminating and promoting ICNP in CEE countries a major concern was to identify the best way to involve a large number of nurses and to make them share ideas and opinions. Besides the dissemination meetings and conferences, Internet and the web offers a friendly and attractive way to approach very serious topics as terminology and classification. The dissemination media we have designed is proving to be not only a valuable documentation and research tool, but also one of the best approaches to connect nurses, to make them get over the psychological barrier of a non IT specialist and perhaps to understand the true meaning of 'to share'.

References

[1] International Council of Nurses. *Nursing's Next Advance: An International Classification for Nursing Practice (ICNP)* A Working Paper (1993). Geneva International Council of Nurses Headquarters. Revised 1996

[2] Assimacopoulos, Andre, *Combining free text and coded nomenclature in an electronic patient record, its application to the nursing process*, Mortensen R.A. (ed) Proceedings of the First European Conference on Nursing Diagnosis, pp. 70-95, DIHNR, Copenhagen, 1995

[3] *** *The International Classification for Nursing Practices ICNP Alpha version with TELENURSE Introduction*, Mortensen R.A. (ed), DIHNR, Copenhagen, 1996

[4] McKormick, K.,*Toward standard classification schemes for nursing language: Recommendations of the American Nurses Association Steering Committee on databases to support clinical nursing practice*, JAMIA, 1(6):422-427, 1994

[5] Saba, V., *A new nursing vision. The information highway*, Nursing Leadership Forum, 1(2):44-51, 1995

[6] Nielsen, G.H., Mortensen, R.A., *The Architecture of ICNP: Time for Outcomes—Part I*, Int. Nurs.Rev.44, 6, 1997

[7] Tallberg, M., *Standardization and Terminology Projects. Implications for Nursing Professional Practice*, speach heald in Barcelona, May, 1997

[8] Moisil, I., Tieru, C., Telman, M., Cioara, E., *Strategic Plan for Promoting ICNP in Romania*, Medical Informatics Europe'97, IOS Press, Technology and Informatics, 43: 691-693,1997

[9] Moisil, I., *Preparing Nursing Information Systems through Education*, workshop at the 6th International Congress on Nursing Informatics NI'97 Stockholm Proceedings, IOS Press, 1997

[10] Nielsen, G.H., Mortensen, R.A., *The Architecture of ICNP: Time for Outcomes—Part II*, Int. Nurs.Rev.45, 1, 1998

[11] Rossi Mori, A. *ICNP: Towards second and third generation terminology systems*, Mortensen R.A. (ed) ICNP in Europe:TELENURSE, IOS Press, 1997

[12] Read, J.D., The READ Clinical Classification, Medical Informatics Course, EuroMISE , Prague, 1998

[13] Moisil, I., *Communication in Medicine and Health Care. Information Sources on Internet*, Medical Informatics Course, EuroMISE , Prague, 1998

[14] *** *Handbook of Medical Informatics*, J.H. van Bemmel (ed), Bohn Stafleu Van Loghum, Houten, 1996

[15] Rossi Mori, A., Consorti, F., Galeazzi, E., *Standards to support development of terminological systems for healthcare telematics*, Paper to IMIA WG6

[16] Hardiker, N., *Proposed Short Strategic Study: "Systems of concepts for nursing: a strategy for progress"*, ACENDIO Newsletter, no.4, August, 1998

[17] *** *WHO – International Classification of Impairments, Activities and Participation (ICIDH-2)*, http://www.who.int/msa/mnh/ems/icidh/brochure/howuse.htm

[18] Jorgensen, H.D., Nielsen, T.M., *TELENURSE – Nursing Classifications, Quality Indicators and the Electronic Nursing Record*, Medical Informatics Europe'97, IOS Press, Technology and Informatics, 43: 133-137,1997

Medical Informatics Europe '99
P. Kokol et al. (Eds.)
IOS Press, 1999

The development and testing of information system for community nursing

Robert LESKOVAR[1], Olga ŠUŠTERŠIČ[2], Vladislav RAJKOVIČ[1], Iztok BITENC[1], Igor ZELIČ[3]
[1]*Faculty of Organizational Sciences, Kidričeva 55a, 4000 Kranj, Slovenia*
[2]*University College of Health Care, Poljanska 26a, 1000 Ljubljana, Slovenia*
[3]*"Jozef Stefan" Institute, Jamova 39, 1000 Ljubljana, Slovenia*

Abstract. The paper presents the development and testing of information system (IS) for community nursing (CN). The goal of IS is to support CN practice and to encourage research and developement in the field. The development was based on analysis of CN process. Principal functions of CN were analysed. The logical data model and corresponding user interface were designed. A special emphasis in the development process was put on testing in practice and users' training. The developed IS will: increase work efficiency, introduce process-oriented nursing doctrine, support integrated treatment of the subjects and enable data comparison and exchange. An important subsidary goal of the IS development and usage is the harmonisation of concepts and terminology used in Slovenia with those used in the EU. In this framework International Classification of Nursing Practice (ICNP) which was translated into Slovene was introduced and tested.

1. Introduction

CN is defined as a special form of health care that ensures an active health and social care of clients (individuals, families and communities) that are, due to their biological features or a particular disease, more exposed to harmful effects from the environment. Community nurse helps clients to better perform daily living activities in various health conditions from birth to death. The role of the community nurse is to support activities in primary health care, prevention and health education (for example Salvage, 1993). According to the Resolution WHA49.1 (World Health Assembly) »nursing/midwifery service development is an integral part of health development. To maximize the contribution of nurses and midwives to the achievements in the field of health country-specific approach must be adopted. Active involvement of nurses at all levels of the health care system, together with the recipients of health care, policymakers, the public and private sectors, representatives of professional associations and educational institutions, and those who have responsibility for social and economic development must be assured«.

The goal of an IS for CN is not only to help in performing the routine work in pratcise. The use of information tools is also a challenge and opportunity for new ideas and solutions leading to a higher level of quality of work and life. The interdisciplinary approach is herewith a prerequisite as it enables co-operation of various experts from different institutions. The IS will move the community nurse's work away from a task-oriented approach to a more client-oriented one using problem-solving strategy covering the following major steps: identification of needs for nursing care, decisions on nursing interventions and outcome evaluation (Šušteršič, Rajkovič, 1996).

The IS was developed in the frame of EU project INCO Copernicus: Co-operative Research in Information Infrastructure. The project linked the efforts of several public and private research/government /industry partners: University of Maribor, Faculty of Organizational Sciences, University of Ljubljana, University College of Health Care, INFONET company, Health Centre Ljubljana-Bežigrad, Health Centre Radovljica and Danish Institute for Health and Nursing Research . Summary of the project is available on Internet page (http://lopes1.fov.uni-mb.si/patro/index.htm). In the process of IS development prototyping approach with the on-line verification in practice was used. This methodology is suggested in the literature (for example Martin, 1991). Such approach does not only ensure greater functional adequacy of the system, it also stimulates the user, i.e. the community nurses, to exhibit a higher degree of creativity. The program is written in Borland Delphi and runs under Microsoft Windows. Users' manual with program documentation is already available. IS supports the following main functions of CN process: identification of needs for CN care, treatment and evaluation, including statistics and costs. Clients' treatment includes follow-up of daily activities (nursing anamneses), nursing diagnoses, nursing interventions (actions) and evaluation of outcomes. Program is designed to be used as a client-server application on local area network in health centres. It offers the possibility for the nurse to use a portable PC, for example Toshiba Libretto, on home visits and use it for updating the client's record immediately on site.

In the paper the function of CN will be described, followed by the data model and user's interface description. Special emphasis will be laid on implementation and testing of the proposed of prototype.

2. Functional model of community nursing

The process of CN enables systematical, individualized and holistic approach in solving nursing issues relevant to healthy or sick client, family and community. There are four phases: a) need assessment which covers nursing problem and making of diagnosis, b) goal and intervention planning, c) performing nursing interventions and d) evaluation of outcome (Ellis, 1989). The data flow diagrams showing the detailed functional decomposition is reported in the proposed project documentation (Jereb, 1997). The need assessment function consists of five subfunctions: information gathering, interpreting, recognizing, ranking and checking. The planning gives detailed CN plan, which includes decision making, what to do and how to do. The subprocess of planning are: joint goal settings, selecting nursing interventions, preliminary contact with client in order to get confirmation of the plan, dissemination of the CN plan to other relevant recipients (co-workers, relatives). Implementation of planned interventions includes nursing and technical procedures. These procedures are adjusted according to the current state of the client and unpredictable developments. Performed interventions are recorded in CN plan. Evaluation is the most important phase in CN. It enables process improvement for the benefit of the client and cost effective treatment. Feedback information can contribute to better need assessment.

The analysis of the current practice in two health centres was performed. It was determined that current practice differs among health centres and that practice deviates from proposed theoretical education process. Duplicated, incomplete and inaccurate paper documentation on clients are kept on various locations. Several problems related to data gathering, data updating, and data deletion were identified. Personal data security problem was generally inadequately treated. Scheduling of the CN process, planning and evaluation were neglected either because of shortage of time or because of inaccessibility of relevant data. On the other hand the administrative tasks proposed by theoretical model would significantly decrease the time that a nurse devotes to a client. The »unified nursing language« described in (Mortensen, 1993, Wake et al, 1993, Mortensen, 1997) and proposed by ICNP is hard to use without computer support. Extensiveness of the language on one side and semantic deficiency on the other side are identified as serious problems. The conclusions made by system analysts were not black/white. It was decided to design open-ended system, to implement theoretical model where it is reasonable, and to support good practice where necessary.

3. Data model

Data model was developed gradually during the research project. The first preliminary models were more medically oriented (for example Milavec et al, 1995) and proposed mainly logical-semantic approach (Šušteršič, Rajkovič, 1996). The later one included more or less complete data support for CN. The core of the current data model is described in Leskovar et al (1998). Complete data model includes more than 60 relational tables. The most important relational tables are *Client*, *Family*, *Community* and *Nurse*. Each *Family* can be include many Clients; each family member is a potential *Client*. The new *Order* issued by *Order Issuer* triggers one or more *CN Processes*. Each *Process* corresponds to one of the states of the *Client* (for example newborn, child, teenager, adult, elderly person). The *Process* triggers *Visit*. Each *Visit* is scheduled by *Calendar*. The *Process* links different states of the same person while *Visit* links different activities during the visit. *Properties* are measured and each property has its own set of agreed values (*Domain*). *Instances of CN diagnoses* are confirmed during the visit. *Instances of CN interventions* are executed during the visit. Table *Property* stores all nursing anamneses. Additional classification of properties enables testing various coding schemes (for example complete or reduced ICNP, user proposed properties etc.). Tables *Insurance Company* and Instance of *Other intervention* will serve to demonstrate the financial aspect of CN.

4. User interface

Borland Delphi was the chosen implementation tool. The application was designed as multiple document interface (MDI). Main window controls one or more child windows as presented in Figure 1. Standard Windows entry/transition controls are used (drop down menus, combo boxes, ALT+character, toolbars etc.). After successful authorization, the application permits the user to perform granted functions. Three classes of users can simultaneously use the programe: Administrator, Head Nurse and Nurse. The user interface keeps a significant degree of similarity with theoretical model of community nursing described in chapter 2. Report section of the application is opened for new tools such as statistical package or expert system.

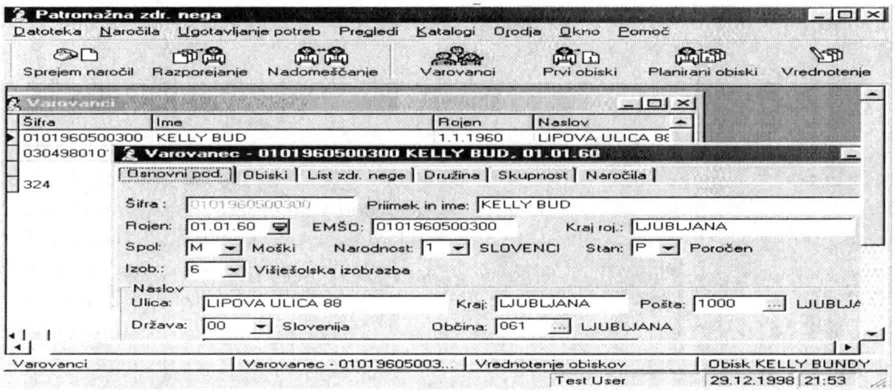

Figure 1: Main window of community nursing IS with four child windows.

5. Implementation of the information system

The information system architecture is schematically presented in figure 2. Servers in different municipals are connected via routers and public or private network. Alternatively, fast modems can be used. It is expected that the link between servers will support e-mail and client migration mainly. The proposed minimum configuration of the server is: processor speed 166MHz, memory 32MB, disk capacity 2Gb, DAT backup unit 4/8Gb, Windows NT operation system and Access/Paradox/Oracle/MS SQL database system. Work stations and portable PCs are Windows 95/98 based systems. The communication between server and client is enabled via LAN preferably Ethernet. Portable PCs and personal digital assistants without network interface card will receive and send data through RS 232 or infrared interface. Personal digital assistants require data conversion from chosen database format to ASCII and vice versa. Preliminary tests with Apple Newton PDA and cable showed relatively fast conversion and transmission but at present too complicated for target users (nurses).

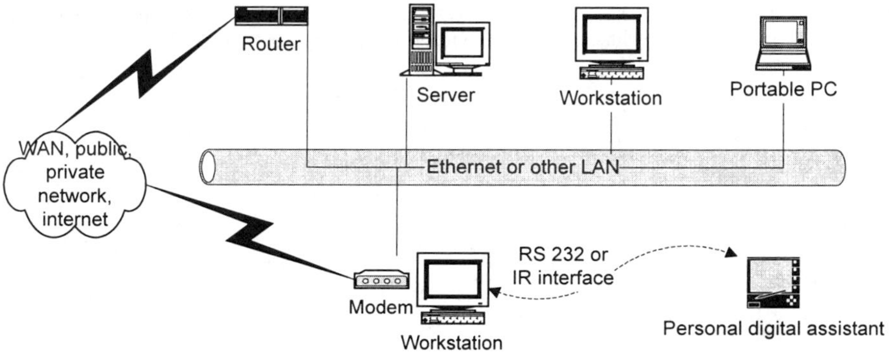

Figure 2: Information system architecture for community nursing.

6. Conclusion

The proposed information system integrates nursing practice with modern information technology. Information system for community nursing can serve operational, administrative, research and educational purposes. Theoretical model of the process approach to community nursing is effectively applied and adapted for the practice. Modular structure enables flexibility and adaptability. User-friendly interface also enabled several testings including ICNP. The extensiveness of the language and semantic deficiency were identified as serious obstacles in practical usage. Various adds-on like financial module, statistical package or expert system, could be easily connected. Some supplementary functions will be added in the final release until mid of 1999.

References

[1] Ellis J.R., Nowlis E.A. (1989): Nursing: A Human Needs Approach (fourth edition), Boston: Houghton Mifflin Company.
[2] http://lopes1.fov.uni-mb.si/patro/index.htm
[3] Jereb B. (1997): The software requirement specification for community nursing (English abstract, Slovene: Opredelitev zahtevanih lastnosti programske opreme za področje patronažne zdravstvene nege), Faculty of Organizational Sciences, university diploma work, Kranj.
[4] Leskovar R., Šušteršič O., Rajkovič V., Bitenc I., Zelič I. (1998): The development of information system for community nursing (English abstract, Slovene: Razvoj informacijskega sistema patronažne zdravstvene nege), Organizacija, (31), št. 6.
[5] Martin J. (1991): Information Engineering: Introduction, Prentice Hall, ISBN:013464462X.
[6] Milavec M, Šušteršič O, Rajkovič V. (1995): Data model for community nursing (English abstract, Slovene: Podatkovni model patronažne zdravstvene nege), Obzornik zdravstvene nege, št. 29, str: 143-147.
[7] Mortensen R.A., editor (1997): ICNP in Europe: Telenurse, Volume 38 in Studies in Health Technology and Informatics , IOS Press, ISBN: 90 5199 321 8.
[8] Mortensen, R.A. (1993) A common language for nursing practice: a persistent dilemma, A European viewpoint. Vard Nord Utveckl Forsk, 13, 18-24.
[9] Salvage J., editor (1993): Nursing in Action, Strengthening Nursing and Midwifery to Support Health for All, WHO Regional Publications, European Series, No. 48, ISBN 92 890 1312 5.
[10] Šušteršič O., Rajkovič V. (1996): An information system for community nursing support. In: Technology and informatics 34, Medical informatics Europe 96, Amsterdam.
[11] Wake, M.M., Murphy, M., Affara, F.A., Lang, N.M., Clark, J., Mortensen, R. (1993): Toward an International Classification for Nursing Practice: a literature review & survey. Int Nurs Rev, 40, 77-80.

Medical Informatics Europe '99
P. Kokol et al. (Eds.)
IOS Press, 1999

Plea for a Standardised Detailed Clinical Nomenclature

Shahan MOMJIAN[1,2], François BORST[1], Nicolas de TRIBOLET[2]
[1]*Division of Medical Informatics, University Hospital of Geneva*
[2]*Division of Neurosurgery, University Hospital of Geneva*
Hôpital Cantonal Universitaire de Genève, Rue Micheli-du-Crest 24, CH - 1211 Genève 14, Switzerland

Abstract. The choice of a nomenclature for the encoding of the medical information to be stored in an electronic patient record (EPR) is a critical issue. As we are currently developing a neurosurgical EPR, we evaluated three nomenclatures or classifications, Read, ICD-10 and Quick Medical Reference (QMR) for the capture of the detailed concepts referenced in the EPR. We scored the correspondence with 2 for a good match, 1 for a fair match and 0 for no match. The Read nomenclature ranked first with an overall score of 1.21 (max. 2.0), the ICD-10 obtained 0.88 and the QMR 0.74. Some groups of items such as the neurosurgical history and examination were fairly well represented in the three systems. On the opposite, others such as the various neurosurgical clinical and radiological scoring and grading systems and the outcome descriptors were not correctly referenced in any coding system. Although the Read coding system has been advocated to represent the clinical activity in neurosurgery, it still needs an enrichment before being able to completely cover the concepts present in a neurosurgical record. Moreover the development of an international, standardised, detailed nomenclature and classification collecting the advantages of the various coding systems currently in use should be encouraged to be able to exchange and compare medical data.

1. Introduction

In the process of the design of an electronic patient record (EPR), one always faces the problem of the choice of the nomenclature for the encoding of the medical information. In order to have an EPR that allows for clinical studies as well as quality of care or financial analysis like resources consumption, one has to use a detailed vocabulary to fully describe all the aspects of the care of a patient. Most of the internationally used classifications such as the ICD-10 were primarily designed to record diagnoses, causes of death and to characterise the treatment, but numerous other variables are relevant in the practice of clinical medicine. Those are information concerning the state of the patient prior to the diagnosis and treatment (type of admission, symptoms and findings, various clinical or radiological grading and scoring systems, social or professional conditions, ...) and after the diagnosis and treatment (change in subjective or objective state, change in pain, outcome, change in health, ...). These items are not detailed in these classifications. Thus there is a tendency towards more comprehensive coding systems, like the « clinical modification » of the ICD-9 CM or the Read coding system.

As we are currently developing a detailed neurosurgical EPR in our institution, we decided to evaluate the comprehensiveness of three classifications or nomenclatures (QMR, ICD-10, Read) in capturing the concepts we chose to be encoded in the neurosurgical EPR. We present the results of this comparison.

2. Brief description of the neurosurgical EPR

The developed EPR is integrated in the DIOGENE hospital information system [1]. This EPR allows the collection and storage in an encoded form of detailed clinical data about the patient. It contains several screens displaying the headings found in the presently used paper neurosurgical medical record. We stressed a detailed and encodable description of the patient with a limited use of free text fields. We included numerous scores and scales to better qualify and particularly quantify the patient state (e.g. WFNS and Hunt-Hess [2], MOS SF-36 [3], Karnofsky [4], ...).

The screens have been manually tested on a sample of 20 randomly selected paper neurosurgical records and they fitted well. One difficulty was to find the level of detail that has to be encoded for all inpatients without making the data entry too fastidious.

3. Materials and methods

We listed all the items of interest in our neurosurgical EPR and excluded those that were diagnoses, procedures, dates, free text descriptions or too specific to our country. The diagnoses and procedures were not included because the goal of this study is to evaluate a less traditional use of the classifications than the coding of diagnoses and procedures. For each of the remaining 359 enumerated items we looked for a corresponding qualification in the Quick Medical Reference (QMR) findings and diagnoses [5], the Read 3 nomenclature [6,7,8] and the ICD-10 [9] classification.

We used an electronic file of the QMR findings, the Read Version 3 browser and the printed form of the ICD-10.

We employed the scoring system described by Chute et al. [10] and subjectively scored the correspondence as follows : 0, no match; 1, fair match; 2, good match. For us, the score 0 means that no correspondence was found and that one would definitely expand the particular classification or nomenclature with the desired item in order to fit the desired concept. The score 1 means that an approximate representation was found, i.e. lacked in precision (e.g. when the desired concept was sonophobia and the best match was hearing problem). Moreover the score 1 was attributed when the desired item was a generic concept and when one could only find in the coding system a particular concept of this class (e.g. when the desired concept was behaviour disorders and the best match was aggressive behaviour). Generally speaking, the score 1 means that one would add a precision to the classification. The score 2 means that the item was found in the nomenclature or classification in the desired form and thus requiring no addition to the coding system.

4. Results

The results of the evaluation are presented in the Table 1. On the whole list of items, the Read nomenclature scored first with an average score of 1.21. This position was found in all the groups of items, as well.

Table 1. Results

		Read				ICD-10				QMR			
		Scores (%)			Average	Scores (%)			Average	Scores (%)			Average
	Number of items	0	1	2		0	1	2		0	1	2	
TOTAL	359	9	61	30	1.21	31	50	19	0.88	39	48	13	0.74
Admission	9	0	67	33	1.33	100	0	0	0	100	0	0	0
History and examination	108	3	41	56	1.53	5	57	38	1.33	18	55	27	1.09
Socio-professional	8	63	0	37	0.74	88	12	0	0.12	88	12	0	0.12
Clinical and radiological scales	48	0	98	2	1.02	33	67	0	0.67	35	63	2	0.67
Pre-op. investigations	106	0	77	23	1.23	20	27	13	0.53	25	66	9	0.84
Complications	22	0	32	68	1.68	0	41	59	1.59	36	36	28	0.92
Outcome	58	41	59	0	0.59	93	7	0	0.07	93	7	0	0.07

The best scores for this coding system were for the concepts regarding neurosurgical history and examination (average score 1.53) and those concerning the complications (average score 1.68). The worse scores were obtained for the groups of neurosurgical clinical and radiological scales (average score 1.02), socio-professional (average score 0.74) and outcome (average score 0.59) items.

The ICD-10 obtained an overall score of 0.88. However, although being a classification and not a nomenclature and not « clinically modified » like the ICD-9 CM, it did relatively well in the groups of concepts were the Read classification scored best. Thus it almost reached the Read system with an average score of 1.33 for the concepts concerning neurosurgical history and examination and 1.59 for those on the complications. As expected the other domains were much less well captured, because they concerned concepts not expected to be included in a classification containing essentially diagnoses.

The QMR is intended to help in the diagnosis in the field of internal medicine. It was included in our evaluation because it clearly refers to clinical findings. Nevertheless it scored worst for the whole list of items and in the group concerning detailed neurosurgical history and examination, as well. It is partly because it is designed for internal medicine and therefore does not describe with enough details concepts for neurosurgery. Moreover as it has been designed as a diagnostic tool it essentially contains particular concepts and lacks some general concepts, as for example « presence of a neurological deficit ». As expected too, the domains like the admission parameters, the socio-professional characteristics, the neurosurgical clinical and radiological scales and the outcome descriptors were not correctly covered. The scores for the whole list of items are represented in the Figure 1.

5. Discussion

We designed an EPR which has two goals. Primarily, to retrieve documents patient by patient for day to day decision support on the specific patient. Secondly, to build a clinical database allowing to extract information on a set of patients, such as outcome analysis, quality of care or costs analysis. This database may serve clinical decision support and research, as well. These features make the process of encoding the information mandatory and crucial.

Few studies have compared the content coverage of various classifications and nomenclatures [10] and the field of neurosurgery has not been specifically addressed.

As mentioned earlier, we focused our study on the detailed concepts found in ICD-10, Read and QMR beyond diagnoses and procedures. Our evaluation showed that the items referring to the neurosurgical history and examination are relatively well represented. Others such as quantified pictures of the patient state, the various neurosurgical clinical or radiological grading and scoring systems, the social or professional conditions, the change in subjective or objective state, the change in pain, the outcome, the change in health or quality of life are not.

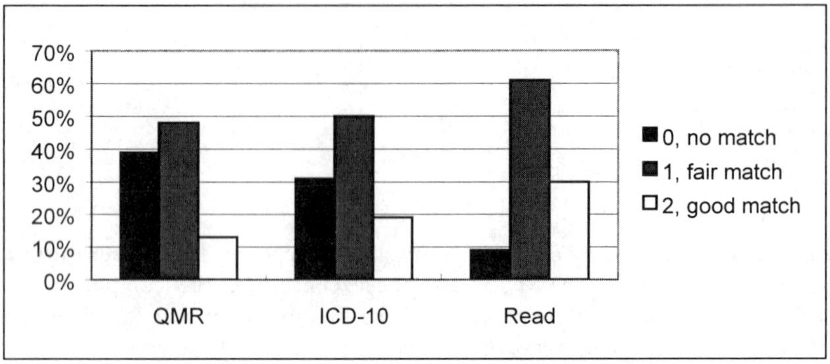

Figure 1. Scores for the whole list of items

These variables are mandatory in the analysis and comparison of groups of patients in terms of outcome, quality of care or efficacy of treatment.

In addition, a classification or nomenclature must have a hierarchical structure with several levels of detail in its items to face various requirements like the simple recording of diagnoses or the drawing of a detailed picture of the clinical, social, economical aspects of the patient care. This issue is quite well addressed in the Read nomenclature and to a lesser extent in the ICD-10.

The Read nomenclature has been designed to fully describe the clinical activity with the goal of being able to associate a code to every relevant information found in a medical record [7,8] and it has been recommended for this purpose in neurosurgery by some authors [11]. Moreover it satisfies for instance in the fields of anaesthesia [12] and plastic surgery [13]. Although our results showed that the Read system captured best our desired concepts, there is still improvement to be done, notably in the field of neurosurgical clinical and radiological scales or scores. Moreover the Read nomenclature is only available in English, thus reducing its international use. As the Read nomenclature is already mapped to the ICD-10 and thus gaining international acceptance, the translation in various languages and the enrichment of the Read nomenclature with the concepts previously mentioned would be a good base for the encoding of the concepts present in a neurosurgical EPR.

As previously mentioned, the ICD-10 did relatively well in the field of history and examination (average score 1.33) and one could suggest that the « clinical modification » of the ICD-10 with an emphasis on the inclusion of qualitative and quantitative variables about the patient state would be a worthy alternative to the Read nomenclature. The base for the improvement of this ICM-10 CM may partly come from the Read nomenclature and, as outlined by Chute et al. [10], from SNOMED [14]. This process would merge the most detailed nomenclatures currently available (Read and SNOMED) with an internationally recognised and used classification (ICD-10) and therefore giving birth to a unified, standardised international medical coding system.

6. Conclusion

The conclusion of this small survey is that the studied classifications and nomenclatures do not correctly reference the essential concepts which have to be mentioned in a clinical neurosurgical medical record. Moreover a standardised detailed nomenclature with generalised acceptance and use does not currently exist. The development of an international, detailed and comprehensive, standardised coding system encompassing all the aspects of medical practice is mandatory to increase the resolution of the patient state's picture which has to be stored in an EPR if one has the goal of exchanging and comparing medical data.

References

[1] Scherrer JR, Lovis C, Borst F : DIOGENE 2, a distributed hospital information system with an emphasis on its medical information content. In Yearbook of Medical Informatics The Computer-based patient record, van Bemmel, McCray (eds), IMIA Schattauer, Stuttgart, 86-97, 1995.
[2] Ducati A : The clinical grading of subarachnoid hemorrhage. Minerva Anestesiol 64(4), 109-112, Apr 1998.
[3] Ware JE et al. : The MOS 36-Item Short-Form Health Survey (SF-36) I. Conceptual Framework and Item Selection. Medical Care, Vol. 30, No. 6, June 1992.
[4] Mor V, Laliberte L, Morris JN, Wiemann M : The Karnofsky Performance Status Scale. An examination of its reliability and validity in research setting. Cancer 53(9), 2002-2007, 1984
[5] Aliferis CF, Cooper GF, Buchanan BG, Miller RA, Bankowitz R, Giuse N : Temporal reasoning abstractions in QMR. MEDINFO 95 Proceedings, 847-851, IMIA, 1995.
[6] Read Version 3 Browser. NHS Centre for Coding and Classification, 1998.
[7] Saint-Yves IFM : The Read clinical classification. Health Bulletin 50(6), 422-427, 1992.
[8] Stuart-Buttle C, Sutton Y, Walters P : The facts about the Read codes. British Journal of Healthcare Computing and Information Management, 1996.
[9] International statistical classification of diseases and related health problems-10th revision. World Health Organization, 1992.
[10] Chute CG, Cohn SP, Campbell KE, Oliver DE, Campbell JR : The content coverage of clinical classifications. JAMIA, Vol. 3, 224-233, 1996.
[11] Brocklehurst G : Classification and coding in neurosurgery. Zent bl Neurochir 53, 185-188, 1992.
[12] Banks IC : The application of Read Codes to anaesthesia. Anaesthesia 49(4), 324-327, Apr 1994.
[13] James NK : The Read clinical classification and its use in plastic surgery. Ann R Coll Surg Engl 76(3), 164-168, May 1994.
[14] Cote RA, Rothwell DJ, Palotay JL, Becket RS, Brochu RS, Brochu L, eds. The Systematized Nomenclature of Human and Veterinary Medicine : SNOMED International. Northfield, IL : College of American Pathologists, 1993.

Medical Informatics Europe '99
P. Kokol et al. (Eds.)
IOS Press, 1999

A Computerised Guideline for Pressure Ulcer Prevention

Silvana QUAGLINI*, Manuela GRANDI**, Paola BAIARDI**, M.Cristina MAZZOLENI**, Clara FASSINO*, Giorgio FRANCHI**, Stefania MELINO**
**Dipartimento di Informatica e Sistemistica, Università di Pavia*
***IRCCS Fondazione "S. Maugeri", Clin. del Lavoro e della Riabilitazione, Pavia, Italy*

Abstract. This work illustrates the implementation of a computerised guideline for the pressure ulcers prevention. In particular, we describe the site-specification of a guideline delivered by the Agency for Health Care Policy Research, its integration with the electronic patient record, and its introduction within the clinical routine. The system facilitates trained nurses in the patient management by producing daily work-plans, and novice nurses by running as an educational tool.

1. Introduction

Despite the great emphasis that medical communities put on clinical practice guidelines (GLs) during last years, several problems are associated with diffusion and implementation in clinical setting: "official" GLs often do not fit the organisational constraints, health care operators often do not fully comply with GLs, and physicians rarely are provided with instruments for evaluating the benefits of a GL introduction, in such a way to be convinced by the evidence of improved outcomes. Information technology may help to overcome these difficulties. Formalisms for computerized GL representation have been developed [1,2], and connection of the GL with the electronic patient record has been shown to enhance compliance. Very important, different inference engines may be applied to the same GL in order to achieve a user interaction tailored to the specific clinical setting. As for any other information tool or decision support system, it is very important that the GL do not badly interfere with the clinical routine. Thus, we focussed our attention on the GL/user interaction, and we distinguished three key aspects:

- The *advice production*: it can be "explicit", i.e. the GL suggests actions in real time (suitable for beginners), or it can be "silent", i.e. the user is advised only when a non-compliance is detected (worth for expert users).
- The *compliance*: the GL proceed to the next task(s) only if the user fully complied with it concerning the previous tasks; or the GL proceeds also in case of non compliance, but only if the user provides a justification for that; finally the GL proceeds in any case, storing the non-compliance in a silent mode.
- The *intervention time*: the GL reacts in real time to the users actions: this implies the possibility of interacting very frequently with the computer and thus assumes the existence of a very efficient and distributed information system; on the contrary, the user could access the GL only in specific time slices.

In this work, we illustrate the implementation of a GL for the prevention of pressure ulcers, and motivate our design choices according to the framework illustrated above.

Pressure ulcers are defined as any lesion caused by unrelieved pressure that results in damage to underlying tissue. They are serious problems that can lead to pain, a longer hospital stay, a lower recovery, and additional pharmacological treatment, all factors affecting both quality of life of the patients and economic costs. Pressure ulcers prevalence surveys point out percentages from 9.2% to 47% [3,4]. Prevention plays an essential role: risk evaluation and preventive care plan are needed since the first days of hospitalisation. In fact about 50% of pressure ulcers occurring during the stay appear within the first week. Nurses, who are traditionally sensitive to this problem, often lack of precise and standardised procedure to approach it. The Agency for the Health Care Policy Research (AHCPR) [5] delivered a GL for the pressure ulcers prevention, that has been the starting point for our study, as well as for past implementation [6].

2. The site-specification of the GL

The AHCPR recommendations were tailored according to the proposal of both the Italian Nurse Association for the Study of Cutaneous Lesions and our hospital physicians and nurses [7], in order to make GL usable on all the hospitalized patients with efforts and resources maintained within acceptable limits. Site specifications concern risk assessment and actions to be taken. In particular: age over 65 was locally considered sufficient to include the patient into at risk population (absent in the AHCPR GL); nutritional deficit is inspected through different variables; some predisposing pathologies together with the presence of an existing pressure ulcer are included in the evaluation of risk; the frequent (every two hours) reposition of the patient proposed by AHCPR with strength of evidence=B (high) was not accepted due to excessive induced overburden for nurses; skin evaluation every two days, instead of once a day; finally, more details are provided on medications to be used in order to reduce friction injures.

3. The GL formal representation

Figures 1 shows the site-specified GL through a graphical editor [6], that allows to represent GLs at different hierarchical levels. The editor, written in Java, produces an internal representation of the GL in terms of relational tables and is associated to an inference engine that generates advises according to the stored patient data. It is very useful for educational purposes, because the user can simulate patients and obtain suggestions in real time. Graphical facilities have been designed such as different colours indicating different task states and different bullets indicating levels of scientific evidence supporting that task: red for a *strongly recommended* task, yellow for a *recommended* task and green for a *suggested* task. Pointers to literature may be associated to bullets as a GL documentation.

4. The functional architecture

As mentioned above, the GL implementation took into great account possible bad interference with daily work. Figure 2 shows the system functionality. At the beginning of their shift, nurses ask for a printing of the workplan for the day. The workplan is produced by the GL inference engine, according to the GL rules, fired with data stored in the EPR. At the end of their shift, nurses store data about the executed workplan, using the same interface they are using since many years for the HIS. Of course nurses adopting the GL are not the only users accessing the EPR. Additional information is stored also by physicians and laboratorists. The difference lie in the fact that nurses *must* fill the EPR, because the GL will not produce the next day workplan if the previous one has not been discharged. Also

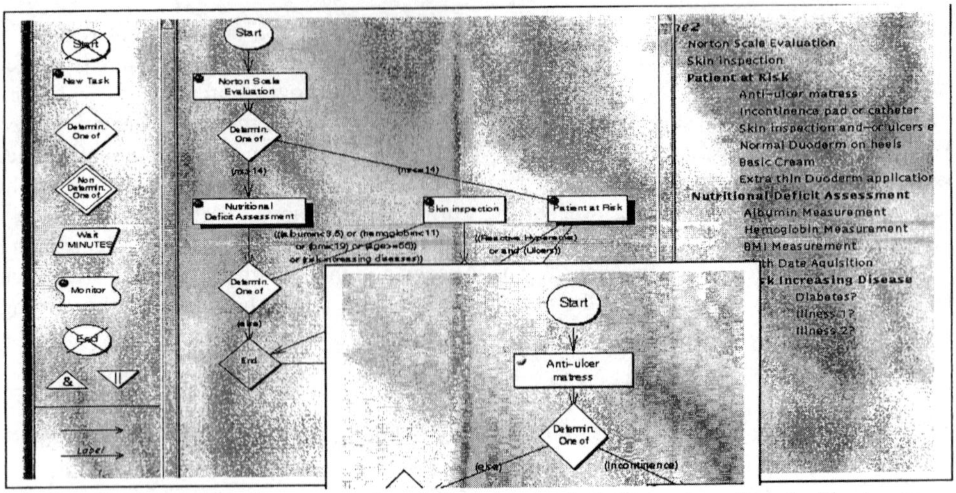

Figure 1- The graphical GL representation: shadowed rectangles indicate composite tasks. The pop-up window is a scratch of the expansion of the "patient at risk" task

storing the non-compliance is mandatory, in order to continue with next workplans: if some of the suggested actions have not been performed, nurses must give a justification, and the same actions will be suggested again the day after.

A scratch of a printed workplan is shown in Table II (bold items are filled by nurses). The interaction with the system is then at specific time slices, at the beginning and at the end of the daily work. All day long, nurses annotates information on the paper workplan. This has been considered as the optimal system/user interaction in our environment, because a real time storing of data about actions performed on the patient is impossible for logistic reasons.

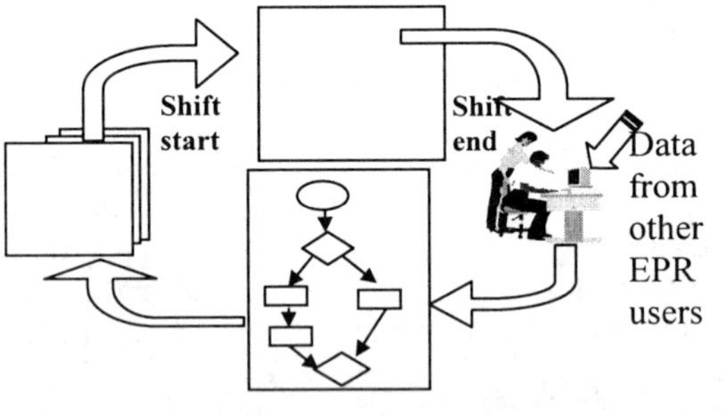

Figure 2 – The system-user interaction

5. The interaction with the EPR

Figure 3 shows the compilation of the ulcer risk assessment form. This task is mandatory for every patient admitted to the ward. Weight and height data, as well as information about diseases that increase the ulcer risk, are retrieved from the EPR, because this form is filled after objective examination and anamnesis. Other fields, namely the Norton scale and the feeding type, are filled by the nurses. The GL *imposes* the compilation of this form at pre-defined time intervals, that vary according to the patient condition. As a matter of fact, to each item stored in the EPR, a time stamp is associated, that is compared with the *persistence* time stored in the GL. Figure 4 shows the form that nurses fill at the end of their shift. It is a copy of the workplan that they should have used during the day. The pop-up window illustrates the input of the motivation of a non compliance.

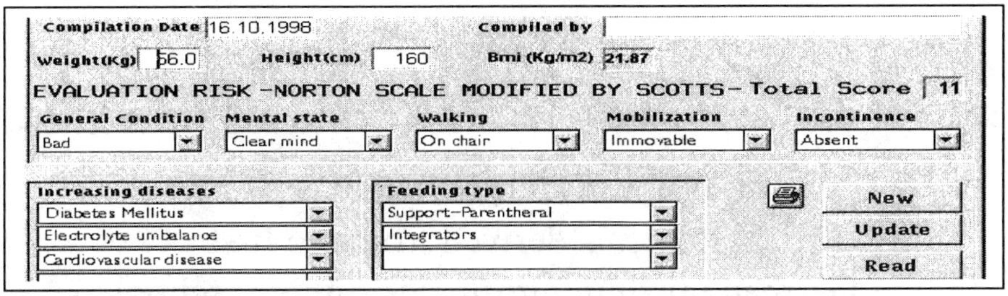

Figure 3 – Filling the form for the patient risk evaluation

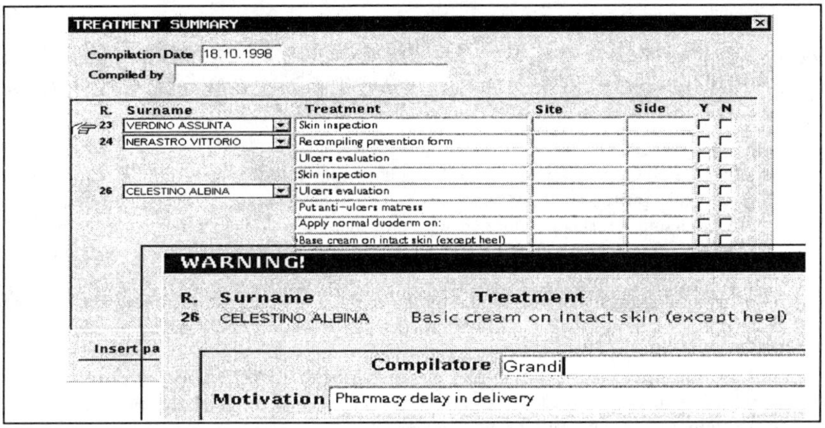

Figure 4 – Filling the workplan at the end of the shift: non-compliance must be justified

6. Conclusion and future development

We have designed and implemented a decision support system for the pressure ulcer prevention, integrating it into the existing electronic patient record of a general medicine ward. During next months data will be collected with two aims: to evaluate the user satisfaction and to evaluate the benefits of the GL introduction on patient outcomes. Comparisons with previous ulcer incidence in the same ward and with other wards where the GL has not been adopted will be performed. Data about non-compliance will be used as a feedback for improving the GL implementation.

References

[1] S. Quaglini, L. Dazzi, L. Gatti, M. Stefanelli, C. Fassino, C. Tondini. Supporting tools for guideline development and dissemination, Artificial Intelligence in Medicine (1988), 14:119-137

[2] S.W. Tu, M.A. Musen, The EON Model of Intervention Protocols and Guidelines, in: J.J. Cimino ed.,Journal of the American Medical Informatics Association, Proceedings of the 1996 AMIA Annual Fall Symposium, (Hanley and Belfus Inc., Philadelphia, 1996) 587-591.

[3] P. Di Giulio, La prevalenza delle lesioni da decubito nei pazienti ospedalizzati. Rivista dell'infermiere 2, (1985).

[4] M. Meehan, National Pressure Ulcer Prevalence Survey, Advances in wound care, Vol.7, n° 3, May 1994

[5] U.S. Department of Health and Human Services. Pressure Ulcers in Adults: Prediction and Prevention (AHCPR 92-0047). Rockville, MD. Agency for Health Care Policy and Research (1992).

[6] R.D. Zielstorff, G.O. Barnett, J.B. Fitzmaurice, G. Estey, G. Hamilton, A Vickery, E Welebob, C Shahzad. A decision support system for prevention and treatment of pressure ulcers based on AHCPR guidelines, JAMIA, Symposium supplement (1996) 562-566

[7] AISLEC, Profilassi delle lesioni da decubito e cambio posturale: ricerca multicentrica, linee guida. ANIN-NEU 1995

Medical Informatics Europe '99
P. Kokol et al. (Eds.)
IOS Press, 1999

How can we improve informatics education for German nurses ?

Statements derived from the first German nursing informatics summer school

Thomas BÜRKLE[1], Ulrich SCHRADER[2]
[1]*Department of Medical Informatics, Heinrich-Buff-Ring 44, D-35392 Gießen, Germany*
[2]*University of Applied Sciences, Nibelungenplatz 1, D-60318 Frankfurt a. M., Germany*

Abstract. For German nurses it is difficult to join training in health informatics besides their professional activity. The authors have successfully established a German nursing informatics summer school in shape of a 5 day intensive curriculum which they offer to German nurses during the summer hollidays. The summer school introduces nurses into health informatics and nursing informatics. It targets interested nursing staff, nurse executives, and nurse teachers. It promotes self learning abilities for continued self education of the participants. One of its goals is to enable participants to formulate their own requirements in health information processing and to influence system design and system introduction. The paper presents the curriculum, talks about first experiences, and demonstrates the results of an evaluation among the participants. Conclusions are drawn in a set of statements on informatics education of nurses.

1. Health informatics education in Germany

Several medical informatics programs have been established in Germany, e.g. a 4.5 year curriculum for *Diplominformatiker der Medizin* that is roughly equivalent to a master of science (MS) [1,2]. Post graduate certificates *Medical Informatics* can be obtained from the German Informatics (GI) and the German Medical Informatics (GMDS) associations.

However fewer opportunities exist for non-university graduates such as German nurses to receive training in medical informatics. Some institutions offer 2 or 3 year undergraduate curricula for *Medical Documentalists* [3]. Indeed those fulltime courses often attract nurses who had to quit their old profession. But they are not suitable for nurses who keep working in their profession.

Besides that few training opportunities in nursing informatics exist for German nurses. To become a registered nurse in Germany one must complete a three year undergraduate training in a school of nursing (some 800 exist). But there nursing informatics is no regular topic. Some schools may teach computer literacy, but even the comprehensive nursing curriculum of Hessen [4] does not contain an explicit teaching unit for nursing informatics. Recently few university based nursing curricula have been established in Germany. Graduates may obtain a diploma, e.g. as *Diplom-Pflegewirt* after 4 years. Fortunately some of those curricula now include explicit modules on medical informatics [5].

2. Is there a need for additional health or nursing informatics training in Germany ?

Under these circumstances one is inclined to ask „Do German nurses need additional informatics and computer training?“. Today few comprehensive nursing information systems are in active use in German hospitals. However, German nurses are increasingly confronted with clinical information systems [6,7]. Furthermore, many nurses use standard software like text processors and spread sheets to organise their working environment. Effectively they do ask for computer training. Large hospitals have recognised this need and organise computer training for their employees. A study at Giessen University Hospital revealed that even on a ward where no computer applications existed, nearly a third of the nurses possessed computer knowledge and one fifth had taken computer lessons already [8]. This implies that a significant percentage of nurses possesses basic computer knowledge. But medical informatics is more than just computer literacy. Many German hospitals are in the process to implement clinical networks and clinical information systems [9]. In this process it is essential that nurses formulate their requirements, that they are able to influence system design and that they can contribute to system introduction. This requires deep knowledge in nursing informatics.

3. The German nursing informatics summer school

For more than 9 years the European Summer School of Nursing Informatics, sponsored by the Erasmus programme, has been held at various European sites (e.g. 1999 Horn / Vienna, Austria). It's disadvantage from the point of German nurses however is that it is conducted in English language only, so that the participants have to be more or less fluent in English. We note that German nurses hardly participated in this event which rather attracted informatics specialists from Germany.

Thus the authors decided to adapt the approach of the European Summer School of Nursing Informatics and to establish a German nursing informatics summer school likewise. The first German summer school took place July 20th to July 24th, 1998 at the castle Rauischholzhausen, a conference site of Giessen University. We were not able to accommodate all applicants. The German summer school offered 3 different tracks:

1. *Nursing classifications (G. Nielsen)*
2. *Nursing informatics and education (W. Goossen)*
3. *Information systems in nursing and their introduction (T. Bürkle / U. Schrader)*

The first track dealt with nursing taxonomies and classifications such as NANDA, OMAHA, UNLS and ICNP. Track 2 introduced into nursing informatics and it's integration into the nursing curriculum. Teaching strategies have been compared and at the end participants designed a complete nursing informatics workshop. Track 3 dealt with nursing requirements for a clinical information system. Requirement's analysis, selection criteria and system introduction have been discussed.

During five work days plenary sessions were given each morning. In three plenaries the tutors gave an introduction into the essentials of their respective track. One plenary was dedicated to an invited speaker, Dr. Antes from Freiburg who gave a lecture on evidence based medicine and the German Cochrane Center. The last plenary was filled with presentations produced by the participants, who demonstrated what they had learned in their respective track. The afternoon has been divided in two regular teaching blocks and one late night block after dinner. Those blocks started with an introduction into a specific problem, given by the respective tutor, and continued with tasks for the participants to solve this problem. Appropriate learning materials have been supplied to promote cooperation among the participants and to enable them for continuous self teaching. One block was dedicated to an introduction and practice with Microsoft's Powerpoint presentation software. For this task a small computer lab had been established using seven portable computers.

4. The evaluation

A questionnaire was distributed the last day of the summer school to evaluate the participant's reaction to this event. 88% of our participants returned the questionnaire. Here we present just a few highlights:

How did you find out about the summer school ? (multiple answers possible)	
– I read the paper leaflet	9
– I found it on the internet	9
– I heard about from other persons	12
– others	5

How did you pay for the summer school ?	
– my employer paid	25
– I paid myself	3
– others (e.g. partial subsistence)	2

How would you rate the summer school ?	
– excellent	23
– good	6
– satisfying	1
– sufficient	0
– insufficient	0

How would you rate the summer school plenary sessions ?	
– excellent	26
– good	5
– satisfying	0
– sufficient	0
– insufficient	0

Would you recommend the summer school to your colleagues ?	
– yes, I would	30
– I would recommend it partially	1
– no, I would not	0

5. Statements on health and nursing informatics training

Considering the mentioned observations and evaluation results we would like to establish the following statements for nursing informatics training in Germany:

1. *There is a need for nursing informatics training among German nurses*
2. *The training has to be extended beyond teaching merely computer literacy*
3. *The training has to enable nurses to participate actively in decision groups and task forces concerned with introduction of computer applications in healthcare. They must:*
    - be able to select systems and adapt them to nursing requirements
    - be able to prepare local nursing standards and nursing terminology
    - be able to organise computer training for their colleagues
4. *A condensed summer school teaching program enables actively working nurses to participate and to become involved with nursing informatics.*
5. *The curriculum contents of the first German summer school met the interest of the participating nurses.*

6. Discussion

In this paper we have pointed out that it is difficult for German nurses to receive appropriate training in nursing informatics if they are not enrolled in qualification programs for nurse executives or specialising in health informatics. However those „normal" nurses who keep working in their profession, are the ones who need to cooperate in task forces and decision groups to enable the introduction and spreading of informatics applications in healthcare. Many of them know how to use a computer and we would like to point out specifically that more than a fourth of our participants found the invitation to the first German summerschool on the internet. But for the mentioned tasks comprehensive health informatics knowledge extending beyond simple computer literacy is required. It was interesting for us to notice that nurse employers have recognised this need for more knowledge. More than 80% of them resumed the full costs of the summer school for their employees.

However, the barrier of a foreign country and a foreign language, e.g. in the European Summer School program is too high for many German nurses willing to acquire health informatics and nursing informatics knowledge. In an attempt to overcome those barriers we have successfully established a German nursing informatics summer school. The response to this five day event exceeded our expectations by far. Considering our evaluation results we can conclude that a mixed curriculum dealing with nursing terminology and classifications, nursing informatics education and introduction of clinical information systems does satisfy the information needs of our participants. The last of those topics met the strongest interest. We will continue offering similar events to help nurses to formulate their own requirements in health informatics. This should enable our participants to influence their future working environment successfully. Finally the German nursing informatics summer school might help to establish aspects of health and nursing informatics in the nursing curricula.

Accomplishments

The authors thank especially William Goossen and Gunnar Nielsen for their activities in the German summer school. The event has been supported nominally from the German Medical Informatics Association GMDS.

References

[1] R. Haux *et al.*, Recommendations of the German Association for Medical Informatics, Biometry and Epidemiology for Education and Training in Medical Informatics. In: A. Hasman *et al.*(eds) Education and Training in Health Informatics. IOS Press Amsterdam (1995) 111-129.

[2] F. J. Leven, Curriculum for Medical Informatics at the University of Heidelberg / School of Technology Heilbronn. *Meth. Inform. Med.* **33** (1994) 262-267.

[3] H. J. Trampisch, Praxis- Studien- und Forschungsführer Medizinische Informatik, Biometrie und Epidemiologie, 2. Aufl. Gustav Fischer Verlag Stuttgart (1995).

[4] Hessisches Ministerium für Jugend, Familie und Gesundheit, Hessisches Curriculum Krankenpflege. 1.&2.Ausbildungsabschnitt. Deutscher Berufsverband für Pflegeberufe e.V. (eds) Eschborn (1990/91)

[5] W. Goossen *et al.*, Informatik in der Aus- und Weiterbildung. In: J. Beier *et al.* (eds) Jahrbuch der Pflege- und Gesundheitsberufe 1997. LAU-Ausbildungssysteme (1997) 549-568.

[6] T. Bürkle *et al.*, Pflegeinformationssysteme Eine Literaturübersicht. *Informatik, Biometrie und Epidemiologie in Medizin und Biologie* **25** (1994) 199-215.

[7] E. Opitz, Informationsverarbeitung im Pflegebereich - Checkliste und Marktlage. In: P. Haas *et al.* (eds) Praxis der Informationsverarbeitung im Krankenhaus. Ecomed Landsberg (1996) 123-130.

[8] T. Bürkle *et al.*, Stepwise evaluation of information systems in an University Hospital. *Meth. Inform. Med.* **38** (1999) 9-15.

[9] U. Schrader *et al.*, Klinische Arbeitsplatzsysteme Checkliste und Marklage. In: P. Haas *et al.*(eds) Praxis der Informationsverarbeitung im Krankenhaus. Ecomed Landsberg (1996) 131-138.

Medical Informatics Europe '99
P. Kokol et al. (Eds.)
IOS Press, 1999

A Tutor For Nursing Process Education

Ana Habjanic, Viljem Brumec
University of Maribor, University College of Nursing Studies
Maribor, Zitna 15, Slovenia
Peter Kokol, Milan Zorman
University of Maribor, FERI
The Laboratory for System Design
Maribor, Smetanova 17, Slovenia

Abstract: Computer managed instruction (CMI) has been used in nursing education since the late 1960's. It is due to the accessibility and self paced format that CMI is very well suited for both students and practicing nurses, while learning can occur at the learner's own pace and time. In addition CMI supports also continuing education and distant learning. The aim of this paper is to present CArE – a software package for **C**omputer **A**ided Nu**r**se **E**ducation in particular for teaching the basics of the nursing care process, developed as a result of the Phare TEMPUS project called NICE (Nursing Informatics and Computer Aided Education).

1. Introduction

Computer and information processing sciences were applied initially to support medical practitioners, health service administrators and governments during the late 1960's. The nursing informatics began during the1970s as is evident by the first World Congress on Medical Informatics (Medinfo) held in Stockholm in 1974. This was organised by the International Medical Informatics Association which began as a special interest group of the International Federation of Information Processing (IFIP) [1].

Computer managed instruction (CMI) has been used in nursing education since the late 1960's [3, 4]. It is due to the accessibility and self paced format that CMI is very well suited for both students and practicing nurses [3, 4], while learning can occur at the learner's own pace and time. In addition CMI supports also continuing education and distant learning.

The aim of this paper is to present CArE – a software package for **C**omputer **A**ided Nu**r**se **E**ducation in particular for teaching the basics on the nursing care process, which was developed as a result of the Phare TEMPUS project called NICE (Nursing Informatics and Computer Aided Education) [14, 15].

2. Computer Managed Instruction In Nursing

In the educational process, especially in some specific areas, where students cannot practice in vivo, the computer support can be invaluable. The computer simulation and computer based models provide an opportunity for students to exercise skills which can be otherwise obtained only in real world situations.

The early applications of CMI employed room sized mainframes at large institutions, but the proliferation of microprocessors in the 1990 expanded the depth and breadth of instructional computing [5, 6]. Recent studies [4, 7 - 9] shows that students using CMI have better average examination scores, improved ability for critical thinking [5] and enhanced computer literacy, facilitated decision making skills and positively affected achievements [12]. In spite of these advantages still many students and faculty [12] are reluctant to utilise CMI, but Haus [11] reports that the perception and attitude towards computer managed instruction positively changes after actual use of CMI software packages.
Athappilly [10] list three benefits for using CMI and multimedia tools in the educational process:

1. quality multimedia presentation reduces the cost, in spite that initial investments are large the reduction of participants and instructors time are significant;
2. the effectiveness of the teaching and learning is improved because of greater motivation, retention, and mastery of learning;
3. production is improved because of increased satisfaction and enjoyment of learning.

3. Care – A Brief Description

CArE is a program aimed to facilitate learning of the nursing care process based on the theory of Virginia Henderson presented in previous chapters. Our aim was to develop an application that would overcome the weaknesses of CIM software presented before but at the same time poses the advantages that would help students to learn and improve their knowledge about nursing diagnosing process. Working with CArE is divided into two phases. In the first phase the students have the opportunity to browse through the database of nursing diagnoses and learn, but without any feedback. In the second phase the students can prove or test their knowledge about the nursing diagnosing process – this phase employs the learning with feedback. Based on the nursing assessment, randomly selected from the database, the students have to choose the correct nursing diagnosis, related factors, defining characteristics, goals and nursing interventions. The results of the tests are saved in form, which

- enable students to analyse the questions and answers and review their knowledge, and
- enable teachers to evaluate the quality of student's knowledge – the computer managed exams.

To implement the CArE according to our needs (we have had to find a tool, that was able to work with databases, had possibility to build a friendly and easy-to-use user interface, was running under MS Windows and was cheap and widely spread) we decided to use MS Access 97, a part of MS Office package.
The main menu appears (shown in figure 1) when we start the application. The window is divided in three parts:

- **Database administration**
  In the upper right part there is a set of buttons, that start different actions in the database administration. Here we can add, update and delete nursing diagnoses and their attributes. If we are dealing with an empty database or we want to add a new nursing diagnosis, we must first check if there are all the attributes in the database. For checking the related factors, we just click the "Related factors" button and the window opens, where we can add, modify or delete the related factors. The procedure is similar for definitions, defining characteristics, patient goals, nursing

interventions and expected outcomes. After that we click the button "Diagnoses" and next window appears.
With buttons at the bottom of the window we can navigate through the records. For adding a new nursing diagnosis we move to the last record, which is empty. We type in the name of the diagnosis and the assesment (if the nursing diagnosis is individual). Then we select from a drop-down menu the definition, related factors, defining characteristics, patient goals, nursing interventions and expected outcomes.

- **Learning and testing of knowledge**
  This part is meant for students (learning and testing) and teachers (statistics). Clicking on the "Learning of diagnoses" button opens a window, similar to the window for adding new nursing diagnoses. Students can browse through all the nursing diagnoses in the database and learn about the diagnoses, without having the possibility to make changes to the records.
  Button "Testing of knowledge about diagnoses" is also meant for the students. The upper part of the window is similar to the one for adding new nursing diagnoses.

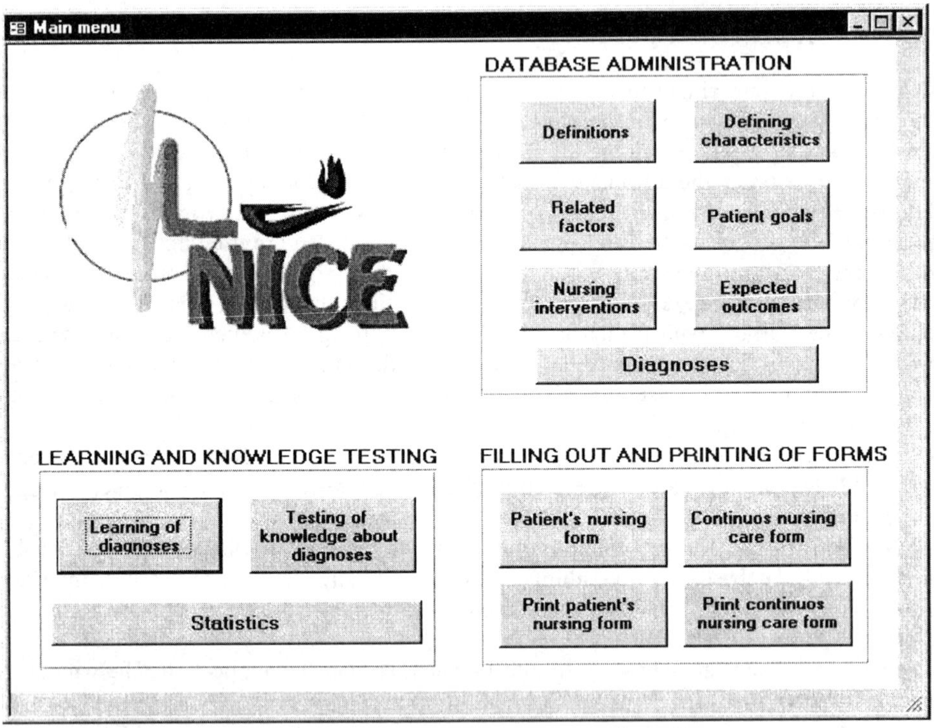

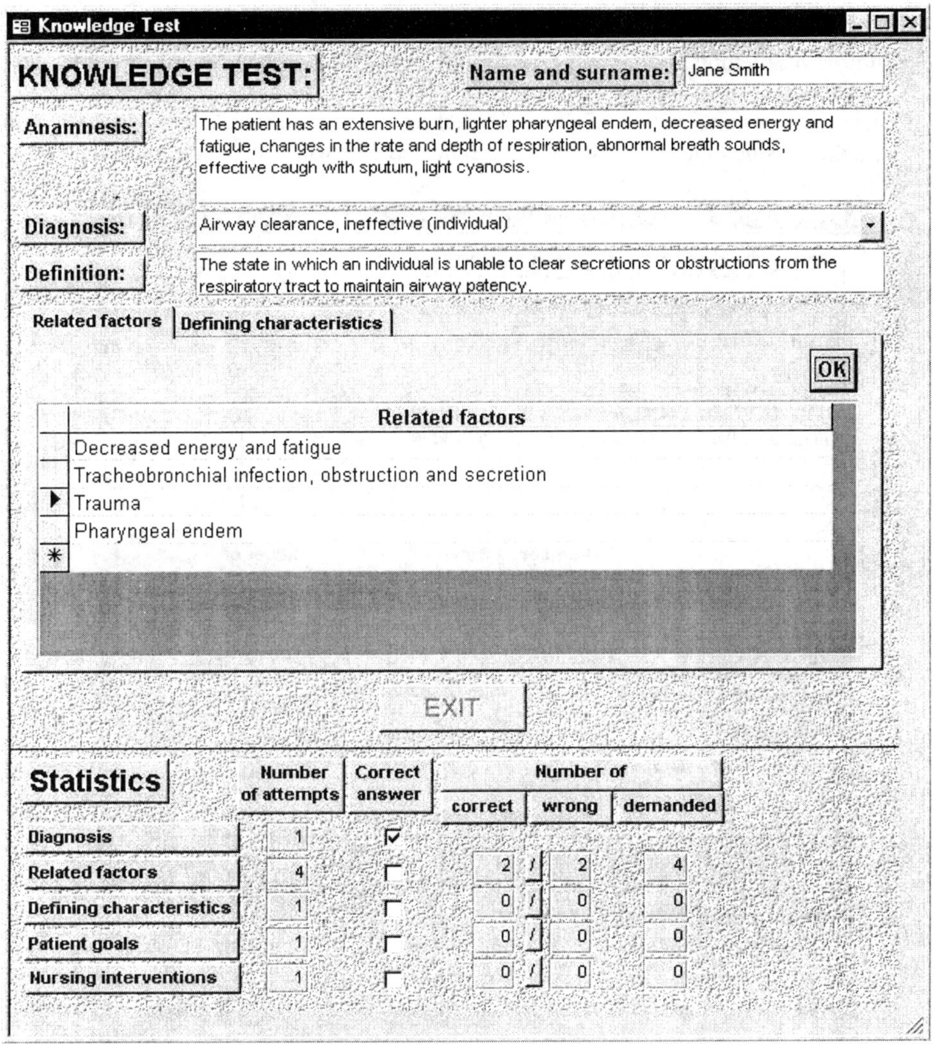

Students must write their name and surname, before they start with the test. Based on the randomly selected anamnesis, they must find the correct diagnosis from the list of all the diagnoses in three attempts. If the correct diagnosis is not found in three attempts, then the right diagnosis is written automatically and student can proceed with finding the related factors. They can be chosen from the list of all the related factors in the database. When the student thinks that all the related factors are found, he clicks the "OK" button. If there are the correct factors chosen, he can proceed with finding the defining characteristics, otherwise he gets the error warning with the short description of the error (e.g. "Not enough related factors chosen!"). After three unsuccessful attempts, the correct answer is provided by the application and the student can proceed with finding defining characteristics. The procedure for finding the defining characteristics, patient goals and nursing interventions is exactly the same.

At the bottom of the window there is the statistics of each test, where the student can see, the number of attempts, how many answers are correct, how many wrong and how many demanded.
Teachers get the same statistic figures for each test, including name and surname of the student, the nursing diagnosis and the exact time and date when the test has taken place.

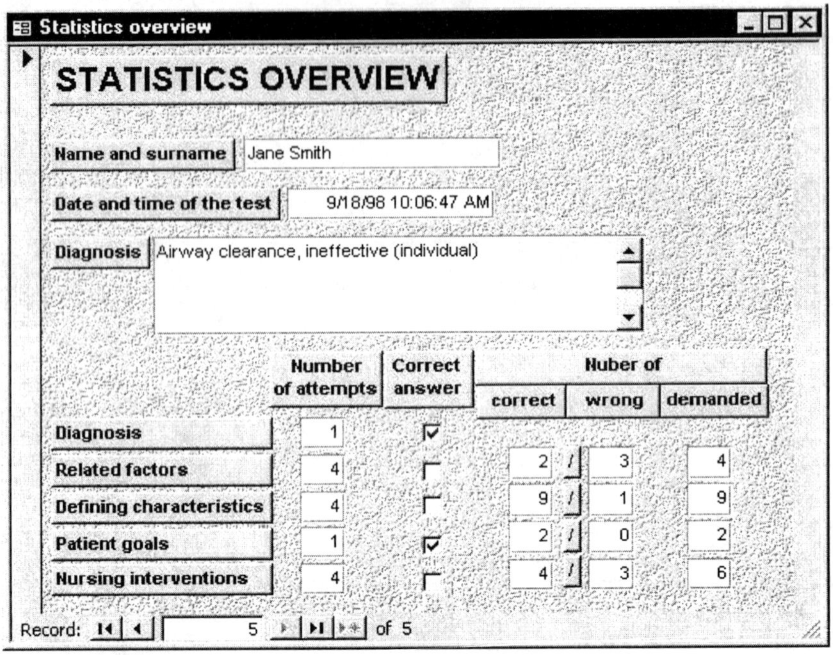

Those figures can be used to evaluate student's knowledge for the grading purposes.

- **Filling out and printing of forms**
  By clicking the "Patient's nursing form" and "Continuos nursing care form" buttons, you can enter data to those two forms. It is also possible to print both forms.

4. Care – An Empirical Study Of It's Use

The CArE was evaluated at the School of Nursing, University College of Maribor, in the multimedia learning center with both:

1. second year students having the theoretical knowledge of the nursing care process; and
2. nursing professors/lecturers.

The purpose of this research was to conclude if CArE can be used for educational purposes and as a tool for the individualised examination of the student's knowledge.
In testing we used qualitative analysis in the form of two survey questionnaires. Both of the above stated groups answered the same questionnaires. In the first survey questionnaire we wished to ascertain if the CArE is an appropriate teaching method compared with the classical one, and if students are willing to utilise such a learning method. In the second questionnaire we wished to ascertain if CArE is user friendly, if the response time is fast enough, and if such a program can be used in daily practice. Both the majority students and the majority of lecturers found the program very or good and would like to use it in

learning, lecturing and also in the clinical practice with the distinction that students were a bit more critical in evaluating it's use.

References

[1] B. Cesnik , History of Health Informatics in: E.Hovenga, M.Kidd, B.Cesnik (Eds) Health Informatics – an Overview, Churchill Livingstone, Melbourne 1996.

[2] E. Hovenga, Global Health Informatics Education., Proceeding of THE 98, Edited by J. Mantas, University of Athens, 1998.

[3] J. M. Belfry, A Review of the Effect of Computer Assisted Instruction in Nursing Education, Computers in Nursing, March 1988. (http://www.nursing.ab.umd.edu/students/~jkohl/cai.htm).

[4] C. M. Curtis, M K Howard, A Comparison Study of the Effectiveness of Computer Assited Instruction and Traditional Lecture Techniques as Methods of Staff Development for Nurses, Research report, 1990. (http://www.widomaker.com/~ccurtis/cai.study.html).

[5] J.E. Kohl, M. C. Su, Computer Assisted Instruction: Implications for Achevement and Critical Thinking, Research report, 1995.

[6] T. Hebda, A Profile of the Use of CAI within baccalaureate nursing education, Computers in Nursing, November 1988.

[7] M. Williamson, High teach training, Byte, December 1994,

[8] M. Cambre, L. J. Castner, The status of interactive video in nursing education environments, FITNE 1993, Atlanta, 1993.

[9] F. R. Jelovsek, Abebonojo, Learning principles as applied to computer – asssisted instruction, MD Computing, October, 1993.

[10] K. K. Athappilly, C. Durben, S. Woods, Multimedia Computing. Multimedia Computing edited by S. Reisman, Harrisburg 1994.

[11] K. Haus, Changes in Perception of Computer Aided Instruction, Research report, 1996 (http://parsons.ab.umd.cdu/~khaus/paper.html

[12] Gleydura, J. Michelman, C. Wilson, Multimedia Training in Nursing Education, Computers in Nursing, July, 1995.

[13] F. Khoiny, Factors that contribute to computer assisted instruction effectiveness, Computers in Nursing, July 1995.

[14] Kokol P, Brumec V: The first report about the NICE Project -Nursing informatics and computer aided education. Nursing informatics / edited by U. Gerdin, M. Tallberg and P. Wainwright, IOS Press : Ohmsha, 1997. p.p. 591.

[15] Kokol P, Zazula D, Brumec V, Kolenc L, Šlajmer Japelj M: New Nursing Informatics Curriculum – an Outcome from the NICE Project, HTE 98, University of Athens, 1998.

Medical Informatics Europe '99
P. Kokol et al. (Eds.)
IOS Press, 1999

Towards a Nursing Information System in Slovenia

Bojana Filej[1], Petra Kersnič[2], Veronika Pretnar Kunstek[2], Majda Šlajmer Japelj[3]
[1]WHO Collaborating Center for Primary Health Care Nursing, Ul. talcev 9, 2000 Maribor, Slovenia
[2]Nurses Association of Slovenia, Vidovdanska 9, 1000 Ljubljana, Slovenia
[3]WHO Collaborating Center for Primary Health Care Nursing

Abstract. In the paper are described the starting points of health informatic system developement in Slovenia as also the situation in nursing. There are presented the goals, which nurses want to achieve with informatic system development and the activities for their attainability.

Health care is a highly specific and complex system going through a constant process of change and development. This is also true of nursing as an integral part of the health care system. In Slovenia, nursing has only developed at an increased rate for the past fifteen years, making nurses realise that as nursing develops they must take full professional responsibility for their work. It is for this reason that they must strive to make nursing visible. The only instrument of visibility is documentation, which at the same time provides a basis for the evaluation of the care delivered and a means of legal protection for nurses. A systematic, comprehensive and continued approach to the treatment of their clients dictates the need for nurses to collect large amounts of information, so consequently they spend much of their working time collecting, managing and conveying information. In order to make data comparable not only at national but also at international level, a uniform format must be adopted to maka data equally understandable and useful for all.

The idea of a unified body of nursing terminology first appeared while the Unit for Nursing of the WHO Regional Office for Europe was conducting a multinational survey »People's Needs for Nursing Care« between 1976 and 1985. A milestone in the history of nursing in Europe, the survey was the most comprehensive survey on nursing ever to be conducted in Europe and probably the world as well. It covered 11 countries, including Slovenia. The purpose of the survey was to develop, through research, better working methods in nursing, to improve planning and to provide for better evaluation of the results of work. Analysis of huge amounts of data from various countries was required and same interpretation of answers were needed. This dictated the need for a simplified professional nursing terminology.

In Slovenia, an Expert Preparatory Commission for a Health Care Information System was set up at the Ministry of Health in 1992. However, it only formulated general guidelines for a national strategy for the field and drafted the national health care information system programme. The strategy was based on the premise that a health care information system should meet the needs of both the health care system and the population, it should secure information privacy and provide for the fastest possible data access. In addition, the strategy underlined the need for uniform organisation and content at the national level and the need for communication between subsystems that should be designed so as to serve the needs of the health institutions and to collect and store all data at regional and state levels.

The 1992 Health Insurance Amendment Act required health institutions to introduce computerised data management. This was necessary as it became impossible for health care institutions to deal with all of the data flow, invoicing in particular, using the old, most often »manual«, methods. For this reason the national Health Insurance Company donated large numbers of computers to health institutions around Slovenia. Certainly, these computers alone were not enough to effectively computerise the entire health care system, given that a comprehensive information system must meet not only business and statistical requirements but also those of a more professional nature.

Health care is a sector known for its variety and size, but also rigidity and lack of flexibility. This is why there is still so much chaos in the health care information system in Slovenia. Virtually every health institution has its own information system, and communication between them is yet to be established. Even though considerable funds are spent on nursing, this sector is not recorded neither from the statistical nor the professional point of view and nursing in most cases is not included in the health care information system. Unfortunately, no consensus has yet been reached in the nursing profession about what data are needed to make nursing visible in Slovenia's health care system and comparable in European frameworks.

Nevertheless, first attempts have been made in certain health institutions and social-welfare institutions as nurses come to realise it is not only computer experts and professionals but nurses as well who should decide the nursing information system development.

The WHO Collaborating Center for Primary Health Care Nursing, whose responsibilties also include monitoring the health care information system development in Slovenia, conducted a survey in year 1998 to establish the overall situation in the field and to find out whether individual health care institutions had computer-supported information systems and whether these included nursing.

The survey included 12 hospitals (out of 22), 30 health centres (out of 53) and 25 old people's homes (out of 54), which makes 67 institutions althogether. Data analysis produced the following findings:

1. Nursing is included in the computer-supported information systems of 35 institutions, chiefly old people's homes, followed by health centres and only two hospitals. We believe this is mainly due to the desire of the funding-providing institutions (Health Insurance Company, Ministry for Labour, Social Affairs and Family) to control spending.
2. In most cases computer software in the said institutions is designed so as to include nursing as an integral part of the system. Nursing is most often included in the information software in old people's homes where actitivities are funded through nursing services in that these provide categorisation of clients in terms of their basic needs and the level of dependency in meeting the latter. Health centres mainly include community nursing delivered by community nurses as the sole providers of this kind of service.
3. Institutions primarily use their information systems for accounting purposes, followed by statistical data processing, and work flow organisation in both health centres and hospitals. On the other hand, areas of nursing practice range third ahead of work flow organisation in old people's homes.
4. Nearly all institutions use software developed by IT companies, only 10 institutions rely on software developed by in-house IT staff.

5. The range of information covered by nursing software varies from instititution to institution, depending on specific requirements of individual institutions and the availabilty of appropriate software for the nursing practice in Slovenia.
6. Old people's homes are specific in that nurses are far more independent in their work from their counterparts in hospitals, out patients' departments or dispensaries (but not in community nursing). Doctors are responsible for treatment and therapy and are usually present in the old people's homes in the morning and not necesserily every day. Another important characteristic is that the elderly usually live in the homes for very long time so nurses get to know them very well.
7. Old people's homes are also specific in that the need to order data emerged at a very early point. To be able to conduct their work effectively, old people's homes must keep a number of records and collect huge amounts of data that are often untransparent without an appropriate computer-supported information system. This is why as early as 1991 they started developing the Social Welfare and Health Application that is now used by 35 out of 54 old peoples' homes across Slovenia. The software's major shortcoming is that it is not based on the nursing process as the key method of work for nurses.
8. Hospitals, the Ljubljana Clinical Centre in particular, also started developing nursing information systems. Here, nursing forms a subsystem within the integrated health care information system that also comprises medicine, administration and management, and statistics. The nursing subsystem is further divided to the administration and management section and the section dealing with professional nursing matters.
9. Computer-assisted data management is also present in community nursing, but it essentially remains restricted to accounting and statistics. A community nurse keeps records of her visits to patient's homes, feeding data into the computer. Existing applications are deficient in that they are based on the old record-keeping system, consequently failing to include all aspects of community nursing practice and observe the modern process-based method of work in community nursing.

Conclusions

In Slovenia with the support of computerised informatic system we present only the financial evaluation of our work and we get the data for statistical and analytical report. Nurses are aware that informatic system is necessary for rationality of nursing work what mean:

- unitary terminology development,
- unitary naming of nursing problems or needs or nursing diagnoses,
- unitary system for data collecting,
- quicker documentation of data,
- possibilities for controlling of done work,
- possibilities for measuring of done work, collecting data for statistical and analytical reports,
- financial evaluation of done work,
- preparing the basis for nursing research,
- evidencing proportion of nursing at the whole client treatment.

To reach these goals it is necessary:

1. Nursing in Slovenia has to be included into national health informatic system, especially of two reasons - because of complete participation in health team and because of continuing nursing treatment, when client passes from one to another health care level.

2. Nursing in Slovenia has to be included into international collaboration and multilateral research work, which allow quick and complete informations (ICNP - International Classification of Nursing Practice, Telenurse ID).
3. The informatic system development in nursing is also necessary because of synchronisation with the European union documents, what mean that we have:
- to develop professional language, which will be useful for classification and for coding;
- to prepare the software (translation or our own);
- to educate nurses about informatic systems and how to work with computers;
- to change the basic nursing curricula;
- to develop nursing legislation and other regulations about obligatory nursing documentation.

References

[1] Ashworth P., Bjorn A., Dechanoz G. et al. Potrebe ljudi po zdravstveni negi, študija evropskega urada Svetovne zdravstvene organizacije. Maribor: Kolaborativni center Svetovne zdravstvene organizacije za primarno zdravstveno nego, 1988

[2] Bigec M. Pogovor s prim. Dunjo Piškur Kosmač, dr.med., sekretarko Ministrstva za zdravstvo Republike Slovenije. INFORM. MED. SLOV. 1994; 1: 9-11.

[3] Danish Institute for Health and Nursing Research. Telenurse, The Nursing Research Potential of Electronic Health Care Records and the Role of Nursing Research Centres in Europe.Copenhagen: DIHNR, 1995

[4] Filej B. Predstavitev novosti v okviru evropskega projekta Telenurse. Ljubljana: Psihiatrična in nevrološka sekcija pri Zbornici zdravstvene nege Slovenije, 1997

[5] Gašparovič M. Računalniški program v socialnih zavodih - domovih starejših občanov. Teorija in praksa zdravstvene nege: zbornik posvetovanj o teoriji in praksi zdravstvene nege. Ljubljana: psihiatrična in nevrološka sekcija pri Zbornici zdravstvene nege Slovenije. 1997; 160-161.

[6] Habjanič A., Vuga S., Kokol P., Zorman A. Računalništvo v zdravstveni negi. INFORM. MED. SLOV. 1995; 2: 25-27.

[7] International Council of Nurses. International Classification of Nursing Practice (ICNP), update - ICNP, emerging beta version. Geneva: ICN, 1998

[8] Milavec M., Šušteršič O., Rajkovič V. Podatkovni model patronažne zdravstvene nege. Obzor Zdrav n 1995; 29: 143-147.

[9] Mortensen R. A. Mednarodna klasifikacija prakse zdravstvene nege. Kranj: Moderna organizacija, 1998

[10] NANDA. Uvod v študij negovalnih diagnoz. Maribor: Kolaborativni center Svetovne zdravstvene organizacije za primarno zdravstveno nego, 1993

[11] Nielsen G. H., Mortensen R. A. Telenursing, Definition, Classification, and Coding of the Nursing Process in Hospitals in Europe. Copenhagen: The Danish Institute for Health and Nursing Research, 1994

[12] Pavčič Trškan B. Informacijski sistem zdravstvene nege v Kliničnem centru. Teorija in praksa zdravstvene nege: zbornik posvetovanj o teoriji in praksi zdravstvene nege. Ljubljana: psihiatrična in nevrološka sekcija pri Zbornici zdravstvene nege Slovenije. 1997; 162-165.

[13] Šušteršič O., Rajkovič V., Leskovar R., Bitenc I. Zasnova informacijskega sistema v patronažni zdravstveni negi. teorija in praksa zdravstvene nege: zbornik posvetovanj o teoriji in praksi zdravstvene nege. Ljubljana: psihiatrična in nevrološka sekcija pri Zbornici zdravstvene nege Slovenije. 1997; 155-159.

Medical Informatics Europe '99
P. Kokol et al. (Eds.)
IOS Press, 1999

Internet provides fast and inexpensive information to home care

Nils Bjørn
Danish Centre for Health Telematics, Heden 18, DK-5000 Odense C, Denmark

In Denmark the communities are responsible for home care services to elderly people. Many of the smaller Danish communities don't use patient record systems in home care, but manage with paper-based system or they use text-processing to do their reporting.

When people are admitted to hospital, the hospital nurse would contact the district nurse. Most of this information would go by phone or fax, and is not formalised. When it is evident, during a hospital admittance, that a patient will need home care services, the hospital nurse will write a 'notification of discharge', which describes the specific needs required from home care. At the actual time for the discharge, a similar – but updated - report is sent from hospital to home care.

A web-based service can now be offered to home care units, because the aforementioned nursing documents can be sent electronically to home care and be presented on the Internet.

The background is that the Danish hospitals over the past years has sent EDIFACT messages to GPs such as discharge letters and laboratory results. Now time has come to continue with messages to the municipality. The two messages are sent as EDIFACT using MEDDIS and they can be received on the Internet solution called EDI2WEB.

The target group for a web-based service will typically be partners that has little traffic, so the investment in an integrated solution is too expensive. These organisations can use this Internet solution as a temporary solution, and can always change to an integrated solution without changing any procedures in the way you are sending and/or receiving messages. The advantages for the sender are that you don't have to think about what system is used and which platform data is received on. For the receiver the advantage is faster communication, no handling of paper, and no distribution in the organisation. The communication uses the technical communication standards of the Danish healthcare data network.

A number of nurses have been involved in the design of the HTML based screens for notifications of discharge and the nurses discharge letter.

This project has co-operated with a hospital in the County of Funen, Rudkoebing hospital. This hospital is a geriatric hospital, which uses an electronic patient-record-system, developed by RAMBOLL Data systems. This system is a client-server solution, driven in a Novell Network on IBM equipment.

The systems address their own electronic mail box at one of the two VANS-providers in Denmark and from there the messages are distributed to the mail box of the relevant receiver of the message, according to the receiving EAN-number. From here the IT-system in the different organisations receive their messages. The receiving part, the home care in the small communities, will communicate with the mailbox through an ISDN line.

The home care personnel will connect to the Internet, call the homepage www.edi2web.dk, will perform an authorised login procedure, and can then view and archive messages. When optimising the messages being sent, the typical cost of a message is less than 25% of the cost of sending a letter.

All the users were given a short course in using a browser; they had to be able to log on to the system, identify the new messages, print the messages and log out of the system. It takes about 2 hours for a nurse that is not familiar with the Internet.

Below you can see a number of messages to the home care unit.
It is possible to sort the documents according to the shown columns - document number, action
on the document (show, archive), type of document, date of document, name of hospital.

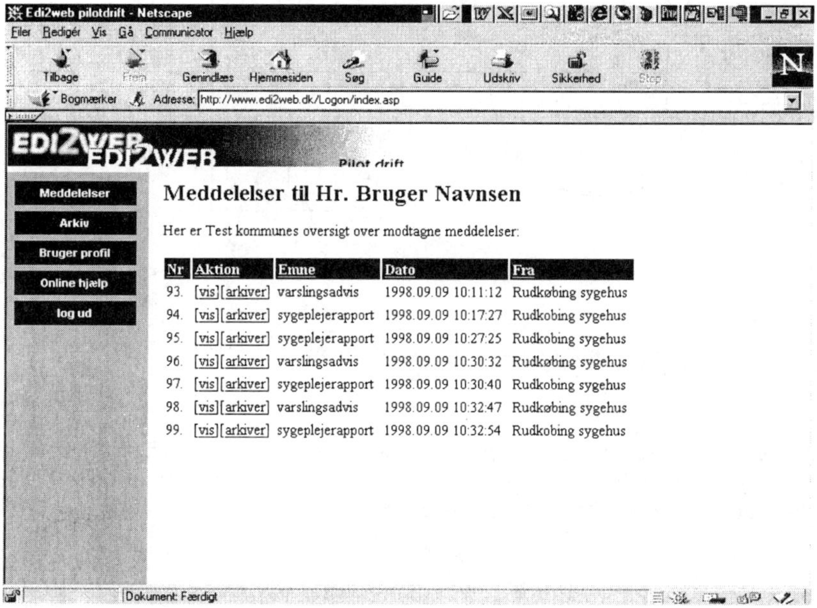

Since this is an Internet solution - no additional software has to be bought - except for the presence of a browser.
You can use any Internet service provider for this solution.

When using this service, you need to have a telephone line by any provider, probably an ISDN line. Since you are receiving & sending EDIFACT messages, you need to have a 13-digit EAN number. You must pay for a license to use the product. The price depends on the type of customer (hospital, home care) and the size of the home care.

When you buy a license to the EDI2WEB service, you receive a user ID and a password. You see the messages meant for the relevant organisation only.

For maximum security this solution uses secure socket layer, SSL, to achieve three things:

1) Server authentication so that the user has a security that it is the correct web-server that is being used.
2) Encryption, the communication between the web/server and the web service is encrypted.
3) Data integrity, securing that the EDI messages can not be changed between the health care data network and the web service.

On the diagram below, one can follow the messages from hospital. They leave as normal EDIFACT messages, and it is the receiving EAN-number that distinguishes normal messages from messages that has to be converted into HTML. These messages are removes from the Danish health care data network, sent to the Internet server where the message is converted and stored on the internet server until home care will log on to this service.

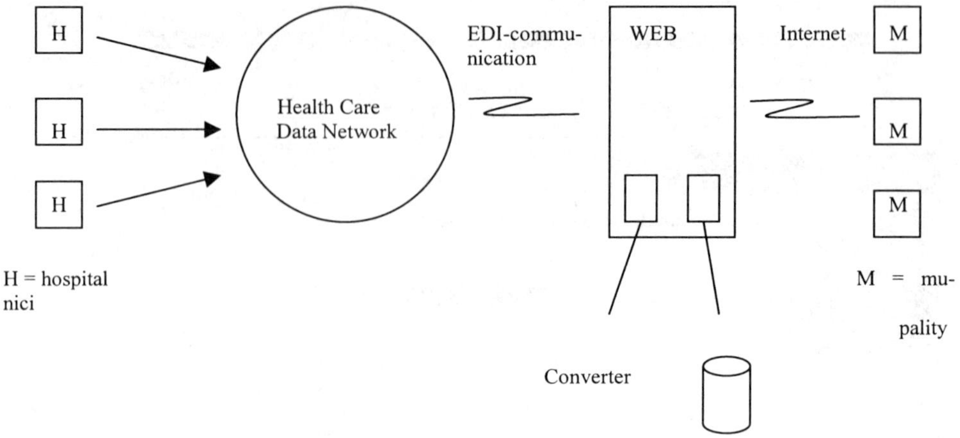

The nurses in the home care unit are happy with the Internet solution. They are looking once or twice a day and they have a feeling of being updated a lot faster than before. The reports are now more structured than before and readable.

Posters

Medical Informatics Europe '99
P. Kokol et al. (Eds.)
IOS Press, 1999

Interdisciplinary Dialogue Center – a model for collaborative work

http://www.cdi.pub.ro

Floriana Filip[1], Alexandru Trica[2], Elena Jitaru[2], Mihai Cristian Jitaru[1], Radu Dop[4], Ion Gutiu[3], Ion Dumitrache[1], Bernard Richards[5], Costas Pappas[6]

[1] *POLITEHNICA University of Bucharest, Faculty of Automatics and Computers, RO*
[2] *Institute for Research in Informatics, Bucharest, RO*
[3] *University of Medicine and Pharmacy Bucharest, RO*
[4] *Romanian Medical Association, RO*
[5] *UMIST, Manchester, UK*
[6] *School of Medicine, Thessaloniki, GR*

Abstract. The paper describes the adopted concept in the design of an interdisciplinary center aiming to be a frame for a collaborative work between practicing clinicians, health service managers, those involved in the use and management of health care information, the design and implementation of health care systems, including commercial suppliers, research into these areas and NGOs.

Keywords: communication, Internet, dynamic database, interactive forms, multidisciplinary team, Medical Informatics and Bioengineering education, Web Server, Active Server Pages

1. Introduction

Virtuality and *communication (dialogue)* are two main concepts of the contemporary information society that need to share information and experience bringing people together. These communication links open up new ways for personal and group interaction and support and provide access to a global network of distributed personal knowledge and expertise.

History: The Bioengineering Department of the Faculty of Automatics and Computer Science of the "POLITEHNICA" University of Bucharest, together with the "Carol Davila" Medicine and Pharmacy University of Bucharest, the Romanian Society for Control Systems and Technical Informatics, the Romanian Medical Association and the foreign partners the University Manchester Institute of Science Technology- United Kingdom and the University of Medicine Thessaloniki - Greece have initiated the TEMPUS - Phare project entitled: **Interdisciplinary Dialogue Center (IDC)**. The project is based on a previous Tempus project entitled "Regional Network for Healthcare Management" [1].

2. Goal and objectives

The goal was to establish an interdisciplinary center for the Medical Informatics domain aiming to support the health care system by improving the communication between human factors from health care, education, research and industry. So this project can support the health care field that is passing through major changes in Romania now.

The Interdisciplinary Dialogue Centre aims to become an infrastructure for information services dedicated to the medical domain using network information management. IDC aims to act as an integration mechanism by identifying the information needs and resources in the health field. It uses a computing platform offering:

- a health care information management infrastructure
- a dialog framework for technicians, physicians and health care managers
- catalysis for interdisciplinary cooperation
- catalysis for co-operation with international organizations: WHO, EU, EFMI
- promotion of the facilities offered by the European integration programs
- support for implementation of reform in higher education and health care
- curricula development for Medical Informatics and Bioengineering
- IT support for health care education
- development of professional skills in Medical Informatics
- framework for medical profession and health practice development
- faster information access
- a teamwork model

3. Achievement

The Interdisciplinary Dialogue Center is hosted by the POLITEHNICA University of Bucharest - Faculty of Automatics and Computers. We created an Internet site (http://www.cdi.pub.ro) able to share and to receive **on-line** precious information in the health care domain. The Interdisciplinary Dialogue Center offers services by Internet and direct contacts.

4. Services

The Interdisciplinary Dialogue Center tries to achieve its main purpose - *a mechanism of integration through health care needs and resources identification* - by offering the following services :

- access to the specific information concerning: organizations, projects, people

  This information allows people who are interested to be informed of the specialists' activities and their expertise gained during the projects' implementation. The contact persons mentioned can give additional information about their achievements and implementation methods - practical factors for the success or failure of an activity.
- access to the university offer represented by:

  national description of academic departments
  the analytic programs of the university lectures
  the analytic programs of the post-university lectures
  activities concerning: distance and computer-aided learning
  joint diploma projects and a list of graduates

  The sustained presence of departments and academic centers from this field at national level can be a support for:

  - professional guidance for high-school graduates
  - specified lectures chosen by any interested individual without necessarily being a student of the particular section.

  The institutions which are interested can obtain also the list of graduates in this field.

- dialog framework for creating a multidisciplinary workteam by knowing: partnership offers based on specific proposed projects and individual collaboration requests
  The corresponding designed forms (interfaces) request to express the necessary skills -as own and outside contribution – for the good running and achievement of the project.
- advertising - requests and offers - for services, software and medical equipment
- job demands and offers
- access to specific news
- self-advertising of news
- medical sub – site (news, events, associations, emergency medical assistance, etc.)

5. Technical platform

We developed a computer network based on the Microsoft solution - Windows NT Small Business Server: a web server (Internet Information Server version 4.0), a search engine for finding information on our web site (Microsoft Index Server 2.0), an e-mail, Discussion and News server (Microsoft Exchange Server 5.0), a firewall for protecting our network (Microsoft Proxy Server 2.0).

To achieve a competitive interactive and dynamic web site we used:

a. Microsoft Access database accessed by the Web procedure via ODBC;

The IDC database is composed of 10 linked and independent tables and some queries designed to ensure the access to the complex data.

The database has a security mechanism able to control the rights to access the records in order to up-date them. It was implemented also a mechanism for verifying all information entered in the database, before permitting the public access to them, so the Web administrator can have the control of the new date proposed for presentation on the IDC site.

b. Active Server Pages (ASP) procedures managing the database interface for handling dynamic data;

The data are input via INTERNET by the registered users who receive an individual login name and password. Only the registered users can add and update the database information. The Internet programming language JavaScript is used to perform plausibility checks before the data are sent to the server and entered into the database. Every user (not only a registered one) can view the database information via queries from the Web.

The heart of the interface is written using ASP (Active Server Pages) technology. The ASP procedures ensure the interface of the Web users with the database engine offering a number of functions for adding and editing data and also for viewing the information stored in the IDC database. For retrieving specific records that meet appropriate search criteria single or in combination, according to a number of different variables, we implemented a search facility by using SQL language.

The interface is a user friendly one, and is designed to be easy used by the people without a computer literacy like the physicians. The IDC Web site has interactive features thoroughly verified at the level of each item of available information.

c. HTML pages for presenting static information

The information stored as HTML pages are linked using the standard hyperlinks, ensuring in this manner a lot of connections between different pages. Different ways of navigation inside the IDC Web server facilitate the access to the interest information.

In order to retrieve the desired data on the IDC Web server, it was developed a search engine able to search in the static data

6. Other experiences

The last years many projects have focused on collaboration work in different fields. Please note several interesting projects in the domain of health. **InterMed collaboratory** is an interdisciplinary complex project involving six participating medical institutions from USA and providing a broadly applicable model for shared component-based collaborative development. **EHTO** (European Health Telematics Observatory) is a meeting place for persons wanting to find and/or display multimedia information on what is going in the field of Health Telematics [2]. The **Center for Clinical Informatics** encourages collaboration by stimulating joint research projects between members of the Center and clinicians and academics working elsewhere in the field of clinical informatics, encourage co-operation between relevant departments of the University and other users of health service information and provide a source of expertise for advising on efficient dissemination of best current knowledge for patients and clinicians [3].

Regarding the partner search mechanism we could quote the Partner Search Databases belonging to the Finnish Leonardo Center (http://www.leonardocentre.fi) and to the Community Research and Development Information Service (CORDIS) (http://www.cordis.lu).

7. Traffic analysis

We analyzed the IDC Web site traffic using Microsoft Site Server Express 3.0 over a period covering 9 months. The analysis tracked the Web site hits - visits and visitors, average time visit on an hourly, daily, and weekly basis, countries, browsers, referring Web sites, organizations, bandwidth, most and least requested documents over time and by directory, the number and distribution of media type categories (i.e., documents, applications, and scripts) and media types (i.e., HTML, pdf, and CGI scripts) and other interesting information. The results show a linear increase in the access to the IDC web site.

8. Conclusion

The demand for knowledge and co-operation should be met by well managed, intuitively structured and accessible information frame.

The Interdisciplinary Dialogue Center Web site promotes the concept of *co-operation through Internet* and we consider the way we implemented this concept to be the first in Romania. The partnership offer is initiated by organizations (offering specific projects) and individuals (offering own skills).

The health services and information users and providers meet each other hosted by the Interdisciplinary Dialogue Center. We must work together to make this center as efficient as possible. The co-operation and communication are vital for its success. The adopted concept could represent a major change in the Romanian co-operation mentality.

References

[1] F. Filip *et al.*, An Approach to Establishing a Health Information Market, IOS Press, Medical Informatics Europe '97, pp.869 -73

[2] M. Laires - New EHTO policy on satellite sites. In: EHTO Journal, vol.1, no. 4,February 1997, pp.12-13

[3] The Centre for Clinical Informatics - http://www.medinfo.cam.ac.uk

[4] J. Murphy *et al.*, Designing, implementing and evaluating a Web site for health informatics. In: Current perspectives in healthcare computing HC98 - UK, pp.189 –99

Medical Informatics Europe '99
P. Kokol et al. (Eds.)
IOS Press, 1999

Establishment Of National Information Infrastructure Program

Ihor Tchaklosh, Yury Tchaklosh, Ivan Luchechko, Jaroslav Lubinets
Dept. of Health Care Administration of L'viv Medical University.
80/4 Tarnavsky St., L'viv 290017 Ukraine
Fax:38-0322-76-77-76, e-mail: tch@ipm.lviv.ua

Abstract: This article presents main principles and ideology of establishment of national information infrastructure program and describes experience of the implementation of the pilot project in L'viv Region. The project primary goal is to improve the quality management of three major health care segments - financial management, medical personnel performance evaluation and health condition of population monitoring. System provides informational basis for decision-making support systems. The problems of system implementation and ways of their solutions have been presented in the article as well.

1. Background information

Cost of services, their efficiency and quality are still the most important issues for Ukrainian health care. It is impossible to find any solutions without appropriate information infrastructure.

Our opinion is that the first step in health reform is the establishment of national information infrastructure, which would join all health care providers via global computer network.

Establishing computer database on health condition of every patient will provide an opportunity to store, generate, transfer and analyze data through decision-making support system which will consequently improve quality and effectiveness as well as provide control over budget expenditures.

The National Information Infrastructural Program requires design and development various analytical-information system for different types of medical institutions from family medicine ambulatory to large multi-profile hospitals. Principle distinction of these systems is unified ideology and database architecture for institutions of different type of specialization and different administrative hierarchical level. It allows receive information from medical institutions of different specialization in unified format and to store or transmit the data to electronic patient record.

Now we build Regional Information Infrastructure Program as a pilot project of implementation above-mentioned system in Ukraine. Unfortunately implementation of this system in all regional medical institutions is impossible because of limit of finance. So the Program realization was performed on step by step basis starting from 1995. At this time we have implemented several prototypes of analytical-information system: ambulatory (polyclinic), hospital, children hospital, maternity hospital, dentist clinic. It works in L'viv Central Clinic Hospital, L'viv Region Prenatal Center, L`viv Regional War Weterans

Hospital, L'viv Regional Psychiatry Hospital, L'viv Regional Diagnostic Center, some large polyclinic and dental clinic of L'viv Region

2. System description

The project primary goal is to improve the quality management of three major health care segments - financial management, medical personnel performance evaluation and health condition of population monitoring; and to provide informational basis for decision-making support systems.

Establishment of national informational health infrastructure allows:

1) To provide account of all the diagnostic and treatment procedures for determining their efficiency, cost and for planning needs for medical equipment, drugs, etc.;

2) To establish database on health condition of every patient in the region to work out the implementation of per capita financing adjusted to health indicator and environment;

3) To develop a system of performance indicator for every health employee by means of quality standards to establish salary incentive system based on rating indicators;

4) To determine a priority list for health financing starting with family physician level up to the national level;

5) To implement market research system and to develop financial projections including budget utilization projection, revenue and expenditure budget, balance report, money sources and their utilization as well as description of potential risks and problems;

6) To identify optimal financing mechanisms and to determine it's guaranteed minimum;

7) To start health care provision based on health insurance principles.

All above-mentioned prototypes of analytical-information systems consist from two main parts: gathering information and information analysis with using decision-making support. Gathered information has been stored in patient database, medical staff database, resources and cost database. Information retrieval have been performed in three directions:

- Health assessment and health policy making
- Health economics, cost effectiveness, resource allocation
- Health care quality assurance, improvement and clinical audit

Technically the information system has been operating in multi-organization / multi-location environment. The application has been performed in 3-tiered system architecture with optional DB back-end. Information system allows connection from local network, via Internet and also makes possible work in off-line mode with next data replication. Application was designed to work in minimal configuration – it requires Windows 95/98/NT operating system, PC with 16 MB RAM. The application shell size does not exceed 6 MB.

3. Evaluation

The experience of implementation showed that during a year the quality and efficiency evaluation indicators increased by 5-15%. Also, the patient and health personnel satisfaction is gradually increasing. It has been identified through sociological surveys.
Planning the need for resources, control over the appropriateness of the provided services allows saving up to 10% of the budget that can be reallocated for current priorities.
The part of medical data should be available for publicity and government officials. For example, we can provide detailed data on health monitoring from 0 to 100 years, find all morbidity peaks, their structure and changes' dynamics for districts, villages, employers or professional groups. This kind of information should be basic for prophylactic programs development not only for health care services but for government, mass media, social and politic organisations as well.
During the project implementation we have got several quite serious problems, that were solved after additional investigation. There are some of the issues and the ways of their fixing:

1. Poor modem communications via telephone lines, especially during long packages transmission. – Have been developed algorithms for representing data to be transmitted in compact form. Also have been developed procedures for automatic data transmission during night.
2. Insufficient database server performance for database containing large amount of data while generating analytic reports. – We designed special data structure for representing data used in analytical reports as well as optimised data retrieving algorithms.
3. Medical documentation has not been organised properly, the datasheets were duplicating each other and were not prepared for automated processing. The documentation standards were different in different clinics. - We developed unified medical documentation standards that allowed electronic processing with sophisticated saving, transmitting, storing and retrieving capabilities.
4. Impossibility to work without unified catalogue of the manipulations, procedures and operations. - We use 9 ICD-CM with our additions of laboratory diagnostics, radiology, paraclinic and dental procedures.
5. Users have not been able to analyse complex data properly. The managers are ready to analyse just the forms required by Health Care Ministry. However, these forms are not displaying the funds expenditure particularly for some diseases or treatment technique or for some physician. The information about medical staff work quality and efficiency has been provided poorly as well. – We implemented evaluation system of quality and efficiency of medical staff as well as manager work in rating form.

4. Conclusions

Thus, we can conclude that the implementation of computer databases in each Region of Ukraine is a priority for establishing health issue information exchange.
This information could be utilized as basic one when determining priorities, doing strategic planning, making financial decisions, and implementing random control. So, establishing and utilizing informational system is the best way to increase effectiveness of the management, to provide an opportunity of training, and convicting people as well as making political decisions.

Medical Informatics Europe '99
P. Kokol et al. (Eds.)
IOS Press, 1999

Hierarchical multi-attribute models for decision support in the management of diabetic foot syndrome

Gorazd Plaper[(1)], Milivoj Piletič[(2)], Marko Bohanec[(3)], Vladislav Rajkovič[(4,3)], Božo Urh[(5)]
(1) Ministry of Interior Affairs of the Republic of Slovenia, Štefanova 2, SI-1000 Ljubljana, Slovenia,
gorazd.plaper@guest.arnes.si
(2) General Hospital Novo mesto, Slovenia
(3) Jožef Stefan Institute, Ljubljana, Slovenia
(4) University of Maribor, Faculty of Organizational Sciences, Kranj, Slovenia
(5) Infonet d.o.o. Kranj

1. Background

To reduce the number of amputations in diabetic population, a comprehensive diabetic foot care program started in diabetic out-patient clinic in General Hospital Novo mesto in 1995 (Piletič 97). All diabetics are screened for risk factors for developing foot pathology (Larsson, Apelquist 95), namely: history of foot ulceration and amputation; symptoms of diabetic neuropathy; loss of protective sensitivity (S-W monofilament); angiopathy (palpation of pulses); and high plantar pressure (foot deformities). After the screening the patients are classified in risk group 1 (no pathology is found), risk group 2 (insensate for monofilament), risk group 3 (no pulse palpated), and in risk group 4 for any combination of findings or positive history for amputation/ulceration. Doctors found the group 4 quite heterogeneous but difficult to split into subgroups without risking some mistakes in more complicated categorization of patients.

2. Aim

The long-term goal of our research is to help doctor in reassessing the risk status for the patients from group 4 and make subgroups of patients with similar characteristics. We present an attempt to solve this problem using an approach based on hierarchical multi-attribute decision modeling. The role of such models in supporting medical doctors in management of diabetic foot syndrome is shown.

3. Methods

We analyze data from screening test of 2925 diabetic patients, attending diabetic out-patient clinic in General Hospital Novo mesto since January 1995 to October 1998. The following data of each patient were collected: history of foot ulceration and amputation, symptoms of diabetic neuropathy (pain, parastesy, burn sensation, restless feet, numbness), loss of protective sensitivity (S-W monofilament); angiopathy (palpation of pulses); presence of foot deformities (hallux valgus, atrophy of plantar fat, claw toes, Charcot foot, callus, changes in skin color).

A decision model for the assessment of risk factors for developing foot pathology was developed using DEX, an expert system shell for decision support (Bohanec, Rajkovič 90). DEX facilitates the development of qualitative multi-attribute decision models and the evaluation of options. It is aimed at the support of decision-makers in complex decision-making problems: given a set of options (alternatives), the task is to select the option that best satisfies the goals of the decision-maker. The decision model consists of (1) a hierarchy of qualitative attributes and (2) decision rules that define the aggregation of lower-level attributes into the higher-level ones. Particularly important features of DEX are its ability to check the decision rules for consistency and provide a detailed explanation of the evaluation results.

On the basis of expert knowledge, attributes important for developing the diabetic foot syndrome were determined, namely: *history* (data of previous *ulcers* or *amputations*), *present status* (data of *symptoms, deformities, other changes*), and *test* results (*loss of protective sensation, no pulse palpated*). Each attribute consists of different values gradated in hierarchical manner. The structure of decision model was designed as a semantic tree whose leaves represent the above mentioned attributes, and its root represents the final *classification* of patient's risk status (Figure 1). With this model, patients are evaluated by an aggregation that is carried out from the leaves towards the root of the hierarchy. Decision rules were defined by the expert according to the influence of a particular attribute on diabetic foot syndrome development.

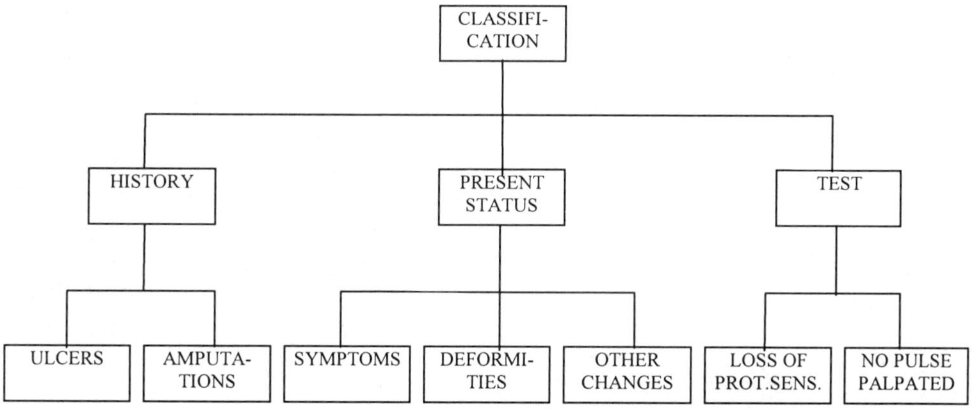

Figure 1: Hierarchical structure of decision model

4. Conclusion

The model was evaluated on data of 2925 diabetic patients. The highest risk group 4 was split into 6 subgroups with different risk levels. These subgroups are considerably more homogeneous than the original group 4, and are thus more appropriate for the planning of further diagnostic procedures and treatment. This brought a new quality in the experts' further management of the patients at greatest risk. In summary, it was confirmed that the approach that uses hierarchical qualitative decision models was appropriate for this type of task and brought some important improvements in terms of the comprehensibility and transparency of the model, and explanations and verifications of decisions. The approach is promising for future development. We propose a further improvement of its sensitivity and specificity using machine learning methods.

References

[1] Bohanec, M., Rajkovič, V., DEX: An expert system shell for decision support, *Sistemica* 1(1), 145-157, 1990.

[2] Larsson, J., Apelquist, J.: Towards less amputations in diabetic patients, *Acta Orthop. Scand.* 66, 181-192, 1995.

[3] Piletič M.,: *Oskrba diabetičnega stopala*, Priročnik za medicinske sestre in zdravstvene tehnike Lj. 23-30, 1997.

Medical Informatics Europe '99
P. Kokol et al. (Eds.)
IOS Press, 1999

Failure Analysis of Thyroid Laboratory Diagnostic Module

Zdenko SONICKI[1], Tomislav PLASAJ[2], Josipa KERN[1], Davor IVANKOVIĆ[1], Zvonko KUSIĆ[2]

[1] *Andrija Štampar School of Public Health, Medical School, University of Zagreb, HR-10000 Zagreb, Rockefellerova 4, Croatia*

[2] *Sestre Milosrdnice University Hospital, HR-10000 Zagreb, Vinogradska 29, Croatia*

E-mail: Zdenko.Sonicki@snz.hr

Abstract. The aim of this paper is to analyse the misclassification patterns of the diagnostic module of Laboratory Information System for thyroid function diagnosis at the Sestre Milosrdnice University Hospital. In order to select misclassified patients the diagnosis of an experienced physician and the diagnostic module were compared. According to the pattern of the laboratory test results, misclassified patients were described and grouped. In conclusion, we have found one obvious module's mistake but the other misclassification patterns have shown more dubious problem in the thyroid function classification.

Keywords: thyroid, diagnosis, diagnostic module, misclassification patterns

1. Introduction

At the Sestre Milosrdnice University Hospital in Zagreb, Laboratory Information System for Thyroid Clinical Laboratory requirements has been designed and developed since 1990. In the early period, this Information System has been used only for collecting data, printing test results, and for scientific research. Over the period of several years considerable quantities of data have been collected.

An idea to develop a kind of an expert system for making thyroid function diagnosis emerged. The purpose of such a system was to make a diagnosis hint for GPs and for laboratory quality control to determine more precise normal cutoff values for laboratory tests. To obtain diagnostic rules, inductive learning algorithm was applied to data collected by 1992[1]. It was the Assistant-algorithm, Quinlan's ID3 algorithm modified by Kononenko and collaborators based on Shannon's expression for information amount necessary to classify an example [2]. The result was a decision tree for thyroid function diagnosis.

In order to implement this knowledge in the existing Laboratory Information System, diagnostic rules have been constructed from the decision tree, and diagnostic module developed [3]. It was a classical system based on rules with the possibility to explain the decision path. Classification was forced with the appropriate probability of belonging to a diagnostic class. Diagnostic module takes data from the Information System - total triiodothyronine (T3), total thyroxine (T4), thyroid stimulating hormone (TSH), its referent values, and other data.

It applies decision rules and returns thyroid function diagnosis. Possible outcomes are Euthyreosis, Hyperthyreosis and Hypothyreosis (Eu/Hyper/Hypo). This diagnostic module was implemented as a background knowledge generator in 1995[4]. Because of its characteristics it was used on backup data in order to evaluate its function [5].

The aim of this paper is to analyse the misclassification patterns of the diagnostic module.

2. Sample and methods

From 1990 to 1998, more than 118.000 test results for over 24.000 patients with over 42.000 visits were recorded in the information system. For the misclassification pattern analysis a random sample of the first-visit thyroid hormones measurements was taken. Patients with physiological and pathophysiological conditions like thyroidectomy, kidney function disorders, pregnancy, oral contraception, etc. which may have an influence to the thyroid function, were excluded. The random sample size was 1.101 examinees. Incomplete records had 203 examinees, so it was not possible to obtain a diagnosis from the diagnostic module.

In order to select misclassified patients, the diagnosis of an experienced physician and the diagnostic module were compared. According to the pattern of the laboratory test results, misclassified patients were described and grouped.

3. Results

The frequencies of the module's diagnosis are shown in Table 1. Misclassification occurred in 15 records (1.67%). Absolute predictive accuracy was 98.33%.

Table 1. Frequencies of the module's diagnosis

Diagnosis	Frequency	%
Eu	841	93.64
Hyper	27	3.01
Hypo	26	2.90
Hyper/Hypo	4	0.45
Total	898	100.00

Misclassifications may be described in 6 logically different patterns of the laboratory test results and a possible therapy. Characteristics of misclassifications, difference between physician's and module's diagnosis with the corresponding number of cases and T3, T4, TSH and therapy pattern, could be seen in Table 2.

Table 2. Misclassification patterns

Pattern No.	Doctor's Dg.	Module Dg.	Number of cases	T3	T4	TSH	Therapy
1	Hypo	Eu	1	Low	Normal	High	Without
2	Hypo	Eu	1	Low	Low	Normal	Without
3	Eu	Hyper/Hypo	1	Normal	Normal	Normal	Thyreostatic
4	Hyper	Eu	4	High	Normal	Normal	Without
5	Hyper	Eu	5	High	High	Normal	Without
6	Hyper	Eu	3	Normal	High	Normal	Without

4. Discussion

Absolute predictive accuracy in this random sample was slightly higher than the accuracy calculated on test data set during inductive learning, i.e. 2.33% higher. Misclassification patterns have shown some obvious mistakes made by diagnostic module and some problems based on the hormone dynamics and classification definition.

Pattern number 1 is Hypothyroid patient misclassified as Euthyreosis. It is an obvious module's mistake.

Pattern number 2 is more dubious, because the module's diagnosis is based on normal TSH level, and at that point it is correct, but T3 and T4 concentrations which are low are indicating *subclinical* Hypothyreosis or Hypothyreosis with the tendency in time towards Euthyreosis. In other words, the doctor's diagnosis is more laboratory-based diagnosis, and the module's diagnosis is more clinically oriented.

Pattern number 3 shows the same problem but the module's reasoning is proposing some kind of dysfunction diagnosis based on the information of drug therapy although laboratory test results are normal. The physician's diagnosis is again laboratory tests based.

Patterns number 4, 5 and 6 show misclassification based on TSH level which is normal and indicates Euthyreosis as the module suggests. The physician's diagnosis of Hyperthyreosis is based on laboratory information of high concentrations of T3 or/and T4. It is again like the dubious Hypo/Eu misclassification problem. Patients are *subclinicaly* Hyperthyroid or Hyperthyroid with the tendency towards Euthyreosis.

The physician's diagnosis is more laboratory based and the module's diagnosis is more clinically sound. It is difficult to say what is correct. It depends on classification attitudes – laboratory or clinical signs. There is a time delay between hormone concentrations in blood and the effects on tissues. The former can be measured from blood samples and the latter could be seen during the physical examination. Also it should be stated that these test results patterns are very rare in our database records.

In conclusion, we have found one obvious module's mistake but the other misclassification patterns show a more dubious problem in thyroid function classification. It suggests that we should introduce two new categories into the classification process – *subHypo* and *subHyper*. Our plans are also to use several diagnostic modules based on various paradigms to compare the outcomes and to reinforce the classification process.

References

[1] Z Sonicki *et al.*, The use of induction in routine laboratory diagnostics of thyroid, (In Croatian), Liječnički vjesnik, 115, 306-309, 1993.
[2] I Kononenko *et al.*, A System for Inductive Learning ASSISTANT, Informatika, 10, 43-52, 1986.
[3] AS Houston *et al.*, The use of induction in the design of an expert system for thyroid function studies, Nuclear Medicine Communications, 12, 497-506, 1991.
[4] T. Plasaj *et al.*, Dijagnostički modul informacijskog sustava laboratorija za bolesti štitnjače, Med. Inform. 2,31-35, 1995.
[5] PE File *et al.*, Evaluation of the Use of Induction in the Development of a Medical Expert System, Computer and Biomedical Research, 27, 383-395, 1994.

Medical Informatics Europe '99
P. Kokol et al. (Eds.)
IOS Press, 1999

A Software Tool to Assist the Planning of Electrophysiological Experiments on Rat Brain Slices

Alexandra BOCIOACA, Cristian BADEA, Costas PAPATHEODOROPOULOS, George KOSTOPOULOS
Department of Physiology, Medical School, University of Patras, 26500 Patras, Greece

Abstract. We propose an interactive software tool for finding the plane which can be cut through the rat brain so as to contain maximum cross-section with a selected brain structure or combination of structures, i.e. a path of nerve fibers and the area they are known to connect to. A set of digitized coronal images from a stereotactic rat brain atlas is preprocessed: the images are registered, and the structures of interest plus the bulk of the brain are assigned specific gray levels. The Interactive Data Language (IDL) computing environment is used for volume reconstruction, visualization, and implementing the search procedure. Selected rat brain structures can be analyzed with our method, provided that the preprocessing of the atlas images is performed. As a first application of this method we have identified a set of parameters for which a plane (0.4 mm slice thickness) cut through the rat brain includes as many as possible intact connections between the fornix fibers and the mammilary bodies. Further development of the application will focus on automating the process and extending it to visualization of histochemical and autoradiographic data.

Keywords: Visualization; Reconstruction; Rat brain slices; 3D brain images.

1. Introduction

In vivo studies have established the excitatory nature of the fornix (F) fibers, originating from hippocampus (H), to the mammilary bodies (MB) but were unable to investigate the detailed synaptic mechanisms and possible plasticity of this connection [1]. Such precise studies demand the experimental convenience of brain slices maintained in vitro.

Experimental studies on rat brain slices maintained in vitro make use of rat brain atlases, which provide images at either coronal, sagittal, or horizontal orientation. Frequently a different orientation of sectioning is desired for optimal visualization of specific brain areas and pathways stained with specific markers. For example, the study of synaptic relationships between the fornix and the mammilary bodies, needs to be done in a plane different than the three conventional stereotactic planes, in order that the functional connections between these structures are maintained. The computer aided three-dimensional reconstruction of anatomical data is advantageous over past methods, like wax or plastic models of a definite scale, since it allows to visualize the data in any desired modality. Starting from these needs, an interactive software tool for the determination of the plane of cut through the rat brain, which yields the maximum section through selected brain structures, was designed. Such a tool assists in the planning of in vitro electrophysiological studies in brain slices, by determining and graphically illustrating the optimal plane of brain sectioning.

2. Methods and Materials

The present approach involves the preprocessing of the atlas images and the volume reconstruction in order to determine the proposed plane of cut, offered to the experimenter for further interactive refinement in the search of the optimal plane.

The resources employed consist of a stereotactic rat brain atlas [2], an image processing software (Paint Shop Pro) and the IDL computing environment. The application runs on a PC, Pentium II, 333 MHz, 64 M RAM, under Windows platform. The input data consists in 76 coronal images, digitized, spaced at an average distance of 0.3 mm along the anterior to posterior axis, taken from the Paxinos and Watson rat brain atlas. The image registration was achieved with reference to an arbitrary point, identified to be present in all images. In the next preprocessing step the brain contour and the structures of interest: mammilary bodies (MB), fornix (F), and hippocampus (H), were manually segmented and specific gray levels were assigned to each of them.

The proposed software tool was written in IDL and includes three-dimensional reconstruction and visualization, based on isosurfaces of the brain and selected structures: MB, F and H, providing visual clues about their spatial position and orientation. The volume reconstruction was done twice, with a high resolution in the region of interest, containing MB and F, and with a coarse resolution for the whole brain volume. To compensate for the unequal spacing between the original image slices, interpolated slices were generated.

The problem of finding the optimal plane is reduced to finding the plane that: (a) contains the maximum area of continuous F fibers and (b) intersects the MB.

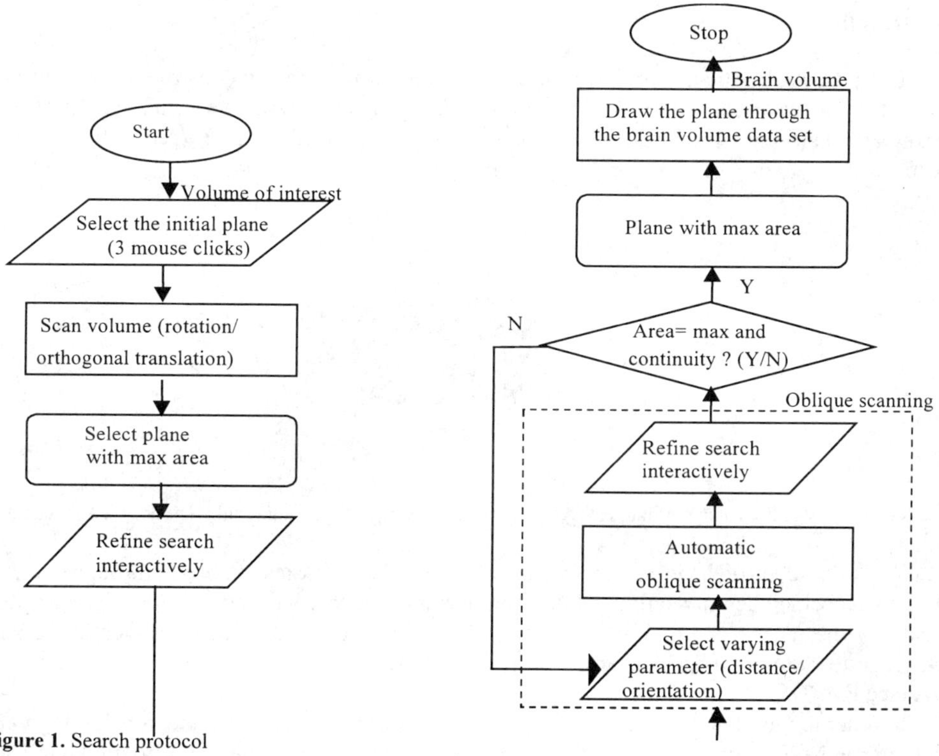

Figure 1. Search protocol

The search protocol (Fig. 1) involves the selection of the initial cut plane and the determination of the optimum plane. The coronal images are loaded one by one and the initial plane is defined by three mouse clicks on these images. This first step of the search protocol should be done for increased precision in the small volume, containing only the details. In the case of structures present in both brain hemispheres, and positioned symmetrically relative to the middsagittal plane a bilateral search is performed. The first two points are selected on the MB and define the rotational axis, calculated to be parallel to the left-to-right axis. The third point is marked on the fornix. The search for the desired plane is performed rotating the initial plane around the axis passing through MB. For each plane the cut areas are calculated and compared with the maximum value; the plane with maximum area and preserving the continuity of F is stored in memory for future reference.

In case the suggested sectioning plane is considered inconvenient by the experimenter for practical reasons, he can either adjust manually the plane parameters or restart the search procedure. For improved results, the search can be done in a similar manner, in one hemisphere, the first two points marked by mouse clicking defining the rotation axis, while the third point marked is needed for the initial estimation of the cut plane. The optimum plane found in the small volume of interest is reconstructed through the volume containing the whole brain.

The software returns the plane parameters with reference to the bregma, a landmark on the skull. These parameters are the three coordinates of the plane normal origin, and the angles made by the plane normal with the axes.

3. Results

The proposed software tool was used for three-dimensional reconstruction of the rat brain from a set of coronal images from a stereotaxic atlas, interactive visualization of the brain and selected structures within the brain, i.e. MB, F and H (see Fig. 2), and reconstructing planes of given orientations and positions.

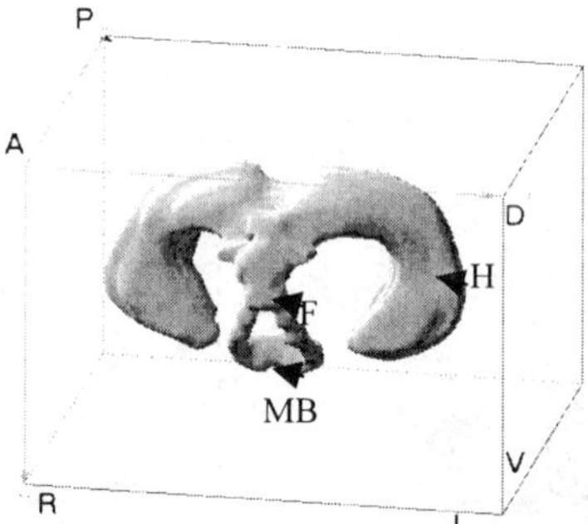

Figure 2. View of the volume of interest (A= anterior, P= posterior, L= left, R= right, D= dorsal, V= ventral)

We have identified the parameters of a plane (slice thickness 0.4mm) through the rat brain which includes a relatively long, uninterrupted area of F and the MB. The angles made by the normal to the cut plane with the right-to–left (RL), dorsal-to-ventral (DV), posterior to–anterior (PA) axes are: 113° relative to RL, 148° relative to DV, 71° relative to PA (see Fig. 3).

In order to facilitate the precise sectioning at the desired orientation and considering that cutting can be done only in the vertical plane it was constructed a Plexiglas prism having an angle of 32^{0} degrees used to bring the cut plane in vertical position. The prism's angles were deduced from the values of the angles between the cut plane and the stereotactic planes. Initial cuts are made midsagittaly and parasagittaly. The right brain hemisphere is laid on a prism, the midsagittal plane facing upwards, and the parasagittal plane downwards. The resulting brain slice is rotated around the left to right axis by 90° minus the angle the sectioning plane makes with the anterior to posterior axis, that is19 °.

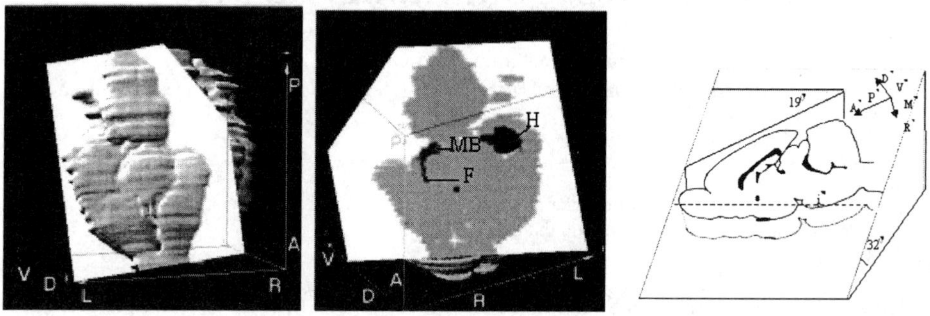

a) b) c)
Figure 3. Suggested cut plane containing MB and the maximum area of the right fornix column connected to MB: **a)** ventral view, **b)** dorsal view; **c)** experimental arrangement used to bring the cut plane in the vertical orientation, the dashed line indicates how the sectioning is done.

4. Discussion and Conclusion

An interactive software tool is proposed to assist the planning of electrophysiological experiments on the synaptic relationships in brain slices maintained in vitro. Specifically it aims to find the cut plane through the rat brain, which would preserve as much as possible intact connections between the F and the MB. Before the experiment, the cut plane would be determined and illustrated. Planes of arbitrary orientations can be reconstructed, offering visual clues not evident in classical atlases. It would be best to characterize the sectioning plane relative to anatomical landmarks on the brain surface, and not relative to bregma, since this is not visible after extracting the brain from the skulls. The interactivity is advantageous since there is no unique solution to this problem, at least for symmetry reasons. Insufficient data and unequally spaced images provided by the atlas have been identified as sources of inaccuracy. Actual experiments on rat brain slices are planned in order to validate the approach.

Any rat brain atlas can be used to provide the set of two-dimensional data used to reconstruct the brain volume. Evidently, other selected rat brain structures can be analyzed with this tool, if the preprocessing of the atlas images is performed. We plan to extend the use of this software tool to visualization of combined histochemical and receptor autoradiography data. Further development of the application will focus on automating the process.

Acknowledgements

Alexandra Bocioaca and Cristian Badea are supported by scholarships from the Greek State Scholarships Foundation.

References

[1] Kostopoulos G. K. and Phillis J.W., "Mammilothalamic neurons activated antidromically and by the stimulation of the fornix", Brain Research, 122, pp. 143-149, 1977.

[2] Paxinos G., Watson Ch., "The rat brain in stereotactic coordinates", Academic Press, San Diego, Ca, USA, 1997.

Medical Informatics Europe '99
P. Kokol et al. (Eds.)
IOS Press, 1999

A National Society for the Medical Informatics Community: BMiS

Tita McCart and Colin Gordon
Information Services, Royal Brompton & Harefield NHS Trust, Sydney Street, London SW3 6NP, UK

Abstract. The poster describes the aims and activities of a national society for the medical informatics community in the UK.

The British Medical Informatics Society ('BMiS') was formed in 1986 as the equivalent of Medical Informatics societies in North America and other European countries.

The broad objectives of BMiS are:

- To promote research and development of information systems to support patient care
- To promote the application of information technology in medical education and biomedical research;
- To assist in the education of Medical Informatics and healthcare professionals;
- To act as an open forum and focal point for professionals from all disciplines and across all sectors;
- To publish ***Biomedical Informatics Today***, a newsletter which aims to keep its membership informed of current issues in Medical Informatics;
- To arrange open workshops, conferences and other meetings addressing both introductory and research areas;
- To set up local and special interest groups, electronic bulletin boards and other mechanisms to further the above objectives.

Medical Informatics is the discipline concerned with the application of information technology and telecommunications techniques in acquiring, processing and disseminating biomedical patient data and clinical knowledge. The optimal use and availability of such information is an essential part of problem solving in clinical practice.

The emergence of Medical Informatics as a new discipline is due in large part to advances in computing and communications technology and to an increasing awareness that the knowledge base of medicine is essentially unmanageable by traditional paper-based methods. Medical Informaticians recognise that the process of retrieving clinical knowledge and making expert decisions is as important to modern biomedicine as the fact based on which clinical decisions or research plans are made. A focus on the IT infrastructure and algorithms needed to manipulate the information separates Medical Informatics from other medical disciplines, where information content is the focus.

The widespread introduction of computers into clinical practice offers new methods of storing, manipulating and communicating medical information which are more flexible and more powerful than paper based systems. Medical Informatics focuses on the following issues:

- Clinical information and decision support systems
- Medical bibliographic information systems

- Medical terminology, coding and classification
- Evaluation of the impact of IT systems on the clinical process, clinical patient outcome, organisations and resources
- Developing methodologies for systems design and evaluation
- Education of healthcare professionals and Informatics specialists
- Objectives, strategies and priorities for IT in healthcare
- Confidentiality and authentication of electronic patient data

With the establishment of Medical Informatics Departments an research groups throughout Europe and North America, Medical Informatics has become an accepted discipline worldwide. The last two decades has seen the emergence of a number of major conferences and journals devoted to the topic of Medical Informatics. As well as the introduction of taught courses. In the UK, the existing MSc courses in medical or healthcare informatics are all well subscribed.

Membership of BMiS is open to all those interested in Medical Informatics, including medical informatics academics and professionals, healthcare professionals and managers, computer scientists, librarians and information managers.

Activities

List Server. BMiS maintains an electronic list server, which provides a forum for active debate and discussion about Medical Informatics in the UK.

Fellowship. In 1995 BMiS has amended its constitution to establish a new class of membership, that of Fellow of BMiS (FBMIS). Fellowship may be applied for by members and non-members, and where awarded will indicate educational background and practical experience expected of a competent medical or health informatics professional.

BMIT. BMiS publishes a newsletter two or three times a year, titled Biomedical Informatics Today (BMIT). BMIT is posted to members of BMiS.

The newsletter typically contains a diary of forthcoming BMiS events, and of Medical Informatics events generally in the UK and abroad. News is also given of activities sponsored by BMiS. The greater part of the newsletter, however, contains articles, review and opinions on all aspects of Medical Informatics.

Web Site. BMiS has its own web site which publicises details of BMiS ordinary and fellowship memberships, newsletter, future and past meetings / events, useful links, UK jobs and the Executive Committee members.

The BMiS URL is *http://www.cs.man.ac.uk/mig/people/medicine/bmis*

Meetings

Making Medical Informatics Work Conferences (MMIW). This conference is jointly organised by BMiS and the Manchester Metropolitan University. It has been held in 1995, 1997 and 1998 and will again be held in 1999. The conference is becoming a major event in the Medical informatics calendar. In 1998 it was featured on BBC Radio 4's 'Medicine Now' programme reflecting public concern over the use, and misuse, of medical computer systems as we approach the millennium. The first day concentrated on 'Doing Medical Informatics in NHS Trusts'.

The 1999 conference will continue to encourage the commercial sector to add to what has mainly been a health service, research and academia based forum. MMIW99 details are available at: *http://www.doc.mmu.ac.uk/Conferences.html*

Knowledge Resource Meeting 1997. This meeting was about the 'Proposal for universal access to essential information resources for healthworkers'. The goal of this meeting was to make participants aware of the possibilities and to obtain an informed view of the basic requirements. Presentations were held by informatics workers and potential providers of networking, e-mail, literature retrieval and directory links, and an expert in human computer interface design.

Postgraduate Education in Medical Informatics Meeting 1998. The third in a series of BMiS Workshops on postgraduate education in Medical Informatics took place at City University, London. The aim of this series is to provide a forum in which to explore and discuss current issues; issues that include changing needs and the way in which educational providers are responding to those needs. Courses are now available on full-time, part-time and distance learning patterns and institutions offering each of these were represented. The participants also included both current students and successful graduates of Masters programmes in medical and health informatics.

The meeting will again take place in 1999.

Advances in Clinical Knowledge Management Meeting 1998. This meeting was jointly organised by BMiS and Health Libraries Group and held for the first time in 1998. The aims of the meeting were: 1) to explore practical advances in methods for capturing, processing, distributing, finding and using knowledge for the benefit of clinical professionals and patients; and 2) to bring together professionals form the disciplines of Medical Informatics, information retrieval, clinical, library, computer, cognitive and information sciences to share techniques & insights.

A follow-up of the meeting will take place in 1999.

Information for Health in the New NHS: the New Strategy and Medical Informatics in the NHS 1999. In 1998 the **New NHS** White Paper and the strategy document *Information for Health* have set out the prospect of radical change and expansion in the role of medical informatics in the NHS. In response, BMiS organised a major one-day meeting designed especially for the community of IM&T professionals working in NHS Trusts.

The purpose of this meeting was to bring together members of the Medical Informatics community in the NHS Trust sector, domain experts and clinical IT users to discuss how to respond to the challenges and opportunities ***Information for Health*** will be offering over the coming period. A outstanding and varied panel of speakers was assembled; they provided authoritative insight into aspects of the ***Information for Health*** strategy, as well as first-hand reports from IM&T work in NHS Trusts on what has been achieved so far, strategies for next steps and insight into key obstacles and challenges. The meeting was very well attended by more than 120 delegates from various areas in the NHS.

Following this initiative, BMIS has been invited to assist in coordinating the 'Informatics' section of the UK NHS's new National Electronic Library of Health, one of the major components of the national ***Information for Health*** strategy. The web proceedings of the conference are available at **http://www.rbh.nthames.nhs.uk/bmis/index.htm**.

Medical Informatics Europe '99
P. Kokol et al. (Eds.)
IOS Press, 1999

TeCoMed
Online Consulting of Acute Health Risks

G. Greiner, G. Kundt, L. Gierl
University of Rostock
Institute for Medical Informatics and Biometrics
Rembrandtstr. 16/17
18055 Rostock
Germany

Abstract. Geomedical systems are information systems used to monitor the health situation in geographically distributed populations. Both are used to detect and to forecast health risks. In this paper, we present the system TeCoMed, which fulfills the following tasks: (1) discovering health risks; (2) forecasting temporal and spatial spread of epidemics; (3) estimating consequences of an epidemic; (4) presentation of the results via Internet.
Keywords: medical informatics, information system, case-based reasoning

1 Introduction

Physicians, hospitals, and health authorities need sufficient information on current health risks including outbreak and spreading of diseases with a high contagion level to ensure a high level of human health protection. The TeCoMed Project provides an application for medical informatics, which empowers MDs, those heading medical institutions, health insurance companies, and health authorities as future users to engage in a decision-making process regarding the early combat of contagious diseases. It is geared to accomplish the following tasks: Reflecting the general state of health, early discovery of acute health risks and outbreaks of infectious epidemics, detection of hitherto unknown diseases, forecasting of the temporal and spatial spread of epidemics as well as the economic and constitutional consequences of a given epidemic.
Our Online Consulting System consists of three fundamental, mutually engaged components:

- Data capturing
- Information processing
- Presentation and visualization on the Internet

2 Data capturing

In our system digitized health data of the AOK in Mecklenburg-Vorpommern* can be used. The AOK sends patient records, which contain information about medical treatment of insurants. More precisely, the following items are contained: decade of birth, sex, encoded profession, postcode of the domicile, date of fall ill, emergency, convalescence, death, and the diagnose given by ICD (International Statistical Classification of Diseases and Related Health Problems). A comprehensive data-pool is available, because about 40% of the Mecklenburgian

* AOK: General Health Insurance Company; Mecklenburg-Vorpommern: state in north-east Germany

population are registered under the roof of the AOK Health Insurance Company. The data is rendered anonymous in accordance with the law of the land, and the capturing process takes place largely on a self-induced basis via ISDN transfer. It is kept on a database for further processing.

In addition, data of the state health authorities is included. We receive weekly reports about notifiable diseases, which include microbiological data.

3 Information processing

The considerable quantity of acquired health data provides material for sequences of health situations to discover health risks. Although we have a large and rich data source, we have to notice that these data can not be considered as a representative sample within the meaning of statistics. The social structure as well as the age distribution of the insurants and of the whole population does not correspond. Consequently parametric statistical methods are not applicable. Therefor we combine various geostatistical methods and case-based reasoning to evaluate the collected data.

3.1 Case-based Reasoning

Case-based reasoning (CBR) is a cyclical paradigm of artificial intelligence for solving problems by analogical reasoning and for learning new problem-solution pairs through experiences. CBR is an approach based on the presupposition: similar problem instances have similar solutions. The CBR-cycle consists of four stages (due to Aamodt and Plaza [1]): *retrieve* the most similar case or cases; *reuse* the information and knowledge in that case to solve the problem; *revise* the proposed solution; *retain* the parts of this experience likely to be useful for future problem solving.

We apply the CBR-techniques to answer mainly the following question: What could be the further development of a conspicuous health situation?

By a *case* we understand a concept which describes the public health situation in the considered area (state Mecklenburg-Vorpommern) during a time period, such a description is called a *scenario* Σ. Because we examine the health situation during a time period a scenario is a sequence of separate *situations*, $\Sigma=(\sigma_1,\ldots,\sigma_n)$. Here a *situation* reflects the public health state for a certain week.

For each postcode unit we accumulate the information about new cases of disease and construct scenarios. All scenarios are stored in a case-base Σ^*. Given a current scenario Σ, the system retrieves all scenarios $\Sigma'\sigma'_{n+1} = (\sigma'_1,\ldots, \sigma'_n,\sigma'_{n+1})$ from the case-base Σ^* so that the differences between Σ and Σ' are minimal. By using the retrieved scenarios $\Sigma'\sigma'_{n+1}$ the system adapts the situation σ'_{n+1} to a forecast situation σ_f. The result will be stored in the case-base and will be available for graphical presentation. After a time period we know the situation σ_{n+1}. In comparing the forecast situation σ_f with the situation σ_{n+1} the system evaluate the forecast mechanism. If there are too many differences between these situations the system has to integrate the new scenario $\Sigma\sigma_{n+1}$ in the case-base or the inference mechanism must be changed.

3.2 *Geostatistical Methods*

A given situation σ is analyzed with geostatistical techniques, such as the G Test developed by Getis and Ord (see [2], [3]), to diagnose constitutional risks. The G-statistic is based on a permutation test, which measures the concentration or the lack of concentration of the sum of considered values in an area. The area (state Mecklenburg-Vorpommern) is subdivided into

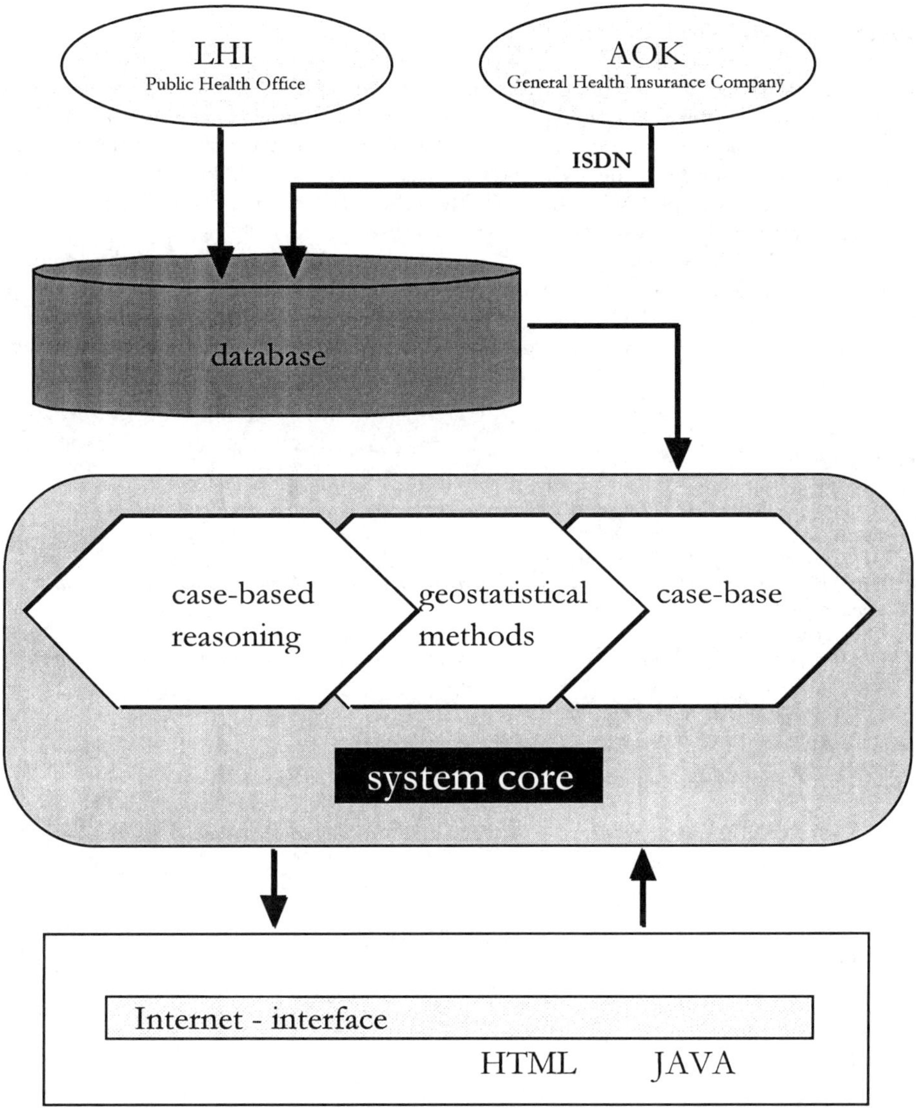

Figure 1. Structure of the System TeCoMed

regions (postcode units). Each region is associated with an incidence value for every disease. We fix the value for a certain region and consider all permutations of the remaining values. The statistic is subsequently calculated as the proportion of the sum of all values that are within a certain neighborhood of the region to the total sum of the area. Under the null hypothesis of spatial independence, the permutations are equally likely, and the statistic is approximately normal distributed. By testing the null hypothesis we detect regions with a conspicuous concentration of either high or low values in the environment.

4 Presentation and Visualization on the Internet

The informational content of the health data captured will be visually represented on the TeCoMed Web Site. Depiction of graphics allows a quick and intuitive recognition of the data results for the respective user groups. In particular, geomedical maps allow, in the given case, an individual evaluation by the user without need to presuppose knowledge of the data structure. In an initial phase of the TeCoMed Project, two independent prototypes for visualization were designed, which can be used as well.

Visualized health data and constitutional scenarios are made available on the Internet to conform to individual needs of respective user classes. In addition, HTML pages and Java applets (for instance on the basis of one of the above prototypes) will be presented on the net page. The access of the system shall be possible without prior knowledge of data processing on a WWW interface.

References

[1] Aamodt, A., Plaza, E. (1994) *Case-Based Reasoning: Foundational Issues, Methodological Variations, and System Approaches.*
AI Communications, IOS Press, 7:1, 39 – 59.

[2] Ord, J.K., Getis, A. (1995) *Local spatial autocorrelation statistics: Distributional Issues and an application.*
Geographical Analysis, 27, 286 – 306.

[3] Ord, J.K., Getis, A. (1995) *Local spatial autocorrelation statistics: Distributional Issues and an application.*
Geographical Analysis, 27, 286 – 306.

Medical Informatics Europe '99
P. Kokol et al. (Eds.)
IOS Press, 1999

Site Specific Outcomes Analysis: Inducing Knowledge from a Limited Set of the Cardiac Assist Support Data

Ankica Babic[1,2], Ph.D.
1 Department of Biomedical Engineering, Medical Informatics, Linköping University, Sweden
2 Faculty of Electrical Engineering, University of Ljubljana, Slovenia

Abstract. Introducing a new mechanical cardiac support into a surgical practice assumes, among other things, the risk stratification. However, the favourable outcome would not relate barely to the performance of device, but would rather concern all other risk factors that could be identified in clinical data sets.
A pilot study on the 24 patients undergoing coronary artery bypass surgery (CABG) addressed the performance and features specific of the Hemopump (HP). A comparative analysis of 36 patients was done to compare the new device (HP) to commonly used Intra-Aortic Balloon Pump (IABP). Results of multivariate discriminant analysis showed that the choice of the assist device did not affect survival. Operative mortality related to a greater number of the bypass grafts, increased age, and the Higgins score, which is a risk factor extracted from the large clinical data sets of several thousand patients in North America.
Regression analysis predicted that an early surgical intervention is favourable of the positive patient outcome.
Risk factors identified by the study could be seen as a part of a wider theoretical framework, and could be forwarded into the clinical practice using electronic patient record system.

1. Selection of the Risk Factors

Mortality and morbidity are most common outcomes relating to the perioperative risk factors. They can be easily obtained by simple calculations, but could be also described in more structured clinical terms as results of univariate and multivariate statistical analysis. According to the research by Higgins [1] perioperative factors connected with mortality are preoperative creatinine levels higher than 168 mmol/L, severe left ventricular dysfunction, preoperative hematocrit of less or equal 0.34, increasing age, chronic obstructive pulmonary disease, prior vascular surgery, re-operation, and mitral valve insufficiency. In addition to these, diabetes mellitus, body weight of 65 kg or more, aortic stenosis, and cerebrovascular disease relate to morbidity. These preoperative factors were found significant by univariate statistics, and were assigned weights in regression analysis for a precise predication. Data of over 5000 consecutive patients was used for this purpose which provided knowledge base superior to simple models of predicting the same risk factors. The validation would be however needed in more demanding clinical decisions and in relation to pertinent patient groups.

As predictors in immediate and long term inotropic drug support Royster et al. [2] had used intraoperative factors, duration on bypass, aortic cross clamp time, ejection fraction function, demographic factors and New York Heart Association Classification (NYHA).

Similar set of factors was used by Murakami et al. [3] and Clark et al. [4] to predict quality of surviving and intolerance to the exercise test.

More general sources of the risk were specified in [5]. List of risk factors is long and concerns data items such as *age, gender, acute clinical instability, principal diagnosis, extent and severity of principal diagnosis.* Of importance and value are additionally *extent and severity of co-morbidities, coexisting disease, physical functional status, psychological, cognitive, and psychosocial functions, cultural, ethnic, and socio-economic attributes and behaviours, health status and quality of life, patient attitudes and preferences for outcomes.* The outcome could be defined as longevity, death; acute physiologic stability, complications of medical care, chronic disease and physiologic dysfunction, physical functional status, psychosocial functioning, role function (e.g. return to work, quality of life) costs of care service use (e.g. hospitalisation and readmission, length of stay).

2. Theoretical Premises

Improvement in predicting the outcomes progressed from clinical models based on an expert opinion to multivariate models [6,7]. Any methodological approach used should enable care providers a general orientation to risk and outcomes data issues, as well as possibilities to discuss the techniques applied and potential interpretation in a clinical practice setting [8]. Importance of the data in clinical decision making is a shift from a clinical judgement to the risk adjustment. This should help predicting outcomes and informing patients at the earliest stage of their symptoms.

Specialised systems have routines for the prediction thus enabling a regular patient follow up. Their risk adjustments are to be discussed with respect to a clinical, regional and all other settings [9].

3. Statistical Insights into Outcomes of the HP and IABP Assist Devices

During a period from 1989 to 1994, the intra-aortic balloon pump (IABP) was used in 36 and Hemopump (HP) in 24 patients at Linkoping Heart Center, Sweden. Multivariate discrimination and logistic regression were applied only on perioperative data. That included Higgins score and New York Heart Association class (NYHA) to estimate preoperative risk. The patient groups statistically differentiated with respect to diabetes mellitus (more in the HP group), gender (more males among the HP patients), indication for the surgery (more biventricular failures in the HP group), Body Mass Index (BMI) (higher in the HP group), assist related complications (more in the IAPB group). Age and Higgins were best preoperative items to separate survivors (age: 62.6+/-8, Higgins: 5.2 +/-3.8) from nonsurvivors (age: 69.8+/-6.8, Higgins: 7.9+/-4.3) [10].

Maximal levels of serum creatinine, aspartate aminotransferase and platelet count measured after the surgery, and a high number of the grafts, were additionally characteristic of nonsurvival patient subgroup. A choice of assist device did not affect survival, but considerably fewer complications occurred in the HP patient group even if it could be judged as more demanding to treat according to the risk factors [10].

The time of HP insertion significantly reflected in the blood transaminases [11]. In particular, a maximum average level of aspartate aminotransferase (AST) is lower in patients with early intervention (4.57 μkat/l) than in those with late intervention (10.1 μkat/l). At the time of discharge, lower alanine aminotransferase (ALT) values correspond to the patients with early intervention (0.89 μkat/l), as compared to the group of the late intervention (1.83 μkat/l). Thus, an early HP insertion seems to be beneficial.

4. Discussion and Conclusions

The presented research included a great number of the risk factors, hemodynamic and laboratory data. As no guidelines regarding the mechanical circulatory support were available, an elaborate literature search was done to select risk factors of interest. It was unavoidable to limit the number of findings to those pointed out in other studies and measured during the surgery. This enabled outcome results which were informative and useful.

The time of insertion, which provides an important classification definition in this particular patient material, was determined retrograde and according to the clinical experience of the two surgical teams. That can be seen as a vogue point in estimating outcomes, but an early insertion of the instrument could be recommended in any case.

The Summit [12], a patient electronic record system at the Heart Center in Linköping, enables a fast and simple implementation of this knowledge, which must be completed by recommendations on the drug administration.

Acknowledgement

The author would like to thank Henrik Casimir-Ahn, MD, Ph.D., Hans Rutberg, MD, Ph.D., Urban Lönn, MD, Ph.D., and Bengt Peterzen, MD, for the research initiative.

This research has been supported by the Swedish Research Council for Engineering sciences (TFR).

References

[1] Higgins T. L., Estafanous F.G., Loop F.D., Beck G.J., Blum J.M., Paranadi L., Stratification of Morbidity and Mortality Outcome by Perioperative Risk Factors in Coronary Artery Bypass Patients. A clinical Severity Score, JAMA 1992, 267:2344-48

[2] Royster R.L., Butterworth J.F., Prough D.S., Johnston W. E., Thomas J.L., Hogan P.E., Case D.L., Gravlee G.P., Perioperative and Intraoperative Predictors of Inotropic Support and Long-Term Outcome in Patients Having Coronary Artery Bypass Grafting, Anesth Analg 1991, 72:729-36

[3] Murakami T., Nakayama H., Irie H., Kino K., Hisamochi K., Koomoto T., Takagaki M., Sugawara E., Senoo Y., Teramoto S., Circulatory Support for Patients Experiencing Postcardiotomy Cardiogenic Shock: Analysis of Risk Factors for Death and Long-Term Follow-up, Artificial Organs 1993, 17(7): 634-9

[4] Clark R.E., Edwards F.H., Schwartz M., Profile of Perioperative Characteristics of Patients Having CABG Over the Past Decade, Ann Thorac Surg 1994, 58:1683-5

[5] Iezzoni L.I., Using Risk-Adjusted Outcomes to Assess Clinical Practice: An Overview of Issues Pertaining to Risk Adjustment, Ann Thorac Surg 1994, 58:1822-6

[6] Steen P.M, Apporaches to Predictive Modeling, Ann Thorac Surg 1994, 58:1836:40 (Hammermeister 1994) Hammermeister K.E., Participatory Continuous Improvement, Ann Thorac Surg 1994, 58:1815-21

[7] Shroyer A.L.W., Dauber I., Jones R.H., Daley J., Grover F.L., Hammermeister K.E., Provider Perceptions in Using Outcome Data to Improve Clinical Practice, Ann Thorac Surg 1994, 58:1877-80

[8] Ebert P.A., The Importance of Data in Improving Practice: Effective Clinical Use of Outcomes Data, Ann Thorac Surg 1994, 58:1812-4

[9] Daley J., Criteria by Which to Evaluate Risk-Adjustment Outcomes Programs in Cardiac Surgery, Ann Thorac Surg 1994, 58:1827-35

[10] Babic A, U Lönn, B Peterzén, H Rutberg, H Casimir-Ahn. Risk factors in patients requiring mechanical circulatory support after open heart surgery: Intra-aortic balloon pump and the hemopump. In Proceeding of the 4th World Congress on Heart Failure, Israel, May. 1996.

[11] Lönn U., Peterzen B., Granfeldt H., Babic A., Casimir-Ahn H., Hemopump treatment ni patients with postcardiotomy heart failure. Ann Thorac Surg, 60:1067-71, 1995.

[12] (Summit Medical Systems, Minneapolis, Minnesota 55447).

Medical Informatics Europe '99
P. Kokol et al. (Eds.)
IOS Press, 1999

Application of Thanatos in Creating Thyroid Cancer Registry

Tomislav Plasaj[1], Mirna Lechpammer[1], Dalibor Šimunović[1], Ivan Cvjetko[1], Marija Strnad[2], Zvonko Kusić[1], Mladen Belicza[1]
[1]*Sisters of Mercy University Hospital, Zagreb, Croatia*
[2]*Croatian Institute of Public Health, Zagreb, Croatia*

Abstract. The aim of this paper is to present the practical results of processing data from biopsy findings by Thanatos the Information System developed for Department of Clinical Patology Sisters of Mercy University Hospital, Zagreb, Croatia. After completing the Thyroid Cancer Registry which is a part of the Hospital Cancer Registry we are able to make distribution of histological representation of each type od thyroid cancer. From age distribution at diagnosis advansed informations are gained souch as increasing of average age for patients with follicular cancer. By comparing data from our Thyroid Cancer Registry wiht Croatian Cancer Registry for follow up purposes it is possible to calculate 5-year survival rate. We expected that all these advanced informations will makes possible to better predict behavior of thyroid diseases and to use more efficient prevention or cure.

Key words: information system, pathology, thyroid cancer

1. Introduction

Thanatos is an Information System (IS) developed for the "Ljudevit Jurak" Department of Clinical Pathology Sisters of Mercy University Hospital. Thanatos allows creation, processing and printing of Death Report, Death Certificate, Autopsy Report and Biopsy Report. Diagnoses are in Latin, based on ICD-10 and pathological classification of malignant tumours (pTNM) and gathered in a separate module.
It is programmed in Borland's Paradox 7 for Windows/95 and NT environment. It was implemented in September 1997.

For now, Thanatos consists of five separate modules: Coronary-Inquest, Autopsy, Biopsy, Cytology and Diagnoses. These modules make an entity that enables data processing for all activities in the Department of Clinical Pathology.
Besides, there are a few functions that are common to all modules:

1. Controlled data entry
2. Statistics for modules: Coronary-Inquest, Autopsy, Biopsy and Cytology
3. On line help

Thanatos is designed as a part of hospital Cancer Registry and for this reason it contains typical clinical data, such as therapy, surgery protocol and all relevant clinical reports. Thanks to the fact that data from the Croatian Cancer Registry are included, it is possible to conduct the survival and retrospective studies.

The desired characteristic of Thanatos to be a part of the hospital Cancer Registry was checked in practice by making specific Thyroid Cancer Registry. Beside the possibility to memorise data, Thanatos memorises images like microscopic pictures, histology reports or CT reports, so patient's medical record can be used for routine, education and medical research.
By linking all the above mentioned characteristics inside Thanatos, it becomes a very strong information tool.

2. Methods

Hospital Cancer Registry including Thyroid Cancer Registry was filled with data from biopsy findings after surgery in University Hospital and clinical data both preoperative and postoperative. Contribute data was reached after connecting with Croatian Cancer Registry for follow up purposes. Modules for automatic search through Croatian Cancer Registry of any patient added in Thyroid Cancer Registry are just now being implemented in Thanatos.

3. Results

After completing Thyroid Cancer Registry using statistical modules we came up with some practical results. Total of 3815 patients is now present in our Hospital Thyroid Disease Registry that recived treatment in our hospital from 1980 to 1999. Of those 2403 (or 63 %) patients were with non-tumour disorder, while 1412 patients (37 %) had thyroid tumour.

Goiter is most common with 2021 patients (53 %) in non-tumour section, then Morbus Basedow with 156 patients, Hashimoto thyreoiditis with 138 patients. Female to male ratio and average age at the time of diagnosis for these patients was calculated as shown on table 1.

Table 1. Female to male ratio and average age at diagnosis for non-tumour disorders

	F:M	AA*
Goiter	6,8	NA
Mb. Basedow	8,1	39,8
Hashimoto	14,3	48,4

* AA – average age in years

In patients with tumours (1412 patients) adenomas were most common making total of 979 patients (or 69 % of all thyroid tumours). Female to male ratio was 6,1 to 1, and average age of patients was 44,5 years.

In Thyroid Cancer Registry we found 433 patients with thyroid cancer. Histological representation of each type is shown on picture 1.

Picture 1. Thyroid cancer by histological types in our sample

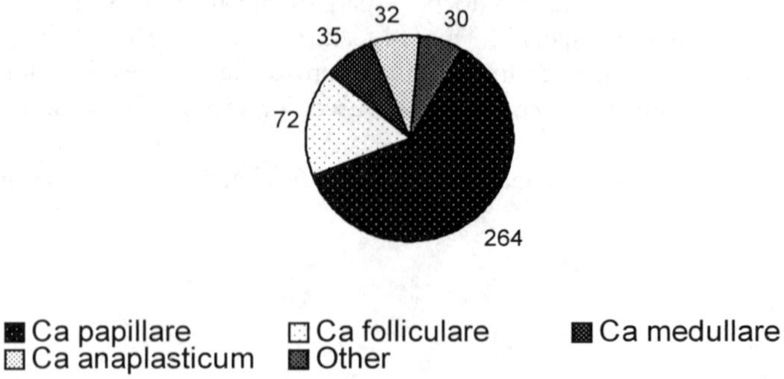

Most patients with thyroid cancer had papillary cancer, 61% of them and female to male ratio was 3.3:1. Follicular cancer was found in 16,6% cases with female to male ratio of 2:1. Medullar cancer was found in 8,1% cases with F: M of 1,3:1. Smallest group of patients had anaplastic cancer 7,4% of them with F: M ratio 1,9:1.

Average age and eventual changes were of our special interest because of long time period that we used for observation. So to gain advanced information considering age distribution we compared average age at diagnosis of our patients in two different 2-year periods (1980-81 vs. 1997-98). In most cases no significant change was found, except follicular cancer were average age was increased from 45,5 years in 1980-81 to 61,3 years in 1997-98. Also pointing more to that fact we observed that number of cases of follicular cancer has been decreasing through years. So in 1980th 15 patients with follicular cancer was reported, in 1997 only three, and in 1999 so far none.

As mentioned follow up of our patients is one of primary objectives. By comparing data from our Thyroid Cancer Registry with Croatian Cancer Registry we calculated this next figures. Survival rates are as follows: 5-year survival for papillary cancer is 97%, for follicular cancer 93% and for the medullary carcinoma 78%. Extended 10 and 15 year survival studies are in progress.

4. Conclusion

Sex distribution in our registry is as quoted in literature. Follicular cancer is on the lower border of distribution for countries with abnormal iodine uptake what is in correlation with presence of endemic goiter in Croatia, but with decreasing number of follicular cancer cases from 15 in 1980 to 3 in 1997 and none in 1998 overall. By comparing two different 2-year periods we found that average age of patients with follicular cancer was increased form 45,5 years (1980-81) to 61,3 years (1997-98).

Valuable data received from registry will make possible to better predict behavior of thyroid diseases and thus making prevention or cure more efficient, especially when combined with other clinical data (levels of calcitonin, thyreoglobulin etc.)

References

[1] Raue F, Spath-Roger M, Winter J, Benker G, Buhr P, Dorn R, Dralle H, Frilling A, Herrmann J, Hornig I, et al. A registry of medullary thyroid cancer in West Germany. Med Klin 1990; 85(3): 113-116.

[2] Delisele MJ, Hannequin P, Liehn JC, Gibold C, Maes B, Vaudrey C, Pochart JM, Morel M, Thyroid cancer in Champagne - Ardenne: 1967-1984. Epidemiologic findings in a regional register. Bull Cancer 1986; 73(2): 165-170.

[3] Meurisse M, Claeys N, Paesmans M, Nguyen Dang M, Degauque C, Delmelle M, Larismont D, T'Hooft-Andry M, Verhest A, Hamoir E, Andry G, Squifflet JP. Belgian registry of thyroid cancer. Preliminary epidemiological characteristic revealed by retrospective study (1988 - 1995). Belgian Thyroid Cancer Study Group. Ann Endocrinol (Paris) 1997; 58: 163-171.

[4] Plasaj T, Belicza M. Dometi uporabe Thanatosa informacijskog sustava za kliničku patologiju. Medicinska informatika (Zagreb) 1997; 3: 1-4.

[5] Bleich HL, Stack WV. Designing a hospital information system: a comparison of interfaced and integral systems. M.D. Computing 1991; 8: 291-299

[6] Pagliara S et al., Ann Ist Super Sanita 1998; 34(3): 417.

[7] Lind P et al., Thyroid 1998; 8(12): 1179.

[8] Teppo L et al., Eur J Cancer 1998; 34: 2248.

[9] Hundahl SA et al., Cancer 1998; 83: 2638

[10] Kusić Z et al., Endocrinol Invest 1996; 19: 204.

Medical Informatics Europe '99
P. Kokol et al. (Eds.)
IOS Press, 1999

Can humoral factors help to predict hypertension?

J. Peleška, J. Reissigová*, D. Janeba*, J. Zvárová*, K.Horký, M. Jáchymová, A. Jindra, S. Heller, Z. Marečková, V. Umnerová
2nd Dept. of Medicine, 1st Faculty of Medicine, Charles University, Prague, Czech Republic
** EuroMISE Center, Charles University and Academy of Sciences, Prague, Czech Republic*

Abstract. The aim of the study was to compare a set of plasma humoral factors, age and body mass index between normotensive sons from hypertensive (SH, n=101) and normotensive (SN, n=100) families. The sons were at the age of 18-40 years. Comparing individual variables, the significant differences were found in basal adrenalin load, noradrenalin before (basal) and after glucose load, basal dopamine, basal endothelin and fibrinogen between SH and SN. Moreover, SH was significantly older by two years than SN. The linear discriminant analysis and neutral network were applied to find the best classifying variables between SH and SN. Basal noradrenalin, fibrinogen, basal glycemia and age were the best discriminating variables between SH and SN using the discriminant analysis. The neural network used, in addition, basal aldosterone, relative plasma viscosity, glycated hemoglobin to estimate family status (SH or SN). There were no essential differences between those methods in predicting family status in the test set (66% of correct classification), even if the results in the training set were far better for the neural network (83% of correct classification) than for the discriminant analysis (69% of correct classification). Simultaneous using of several humoral factors can serve as intermediate phenotype that could improve identification of hypertension.

1. Introduction

For the blood pressure as a phenotype is not suitable for genetic studies due to its instability and the genuine genetic markers for essential hypertension are not known, the research interest turned to so called intermediate phenotypes, such as changes of membrane transport or concentration of humoral factors, and their relation to polymorphism of candidate genes [1].

The objective of this study was to compare humoral factors, age and body mass index (BMI) between normotensive sons from hypertensive (SH) and normotensive (SN) families, and to predict family status (SH, SN) from these variables. The following plasma humoral factors were compared: glycemia, adrenalin, noradrenalin, dopamine, aldosterone, atrial natriuretic peptide, endothelin and plasma renin activity - all under basal conditions and then 90 min. after a 75 g oral glucose load. Furthermore, relative plasma viscosity, fibrinogen concentration and glycated hemoglobin were measured only under basal conditions.

2. Methods

Two samples from SH (n=101) and SN (n=100) were sons of patients of 2nd Department of Medicine or volunteers. The study was not randomized. Normotensive sons were at the age

of 18-40. Normotension of sons was defined as systolic blood pressure of ≤ 140 mmHg and diastolic blood pressure of ≤ 90 mm Hg.
The differences in the individual variables between the groups were tested by the independent t-test. The equality of variances of the variables in SH and SN was analysed by Leven's test.
The linear discriminant analysis was applied to find the best discriminating variables between SH and SN among the variables. A priori probabilities were assumed to be equal. Box's M test was used to assess whether the variance matrices are homogeneous across the groups. The stepwise procedure (using Wilks' lambda) was employed to identify the best discriminating variables [2]. Apart from the discriminant analysis neural networks were also used to predict the family status from the humoral factors, age and BMI.
In the t-test and the discriminant analysis the variables not following normal distribution were log-transformed to meet assumptions of these tests. The normality was verified by Shapiro-Wilk's W test.
The software packages STATISTICA (StatSoft 1995), StatXact (Cytel Software Corporaion 1995) and STATISTICA Neural Networks (StatSoft 1998, [3]) were used in all the calculations.

3. Results

The majority of the variables did not follow the normal distribution. After log-transforming the distribution of these variables followed the normal type, or approached to it. Only the distribution of viscosity highly significantly differed from the normal distribution.
The significant differences were found in age, basal adrenalin, noradrenalin before and after glucose load, basal dopamine, basal endothelin and fibrinogen between SH and SN. The group SH was significantly older (by 2 years) than SN. These results are presented in Table 1.

Table 1. Comparison of age, basal adrenalin (ADR), noradrenalin before (NA1) and after (NA2) glucose load, basal dopamine (DOP), basal endothelin (END) and fibrinogen (FIB) between SH and SN for the cases with no missing observations (log means that the variable was log-transformed, SD = the standard deviation, p = the attained level of significance).

Variables	Group				p
	SH (n=70)		SN (n=87)		
	Mean	SD	Mean	SD	
log(AGE)	3.28	0.21	3.20	0.19	0.008
log(ADR)	-1.17	0.72	-1.49	0.69	0.005
log(NA1)	0.37	0.59	0.03	0.55	0.000
log(NA2)	0.42	0.58	0.19	0.45	0.005
log(DOP)	-0.94	0.93	-1.32	0.78	0.007
END	17.33	6.05	15.38	5.24	0.032
log(FIB)	0.87	0.21	0.79	0.20	0.011

Basal noradrenalin, fibrinogen, basal glycemia and age were the best discriminating variables between SH and SN (basal noradrenalin, fibrinogen and age were log-transformed). They were selected by the stepwise procedure on the basis of 157 cases with no missing values of all humoral factors, age and BMI. It should be noted, there was no significant difference in basal glycemia between groups (5.20±0.61 for SH, 5.02±0.52 for SN), however, the attained level of significance approached to 5% (p=0.06). The discriminant function classified correctly 68% (95% c.i. (60%,75%)) of cases. The specificity of 74% (95% c.i. (63%,82%)) was higher than the sensitivity of 60% (95% c.i.

(48%,72%)). If age, chosen by the stepwise procedure using Wilks' lambda as a decisive rule for a choice of the best predicting variable, was not in the discriminant function, the percentage of correct classification went up to 71%.
We divided the cases (with not missing values of basal noradrenalin, fibrinogen, basal glycemia and age) randomly in the ratio 3:1 into training (n=131) and test (n=47) sets. After developing a discriminant function with the best discriminating variables derived from all cases in the training set we applied it to the test set. The accuracy of classification in both sets shown in the Table 2 was comparable.

Table 2. Percentage of correct classification with 95% confidence interval according to the discriminant analysis in the training and test sets.

Correct Classification	**Training set**			**Test set**		
	SH (n=67)	**SN (n=64)**	**Total (n=131)**	**SH (n=19)**	**SN (n=28)**	**Total (n=47)**
%	63	75	69	68	64	66
95% c.i	(50,74)	(63,85)	(60,77)	(43,87)	(44,81)	(51,79)

The whole set of 201 patients was randomly split in the ratio 3:1 into training (n=151) and test (n=50) sets. Several neural networks have been suggested with the architecture 7-7-5-1, 7-6-4-1, 7-5-3-1, all of them with the prognosis rate about 65%. The input parameters were fibrinogen, basal glycemia, basal noradrenalin, basal aldosterone, viscosity, glycated hemoglobin and age. The results of the neural network with the architecture 7-5-3-1 are shown in the Table 3. The neural network worked with missing values in the contrary to the discriminant analysis.

Table 3. Percentage of correct classification with 95% confidence interval according to the neural network with the architecture 7-5-3-1 in the training and test sets.

Correct Classification	**Training set**			**Test set**		
	SH (n=76)	**SN (n=75)**	**Total (n=151)**	**SH (n=25)**	**SN (n=25)**	**Total (n=50)**
%	70	96	83	68	64	66
95% c.i.	(58,80)	(89,99)	(76,88)	(47,85)	(43,82)	(51,79)

4. Discussion

The differences in basal adrenalin, noradrenalin before and after glucose load, basal dopamine, basal endothelin and fibrinogen were found out between SH and SN. Some differences in a smaller sample were already described earlier [4].
In our study, the discriminant function classified correctly 68% of cases. However, the sensitivity of 60% was not sufficiently high compared to the specificity of 74%. The result can be biased because of the discriminant analysis sensitivity to the ratio of sample size to the number of independent variables. Our ratio of 7 cases for each independent variable could impact the selection of the best discriminating variables by the stepwise procedure. Furthermore, we should remark that the linear discriminant analysis we used for classification does not reflect nonlinear relationships among variables. Despite of it the results of classifications by means of the discriminant function with basal noradrenalin, fibrinogen, basal glycemia and age were comparable in the training and test sets. As regard of age, prevalence of hypertension increases with age. The difference in age between SH and SN can partly result from this dependency and can be partly caused by admission of some SH – offspring of older hypertensives from our out-patient clinic. When we excluded age from the discriminant function, the percentage of correct classification was close to that deriving from the discriminant function using age.

There were not found essential differences between the discriminant analysis and the neural network in predicting family status in the test set, even if the results in the training set were far better for the neural network than for the discriminant analysis. The accuracy of classification in the neural network can be also biased by a small number of observations. According to epidemiological studies, hypertension develops only in about 65% cases in SH. Therefore, the correct prediction of family status SH and SN, respectively, does not mean the prediction of hypertension. The prediction of hypertension can be confirmed only by a longer follow-up. On the contrary, some of normotensive parents and their offspring can become hypertensive in future.

5. Conclusions

There were no essential differences between the linear discriminant analysis and the neural network in predicting family status, i.e. hypertnesive family or normotensive family, in test set (66% of correct classification for both the discriminant analysis and the neural network). Simultaneous using of several humoral factors can serve as an intermediate phenotype of essential hypertension that could improve its prediction.

References

[1] Soubrier, F.: Search for the genes of human essential hypertension, Journal of Hypertension, 1993, 11, Suppl. 5, 20-26

[2] Rao, C. R.: Linear statistical inference and its application. NewYork, Wiley 1965

[3] STATISTICA Neural Networks Users Guide, StatSoft 1998

[4] Horký K., Jáchymová M., Jindra A., Šavlíková J., Peleška J., Umnerová V., Linhart A.: Metabolic, humoral and haemodynamic characteristics of normotensive offspring from hypertensive families, Journal of Human Hypertension, 1996, 10, Suppl. 3, 85-87

Medical Informatics Europe '99
P. Kokol et al. (Eds.)
IOS Press, 1999

A survey on the current state of development, dissemination and implementation of guidelines of clinical practice in European countries

Sonja Courté-Wienecke, Markus Struppe, Rolf Engelbrecht
GSF - National Research Center for Environment and Health,
medis Institute for Medical Informatics and Health Systems Research,
Ingolstädter Landstr. 1, 85764 Neuherberg, Germany

Abstract. In the context of ProGuide, a support action in the EU Telematics Application Programme, a survey was conducted in summer 1998 to collect information on the current state of the development, dissemination and implementation of guidelines of clinical practice in European countries. A survey questionnaire was mailed to a total of 292 organisations in all EU member countries and five Non-EU-member countries. A follow-up survey was conducted in April 1999 with a reduced set of questions and an altered questionnaire dissemination strategy relying more on telephone and fax communication. By May 1999, 69 organisations had answered and 43 questionnaires could be evaluated. Preliminary results suggest that in most of the responding countries, a wide range of organisations is involved in development, dissemination or implementation of guidelines. Paper-based ways of guideline dissemination still play a major role, although this may change in the future. Obstacles to guideline implementation range from policy issues to practical challenges of integrating guidelines into the care process.

1. Background

Clinical guidelines are seen as a tool for improving the quality and efficiency of care in an increasingly complex health care delivery environment[1,2,3]. Recent publications have provided additional evidence that use of guidelines is much facilitated when they are computer-based - partly this is due to the sheer number of guidelines in existence[4,5]. An electronic environment opens up the possibility to develop telematics applications that not only support the use of guidelines but also enable their development and dissemination.

ProGuide (Promoting the development, dissemination, and implementation of guidelines of clinical practice) is a support action conducted in the Fourth Framework of the Telematics Applications Programme for Health Care in the European Union. ProGuide focuses on computer-based guidelines of clinical practice and aims to develop an infrastructure that supports the development, dissemination and implementation of evidence-based clinical guidelines.

Project activities in the first phase of the project concentrated on researching the empirical basis, i.e., the state of the art of guideline development, dissemination and implementation, the role of telematics tools, presence of guidelines on the Internet, and the exploration of users' requirements concerning a WWW-server providing guideline-relevant information. As one of these activities, in summer of 1998, a survey was conducted to compile information for a report on the current state of development, dissemination, and implementation of guidelines of clinical practice in European countries.

2. Method

Countries surveyed included all EU member countries. In addition, Norway, and Switzerland as non-EU member countries, and the Czech Republic, Hungary and Poland as examples of candidates for future member countries were surveyed.

Due to the anticipated diversity of organisations involved in the field in the different countries, 4 categories of organisations to be surveyed were identified: 1. national organisations (e.g., departments of health), 2. medical associations and scientific societies of medical specialties, 3. associations of health care delivery organsiations and health care financing organisations, 4. other organisations, e.g., research organisations. A total of 292 organisations in the above countries were thus identified. In order to be inclusive with regard to the potential information base to use, all of these organisations were contacted in the survey.

A survey questionnaire addressing the following issues was developed:

- organisations involved in the field and their particular role,
- common ways of dissemination of guidelines,
- quality assurance of guidelines,
- financial and legal implications of compliance with guidelines
- efforts to assess physicians' compliance with guidelines,
- benefits and problems of compliance with guidelines perceived by physicians
- exploration of requirements for guidelines

The survey was mailed to the above organisations in July/August 1998. In April 1999, a follow-up survey was conducted with a reduced set of questions and an altered questionnaire dissemination strategy relying more on telephone and fax communication. By May 1999, a total of 69 organisations had answered. 43 questionnaires could be evaluated. Other replies suggested that several responding organisations did not feel involved enough in the field to answer the questionnaire with confidence, or that the field was much in transition, thus it was difficult to answer some questions.

3. Results

At the time of submission of the manuscript, the follow-up survey has not been concluded. Preliminary results of the survey suggest that in most of the responding countries, a wide range of organisations, including governmental and non-governmental policy-makers, government agencies in health care, scientific organisations and medical societies of specialties and subspecialties are involved in efforts relating to one or more functions in the development, dissemination and implementation of guidelines. Health care delivery organisations, particularly hospitals develop and implement guidelines in several countries, while health care financing organisations such as health insurances appear to play a role in fewer countries. For each country, an inventory of organisations engaged in the field was created, listing their particular relevant functions. An example of such an inventory (Germany) is shown in Table 1.

Table 1: Survey results: Organisations involved in guideline development, dissemination and implementation in Germany

Organisation	Function			
	guideline developm ent	**guideline dissemina tion**	**guideline implemen tation**	**other function**
Policy makers (governmental and non-governmental):				
Federal Ministry of Health				framework, material support, if necessary
Federal and State Medical Associations	x	x	x	
Agency for Quality in Medicine		x		development of a clearinghouse for guidelines, appraisal of the quality of guidelines (joint effort of the Federal Medical Assoc., the Federal Assoc. of Sickness Fund Physicians, the Assoc. of Statutory Sickness Funds, and the German Hospital Assoc.)
AkdÄ, Drug Commission of the German Medical Association	x	x		
Government agencies in health care:				
Organisations subordinate to the federal ministry of health (e.g., Robert-Koch-Institut, Paul-Ehrlich-Institut)	x			supply of expertise
DIMDI, German Institute for Documentation and Information		x		
Scientific/research organisations and medical associations of specialties and subspecialties:				
AWMF, Association of the Scientific Medical Societies in Germany	x	x		
Scientific medical societies (specialty societies, e.g., German Society of General Practice, German Cancer Society, German Society of Medical Education)	x	x	x	
Professional societies	x	x	x	
Institute for Health Economics, Cologne	x	x	x	economic appraisal of guidelines
Health care delivery organisations:				
Hospitals			x	some hospitals, e.g., the university hospital, Cologne, are developing and implementing internal guidelines.
Association of Sickness Fund Physicians			x	quality circles, special projects
Health care financing organisations:				
Several sickness funds, e.g., AOK, VdAK		x	x	use of guidelines in special projects
Other organisations:				
Pharmaceutical manufacturers	x	x	x	

Scientific journals, professional newsletters and periodicals/handbooks were indicated as the most important modes of dissemination of guidelines to physicians, suggesting that paper-based ways of guideline dissemination still are widely relied on, although this may change in the future: In most of the responding countries, guidelines are also distributed via Internet and/or CD-ROM.

The quality of guidelines is assured, among other means, by developing and publishing standards of guideline development, appraising existing guidelines and revising guidelines based on comments from the professional community. Examples of these activities include the methodology for guidelines development published by the Scottish Intercollegiate Guidelines Network SIGN, the consensus development program established by the National Organisation for Quality Assurance in Hospitals CBO in the Netherlands[6], and the methodological recommendations and quality criteria published by the Association of the Scientific Medical Societies AWMF and institution of a guidelines clearinghouse by the Agency for Quality in Medicine in Germany[7]. In some countries, no systematic assessment of clinical guidelines has been established so far. In several of the responding countries, efforts to assess physician compliance with guidelines have been conducted, mostly by scientific medical societies or governmental organisations. Examples are a study on health care providers using computerised guidelines for primary care in Finland[8] and efforts by the Ministry of Public Health and the Scientific Society of General Practitioners in Belgium.

Respondents' answers confirm that guidelines are very widely credited with being tools of improving the quality of care provided, particularly through standardising care and assisting practitioners by summarising current knowledge on particular topics. Financial savings and protection of providers were only mentioned by few respondents. These benefits are counterbalanced by a number of perceived problems: the high number of guidelines, problems surrounding their format and presentation and a lack of their integration into the care process, health care providers' reservations because of fear of loss of clinical independence, concerns regarding the applicability of guidelines to individual patients/situations or environments, and the resource implications both of developing and implementing guidelines. Respondents recommendations for actions to improve the utility of guidelines in health care centered around the following issues:

- There is a strong perception that physicians must play a prominent role in guideline development. Objective criteria of validation of guidelines should be developed and timely revision of guidelines should be assured. This is both in order to assure the quality of guidelines and to increase acceptance among practitioners.
- To increase accessibility of guidelines and facilitate their integration into care, the use of electronic media and in particular internet technology should be enhanced.
- Guidelines should be integrated into medical education, with other quality assurance systems and activities, and there should be incentives to use guidelines.
- More attention needs to be paid to the (local) implementation of guidelines. E.g., guidelines compliance should be monitored in order to understand what the effect is and what changes are needed.
- Patients' needs need to be taken more into account both in development and presentation of guidelines.
- Funding for the development, dissemination and implementation of guidelines needs to be available.

4. Discussion

Surveys on development, availability and use guidelines have been conducted, (e.g.,[2, 9]), but an effort to assess the current state of guideline development, dissemination and implementation in a number of different countries poses additional challenges. Due to the expected diversity of organisations engaged in the relevant fields in different countries, a very inclusive approach was chosen with regard to the audience surveyed, taking into account that possibly several of the addressees would not be involved enough to answer all questions. The response rate to the survey has to be seen in light of this. In addition, it turned out that in several countries guideline-related activities are diverse, thus it was challenging even for persons involved to give an overview.

Our survey confirms that widespread activities relating to guidelines development, measures to assure their quality and to gain insight into their implementation are taking place in numerous countries. Questions surrounding guideline development, distribution and implementation by health care providers range from policy issues to technical aspects. Some of these challenges, e.g., improving the availability of guidelines and possibilities of use at the point of care can be addressed by developing suitable electronic infrastructure, which is the aim of ProGuide. The information gained in this survey will be used and built on in the project and further related activities.

References

[1] M. Field, K. Lohr, Guidelines for Clinical Practice: From Development to Use. Washington DC: National Academy Press, 1992

[2] H. Varonen, M. Mäkelä, Practice Guidelines in Finland: Availability and Quality. *Quality in Health Care* 6 (1997) 75-9

[3] C. Huttin, The Use of Clinical Guidelines to Improve Medical Practice: Main Issues in the United States. *International Journal for Quality in Health Care* **9**: 3 (1997) 207-214

[4] A. Hibble, D. Kanka, D. Penheon, F. Pooles, Guidelines in General Practice: The New Tower of Babel? *British Medical Journal* **317** (1998) 862-863

[5] R. Zielstorff, Online Practice Guidelines: Issues, Obstacles and Future Prospects. *Journal of the American Medical Informatics Association* **5**: 3 (1998) 227-236

[6] N. Klazinga, K. Lombarts, J. v. Everdingen, Quality Management in Medical Specialties: The Use of Channels and Dikes in Improving Health Care in The Netherlands. *Journal of the Joint Commission for Accreditation in Health Care* **24**: 5 (1998) 240-250

[7] Leitlinein-In-FO, Schriftenreihe der Ärztlichen Zentralstelle Qualitätssicherung, Band 1, 1. Auflage, Oktober 1998. W.Zuckschwerdt Verlag München

[8] J. Jousimaa, I.Kunnamo, M. Mäkelä, Physicians' patterns of using a computerized collection of guidelines for primary care. *International Journal of Technology Assessment in Health Care* **14**: 3 (1998) 484-493

[9] A-M. Audet, S. Greenfield, M. Field, Medical Practice Guidelines: Current activities and future directions. *Annals of Internal Medicine* **113** (1990) 709 - 714

Author Index